Practical Clinical Oncology

Human Values, Therapeutic Equipoise
Science & Technology
IS
At the Core of Clinical Medicine

Practical Clinical Oncology

Editor-in-Chief

Praful Desai

Associate Editors

Suresh Advani

Rajendra Badwe

Anita Borges

Nagraj Huilgol

Bhavin Jankharia

Co-ordinating Editor

Ratna Parikh

Editorial Assistant

Ishan Thakkar

Foreword

Farokh Udwadia

JAYPEE

JAYPEE BROTHERS MEDICAL PUBLISHERS (P) LTD

New Delhi • London • Philadelphia • Panama

Jaypee Brothers Medical Publishers (P) Ltd

Headquarters

Jaypee Brothers Medical Publishers (P) Ltd
4838/24, Ansari Road, Daryaganj
New Delhi 110 002, India
Phone: +91-11-43574357
Fax: +91-11-43574314
Email: jaypee@jaypeebrothers.com

Overseas Offices

J.P. Medical Ltd
83 Victoria Street, London
SW1H 0HW (UK)
Phone: +44-2031708910
Fax: +02-03-0086180
Email: info@jpmedpub.com

Jaypee-Highlights Medical Publishers Inc
City of Knowledge, Bld. 237, Clayton
Panama City, Panama
Phone: +1 507-301-0496
Fax: +1 507-301-0499
Email: cservice@jphmedical.com

Jaypee Medical Inc
The Bourse
111 South Independence Mall East
Suite 835, Philadelphia, PA 19106, USA
Phone: +1 267-519-9789
Email: jpmed.us@gmail.com

Jaypee Brothers Medical Publishers (P) Ltd
17/1-B Babar Road, Block-B, Shaymali
Mohammadpur, Dhaka-1207
Bangladesh
Mobile: +08801912003485
Email: jaypeedhaka@gmail.com

Jaypee Brothers Medical Publishers (P) Ltd
Bhotahity, Kathmandu, Nepal
Phone: +977-9741283608
Email: kathmandu@jaypeebrothers.com

Website: www.jaypeebrothers.com
Website: www.jaypeedigital.com

Inquiries for bulk sales may be solicited at: jaypee@jaypeebrothers.com

Practical Clinical Oncology

First Edition: **2014**

ISBN 978-93-5152-205-8

Printed at Replika Press Pvt. Ltd.

This compilation is gratefully

Dedicated to

The Tata Memorial Centre

and

The Legions of its patients

The driving forces

responsible for this effort

Contributors

Advani SH MD FICP FNAMS
Director, Medical Oncology
Jaslok Hospital
Mumbai, Maharashtra, India

Agarwal Jai Bakash MD
Department of Radiation Oncology
Tata Memorial Hospital
Mumbai, Maharashtra, India

Agarwal-Joshi Geetanjali MS
Consultant Surgical Oncologist
Galaxy Care Laparoscopic Institute
Pune, Maharashtra, India

Arneja Sarabjeet Kaur MD
Head, Department of Surgical Pathology and Cytology
Breach Candy Hospital
Mumbai, Maharashtra, India

Arora Brijesh MD DM
Professor, Department of Medical Oncology
Tata Memorial Hospital
Mumbai, Maharashtra, India

Atreya Shrikant MD
Consultant, Department of Palliative Medicine and Psycho-oncology, Tata Memorial Hospital
Mumbai, Maharashtra, India

Badwe Rajendra MS
Director and Chief of Surgery
Tata Memorial Hospital
Mumbai, Maharashtra, India

Bakshi Ganesh K MS MCh (Urology)
Associate Professor and Surgeon
Department of Uro-oncology
Tata Memorial Hospital
Mumbai, Maharashtra, India

Balasubramaniam Ganesh PhD (Epidemiology)
Assistant Professor
Tata Memorial Hospital
Mumbai, Maharashtra, India

Borges Anita MD FRC Path
COE Histopathology, Consultant Histopathologist
Asian Institute of Oncology, S L Raheja Hospital and SRL Diagnostics
Mumbai, Maharashtra, India

Buch Harikesh MS FRCS (Eng) FRCS (Ed)
Consulting Surgeon and Vice-President – Asian South Pacific Ostomy Association
Asian Institute of Oncology and
Bharatiya Arogya Nidhi Hospital
Mumbai, Maharashtra, India

Chauhan Madan MD
Medical Superintendent
Barshi Cancer Research and Treatment Center
Solapur, Maharashtra, India

Chhabra Deepak MS DNB MRCS (Edin UK)
Consultant Gastro-Intestinal and Hepato-Pancreato-Biliary Surgeon, Department of Surgical Oncology
Dr L H Hiranandani Hospital and Bombay Hospital
Mumbai, Maharashtra, India

Choudhary Devendra MS
Senior Resident
Bombay Hospital
Mumbai, Maharashtra, India

Deodhar Jayita
MD (Psy) DPM DNB (Psy) DMH (UK) MRC Psych
Associate Professor
Tata Memorial Hospital
Mumbai, Maharashtra, India

Desai Neil PhD
Vice President, Strategic platforms
Abraxis Biosciences
Los Angeles, USA

Desai Praful MS FRCS FACS
Senior Surgical Oncologist
Former Director and Chief of Surgery
Tata Memorial Hospital
Breach Candy Hospital and Bombay Hospital
Mumbai, Maharashtra, India

Deshpande Ramakant MS FICS FAIS DHA
Consultant Surgical Oncologist
Asian Institute of Oncology
Breach Candy Hospital and Jaslok Hospital
Mumbai, Maharashtra, India

Dhale Abhijit MS
Senior Resident
Bombay Hospital
Mumbai, Maharashtra, India

Gite Nasreen MS
Senior Resident
Bombay Hospital
Mumbai, Maharashtra, India

Goyal Gautam MD DM ECMO
Consultant Medical Oncologist
SPS Apollo Hospital
Ludhiana, Punjab, India

Gunavanthe Varun MS
Senior Resident
Bombay Hospital
Mumbai, Maharashtra, India

Gupta Sudeep MD DM (Medical Oncology)
Professor, Medical Oncology and Deputy Director
Advanced Centre for Treatment Research and Education in Cancer (ACTREC), Tata Memorial Hospital
Mumbai, Maharashtra, India

Gupte Sateesh DA (Lon) FRCA (Eng)
Anaesthesiologist
Bombay Hospital
Mumbai, Maharashtra, India

Haribhakti Vijay MS
Consultant Surgical Oncologist
Head, Department of Surgical Oncology, Saifee Hospital
Jaslok Hospital and Breach Candy Hospital
Mumbai, Maharashtra, India

Huilgol Nagraj G DGO MD
Chief, Div. of Radiation Oncology
Dr. Balabhai Nanavati Hospital, Cancer Centre
Mumbai, Maharashtra, India

Jagannath Palepu MS FACS FICS FIMSA FAMS
Chairman, Department of Surgical Oncology
and Chief of Gastrointestinal Oncology
Lilavati Hospital and SL Raheja Hospital
Mumbai, Maharashtra, India

Jain Parmanand MD MNAMS
Head, Division of Pain
Professor, Department of Anaesthesiology
Critical Care and Pain, Tata Memorial Hospital
Mumbai, Maharashtra, India

Jalali Rakesh MD
Professor, Radiation and Neuro-Oncology Group
Tata Memorial Hospital
Mumbai, Maharashtra, India

Jambhekar Nirmala MD
Professor and Head, Department of Pathology
Tata Memorial Hospital
Mumbai, Maharashtra, India

Jankharia Bhavin MD
Consultant Radiologist
SRL – Jankharia Imaging
Mumbai, Maharashtra, India

Joshi Amit MD DM
Associate Professor, Department of
Medical Oncology
Tata Memorial Hospital
Mumbai, Maharashtra, India

Joshi Saurabh MS
Consultant Surgical Oncologist
Galaxy Care Laparoscopic Institute
Pune, Maharashtra, India

Kalyani Nikhil MD
Department of Radiation Oncology
Tata Memorial Hospital
Mumbai, Maharashtra, India

Kelkar Rohini MD DPB
Professor and Head, Department of Microbiology
Tata Memorial Hospital
Mumbai, Maharashtra, India

Krishna BA DRM MNAMS
Head, Department of Nuclear Medicine and PET Imaging
Bombay Hospital
Mumbai, Maharashtra, India

Krishna Uday MD DNB
Neuro-oncology Fellow
Tata Memorial Hospital
Mumbai, Maharashtra, India

Kuchekar Mridula DNB (General Surgery)
Clinical Assistant
Global Hospital
Mumbai, Maharashtra, India

Kulkarni Jagdeesh MS MCh MNAMS FCPS FICS
Professor Uro-oncology
Bombay Hospital
Mumbai, Maharashtra, India

Kurkure Purna MD DCH FIAP
Professor Emeritus, Paediatric Oncology
Tata Memorial Hospital
Mumbai, Maharashtra, India

Lalande Louise Forest
Entero Stomal (ET) Nurse, President World Council of Entero Stomal Therapist (WCET)
CHU Sainte-Justine, Mother-and-Child University Health Centre, Montreal, Canada

Lawande Akhil MS
Laparoscopic Gynaecologist
Galaxy Care Laparoscopic Institute
Pune, Maharashtra, India

Majeed Tanveer Abdul MS DNB MRCS (Ed) MRCP (Glas)
Consultant Surgical Oncologist
Joy Hospital and Asian Institute of Oncology
Mumbai, Maharashtra, India

Menon Santosh MD DNB
Associate Professor, Department of Pathology
Tata Memorial Hospital
Mumbai, Maharashtra, India

Muckaden Mary Ann
MD (Rad Onco) Diploma (Palliative Medicine)
Professor and Head, Department of Palliative Medicine
Tata Memorial Hospital
Mumbai, Maharashtra, India

Nene Bhagwan MD MRCP
Senior Physician and Director
Barshi Cancer Research and Treatment Centre
Solapur, Maharashtra, India

Parikh Bhavna MD
Consultant Medical Oncologist
Bombay Hospital, Dr Balabhai Nanavati Hospital and Holy Family Hospital
Mumbai, Maharashtra, India

Parikh Ratna MS FACS FAIS
Consultant Surgical Oncologist
Breach Candy Hospital, Saifee Hospital and Bharatiya Arogya Nidhi Hospital
Mumbai, Maharashtra, India

Parikh Samir MD DM DNB (Gastroenterology)
Consultant Gastroenterologist
Lilavati Hospital and Dr. Balabhai Nanavati Hospital
Mumbai, Maharashtra, India

Patel Keyuri MD (Pathology)
Histopathologist and Cytologist
Bombay Hospital
Mumbai, Maharashtra, India

Patil Vijaya MD DA (CPS – Anaesthesiology)
Professor, Department of Anaesthesiology
Critical Care and Pain, Tata Memorial Hospital
Mumbai, Maharashtra, India

Pezcoller Carlo MS
Consultant Colorectal Surgeon
Former Professor of Surgery – Postgraduate School of Surgery and Oncology – University of Modena and Reggio Emilia, Italy, Hesperia Hospital
Modena, Italy

Prabhash Kumar MD DM
Professor, Department of Medical Oncology
Tata Memorial Hospital
Mumbai, Maharashtra, India

Pramesh CS MS FRCS
Professor, Thoracic Surgery
Tata Memorial Hospital
Mumbai, Maharashtra, India

Puntambekar Shailesh MS
Medical Director
Galaxy Care Laparoscopic Institute
Pune, Maharashtra, India

Puri Ajay MS
Professor and Chief, Orthopaedic Oncology
Tata Memorial Hospital
Mumbai, Maharashtra, India

Roy Mukul DNB
Clinical Assistant
Dr Balabhai Nanavati Hospital
Mumbai, Maharashtra, India

Sarin Rajiv MD FRCR
Professor of Radiation Oncology and Chief Cancer Genetics Unit, ACTREC
Tata Memorial Hospital
Mumbai, Maharashtra, India

Savant Dhairyasheel MS FICS
Consultant Surgical Oncologist and Reconstructive Surgeon
Asian Institute of Oncology and S L Raheja Hospital
Mumbai, Maharashtra, India

Sengar Manju MD DM
Professor
Adult Hemato Lymphoid Disease Management Group
Tata Memorial Hospital
Mumbai, Maharashtra, India

Sharma Kailash MD DA (Anaesthesiology)
Director
Academics and Professor, Department of Anaesthesiology, Critical Care and Pain
Tata Memorial Hospital
Mumbai, Maharashtra, India

Shastri Aditi MD
Senior Fellow, Medical Oncology and Hematology
Montefiore Hospital, Albert Einstein College of Medicine
New York, USA

Shastri Surendra MD DPh DHA
Head, Department of Preventive Oncology
Tata Memorial Hospital
Mumbai, Maharashtra, India

Shrikhande Shailesh V MS MD
Chief, Gastro-Intestinal and Hepato-Pancreato-Biliary Service
Professor, Department of Surgical Oncology
Tata Memorial Hospital
Mumbai, Maharashtra, India

Sondhi Vishal MD DNB
Assistant Professor
Department of Pediatrics
Armed Forces Medical College
Pune, Maharashtra, India

Tongaonkar Hemant B MS
Consultant Urologic and Gynaecologic Oncologist
P D Hinduja National Hospital and Research Centre
Mumbai, Maharashtra, India

Udwadia Tehemton E MS FRCS (Eng) FRCS (Edin) FACS, FAMS
Emeritus Professor of Surgery
Grant Medical College and J J Hospital
Consultant Surgeon
Head Department of Minimally Access Surgery
Hinduja, Hospital and Breach Candy Hospital
Mumbai, Maharashtra, India

Foreword

Cancer indeed has been rightly termed "The Emperor of All Maladies". Extensive research coupled with the clinical experience of oncologists all over the world for several decades has helped to unravel some aspects of the problem. The disease however continues to beguile and mock the medical profession.

The present text on "Practical Clinical Oncology" is welcome, important and necessary. This is the first composite Indian text on cancer, written by numerous well-known oncologists and other distinguished doctors associated with the diagnosis and management of cancer, working in our country. It has been admirably compiled and edited by Dr. Praful Desai (Editor-in-Chief), one of the most eminent oncosurgeons of India, together with the help of Associate Editors and a Coordinating Editor and an Editorial Assistant, each well known in his or her specialized field. They all deserve our heartiest congratulations.

The incidence, causative factors and epidemiology of various cancers in our country, their natural history and the problems in diagnosis and management in a socio-economic milieu so different from the West have been adequately high-lighted. Ours is a country of over a billion people, riddled with social inequity and abject poverty. Tertiary and academic cancer centers in India are of help but cannot cope with the magnitude of the problem. A great deal of the fight against cancer in our country will be waged outside these centers. The present text provides a practical approach to oncologists, surgeons, physicians, pathologists, radiologists treating common cancers outside tertiary centers. The text also stresses the importance of a team effort involving various disciplines in the management and care of each cancer patient. The timing of different modalities of treatment for different cancers at different stages of the disease is important and has been well emphasized. The role of genetics in cancer has also been included. The disease leaves its genomic fingerprints in the DNA of a cancer patient, and the fingerprints are different for different cancers. The early recognition of these fingerprints may help towards prevention, diagnosis and management of the disease.

The struggle against cancer will continue unabated. It is implicit within the text that there will never be a magic bullet that will cure all cancers. One foresees in the near future some more cancers being cured and some more contained. The cycle of treatment, recurrence, retreatment will almost certainly be more stretched out over time so that patients with different cancers will live longer than they do today. Will the disease be ever eradicated in the distant future? Cancer seems to be embedded, hidden (ever ready to erupt) within the genome of the human race. If this is needed, it will require many quantum leaps in genomic science for this hope and dream to be realized.

Being smitten by cancer is invariably traumatic, devasting, soul-shattering experience for the patient. Doctors should therefore not just treat cancer, but more importantly treat the patient who has cancer, "Cancer begins and ends with people. In the midst of scientific abstraction, it is sometimes possible to forget this basic fact." (June Goodfield)
This book should not only be useful to all oncologists, but to surgeons, pathologists, radiologists, postgraduate trainees and to all those interested or involved in the care and management of cancer patients. "*Practical Clinical Oncology*" is indeed an important landmark in the history of medicine in our country.

Farokh Udwadia

Prologue

Majority of health care problems are often entwined with socio-economic conditions and lifestyle issues. Cancer is no exception. Demographic factors show a continuing rise in its frequency and incidence. In an era of information overload and practice changing paradigms in cancer, a sense of equipoise needs to be maintained. One more text on "CANCER" may appear superfluous and yet the authors contend that the vast majority of our busy oncologists, surgeons, physicians and pathologists working beyond the academic and tertiary cancer centers need a practical approach to the commonly occurring cancers in our country. This, in essence, is the primary objective of this compilation. The authors therefore address only commonly occurring solid tumors, the lymphoproliferative disorders and common neuro-oncology problems. Rare and uncommon cancers have been excluded. This book, therefore, is indeed not a treatise on cancer.

We live in an era of genomics, evidence based and 'personalized' medicine for every cancer. The paucity of modern medical facilities, trained professionals, our socio-economic environment and the failure to address fundamental issues makes it imperative that a practical approach be charted out to meet our current therapeutic needs for the cancer afflicted in an urban, and more particularly in a rural setting. We therefore hope that this book will be useful as a practical guide and approach not only to all oncology trainees but to all consultants in general medicine and surgery, who may be called upon to manage or advise a cancer patient. The authors of this compilation represent experts in various oncology disciplines and are deeply committed to the subject. The vast majority of them represent the past and the present faculty of the Tata Memorial Hospital, the country's largest and oldest cancer facility over the past seven decades. This work is not a treatise on cancer and therefore, is not meant to encompass all aspects of oncology in great details. Apart from standard of care, alternatives and controversies in management, where it exists, have been alluded to. The science of medicine has moved from an era of a clinical bedside art to an innovative technologic craft and more recently into a genomic science due to our increased understanding of human biology in health and disease; and yet cancer continues to be the most complex and feared disease which afflict human civilization today. The magic cure bullet is not yet at hand and one wonders whether it will ever be so.

In the new millennium we are witnessing changing paradigms in our approach to oncology due to fundamental research as well as technologic and therapeutic innovations. With increasing connectivity via information technology, we live in an era of hyper-information, occasionally even misinformation, due to plethora of scientific publications for every given cancer. 'One size does not fit all,' "Evidence based medicine" are the modern buzz words signifying some progress towards a standard of care for cancer control and cure. Real progress in science and medicine is a painfully slow process and no quantum jump can be expected towards a cancer cure. Fundamental principles of complementary cancer management has remained steadfast; however, conservation surgery, morbidity reduction, greater attention to quality of life issues and palliation for terminal care must receive due consideration. The book addresses these issues in a comprehensive manner. We need to show patience towards alternative medicine and greater scientific ethos, as nearly 50% of patients seek alternative medicine along with the current standard of care.

President John F Kennedy vowed to place a man on the moon in 1963 and so he did in 1970. Likewise, President Nixon in 1972 proclaimed a 'cure for cancer' by 1980 in the US Congress. Billions of dollars and 40 years later the call for 'cancer cure' eludes us and continues to test the skill and ingenuity of the human mind. Cancer cure is obviously harder to crack than placing a 'man on the moon.' Medicine must remain a harmonious blend of the clinical art of medicine and scientific technology. We must weigh our successes against our failures, the benefits versus the risks and the value of old treatment versus new practices. Only then can we practice medicine with a conscience.

This is a miniscule attempt to complement our slow and steady march towards the control and understanding of this fascinating but frustrating disease. Hopefully this compilation will offer practical guidelines for understanding cancer and help in its management by concerned professionals across our country and elsewhere. Indeed, cancer is not a disease or a phenomenon to be exorcised; it is an abnormal physio-pathologic aberration which needs to be understood. The human mind will slowly and steadily unravel the enigma of cancer. Aided and abetted by the forces of medicine, science and technology mankind will slowly proceed towards the ultimate destination—"The Conquest of Mortality? To understand cancer is to understand life itself."

Praful Desai

Acknowledgments

It is a matter of great privilege, pride and pleasure that together we have reached a stage when I have to gather my thoughts to pen down my sincere debt of gratitude and thanks to all who have made this compilation possible. The idea to embark upon this journey was not sudden but a very gradual process germinating for more than a decade. It is incumbent and obligatory on our part to return to the society or to the profession - what we have received from them; it is in this humble spirit that I write this brief connotation.

First and foremost, my gratitude reaches out to my Alma Mater, The Tata Memorial Hospital and legions of its patients which helped me to evolve into an oncology professional. It cannot be measured in words and the feelings cannot be translated on paper.

Evolving ideas like this one into action and reality is a multistep and a very gradual process; friends, colleagues - critical colleagues and family form the core of this pyramid. I have been very deeply blessed in this regard. My dear wife, Meena and my sons Jay and Neil - each one of them authors of repute, always looked at me askance as to when will I ever follow their lead. Generally it should have been the other way around; I should have inspired them; however, their respective contributions spurred me into activity, however delayed.

I cannot but specially mention Dr Rajendra Badwe, the current Director of the Tata Memorial Hospital, for his critical inputs and Dr Rakesh Jalali, Neuro-Radiotherapist at the Tata Memorial Hospital, for his enthusiasm which spurred colleagues at the Tata Memorial Hospital into activity. Dr Rajendra Badwe's gracious permission to the present faculty of Tata Memorial Center to participate in this venture has been of critical importance. Nearly 80% of the contributing authors represent the past and present faculty of the Tata Memorial Center. Words cannot measure or evaluate their contribution.

My sincere appreciation and thanks to all my co-editors for frequent brain-storming sessions and their time, which gave shape and form to this book.

I owe a very special thanks and gratitude to Dr Ratna Parikh, my close colleague and a young surgical oncologist who has diligently worked as a co-ordinating editor for this effort. She is indeed the mind, the soul and the heart of this book. In fact, this is her book, which would not have been possible without her. Coaxing, cajoling and gently reminding in her own persuasive style, she managed to get most manuscripts in reasonable time from all participating colleagues. I cannot thank and applaud her enough.

I have no words to evaluate the enthusiasm and hard work of Dr Ishan Thakkar. A young homoeopath with a gentle smile conveyed everything. He went beyond the call of duty for the project. A net savvy and computer expert who along with Dr Ratna truly and literally put everything together. Both of them spent hours and days together to bring this effort to a successful fruition.

My special gratitude and thanks to Shri Jitendar P Vij (Group Chairman), Mr Ankit Vij (Managing Director) and Mr Tarun Duneja (Director-Publishing) of M/s Jaypee Brothers Medical Publishers (P) Ltd, New Delhi, India, for their enthusiasm and encouragement at every level enthused us to expedite the collection of manuscripts. To all others at Jaypee's who have revised, reviewed and added their artistic inputs, I am deeply grateful for their support.

Last but not the least, Dr Farokh Udwadia, probably the most prolific medical author of our times and an icon in the profession, whom I regard as one of my mentors, my deepest regards, salutation and thanks for penning the Foreword.

Contents

1. **Cancer – Reflections from the Past** 1
Praful Desai
Radiotherapy 3
Chemotherapy 4
Biological (targeted) therapy 5
The Indian scenario 5
The future 6

2. **Surgical Oncology: An Overview** 7
Praful Desai

3. **Geographic Variations in Frequency and Incidence: A Global Perspective** 9
Ganesh Balasubramaniam
Geographic variations in incidence 10
Incidence rates based on economic development 10

4. **Primary and Secondary Prevention of Common Cancers** 15
Surendra Shastri, Aditi Shastri
Cervical cancer screening and prevention 15
Breast cancer screening 18
Oral cancer prevention and screening 20

5. **The Changing Face of Surgical Pathology** 24
Anita Borges

6. **Current and Future Imaging Techniques: Therapeutic Impact on Treatment Planning** 35
Bhavin Jankharia
Plain radiographs 35
Mammography 35
Ultrasound 36
Computed tomography scan 36
Magnetic resonance imaging 37
Positron emission tomography/computed tomography 37
Positron emission tomography/magnetic resonance imaging 39
Interventional radiology 40

7. **Role of Nuclear Medicine in Oncology** 42
BA Krishna
Principle of nuclear imaging 43
Diagnostic role 43
Types of nuclear scans in oncology 43
Clinical applications 44
Breast cancer 46
Lung cancer 48
Gastrointestinal cancers 50
Genitourinary cancers 52
Head and neck cancer 53
Bone and soft tissue tumors 53
Positron emission tomography-computed tomography in radiotherapy 53
Infections in oncology 54

Evolving applications of positron emission tomography scan with new tracers 54
Therapeutic nuclear oncology 55

8. Tumor Markers in Cancer: Therapeutic Impact **59**
Praful Desai
Therapeutic impact of tumor markers in cancer 59

9. Cancer Chemotherapy: Future Perspectives **61**
SH Advani
Supportive care 62
Introduction of hormone therapy 63
Biological therapeutics 63
Growth signal inhibitors 63

10. Radiotherapy: Prospects and Retrospects **65**
Nagraj G Huilgol, Mukul Roy
Biological basics of radiation therapy 67
Rationale for combination chemoradiotherapy 68
Brachytherapy 70
Development of new radionuclides and radiation physics 70
Brachytherapy types based on dose rate 71
Types of brachytherapy based on sources placed 71
Intensity-modulated radiotherapy 71
Future of radiation oncology 72

11. Hormonal Dependence of Malignant Cells **74**
Rajendra Badwe, Sudeep Gupta, Gautam Goyal
History 74
Pathophysiology 74
Molecular effects of hormonal therapies 75
Breast cancer 76
Hormones in prostate cancer 79
Hormonal use in other tumors 81
Newer perspectives 82

12. Genetics and Cancer **84**
Rajiv Sarin
Genetics of sporadic and hereditary cancers 84
Burden of hereditary cancers 84
Genetic mechanism of cancer development: multistep carcinogenesis and genomic instability 85
Tumor suppressor genes and oncogenes 86
The two-hit model of Knudson and hereditary retinoblastoma 86
Epigenetics and cancer 87
Clinical presentation and evaluation of hereditary cancers 87
Ascertaining family history 88
Genetic testing, its indications and interpretation 91
Cancer screening and prevention in high-risk individuals/mutation carriers 92
Molecular taxonomy of cancers and its clinical relevance 93
Molecular diagnostic techniques in cancer 94

13. Nanotechnology in Cancer Diagnosis and Treatment: A New Frontier **98**
Neil Desai
Nanotechnology application in cancer diagnosis 100
Nanotechnology application in cancer therapy 102

14. Translational Research in Oncology **112**
CS Pramesh, Rajendra Badwe
Research in cancer 112
A brief history of cancer research 112
Translational research 113

15. The Impact of Minimally Invasive Surgery in Oncology 120
Shailesh Puntambekar, Geetanjali Agarwal-Joshi, Saurabh Joshi, Akhil Lawande
Laparoscopy in oncology 121
Esophagus 122
Colon and rectal cancer 125
Hysterectomy 130

16. Toward the Future of Minimal Access Surgery: A Personal Perspective 135
Tehemton E Udwadia
Training 135
Simulator training 136
Technology 137
Pragmatic evaluation 138
The future 138
Socioeconomic reality 139

17. Oral Premalignant Lesions 142
Vijay Haribhakti
Definitions and terms 142
Leukoplakia 142
Erythroplakia 143
Submucous fibrosis (SMF) 143
Oral lichen planus (OLP) 144
Approach to a patient 144
Biopsy interpretation 145
Management 146

18. Oral Cancers 147
Vijay Haribhakti
Anatomical boundaries and subsites 147
General features 147
Approach to treatment 149
Surgical approaches 149
The lips 153
Cheek and gum 153
The mandible 154
Retromolar trigone 157
Floor of mouth/tongue 157
Radiotherapy 159
Chemotherapy 159

19. Cancer of the Larynx 160
Vijay Haribhakti
Diagnosis 161
Staging of cancer of the larynx 162
Management of laryngeal cancer 162

20. Cancer of the Pharynx 168
Vijay Haribhakti
Surgical anatomy 168
General features 168
The nasopharynx 169
The oropharynx 171
The hypopharynx and cervical esophagus 174

21. Salivary Gland Tumors 180
Vijay Haribhakti
Surgical anatomy 180
Clinical features and diagnosis 181

Classification of salivary tumors 183
Mucoepidermoid carcinoma 183
Adenoid cystic carcinoma 183
Adenocarcinoma 183
Others 183
Treatment goals and alternatives 184
Superficial parotidectomy—technique 184
Management of the neck 184
Issues in salivary gland surgery 185

22. Carcinoma of the Thyroid **186**

Praful Desai, Sarabjeet Kaur Arneja

Etiology 186
Pathology 186
Staging 188
Clinical features and investigations 188
Fine needle aspiration cytology 188
Treatment 188
Management of neck nodes 190
Adjuvant radioactive iodine 191
Lobectomy versus total thyroidectomy in thyroid cancers 191
Solitary thyroid nodule—management algorithm 191

23. Parathyroid Tumors **194**

Praful Desai

24. The Metastatic Neck **197**

Vijay Haribhakti

Anatomy of the fascia and spaces of the neck 197
Triangles of the neck 197
Neck levels 198
Determinants of nodal metastasis 199
Clinical features 199
Staging 199
Management of the metastatic neck 200
Nomenclature of neck dissections 200
The surgical pathology report 201

25. The Role of Diagnostic and Therapeutic Endoscopy in Digestive Tract Malignancies **202**

Samir Parikh

Premalignant/dysplastic lesions of digestive tract 203
Diagnosis and staging of digestive cancers 206
Endoscopic treatment 210
Endoscopic resection 211
Laparoscopic surgery 213
Natural orifice transluminal endoscopic surgery 213
Endoscopic palliative treatment 214
Endoscopic treatment of postoperative/postradiotherapy complications 216

26. Cancer of the Esophagus **222**

Praful Desai, Ganesh Balasubramaniam

Associated factors 223
Pretherapy work-up and investigation 223
Surgical approach 224
Localized (locoregional) esophageal cancer 224
Nodal dissection (two-field/three-field) 226
Type of anastomotic disruptions 228
Chemoradiotherapy as definitive treatment 229
Palliation 229

Chemotherapy 229
Tracheoesophageal fistula 231

27. Carcinoma Stomach 233
Praful Desai, Bhavna Parikh, Nagraj G Huilgol, Ganesh Balasubramaniam
Epidemiology 233
Diet 234
Tobacco 234
Alcohol 234
Obesity 234
Ethnicity 235
Genetics 235
Pathology 235

28. Tumors of the Small Bowel 245
Ratna Parikh, Praful Desai
Etiology 245
Clinical presentation 245
Diagnostic work-up 245
Carcinoid tumors 245
Treatment 246

29. Cancer of Colon, Rectum and Anal Canal 250
Praful Desai, Sarabjeet Kaur Arneja, Bhavna Parikh
Carcinoma of the Colon 250
Pathology 250
Diagnosis/investigations 252
Staging 253
Treatment planning 254
Complications of colonic surgery 255
Neoadjuvant chemotherapy in colonic cancers 255
Carcinoma of the Rectum 255
Etiology 255
Clinical presentation and investigations 256
Fundamental principles of therapy 256
Cancers of the Anal Canal 264
Introduction and etiology 264
Diagnosis and pretherapy workup 264
Pathology 265
Treatment 265

30. Pseudomyxoma Peritonei 269
Ratna Parikh, Praful Desai, Sarabjeet Kaur Arneja
Pathology 269
Diagnosis 269
Treatment 269
Chemotherapy 271

31. Gastrointestinal Stromal Tumors 273
Praful Desai, Keyuri Patel
Pathology 273
Clinical 274
Investigations 275
Management 275

32. Hepatic Malignancies 277
Deepak Chhabra, Palepu Jagannath
Hepatocellular carcinoma 277

Surgical treatment of hepatocellular carcinoma 281
Liver transplantation 285
Locoregional therapy 285
Targeted therapy 287
Prevention and surveillance 287
Other primary malignant liver tumors 287
Rare primary liver tumors 288

33. Biliary Malignancies 291
Deepak Chhabra, Palepu Jagannath

Gallbladder Carcinoma 291
Epidemiology and risk factors for gallbladder carcinoma 291
Clinical presentation 292
Pathology and patterns of spread 292
Staging 293
Investigations 293
Management 295
Extent of liver resection for gallbladder cancers 296
Extent of lymphadenectomy 299
Bile duct resection 299
Neoadjuvant and adjuvant treatments for GBC 299
Palliative care 299

Hilar 299

Cholangiocarcinoma 299
Epidemiology and risk factors for cholangiocarcioma 300
Pathology and patterns of spread 300
Staging 301
Preoperative evaluation 303
Management 304
Principles of surgical resection in hilar cholangiocarcinoma 304
Palliation 306
Systemic and other treatments 306

34. Pancreatic Malignancies 310
Shailesh V Shrikhande, Palepu Jagannath

Risk factors and molecular biology 310
Clinical features 310
Pretherapy investigations 311
Confirmation of diagnosis 312
Obstructive jaundice in resectable pancreatic head and periampullary cancer: management approach 312
Treatment 312
Adjuvant therapy in pancreatic cancer 319
Neoadjuvant approaches in pancreatic cancer 319
Palliation in pancreatic cancer 319
Uncommon pancreatic tumors 319

35. Breast Cancer 325
Ratna Parikh, Praful Desai, Anita Borges, Sarabjeet Kaur Arneja, Nagraj G Huilgol, Bhavin Jankharia, Bhavna Parikh, Ganesh Balasubramaniam

Epidemiology 325
Pathology 326
Grading of breast carcinoma 328
Hormone receptor 329
HER2 neu 329
Molecular classification 329
Screening 330
Prevention 330

Diagnosis 330
Noninvasive breast cancer 336
Invasive breast cancer 339
Sentinel lymph node retrieval in breast cancer 343
Locally advanced breast cancer 344
Inflammatory breast cancer 345
Bilateral breast cancer 346
Mucinous breast cancer (colloid or granulomatous carcinoma) 346
Tubular carcinoma 346
Papillary carcinoma 346
Medullary carcinoma 346
Male breast cancer 347
Phyllodes tumor (cystosarcoma phyllodes) 347
Paget's disease 347
Breast cancer and pregnancy 349
Recurrent disease 350
Metastatic breast cancer 350
Systemic therapy of breast cancer 352
Radiation therapy 355

36. Ovarian Cancer **363**

Ratna Parikh, Praful Desai, Ganesh Balasubramaniam, Bhavna Parikh, Sarabjeet Kaur Arneja

Epidemiology 363
Associated factors 363
Surveillance 365
Chemoprevention 365
Prophylactic surgery 365
Pathology 365
Clinical features 368
Investigations 368
Mode of spread 369
Surgery 370
Systemic therapy of epithelial ovarian cancer 371
Management of recurrent disease 372
Common protocols 373

37. Carcinoma of the Cervix **379**

Praful Desai, Keyuri Patel, Bhavna Parikh, Nagraj G Huilgol, Ganesh Balasubramaniam

Epidemiology 379
Human papilloma virus infection 379
Pathology 381
Screening for cervical cancer 383
Papanicolaou smears 383
Problems and challenges 384
Clinical features and pre-therapy work-up 385
Invasive carcinoma of the cervix: surgical management 385

Chemotherapy 389

Neoadjuvant chemotherapy 389
Adjuvant chemotherapy 390
Salvage chemotherapy for metastatic and recurrent disease 390
Standard protocols 390

Radiotherapy 391

Stage IA–C FIGO 391
Stage IA 2 391
FIGO–stage IBI, and IIA A 391
Adjuvant postoperative radiation therapy 391
Acute side-effects 392
Late side-effects 392

38. Endometrial Cancer 394

Praful Desai, Keyuri Patel, Bhavna Parikh, Nagraj G Huilgol, Ganesh Balasubramaniam

Epidemiology 394
Pathology 396
Clinical features 397
Treatment 398
Radiotherapy (RT) 399

39. Management of Lung Cancer 403

Ramakant Deshpande, Tanveer Abdul Majeed

Epidemiology 403
Etiology 404
Pathology 405
Modes of dissemination 405
Clinical features 407
Diagnosis of lung cancer 407
Treatment of lung cancer 409

40. Mediastinal Tumors 424

Ramakant Deshpande, Tanveer Abdul Majeed

Surgical anatomy of mediastinum 424
Incidence and pathology 424
Diagnosis 424
Symptoms and signs 425
Paraneoplastic syndrome 425
Thymus 426
Thymoma 426
Germ cell tumors 428

41. Tumors of the Chest Wall 436

Ramakant Deshpande, Tanveer Abdul Majeed

Histological types 436
Clinical features 439
Diagnosis 440
Chest wall resections and reconstructions 440

42. Tumors of the Adrenal Gland 444

Varun Gunavanthe, Jagdeesh Kulkarni

Clinical presentation 444
Etiopathology of adrenal mass 445
Surgical indications for adrenalectomy 446
Differential diagnosis of adrenal tumors 446
Illustrative case reports 451

43. Renal Cell Carcinoma 454

Hemant B Tongaonkar, Ganesh K Bakshi, Santosh Menon, Kumar Prabhash, Amit Joshi

Epidemiology 454
Etiology 454
Pathology 455
Pathogenesis 456
Diagnosis and staging 456
Treatment of localized renal cell carcinoma 462
Management of tumor extension to renal vein or inferior vena cava 464
Metastatic renal cell carcinoma 466

44. Prostate Cancer 474

Jagdeesh Kulkarni, Varun Gunavanthe, Nasreen Gite, Abhijit Dhale, Devendra Choudhary

Epidemiology 475
Primary chemoprevention 476

Pathology 476
Diagnosis 477
Staging and risk stratification 480
Treatment options and optimum management 480
Castration resistant prostate cancer 484

45. Bladder Cancer 488
Jagdeesh Kulkarni, Varun Gunavanthe, Nasreen Gite, Abhijit Dhale, Devendra Choudhary

Etiology and risk factors 488
Clinical features 488
Pathology 488
Staging 489
Investigations and staging techniques 490
Contemporary management of bladder cancer 492
Metastatic and recurrent tumors 498
Minimally invasive surgery for bladder cancer 498

46. Testicular Tumors 500
Jagdeesh Kulkarni, Abhijit Dhale, Devendra Choudhary, Nasreen Gite, Varun Gunavanthe

Epidemiology and risk factors 500
Classification 500
Germ cell tumors 500
Classification of germ cell tumors of testis 501
Clinical features 502
Investigations 502
Treatment of primary tumor—orchiectomy 503
Testes sparing surgery 504
Staging, stage grouping and risk stratification 504
Management of germ cell tumors of the testis 504
Growing teratoma syndrome 508
Salvage therapy 509
Fertility in testicular tumors 509
Tumors in undescended testis 509

47. Stoma Care 512
Harikesh Buch, Carlo Pezcoller, Louise Forest Lalande

Development of stoma appliance and stoma care 512
Incidence of stomas 512
Marking the stoma site and creation of ideal stoma 512
Indication for intestinal stoma surgery 515
Preoperative preparations 515
Technique of creation of stoma 516
Preoperative and postoperative counseling 520
Common stoma complications and its management 520
Complications related to urostomy 522
Psychosocial issues of ostomates 524
Other common problems that patient will have 525
Management of different types of stoma 526
Stoma support groups 527

48. Neuroendocrine Tumors (Carcinoids) 529
Praful Desai, Keyuri Patel

Pathology 529
Investigations 532
Gastrointestinal carcinoids (NETs) 533
Molecular based therapy 535

49. Bone Tumors and Soft Tissue Sarcomas 536
Ajay Puri, Nirmala Jambhekar

Primary bone tumors 536

Osteosarcoma 538
Ewing sarcoma 541
Chondrosarcoma 542
Principles of surgical treatment and reconstruction after wide excision in bone tumors 543
Soft tissue sarcomas 545
Management of metastatic disease from bone and soft tissue sarcomas 547

50. Retroperitoneal Sarcomas **550**
Praful Desai

Etiology 550
Pathology 550
Clinical features 550
Investigations 550
Treatment 550

51. Management of Skeletal Metastases **553**
Jai Prakash Agarwal, Nikhil Kalyani

Clinical presentation and diagnosis 553
Treatment 555

52. Management of Primary Brain Tumors **560**
Rakesh Jalali, Uday Krishna

Epidemiology 560
Imaging of primary brain tumors 561
Histology of CNS tumors 561
Management of common symptoms and complications of CNS tumors 564
Management of individual tumors 565
Management of pediatric CNS tumors 568
Management of benign tumors and intracranial extra-axial tumors 570
Palliative and supportive care 572
Hospice/end of life care 572
Quality of life 573

53. Management of Brain Metastasis **577**
Rakesh Jalali, Uday Krishna

Epidemiology 577
Clinical presentation 577
Diagnosis and evaluation 577
Pathogenesis and spread of metastases to the brain 578
Prognostic factors and staging 578
Medical management of brain metastasis 579
Radiotherapy 580

54. Cancers from an Unknown Primary Site **585**
Praful Desai

Clinical presentation 585
Clinical approach and investigations including histologic studies of the metastatic lesion 585
Treatment 586

55. Paraneoplastic Syndromes in Cancer **588**
Praful Desai

56. Reconstructive Surgery in Oncology **590**
Dhairyasheel Savant, Mridula Kuchekar

Reconstruction techniques in head and neck cancers 591
Reconstructive options for various sites in the head and neck region 593
Mandibular reconstructions 595
Chest wall reconstruction 598
Abdominal wall reconstruction 601
Breast reconstruction 603

57. Emergencies in Oncology 609
Vijaya Patil, Kailash Sharma
Neutropenic sepsis 609
Tumor lysis syndrome 609
Hypercalcemia 610
Anaphylactic reactions due to chemotherapeutic agents 610
Pheochromocytoma 611
Tumor-induced hypoglycemia 611
Superior vena cava syndrome 611
Airway obstruction 611
Cardiac tamponade 612
Cardiac failure 612
Spinal cord compression 612
Hyperviscosity syndrome 612
Hyponatremia 613

58. Pediatric Oncology: A Journey from Nihilism to Cautious Optimism 614
Purna Kurkure
Burden of childhood cancers 614
Neuroblastoma 617
Wilm's tumor 619
Retinoblastoma 620
Barriers to optimal treatment of childhood cancers in India 621

59. Lymphomas in Children 624
Brijesh Arora, Vishal Sodhi
Lymphomas in children 624

60. Adult Lymphomas 644
Manju Sengar
Non-Hodgkin lymphoma 644

61. Evidence-based Medicine in Oncology: Problems, Challenges and Opportunities 653
Praful Desai
Problems and challenges 653

62. General Principles in Oncologic Anesthesia 657
Sateesh Gupte
Gastrointestinal 657
Fever 658
Hematological abnormalities 658
Hypoglycemia 658
Hypercalcemia 658
Renal dysfunction 659
Endocrinologic 659
Neurologic 659
Lactic acidosis 659
Anesthetic problems in specific operations 660
Tumors of endocrine gland 661
Adrenal 661
Cancer chemotherapy 662

63. Cancer Pain Management 666
KS Sharma, PN Jain
Epidemiology 666
Definition and types of pain 667
Practical approach to a patient with cancer pain 668
Pharmacological management of cancer pain 668
Interventions in pain management 672

64. Palliative Care and Quality of Life in Advanced Cancer **674**
Mary Ann Muckaden, Jayita Deodhar, Shrikant Atreya
Incidence of advanced cancers 674
Definition of palliative care 675
Goals of care 675
Physical symptoms and their control 675
Gastrointestinal symptoms 675
Psychological care 679
Place of care 680
Spiritual care 680
Ethics and palliative care 681
End-of-life care 681
Ethics in end-of-life care 681
Bereavement support 682
Research and palliative care 682
Pediatric palliative care 682
Community-based palliative care 682
Epilogue 683

65. Microbial Pathogens and Infection Control in Immunocompromised Cancer Patients **685**
Rohini Kelkar
Etiology 685
Epidemiology 687
Laboratory diagnosis 687
Viral infections 688
Fungal infections 689
Mycobacterial infections 693
Cytomegalovirus infections 693
Infections in surgical oncology: surgical site infections 694
Multidrug-resistant organisms: current scenario 694
Principles of antimicrobial prophylaxis in surgical oncology 696
Infections in hematopoietic cell transplant recipients 697
Management principles 698
Guidelines for antimicrobial therapy 698
Prevention and control of infectious complications 699
Prevention of surgical site infections 700

66. Cancer Control in Developing Countries **706**
Praful Desai, Bhagwan Nene, Manoj Chauhan
Methodology—low cost/low technology effort—a replicable module 706
Comprehensive cancer centers 707
Community cancer centers 707

67. The Future: Cure, Control or Peaceful Coexistence? **711**
Praful Desai

68. The Conquest of Mortality: Science, Medicine and Technology's Final Destination? **714**
Praful Desai

Index ***719***

1 Cancer – Reflections from the Past

Praful Desai

INTRODUCTION

History is merely a collation of events and facts based on human endeavors of the past which impacts and modifies the lives of the present generation with a positive or negative outcomes. Medicine, science and technology aim to confer health, comfort, increasing knowledge and communications to make the world a better place to live in. There is hardly any subject which illumines the human mind more than the perusal of history as our past shapes the present which guides us towards the future. Above all, lessons learnt from history are a source of inspiration, helps us to inculcate a sense of humility, makes us realize the limits of medicine and the fact that any truth is relative, never absolute. If we do not learn the lessons from the past we are bound to repeat the fallacies of the yore.

The history of cancer is the history of life itself. Cancer probably existed ever since civilization began. Life began as a unicellular unit-organism which had the inherent potency to replicate to reach its present form. Cancer, indeed, has the identical propensity to replicate and grow even more rapidly than the normal cells. Regulated cellular proliferation and apoptosis is at the core of normal human existence; while dysregulation of the same, for whatever reasons, is at the core of cancer genesis.

Hippocrates, almost 2,500 years ago (400 BC) coined the Greek word: "karkinos"—swelling—or "onkos" (load mass) on one of the islands of Greece (Cos). It signified a crab-like form of the abnormality he saw in the human system. Hippocrates felt cancer "karkinos" is best left untreated as patients live longer that way. This was probably the first reference to appear in literature, credited to Hippocrates. He also described the four famous body fluids, "humors" as he called them; blood, yellow bile, black bile and phlegm responsible for disease states in the human body.

Following Hippocrates, Galen—the famous Greek and Roman physician, attributed cancer to "black bile", a fluid which flows in the body and stagnates and forms "masses" (cancer). Since the black bile flows everywhere, the masses (metastasis) are the natural consequences. Famous as he was, Galen's theory of black bile persisted for nearly fifteen centuries long after he passed around 200 AD. A vividly and deftly sculptured Roman female stands in a museum in Florence, Italy. The sculpture has vividly brought to life, breast cancer on the left side with a mass and retraction of the breast, probably dated around 14th or 15th century. Known since the time of Hippocrates and Galen, this sculpture is probably the first graphic representation of cancer. The "humoral" black bile and fluid theory of Galen was finally put to rest by a brilliant French anatomist of the yore (1533) Andreas Vesalius (Fig. 1), who dissected all the nerves, blood vessels and muscles in the human body. He found no evidence of the black bile theory of Galen.

One of the earliest observation as early as 1775 regarding the causation of cancer due to external environmental factors came from London surgeon Percivall Pott who hypothesized that the high incidence of scrotal cancers in chimney sweeps could be due to the effect of soot, as a chemical carcinogen constantly affecting the scrotal area (Fig. 2).

There are always times in history when human intellect pursues an untrodden path. The fundamental understandings of the normal and abnormal cells were studied first by the brilliant German pathologist Rudolf Virchow (Fig. 3) in 1855 at the University of Wurzburg in Germany. The lives of all cells and changes therein are due to external and internal stimuli. These principles

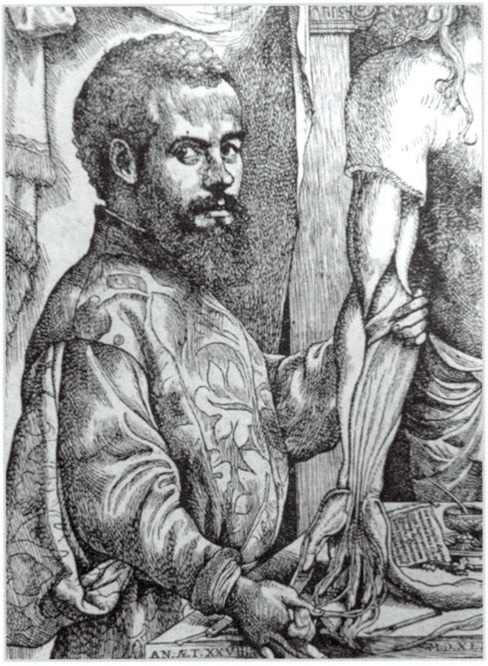

Fig. 1: The anatomist Andreas Vesalius (1514–1564) tried to discover the source for black bile, the fluid thought to be responsible for cancer. Unable to find it, Vesalius launched a new search for cancer's real cause and cure

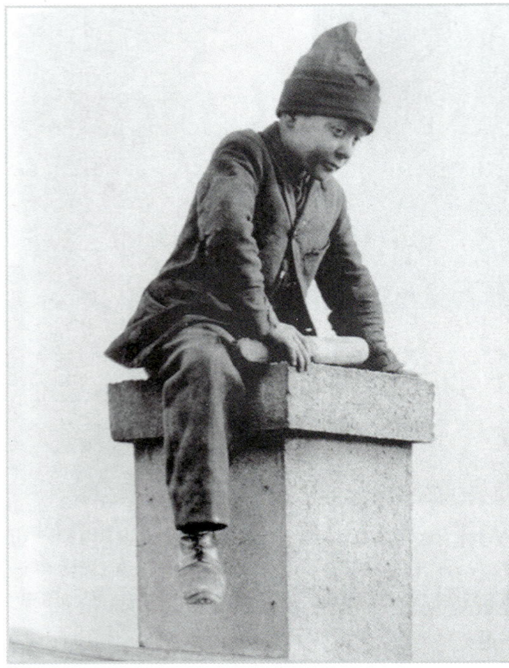

Fig. 2: Chimney—in 1775, the London surgeon Percivall Pott, observed that scrotal cancer occurred disproportionately in adolescent chimney sweeps and proposed a link between soot and scrotal cancer, launching the hunt for preventable carcinogens in the environment

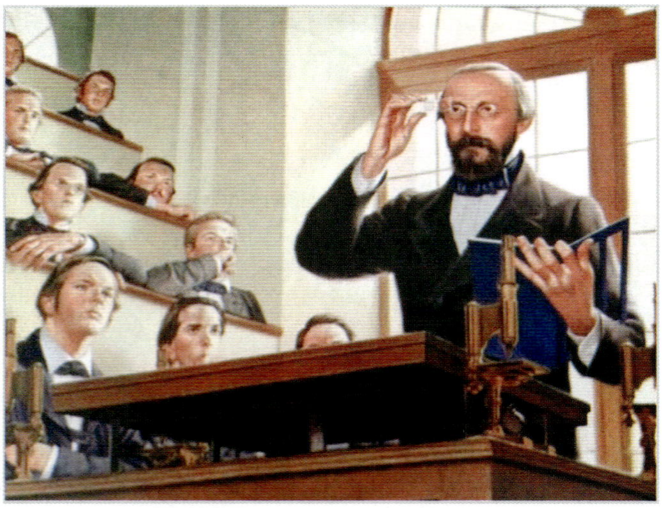

Fig. 3: Rudolph Virchow and cellular pathology

enunciated by Virchow have dominated cellular biology ever since. Indeed, the diagnosis, therapy and prognostication of a given patient squarely rests on the fundamental histopathologic studies of a given lesion. This was and is the major bedrock of cancer diagnosis and therapy.

Surgery has been the oldest method recorded in history for the treatment of cancer. Bereft of anesthesia, devoid of any idea of sepsis or antisepsis, it was the speed and the courage of the "surgeons" of the time coupled with even greater determination and courage of the patients to get rid of the pain and misery of the affliction by cancerous growths in their body. Cocaine, alcohol and tincture of opium were substitutes for anesthesia and leather belts strapping and manual "hold" were used to keep the patients on the table for "amputations" (within 10-15 minutes) and other procedures to hack the tumor out of the body. Control of bleeding was manual pressure and huge covering by clothes and bandages were the dressings.

The scenario suddenly changed in the second half of the 19th century; in October 1846, William Morton, an American dentist, successfully used ether vapor spray to successfully "anesthetise" a patient in the amphitheater at the Massachusetts General Hospital in Boston to remove a neck mass in the presence of a packed audience. This was a seminal event in the history of surgery and opened up new vistas of surgical treatment. Joseph Lister, a Scottish surgeon, in 1865 carefully studied the angry wounds and the infected necrotic material (pus) when the wounds were left open. Louis Pasteur, a French chemist, in Paris postulated that organisms—bacteria in the air are responsible for wound infection. Joseph Lister and Louis Pasteur together revolutionized surgery by understanding sepsis and antisepsis, the fundamentals of any surgical procedure. Lister began to cover the wounds after surgery to avoid bacterial contamination. Surgical procedures became easier as the wound began to heal quickly without infections.

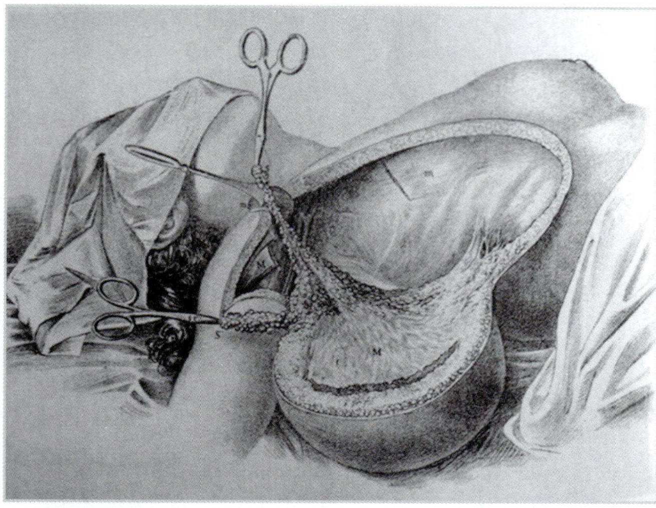

Fig. 4: "The patient was a young lady whom I was loath to disfigure," Halsted wrote. In this etching, Halsted presented an idealized patient. Real cancer patients tended to be older women with larger tumors, far less able to withstand this radical attack

The legendary names of Theodor Billroth and William Halsted dominated the surgical arena of the later part of the 18th century and can be justifiably known as the beginning of oncologic surgery; their techniques and teachings smoothly transitioned into the 19th century with ever increasing radical surgical procedures devised for "curing" cancer. Surgical "radicality" (going to the roots) for cancer gained a strong foothold and the "bigger the better" became a watchword particularly for Halsted in surgically curing breast cancer (Fig. 4). Recurrences after a smaller surgery haunted Halsted and he continued to enlarge the scope and width of his surgery by removing axillary and neck nodes, even including mediastinal nodes. "Cures" eluded even supraradical surgery due to distant metastasis, the hallmark of any cancer. A great surgical teacher and a formidable personality William Halsted and Billroth left behind stalwarts like Harvey Cushing, Hampton Young, Joseph Bloodgood, to name a few. Halsted remains, apart from his "radical mastectomy" the architect of residency training programs at the Johns Hopkins which, today remains a landmark of surgical training anywhere.

The concept "radicalism" in cancer surgery spilled over the 20th century and was followed by the Wertheim-Meigs procedure (1903) for cancer of the cervix, esophagectomy (Torek,1913), pneumonectomy (Graham, 1933) and abdominoperineal resection for cancer of the rectum (Miles). Soon Brunswick (pelvic exenteration) followed suit. The first half of the 19th century, can rightly be called as an incandescent era of "radical surgery" for the control and cure of cancer (1880–1950). The Billroth–Halsted era of megasurgical approaches continued almost for more than half a century.

Progress in science, medicine and technology, admittedly, is due to those who "believe" in proving a point; however, the contribution of the "naysayers" is no less important and may be even more important than the believers. George Crile Sr and Jr, the famous father and son duo in American surgery, were poles apart in praise for Halsted's radical mastectomy. Crile Jr was one of the leading opponents of radicality in surgery for all cases in view of frequent distant metastasis in breast cancer. Geoffrey Keynes, at St. Barts Hospital in London, treated a frail lady in poor health with breast cancer with radium insertion; the lesion shrunk significantly and he excised the lesion locally which resulted in a long-term control. Not entirely convinced about the "radical", he continued to do local removal with radiation and gathered a fair number of patients. George Crile Jr, in America, doubting about the radicality veered towards a simple mastectomy. Distant recurrences within a short time (2–5 years) even after radical mastectomy was enough to convince surgeons and radiotherapists that occult metastasis could exist even before surgery and can occur even after the most supra-radical mastectomy. Geoffrey Keynes in Britain and Crile Jr in the USA led the way towards conservative surgical approach to breast cancer. Combination of conservative surgery (simple mastectomy) and radiotherapy (McWhirter) came into vogue and results appeared to be comparable. Though the results of this seemingly smaller procedures appeared similar there was no way to prove it for lack of numbers or a randomized trial. Doubts, were however, beginning to arise in the minds of large number of surgeons and oncologists the world over, about the theory of "centrifugal" local spread of breast cancer and "the bigger the better" procedures for breast cancer of the Halstedian era.

RADIOTHERAPY

The discovery of X-rays by Wilhelm Roentgen (1895) and Radium by Marie Curie (1902) heralded yet another dimension for cancer therapy. Emil Grubbe, a 21-year-old medical student with a brilliant intellect and restless mind had a notion to use X-rays for treating cancer. He started with breast cancer and noticed shrinking, fibrosis and ulceration as a result of shining X-rays on breast cancer lesions. This is probably the first instance of documented response by X-ray therapy. Geoffrey Keynes in Britain treated a number of breast cancers by using X-ray radiation with satisfactory results; surgery and X-ray radiation thus became two important modalities for local therapy of cancer. X-ray radiation therapy was a powerful tool, patients developed over a time (10 to 20 years), new cancers because of radiation therapy, a lesson which was quickly learnt by careful case analysis.

Refinements of radiotherapy were evident in the 1950s and 60s with the advent of Cobalt-60 and the linear accelerator. McWhirter, a radiation therapist, ran trials advocating only simple mastectomies and postoperative radiotherapy. This was slowly and logically extended to breast conservation surgery and postoperative radiation. Careful analysis and trials showed equivalent results and overall survivals. Radical mastectomies slowly began to recede from the scene. Progress in radiotherapy through radiosensitizers, conformal radiation, brachytherapy, intensity modulated radiation therapy (IMRT) and image-guided radiation therapy (IGRT) are recent innovations; progress of radiotherapy continues unabated.

It needed yet another surgeon, 'Bernard Fisher', to rise like a colossus to challenge and prove that the Halstedian concept was erroneous. The only way to contain distant occult disseminated cancer metastasis was obviously by chemotherapy. The initial moderate successes of chemotherapy by the use of antifolates by Sidney Farber (1948) for leukemia had heralded the era of chemotherapy around 1947-48.

CHEMOTHERAPY

The conceptual thought of a specific drug for destroying an organism or a cancer cell reverberated in the mind of Paul Ehrlich; working with Robert Koch he developed a specific chemical-stain for *Mycobacterium tuberculi*. He also worked on certain dyes and noted its specificity to stain only a part of the cell—a kind of molecular specificity. This thought veered towards the fact that some chemicals would discriminate between bacterial cell (bacterium) and animal cell and destroy the former without affecting the normal cell. Ehrlich won the Nobel Prize for this discovery; the paradox was that the normal and cancer cell are generally similar and distinguishing the two was a major issue. This has, ever since, remained a major issue in cancer chemotherapy—the destruction of normal cells and the bone marrow. The idea of a drug selectively destroying a bacterium or a cancer cell continued to haunt Ehrlich; indeed, he discovered "Salvarsan", a specific drug for syphilis selectively destroying *Treponema pallidum*, responsible for syphilis.

The earliest reported successes in chemotherapy is attributed to Sidney Farber, a pathologist turned leukemia doctor, who started chemotherapy treatment of leukemia with antifolates—aminopterin with reasonable success for a short period of time. Prior to this, mustard gas used in chemical warfare in the First World War, fortunately, burst upon the scene during the Second World War when the use of mustard gas through bombarding in the European zone created severe sicknesses and death in soldiers affected by the poisonous gas. Studies revealed a severe depression of the bone marrow which selectively damaged the white blood cells. The initial use of nitrogen mustard was utilized for the treatment of lymphomas with excellent responses. It is paradoxical that the substance used for warfare and death was now being effectively used for saving lives. A systemic chemical treatment (chemotherapy) for most cancers to control dissemination was thus initiated in the late 1940s (1948) by Sidney Farber for acute leukemia and the use of nitrogen mustard for the treatment of lymphoma. Massive mediastinal lymphomas melted away with drips of nitrogen mustard.

Notwithstanding the above limitations, Bernard Fisher—a surgeon from Philadelphia, USA, initiated a large number of clinical trials as the Chairman of the National Surgical Adjuvant Breast and Bowel Project (NSABP) from 1967. Name any combinations; radical mastectomy versus simple mastectomy, surgery versus surgery followed by adjuvant chemotherapy, neoadjuvant (upfront) chemotherapy followed by surgery; the use of Tamoxifen for prophylaxis against development of breast cancer in high-risk patients with positive receptors and a host of other trials generated evidence-based collated data that changed the face of cancer chemotherapy not only in breast cancer but almost all the cancers worldwide. Fisher used to say, "In God we trust; all others must have data." A major trigger to this was the Classic trial of Bonnadona (The CMF Trial—1970), which opened up major vistas. Bonnadona and Veronesi soon proved equivalency and superior results with CMF (cyclophosphamide, methotrexate, fluorouracil) chemotherapy given after surgery in node positive patients. It would be interesting to recall that the first solid tumor known to have responded to chemotherapy was Wilms' tumor with actinomycin D. As years and decades rolled by, the ever increasing number of chemotherapy drugs appeared on the scene and continues to do so. Cisplatin in 1976, (NSABP 04 Trial), adriamycin 1969, taxol 1985; bleomycin, vinca alkaloids, etoposide were drugs of the earlier era.

Permutations and combinations, dose intensifications, methods of administration makes a fascinating read; the diehard radical surgeons of the 1950s and 60s used to deride chemotherapy as "poison of the month". Medical oncologists had the last laugh. Major successes in chemotherapy—albeit at a high price—has been and is a major factor in our slow and steady progress toward the control, increasing remissions and cure of cancer. It is not that aggressive chemotherapists of the 1960s and 70s did not pursue the same Halstedian methods. Emil "Tom" Frei III and Emil Freireich's aggressive approach to cure breast cancer led to very intensive chemotherapy schedules to the point of destroying the bone marrow in order to kill the last cancer cell. The autologous bone marrow transplant (ABMT) for breast cancer captured the imagination of oncology community in the early 1980s and minor improvements were reported at a high cost of severe morbidity and significant mortality. Scientific frauds were reported from South Africa which were ultimately revealed and exposed. The futility of the Halstedian approach in chemotherapy attained the same fate. Cancer cells do not distinguish between surgery, radiotherapy or chemotherapy. We need to understand the heterogeneity of the cancer cell.

BIOLOGICAL (TARGETED) THERAPY

The latest buzzword now is targeted or biological therapy, much similar to the original idea of Paul Ehrlich; many other names who made seminal contributions can be added. The adage "bigger the better" as it was in surgery once (proved wrong) was also true in medical oncology, e.g. the ABMT (after very intensive chemotherapy taking marrow activity to zero in breast cancer) also went the Halsted way. The steadily increasing knowledge about tumor biology and pharmacokinetics of the newer cytotoxic agents, and the understanding of tumor pathways of growth, proliferation, angiogenesis and subsequent metastases have heralded targeted therapies at each step on the way to prevent growth and angiogenesis by deciphering the epidermal growth factor receptors (EGFR) and the vascular endothelial growth factor (VEGF). Targeted biologic agents like Herceptin, bevacizumab (Avastin), Gleevac, cetuximab (Erbitux) are now in routine clinical use which has shown steadily increasing incremental benefits and moderate disease free and overall survival rates. Biological targeted therapies are not without risk; toxicities and difficult cost factors; nevertheless, it has opened up a new era of biologic understanding of the inherent mechanisms of carcinogenesis. The present era, therefore, is of cautious optimism in the increasing control of cancer, hopefully leading towards converting cancer into the category of a chronic controllable disease like many other human illnesses.

THE INDIAN SCENARIO

The scientific history of cancer in India undoubtedly began in February 1941 with the founding of the Tata Memorial Hospital in Bombay (now Mumbai) (Fig. 5). A direct outflow of the philanthropic and societal commitments of the TATA Group, it was triggered by leukemia in the matriarch of the family. It was indeed the first super specialty in medicine— "Oncology" ever to take off in India; specialists from New York Memorial Sloan-Kettering Cancer Institute provided the much needed technology transfer in cancer medicine which was even then in its infancy overseas. During the three years of their time spent at the Tata Memorial, our own medical youngsters in surgery, radiotherapy, research and chemotherapy, imbibed the nuances of cancer; in a superb manner. The rest is history. The initiation of "cytologic diagnosis" in the year 1958 by Ms Hannah Peters and chemotherapy by Dr Jussawalla were landmarks in cancer diagnosis and new vistas in therapy. Many other landmark cancer institutes, the Adyar Cancer Institute in Madras (now Chennai), the Kidwai Memorial Institute of Oncology in Bangalore, the Regional Cancer Centre in Thiruvananthapuram, the Chittaranjan National Cancer Institute in Calcutta (now Kolkata) and Dr B Barooah Cancer Institute in Guwahati spread their expertise across the nation. The Rotary Cancer Institute at the All India Institute of Medical Sciences (AIIMS), New Delhi, was a later and a major landmark in North India. Many other private and public cancer institutes across the country attempt to control and cure cancer which is indeed like a drop in the ocean for the cancer problem in India.

A major effort by the Government of India through the Ministry of Health and the ICMR (Indian Council of Medical Research) made significant contribution. A major component of the ICMR—"Non-Communicable Disease Group" played a very significant role in the development of cytology across the country. The "Cancer Control

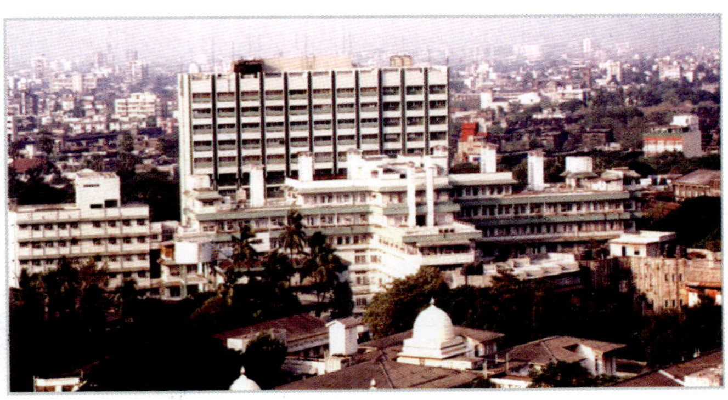

Fig. 5: Tata Memorial Hospital, Mumbai

Programme" for the country was envisioned by the Health Ministry through the ICMR. Dr Ms Usha Luthra led this project.

The Tata Memorial Centre (Hospital and Cancer research institute) has acted as a catalyst in technology transfer across the country aided by all other major cancer organizations. Professionally trained colleagues at the Tata Memorial and other centers now occupy high academic positions in therapy and research not only at cancer institutes in India but many overseas stations.

Prof VR Khanolkar, the first Director of the Cancer Research Institute and Chief of pathology at Tata Memorial went on to become the President of the Union for International Cancer Control (UICC) (previously named International Union Against Cancer). The 1994 International UICC Congress was held in New Delhi for the first time attended by 4,500 delegates, which acted as a catalyst and stimulated the cancer effort in the country.

Oncology is now a much sought after medical specialty. The cancer effort has even been transferred to the semi-urban and rural areas. Though these are miniscule efforts for a country of 1.2 billion population the outlook for a cancer patient in India is significantly better now than even 5 or 10 years ago. It is for the current oncology community to make certain that the science, medicine and technology for cancer control and cure makes an appropriate forward transmission to the future ages across the country for the benefit of all, irrespective of their financial background, caste, creed or community.

The cure and control of any disease necessitates a multipronged approach. Scientists, doctors and nurses are at the base of the pyramid; nevertheless together they can achieve a miniscule of what needs to be done. Science, politics and society need to work in a tandem to achieve the objectives of prevention, early diagnosis, access to appropriate therapy and adequate rehabilitation.

Major advances in cancer research and treatment, therefore, has to have a public visage. Education (public and professional) has to be at the core of this effort. The cancer effort in the United States got a major boost from Sidney Farber and the socialite Mary Lasker; together they made a major impact on the powers that are and that be, to reach right up to the apex of political power which culminated in President Richard Nixon passing a bill to wage a war on cancer in 1972. The objective was to conquer and cure cancer by 1980 which did not materialize due to its complexity—obviously more complex than putting the man on the moon; yet the cancer effort received a major boost through Government agencies —the NCI (National Cancer Institute) and the NIH (National Institute of Health). Likewise in India the support of politics, media and the NGO (Cancer Societies) effort should be strengthened.

It is only from the wisdom of the past that we can weave the fabric of the future. Let us, therefore, not relegate the past into the crucible of history as it is history which drives our enthusiasm to continue to fight and conquer cancer, regardless.

THE FUTURE

The last millennium changed the way we practice medicine from the clinical era of the 1950s, technologic innovations of the 1960s and 70s, and the biologic era of the 1980s and 90s; medicine has become—or should become a harmonious blend of the art of clinical medicine and the power of scientific discoveries and technologies.

"The bigger the better" philosophies of the surgeons (1880 to 1950) and the chemotherapists (1970 to 1990) has not stood the test of time. Supra- and ultra-radical surgeries (radical mastectomies, radical pneumonectomies, massive pelvic operations which sacrifice vital organs), avoiding unnecessary lymph node dissections, etc. have paved way for a conservative approach—without sacrificing the principles of therapeutic oncology.

Massive autologous bone marrow transplants for cancer breast and very aggressive chemotherapies have met the same fate. The hope and the hype of cancer therapy successes needs to be tampered by integrity, humility and truth. Medicine still remains a contact sport and the power of market forces forcefully influence science and medicine.

Success enthrals the mind but the discovery of failure strengthens our resolve and persistence to seek a new path, a new vision, to succeed nevertheless. We and the society will risk a stagnant science, if our resolve weakens and we do not take risks of new ideas and new ventures. The art of medicine lies in evaluating our success against our failures, benefits versus the risks and evaluation of old practices with newer technology. Science and medicine needs to be practiced with conscience. The essential ingredients of humanity, integrity and honesty should not be lost on a long path we have charted ourselves to contain the most serious disease which afflicts our civilization today.

2 Surgical Oncology: An Overview

Praful Desai

The emergence of significant practice changing paradigms in the surgical management of solid tumors in the new millennium makes it mandatory that today's surgical oncologist must function as an integral component of a therapeutic team. The current approach to cancer therapeutics is indeed based on a large number of randomized clinical trials and follow-up studies the world over. Organ preservation, reducing treatment morbidities, combined treatment modalities, redefining our approach to the lymphatic system, appropriate use of new surgical technology and evidence-based medicine are few of the tenets on which modern surgical oncology is soundly based.

Until the middle of the last century, surgery was the mainstay in cancer treatment and has remained steadfast as the therapy of choice for a solid tumor localized to its site of origin. Historically, it was the advent of anesthesia and antisepsis which consolidated surgery in the last and previous millennium. The seminal contributions of outstanding surgical pioneers, whose work and principles, which still form the bedrock of modern surgical oncology is shown in Table 1. These procedures are still in vogue, albeit with modifications, based on our current knowledge of tumor biology. The most complete operation for cancer was devised by Halsted (Radical mastectomy) in 1890 based on the lymphatic spread of cancer. Modifications have surely occurred but the principles of cancer surgery have remained steadfast despite the advent of chemotherapy and radiotherapy. It is therefore mandatory that a good surgical oncologist have sound perceptions about the current state of chemoradiotherapy to plan a combined therapeutic approach as and when indicated. This will remain the "*sine qua non*" in cancer therapy for the most optimum outcomes in terms of its control and cure. The second half of the last century opened up an era of complimentary therapy in cancer as our knowledge in chemotherapy/radiotherapy gained momentum.

The essential basis of all surgery starts with appropriate and adequate training. One is always a better surgical oncologist with a good grounding of general surgery; specialization in an anatomic site is now the rule rather than an exception and postgraduate qualifications in ENT, gynecology, urology, chest, orthopedics will ensure outstanding quality of surgical oncologists, attuned to service, education and research. Residency training at a junior and senior level for at least 3–4 years in a tertiary cancer center or a teaching institution will complete a well thought out training schedule for a surgical oncologist. During the training period sufficient importance should be given to academics, developing research ethos, and instilling the instinct to teach as only by teaching do we learn. Leadership qualities in a budding surgical oncologist will be a natural consequence of such a well-rounded training program. The ability to write projects, working together and to be able to lead a team are essential qualities for an outstanding surgical oncologist.

Apart from honing skills in service, education and research, the current practice changing paradigms in surgical oncology like the impact of conservation surgeries, morbidity reduction, combined therapeutic modalities, practice of evidence-based medicine when feasible and its pros and cons must be well within the grasp of the surgical oncologist. A balanced overview of technology and its use, overuse and misuse should carefully engage his attention. Medical technology has accrued great benefits to the society, but it would be naive to think that there are no

TABLE 1: Pioneers in the field of surgical oncology

Year	Pioneer	Procedure
1809	E McDowell	Elective abdominal surgery (ovarian tumor)
1846	John Warren	Use of ether anesthesia
1867	Joseph Lister	Antisepsis
1860–1890	Theodor Billroth	Gastrectomy, laryngectomy, esophagectomy
1878	Theodor Kocher	Thyroid surgery
1890	Halsted	Radical mastectomy
1896	Beatson	Oophorectomy (for breast cancer)
1904	Hugh Young	Radical prostatectomy
1906	Ernest Wertheim	Radical hysterectomy
1908	W Ernest Miles	Abdominoperineal resection for rectal cancer
1910–1930	Cushing	Brain tumors
1913	Torek	Esophagectomy
1933	Evarts Graham	Pneumonectomy
1935	AO Whipple	Pancreatectomy
1945	C Huggins	Adrenalectomy
1958	B Fisher	NSABP randomized trials

negative spin-offs of improper use of technology. Lives have been lost due to inadequate training and misuse due to improperly indicated technology.

Institutional working background always has a positive impact on overall patient outcomes after therapy; however, it is difficult for every practicing surgical oncologist to have this privilege. Institutional practices and protocols relevant to the environment needs to be devised like clinical trials, technology transfer programs, organization of seminars and conferences and to act as a catalyst are the hallmarks of an outstanding surgical oncologist in an institute. The ability to say "we" instead of "I", being able to ask the right questions and the strength to say "I do not know" will carry a surgical oncologist far and will make him stand apart from his colleagues in his stature, eminence and expertise. It is the journey, not the destination which matters in the end. A well-planned roadmap to learn surgical oncology will ensure a destination which his colleagues will envy and aspire to emulate.

The role of the surgical oncologist is therefore multitasking and multifaceted. Apart from his own education in general surgery and the finer nuances of surgical oncology, his knowledge about the principles of radiation therapy and chemotherapy will allow him to make appropriate therapeutic decisions in a given clinical setting for a cancer patient. It is an old adage and comes out very strongly for surgery in general and surgical oncology in particular that "he is a surgeon, who knows when not to operate". A year spent in chemotherapy and radiotherapy or even a shorter stint should be mandatory. He needs to understand the strength and weaknesses of each of the three therapeutic disciplines and appropriately combine them for the optimal outcome for a given patient. He should also propagate the fact that patients treated in a tertiary cancer center by a team of oncologists have better survival outcomes with significantly less morbidities and mortality. Apart from these therapeutic objectives, he should possess leadership qualities in arranging educational and research programs, ability to raise intramural and extramural funds for appropriate projects to raise the academic standards of his department. Coordination with other divisions and specialties in the institution are of prime importance. Burnouts are high in a surgical oncologist leadership and above all he must have wide-ranging interests and hobbies beyond his professional interest to maintain his life on an even keel.

Needless to state that the discipline of "Surgical Oncology" though arduous and stressful, is exciting, challenging and importantly, often a humbling experience and teaches us that the journey toward the control and cure of cancer is unending, difficult but indeed a very rewarding one.

3 Geographic Variations in Frequency and Incidence: A Global Perspective

Ganesh Balasubramaniam

INTRODUCTION

Cancer forms one of the major components amongst noncommunicable diseases with increase in life expectancy, better control of communicable diseases and an aging population, demographic data shows a significant increase in frequency and incidence of cancer globally. As per the recent GLOBOCAN estimates, approximately 12.6 million new cancer cases (approximately 188 per 100,000 people) and 7.6 million cancer deaths occurred worldwide in 2008.[1] Figure 1 shows the number of common cancers and deaths estimated in men and women.[1] It

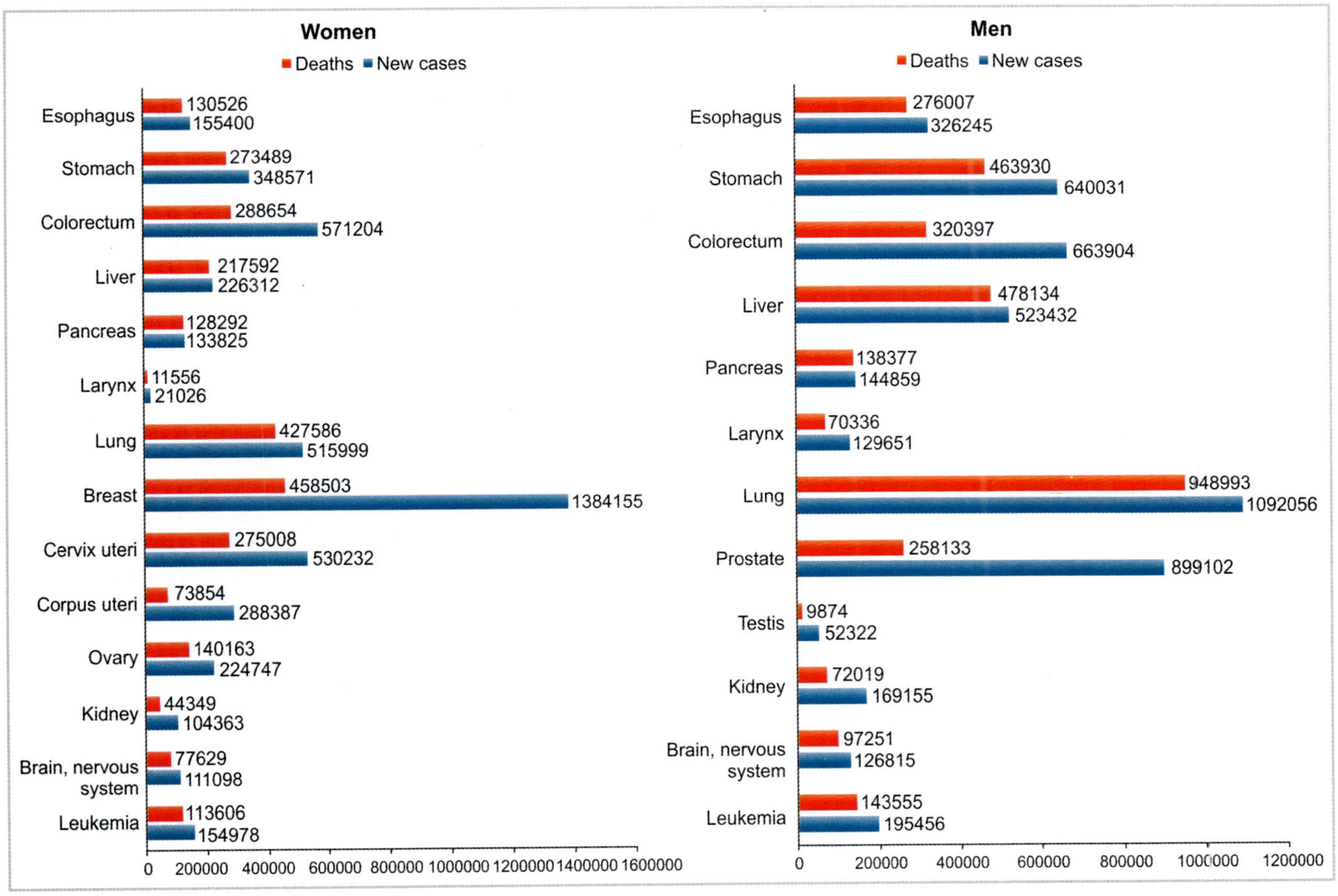

Fig. 1: Estimated annual number of new cancer cases/deaths in the world

is seen that among the males, lung, prostate, colorectum and stomach cancers are leading cancers, whereas among the females, breast, colorectum, cervix uteri and lung cancers are the leading cancer sites. It is known that cancer incidence varies by age, gender, geographic region, race and ethnicity.[2] This overview reviews data from the USA, UK, Japan, India, Europe and China, which covers a major portion of the world population and is also representative of the cancer burden in general.

GEOGRAPHIC VARIATIONS IN INCIDENCE

Cancer incidence worldwide is more than a fifth higher in men than in women, with world age-HYPERLINK "http://www.cancerresearchuk.org/cancer-info/cancerstats/world/the-global-picture/ssLINK/news-age-standardised"standardized incidence rates of 203 and 164 per 100,000, respectively, in 2008 (Fig. 2).[3] Male incidence rates vary almost four-fold across the different regions of the world.[3]

INCIDENCE RATES BASED ON ECONOMIC DEVELOPMENT

There are differences in age-standardized rates of cancer between developed and developing countries. Although cancer is often considered to be more of a developed world issue, in fact, 56% of all cancers occur in developing countries and 44% in developed countries.[3] Due to larger population, there are more cancer cases in the developing regions than in developed regions of the world; however, cancer incidence and cancer deaths estimated in China are three-fold more than in India. There were 256 cases of cancer diagnosed per 100,000 in developed countries, compared to 148 in developing countries in 2008.

The rates of cancer of the cervix uteri in developing countries are twice than in developed countries, while breast cancer rates in more developed countries are three times higher than seen in less developed countries (Fig. 3).[3] For nasopharyngeal cancer, the rate was nearly four times higher in developing than developed countries. Lung, colorectum, breast, prostate, stomach, pancreas and kidney cancers are higher in developed countries while esophagus, larynx and liver cancers are higher in developing countries. Among both sexes the rate for all cancers was 1.7 times higher in more developed as compared to less developed countries (Fig. 4).

Comparison of incidence rates seen in different countries, viz., USA, UK, China, Japan, India and Europe reveals that the incidence rates in India are the lowest and they are one-third of that seen in USA, UK, Europe and Japan, while it is double than China among men and there are no remarkable differences among women between these locations; nonetheless there are distinct differences in rates with regard to the leading cancer sites (Fig. 4).[3]

Figures 5A to F show the age-standardized incidence rates (ASR) of different countries among men;[3] it is seen that lung, prostate, stomach and colorectum are the top-ranking sites in USA, UK, Europe and Japan except in India and China, where lung, esophagus and stomach are among the leading sites.

Similarly, among females, breast is one of the leading sites in all locations except in India, where cervix uteri is the leading cancer site; current registry data reveals that incidence of breast cancer has overtaken that of cervix in

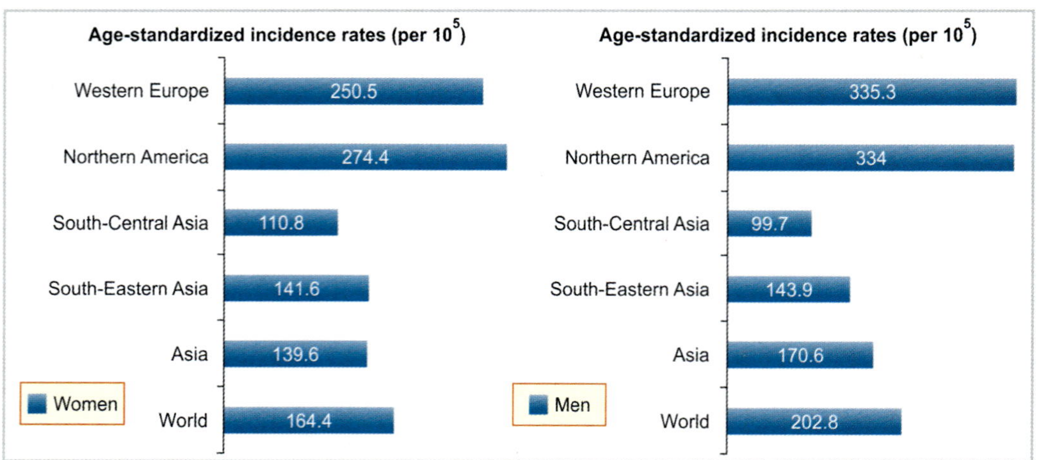

Fig. 2: Age-standardized incidence rates (ASR per 10^5) by geographic locations in the world

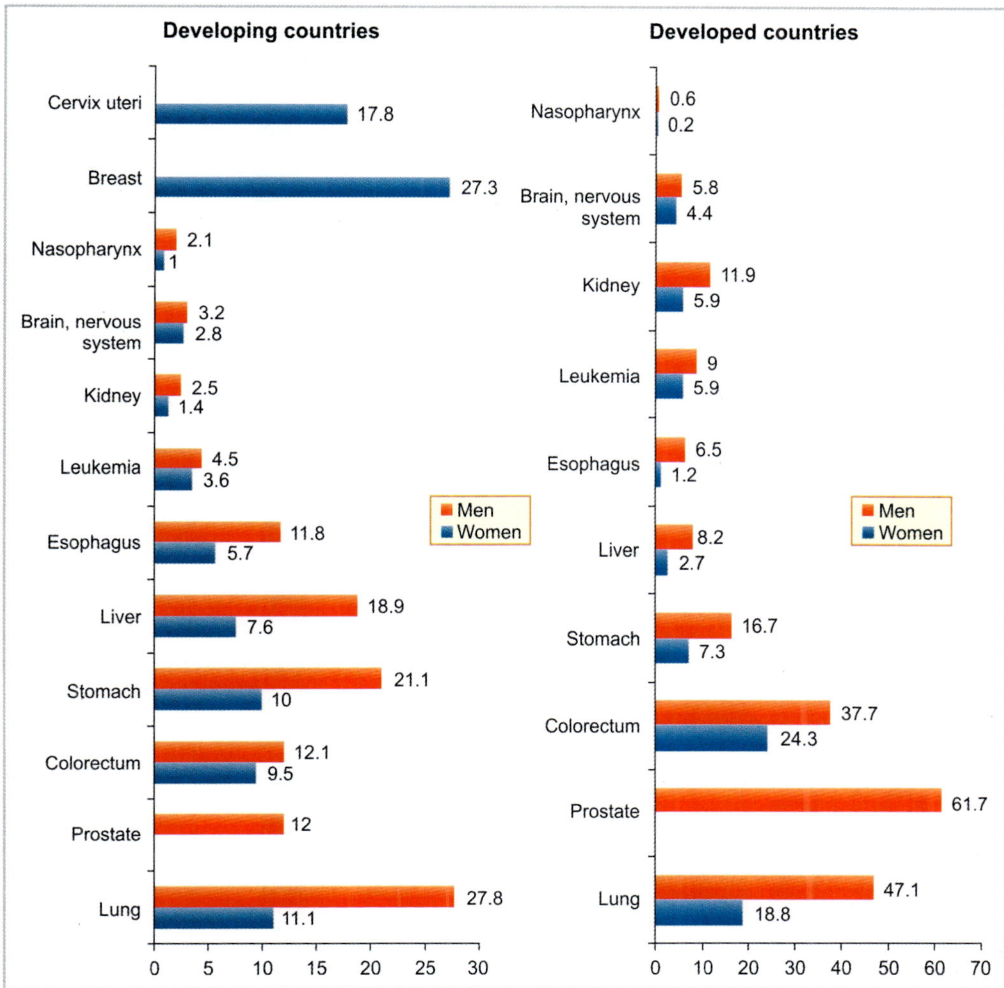

Fig. 3: Comparison of age-standardized incidence rates (ASR per 10^5)—developed and developing countries

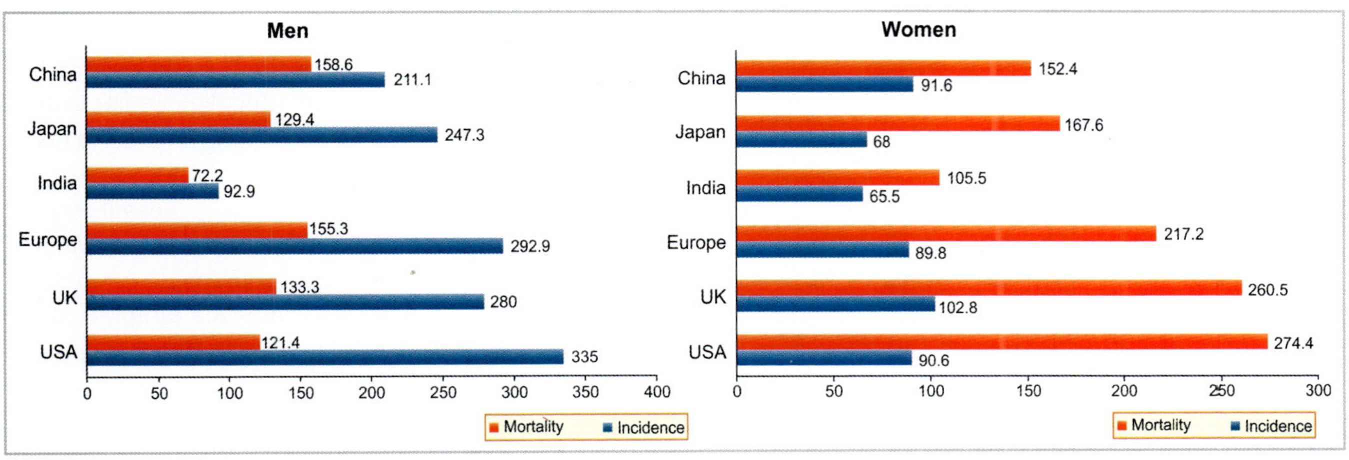

Fig. 4: Age-standardized incidence rates (ASR per 10^5) for selected countries across the world—men and women

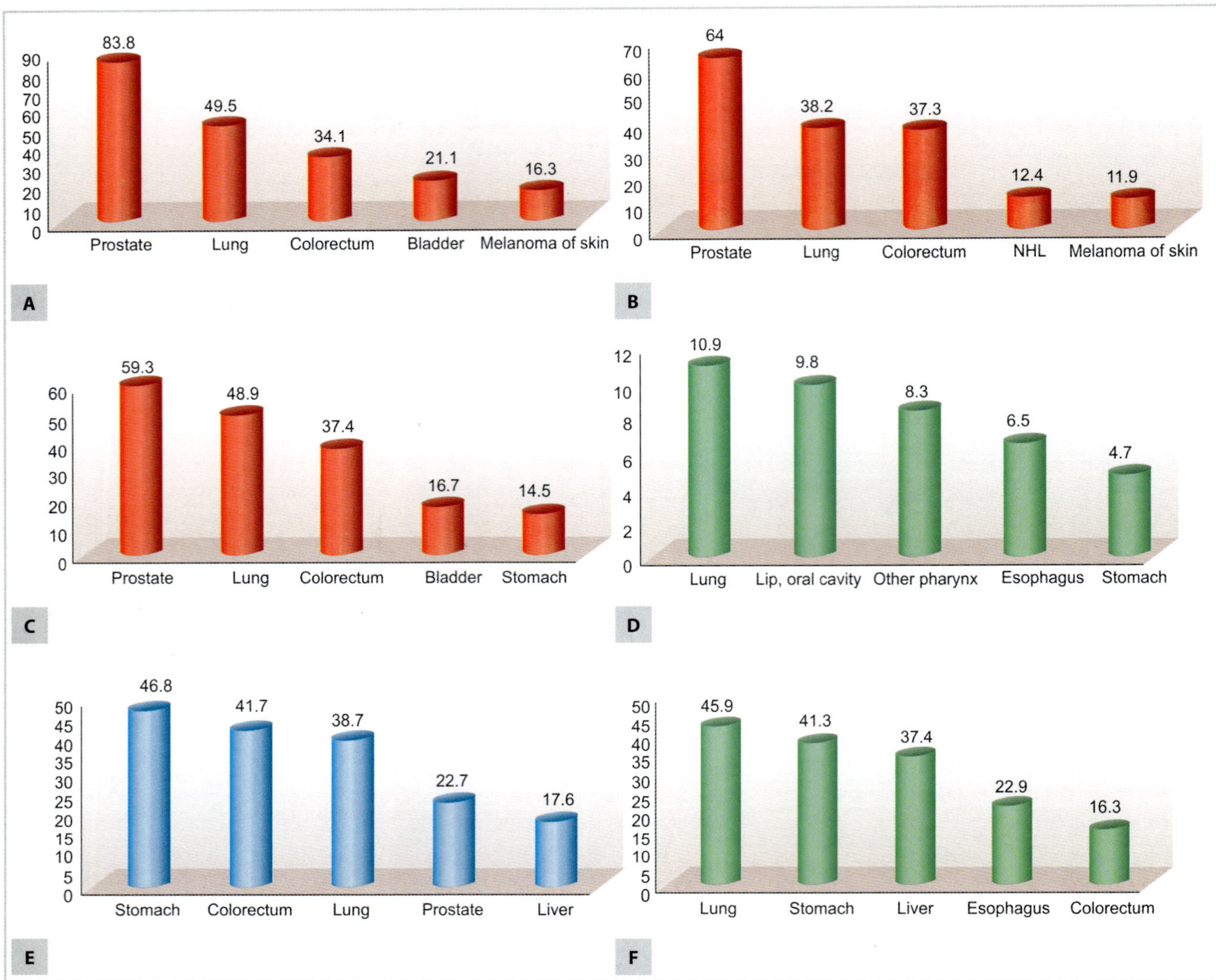

Figs 5A to F: Age-standardized incidence rates (ASR per 10^5) of leading cancers in men for selected geographic locations

the metropolitan regions of India. However, other sites as lung, colorectum and stomach are seen in all locations (Figs 6A to F);[3] however, lip, oral cavity, esophagus and ovary figure in the leading sites of cancer among women only in India.

Variation in Indian Registries

Indian national cancer registries established by the National Cancer Registry Programme (NCRP) under the Indian Council of Medical Research (ICMR), started reporting in the 1980s on cancer incidence from major urban areas; however, over a period of time, several population and hospital registries have been set up. There are distinct variations in incidence rates seen across India.[4] In Figure 7, it is observed that overall there are no remarkable differences in the age-adjusted rates between registries;[4] nonetheless, the occurrence of cancers within India itself has many variations, which is unique to its geographic location.

Incidence rates of three major Indian registries are reported here since they are the oldest registries in India.[4] It is observed from Figure 8 that incidence rates among men are higher for prostate, lung and mouth caners in Mumbai;[4] however, the rates in Chennai for lung cancer and prostate cancer in Bangalore (now Bengaluru) are higher than Mumbai rates. In gastrointestinal (GI) cancers, esophagus and stomach are highest in Chennai. Similarly, among women, breast cancer stands out uniquely as the leading cancer in all registries followed by cervix cancer; cervix cancer is still predominant in rural setup and breast cancer is emerging as the leading cancer in urban registries. These differences between the registries within a country provide unique opportunities to identify the causes by conducting epidemiological studies.

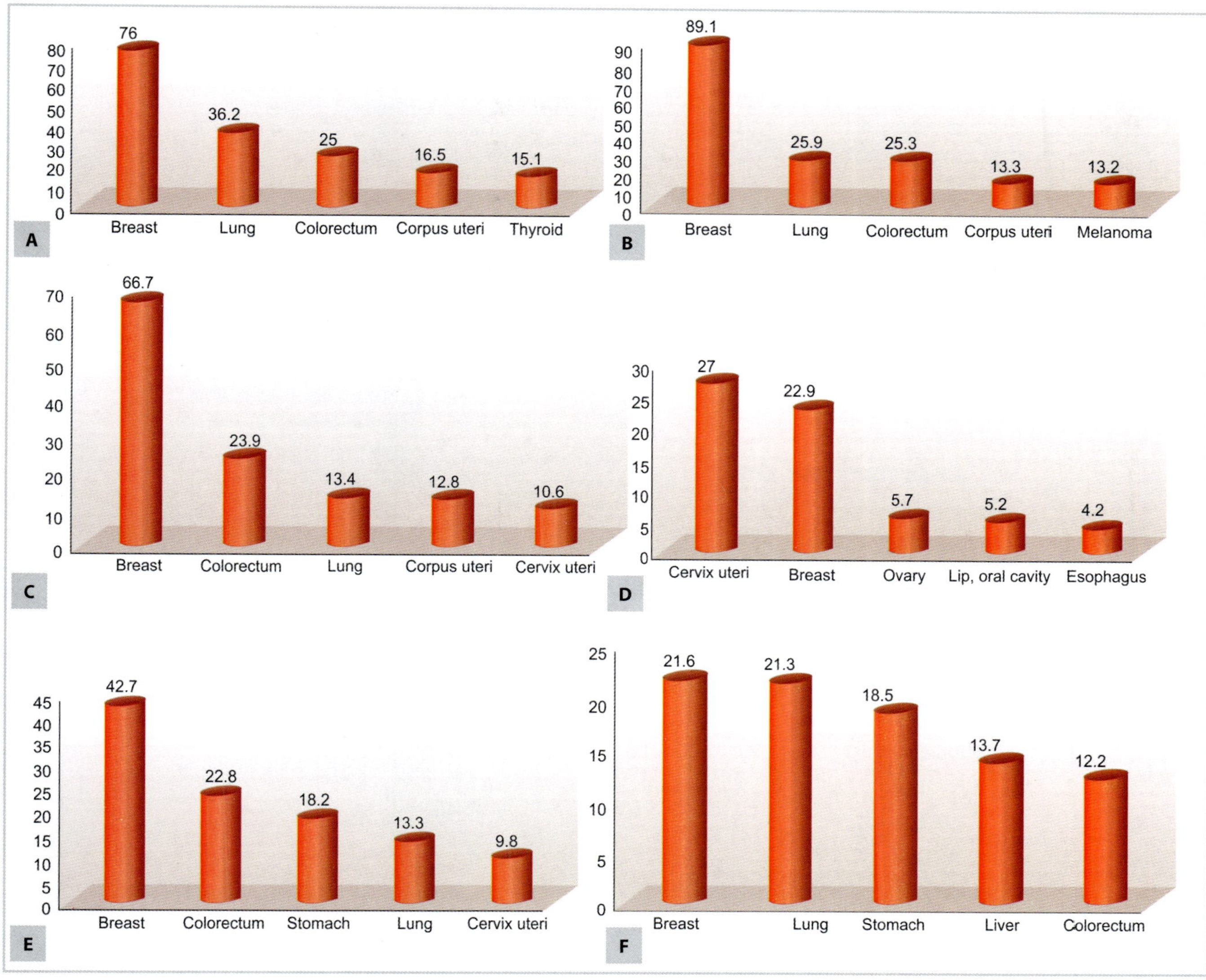

Figs 6A to F: Age-standardized incidence rates (ASR per 10^5) of leading cancers in women for selected geographic locations

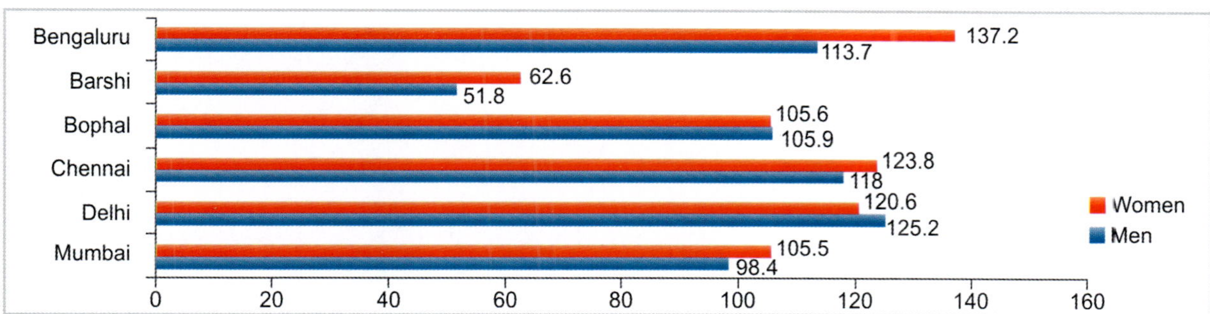

Fig. 7: Age-adjusted incidence rates (AAR per 10^5) observed in Indian registries

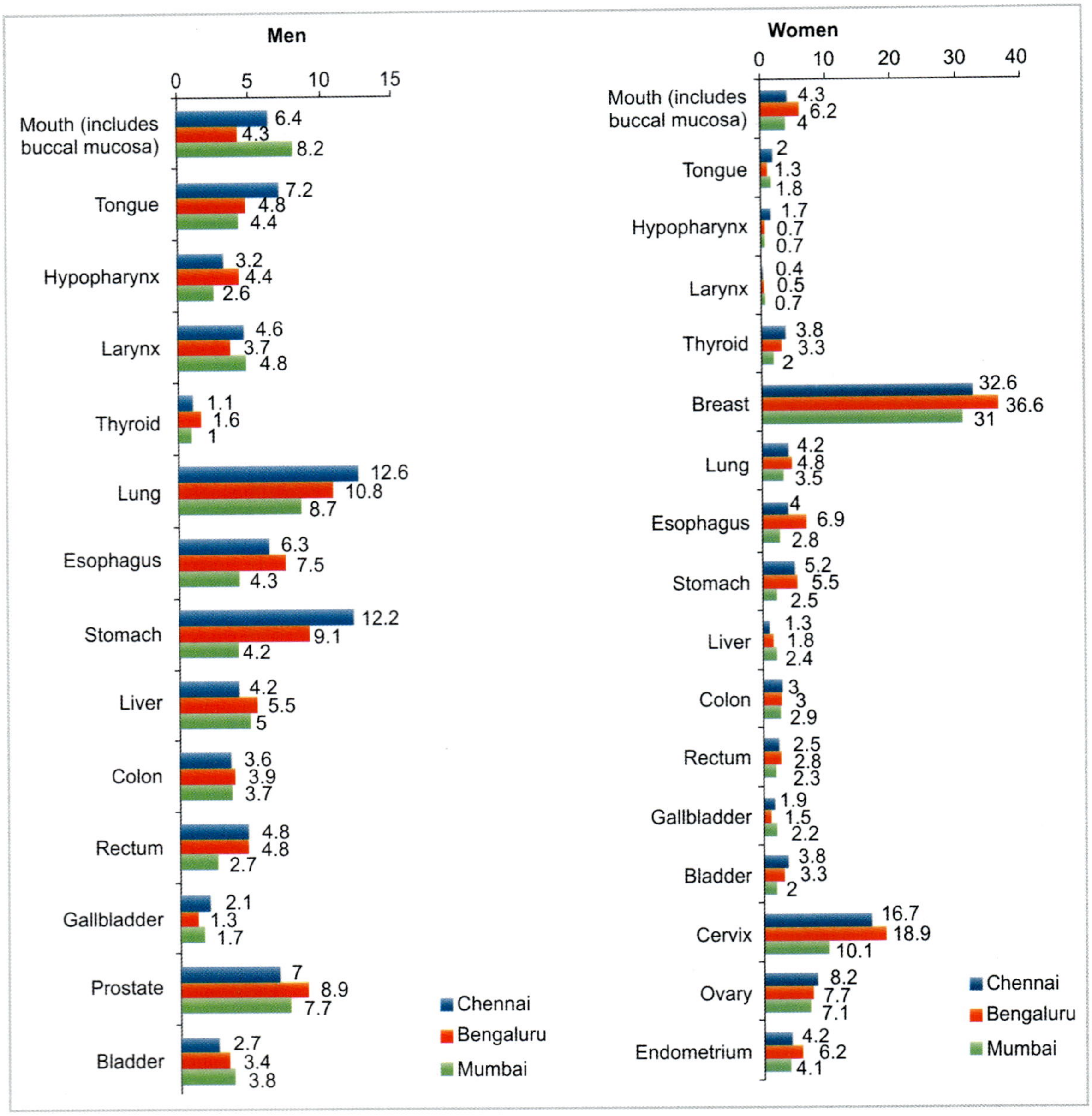

Fig. 8: Age-adjusted incidence (AAR per 10^5) rates in Indian registries

REFERENCES

1. Ferlay J, Shin HR, Bray F, et al. Estimates of worldwide burden of cancer in 2008: GLOBOCAN 2008. Int J Cancer. 2010;127(12): 2893-917.
2. Doll R, Payne P, Waterhouse JAH, (Eds). Cancer Incidence in Five Continents, Volume 1. A Technical Report. Geneva, UICC; Berlin, Springer-Verlag; 1966.
3. GLOBOCAN (2010). Ferlay J, Shin HR, Bray F, et al. GLOBOCAN 2008 v1.2: Cancer incidence and mortality worldwide: IARC Cancer Base No. 10 [Internet]. Lyon, France: IARC Press; 2010. Available from: http://globocan.iarc.fr [Accessed: January, 2014].
4. NCRP (2013). Three-year Report of Population-based Cancer Registries: 2009-2011. National Cancer Registry Programme, ICMR, Bengaluru, India; 2013.

4 Primary and Secondary Prevention of Common Cancers

Surendra Shastri, Aditi Shastri

INTRODUCTION

Cervical and breast cancer among women, and oral cancer among women and men together form 36% of the cancer burden in India.[1] Fortunately, cervical and oral cancers are preventable and can be screened for pre-invasive stages of the disease, while breast cancer can be detected in early stages leading to a cure. Cancer incidence and mortality data of good quality is regularly collected, compiled, analyzed and published by existing cancer registries in India. These registries will however have to be strengthened to increase coverage and further improve the data and reporting quality. The International Agency for Research on Cancer (IARC) has already set up a "Cancer Registry Hub" at the Tata Memorial Centre in Mumbai, India for increasing and improving cancer registries in the region.

CERVICAL CANCER SCREENING AND PREVENTION

Disease Burden

Cervical cancer is the third most common cancer in women worldwide with an estimated 550,700 new cases and 286,823 deaths each year (GLOBOCAN 2008 projected to 2010). Over 85% of the global burden occurs in developing countries, where it accounts for 13% of all female cancers. India diagnoses an estimated 141,768 new cases and 77,096 deaths occur each year from cervical cancer, contributing to over 27% of the global burden of the disease (Fig. 1).[1]

Evidence for Screening

Pap Smear

Cervical cancer is the most preventable cancer and large population-based Pap smear screening programs have been in place for several years in Nordic countries, UK, USA, Australia and New Zealand leading to a significant reduction in cervical cancer incidence and mortality in these countries (Figs 2 and 3).

Although screening using the Pap smear has never been rigorously tested in a randomized clinical trial in developed countries, the marked differences in the cervical cancer incidence and mortality figures, before and after the introduction of screening has been interpreted as "robust" evidence favoring the efficacy of Pap smear screening programs. The success of Pap smear screening programs is strongly influenced by the percentage of coverage of eligible women, the quality control of laboratory procedures, frequency of screening and compliance with regular follow-up. Pap smear screening has however failed to significantly reduce the cervical cancer burden in the Latin American countries due to a combination of several factors including poor coverage, suboptimal follow-up/treatment of screen-positive women, inadequate infrastructure and quality assurance issues. In India, organization of population-wide Pap smear screening programs is not feasible for economic and sociodemographic reasons. An expert committee constituted by the Government of India in 2006, to develop national guidelines for cervical cancer screening in India observed that for the large population of eligible women in India, the infrastructure and resources do not permit Pap

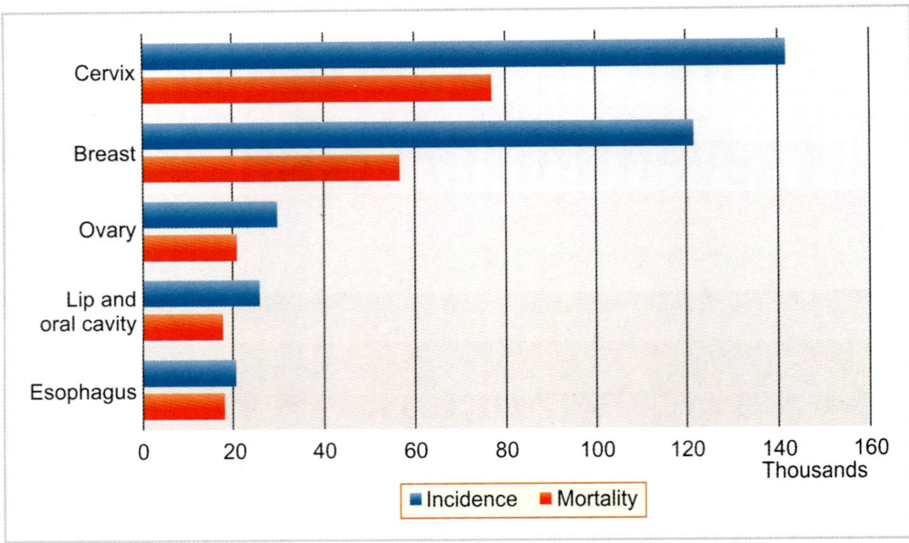

Fig. 1: Top five cancers among women in India

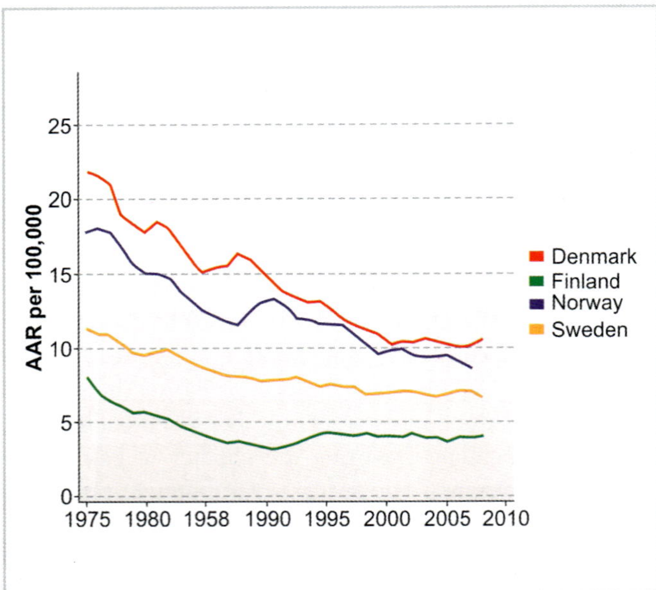

Fig. 2: Cervical cancer incidence trends in NORDIC countries
Source: IARC (International Agency for Research on Cancer)

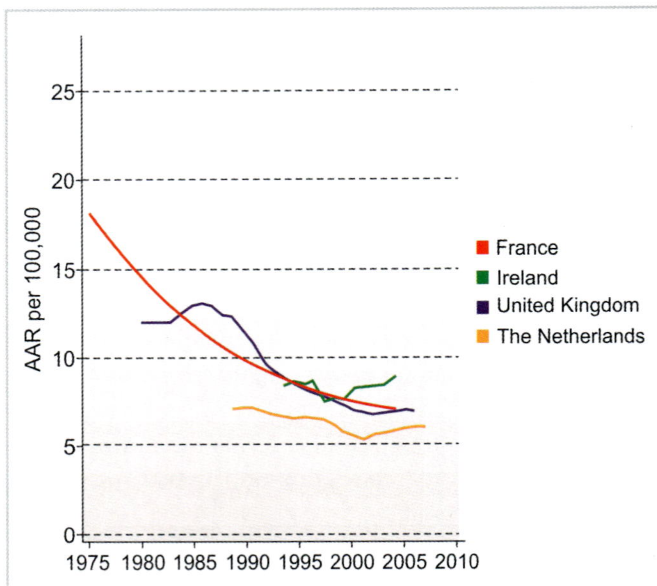

Fig. 3: Cervical cancer incidence trends in other parts of Europe
Source: IARC

smear based national screening programs, and alternative strategies that are feasible and scientifically valid should be identified.

A large randomized controlled trial conducted in rural India tested the effect of a single round of screening by HPV DNA test (Hybrid Capture II), Pap smear, or VIA (Visual inspection with acetic acid) on mortality from cervical cancer. This study reported that there was no reduction in cervical cancer mortality in the group undergoing screening by Pap smear despite the strict quality control and follow-up procedures adopted in the study.[2]

Visual Inspection with Acetic Acid (VIA)

Visual inspection of the cervix after application of acetic acid has emerged as the optimal screening tool for India, since it is economical and provides immediate results. The test characteristics of VIA have been evaluated in several cross-sectional studies in developing countries including India. The results of these studies strongly suggest that VIA screening would be a useful alternative to Pap smear. The pooled estimates of VIA sensitivity to detect high-grade cervical intraepithelial neoplasia (CIN) vary from 62% to 80% and specificity from 77% to 84%.[3-7]

A large randomized controlled trial in Southern India, where VIA was performed by trained nurses, showed that a single round of screening with VIA reduces cervical cancer incidence and mortality by 25% and 35% respectively.[8] Another large randomized controlled study in low socioeconomic populations in Mumbai, India recently reported, that four rounds of biennial VIA screening performed by trained primary health workers reduced cervical cancer mortality by a significant 31%. The study had an interobserver variability (kappa) coefficient of 0.84 between the primary health workers and an expert, suggesting that trained primary health workers are able to provide good quality VIA screening. This study also reported an almost zero overdiagnosis rate, which is very crucial for our overburdened public health system. VIA chart developed by IARC is shown in Figure 4.

Cost effectiveness studies based on data from India, Kenya, Peru, South Africa, and Thailand indicate that the most cost-effective strategies for cervical screening are those approaches which require the fewest visits, leading to improved follow-up and treatment. The analysis reports that screening women once in their lifetime, at the age of 35 years, with a one or two-visit screening strategy involving VIA or HPV testing reduces the lifetime risk of cervical cancer by approximately 25–36%, and costs less than 500 dollars (USD) per year of life saved.[9,10]

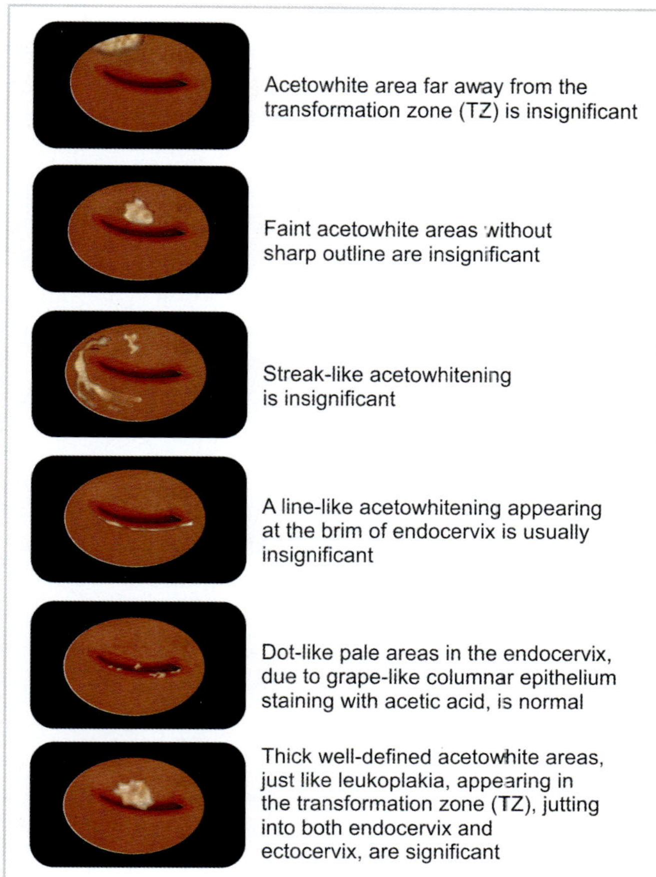

Fig. 4: Visual inspection with acetic acid (VIA) chart developed by IARC

Human Papillomavirus (HPV) Testing

Human papillomavirus causality for cervical cancer is now firmly established. HPV 16 and 18 account for 70% of cervical cancer cases. All reviews of HPV-based screening studies have shown a significantly improved sensitivity (by 30–35%) and a slightly reduced specificity (by 8–12%) compared to Pap smear.[11,12] A large randomized controlled trial from rural India showed that a single round of HPV screening can reduce mortality from cervical cancer when compared to controls that received only health education. Mortality reduction was not seen in the groups that received one round of Pap smear or one round of VIA.[2] Similar results were reported by a large trial in Italy, where the first screening round identified almost double the number of CIN 2+ lesions in the HPV arm as compared to the Pap smear arm, with an almost equal number of invasive cancers in both arms. In the second screening round (at 3-year interval), the number of CIN 2+ lesions in the HPV arm was significantly less as compared to the Pap smear arm. In the second round, the Pap smear arm had incident cases of invasive cancers, while the HPV arm showed no incident cases.[13,14] Studies suggest that when women over 30 years are offered HPV based screening, there is minimal overdiagnosis and that HPV screening is useful even when carried out less frequently.[11]

Early results from E6/E7 screening (RNA test) and triage studies have shown a further gain (over HPV DNA test) of 5–6% in specificity for CIN 2+ lesions at same levels of sensitivity. Both assays showed 20% superiority compared to liquid-based cytology.[15,16]

A more recent entry to the repertoire of cervical cancer screening tools is the "Care HPV" test. This is a HPV DNA test adapted for use in developing countries for primary screening and triage. Care HPV has the benefits of low cost, simple technology and short reporting period that allows for strategies incorporating the see-and-treat approach.[17,18]

Evidence for HPV Vaccination

Currently, two HPV vaccines are commercially available, namely the Quadrivalent (HPV 16, 18, 6 and 11) vaccine and the Bivalent (HPV 16 and 18) vaccine. The results of phase

III clinical trials are now available and these two vaccines are now licensed in over 120 countries. Many developed countries have introduced HPV vaccines into routine vaccination programs. The majority of the critical phase III results for both vaccines are available among women in the age group of 15 to 26 years.[6,19] Several supplementary studies have been completed or are under way, including immune-bridging studies in 9–15 year old girls and boys and efficacy studies in 26–45 year old women, as well as studies in adult men and special populations (immune-suppressed and others).

These two vaccines have so far shown high efficacy with reference to the predefined end point lesions (HPV 16 or 18 related CIN 2+ lesions), adequate safety, tolerability, high immunogenicity, long-term protection (currently 10 years) and strong indications of its ability to induce immune memory. Some degree of cross-protection against CIN related to HPV types 31 for both vaccines and HPV 33 and 45 for the bivalent vaccine has been documented. None of the vaccines have shown therapeutic activity. Very high coverage rates (65–70%) are seen in Australia and in UK.[20]

The limitations of current vaccines, i.e. the lack of therapeutic effect and the limited impact of cross-protection effect requires the continuation of screening programs in the vaccinated women. The cost of the vaccine is currently very high and hence unaffordable in India.[21-26]

Recommendations

On the basis of available evidence it is recommended that cervical cancer screening should be included and implemented on a priority basis in India with the following strategies, indicators and targets.

Screening

Primary cervical cancer screening should be conducted using VIA by primary health workers, one or more times in women aged 30–49 years, with a screening coverage target of 70–80% of the eligible women.

Women who screen positive by VIA should be triaged using either HPV DNA test or Pap smear and those who test positive by the triaging test should be directed for colposcopy and necessary treatment, i.e. cryotherapy/loop electrosurgical excision procedure (LEEP)/conization or hysterectomy. If the triaging tests are not available then all VIA positive women may be directly sent for colposcopy. A target of 30% reduction of cervical cancer mortality by 2025 should be set for India.

Vaccination

Studies on safety, efficacy and feasibility of different dosage schedules of the available vaccines, in girls aged 9–15 years, should be carried out in India before considering countrywide vaccination programs.

Referral in the Absence of Screening

Women who present with abnormal vaginal bleeding, persistent foul-smelling discharge or pain during vaginal intercourse (suggestive of pre/early stage cervical cancer) should undergo a speculum examination. If a cervical growth or ulceration is noticed then they should be referred to a gynecologist for confirmation of diagnosis and further management. Women with confirmed nonmalignant lesions should be included in routine follow-up or re-examined as frequently as advised by the gynecologist. Women presenting with severe abdominal pain, abdominal distention, severe back pain, neck swelling, or symptoms of urethral and rectal fistula (suggestive of advanced cervical cancer) should be referred to a specialized cancer center for confirmation diagnosis and management.

BREAST CANCER SCREENING

Disease Burden

Breast cancer is the most frequent cancer among women worldwide (including developing countries) with an estimated 1,443,421 cases and 478,888 deaths each year (GLOBOCAN 2008 projected to 2010). India diagnoses around 121,226 new cases and 56,754 deaths occur from breast cancer, contributing to over 8% and 12% to the global incidence and mortality burden from the disease (Fig. 5).[1]

Evidence for Screening

Mammography

Mammography screening has been widely used in the developed countries for detecting early signs of breast cancer before lesions become palpable. The objective of mammography screening is to detect and treat breast cancer at significantly earlier stages of the disease when cure is more likely. Earlier studies led us to believe that mammography screening results in reduced breast cancer mortality in the screened women.[27-33] There is however emerging evidence that mammography screening does not reduce breast cancer mortality.[34] Recent studies also

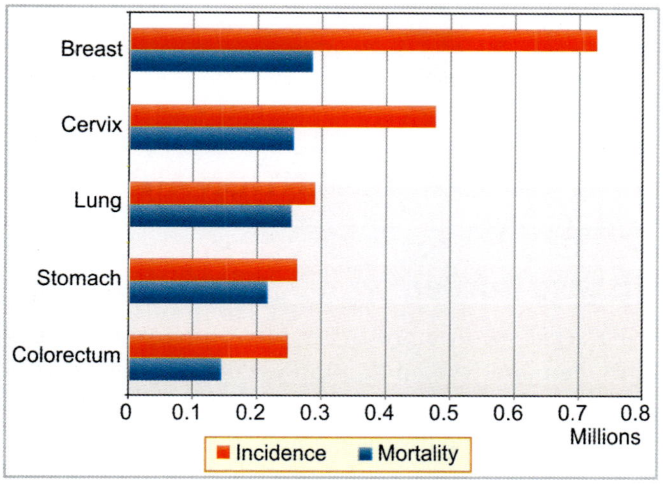

Fig. 5: Top five cancers among women in developing countries (GLOBOCAN 2008 projected to 2010)

show that there is more overdiagnosis and very little or no reduction in the incidence of advanced cancers with screening. Introduction of population-wide breast cancer screening is seen to increase the breast cancer incidence, particularly that of low-risk disease and ductal carcinoma in situ (DCIS).[35-40] Studies from the United States and the United Kingdom demonstrate an increased incidence of DCIS and invasive breast cancer attributable to population-wide mammography screening and use of hormone replacement therapy (HRT).[41,42] After significant reduction in the use of HRT a reduction in breast cancer incidence has been seen. However, it is yet to reach the prescreening levels.[43]

Since screening identifies asymptomatic disease, we should expect a decline in breast cancer rates after some years of regular screening. However, no such reduction in incidence rates has ever been reported following the introduction of mammography screening, clearly pointing to substantive screening related overdiagnosis. Overdiagnosis results in overtreatment, which is a screening related harm that we impose on the population.

Breast Self-examination (BSE)

Two randomized trials of BSE showed no reduction in mortality.[44,45] Nonetheless, BSE is often recommended for resource-poor countries with the expectation that it might help to increase breast cancer awareness.[46]

Clinical Breast Examination (CBE)

The Canadian National Breast Screening Study (CNBSS) randomized over 90,000 women to compare the efficacy of mammography + CBE versus CBE alone in reducing mortality from breast cancer among women aged 40–49 and 50–59 years. In both age groups, the cancers in the control (CBE) groups tended to be diagnosed at an early stage and no significant benefit was found in women aged 40–49 years.[47] Although in women aged 50–59 years, mammography + CBE detected considerably more node-negative and small breast cancers than screening with CBE alone, this had no impact on breast cancer mortality.[48]

A study comparing CBE versus no-screening in Thailand had to be abandoned due to the refractory attitude of the women to clinical follow-up, diagnosis and treatment.[49] An ongoing trial in Thiruvananthapuram, India has randomized 115,652 women aged 30–69 years living in 275 clusters to "CBE screening" versus "no-screening" groups. This study which is evaluating the efficacy of 3 rounds of triennial CBE in downstaging breast cancer disease and reducing breast cancer mortality, reported preliminary results for incidence till May 31, 2009 (after completion of one screening round). This study reported the sensitivity, specificity, false-positive rate, and positive predictive values of CBE as 51.7% (95% confidence interval [CI] = 38.2% to 65.0%), 94.3% (95% CI = 94.1% to 94.5%), 5.7% (95% CI = 5.5% to 5.9%), and 1.0% (95% CI = 0.7% to 1.5%), respectively. The study also reported significant downstaging of invasive breast cancer disease in the screening group when compared to the control group.[50]

Another ongoing randomized controlled trial, which has recruited 151,538 women aged 35–64 years from 20 low socioeconomic housing clusters in Mumbai into "Cancer education + CBE screening" versus "only Cancer education" groups, is investigating the efficacy of four rounds of biennial CBE screening performed by trained primary health workers in downstaging invasive breast cancer disease and reducing mortality from breast cancer. This study reported significant downstaging after the completion of three rounds of screening.[51]

Recommendations

Population-wide breast cancer screening involves significant financial implications and development of diagnostic and treatment facilities. In a resource poor setting like India the value of gains (i.e. disease-free survival and quality of life) should be carefully evaluated through pilot studies before embarking on population-wide breast cancer screening programs. Breast cancer usually evokes a strong sentimental response, especially when it affects celebrities and families of policy makers.

Additionally, there are strong commercial interests in screening mammography. Cancer specialists should explain the difference between individual/opportunistic screening and population-wide screening to policy makers so that they can make learned policy decisions on the subject.

In urban and semi-urban areas of India, where the paying classes have a fair-to-good access to quality health care, we may consider opportunistic screening for breast cancer alongside cervical cancer screening. Whereas in rural India, with a different set of population demographics, the need for breast cancer screening will have to be carefully assessed and introduced, where needed, after the development of diagnostic and treatment facilities at district centers. Till then, primary health workers may include breast cancer education in the current health programs for women.

Referral in the Absence of Screening

Women aged 30 years and above who present with a breast lump, unilateral nipple discharge, skin changes such as eczematous changes in or around the nipple or areola, skin tethering and skin or nipple retraction should be referred for further investigations to rule out breast cancer. Whereas, women under the age of 30 years with a breast lump should only be referred for further investigation, if the lump enlarges or is fixed or hard or skin changes are present. They should also be referred when there is a strong family history of breast cancer, earlier treated breast cancer or therapeutic chest irradiation. Women found with no abnormalities upon CBE should be educated about the signs and symptoms of breast cancer and should be encouraged to be aware of their normal breast and of any changes by performing periodic BSE.

ORAL CANCER PREVENTION AND SCREENING

Disease Burden

India faces a significantly large burden of oral cancer among both men and women due to the culturally determined practice of habitual chewing of tobacco products. It is the second most frequent cancer among men and fourth most frequent cancer among women in India. With a total of 73,946 (males: 48,074; females: 25,872) cases and 50,540 (males: 32,936; females: 17,604) deaths annually from oral cancer, India contributes 27% to the global incidence and 38% to the global mortality from oral cancer (Fig. 6).[1]

Etiology

Oral cancer is directly linked to tobacco (chewing and smoking) and alcohol use. Additionally, areca-nut (*Supari*) and several chemical carcinogens are included in flavored chewing tobacco (*Pan-Masala* and *Gutkha*) available in India. Several studies conducted in India have confirmed the association between tobacco use and oral cancer.[52-56] The Government of India enacted a comprehensive tobacco control legislation in 2003, the "Cigarettes and other Tobacco Products (Prohibition of Advertisement and Regulation of Trade and Commerce, Production, Supply and Distribution) ACT 2003", abbreviated as "COTPA".

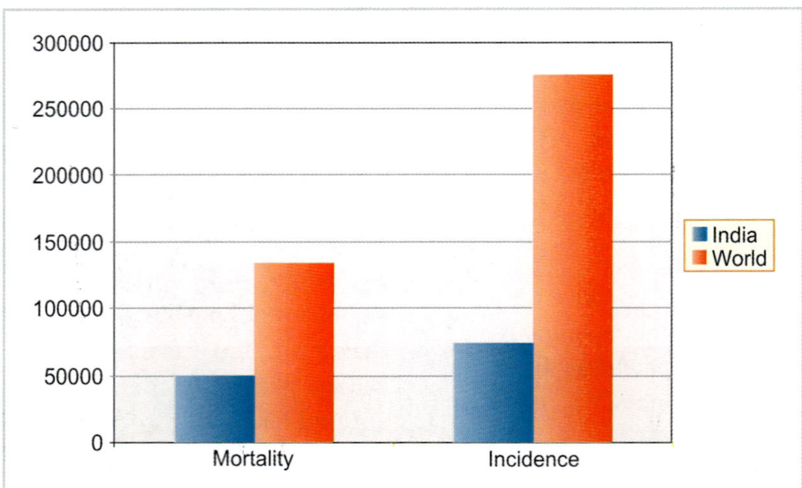

Fig. 6: Oral cancer incidence and mortality in India and world-over (GLOBOCAN 2008 projected to 2010)

There have been significant improvements following the implementation of the ACT, e.g. "smokefree public places" and "ban on advertising". However, important components of the ACT like "ban on the sale of tobacco products in a 100-meters area around educational institutions", "ban on surrogate advertising" and "ban on tobacco use in entertainment media" are yet to be meaningfully enforced. The human papillomavirus is now considered an important part of the process of oral cancer carcinogenesis.

Evidence for Screening

The 5-year relative survival rate for oral cancer is 53% (SEER), 31% in the less-developed countries and 26% in India.[57] Diagnosing oral cancer at an early stage significantly increases the odds of survival, but the evidence in support of routine mass screening to improve early diagnosis of oral cancers is weak.[58] The only randomized controlled trial for oral cancer screening was conducted in Kerala, India. The trial which recruited over 130,000 participants showed improved outcomes, at 3 and 6 years, with reference to surrogate markers like "downstaging" and "3-year survival".[59,60] The same trial at 9 years reported a significant increase in survival in the screened males with high-risk habits such as tobacco and alcohol use, suggesting that oral screening of high-risk individuals might be a useful intervention in India.[61]

Unaided visual inspection of the oral cavity using a normal light source also called "Conventional Oral Examination" (COE) has been the standard method for oral cancer screening in India and world over. There have been reports suggesting that COE based screening may be of limited value in the detection of premalignant and early invasive lesions.[62-64] Sensitivity around 74% and specificity around 99% have also been reported for COE performed by general dentists.[65,66]

India would have to depend on primary health workers for providing population-based oral screening. Studies from Sri Lanka and India, where oral examination was performed by primary health workers, have reported sensitivity ranging from 58% to 97% and specificity ranging from 75% to 94%.[67-70] These results were obtained in rigorous trial settings and may not be easily replicable in general health care settings. Further, COE outcomes are known to vary even at the hands of experienced clinicians. There are other techniques available today, e.g. oral cytology, Toluidine blue staining (TBS), VELscope, ViziLite and MicroLux, to assist oral screening. The usefulness of these aids in the hands of primary health workers has not been established. The application of some of these techniques has been studied in India with varying degrees of success.[71,72]

Recommendations

Tobacco and alcohol control through various strategies coupled with education for improving oral hygiene (particularly in schools) would be the "best buy" strategy for oral cancer prevention in India. Population-wide oral screening involves significant financial implications and development of diagnostic and treatment facilities and hence should be evaluated for efficacy before starting population-wide screening programs.

REFERENCES

1. Ferlay J, Shin HR, Bray F, et al. GLOBOCAN 2008, Cancer Incidence and Mortality Worldwide: IARC CancerBase No. 10. Lyon, France: International Agency for Research on Cancer; 2010. [online] Available from globocan.iarc.fr [Accessed January, 2014].
2. Sankaranarayanan R, Nene BM, Shastri SS, et al. HPV screening for cervical cancer in rural India. N Engl J Med. 2009;360:1385-94.
3. Sankaranarayanan R, Basu P, Wesley RS, et al. Accuracy of visual screening for cervical neoplasia: results from an IARC multicentre study in India and Africa. Int J Cancer. 2004;110:907-13.
4. Sankaranarayanan R, Wesley R, Thara S, et al. Test characteristics of visual inspection with 4% acetic acid (VIA) and Lugol's iodine (VILI) in cervical cancer screening in Kerala, India. Int J Cancer. 2003;106:404-8.
5. Sankaranarayanan R, Shastri SS, Basu P, et al. The role of low-level magnification in visual inspection with acetic acid for the early detection of cervical neoplasia. Cancer Detect Prev. 2004;28:345-51.
6. Sankaranarayanan R, Gaffikin L, Jacob M, et al. A critical assessment of screening methods for cervical neoplasia. Int J Gynaecol Obstet. 2005;89 (Suppl 2): S4-S12.
7. Arbyn M, Sankaranarayanan R, Muwonge R, et al. Pooled analysis of the accuracy of five cervical cancer screening tests assessed in eleven studies in Africa and India. Int J Cancer. 2008;123(1): 153-60.
8. Sankaranarayanan R, Esmy PO, Rajkumar R, et al. Effect of visual screening on cervical cancer incidence and mortality in Tamil Nadu, India: a cluster-randomised trial. Lancet. 2007;370: 398-406.
9. Goldie S, Gaffikin L, Goldhaber-Fiebert J, et al. Cost effectiveness of cervical screening in five developing countries. N Engl J Med. 2005;353:2158-68.
10. Legood R, Gray AM, Mahe C, et al. Screening for cervical cancer in India: How much will it cost? A trial based analysis of the cost per case detected. Int J Cancer. 2005;117:981-7.

11. Cuzick J, Arbyn M, Sankaranarayanan R, et al. Overview of human papillomavirus-based and other novel options for cervical cancer screening in developed and developing countries. Vaccine. 2008;26(Suppl 10):K29-41.

12. Arbyn M, Sasieni P, Meijer CJ, et al. Clinical applications of HPV testing: a summary of meta-analyses. Vaccine. 2006;24(Suppl 3):S378-89.

13. Ronco G, Brezzi S, Carozzi F, et al. The new technologies for cervical cancer screening randomised controlled trial. An overview of results during the first phase of recruitment. Gynecol Oncol. 2007;107(Suppl 1):S230-2.

14. Ronco G, Giorgi-Rossi P, Carozzi F, et al. Efficacy of human papillomavirus testing for the detection of invasive cervical cancers and cervical intraepithelial neoplasia: a randomised controlled trial. Lancet Oncol. 2010;11:249-57.

15. Dockter J, Schroder A, Hill C, et al. Clinical performance of the APTIMA HPV assay for the detection of high-risk HPV and high-grade cervical lesions. J Clin Virol. 2009;45(Suppl 1):S55-61.

16. Monsonego J, Hudgens MG, Zerat L, et al. Evaluation of oncogenic human papillomavirus RNA and DNA tests with liquid-based cytology in primary cervical cancer screening: the FASE study. Int J Cancer. 2011;129(3):691-701.

17. Dockter J, Schroder A, Eaton B, et al. Analytical characterization of the APTIMA HPV assay. J Clin Virol. 2009;45(Suppl 1):S39-47.

18. Blumenthal PD, Lauterbach M, Sellors JW, et al. Training for cervical cancer prevention programs in low-resource settings: focus on visual inspection with acetic acid and cryotherapy. Int J Gynaecol Obstet. 2005;89(Suppl 2):S30-7.

19. Bosch FX, Castellsague X, de Sanjose S. HPV and cervical cancer: screening or vaccination? Br J Cancer. 2008;98:15-21.

20. Bosch FX, de Sanjose S, Castellsague X. Evaluating the potential benefits of universal worldwide human papillomavirus vaccination. Therapy. 2008;5:305-12.

21. Fairley CK, Hocking JS, Gurrin LC, et al. Rapid decline in presentations of genital warts after the implementation of a national quadrivalent human papillomavirus vaccination programme for young women. Sex Transm Infect. 2009;85: 499-502.

22. Markowitz LE, Dunne EF, Saraiya M, et al. Quadrivalent human papillomavirus vaccine: recommendations of the Advisory Committee on Immunization Practices (ACIP). MMWR Recomm Rep. 2007;56(RR-2):1-24.

23. European Center for Disease Prevention and Control (ECDC). Guidance for the introduction of HPV vaccines European countries. [online] Available from http://ecdc. europa.eu/pdf/HPV_report pdf. September 2008. [Accessed January, 2014].

24. World Health Organization. Global Advisory Committee on Vaccine Safety, 17-18 December 2008. Wkly Epidemiol Rec. 2009;84:37-40. [online] Available from http:// www.who.int/vaccine_safety/en/ [Accessed January, 2014].

25. Schiller JT, Castellsague X, Villa LL, et al. An update of prophylactic human papillomavirus L1 virus-like particle vaccine clinical trial results. Vaccine. 2008;26(Suppl 10):K53-61.

26. Centers for Disease Control and Prevention. Reports of health concerns following HPV vaccination. [online] Available from http://www.cdc.gov/vaccinesafety/vaers/gardasil.htm [Accessed January, 2014].

27. Swedish Organised Service Screening Evaluation Group. Reduction in breast cancer mortality from organized service screening with mammography: 1. Further confirmation with extended data. Cancer Epidemiol Biomarkers Prev. 2006;15(1):45-51. PubMed PMID: 16434585.

28. Swedish Organised Service Screening Evaluation Group. Reduction in breast cancer mortality from the organised service screening with mammography: 2. Validation with alternative analytic methods. Cancer Epidemiol Biomarkers Prev. 2006;15(1):52-6. PubMed PMID: 16434586.

29. Kreutzkamp B. Mammography screening. Breast cancer mortality reduction by one fourth. Med Monatsschr Pharm. 2005;28(9):330-1.

30. Giles GG, Amos A. Evaluation of the organised mammographic screening programme in Australia. Ann Oncol. 2003;14(8):1209-11. PubMed PMID: 12881380.

31. Tabar L, Fagerberg CJ, Gad A, et al. Reduction in mortality from breast cancer after mass screening with mammography. Randomised trial from the Breast Cancer Screening Working Group of the Swedish National Board of Health and Welfare. Lancet. 1985 ;1(8433):829-32.

32. Verbeek AL, Hendriks JH, Holland R, et al. Reduction of breast cancer mortality through mass screening with modern mammography. First results of the Nijmegen project, 1975-1981. Lancet. 1984;1(8388):1222-4.

33. Strax P, Venet L, Shapiro S. Value of mammography in reduction of mortality from breast cancer in mass screening. Am J Roentgenol Radium Ther Nucl Med. 1973 ;117(3):686-9.

34. Gotzsche PC, Jorgensen KJ. Screening for breast cancer with mammography. Cochrane Database Syst Rev. 2013;6:CD001877.

35. Coldman A, Phillips N. Incidence of breast cancer and estimates of overdiagnosis after the initiation of a population-based mammography screening program. CMAJ. 2013 Jun 10.

36. Jorgensen KJ. Mammography screening in Norway caused substantial overdiagnosis and did not reduce late-stage breast cancers. Evid Based Med. 2013;18(2):e17.

37. Zahl PH. Overdiagnosis of invasive breast cancer due to mammography screening. Ann Intern Med. 2012;157(3):220-1; author reply 1-2.

38. Haldorsen T, Tretli S, Ursin G. Overdiagnosis of invasive breast cancer due to mammography screening. Ann Intern Med. 2012;157(3):220; author reply 1-2.

39. Jorgensen KJ. Overdiagnosis of invasive breast cancer due to mammography screening. Ann Intern Med. 2012;157(3):219-20; author reply 21-2.

40. Hellquist BN, Duffy SW, Nystrom L, et al. Overdiagnosis in the population-based service screening programme with mammography for women aged 40 to 49 years in Sweden. J Med Screen. 2012;19(1):14-9.

41. Altekruse SF, Kosary CL, Krapcho M, et al. SEER Cancer Statistics Review, 1975-2007. Bethesda, Md: National Cancer Institute, 2010. [online] Available from http://seer.cancer.gov/csr/1975_2007/. [Accessed on October 26, 2013].
42. Johnson A, Shekhdar J. Breast cancer incidence: what do the figures mean? J Eval Clin Pract. 2005;11(1):27-31.
43. Haas JS, Kaplan CP, Gerstenberger EP, et al. Changes in the use of postmenopausal hormone therapy after the publication of clinical trial results. Ann Intern Med. 2004 ;140(3):184-8.
44. Semiglazov VF, Moiseyenko VM, Bavli JL, et al. The role of breast self-examination in early breast cancer detection (results of the 5-years USSR/WHO randomized study in Leningrad). Eur J Epidemiol. 1992;8(4):498-502.
45. Thomas DB, Gao DL, Ray RM, et al. Randomized trial of breast self-examination in Shanghai: final results. J Natl Cancer Inst. 2002;94(19):1445-57.
46. Smith RA, Caleffi M, Albert US, et al. Breast cancer in limited-resource countries: early detection and access to care. Breast J. 2006;12 (Suppl 1):S16-26.
47. Miller AB, To T, Baines CJ, et al. The Canadian National Breast Screening Study-1: breast cancer mortality after 11 to 16 years of follow-up. A randomized screening trial of mammography in women age 40 to 49 years. Ann Intern Med. 2002;137(5 Part 1):305-12.
48. Miller AB, To T, Baines CJ, et al. Canadian National Breast Screening Study-2: 13-year results of a randomized trial in women aged 50-59 years. J Natl Cancer Inst. 2000;92(18):1490-9.
49. Pisani P, Parkin DM, Ngelangel C, et al. Outcome of screening by clinical examination of the breast in a trial in the Philippines. Int J Cancer. 2006;118(1):149-54.
50. Sankaranarayanan R, Ramadas K, Thara S, et al. Clinical breast examination: preliminary results from a cluster randomized controlled trial in India. J Natl Cancer Inst. 2011;103(19):1476-80.
51. Mittra I, Mishra GA, Singh S, et al. A cluster randomized, controlled trial of breast and cervix cancer screening in Mumbai, India: methodology and interim results after three rounds of screening. Int J Cancer. 2010;126(4):976-84.
52. Jayalekshmi PA, Gangadharan P, Akiba S, et al. Tobacco chewing and female oral cavity cancer risk in Karunagappally cohort, India. Br J Cancer. 2009;100:848-52.
53. Jayalekshmi PA, Gangadharan P, Akiba S, et al. Oral cavity cancer risk in relation to tobacco chewing and bidi smoking among men in Karunagappally, Kerala, India: Karunagappally cohort study. Cancer Sci. 2011;102:460-7.
54. Pednekar MS, Gupta PC, Yeole BB, et al. Association of tobacco habits, including bidi smoking, with overall and site-specific cancer incidence: results from the Mumbai cohort study. Cancer Causes Control. 2011;22:859-68.
55. Gupta PC, Ray CS. Epidemiology of betel quid usage. Ann Acad Med Singapore. 2004;33 (4 Suppl):31-6.
56. Znaor A, Brennan P, Gajalakshmi V, et al. Independent and combined effects of tobacco smoking, chewing and alcohol drinking on the risk of oral, pharyngeal and esophageal cancers in Indian men. Int J Cancer. 2003;105(5):681-6.
57. Parkin DM, Pisani P, Ferlay J. Global cancer statistics. CA Cancer J Clin. 1999;49(1):33-64.
58. Brocklehurst P, Kujan O, Glenny AM, et al. Screening programmes for the early detection and prevention of oral cancer. Cochrane Database Syst Rev. 2010;11:CD004150.
59. Sankaranarayanan R, Mathew B, Jacob BJ, et al. Early findings from a community-based, cluster-randomized, controlled oral cancer screening trial in Kerala, India. The Trivandrum Oral Cancer Screening Study Group. Cancer.2000;88(3):664-73.
60. Ramadas K, Sankaranarayanan R, Jacob BJ, et al. Interim results from a cluster randomized controlled oral cancer screening trial in Kerala, India. Oral Oncol. 2003 ;39(6):580-8.
61. Sankaranarayanan R, Ramadas K, Thomas G, et al. Effect of screening on oral cancer mortality in Kerala, India: a cluster-randomised controlled trial. Lancet. 2005;365(9475):1927-33.
62. Shugars DC, Patton LL. Detecting, diagnosing, and preventing oral cancer. Nurse Pract.1997;22(6):105, 109-10, 113-5 passim.
63. Silverman S. Early diagnosis of oral cancer. Cancer.1988;62 (8 Suppl):1796-9.
64. Sandler HC. Cytological screening for early mouth cancer. Cancer.1962;15:1119-24.
65. Jullien JA, Downer MC, Zakrzewska JM, et al. Evaluation of a screening test for the early detection of oral cancer and precancer. Community Dent Health. 1995;12(1):3-7.
66. Downer MC, Evans AW, Hughes Hallet CM, et al. Evaluation of screening for oral cancer and precancer in a company headquarters. Community Dent Oral Epidemiol. 1995;23(2):84-8.
67. Warnakulasuriya KA, Nanayakkara BG. Reproducibility of an oral cancer and precancer detection program using a primary health care model in Sri Lanka. Cancer Detect Prev. 1991;15(5):331-4.
68. Warnakulasuriya S, Pindborg JJ. Reliability of oral precancers screening by primary health care workers in Sri Lanka. Community Dent Health. 1990;7(1):73-9.
69. Mathew B, Sankaranarayanan R, Sunilkumar KB, et al. Reproducibility and validity of oral visual inspection by trained health workers in the detection of oral precancer and cancer. Br J Cancer.1997;76(3):390-4.
70. Mehta FS, Gupta PC, Bhonsle RB, et al. Detection of oral cancer using basic health workers in an area of high oral cancer incidence in India. Cancer Detect Prev.1986;9(3-4) 219-25.
71. Mehrotra R, Singh MK, Pandya S, et al. The use of an oral brush biopsy without computer-assisted analysis in the evaluation of oral lesions: a study of 94 patients. Oral Surg Oral Med Oral Pathol Oral Radiol Endod. 2008;106(2):246-53.
72. Gupta A, Singh M, Ibrahim R, et al. Utility of toluidine blue staining and brush biopsy in precancerous and cancerous oral lesions. Acta Cytol. 2007;51(5):788-94.

5 The Changing Face of Surgical Pathology

Anita Borges

INTRODUCTION

Surgical pathology as a discipline was born in the USA in the early years of the 20th century. It was created by surgeons, some of whom became its first practitioners. The first surgical pathologists were actually hired by departments of surgery to tackle the practical issues that surgeons faced in making clinical decisions. Rapid cancer diagnosis was one of these. Thus was born frozen section diagnosis. Academic pathologists in their ivory towers looked down on these newcomers as upstarts and hacks. They were reluctant to acknowledge this discipline until its viability left them with no choice. George Humphreys[1] wrote of this hybrid discipline "it was born of necessity and out of wedlock...never acknowledged in its infancy". Today in the US, surgical pathology is not only well-ensconced in the bosom of mainstream anatomic pathology, it is mainstream anatomic pathology. The practise of surgical pathology spread slowly across the Atlantic to Britain. Europe, where traditional histopathology was born, was even slower to embrace this discipline. In India, the Tata Memorial Hospital with its strong surgical traditions was perhaps the first center to practise the discipline. Although Dr VR Khanolkar, the doyen of Indian pathology, was the first pathologist at the institute, Dr MV Sirsat is recognized as its first surgical pathologist.

Surgical pathology is best defined as tissue pathology which is relevant to clinical management. It should answer the questions every treating physician asks of a tissue pathologist, only one of which is, "what is the diagnosis?" Oncologists, in particular, demand a great deal from a surgical pathologist. Is this a tumor? How aggressive is it? Where has it spread? What is the p-stage? Will the tumor respond to targeted therapy? Are the margins of resection clear? Has the response to treatment been good? Is the biopsy adequate and if not, how can the yield be maximized?

Traditional surgical pathology consisted of four important issues. Prime among them was a diagnosis. The others were staging, completeness of surgery or evaluation of the therapeutic response and prognosis. However, the age of personalized medicine is upon us. With the advent of targeted therapies, it is becoming imperative that these targets be detected in tissues. Predictive pathology is now an integral part of oncopathology. Surgical pathology is therefore not just histotaxonomy, i.e. a sophisticated way of classifying disease but an important component of therapeutic decision making, offering vital information that will help the treating physician decide what to do next.

Traditional Surgical Pathology

"There is no technique in all of medicine that provides so much information so quickly and for such little cost as the H&E technique"—Juan Rosai[2]

Any surgical pathology exercise starts with a good gross examination and sampling of resected specimens followed by a detailed microscopic examination of well-processed and stained hematoxylin and eosin (H&E) sections. In the exciting era of immunohistochemistry (IHC) and other ancillary molecular techniques, it is often forgotten that without this bedrock much of the advantage of molecular imaging is lost.

Diagnosis and Subtyping

This is the cornerstone of treatment. Without an accurate diagnosis, it is difficult to plan effective treatment in the majority of cases. It is imperative that a carcinoma be separated from a large cell lymphoma or a melanoma. Furthermore, subtyping of tumors, viz. non-Hodgkin's lymphoma or lung carcinoma has become essential. However, there are instances where an accurate diagnosis may be unnecessary for perfectly acceptable management. Many adult soft tissue sarcomas (STSs) of spindle cell or pleomorphic type fall into this category. It is more important in these cases to be able to stage the disease with respect to the size and depth of occurrence, evaluate the completeness of resection (R status), and state the grade of the tumor. It must be noted however, that this is not a blanket recipe for all STS. With the advent of imatinib, it is a serious error to misdiagnose a gastrointestinal stromal tumor (GIST) especially in a metastatic situation. It is also well-recognized that the grade of some STS is implicit in the diagnosis, e.g. alveolar soft part sarcoma is always high grade. All STS in children mandate subtyping, but are not graded as this implicit in the diagnosis, e.g. Ewing's sarcoma.

What if the diagnosis on a biopsy is difficult or impossible? This occurs in two situations: one, in which ancillary techniques can be helpful, e.g. lymphoma versus carcinoma or melanoma; the other, in which no ancillary technique will help. This is where the clinical and imaging findings often help to resolve the issue, e.g. diagnosis of verrucous squamous carcinoma. Pseudoepitheliomatous hyperplasia, on the other hand, is a condition where very little except experience helps. Bone tumors are uncommon and can pose diagnostic problems for pathologists who do not encounter many cases. Making a diagnosis without access to good imaging, especially a plain radiograph, is suicidal because benign bone forming lesions can be mistaken for malignant tumors on histology and vice versa.

Small tissue, big diagnosis

This is the era of "small tissue, big diagnosis". With the advent of interventional imaging and endoscopy, tissue biopsies are getting smaller and smaller, putting a great strain on the diagnostic skills of histopathologists. Ancillary techniques can and do help in some instance as discussed later in this chapter. However, sampling error and the inappropriate use of these biopsy techniques, e.g. needle core biopsy of an accessible cervical lymph node enlargement, may cause serious under or over diagnosis. Low grade follicular lymphomas and Hodgkin's lymphoma may be difficult to diagnose on small or fragmented biopsies, because pattern and a sparse population of Reed-Sternberg cells response may be impossible to discern despite the use of immunostaining. Additional material for diagnosis may be necessary and is not an admission of the pathologist's incompetence.

Box 1: Advantages of core needle biopsy over fine needle aspiration cytology (FNAC)

- Histopathology is generally considered to be the gold standard
- Greater availability of diagnostic histopathologists
- Higher accuracy of diagnosis, viz. presence or absence of invasion, type and grade of cancer
- Sufficient material available for ancillary techniques, especially where neoadjuvant therapies are being utilized, e.g. breast cancer
- Archival material available for reviews and further tests.

Has fine needle aspiration cytology (FNAC) become less relevant in the era of needle core biopsies? In a low resource country where tumors are large, FNAC is ubiquitously available, and core biopsy needles are expensive, FNAC is unlikely to become redundant any time soon especially for superficially located lumps, viz. breast. FNAC is also a quick and efficient diagnostic technique for screening lymph node enlargements for mycobacterial disease. It is also possible to simultaneously obtain material for culture. Having said this, there is no doubt that needle core biopsy offers several advantages over FNAC (Box 1).

In one particular center in the US, the use of FNAC for the diagnosis of breast cancer has declined 10-fold over a decade.[3] This bears testimony to decreasing tumor size due to the increased use of mammography for screening and the use of neoadjuvant therapy. For tumors, viz. lung cancer, which requires several predictive markers for targeted therapy, the amount of tissue is a huge issue as it has to be shared with the diagnostic histopathology laboratory, the molecular biology laboratory for mutation analyses, and the molecular pathology laboratory for fluorescent in situ hybridization (FISH) analyses. A good interventional radiologist can obtain several good cores from a tumor to satisfy all the demands for tissue, demands that will only grow with time. The question "FNAC or core biopsy?" cannot be answered in a one size fits all manner. The choice will depend on what the best method is of obtaining a diagnosis and what are the likely management strategies in a given patient.

Frozen section diagnosis

It always had a special place in the practise of oncological diagnosis. Up until the end of the 1970s, it was impossible to imagine a major cancer center embarking on a mastectomy without the aid of a frozen section (FS) diagnosis. The advent of FNAC changed this practise dramatically. Mastectomies without FS could now be undertaken not only at large hospitals, but were increasingly being performed in many mofussil towns and nursing homes. FS for the primary diagnosis of cancer has declined. However, FS for the control of resection margins and the intraoperative diagnosis of lymph node status is alive and well. A much neglected indication for a FS diagnosis is to judge the representativeness of a biopsy, especially if this is obtained by surgical intervention, e.g. a thoracoscopically obtained pleural biopsy. If the biopsy is not judged representative, another can be obtained at the same sitting. In a busy oncological department, the use of FS diagnosis for routine outpatient biopsies can be very helpful both for judging representativeness and for reducing the turnaround time for management decisions. This was successfully practised at the Tata Memorial Hospital, where the workload justified a dedicated outpatient pathology service. There are many centers that offer FS diagnosis on demand. In several of these centers, very few resections are performed without benefit of a FS diagnosis. There is considerable merit in this practise which helps to increase the experience of the pathologist in FS diagnosis. However, I submit that this practise requires a great deal of maturity on the part of the surgeon and pathologist to recognize those cases where the diagnosis is difficult, but where the impact on intraoperative decision making is negligible. If this maturity is lacking the confidence of the pathologist and that of the surgeon in the pathology service can be seriously eroded. It goes without saying that the best way to build confidence in FS diagnosis is an audit of FS versus final diagnoses.

P-Staging

Several standard protocols for gross examination and sampling of specimens exist. Without adequate sampling of a resected specimen, crucial information for diagnosis and staging is lost. Take for instance the case of a sigmoid colon cancer. The diagnosis of adenocarcinoma of the colon is usually known before the colectomy. However, depending on how the specimen is sampled, the p-stage can vary widely (Figs 1A to C). This will have serious consequences for adjuvant therapy.

Despite the availability of standard guidelines and checklists, gross examination and sampling of tissues is often inadequate in our country. Perhaps, it is the pathologist's lack of the appreciation of the impact this has on clinical management that is responsible for this problem. However, healthy feedback from surgical colleagues is often lacking. Clinicians, especially surgeons, must interact with their pathologists on a regular basis. The value of constructive feedback cannot be over emphasized. Fred Stewart,[4] one of the doyens of surgical pathology in USA, wrote that the surgical pathology exercise is "what the combined intelligence of the surgeon and pathologist makes it". It follows, therefore, that a surgeon gets the surgical pathologist he or she deserves!

Synoptic reporting is the current buzzword in report generation. In many laboratories around the world, the carefully crafted, gross and microscopic descriptions of yore have been replaced by reports that meet the requirements of electronic data storage and retrieval (Fig. 2).[5] It is generally acknowledged that the human brain processes information better in a written form rather than as numbers or symbols. On the other hand, checklists are extremely important and must be consulted in every case. I believe that synoptic reports accompanied by concise written summaries containing all relevant positive and negative information make for an ideal communication to the treating physician. It goes without saying that merely adhering to a checklist does not guarantee good pathology.

Good microscopic examination cannot compensate for an inadequate gross examination and sampling of tissues. This is a situation faced by many consultants when asked for second opinions on slides and blocks. Staging, in such a situation is entirely dependent on the tumor areas and number of lymph nodes sampled by the referring

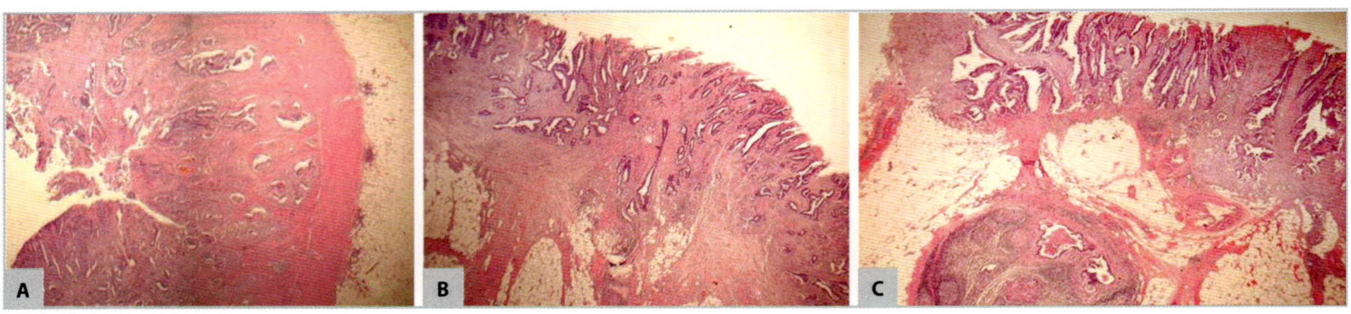

Figs 1A to C: Change of p-stage by three sections through different areas of the same tumor in the sigmoid colon in which all the sampled regional lymph nodes were negative. (A) Modified Astler-Coller B1; (B) Modified Astler-Coller B2; (C) Modified Astler-Coller C2

National Minimum Dataset
Colorectal Cancer Histopathology Report

Surname .... Forenames .... Date of birth .... Sex........

Hospital .... Hospital No .... NHS No....................

Date of receipt .... Date of reporting .... Report No....................

Pathologist .... Surgeon ....

Gross description

Site of tumor..

Maximum tumor diameter...

Distance of tumor to nearer margin (cut end).............

Presence of tumor perforation (pT4) ☐ Yes ☐ No

For rectal tumors

Tumor is ☐ above ☐ at ☐ below
the peritoneal reflection

Distance from the dentate line.......................................

Histology

Type

Adenocarcinoma ☐ Yes ☐ No
(to include mucinous and signet ring adenocarcinomas)

If no, other...

Differentiation by predominant area

☐ Well/moderate ☐ Poor

Local invasion

☐ Submucosa (pT1)
☐ Muscularis propria (pT2)
☐ Beyond muscularis propria (pT3)
☐ Tumor cells have breached the peritoneal surface or invaded adjacent organs (pT4)

Margins

Tumor involvement	**N/A**	**Yes**	**No**
Doughnut	☐	☐	☐
Margin (cut end)	☐	☐	☐
For rectal tumors			
Circumferential margin involvement	☐	☐	☐

Histological measurement from tumor to circumferential margin..........mm

Metastatic spread

No of lymph nodes examined..

No of positive lymph nodes.......................................

(pN1 1–3 nodes, pN2 4 + nodes involved)

	Yes	No
Apical node positive (Duties C2)	☐	☐
Extramural vascular invasion	☐	☐

Background abnormalities

	Yes	No
Adenoma(s)	☐	☐
Synchronous carcinoma(s) *(Complete and separate form for each cancer)*	☐	☐
Ulcerative colitis	☐	☐
Crobin's disease	☐	☐
Familial adenomatous polyposis	☐	☐

Other comments..

....

Pathological staging

Complete resectional all margins ☐ Yes ☐ No

TNM

☐ T ☐ N ☐ M

Dukes

☐ Dukes A (Growth limited to wall, nodes negative)
☐ Dukes B (Growth beyond wall, nodes negative)
☐ Dukes C1 (Nodes positive and apical node negative)
☐ Dukes C2 (Apical node positive)

Histologically confirmed liver mets ☐ Yes ☐ No

Fig. 2: Synoptic report on a colorectal cancer. Modified from the National Minimum Dataset for colorectal cancer in Britain laboratory. For instance, 12 is the minimum number of lymph nodes considered adequate for a colorectal cancer dissection. For obvious reasons, the prognosis of a pN0 tumor varies inversely with the number of lymph nodes examined.

Margins of resection: As surgery for tumors becomes more and more conservative, the importance of margins of tumor clearance at some sites where this has never been an issue has assumed immense importance. A prime example is the breast. As tumor sizes get smaller, lumpectomy for cancer is replacing mastectomy. Resection margins are a very important determinant of local recurrence and must therefore be examined carefully. This is usually done intraoperatively by FS followed by confirmation on paraffin embedded sections. Revision surgery follows a report of "positive margins". A lively debate continues in the literature about the value of intraoperative versus postoperative evaluation of the margins, and the definition of what constitutes a positive margin. This is not only true of the breast, but obtains at other sites, e.g. the head and neck. These debates notwithstanding, the presence of tumor at the cut edge whether it be circumferential soft tissue, skin or mucosa, must be reported so that appropriate action can be initiated. The method of examination, radial or shave depends on the site and grossly estimated distance. An important contribution to the successful evaluation of resection margins is orientation of the specimen by the surgeon. Standard methods of orientation by sutures and colored inks are available.

Evaluation of the therapeutic response: Neoadjuvant ablative therapies are routinely undertaken in modern cancer management. The effectiveness of these treatments is significance for determining prognosis and possible change in management strategy. Each site has a protocol for determining the extent of residual tumor. Osteogenic sarcoma in the long bones is an example of how exhaustive such an exercise can be. At sites such as the breast, esophagus and rectum, if no tumor is found in preliminary sections, the entire tumor bed would have to be microscopically examined to document a complete response (CR). Clinical oncologists and surgical pathologists must be aware of these protocols, so that the patient is given the benefit of the observations. Moreover, studies from different centers cannot be compared if methods of assigning CR vary.

The Changing Face of Surgical Pathology

Modern day surgical pathology serves the same ends as its traditional counterpart. However, the technologies that a pathologist has at his or her command have changed. Imaging has made diagnosis both easier and more difficult. Furthermore, the era of molecular medicine has ushered in the promise of personalized medicine. All these and the rising cost of health care have changed the way surgical pathology is practised (Box 2).

Box 2: **Factors that impact on the practise of modern surgical pathology**

- Ancillary techniques
  - Immunohistochemistry
  - In-situ hybridization
  - PCR and RT-PCR
  - Cytogenetics
  - Gene expression profiling
- Imaging
  - Radiological tissue diagnosis
  - Precise localization for biopsy
  - "Small tissue, big diagnosis"
- Personalized medicine
  - Targeted therapy
  - Predictive pathology
- Evidence based pathology
- Quality assurance in surgical pathology
- Second opinion pathology

Ancillary Techniques on Tissue Sections

The H&E stain has been the backbone of routine histopathology diagnosis. It remains so today. However, there are limitations to morphology which have been overcome by molecular imaging, and other molecular biology techniques, viz. polymerase chain reaction (PCR), reverse transcription polymerase chain reaction (RT-PCR) and gene expressing profiling (GEP) which is commonly referred to as DNA microarray.

Molecular imaging

This is a technique by which the presence of proteins and nucleotide sequences can be visualized within cells and tissues by the binding of antibodies or complementary nucleotide probes respectively. The specific binding can be visualized by attaching reporter molecules to the antibody or probe which will emit a signal that involves color or fluorescence. IHC is the most important ancillary technique in diagnosis, because it is easily integrated into the normal working pattern of a routine histopathology laboratory (Figs 3A and B).

Immunohistochemistry

It has revolutionized diagnosis by making many molecules that are expressed in cells and tissues visible. Yet, it bears reiterating that the choice of what molecules to look for and the interpretation of the stain are still based on the

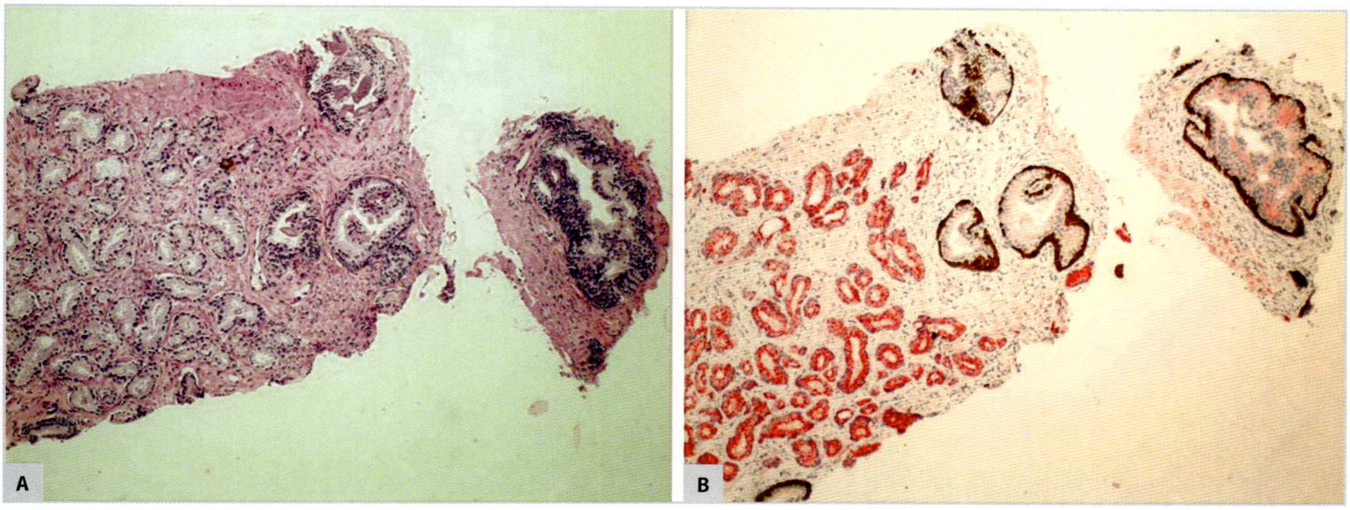

Figs 3A and B: Prostate carcinoma immunostained by PIN4 a "cocktail" containing antibodies against basal cell proteins CK5/14 and p63 and alpha-methylacyl-CoA racemase (AMACR). Prostatic carcinoma cells express AMACR (red) while the normal glands remain unstained. Normal glands retain their basal layer staining (brown), whereas the carcinoma shows absence of staining

gold standard H&E section. For IHC to be of value, it must, like any other laboratory procedure, be standardized, validated and constantly monitored. IHC is not a magic wand. It is exquisitely dependent on antigen preservation in tissues. It cannot undo the crimes perpetrated on tissues by bad fixation or processing. This is particularly true of those antigens which are semiquantitatively analyzed, viz. estrogen receptors (ER), progesterone receptors (PR) and Her2/neu (Her2). Many clinicians and pathologists do not realize that fixation times are of the utmost importance in histopathology in general and IHC in particular. An antibody recognizes an antigen by a binding site called an epitope. If this has been altered or destroyed by poor fixation or processing, a false negative result will be reported. It is difficult to estimate the exact number of false negative ER, PR and Her2 tests that are reported in India as a result of poor antigen preservation. However, the numbers are expected to be high in those cases where specimens are not fixed and processed in-house.

Immunohistochemistry for diagnosis very seldom involves the use of a single antibody. A panel of antibodies based on the possible differential diagnoses in a given case is used in a sequential algorithmic manner. The common practise, in some parts of this country, of a clinician deciding on the number of IHC "markers" to be performed, is mentioned here only to be deplored. On the other hand, if a clinical oncologist is cognizant of the common antibodies employed and the markers tested, a meaningful dialogue can take place between him or her and the pathologist, to the benefit of the patient. Good laboratory practise requires the use of controls and proficiency testing.

In situ hybridization (ISH)

It is similar in principle to IHC except that a probe consisting of a nucleotide sequence complimentary to that which is sought in the tissues is used instead of an antibody. This technique is useful in the diagnosis of tumors which have a unique chromosomal translocation in the tissues which is not reflected in an abnormal protein signal detectable by IHC. Examples of such tumors are Ewing's sarcoma and desmoplastic small round cell tumor. In situ hybridization (ISH) is also used to evaluate gene amplification in cells. The most commonly used test is for Her2 amplification in breast carcinoma. Most ISH is done by using fluorescence-labeled probes. This is usually referred to as FISH.

Genogenic immunohistochemistry

The ability of IHC to reflect changes in the genome has been referred to as genogenic by Alan Gown.[6] Expression of ALK1 protein in ALK1 translocated anaplastic large cell lymphoma and inflammatory myofibroblastic tumor; C-kit expression in KIT mutated gastrointestinal stromal tumors (GIST); loss of mismatch repair (MMR) proteins in some colon cancers; and over expression in breast and stomach cancer of Her2 protein as a result of gene amplification are examples of genogenic IHC (Figs 4 and 5).

Molecular pathology

All techniques that investigate the composition and interactions of subcellular structures and molecules should constitute the field of molecular pathology. Immunohistochemistry in a broad sense is also molecular pathology as it investigates molecular expression in cells and tissues. However, the standard understanding

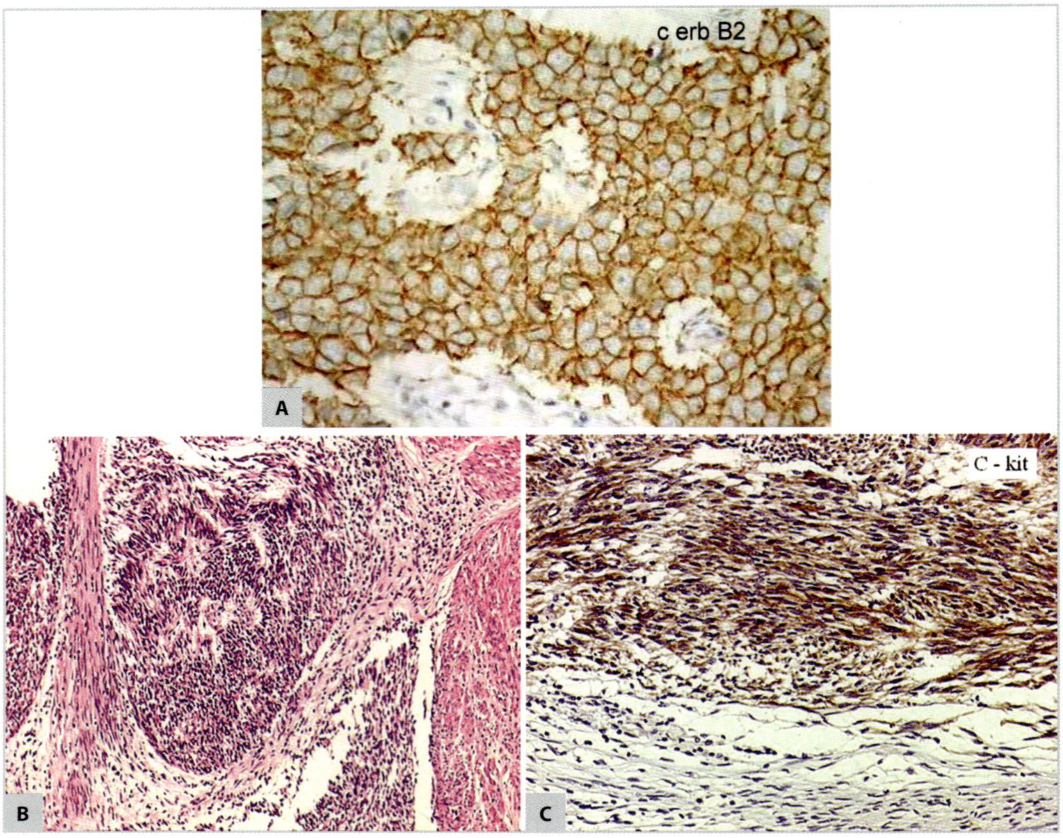

Figs 4A to C: Examples of genogenic immunohistochemistry (IHC). (A) Her2/neu (C erb B2) gene amplification seen as heavy and complete cytoplasmic membrane staining; (B and C) Epithelioid GIST (H&E) and expression of c-kit (CD117)

of molecular pathology is limited to that discipline of anatomic pathology which uses nucleic acid-based techniques such as ISH, RT-PCR, and nucleic acid microarrays for specialized studies of disease in tissues and cells. It encompasses all aspects of patient care from disease diagnosis to prevention and therapeutics. As more and more is known about the genome of normal and diseased cells, the field of molecular pathology can only grow exponentially.

Polymerase chain reaction based techniques

These techniques are used where IHC and ISH cannot be used to establish a diagnosis or have failed to do so. For instance, the clonality of T-cell proliferations cannot be established without the use of gene rearrangement studies that are PCR based. This is also true for gene mutations that are not reflected in a protein product detectable by IHC, or mutations in specific exons that have a clinical bearing on targeted therapy and the diagnosis of familial cancers. Examples are exons 9 and 11 in the KIT gene in GIST and RET mutations in familial medullary carcinoma syndromes.

Gene expression profiling

It also referred as DNA microarray technology, has become a buzzword in molecular pathology. This technology allows the simultaneous analysis of thousands of genes expressed in a tissue. The results are a complex set of expression patterns of red and green fluorescence which require computer analysis and the help of bioinformaticians. From these studies, a new understanding of the relationship between the tumor and its microenvironment, tumor behavior and tumor subtyping has come about. Much of the information pertains to prognosis and indirectly to possible therapeutic modulation of tumor behavior.

Alizadeh et al.[7] in 2000 reported that the heterogeneous group of diffuse large B-cell lymphomas (DLBCLs) could be segregated into two major prognostic groups on the basis of GEP; an activated B-cell type and a germinal center type. Several studies have confirmed that the former is prognostically worse than the latter even in the era of rituximab therapy. It would make sense therefore to use this prognostic classification in prospective trials

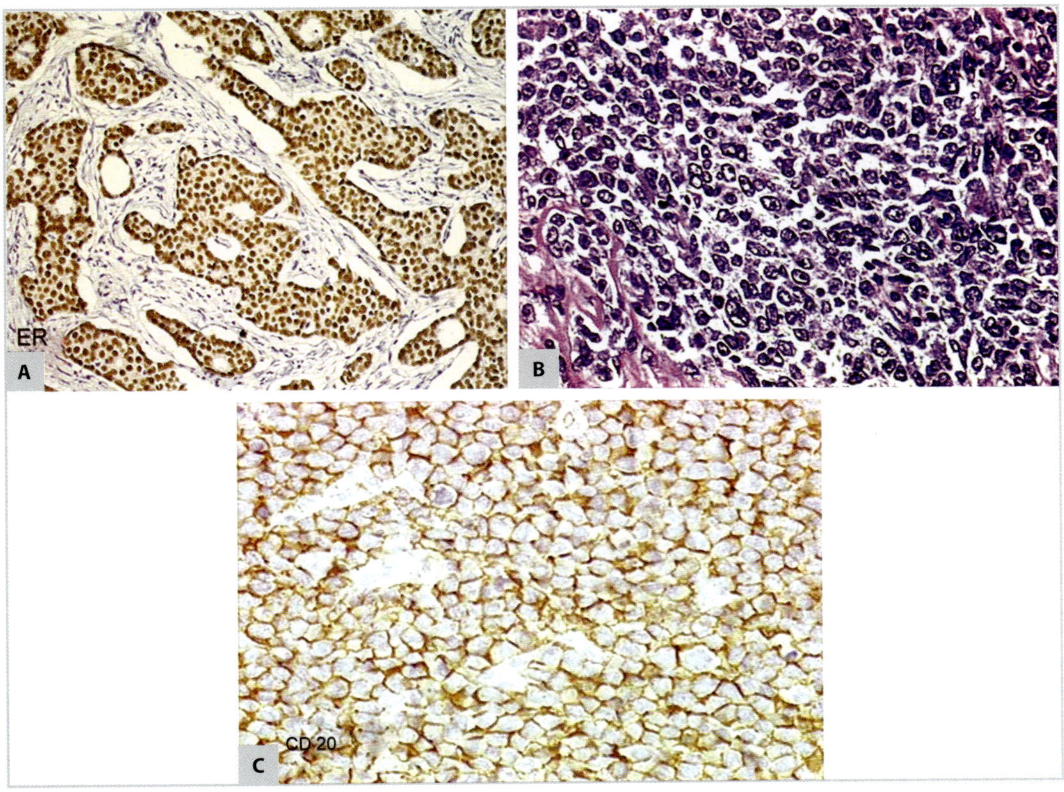

Figs 5A to C: Examples of predictive pathology. (A) Strong and diffuse expression of estrogen receptor (ER) in the nucleus of a breast carcinoma; (B and C) H&E and CD20 immunostained sections of a non-Hodgkin's lymphoma of diffuse large B-cell type

of new therapies for DLBCL. This has proved to be very difficult to do because of the cost and expertise entailed in performing GEP on routine cases in the clinic. Surrogate IHC algorithms for some of the important proteins expressed in the two types have been tried with variable degrees of correlation with GEP. It remains to be seen how this particular exercise in prognostic classification of DLBCL works in the clinic (Figs 5A to C).[8]

Gene expressing profiling of breast cancer, on the other hand, has made its appearance in routine clinical practise, albeit that the tests can only be performed under license from the patent holders. Oncotype DX®[9] and MammaPrint®[10] are of the best known examples. The former is used to predict the risk of relapse in small, ER-positive, node-negative breast cancers. The implication of a high-risk score is that adjuvant chemotherapy would be offered in addition to hormonal treatment. GEP has also been used to classify breast cancer into intrinsic types by Sorlie and Perou et al.[11] These types seem to correlate with the expression profile of ER, Her2/neu, basal cytokeratins (CK5/6) and epidermal growth factor receptor (EGFR). The high-risk group in the Oncotype DX® 22 gene profile seems to correlate with the luminal type B intrinsic subtype and a proliferation fraction greater than 14%. As with DLBCL, until GEP technology becomes clinic friendly, the use of IHC as an imperfect surrogate for GEP in breast cancer will remain.

Predictive Pathology

Pathologists have been prognosticating the behavior of tumors based on tumor type, grade and stage for the longest time. However, the term "prediction" in oncology has come to mean something other than prognosis. Prediction is used in the context of response to a specific drug or line of treatment. Prediction is the base on which is built the promise of personalized medicine, i.e. the right drug, at the right dose delivered to the right individual at the right time. Targeted therapy is the name of the game. The target is a specific molecule or signaling pathway which should be qualitatively or quantitatively identifiable in the clinic and the outcome of therapy should relate to its presence or quantity. Drug toxicity is another area where prediction is important. Although these tests, viz. prediction of sensitivity to fluorouracil (5-FU) and methotrexate save lives, they are beyond the scope of surgical pathology. Targets in tissues, however, are not. They are being actively sought and tested in clinical trials. ACTNOW is an acronym for Accelerating Clinical Trials of Novel Oncologic Pathways.[12] The hope is that the many signaling pathways involved in cancer cell growth, development and apoptosis will be profitably targeted.

The epitome of predictive oncology is ER (Flow chart 1). It is the oldest and most used target in clinical oncology. All breast cancers today must have three targets qualitatively and semiquantitatively analyzed by IHC in tissue sections. These are ER, PR and Her2/neu. Effective adjuvant therapy is based on the results. Triple negative (TN) is now so much a part of the breast cancer lexicon that one fails to realize that it is based on three negative results that preclude the use of adjuvant hormonal and anti-HER2 monoclonal therapy, rather than being a special type of breast cancer.

Other tumors have been successfully treated based on the tissue expression of targets. The two most quoted success stories are rituximab in the treatment of CD20 expressing DLBCL and imatinib in the treatment of c-kit expressing GIST (Figs 5A to C). In fact, the latter is truly a remarkable example of the complete resolution by an oral non-chemotherapeutic agent of a solid tumor that was virtually untreatable when widespread metastasis had supervened.

The story of the role of predictive oncology in lung cancer also bears telling. It reads almost like a fairy tale. Once upon a time, life for a pathologist was simple. Lung carcinomas were either small cell or non-small cell lung carcinoma (NSCLC). The former were chemosensitive, the latter were treated by surgeons. Subtyping of NSCLC was an academic exercise which was undertaken on resection specimens. Then came the need to subclassify NSCLC into squamous and nonsquamous types on small biopsies and cytology smears, because it was shown that some therapeutic agents such as bevacizumab had an adverse and possible lethal effect in patients with squamous carcinoma. Others, such as pemetrexed had no therapeutic effect at all. Adenocarcinomas on the other hand which has seen a dramatic rise in both smokers and nonsmokers have been the subject of much therapeutic research after it was shown that response to tyrosine kinase inhibitors (TKIs) in patients with EGFR mutations produced good responses. Today, it is almost mandatory to subclassify NSCLC. The pressure to do so on very small amounts of tissue has led to a classification of lung cancer that is applicable to

Flow chart 1: One of several immunohistochemistry (IHC) based algorithms for the classification of diffuse large B-cell lymphoma (DLBCL) into activated B-cell (ABC) and germinal center B (GCB) types[8]

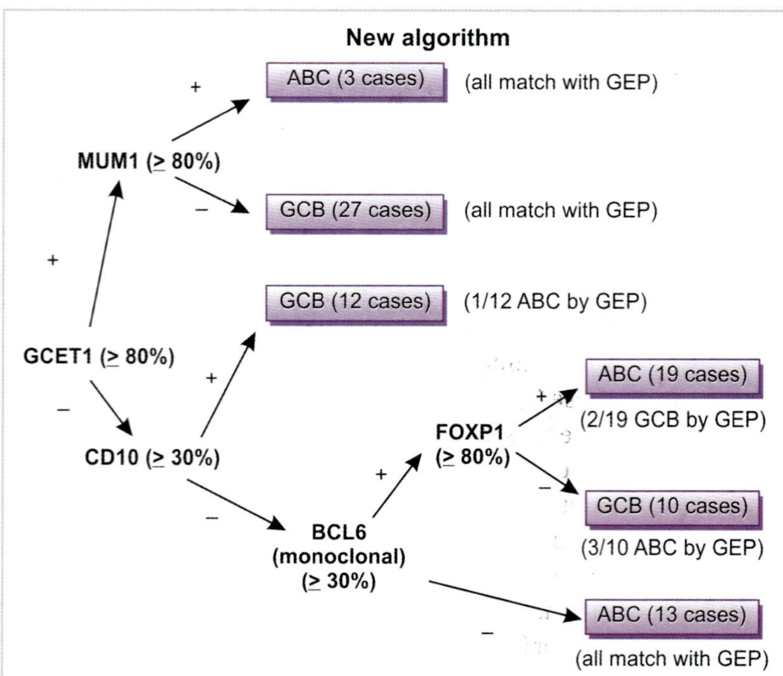

biopsy specimens.[13] Apart from subclassification, tissue is required for molecular analysis of mutations in epidermal growth factor receptor (EGFR), radiology oncology system (ROS) and BRAF genes and ALK-EML4 translocation, each of which have implications for the use of specific targeted agents. Mutations of RAS and genetic polymorphism in ERCC1 and RRM1 genes have a profound impact on whether or what chemotherapy will work in lung cancer. All these investigations require sharing of tissue between the pathologist and the molecular pathology laboratory. "Tissue is an issue" has been the topic of discussion at many symposia on lung and other solid tumors. As the nodal person in this team, the surgical pathologist has a responsibility to coordinate the exercise of tissue sharing and archiving as well as to collate all available information on the tissue biopsy in a comprehensive report.

Evidence-based Pathology

No branch of medicine is immune from practicing the mantra of "evidence-based medicine (EBM)". Surgical pathology is no exception. It is an astonishing fact that histopathology, which is a qualitative discipline, is used as the basis of the majority of clinical trials that result in level 1 evidence in clinical practise. To quote James Crawford "how can it be that morphologic examination of devitalized human tissue that has been fixed in formalin, dehydrated and permeated with paraffin, sliced thinly and stained with biblical era colorizing agents (hematoxylin and eosin), covered in glue and sandwiched between glass, has any bearing on clinical management decisions made for the living patient?" Is it possible to name a single therapeutic trial in head and neck oncology that does not have a histopathologic diagnosis as an inclusion criterion? Yet, there is room for the EBM approach to make diagnoses more clinically meaningful and to refine the way ancillary techniques are used in practise, to name just two areas which have been the subject of published research. A recent publication on the redundancy in the number subcategories of the WHO subclassification of thymomas is a case in point.[14] There are also several reports on the most cost-effective algorithms for the use of IHC and molecular tests in diagnosis of a variety of tumors.[15] Evidence-based pathology has also led to the publication of guidelines for the standardized reporting of semiquantitative tests, e.g. Her2/neu, and categories of prognostic relevance for various parameters in common tumors.

Second Opinions

These form an increasing proportion of the work load of tertiary care centers and busy consultant practises. The most common reason for such consults is the lack of access to IHC facilities at the primary pathology laboratory. This need is most acutely felt in the diagnosis of lymph node disorders and undifferentiated malignancies in children and adults. Soft tissue tumors are also areas of difficulty. Second opinions requested by clinicians are the result of discrepancies between clinical and pathologic diagnoses. The problems faced by those offering second opinions are many and often not appreciated by both the referring pathologist and the clinician. Poor tissue fixation and processing, which impact on the results of ancillary techniques, are the most common. P-staging is also impossible if the original pathologist has inappropriately sampled the tissue. Slides will only reflect what is in a block, which in turn will reflect what has been sampled. I make this specific point because of the oft-heard refrain "but you have the block!" Difficulty in accessing reliable clinical and radiological details, especially a history of past illnesses is another common problem. Quite often the answer is that the information is unobtainable. The information exists, but the will to pursue it is missing. Yet without this crucial piece of the puzzle, a second opinion is no better than a second guess!

Quality Assurance in Surgical Pathology

There is a prevailing misconception that quality assurance applies only to tests which can be quantitated. As a result, histopathology gets short shrift. Needless to say that this attitude must change if good quality practices are to be followed all the way from accessioning specimens to producing well-stained sections for a pathologist to report on in a standardized format. Accreditation of histopathology laboratories is the need of the hour. However, this is unlikely to be generally effective any time soon. Laboratory accreditation in India is a voluntary exercise that is growing slowly. The National Accreditation Board for Testing and Calibration Laboratories (NABL) has accredited over 400 laboratories in India. However, a miniscule number of these have their histopathology services accredited. There is another problem that NABL has only recently started to address. This is the lack of accredited external quality assessment (EQA) schemes. This is particularly true of histopathology and cytopathology, where until recently there were no local or national EQA schemes available. Today, due to the pioneering efforts of certain determined individuals, laboratories can and should avail these programs. The most serious lack of EQA is in the area of semiquantitative testing of ER, PR and Her2/neu. Many laboratories offer these services, but have never had them tested for proficiency. This can lead to under reporting which may have serious therapeutic consequences. Clinicians have an important role in encouraging pathologists to have their testing facilities accredited. A failure of testing standards for hormone receptors in breast cancer set off a country wide alarm and soul searching in Newfoundland, Canada. The inquiry brought to light several lacunae in the system not the least being the casual approach to quality management in the laboratory. We, in this country have a long way to go, but there is light at the end of the tunnel.

Challenges of Surgical Pathology

These are many and varied. They range from training of pathologists to upgradation of pathology laboratories to meet the growing need for ancillary techniques in oncological diagnosis. Research into common cancers in the subcontinent to which a pathologist can contribute is not only possible, but is the need of the hour. Extrapolation of results from the published literature to a different population does not always pay dividends. It is a sad fact that much of our clinical research is pharma-driven for profit. There are clinical questions that can be answered without huge resources. These should be the focus of cooperation between the pathologist and oncologist.

SUMMARY

Surgical pathology is a clinical discipline. It was born out of necessity to cater to the needs of surgeons. Walking with oncologists is both an art and a science. Molecular pathology and molecular imaging have posed new challenges to the way pathology is practised. To keep pace with changing trends, a modern day surgical pathologist must have his/her feet firmly planted in traditional surgical pathology and be willing to embrace with both hands the new advances in the field, all the while keeping a questioning and open mind. If pathologists fail to grasp the opportunities that the new world offers they will have only themselves to blame if the world passes them by.

"In a time of drastic change, it is the learners who inherit the future.

The learned find themselves equipped to live in a world which no longer exists."—Eric Hoffer (1902–1983)

REFERENCES

1. Humphreys GH. The surgeon-pathologists at P&S. In: Fenoglio CM, Wolff M (Eds). Progress in Surgical Pathology. New York: Masson Publishing; 1980. pp. 1-3.
2. Rosai J. Why microscopy will remain a cornerstone of surgical pathology. Lab Invest. 2007;87(5):403-8.
3. Dawson A. Breast lesion diagnosis with FNA and core biopsy: Challenges and Opportunities. Papanicolaou Society of Cytology. USCAP; 2009.
4. Hajdu SI, Melamed MR. Limitations of aspiration cytology in the diagnosis of primary neoplasms. Acta Cytol. 1984;28(3):337-45.
5. Quirke P, Morris E. Reporting colorectal cancer. Histopathology. 2007;50(1):103-12.
6. Gown AM. Genogenic immunohistochemistry: A new era in diagnostic immunohistochemistry. Curr Diagn Pathol. 2002;8(3):193-200.
7. Alizadeh AA, Eisen MB, Davis RE, et al. Distinct types of diffuse large B-cell lymphoma identified by gene expression profiling. Nature. 2000;403(6769):503-11.
8. Choi WW, Weisenburger DD, Greiner TC, et al. A new immunostain algorithm classifies diffuse large B-cell lymphoma into molecular subtypes with high accuracy. Clin Cancer Res. 2009;15(17):5494-502.
9. Paik S, Shak S, Tang G, et al. A multigene assay to predict recurrence of tamoxifen-treated, node-negative breast cancer. N Engl J Med. 2004;351(27):2817-26.
10. van't Veer LJ, Dai H, van de Vijver MJ, et al. Gene expression profiling predicts clinical outcome of breast cancer. Nature. 2002;415(6871):530-6.
11. Sørlie T, Perou CM, Tibshirani R, et al. Gene expression patterns of breast carcinomas distinguish tumor subclasses with clinical implications. Proc Natl Acad Sci USA. 2001;98(19):10869-74.
12. National Cancer Institute, NIH. Accelerating clinical trials of novel oncologic pathways (ACTNOW). [online] Available from http://www.cancer.gov/aboutnci/recovery/recoveryfunding/actnow [Accessed January, 2014].
13. Travis WD, Brambilla E, Riely GJ, et al. New pathologic classification of lung cancer: relevance for clinical practice and clinical trials. J Clin Oncol. 2013;31(8):992-1001.
14. Marchevsky AM, Gupta R, McKenna RJ, et al. Evidence-based pathology and the pathologic evaluation of thymomas: the World Health Organization classification can be simplified into only 3 categories other than thymic carcinoma. Cancer. 2008;112(12):2780-8.
15. Marchevsky AM, Wick MR. Evidence-based guidelines for the utilization of immunostains in diagnostic pathology: pulmonary adenocarcinoma versus mesothelioma. Appl Immunohistochem Mol Morphol. 2007;15(2):140-4.

6

Current and Future Imaging Techniques: Therapeutic Impact on Treatment Planning

Bhavin Jankharia

INTRODUCTION

Imaging has a critical and important role to play in oncology. From diagnosis to treatment, it helps answer the critical questions in oncology related to overall management.

- Diagnosis
- Staging
- Biopsy
- Treatment decisions—radiotherapy/surgery
- Interim and post-treatment surveillance
- Evaluation of recurrence
- Image-guided therapy.

PLAIN RADIOGRAPHS

The utility of plain radiographs is limited. Yet, as an initial modality, they help in diagnosing cancer of the lungs when a nodule or mass is seen initially which helps planning further imaging like the CT scan or a PET/CT as well. For characterization of bone tumors, the role of plain radiographs is still highly significant and important (Fig. 1).[1] Monitoring patients on chemotherapy and radiotherapy; appropriate imaging will indicate progression/regression for a given lesion.

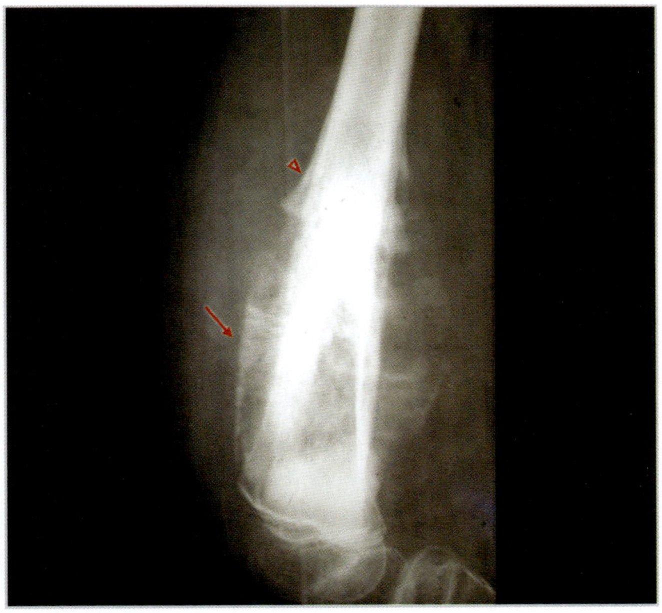

Fig. 1: Lateral radiograph of the femur shows a bone forming neoplasm involving the distal femur, showing typical characteristics of an osteosarcoma with a Codman triangle (arrowhead) and a sun-ray pattern (arrow) of periosteal reaction

Procedures[2]

A simple barium swallow study is useful in giving a global overview of carcinoma of the esophagus and for delineating the distal extent. It has no role now in the evaluation of gastric malignancies; however, a small bowel enema may detect a subtle stricture due to malignancy that can then be evaluated with a CT scan. Similarly with an obstructed colon cancer, a barium enema can delineate the proximal extent of the lesion. None of the other procedures, such as intravenous urography, etc. today have any role in oncology, though in a rural or a semi-urban area it still can help in simple diagnosis.

MAMMOGRAPHY

Mammography is the gold standard for screening and detection of breast cancer.[3] It is now proven to save lives because of early detection of cancer, though there is still some controversy regarding its use as a screening tool except in the group with positive family history.[4]

Mammography can help to characterize a lesion regarding multicentricity and bilaterality. Mammography-guided stereotactic biopsy helps to evaluate lesions which are impalpable and not visualized on ultrasonography (USG).[5] A new technique of breast tomosynthesis has improved the ability to detect cancer, but its utility in overall screening is still unproven.[6] Full-field digital and computed radiography digital mammograms have improved quality in the detection of cancerous lesions.[7]

ULTRASOUND

Ultrasound is an excellent modality in the detection of lesions virtually all over the body except the brain, parts of head and neck, lungs, mediastinum, bones and joints. In many organs, it helps in early diagnosis of lesions which require further evaluation to confirm or exclude malignancy. It is also used for surveillance in patients with hepatitis B cirrhosis, who have a high incidence of hepatomas; USG can be used at regular intervals to delineate a new lesion that may be a potential hepatoma.[8]

The role of USG in characterization of lesions is limited. Color Doppler, power Doppler, elastography, are techniques that help to improve the accuracy of characterization and differentiating benign from malignant lesions; however, most lesions detected on USG still have to be biopsied to obtain histologic diagnosis. USG is a good tool for guided biopsies and aspirations, especially in superficial organs like the thyroid and breast as well as deeper structures in the abdomen, pleura and pelvis.[9] USG guided ablation of thyroid, renal and liver cancers is performed at many centers in the world, using radiofrequency, microwave or laser ablation techniques.[10]

COMPUTED TOMOGRAPHY SCAN

Computed tomography scan is a powerful tool that addresses many issues in oncology. Currently, a typical scanner used is of 16-slice or higher and up to 320-slice scanner are available, which are predominantly used in cardiac imaging. Lung cancer screening is now gaining attention as a modality for use in high-risk individuals with history of smoking and alcohol intake. Characterization of lesions as with all modalities is often difficult and requires cytologic or histologic evidence; however, there are features including the shape of the lesion, the involvement of adjacent structures, the vascularity, etc. that help in therapeutic decisions. For example, in patients with cirrhosis, a typical pattern of vascularity is enough to call a lesion hepatoma, without a biopsy (Figs 2A and B).[11] Similarly in kidney tumors, the mere presence of a solid hypervascular lesion is sufficient to label it malignant.[12] CT perfusion has been used in some centers to help with further characterization of lesions using perfusion curves.[13] While it helps to a certain degree, it does not obviate the need for a biopsy; however, it can help in monitoring response to therapy based on angiogenesis.

The versatility of a CT scan allows its use for radiotherapy planning where a special table top needs to be used to avoid the curvature deformity that can occur with the standard table top. These images are fed into sophisticated computers that then help plan

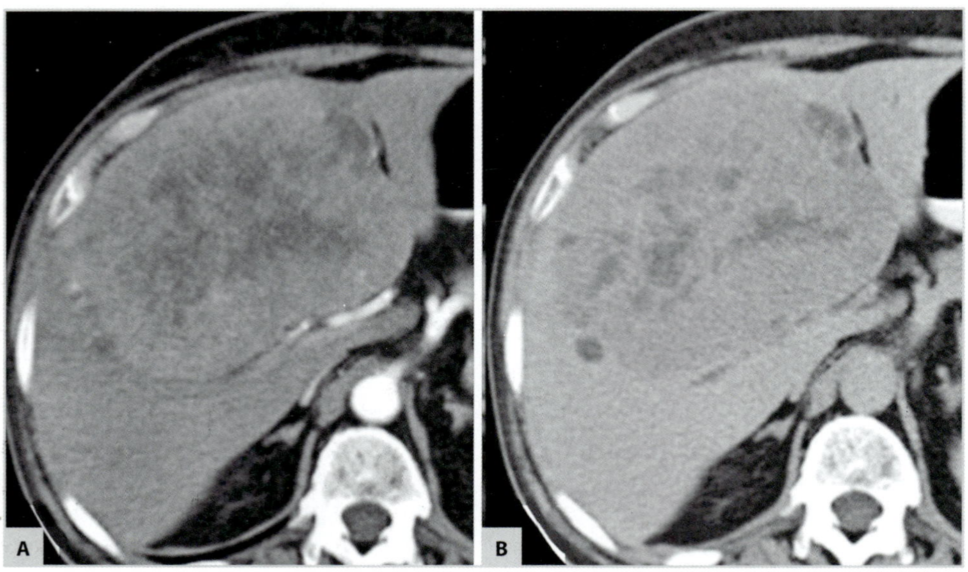

Figs 2A and B: Computed tomography (CT) scan images showing a typical hepatoma in the liver showing (A) Arterial phase and; (B) Rapid wash out

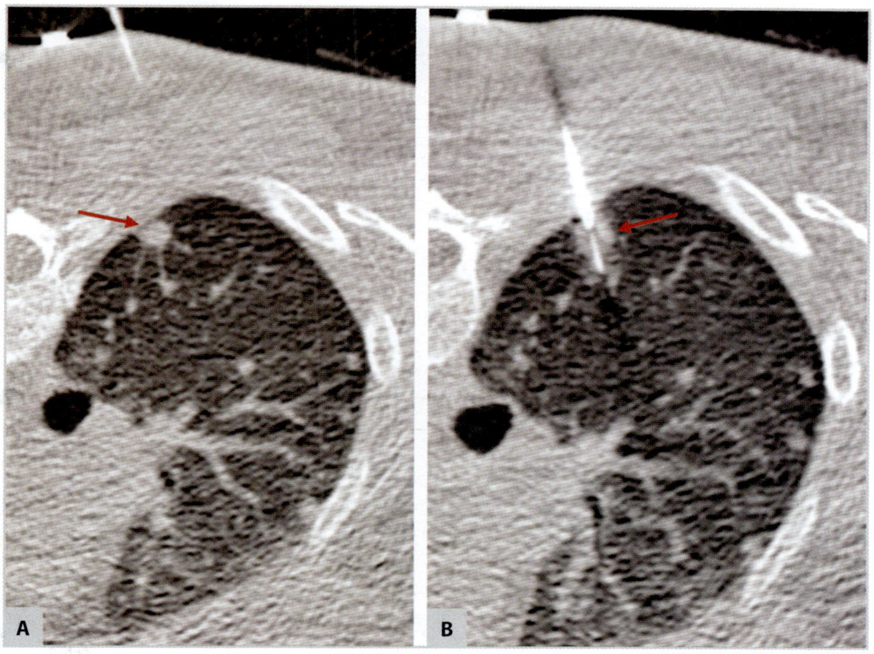

Figs 3A and B: Prone images show a nodule in the right lower lobe measuring 7.2 mm in diameter that was successfully biopsied with the help of CT fluoroscopy

accurate treatment especially with the newer image-guided radiation therapy (IGRT) and intensity-modulated radiation therapy (IMRT) scanners.[14] CT scan is also used for therapy monitoring and for detecting recurrence, especially in situations where PET/CT is not advisable or available. Special dental CT reconstruction programs allow detailed evaluation of the mandible or maxilla in buccal cancer and also help fashion templates if surgery is planned.[15] CT scan data can be used with 3D printers to create models that can help planning complex surgery especially in the head and neck and with bone and joint tumors.[16] CT scan-guided biopsies are now commonplace. The use of CT fluoroscopy further improves accuracy and it is possible to image lung nodules as small as 6.5 mm diameter using virtually real-time guidance (Figs 3A and B). Using various techniques like gantry tilt, contrast examination, etc. it is possible to improve accuracy of biopsy. The same techniques allow CT-guided ablation of lung, liver, renal and adrenal tumors using radiofrequency, microware and laser ablation techniques.

MAGNETIC RESONANCE IMAGING

Magnetic resonance imaging (MRI) is a standard modality for imaging various anatomic regions. In oncology, it is used for specific organ systems. From a screening perspective, MRI is used in the detection of breast cancer, in high-risk patients, especially those who are *BRCA1* and *BRCA2* positive.[17] In the prostate, in patients with high prostate-specific antigen (PSA) and a normal USG, MRI with spectroscopy can help pinpoint abnormal areas that can be targeted for biopsy.[18] Its main role, as with most other modalities, is in staging. It is invaluable for brain and spine tumors and a wide variety of techniques including spectroscopy and perfusion are used to characterize brain tumors.[19] Functional MRI (fMRI) is often used prior to surgery to map out vital areas that need to be spared during surgery (Figs 4A to D).[20] It is invaluable for characterizing head and neck,[21] liver,[22] pancreatic,[23] prostatic, rectal,[24] ovarian and uterine[25] lesions, where it is superior to CT scan for accurate preoperative staging. MRI is also used for mid- and post-therapy surveillance to look for recurrence or control of a given lesion.[26]

POSITRON EMISSION TOMOGRAPHY/ COMPUTED TOMOGRAPHY

This technique has revolutionized oncology management. It is a fusion of CT scanning and PET technology that allows us to fuse function and anatomy. Currently, fluorodeoxyglucose (FDG) is the most commonly available nuclear material, though there are many others including choline, etc. that are under development to target specific tumors.[27] In patients with metastases from an unknown primary, PET/CT is perhaps the best imaging

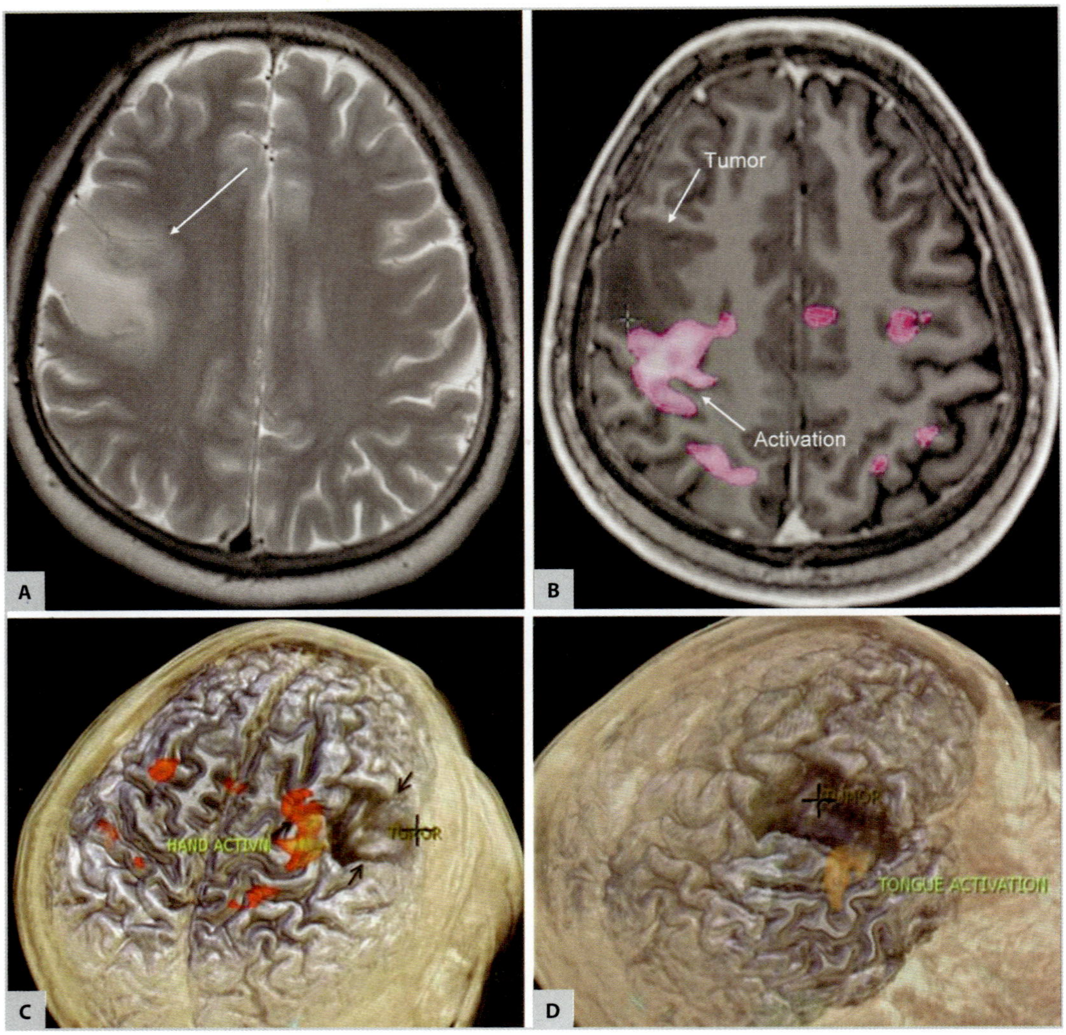

Figs 4A to D: Functional magnetic resonance imaging (fMRI). Tumor involving the precentral gyrus of the right frontal lobe. (A) Axial T2W MRI shows the tumor well (arrow), along the lateral cortex of the precentral gyrus of the right frontal lobe; (B) Axial fMRI image after finger tapping task shows robust activation along the right primary sensory motor cortex, posterior to the tumor with a distance of less than 1 cm from its posterior margin; (C) Three-dimensional fMRI image after finger tapping shows how the activation extends along the posteromedial margin of the tumor, (D) while the 3D fMRI image after tongue movement shows that the activation extends along the inferior aspect of the tumor and within the tumor boundary

tool currently to look for a primary, with a sensitivity rate of about 75% (Figs 5A and B).[28] In patients with unexplained weight loss or abnormal tumor markers, PET/CT could be diagnostic by localizing the primary site of disease. Its main role though is in staging, for lymphomas (Fig. 6),[29] breast,[30] lung,[31] colon[32] and many other cancers, PET/CT is used for staging prior to any definitive treatment. It is necessary to evaluate the CT scan images and to accurately use information from both modalities so as to reduce both the false-positive and the false-negative rates. PET/CT helps guide radiotherapy planning by defining accurately the active area that needs targeting.[33] PET/CT helps with therapeutic monitoring and surveillance for a large number of tumors;[34] commonly lymphoma, breast and colon. Recurrences in the post therapy follow-up by PET/CT at appropriate time can be suspected even in asymptomatic patients or with those with rising tumor markers, e.g. ovary. PET-/CT-guided biopsies are done either in the PET/CT gantry itself to target the most active part of the lesion,[35] or more commonly in a regular CT scanner, by targeting the most active area of the lesion as seen on the fused PET/CT images. This often improves the

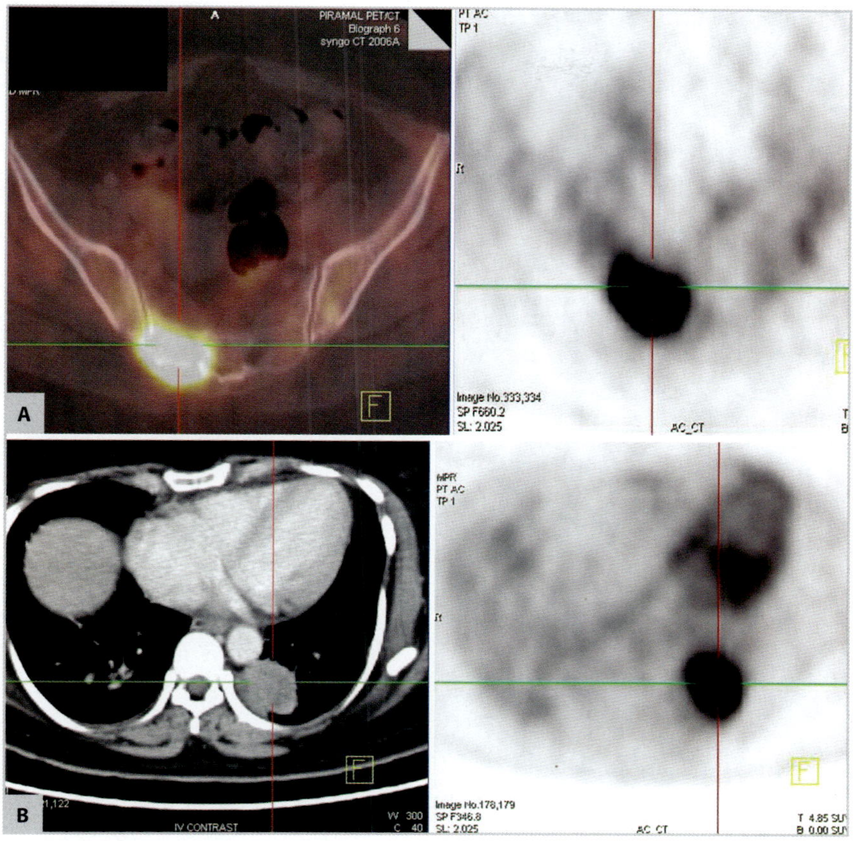

Figs 5A and B: (A) Positron emission tomography/Computed tomography (PET/CT). This patient presented with a lesion in the right pelvis that on biopsy showed adenocarcinoma metastases; (B) The PET/CT shows a lung primary

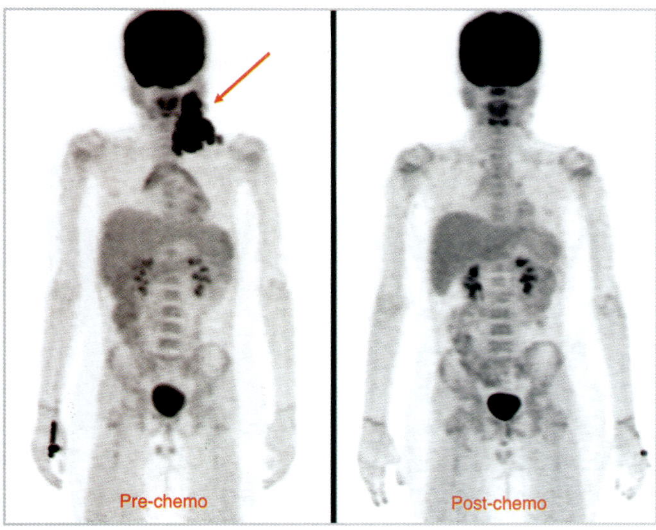

Fig. 6: Positron emission tomography/Computed tomography (PET/CT). This 15-year-old boy presented with Hodgkin's disease of the left lower neck (arrow in pre-chemo). Following chemotherapy, PET/CT shows complete metabolic response (post-chemo)

yield from a biopsy, especially if the first procedure has not yielded adequate material.

POSITRON EMISSION TOMOGRAPHY/ MAGNETIC RESONANCE IMAGING

Positron emission tomography/Magnetic resonance imaging is an upcoming tool that fuses images from PET and MRI to obtain images similar to PET/CT, but with the advantage of the superior soft tissue resolution of MRI and the reduced radiation exposure.[36] Currently, its role is predominant in the brain and breast and for disorders that predominantly affect the marrow.[37] Being expensive, there are few PET/MRIs available in the country and the world and the technology is still evolving and not routinely used. A major disadvantage is the inability to pick up small lung metastases that are inactive, especially since uptake in lung metastases is often size dependent, as nodules less than 10 mm often do not show any uptake even on a high-definition PET scanners.[38]

INTERVENTIONAL RADIOLOGY

Image-guided tumor ablation has already been discussed in the USG, CT scan and MRI sections; however, vascular interventional radiology also has a role to play in oncology. Trans-arterial chemoembolization (TACE) for liver tumors using different materials has now become a common modality for dealing with liver tumors (Figs 7A and B).[39] Embolization of large tumors in the kidney or pelvis or in bone and soft tissue malignancies are common immediately prior to surgery to curtail bone loss.[40] Diagnostic catheter angiography, however, has no role to play currently in oncology.

CONCLUSION

Imaging modalities are of vital importance in oncology. It helps in screening, staging, monitoring, guiding interventions and diagnosing recurrences. Appropriate use of imaging techniques and its correct interpretation is thus a most valuable guide in diagnosis and treatment planning in oncology. Any new technique can also be misused, overused or abused. Special care should therefore be taken to avoid unnecessary use of technology in medicine, simply because of its availability.

ACKNOWLEDGMENTS

I would like to acknowledge the names of Drs Ujwal Bhure, Karthik Ganesan, Aparna Ringe, Khushboo Pilania for help with the figures and references.

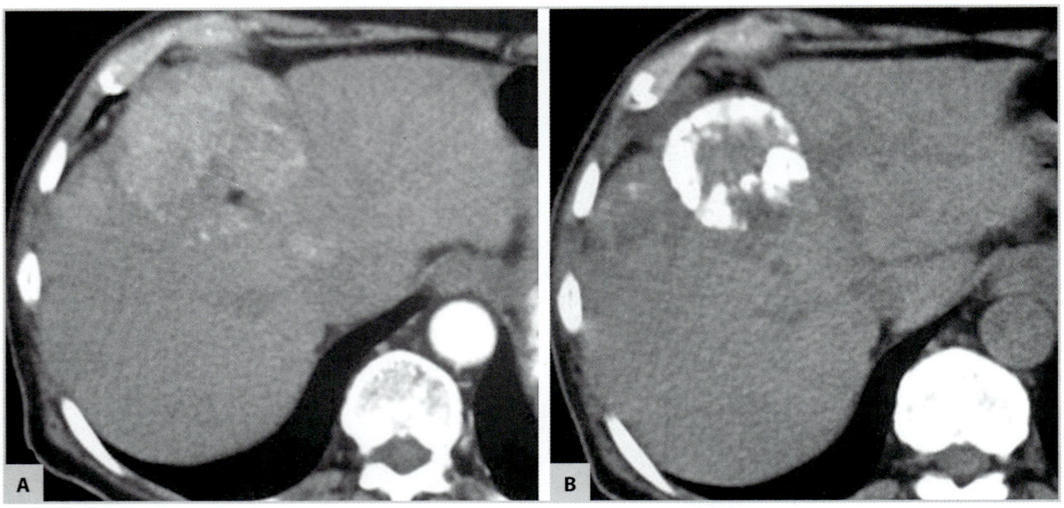

Figs 7A and B: Transarterial chemoembolization (TACE). (A) The arterial phase study shows a typical hypervascular hepatoma that was successfully embolized; (B) Lipiodol marks the tumor rendering it hyperdense on the plain scan performed 3 months after TACE

REFERENCES

1. Hogendoorn PC; ESMO/EUROBONET Working Group, Athanasou N, et al. Bone sarcomas: ESMO Clinical Practice Guidelines for diagnosis, treatment and follow-up. Ann Oncol. 2010;21(Suppl 5):v204-13.
2. Hansmann J, Grenacher L. Radiological imaging of the upper gastrointestinal tract. Part 1. The esophagus. Radiologe. 2006;46(12):1077-87.
3. Smetherman DH. Screening, imaging, and image-guided biopsy techniques for breast cancer. Surg Clin North Am. 2013;93(2):309-27.
4. Gøtzsche PC, Jørgensen KJ. Screening for breast cancer with mammography. Cochrane Database Syst Rev. 2013;6:CD001877.
5. Reynolds A. Stereotactic breast biopsy: a review. Radiol Technol. 2009;80(5):447M-64M.
6. Houssami N, Skaane P. Overview of the evidence on digital breast tomosynthesis in breast cancer detection. Breast. 2013;22(2):101-8.
7. Vinnicombe S, Pinto Pereira SM, McCormack VA, et al. Full-field digital versus screen-film mammography: comparison within the UK breast screening program and systematic review of published data. Radiology. 2009;251(2):347-58.
8. Memon WA, Haider Z, Beg MA, et al. Diagnosis of hepatoma using grayscale and Doppler ultrasound in patients with chronic liver disease. Int J Gen Med. 2011;4:751-4.

9. Phal PM, Brooks DM, Wolfe R. Sonographically guided biopsy of focal lesions. A comparison of freehand and probe-guided techniques using a phantom. AJR Am J Roentgenol. 2005;184(5):1652-6.
10. West JK, Khaja MS. Percutaneous and intraoperative tumor ablation. Ultrasound Clinics. 2012;7:377-97.
11. Parikh S, Hyman D. Hepatocellular cancer: a guide for the internist. Am J Med. 2007;120(3):194-202.
12. Frank I, Blute ML, Cheville JC, et al. Solid renal tumors: an analysis of pathological features related to tumor size. J Urol. 2003;170:2217-20.
13. Jiang T, Kambadakone A, Kulkarni NM, et al. Monitoring response to antiangiogenic treatment and predicting outcomes in advanced hepatocellular carcinoma using image biomarkers, CT perfusion, tumor density, and tumor size (RECIST). Invest Radiol. 2012;47(1):11-7.
14. Aird EG, Conway J. CT simulation for radiotherapy treatment planning. Br J Radiol. 2002;75(900):937-49.
15. Abrahams JJ. Dental CT imaging: a look at the jaw. Radiology Radiology. 2001;219(2):334-45.
16. Esses SJ, Berman P, Bloom AI, et al. Clinical applications of physical 3D models derived from MDCT data and created by rapid prototyping. AJR Am J Roentgenol. 2011;196(6):W683-8.
17. Drukteinis JS, Mooney BP, Flowers CI, et al. Beyond mammography: new frontiers in breast cancer screening. Am J Med. 2013;126(6):472-9.
18. Thompson J, Lawrentschuk N, Frydenberg M, et al. The role of magnetic resonance imaging in the diagnosis and management of prostate cancer.USANZ. BJU Int. 2013; 112(Suppl 2):6-20.
19. Mowatt G, Scotland G, Boachie C, et al. The diagnostic accuracy and cost-effectiveness of magnetic resonance spectroscopy and enhanced magnetic resonance imaging techniques in aiding the localisation of prostate abnormalities for biopsy: a systematic review and economic evaluation. Health Technol Assess. 2013;17(20):vii-xix, 1-281.
20. Petrella JR, Shah LM, Harris KM, et al. Preoperative functional MR imaging localization of language and motor areas: effect on therapeutic decision making in patients with potentially resectable brain tumors. Radiology. 2006;240(3):793-802.
21. Hagiwara M, Nusbaum A, Schmidt BL. MR assessment of oral cavity carcinomas. Magn Reson Imaging Clin N Am. 2012;20(3):473-94.
22. Fowler KJ Brown JJ, Narra VR. Magnetic resonance imaging of focal liver lesions: approach to imaging diagnosis. Hepatology. 2011;54(6):2227-37.
23. Schima W. MRI of the pancreas: tumours and tumour-simulating processes. Cancer Imaging. 2006;6:199-203.
24. Kaur H, Choi H, You YN et al. MR imaging for preoperative evaluation of primary rectal cancer: practical considerations. Radiographics. 2012;32(2):389-409.
25. Brandão AC, Silva AO. Diseases of the female pelvis: advances in imaging evaluation. Magn Reson Imaging Clin N Am. 2013;21(2):447-69.
26. Dias FL. Assessment of treatment response after chemoradiation of head and neck cancer. Curr Oncol Rep. 2013;15(2):119-27.
27. Hara T, Kosaka N, Kishi H. PET imaging of prostate cancer using carbon-11-choline. J Nucl Med. 1998;39(6):990-5.
28. Bohuslavizki KH, Klutmann S, Kroger S, et al. FDG PET detection of unknown primary tumors. J Nucl Med. 2000;41(5):816-22.
29. Allen-Auerbach M, de Vos S, Czernin J. PET/computed tomography and lymphoma. Radiol Clin North Am. 2013;51(5): 833-44.
30. Bernsdorf M, Berthelsen AK, Wielenga VT, et al. Preoperative PET/CT in early-stage breast cancer. Ann Oncol. 2012;23(9): 2277-82.
31. Truong MT, Viswanathan C, Erasmus JJ. Positron emission tomography/computed tomography in lung cancer staging, prognosis, and assessment of therapeutic response. J Thorac Imaging. 2011;26(2):132-46.
32. Cohade C, Osman M, Leal J, et al. Direct comparison of (18) F-FDG PET and PET/CT in patients with colorectal carcinoma. J Nucl Med. 2003;44(11):1797-803.
33. Messa V, Di Muzio N, Picchio M, et al. PET/CT and radiotherapy. Q J Nucl Med Mol Imaging. 2006;50(1):4-14.
34. Rohren EM, Turkington TG, Coleman RE. Clinical applications of PET in Oncology. Radiology. 2004;231(2):305-32
35. Tatli S, Gerbaudo VH, Feeley CM, et al. PET/CT-guided percutaneous biopsy of abdominal masses: initial experience. J Vasc Interv Radiol. 2011;22(4):507-14.
36. Schlemmer HP, Pichler BJ, Schmand M, et al. Simultaneous MR/PET imaging of the human brain: feasibility study. Radiology. 2008;248(3):1028-35.
37. Catana C, Drzezga A, Heiss WD, Rosen BR. PET/MRI for neurologic applications. J Nucl Med. 2012;53(12):1916-25.
38. Aquino SL, Kuester LB, Muse VV, et al. Accuracy of transmission CT and FDG-PET in the detection of small pulmonary nodules with integrated PET/CT. Eur J Nucl Med Mol Imaging. 2006;33(6): 692-6.
39. Vogl TJ, Zangos S, Balzer JO, et al. Transarterial chemoembolization (TACE) in hepatocellular carcinoma: technique, indication and results. Rofo. 2007;179(11):1113-26.
40. Ibrahim WH, Safran ZA, Hasan H, et al. Preoperative and therapeutic embolization of extremities of bone and soft tissue tumors. Angiology. 2013;64(2):151-6.

7 Role of Nuclear Medicine in Oncology

BA Krishna

INTRODUCTION

Nuclear medicine is a functional imaging technique wherein biochemical, physiological, antigenic, receptor and metabolic functions of biological cell can be imaged both in health and disease. In the evolution of disease process, the above constituents of the cell undergo change first eventually leading to structural change in the organ. Hence, nuclear techniques have the unique property of detecting disease in the early phase even before computed tomography (CT), magnetic resonance imaging (MRI) or ultrasonography (USG). This property makes nuclear techniques ideally suited to oncology where detection of disease in the earlier stage would give a chance for curative treatment. However, nuclear scan lacked anatomical details and hence clinical application was difficult. In 2002, there were two major breakthroughs in the technology. Firstly, the nuclear scanner technology was transformed to produce tomographic functional images [single photon emission computer tomography (SPECT)] like tomographic CT images. Secondly, the scientists at Pittsburgh decided to incorporate CT tube on the nuclear scanners. This resulted in production of simultaneous anatomical images, and the computer was used to fuse the anatomical and functional image slices—referred to as SPECT-CT and Positron emission tomography-computed tomography (PET-CT) images as shown in Figure 1. The innovative technological advances gave birth to "fusion imaging" which has revolutionized the role of nuclear imaging in oncology. The PET-CT imaging has enabled the oncologists to diagnose at molecular level which is the initial stage of cancer and has thus impacted the understanding of cancer significantly.

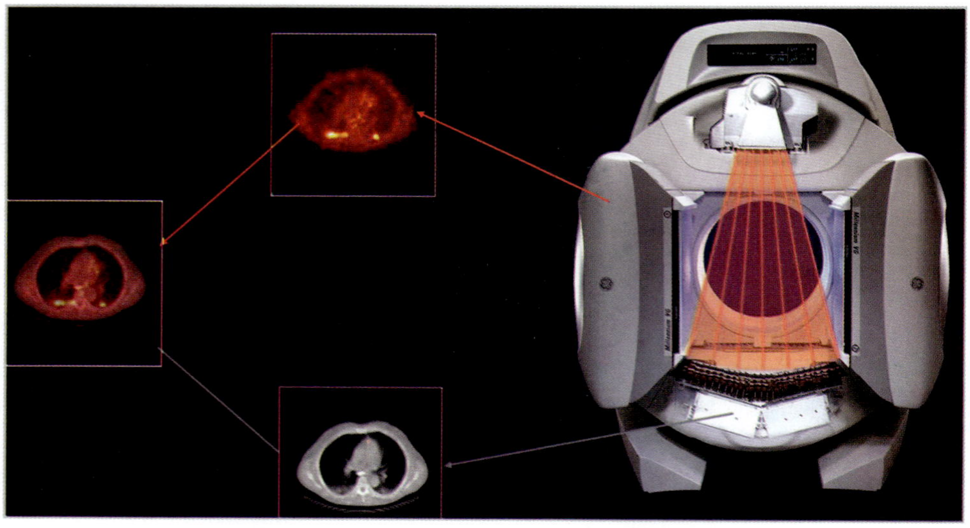

Fig. 1: Fusion imaging technique on gamma and positron emission tomography (PET) scanners

PRINCIPLE OF NUCLEAR IMAGING

The nuclear imaging technique consists of three main components:

1. Radioisotope
2. Pharmaceutical
3. Detecting equipment—gamma camera and PET scanner.

Radioisotope

This is an unstable element [Iodine-131 (^{131}I), ^{99m}Tc] wherein the atom is either deficient or in excess of one of its constituents like electron or proton. The unstable atom reaches its stable form by releasing the excess energy in the form of radiations which are of three types: (1) alpha; (2) beta; and (3) gamma-rays. The gamma rays are used for nuclear imaging while alpha-rays and beta-rays are used for nuclear therapy.

Pharmaceutical

This is a chemical substance which is used to tag to the radioisotope. The choice of the chemical depends upon the organ being imaged, e.g. phosphorus for bone imaging and albumin for liver imaging. When the chemical is labeled to an isotope, it is called radiopharmaceutical. The chemical component leads the isotope to the desired organ and then the gamma radiation from that organ is used for obtaining an image. Hence, the radiopharmaceutical forms the main core of a nuclear scan. The knowledge of biochemistry of each organ in health and disease is useful in developing new tracers for imaging. There is variety of radiopharmaceuticals specific to different tumors which localize in tumors through multiple pathways.

Gamma Camera

This is the main detecting equipment in nuclear imaging which was invented by Anger in 1981. It consists of one or two detectors which receive the gamma-rays emanating from patient's organ and convert it into electronic signals which are then captured on an X-ray plate or color paper in a printer. These signals are called as scintillations which together produce an image which is called nuclear scan. The nuclear images can now be obtained in tomographic slices and these images are called SPECT images which is analogous to CT slices. The SPECT nuclear scans have better resolution and are particularly useful in oncology. The newer gamma cameras have CT tube incorporated in them and two-, four- and six-slice CT images are simultaneously obtained with the nuclear image and these images are called SPECT-CT or FUSION images. The fusion imaging technology came into clinical applications in 2002 and was invented by David Townsend from Pittsburgh. These images are of particular importance to surgeons since they enable anatomic localization of disease focus seen in nuclear scan and thereby appropriate further procedures can be performed accurately.

Positron Emission Tomography-Computed Tomography Scanners

This is a new modality of nuclear imaging (PET) wherein the isotope used for imaging is called "positrons" which emit two gamma radiations simultaneously at 180 degrees apart, and thus help in producing high resolution images of entire body. This new technology has given birth to "molecular imaging" in which biological molecules like glucose, amino acids, fatty acids, are labeled with isotopes like fluorine-18 (18F), carbon-11 (11C), Nitrogen-13 (13N) and Oxygen-15 (15O). These tracers help in understanding tumor metabolism and biological behavior and more importantly in assessing treatment response. This technology has made immense impact in oncology in staging and response assessment in cancer.

DIAGNOSTIC ROLE

The constituents of a biological cell are nucleus comprising of deoxyribonucleic acid (DNA), cytoplasm containing variety of chemical molecules and cell wall comprising of proteins, receptors and antigens. The isotopes target all these different constituents of cell and we can obtain images of each separately. This unique property of isotopes makes it possible to image cancer cell at different cellular level which helps in early detection and staging of disease, predict the biological behavior and determine the optimum therapeutic approach. Based on this concept, there are various types of nuclear scans in oncology.

TYPES OF NUCLEAR SCANS IN ONCOLOGY

Metabolic Scan

In this scan, the isotope localizes in the organ of interest based on the metabolic pathway. The classical example is radioiodine (^{131}I) which is used to scan thyroid gland and the isotope localization occurs through the iodine metabolism pathway.

Receptor Scan

There is variety of receptors expressed by different tumors like somatostatin and catecholamine receptors in neuroendocrine tumors, estrogen receptors by breast cancer, epidermal growth factor receptor (EGFR) in lung cancer. Each of these receptors can be labeled with isotopes (111-indium-octreotide for somatostatin receptors, ^{131}I-metaiodobenzylguanidine (^{131}I-MIBG) for catecholamine receptors and 18F-estrdiol for estrogen receptors). When they are administered intravenously, the respective tumors can be imaged. They will be useful in primary lesion detection, staging and instituting receptor modulated therapies.

Antibody Scan

The tumors express variety of antigens which could be on the cell surface or intracellular [carcinoembryonic antigen (CEA) in colon cancer, cancer antigen-125 (CA-125) in ovarian cancer, prostate-specific antigen (PSA) in prostate cancer]. It is possible to produce monoclonal antibodies to these antigens. These monoclonal antibodies are labeled with isotopes, e.g. ^{131}I anti-CEA antibody, lutetium-177 (^{117}Lu) anti-PSA antibody. When administered intravenously, these tracers bind to tumor antigen and the disease sites images are obtained. This technique is also called as "radioimmunoscintigraphy". This technique is expanding rapidly.

Molecular Scan

Tumors use different types of energy substrates for their growth and to perform different functions. Lymphomas, lung cancer and breast cancers use glucose, prostate cancer uses fatty acids. Based on this concept, there is a new approach to imaging cancer wherein the biological cell molecules like glucose, amino acids, and fatty acids are labeled with isotopes like positrons (18F-flurodeoxyglucose, 11C-methionine and 11C-acetate). These tracers localize in the tumors based upon their metabolic ingredient and whole body image is obtained in 10 minutes. These scans provide information like tumor proliferation rate, tumor necrosis and response to treatment. This approach to tumor imaging is called as PET scan.

Nonspecific Scans

There is variety of nonspecific scans which are used in oncology in selective conditions. They could be for staging (bone scans in prostate and breast cancer), assessing drug toxicity [cardiac multigated acquisition (MUGA) scan, renal glomerular filtration rate (GFR)].

CLINICAL APPLICATIONS

Endocrine and Neuroendocrine Tumors

Thyroid

The first application of isotope imaging in oncology was in 1937 when radioiodine (^{131}I) was used for imaging thyroid cancer. The radioiodine scan shows a "cold" area corresponding to the solitary nodule and this raises suspicion of cancer. The incidence of malignancy in the cold nodule is 25–30%. The other isotopes used for thyroid scan are $^{99m}TcO_4$ (technetium), Iodine-123 (^{123}I) and Iodine-124 (^{124}I). The $^{99m}TcO_4$ and ^{123}I are ideal isotopes because they give low radiation dose and particularly suitable for pediatric patients compared to ^{131}I which gives comparatively higher radiation dose.

The radioiodine scan plays a major postoperative diagnostic and therapeutic role in papillary, follicular and Hürthle cell carcinomas. The differentiated thyroid cancer cells retain the property of trapping radioiodine and this forms the basis of radioiodine role in the post-surgery management. The scan is referred to as "whole-body ^{131}I scan" or "^{131}I dosimetry scan" and has following prerequisites:

- Completion of total thyroidectomy
- Confirmed histology of differentiated thyroid cancer
- Off-thyroxine and iodine containing drugs for 3–4 weeks
- Thyroid-stimulating hormone (TSH) value of 35–40 microunits/mL
- Pregnancy to be ruled out.

The aim of the scan is to detect postoperative residual tissue in neck and functioning metastases.

Patient is administered 5 mCi of radioiodine orally and neck and whole body scans are performed after 48 hours. The neck scan shows amount of residual tissue (Fig. 2) and the whole body scan shows distant metastatic sites. The scan will also help in dosimetry calculations and quantify the dose of radioiodine for therapy.

Neuroendocrine Tumors

These are special types of tumors originating from neural crest and endocrine glands of the foregut, midgut and hindgut. They are characterized by indolent growth and expression of somatostatin (Table 1) and catecholamine receptors (Fig. 3). Majority of these tumors present as metastatic disease in liver and the primary lesion remains undetected in 20% of patients. The conventional diagnostic procedures like endoscopy and CT scans fail to

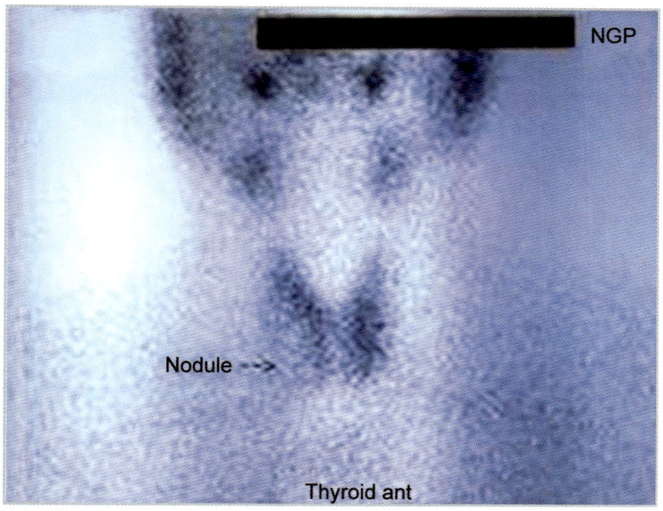

Fig. 2: Radioiodine scan of thyroid, shows a cold area

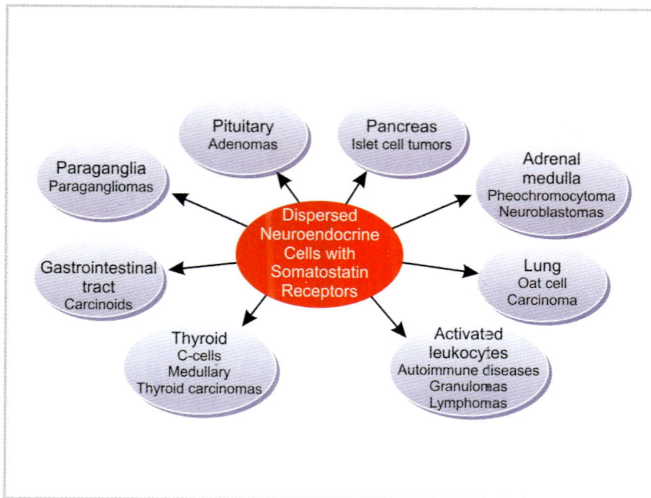

Fig. 3: The APUD/neuroendocrine cell concept

TABLE 1: Incidence of somatostatin receptors in neuroendocrine tumors

Tumor type	*In vivo* scintigraphy*	*In vitro* autoradiography*
Gastrinoma	100% (12/12)	100% (6/6)
Insulinoma	61% (14/23)	72% (8/11)
Carcinoid	96% (69/72)	88% (54/62)
Small cell lung cancer	100% (34/34)	57% (4/7)
Paraganglioma	100% (33/33)	92% (11/12)
Glucagonoma	100% (3/3)	100% (2/2)
Neuroblastoma	89% (8/9)	65% (15/23)
Pheochromocytoma	86% (12/14)	73% (38/52)
Pituitary tumors	75% (21/28)	84% (57/68)
Medullary thyroid carcinoma	71% (20/28)	38% (10/26)
Unclassified apudoma	89% (16/18)	100% (4/4)

*In vivo and in vitro data are from different patient groups

demonstrate primary lesion. In this context radiolabeled-receptor scan is a new imaging approach and two types of receptor scans—somatostatin receptor scan and catecholamine receptor scan are in use in India and worldwide.

Somatostatin receptors are of five types (1–5) and different tumors express different types and degree of expression also varies with tumors. There are many synthetic analogues of somatostatin. These analogues are labeled with different isotopes and variety of tracers is available.

Indium-111 (^{111}In)-octreotide scan[1] was the first receptor scan in neuroendocrine tumors. We established in India for the first time in 1996. After intravenous administration of tracer, whole body images are obtained at 4, 24 and 36 hours. The tracer is taken up by the type II receptors in the active disease sites. The images are obtained in tomographic mode fused with 4-slice CT images (SPECT-CT) on a gamma camera. This tracer has been used for staging and to assess the receptor density in the lesions which would help in therapeutic decision. The disadvantage of the scan is prolonged scanning time and small lesions (< 8 mm) could not be detected. In India, we successfully introduced new scanning agent—(lutetium-177) DOTATATE scan in collaboration with Bhabha Atomic Research Center (BARC) and currently is used in many centers in India to calculate therapeutic dose (Fig. 4).

Gallium 68 (68Ga)-DOTATATE is a PET-CT scan (Fig. 5) technique which uses DOTATATE as the somatostatin analogue seeking type II and V receptors. The image resolution is of 4 mm size and very ideal to pick up small

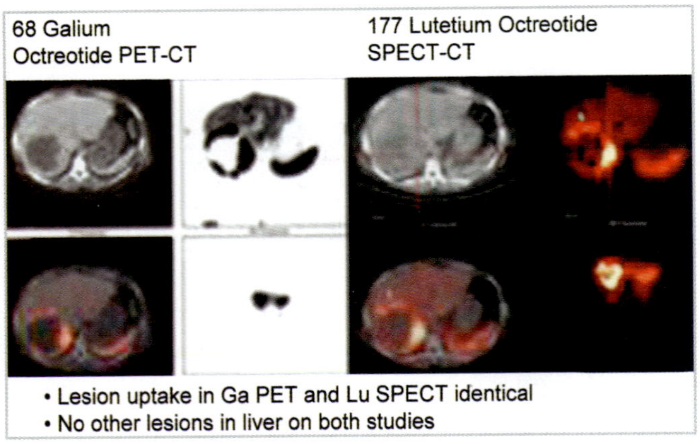

Fig. 4: Comparison of Ga-positron emission tomography (PET) scan and Lu-DOTATATE scan developed at Bhabha Atomic Research Center (BARC), India. Both show same lesions

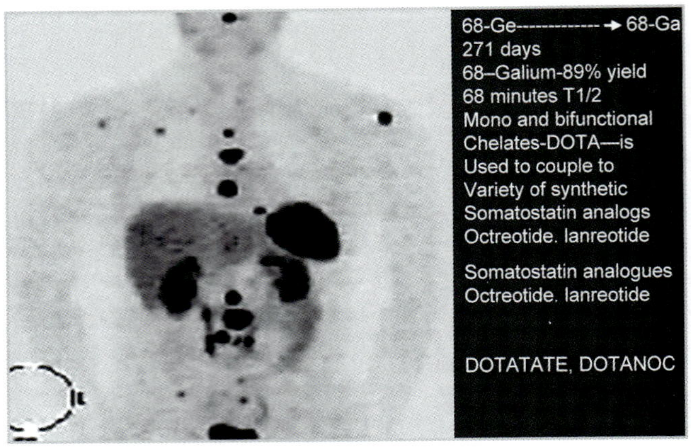

Fig. 5: 68Ga-DOTATATE-PET scan is a high resolution image

undetected primaries. Since high quality CT images are fused with the PET images, the detection sensitivity is almost 90%.[2] The entire scanning procedure is completed in 2 hours and hence it is very patient friendly and rapid diagnosis is achieved.

Catecholamine receptor scanning is used in pheochromocytoma, paragangliomas, neuroblastomas and bronchial carcinoids. These tumors are rich in catecholamine receptors. The tracer ^{131}I-MIBG is a catecholamine receptor seeking tracer. When administered intravenously, they accumulate in myocardium, spleen and liver which have abundant catecholamine receptors. Similarly, the tumors which express these receptors accumulate the tracer and specific diagnosis and staging of disease can be achieved (Fig. 6). The images are taken at 24, 48 and 72 hours after administration of tracer. These scans need 1 week preparation like avoidance of tea, coffee, beta blockers and banana. This scan has sensitivity of 80% and specificity of 95%.[3] In neuroblastoma patients, the scan helps in restaging of disease and also helps in assessing bone marrow involvement.

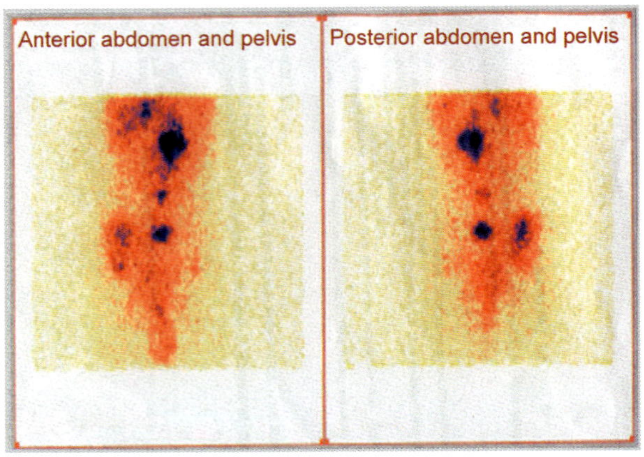

Fig. 6: Metaiodobenzylguanidine (MIBG) scan shows intense catecholamine receptor activity in primary abdominal tumor and nodal metastases

BREAST CANCER

The isotopes plays major role in the diagnosis and management of breast cancer. The various nuclear techniques currently under use are as follows.

- Scintimammography
- Sentinel node mapping
- Bone scans
- Fluorodeoxyglucose-positron emission tomography (FDG-PET) scan
- 18F-fluoroestradiol receptor scan (FES scan)
- Positron emission mammography (PEM)

Scintimammography

This is analogous to mammography and is used in the detection of primary breast lesion in selective situations like inconclusive mammography, dense breasts, recurrence over implants or operated scars.[4] The technique involves intravenous administration of 99mTc-sestamibi isotope and obtain breast images on gamma camera using breast specific table tops. The isotope accumulates in the mitochondria of the cell and lesions up to 8 mm can be detected. In the dense breasts, the focal area can be demonstrated with 85% accuracy. The negative predictive value is almost 100%. We established in India in 2004, and many cancer centers perform it in selected cases.

Sentinel Node Mapping

This technique has gained wide acceptance in the last few years and is performed in stage I and stage IA. The main aim of the test is to decide about axillary node dissection which produces significant morbidity in 40% of patients. The technique helps in identifying the sentinel node for biopsy purpose. The concept is that the sentinel node is the first node to get metastases and hence if sentinel node biopsy is negative then axillary clearance can be avoided. The technique involves administration of isotope 99mTc-albumin colloid in the peritumoral or intratumoral region, and obtains multiple anterior planar and SPECT-CT chest images at different times upto 2 hours. In majority of the patients the node is seen by 30 minutes to 1 hour. In 10–20% of patients, the node may be visualized by 24 hours. The node is marked on the skin and in the operating room the node is excised through a niche after removing primary tumor. If the node is negative then axillary clearance is avoided. This technique has sensitivity of 88% and together with blue dye technique the sensitivity is 95%.[5] We established technique in India in 2007 and currently its use is extended to oral cancers, penile and cancer of cervix.

Bone Scans

There are two types of bone scans. The 99mTc-methylene diphosphonate (MDP) gamma bone scan and 18F bone PET scan. Bone scan was the first staging procedure in breast cancer introduced by Galasko et al. in 1975. The metastatic lesions show high uptake and appear as multiple "hotspots". The bone scan sensitivity is 96%. However, specificity is low (60%) since benign lesions also show high uptake. Hence, radiological correlation with CT scan or MRI is essential to increase the specificity. However in 2002 the fusion imaging technique (SPECT-CT) enhanced the specificity of bone scans by correlating bone scan abnormality to bone changes seen on fused CT scans. The 18F bone PET-CT scan was introduced in 2011 and has a higher sensitivity than MDP gamma bone scan. It shows 30% more lesions missed on MDP bone scan. Moreover, the 18F bone scan has high quality diagnostic CT scans fused with it making it easy to differentiate benign from malignant changes.

18F-Fluorodeoxyglucose Positron Emission Tomography Scan

This is a metabolic scan wherein glucose labeled to isotope 18F is used to obtain whole body images. The concept is that the cancer cells use glucose four to six times more than the normal cell. When radiolabeled glucose is administered intravenously, it is taken up by the cancer cells and then undergoes phosphorylation through hexokinase pathway to 18F-glucose phosphate and does not further undergo glycolysis and remains trapped in the cell and appear as bright areas (hotspot) on the scan (Fig. 7). Lesions as small as 3–4 mm can be detected. The drawback of the CT scan is that lymph nodes upto 1 cm size are considered as normal. This assumption results in false negatives up to 20–30% whereas glucose PET scan characterizes even 4 mm node as disease based on the degree of glucose uptake. The glucose uptake is quantified using a software and expressed as standard uptake value (SUV). The degree of uptake in tumor is directly proportional to tumor proliferation rate. Thus PET scan detects disease much earlier than CT scans. The PET scan

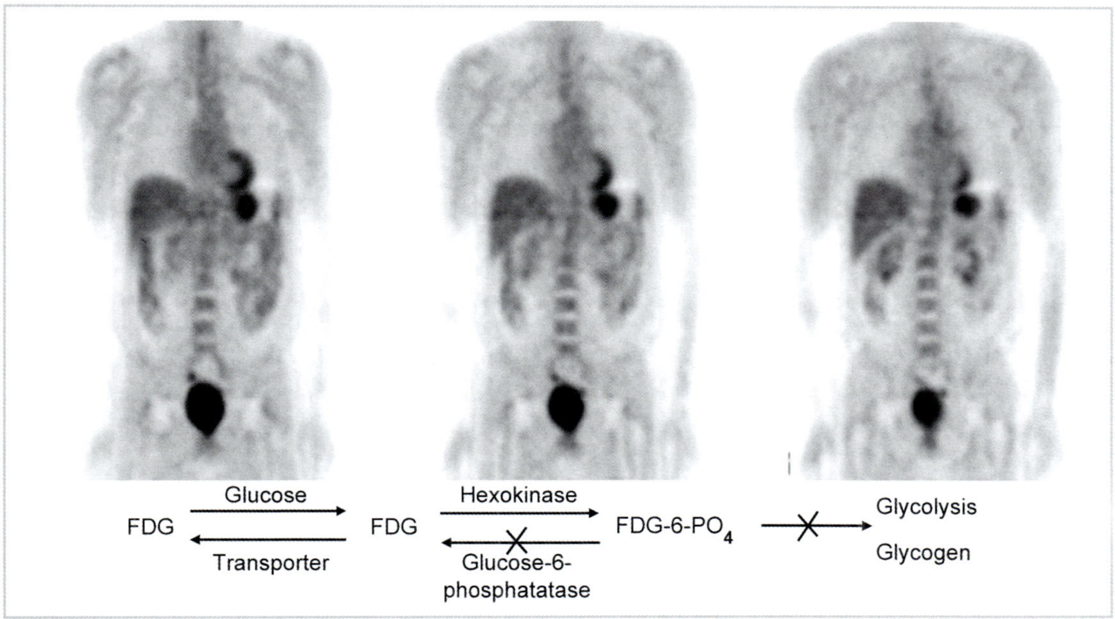

Fig. 7: Concept of fluorodeoxyglucose-positron emission tomography (FDG-PET) scan

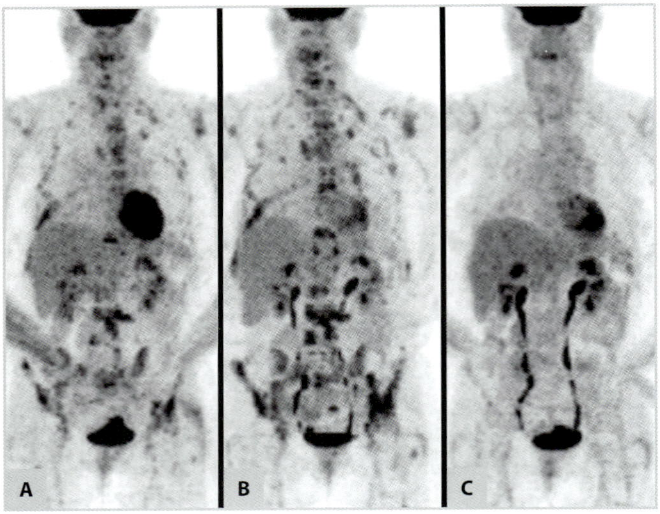

Figs 8A to C: Absence of uptake in the lesions in last scan suggests complete metabolic response

is combined with whole-body contrast CT scan and thus anatomical status of liver, lungs, nodes, skeletal system and brain is simultaneously obtained leading to accurate staging.

In breast cancer, the FDG-PET scan is indicated in stage III and IV for staging and treatment response assessment and for restaging in locally advanced breast cancer (LABC) and in recurrences.[6] The FDG-PET scan upstages the disease in 26–30% of patients and thus impacts in treatment decisions (Figs 8A to C). In treatment response scenario, the follow-up scan is performed 3 months after hormone therapy or after three courses of chemotherapy. The reduction in uptake by 25% is considered as response and the therapy is continued. In nonresponders, the uptake does not change and alternative therapy will be instituted. In patients who are on hormone therapy, the 6 weeks scan shows increase in uptake which is also considered as responder. The FDG uptake in primary breast mass has prognostic impact. If the uptake ratio (SUV) is more than 7.0, then prognosis is poor irrespective of the treatment.

Fluorine-18 Estradiol Receptor Scan (FES)

The estrogen and progesterone receptors have significant bearing on survival of patients with poor prognosis in receptor-negative patients. Till now, the receptor status could be known only after biopsy. However, the FES scan demonstrates estrogen receptors in the primary tumor and metastatic lesions simultaneously which helps in treatment decisions like hormone therapy alone or in combination with chemotherapy. It is also possible to quantify the receptor density pre- and post-hormone therapy.[7] It is an established fact that 30% of metastatic lesions are receptor-negative even though primary lesion is receptor-positive. This has therapeutic implication and FES scan helps in segregating this group of patients. The presence of uptake on FES scan suggests that receptors are active and likely to respond to hormone therapy.

Positron Emission Mammography

The detection of primary breast lesion continues to pose problem. The mammography is not sensitive in dense breast tissue or implant situation. The MRI is a promising technique with better sensitivity and resolution. The positron emission mammography (PEM) is a new technique which uses FDG isotope with dedicated breast collimator and is capable of detecting 1–2 mm lesions with 98% sensitivity. Additionally, the axillary and internal mammary nodes can also be detected in the same image setting. If the primary is detected then simultaneously whole-body staging PET-CT images are obtained providing a comprehensive disease staging.[8] This technique is gaining wide acceptance in major centers of the world and current data is on indeterminate mammography patients. It is being projected as cost-effective compared to MRI since whole-body staging can also be performed in the same setting.

LUNG CANCER

The lung cancer is the most common cancer in men. In non-small cell lung cancer (NSCLC), surgery offers the best chance for cure in the early stages. Hence, accurate staging is very critical in therapeutic decision. Both CT and FDG-PET play important role in diagnosis and staging.[9]

Solitary Pulmonary Nodule

Though CT provides excellent morphological details, it has limitations in differentiating benign from malignant in the primary lesion. In the western literature, FDG-PET is highly accurate (95%) specificity in differentiating benign from malignant.[10] However, the Indian data is not consistent with published data since Koch's lesion also demonstrates varying pattern of high uptake almost similar to malignant lesion (Fig. 9). Hence in our patients, biopsy confirmation followed by staging PET scan will be ideal approach. However, negative predictive value (NPV) is 100% when the lesion shows no FDG uptake. The glucose uptake ratio (SUV) of the primary tumor has been shown to be associated with prognostic significance. If SUV of primary lesion

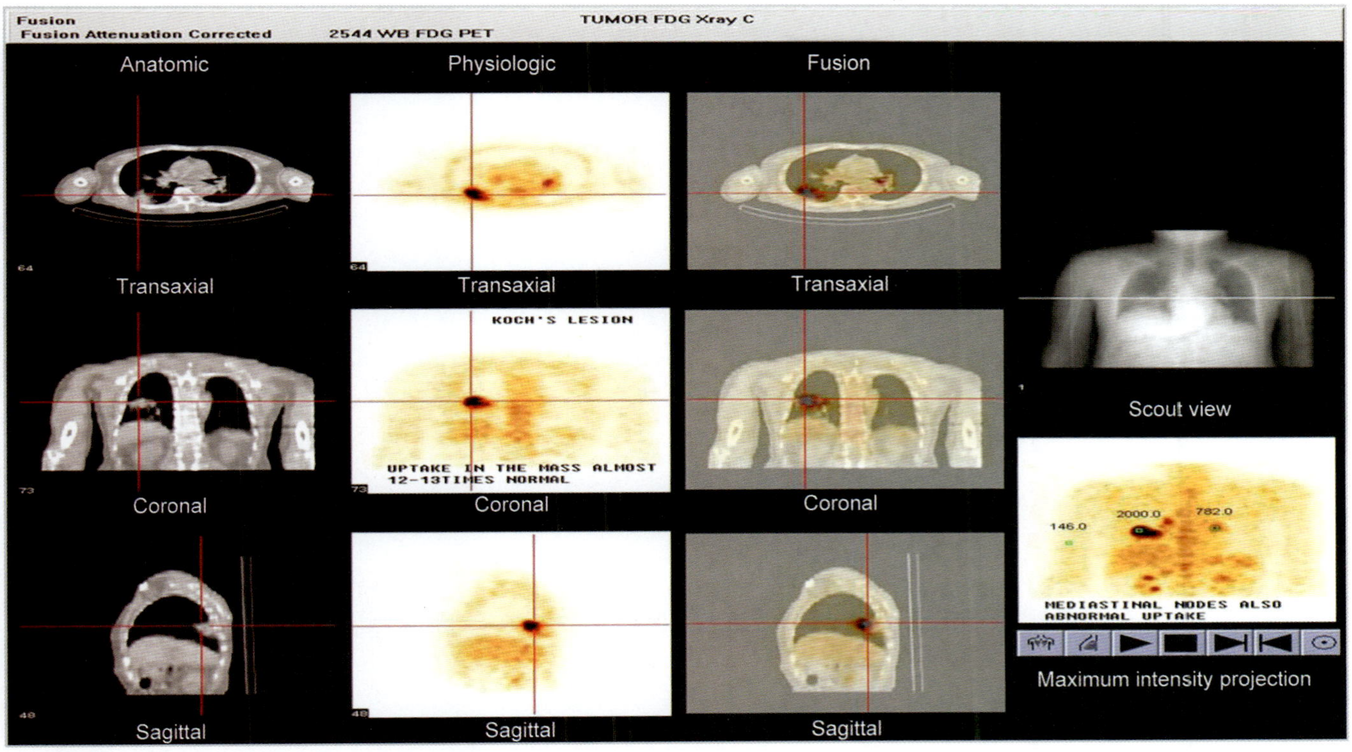

Fig. 9: Koch's lesion also shows high uptake as malignancy

is more than 10.0, then mortality rate is 60% in 6 months irrespective of the stage and treatment. In our study of 75 patients over 2 years, we reproduced this data confirming that glucose uptake ratio of primary tumor is an independent prognostic marker. The PET scan also enhances biopsy yield by accurately pinpointing the most active tumor site in the mass (Fig. 10). In our experience this incidence is around 10%. The integrated PET-CT is useful tool for detection of tumor invasion into chest wall. This is of importance when en bloc resection of primary and contiguous chest wall is under consideration especially in patients with poor cardiopulmonary reserve. Similarly, integrated PET-CT provides accurate information about mediastinal infiltration. The CT has low sensitivity, specificity, accuracy (68%, 72% and 70% respectively). The FDG-PET is also very useful in differentiation between tumoral and peritumoral atelectasis. This is particularly important for the planning of radiotherapy and this information results in change in radiation field in 30–40% of patients.

Nodal Staging and Fluorodeoxyglucose-Positron Emission Tomography

Computed tomography and MRI have substantial limitations in depicting mediastinal nodal metastases. The criteria is purely based on size and shape of nodes and does not take into account that normal sized node may also have metastases. CT sensitivity is 60–70% (Fig. 10) mediastinal nodal disease for while that of PET is 90–95% for mediastinal nodal involvement. FDG-PET also aids mediastinoscopy in detecting additional 6–10% lesions and avoiding mediastinoscopy in 12% of patients where PET is negative. PET limitations include specificity of 73–89% and reduced sensitivity in hilar and subaortic nodes.[11] The American Thoracic Society recommends that all PET-positive nodes need biopsy confirmation.

M Staging

The most common sites of distant metastases from lung cancer are adrenal, liver, bone and brain.

Whole-body FDG-PET is an excellent method to screen for extrathoracic metastases.[12] In a meta-analysis of 581 patients, sensitivity, specificity and accuracy of FDG-PET were 94%, 97%, and 96% respectively. PET detects unsuspected extrathoracic metastases in 10–20% of patients (Fig. 11) and changes therapeutic managements in 20% of patients. FDG-PET is superior (98%) to CT for adrenal metastases (80%) and to bone scan for bone metastases (87%). PET is also superior to CT in liver metastases.

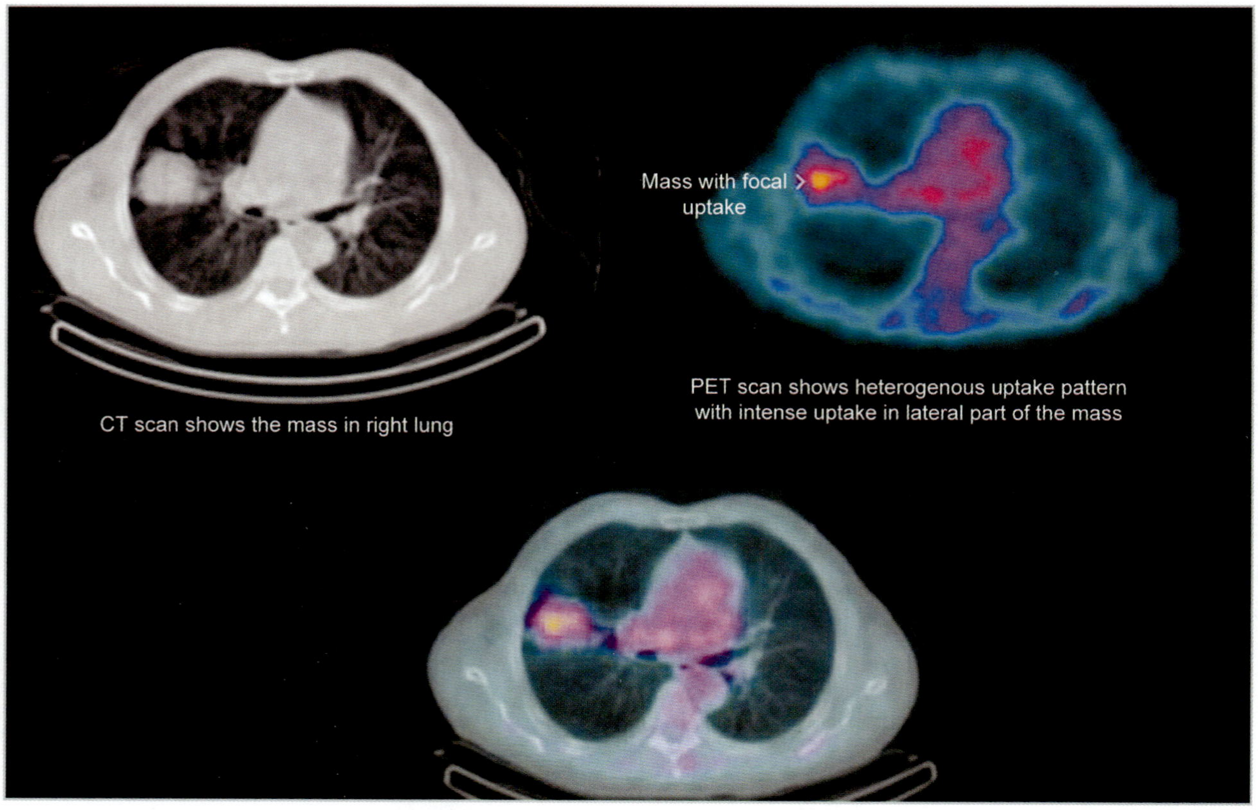

Fig. 10: Computed tomography (CT) based biopsy was negative and positron emission tomography (PET) showed most active site and repeat biopsy was positive

False-negative and False-positive PET in Lung Cancer

False-negative PET results have been reported in pulmonary carcinoids, bronchiole alveolar cell cancers, metastatic nodes lesser than 4 mm in size. False-positive results are due to nonspecificity of FDG. Hence inflammation, tuberculosis, histoplasmosis, aspergillosis and eosinophilic lung disease are the causes of false-positives.

GASTROINTESTINAL CANCERS

Esophageal and Gastric Cancer

The role of FDG-PET in gastrointestinal (GI) cancers is still a matter of debate. The CT and endoscopy form the main investigative approach with high yields and there is no systematic prospective study comparing these modalities with FDG-PET. Currently, the role of PET is limited to response assessment and restaging in recurrences. A significant body of evidence now suggests that FDG-PET has a role to play in response assessment of upper GI malignancies. Weber et al. showed that reduction in metabolic activity after 2 weeks of therapy was associated with subsequent decrease of tumor size, an increased rate of curative resections and histopathological regression. There was also significant correlation between reduction of metabolic activity and patient survival.

Colon and Rectum

There is no conclusive evidence so far for FDG-PET in primary colorectal cancer detection and staging. Recently, the published data suggests that FDG-PET may be used in locally invasive colorectal cancer since 20–30% of these lesions will have metastases at presentation. In the recurrent and metastatic setting, the standard post-treatment surveillance with CEA and CT are not sufficiently sensitive. CEA is 59% sensitive and 84% specific, and CT scan is sensitive for intra-abdominal and pelvic lesions and cannot differentiate benign fibrosis from malignant recurrences. The PET has 95% sensitivity compared to 65% with CT.[13] The clinical context of elevated CEA and normal CT is the most appropriate application of FDG-PET which reveals recurrence site in 90% of patients.[14]

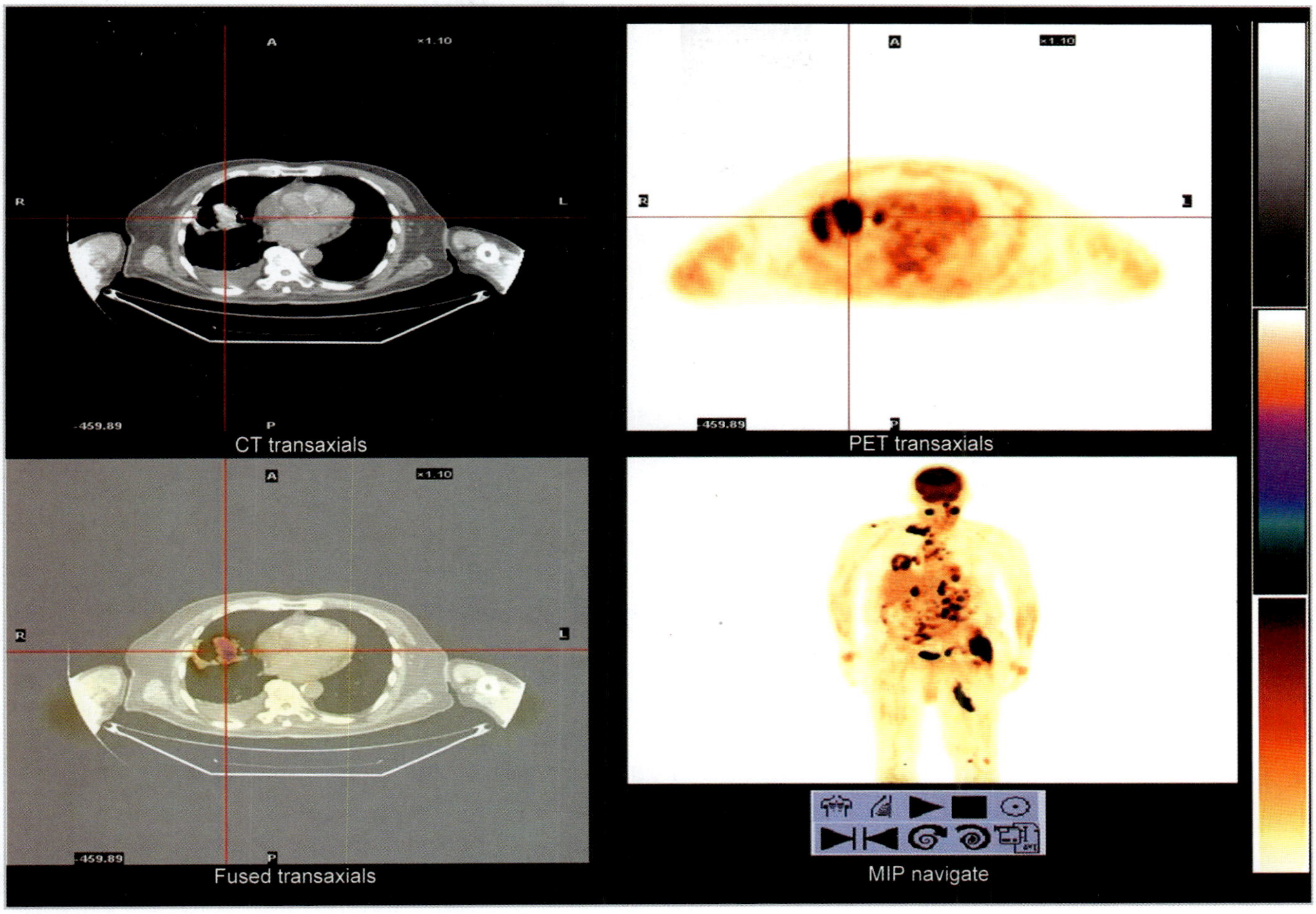

Fig. 11: Extrathoracic metastases on positron emission tomography (PET)

In our study of 60 patients with normal CT and elevated CEA values, FDG-PET detected recurrences in 80% of patients and changed the management strategy in 37% of patients. In patients with resectable liver metastases on CT, the FDG-PET plays a critical role of proper selection of patients by demonstrating additional hepatic lesions and extrahepatic metastases leading to exclusion from surgery. The CT sensitivity and specificity for liver metastases is 74% and 85% and for PET is 95% and 100%.[15] In response assessment after chemotherapy, surgical resection or radiofrequency ablation (RFA) of liver lesions, FDG-PET plays an important role by differentiating responders[16] from non-responders (sensitivity—100%, specificity—90%) and thereby alter the treatment approaches. In radiotherapy to pelvic recurrences, FDG-PET helps in detecting completeness of response and in future will be used to delineate target volume of metabolically active tumor for deciding treatment fields. The PET is particularly of use in differentiating postradiation fibrosis and active recurrence. The negative predictive value is 100%. If the CEA is marginally raised (5–10 ng/mL), the CT sensitivity is very poor while PET detects lesions in 60% of CT negative patients.

Liver and Pancreas

The diagnostic workup of hepatic lesions include dynamic contrast enhanced CT, MRI and ultrasonography. The CT has stood the test of time and hence the use of FDG-PET is still debatable. In hepatocellular carcinoma (HCC), FDG-PET uptake correlated with the tumor activity. The well-differentiated HCC do not show uptake and are associated with better prognosis. HCC with high uptake showed aggressive behavior with poor prognosis. The other tracer used for HCC is 11C-acetate which accumulated in tumors with better prognosis. Further prospective studies are needed to determine the role of these scans. In pancreatic cancer, the FDG-PET role is not defined and is only complementary to three-phase dynamic contrast CT or MRI. However, it can be used in staging and treatment response assessment.

GENITOURINARY CANCERS

The conventional diagnostic techniques like CT, MRI and sonography have high acceptable sensitivity in the primary tumors of entire genitourinary tract. Hence FDG-PET role is limited to indeterminate cases in which it plays complimentary role.

Prostate Cancer

The FDG-PET has no role in the detection of primary tumor since prostate cancer does not utilize glucose as energy substrate. It is known to use fatty acids and hence PET scan using tracers like 11C-choline and 18F-choline have been successfully used for primary tumor imaging. Currently, it is used as complementary test if conventional tests are inconclusive. However in the metastatic setting, FDG-PET is equally sensitive as other cancers in staging, restaging after recurrences and in response assessment.

After the initial local staging of the tumor using conventional procedures, bone scan is routinely performed for skeletal metastases. There are two types of bone scans: 99mTc-MDP gamma bone scan and 18F-PET bone scan. The fluoride bone scan has higher sensitivity and detects 30% more lesions than MDP bone scan. If the PSA is less than 10 ng/mL, then 18F bone scan is the choice while PSA above 10 ng/mL, MDP bone scan would be ideal and cost-effective. In patients with radical prostatectomy and PSA of 2–3 ng/mL, flouride PET bone scan is ideal. Both the scans have poor specificity of 40–60%. However, both the scans are obtained fused with CT which helps in specifying the scan lesions as benign or metastatic. During follow-up these scans are useful in assessing response to treatment.

Box 1: Indications

- All patients with > 20 ng/mL
- All symptomatic patients
- All patients with recurrence
- All patients with PSA of 2.5 ng/mL in postradical prostatectomy context
- Preisotope therapy for pain palliation

Renal and Bladder Cancer

In these cancers also bone scan is the standard staging procedure. In renal cancer, the common occult metastases are seen in ribs (20%) and in vertebrae and pelvic bones (15%) in bladder cancer. They are also used during follow-up and response assessment. FDG-PET scan is used only in metastatic setting as in prostate cancers.

Testicular Cancer

Computed tomography scan along with human chorionic gonadotropin (hCG) and alfa-fetoprotein levels is the diagnostic approach in seminomatous and nonseminomatous tumors. These tumors are highly sensitive to chemotherapy. One of the major issues is indication for surgical removal of residual masses after chemotherapy. In this context FDG-PET is evolving as a major tool with accuracy of 90% and 81% for seminomas and nonseminomatous tumors compared to 79% and 52% for CT.[17] The FDG-PET also detects 40% metastatic lesions at diagnosis not identified by other modalities. Hence, FDG-PET is recommended in the evaluation of postchemotherapy residual masses and in recurrences. The FDG-PET is not useful in teratomas as these tumors do not show significant uptake.

Ovarian Cancer

In the primary tumor detection CT, MRI, sonography, staging laparotomy and FDG-PET have similar sensitivity and hence FDG-PET is not used. However, in the postsurgery recurrences or rising CA-125 values with negative CT, FDG-PET is the ideal indication for detecting local recurrences (80%), peritoneal metastases (90%) and other distant metastases.[18] Today it is the standard of care in the follow-up and response assessment since CA-125 is not specific and does not reflect on the quantum and sites of metastatic disease. In our experience of 60 patients, the FDG-PET sensitivity for local recurrences was 89% compared to 45% for CT. The ability to distinguish postradiotherapy fibrosis from recurrences was 100% compared to 40% for CT. The number of metastatic nodules in the peritoneum was 30% more than CT. A negative FDG-PET is associated with longer survival.

Carcinoma Cervix

This is the most common female cancer in India. One of the major factors in the survival is the local extent of the disease. The CT, MRI and USG have low sensitivity in detecting pelvic (40%) and paraaortic nodes (7%). However, Grigsby et al. showed improved sensitivity by FDG-PET in pelvic nodes (67%) and para-aortic nodes (20%). They also showed that 8% of patients had supraclavicular nodal metastases at presentation thus making a case for staging FDG-PET in all cervix cancers. Currently, bone scan is one of the staging procedures in symptomatic patients.

HEAD AND NECK CANCER

Cancers of upper aerodigestive tract comprise 5% of all cancers in the western world while in India the oral cancers are alarmingly high due to tobacco. Clinical evaluation, CT scan and panendoscopic evaluation for biopsies is the diagnostic approach. However in the last 5 years, FDG PET-CT has become the main staging scan after obtaining histological diagnosis.[19] While PET alone is not ideal for T staging of tumor, integrated PET-CT together accurately stages the T stage of primary tumor. PET is very ideal for N and M staging. The PET and CT sensitivity is 79% and 72% and specificity 92% and 78% respectively for N staging. The MRI has similar sensitivity as PET, but considerably less specificity of 40%. The negative predictive value is almost 100%. However, the causes of false positives for nodal disease include inflammation because activated lymphocytes take up the tracer. FDG-PET is also ideal for distant metastases (M staging) and for detection of second malignancies at presentation which occurs in 10–20% of patients. FDG-PET has prognostic role in head and neck cancers.[20] If the glucose uptake ratio (SUV) of primary tumor is above 10.0, then the survival is poor. This is particularly useful in Thyroid cancers where the glucose uptake in papillary and follicular cancers preoperatively confers poor prognosis—45% versus 85% in those lesions which are negative on FDG-PET. We reproduced this finding in our study of 30 patients. FDG-PET is also the ideal investigation in recurrences for restaging. In response assessment, FDG-PET plays a major role after chemoradiation and surgery. In postradiation setting, the false positives are high in the first 3 months. Hence 6 months postradiation is ideal to minimize false positives. The sensitivity of PET for local recurrence is 80–100%, specificity 57–100% and negative predictive value is 100%. The CT and MRI sensitivity is 58–92% and specificity 50–100%. With increasing evidence in last 2 years, FDG PET-CT is now considered a mandatory staging procedure before any therapy is instituted.

Unknown Primary

This is an important group where detection of primary lesion poses a major challenge. Usually the histological classification of metastatic tissue guides investigative approach. The CT scan, tumor markers and endoscopic evaluation help in the primary detection. However, the sensitivity of clinical examination or CT scan is low in head and neck region. The lesions in tonsils, nasopharynx, palate and pyriform sinuses are difficult to detect clinically. FDG-PET is very sensitive in these areas. In GI areas, endoscopy and CT scan are ideal. FDG-PET detects upto 20% of unknown primary lesions.[21] In patients presenting with tumors in the brain which reveal metastases on biopsy, the search for primary is made easy by FDG-PET scan.

BONE AND SOFT TISSUE TUMORS

They are heterogeneous group of tumors of mesenchymal origin. The anatomical details can be accurately obtained by CT and MRI. The bone scan was used for more than three decades to detect metastases and still is used in certain centers. The histological evaluation faces problems due to intratumoral necrosis since they are large tumors. In this context, FDG-PET is very useful in guiding biopsy site for accurate histological grading which has bearing on treatment planning. In primary bone tumors, the sensitivity is 92% and specificity is 66%. False negative results are seen in low-grade chondrosarcomas while false positives were seen in aggressive lesions like giant cell tumors, fibrous dysplasia and hematogenous osteomyelitis. FDG-PET will be beneficial in asymptomatic lesions wherein increased uptake may lead to further investigations. Some times FDG-PET may show skip lesions and distant metastatic lesions. In response to treatment, FDG-PET is superior to bone scintigraphy. Soft-tissue sarcomas are rare tumors arising from any mesodermal tumors. If they arise from gastrointestinal stroma, they are called gastrointestinal stromal tumors (GIST). The uptake in these tumors is directly proportional to histologic grade and usually they demonstrate a very high uptake and accurate staging is achieved in 90% of patients. These tumors demonstrate remarkable response to the new drug imatinib which is tyrosine kinase inhibitor. The tumor response is remarkable and FDG-PET shows more than 50% reduction in uptake suggesting inhibition of intratumoral metabolism and growth. PET scan at the end of therapy is highly specific for disease free status. In liposarcomas, PET sensitivity is 90% with specificity of 88%.[22] Low-grade soft tissue sarcomas show uptake similar to muscles and benign soft tissue tumors do not show uptake.

POSITRON EMISSION TOMOGRAPHY-COMPUTED TOMOGRAPHY IN RADIOTHERAPY

Radiation is one of the mainstay in treatment of tumors. Currently CT or MRI is used to plan radiation portals. Though fairly accurate, there is significant radiation to the

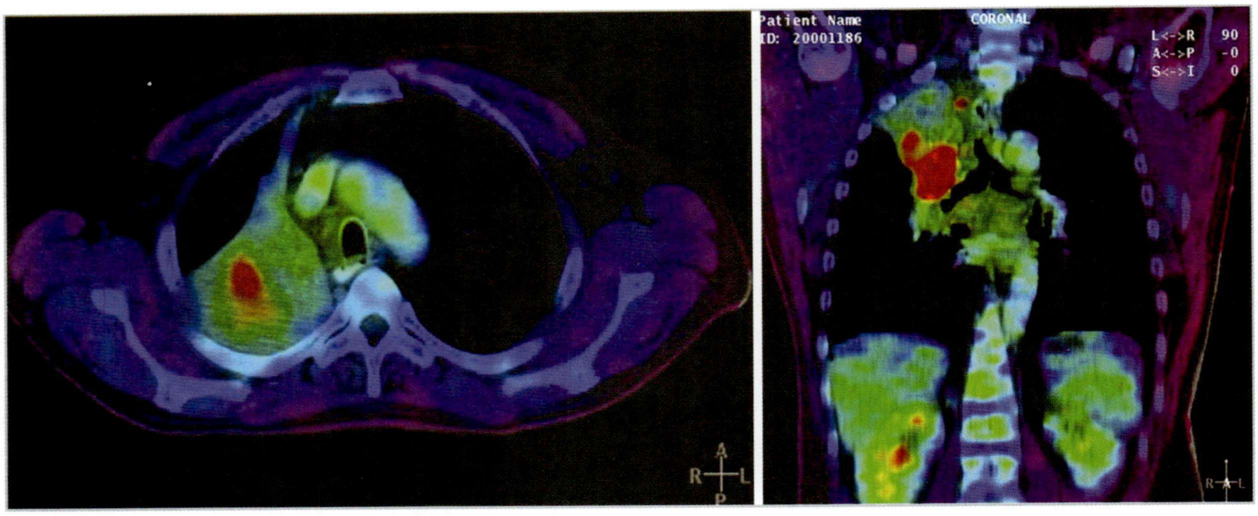

Fig. 12: Active tumor volume (in red color) is 25% of total tumor volume

adjoining tissues resulting in unwanted tissue damage. In breast irradiation, lung and heart receive unwanted radiation and data is emerging of long-term cardiac and lung complications. In pelvic radiation, bowel and bladder complications are well-established in spite of refined radiation techniques. In this context, PET-based radiation concept is emerging. In this approach, the metabolically active tumor volume is determined on FDG PET-CT and major part of the radiation dose is targeted to this active component of the tumor and adjoining inactive component is either spared or given low dose as shown in (Fig. 12). The metabolic active tumor volume[23] is usually less than 60% of the total tumor volume as determined on CT or MRI. Thus significant amount of adjoining normal tissue is spared resulting in lesser long-term complications. This approach is gaining importance in brain and lung tumors. In lung tumors, PET helps in separating atelectasis from active tumor and this is a major contribution for therapy planning. In brain tumors, PET helps in avoiding vital structures in the brain by accurately delineating target volume.

INFECTIONS IN ONCOLOGY

The immunocompromized cancer patient is prone to variety of infections during and after treatment. The infections include port, implant, catheter, drain and stent infections apart from organ infections. Majority of these are diagnosed with conventional techniques like USG, CT, MRI, cultures and X-rays. However, in 2–5% of patients, the source of infection remain unidentified. In such situation, FDG PET-CT is very useful to detect source of infection. The macrophages, which migrate to site of infection, use glucose as energy source to perform phagocytic function. The FDG localizes in macrophages through this mechanism and the source of infection is detected and the CT anatomically localizes the site for biopsy or aspiration for culture purposes. The sensitivity of the technique is 90%. This technique has virtually replaced the earlier techniques like 67Ga scan, 99mTc-leukocyte scan or antigranulocyte antibody scans which were time consuming both in preparation of tracer and imaging. Moreover, the high resolution CT images in PET-CT provide accurate anatomical delineation of structures enabling early interventions like removal of port, catheter, etc. if needed. In our experience, we have been able to demonstrate persistent focus of infections in vascular mesh, chemotherapy port infections, postoperative ileal infections and subacute bacterial endocarditis even when echo was normal.

EVOLVING APPLICATIONS OF POSITRON EMISSION TOMOGRAPHY SCAN WITH NEW TRACERS

The PET scan is expanding its role in oncology in imaging different constituents of cancer cell and these new techniques are likely to have immense impact at therapeutic level.

Imaging Tumor Proliferation

Thymidine is cellular constituent which is associated with cellular division. The 18F-thymidine scan demonstrates tumor proliferation and higher uptake suggests high-grade proliferating tumor. The uptake correlates with Ki index of the tumor with 95% specificity. The proliferation can be quantified and antiproliferative drugs can be instituted and follow-up scan will quantify the therapeutic response. If the scan shows low proliferative pattern then use of anti-proliferative drugs can be avoided.

Tumor Angiogenesis Imaging

Neovascularization is the hallmark of cancer. Accordingly, new drugs have been developed which inhibit tumor angiogenesis. These drugs are expensive and prior knowledge of degree of intratumoral angiogenesis and drug distribution will help using such drugs. Bevacizumab is one such drug which is used in variety of tumors. This drug is now labeled with zirconium-89 (89Zr) and is PET tracer. The images with 89Zr-bevacizumab show high accumulation in the tumor suggesting intense angiogenesis and also confirming drug effect.

Hypoxia Imaging

Tumor hypoxia is one of the resistant factors in radiotherapy. Hence, determination of hypoxia is critical from radiation therapy planning point of view. Mesonidazole localizes in hypoxic tissues. With 18F-mesonidazole (meso scan), the hypoxic area can be mapped out and accordingly planning is altered.

Apoptosis Imaging

Apoptosis is a phenomenon where cells are in the process of death. This is commonly seen after chemotherapy and reflects desired chemotherapeutic effect. This phenomenon can now be imaged using 99mTc-annexin V gamma scans. This compound localizes in apoptotic cells and confirms tumor cell death.

Tumor Drug Resistance Imaging

The tumor develops resistance to drugs after 2–3 courses of chemotherapy. This information will be useful in drug modulation. The gene responsible is p-glycoprotein (Pgp) which is intracellular and usually inactive. As a result of drug, the gene is activated and as a result drug effluxes out of the cell without producing desired effect. This phenomenon is demonstrated on image by scanning with 99mTc-sestamibi which localizes in tumor mitochondrial cell. When the Pgp gene is activated, this tracer is seen in the tumor in 10 minute image and washes out in 2 hour image. This has important therapeutic bearing in future.

THERAPEUTIC NUCLEAR ONCOLOGY

Isotopes have been used as therapeutic agents in cancer for over five decades. The isotope therapy is referred to as internal radiation therapy since the isotopes are administered orally or intravenously or in infusion form and deliver radiation internally to the tumor tissue. For therapy purpose, beta-rays emitted by isotopes are used. They have short track of length (1–3 mm) and intense radiation is delivered since they localize in the tumor cell.

Radioiodine Therapy for Thyroid Cancer

This was the first and highly specific therapy in oncology which came into existence in 1940 when the first patient was treated. The radioiodine ^{131}I is the therapeutic isotope and the beta-rays associated with this isotope produce therapeutic effect. The isotope has 8.4 days half-life and six beta-rays of varying energies. These collectively contribute to desired radiation effect. Total thyroidectomy is essential before radioiodine treatment because metastatic tissues do not pick up radioiodine in the presence of significant thyroid tissue in neck due to competitive inhibition. When surgical ablation of thyroid is not possible due to any reason, then radioablation of the whole thyroid or one lobe can be performed first followed by treatment of metastatic tissues.

The radioiodine is administered orally in liquid or capsule form. The aim of the treatment is to deliver 30,000 rad to the tumor tissue. Accordingly, the treatment doses are as follows:

- Postoperative neck residual tissue: 30–50 mCi
- Neck residue and lymph node metastasis: 150 mCi
- Pulmonary metastases: 150 mCi
- Bone metastases: 200 mCi.

After the radioiodine treatment, post-therapy scans are obtained to document uptake in the disease sites. Patient is put on suppressive dose of thyroxine (keep TSH level in undetectable range).

The treatment with radioiodine enhances the survival either by ablation or stabilization of disease. The pulmonary metastasis patients' survival is up to 20 years is 60% and bone metastasis is 40%. In our experience in 1,000 patients, the incidence of occult pulmonary metastases was 6.8% (^{131}I scan positive and X-ray negative). Such patients achieve complete ablation in 85% with one or two doses of radioiodine. If pulmonary metastases are present on chest

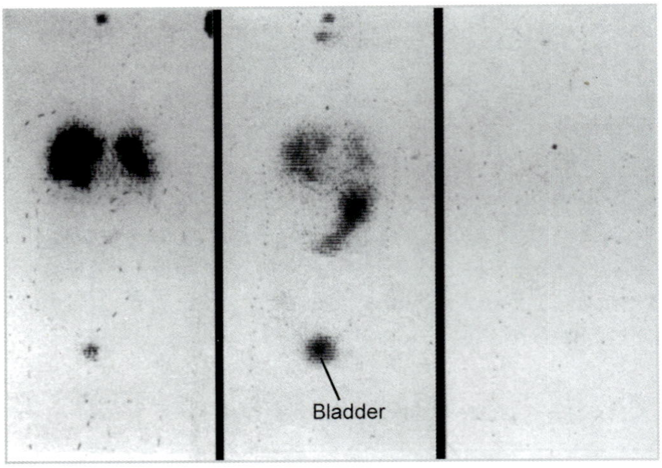

Fig. 13: Complete resolution of pulmonary metastases after radioiodine treatment

X-ray, then total ablation is achieved in about 25–30% patients. Hence, early lesions respond to curative stage.

The radioiodine treatment is well-tolerated by both pediatric and adult patients with minimal side effects like sialadenitis, gastritis and neck pain which usually regress in 2–3 days. The late complications include second malignancies like stomach, bladder, breast cancers, pulmonary fibrosis and hematological malignancies. In our experience of 1,000 patients, there were two breast cancer, three stomach cancers, one bladder cancer and two leukemias. Most of these second malignancies occurred over 15–20 years after radioiodine treatment (Fig. 13).

Isotope Therapy of Neuroendocrine Tumors

The neuroendocrine tumors express variety of receptors like somatostatin, catecholamine receptors. Somatostatin receptors are specific to gastrinomas, insulinomas, carcinoids, VIPomas which are collectively referred as gastroendocrine pancreatic neuroendocrine tumors (GEP-NET). Catecholamine receptors are specific to pheochromocytomas, paragangliomas, neuroblastomas and carcinoids.

These receptor synthetic analogues can be labeled with therapeutic isotopes like yttrium-90 (90Y), ^{131}I and ^{177}Lu which produce radiation effect. This form of therapy is now referred to as peptide receptor radionuclide therapy (PRRT) (radiolabeled receptor therapy) 5, 6, 12. For somatostatin, the synthetic analogues are octreotide, DOTATATE, DOTANOC, hydrazinonicotinyl-Tyr3-octreotide (HYNIC-TOC) and any of these analogues can be labeled with above tracers. For catecholamine receptors, the synthetic analogue is guanidine. Currently available tracers are as follows:

- 90Y/^{177}Lu-DOTATATE—for somatostatin rich tumors
- ^{131}I-MIBG—for catecholamine rich tumors.

Lutetium-177 DOTATATE Therapy

This treatment has gained clinical significance in last 5 years. Its major role is in low grade NET (grade 1 or < 2% Ki) and in drug refractory cases of grade 2 (2–10% Ki) tumors. The existing literature suggests that treatment is more of palliation. However, in the last 2 years, there is convincing evidence that this therapy increases the survival by achieving disease stabilization by arresting tumor growth. The prerequisites for PRRT are as follows:

- Low-grade (< 2% Ki) NET
- Grade 3–4 uptake on Octreoscan™ or DOTATATE scan
- Serum creatinine and creatinine clearance value
- GFR estimation
- Complete hematology profile
- Liver function tests.

Patients with compromised renal function, low platelets and high bilirubin level are excluded from this therapy. The tracer commonly used is ^{177}Lu-DOTATATE which has half-life of 6.7 days and beta-rays (0.5 MeV). Usually 200–300 mCi is administered by infusion over 4 hours. Since major part of the tracer is excreted through kidneys, renal toxicity is a major concern. Hence, prior to and after tracer infusion, patient is administered amino acids to protect kidneys. There are transient side effects like pain at the local site, thrombocytopenia (20%) and leukopenia (60%) which do not need any major treatment. The renal toxicity occurs in 20% of patients. In our own experience, the patients show remarkable symptomatic relief within 2–3 weeks and remain symptom free for 8–12 months. The treatment can be repeated every 3–4 months in responders to achieve tumor regression. In the Basel experience on 1,109 patients, Imhof et al. showed complete and partial response in 34.1%, disease control in 39.3%. The quality of life improves significantly in almost 60% of patients and overall survival benefit is seen 20% of patients.24 This treatment also results in down staging of the disease to make them operable. This treatment could be used as first line therapy in foregut NET, and as second line in bowel carcinoids who fail drug therapy.

Iodine-131 Metaiodobenzylguanidine Therapy

This tracer localizes in catecholamine secreting tumors like pheochromocytoma, paraganglioma, neuroblastomas, medullary thyroid cancer and carcinoids. However, its role is well-established in primary and metastatic neuroblastomas. In inoperable primary tumors, the MIBG therapy downstages the tumor and makes it amenable to surgery. In stage IV disease whole-body MIBG therapy is useful adjunct to chemotherapy in concomitantly irradiating all the metastases. In neuroblastoma stage III and IV patients, MIBG therapy enhances the 5 year survival by 30–40%.[25] Currently, this treatment is administered in conjunction with chemo and immunotherapy. In medullary cancer thyroid, the therapy is palliative but with newer chemotherapeutic drugs the role of MIBG therapy has diminished. In paragangliomas, MIBG therapy is beneficial in controlling the symptoms in 60% of patients. In pheochromocytoma, the role is limited to malignant pheochromocytoma metastases with symptomatic relief.

Metastatic Bone Disease—Phosphorus-32, Strontium-89 Therapy

Bone metastases from carcinoma prostate which are drug refractory pose a major clinical problem. In these patients, hemi body irradiation is one of the options. However, the radiation side effects on extraosseous tissue are considerable. Hence, isotope treatment using strontium-89 (89Sr), phosphorus-32 (32P), and Samarium are currently used to palliate the pain and improve quality of life. The WHO recommends it in patients who need cocktail of analgesics with unremitting pain and have extensive bone disease. The tracer is given intravenously and pain relief occurs by 3rd week in 60% and quality of life improves significantly. In India, 32P is available at low cost from BARC and the International Atomic Energy Agency (IAEA) multicentric study showed that 32P is equally efficacious as 89Sr which is prohibitively expensive. The toxic effects like leukopenia, thrombocytopenia are seen in 20% of patients and can be managed with blood transfusions. With the advent of bisphosphonates therapy recently, the role of isotope therapy in this setting has diminished.

B-Cell Lymphoma—Zevalin® and Bexxar® Radioimmunotherapy

B-cell lymphoma is associated with CD20 antigen. The monoclonal antibody to this antigen is radioconjugated with 131I (Bexxar®) and 90Y (Zevalin®) and systemic administration of radioconjugated antibody results in the delivery of radiation to the tumor directly. Such cytocidal effect also kills neighboring antibody-negative cells, the so-called cross-fire effect. This radio immunotherapy is indicated in follicular lymphoma (FL) relapse and recurrence setting and of late is being considered as first-line therapy in advanced-stage FL. Kaminski et al.[26] showed that when Bexxar® was used in chemotherapy failed FL, 65% showed response and 23% complete remission. 53% of patients had longer duration of response. Bexxar® is also efficacious in those who progressed after rituximab and following transformation of FL. When used alone in newly diagnosed advanced-stage follicular lymphoma, the overall response was 95% with 5-year progression-free survival of 59%. Zevalin® (90Y-ibritumomab tiuxetan) was the first radioimmunoconjugate to receive FDA approval. 90Y is a pure beta-emitter. It is known to produce similar effect as Bexxar®. The toxic effects are similar to chemotherapy.

Radioembolization

In this technique, isotopes like 90Y are conjugated to glass particle and administered into tumor through intra-arterial catheter. The particles trap in the tumor vasculature and the isotope delivers very high radiation directly to the tumor tissue. This treatment is particularly useful in inoperable liver tumors and metastatic liver lesions. The response rate upto 60–80% is documented.

REFERENCES

1. Biscontini G, Massacesi C, Cinti P, et al. PET and Octreoscan in neuroendocrine tumors (NET). J Nucl Med. 2007:48:372.
2. Mittal BR, Agrawal K, Shukla J, et al. Ga-68 DOTATATE PET/CT in neuroendocrine tumors: initial experience. J Postgrad Med Educ Res. 2013;47(1):1-6.
3. Hanson MW. Scintigraphic evaluation of neuroendocrine tumors. Appl Radiol. 2001;30(6):11-7.
4. Palmedo H, Schomburg A, Grünwald F, et al. Technetium-99m-MIBI scintimammography for suspicious breast lesions. J Nucl Med. 1996;37(4):626-30.
5. Newman EA, Newman LA, et al. Lymphatic mapping techniques and sentinel lymph node biopsy in breast cancer. Surg Clin North Am. 2007;87(2):353-64.
6. Kim TS, Moon WK, Lee DS, et al. Fluorodeoxyglucose positron emission tomography for detection of recurrent or metastatic breast cancer. World J Surg. 2001;25(7):829-34.
7. Tsujikawa T, Yoshida Y, Maeda H, et al. Oestrogen-related tumour phenotype: positron emission tomography characterization with ^{18}F-FDG and ^{18}F-FES. Br J Radiol. 2012;85(1015):1020-4.

8. Berg WA, Madsen KS, Tartar M, et al. Breast cancer: comparative effectiveness of positron emission mammography and MR imaging in presurgical planning for the ipsilateral breast. Radiology. 2011;258(1):59-72.
9. Christensen JA, Nathan MA, Mullan BP, et al. Characterization of solitary pulmonary nodule: 18F-FDG PET versus nodule-enhancement CT. AJR Am J Roentgenol. 2006;187(5):1361-7.
10. Lardinois D, Weder W, Hany TF, et al. Staging of non-small-cell lung cancer with integrated positron-emission tomography and computed tomography. N Engl J Med. 2003;348(25):2500-7.
11. Vansteenkiste JF, Stroobants SG, De Leyn PR, et al. Lymph node staging in non-small cell lung cancer with FDG-PET scan: a prospective study on 690 lymph node stations from 68 patients. J Clin Oncol. 1998;16(6):2142-9.
12. Weder W, Schmid R, Bruchhaus H, et al. Detection of extrathoracic metastases by positron emission tomography in lung cancer. Ann Thorac Surg. 1998;66(3):886-92.
13. Metser U, You J, McSweeney S, et al. Assessment of tumor recurrence in patients with colorectal cancer and elevated carcinoembryonic antigen level: FDG PET/CT versus contrast-enhanced 64-MDCT of the chest and abdomen. AJR Am J Roentgenol. 2010;194(3):766-71.
14. Topal B, Flamen P, Aerts R, et al. Clinical value of whole-body emission tomography in potentially curable colorectal liver metastases. Eur J Surg Oncol. 2001;27(2):175-9.
15. Flanagan FL, Dehadasti F, Ogunbiyi OA, et al. Utility of FDG-PET for investigating unexplained plasma CEA elevation in patients with colorectal cancer. Ann Surg. 1998;227(3):319-23.
16. McLeish AR, Lee ST, Byrne AJ, et al. Impact of ^{18}F-FDG-PET in decision making for liver metastectomy of colorectal cancer. ANZ J Surg. 2012;82(1-2):30-5.
17. Chung P, Walker-Dilks C. (2009). PET imaging in testicular cancer. [online] Available from https://www.cancercare.on.ca/common/pages/UserFile.aspx?fileId=43151 [Accessed January, 2014].
18. Prakash P, Cronin CG, Blake MA. Role of PET-CT in ovarian cancer. AJR Am J Roentgenol. 2010;194(6):W464-70.
19. Funk GF. A head and neck surgeon's perspective on best practices for the use of PET-CT scans for the diagnosis of head and neck cancers. Arch Otolaryngol Head Neck Surg. 2012;138(8):748-52.
20. Higgins KA, Hoang JK, Roach MC, et al. Analysis of pretreatment FDG-PET SUV parameters in head-and-neck cancer: tumor SUVmean has superior prognostic value. Int J Radiat Oncol Biol Phys. 2012;82(2):548-53.
21. Pavlidis N, Briasoulis E, Hainsworth J, et al. Diagnosis and therapeutic management of cancer of an unknown primary. Eur J Cancer. 2003;39(14):1990-2005.
22. Early JF, Hawkins DS, Rodler ET, et al. (18)F-FDG PET in sarcoma treatment response imaging. Am J Nucl Med Mol Imaging. 2011;1(1):47-53.
23. Greco C, Rosenzweig K, Cascini GL, et al. Current status for tumor volume definition in radiotherapy treatment planning for non-small cell lung cancer (NSCLC). Lung Cancer. 2007;57(2):125-34.
24. Frilling A, Weber F, Saner F, et al. Treatment with (90)Y and (177)Lu-DOTATOC in patients with metastatic neuroendocrine tumors. Surgery. 2006;140(6):968-76.
25. Bomanji JB, Wong W, Gaze MN, et al. Treatment of neuroendocrine tumors in adults with 131I-MIBG therapy. Clin Oncol (R Coll Radiol). 2003;15(4):193-8.
26. Kaminski MS, Tuck M, Estes J, et al. 131I-tositumomab therapy as initial treatment for follicular lymphoma, N Engl J Med. 2005;352(5):441-9.

8 Tumor Markers in Cancer: Therapeutic Impact

Praful Desai

INTRODUCTION

Increasing biological insights into the complexity of malignant diseases have opened up new vistas and approaches for its diagnosis and management. The exponential advance of science, technology, laboratory medicine and clinical research has impacted in a positive manner on the remissions, control and cure rates in certain types of cancer.

Tumor (bio) markers, essentially, are substances released by tumor tissues which can be measured in body fluids like blood, serum, urine, tumor tissues and lymph nodes. Currently, besides the routine clinical, imaging and histopathologic data, investigations go beyond these morphologic studies towards estimation of tumor markers in most cancers which can help in diagnostic, therapeutic and prognostic implications. As pathways of cancer-understanding increased, the role of tumor markers became more important in the management of cancer patients.

THERAPEUTIC IMPACT OF TUMOR MARKERS IN CANCER

It is important to understand that no tumor marker is 100% specific or sensitive and raised tumor marker does not always indicate malignancy as higher levels are known in inflammatory conditions. Biochemistry has been used for more than a century for measurement of substances in the body fluids to help make a diagnosis. Hardly any biomarker can be used for screening purposes to diagnose early cancer. All tumors do not always secrete a marker and many common cancers may be nonsecretive. Importantly, the significance of tumor markers lies in monitoring the effectiveness of therapy viz—surgery, radiotherapy or chemotherapy, disease progression and control. A large burden or volume of cancer will often have high levels of a tumor marker.

The earliest record of the value of biochemistry in cancer diagnosis was the Bence Jones proteins—IgG for myeloma (1847). Table 1 indicates the utility of biomarkers in diagnosis of common cancers.

TABLE 1: Utility of biomarkers in diagnosis of common malignant tumors

Acid phosphatase	Prostate
Alkaline phosphatase	Osteogenic sarcoma, bone metastasis
β-hCG	Choriocarcinoma
VMA (vanillylmandelic acid)	Pheochromocytoma
Catechol amines	Neuroblastoma
5-HIAA	Carcinoids
Chromogranin	Neuroendocrine tumors
CA 125	Ovary, uterus
CEA	Colon, breast
CA 15.3	Breast
PSA	Prostate
AFP	Liver
CA 19-9	Pancreas
Calcitonin	Medullary thyroid cancer
Cytokines	Lymphoma

(*Abbreviations:* β-hCG, beta human chorionic gonadotropin; 5-HIAA, 5-hydroxyindolacetic acid; CA, cancer antigen; CEA, carcinogenic embryonic antigen; PSA, prostate-specific antigen; AFP, alpha fetoprotein)

Recent insights into tumor biology have increased the range of recent bio (tumor) markers in routine clinical use. It is necessary to reemphasize that none of these markers are useful as a screening tool, but can provide effective information regarding recurrences (in the follow-up period) and monitoring responses to therapy. A very high tumor marker burden usually indicates advanced and disseminated disease. Markers can be identified even in circulation as soluble molecules such as deoxyribo-nucleic acid (DNA), ribo-nucleic acid (RNA) or proteins, e.g. proto-oncogene HER-2, which is a critical target for therapies against breast cancer by targeted monoclonal antibodies like trastuzumab (Herceptin) or lapatinib. A tumor marker can very often be predictive like hormone receptors positivity estrogen receptor, progesterone receptor (ER, PR) which indicates the necessity of hormone therapy. Study of KRAS mutations (colon) and epidermal growth factor receptor (EGFR) mutations (lung) are therapeutically important. Positive KRAS mutation negates the use of Erbitux (Cetuximab) in colon cancers and positive mutations of EGFR indicates its use which may be beneficial in lung cancers.

Tumor markers are, therefore of great significance in management of many common cancers. It indicates the load of cancer burden, can indicate therapeutic efficacy and is helpful in monitoring tumor responses and recurrences in the follow-up period, which may necessitate further management (Figs 1 and 2).

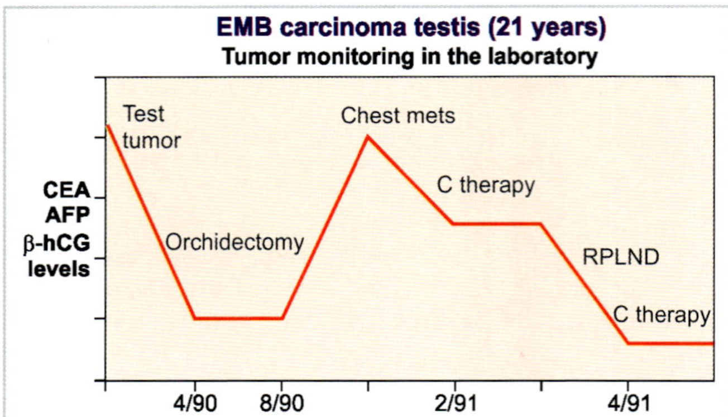

Fig. 1: Testis—embryonal carcinoma—rising tumor markers after normal levels (post-orchidectomy). Response to chemotherapy yet no return to normalcy of marker levels. Retroperitoneal dissection showed lymph node metastasis. Markers return to normal after RPLND

(*Abbreviations:* CEA, carcinogenic embryonic antigen; AFP, alpha fetoprotein; β-HCG, beta human chorionic gonadotropin; RPLND, retroperitoneal lymph node dissection; C, chemotherapy)

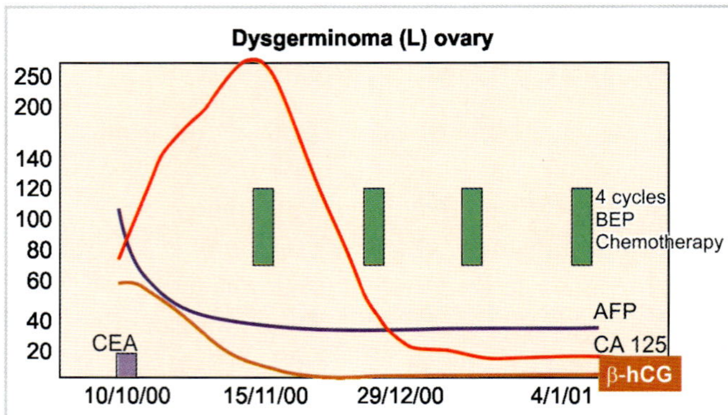

Fig. 2: A young female, 19 years, presented with dysgerminoma of the left ovary. The tumor was resected. Rising tumor markers in the same patient despite being asymptomatic. Appropriate chemotherapy results in markers returning to normal levels. No evidence of disease for 12 years. Normal pregnancy and now a mother of a 6-year-old boy

(*Abbreviations:* CEA, carcinoembryonic antigen; AFP, alpha fetoprotein; BEP, bleomycin, etoposide and cisplatinum)

9 Cancer Chemotherapy: Future Perspectives

SH Advani

INTRODUCTION

The era of cancer chemotherapy started in 1940–50 with nitrogen mustard and methotrexate producing dramatic response in lymphoma and leukemia. Today, cancer drug development has exploded to reach an unprecedented level with discovery of numerous novel chemotherapeutic and targeted agents.

The simple observation of profound lymphopenia in victims exposed to mustard gas helped Goodman and Gilman to use nitrogen mustard in patients with lymphoma with dramatic response. This was the first step suggesting that cancer could be treated with pharmacological agents. Sidney Farber, the father of modern chemotherapy, used folate analogs in acute lymphoblastic leukemia leading to remission in children; Hertz (1956) demonstrated that methotrexate alone can produce complete remission in choriocarcinoma. Joseph Burchenal, working on purine analog, discovered 6-mercaptopurine (6-MP) with good antileukemic effect. Vinca alkaloids, with ability to inhibit microtubule polymerization and cell division, was introduced as an antileukemic agent. Paclitaxel, obtained from bark of Pacific yew tree, showed antimitotic effect promoting microtubule assembly. Camptothecin derived from Chinese ornamental tree was shown to inhibit topoisomerase-1 enzyme responsible for DNA unwinding. Platinum-based compounds were introduced with observation of inhibition of bacterial cell division. Over a period of time, many drugs interfering with DNA synthesis were discovered (Table 1). These drugs are active in different phases of cell cycle (Fig. 1).

Apart from discoveries of newer chemotherapeutic agents, newer concepts in utilization of drugs allowed

TABLE 1: DNA-based cytotoxic agents

Alkylating drug	*Cyclophosphamide*
Antimetabolites	
Folate	MTX
Purine	6MP
Pyrimidine	5FU
Ara-C	Cytosine arabinoside
Cytotoxic antibiotics	Actinomycin D
Platinating agents	Cisplatin
Plant alkaloids	Vinca alkaloids, paclitaxel
Topoisomerase-1 inhibitor	Camptothecin
Topoisomerase-2	Etopoids
Novel drug delivery	nab-paclitaxel

Abbreviations: MTX, methotrexate; 6MP, 6-mercaptopurine; 5FU, 5-fluorouracil

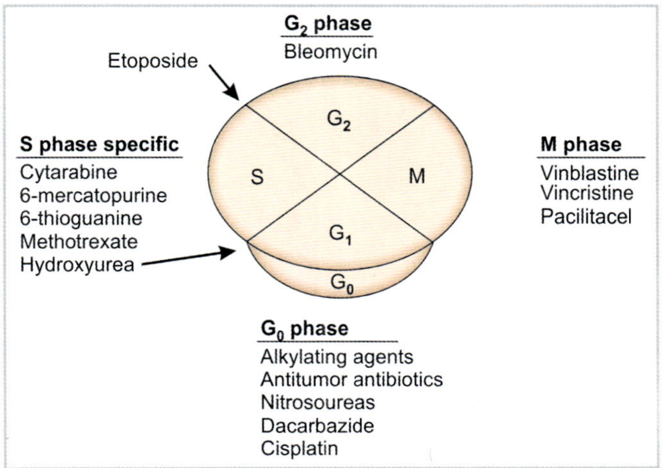

Fig. 1: Cell cycle specific (CCS) and cell cycle nonspecific agents (CCNS)

Box 1: Cancers curable with combination chemotherapy

- Acute lymphoblastic leukemia
- Hodgkin's disease
- Non-Hodgkin's lymphoma
- Choriocarcinoma
- Primary central nervous system non-Hodgkin's lymphoma
- Germ cell tumor
- Burkitt's lymphoma
- Wilms' tumor
- Embryonal rhabdomyosarcoma

Box 2: Expanding role of primary chemotherapy in neoplasms

- Primary chemotherapy
  - Expanding role in neoplasms
    - Non-small-cell lung cancer
    - Breast cancer
    - Esophageal cancer
    - Nasopharyngeal cancer
    - Cancers of the head and neck region
    - Pancreas cancer
    - Gastric carcinoma
    - Prostate cancer (hormones)
    - Cervical carcinoma
    - Ovarian carcinoma

Box 3: Primary chemotherapy can prevent mutilating surgery

- Primary chemotherapy
  - Can prevent mutilating surgery
    - Anal carcinoma
    - Bladder carcinoma
    - Breast cancer
    - Laryngeal cancer
    - Osteogenic sarcoma
    - Soft tissue sarcomas

major thrust in control of cancer. The combination of chemotherapy drugs with different mechanism of action prevented drug resistance. Devita proved that nitrogen mustard, vincristine, procarbazine and prednisolone (MOPP) can lead to cure in Hodgkin's lymphoma; similarly, combination of prednisolone, vincristine, methotrexate and 6-MP (POMP) induced long-term remissions in children with acute lymphoblastic leukemia. Combination chemotherapy can cure many cancers even in advanced stage (Box 1).

Chemotherapy agents can be most effective when tumor burden is small (adjuvant chemotherapy). The strategy of surgery, first to eliminate major tumor burden followed by combination of chemotherapy to eliminate small residual disease has become very successful in many cancers. Adjuvant chemotherapy after complete surgical resection of breast cancer, significantly extended overall survival. High dose methotrexate with calcium leucovorin rescue has shown reduction in recurrence of osteosarcoma following surgical removal of primary tumor. 5-fluorouracil an inhibitor of DNA synthesis alone or in combination with oxaliplatin/irinotecan has prolonged survival following surgery for colon carcinoma (Box 2).

The concept of neoadjuvant chemotherapy (preoperative) was introduced to achieve tumor reduction, thus facilitating surgery. It is extremely useful for organ preservation. It also improves postoperative recovery and long-term outcome. The role of preoperative chemotherapy is being recognized in many tumors (Box 3).

SUPPORTIVE CARE

Improved supportive care has played an important role in the ability to prevent and manage toxicities of cancer chemotherapy. Many chemotherapeutic agents cause profound suppression of the bone marrow. Prevention of leukopenia with G-colony stimulating factor (G-CSF) and support with red cell and platelet transfusion along with broad spectrum antibiotics in case of infection are crucial for recovery of patients.

Chemotherapy induced nausea and vomiting (CINV) was a major limiting factor following emetogenic drugs. The new drugs utilizing 5-HT3 receptor antagonist ondensetron, granisetron and palanosetron can effectively prevent nausea and vomiting during the first 24 hours after chemotherapy. Neurokinin-1 (NK-1) antagonist (aprepitant: substance P inhibitor) is highly efficacious in preventing both acute and delayed emesis. NK-1 antagonists are often used along with 5-HT3 inhibitors and corticosteroids to form a potent cocktail in controlling nausea and vomiting associated with cancer chemotherapy. Dulexetine, an antidepressant has helped to reduce painful peripheral neuropathy caused by neurotoxic chemotherapy.

Indwelling central line and peripherally inserted central catheters (PICC) have allowed safe administration of chemotherapy as well as support therapy.

One important contribution during the last three decades has been the discovery of hematopoietic stem cells obtained from either bone marrow, peripheral blood or umbilical cord blood. The use of hematopoietic blood progenitor cells allows administration of lethal dose of chemotherapy. The patients' stem cells are first harvested, chemotherapy given followed by return of harvested cells to patients. This approach termed as autologous stem cell transplantation has shown curative benefit in Hodgkin's and non-Hodgkin's lymphoma. Allogeneic stem cell transplant has shown success in eradicating acute myeloid leukemia, chronic myeloid leukemia and myelodysplastic syndrome by high-dose chemotherapy and graft versus host response.

INTRODUCTION OF HORMONE THERAPY

During the 19th century, observation of benefit with oophorectomy in advanced breast cancer and dramatic regression of metastatic prostate cancer after removal of testis, laid the ground work for hormone therapy. This work has provided a foundation for use of hormone therapy such as estrogen analog (tamoxifen) and aromatase inhibitors to treat or prevent breast cancer. Similarly, LHRH (luteinizing hormone-releasing hormone) analog and inhibitor have produced control of prostate cancer.

Abiraterone (inhibitor CYP17), is an enzyme expressed in testis, adrenal and prostate tumor catalyzing pregnenolone to androstenedione, the precursor of testosterone. Thus, inhibitor of CYP17 activity by abiraterone decreases circulating level of testosterone. It has been approved for treatment of hormone resistant prostate cancer.

BIOLOGICAL THERAPEUTICS

Unfolding of cell biology has revealed oncogene, suppressor genes and signaling networks regulating cell proliferation and survival. During malignant transformation, cells acquire numerous aberrantly expressed molecular moieties. Many of the signaling networks are radically altered in cancer cells caused by somatic mutation. This knowledge has identified new drug targets for cancer drug development.

GROWTH SIGNAL INHIBITORS

Growth factors and its network-chain responsible for recognizing and responding to growth factors are products of oncogene. Change in these signal pathways have been identified as a cause of abnormal behavior of cancer cells. Molecularly targeted therapy is a type of medication that blocks the growth of cancer cells by interfering with specific targeted molecules needed for carcinogenesis. Identification of targets and the corresponding genes has helped to develop agents which can modify the target to function favorably either at DNA, RNA and protein expression.

TABLE 2: Targeted therapy: monoclonal antibody

Drug	*Target*	*Disease*
Rituximab	CD 20	Non-Hodgkin's lymphoma
Trastuzumab	HER2	Breast cancer
Cetuximab	EGFR	Colon cancer, head and neck cancer, stomach cancer
Bevacizumab	VEGF ligand	Colon cancer
Ipilimumab	CTLA-4	Malignant melanoma

Abbreviations: EGFR, epidermal growth factor receptor VEGF, vascular endothelial growth factor; CTLA-4, cytotoxic T-lymphocyte antigen-4

There are targeted therapies for breast cancer, lymphoma, chronic myeloid leukemia, chronic lymphatic leukemia, multiple myeloma and malignant melanoma, and other cancers. The availability of monoclonal antibody against the identified target in malignant cell allowed the development of rituximab in non-Hodgkin's lymphoma, trastuzumab in HER2-positive breast cancer and cetuximab and bevacizumab in colorectal cancer (Table 2).

Trastuzumab is used to treat HER2-positive breast cancer both as an adjuvant in early breast cancer and advanced breast cancer. In fact, trastuzumab has altered the life history of HER2-positive breast cancer. Pertuzumab is a monoclonal antibody that prevents HER2 from dimenizing with other ligand activated HER3 receptors. Double receptor blockade has shown greater antitumor activity. Trastuzumab emtansine (T-DM1) is another agent with antibody drug conjugate maytansine (microtubule inhibitor). This allows specific delivery to HER2 over expressing cells.

The discovery of large numbers of small molecules targeting gene and gene products has shown great success (Table 3).

In chronic myeloid leukemia, 9:22 chromosome balanced translocation leads to abnormal fusion protein, activated tyrosine kinase Bcr-Abl responsible for aberrant signal and uncontrolled proliferation of the leukemic cells. Imatinib, a small molecule, precisely inhibits this kinase. In chronic myelogenous leukemia (CML), imatinib achieves 90% complete hematological remission and 50–60% molecular remission.

Nilotinib and dasatinib are second-generation Bcr-Abl inhibitors with great potency and selectivity. It also reduces the emergence of Bcr-Abl mutation. The new tyrosine kinase inhibitor ponatinib appears to work for patients not responding to prior therapies.

TABLE 3: Targeted therapies: small molecules

Name	*Target*	*Disease*
Imatinib	Bcr-Abl	Chronic myeloid leukemia
Imatinib	Bcr-Abl	Gastrointestinal stromal tumor
Geftinib	EGFR	Non-small-cell carcinoma
Erlotinib	EGFR	Non-small-cell carcinoma
Bortezumib	Proteasome inhibitor	Multiple myeloma
Janus kinase inhibitor	Jack mutation	Myelofibrosis
Crizotinib	ALK	Non-small-cell carcinoma
Ibrutinib	P13K inhibitory	Chronic lymphoblastic leukemia
Vemurafenib	B-RAF	Melanoma
Vandetanib	EGFR/RET/VEGFR-2	Medullary thyroid cancer
PARP inhibitor	Poly (ADP ribose polymerase enzyme)	Breast cancer with BRCA-1/BRCA-2 mutation

Abbreviations: EGFR, epidermal growth factor receptor; VEGFR-2, vascular endothelial growth factor receptor 2; ALK, anaplastic lymphoma kinase

A potential new drug Ibrutinib in chronic lymphocytic leukemia (CLL) binds and blocks activity of Bruton's tyrosine kinase (BTK) which plays an important role in helping immune cell tumors. Bruton's tyrosine kinase, an essential component of B cell receptors signaling, mediates interactions with tumor microenvironment and promotes the survivors and proliferation of CLL cells. Ibrutinib is beneficial even in patients with most aggressive type of chronic lymphocytic leukemia driven by genetic mutation. Responses were also observed in patients with poor prognostic risk as in cytogenetic subtype del (17p) and del (11q).

The treatment of renal cell carcinoma (RCC) has undergone a paradigm shift from immunotherapy to targeted treatment. Von Hippel-Lindau (VHL) factor, negatively regulates hypoxia inducible factor (HIF). Defects in VHL function are predominant in familial and sporadic RCC. Inactivation of VHL results in increased HIF and upregulation of vascular endothelial growth factor (VEGF) and platelet derived growth factor (PDGF). Inhibition of mammalian target of rapamycin (m-TOR) also leads to HIF production. The success in treatment in RCC has been achieved with small molecular sorafenib, sunitinib, pazopanib by inhibition of VEGF receptors. The monoclonal antibody bevacizumab can achieve tumor inhibiting by VEGF blockade. One more signaling pathway involved in development of renal cell carcinoma is P13K/AK/m-TOR. m-TOR—a target of rapamycin protein, regulates growth factors and regulating proteins. Inhibition of m-TOR essentially stops growth factors and alters regulatory protein favorably. Inhibition of m-TOR offers the potential to block disease progression in renal cell carcinoma.

Today and in future, we will see precision in cancer treatment based on the concept that specific observation within tumor will help to select aberration specific treatment.

Personalized cancer therapy includes molecular information of patient's tumor, its microenvironment characteristic of patient to enable us to deliver tailored therapies with improved outcome and reduced toxicity. Several biomarkers have shown pathway for treatment selection. B-RAF V600E mutation allows treatment selection of melanoma with vemurafenib with 48% response rate.

The identification of driver aberrations has allowed development of therapies targeting aberrant genes a pathways dysregulated by aberrant gene. Thus, future lies with patient selection based on molecular profile and in vitro testing.

Recently, immunotherapeutic approaches seem to alter the negative regulator of immune system by the tumor. Ipilimumab, a humanized monoclonal antibody against programmed cell death protein 1 (PD 1) acts by activating immune system by binding to CTLA-4. Normally, cytotoxic T lymphocyte associated antigen (CTLA-4) turns off the cytotoxic reaction. Ipilimumab blocks CTLA-4 inhibitory signal and allows CTL to destroy the cancer cells. Ipilimumab has shown a marked response in malignant melonama. CTLO19 cell therapy has opened new approach to us, our body's own immune cells to kill cancer cells. Adoptive cell therapy with in vitro expansion activated T-cell, NK cells and dendritic cells appears to have great future in maintaining remission.

10 Radiotherapy: Prospects and Retrospects

Nagraj G Huilgol, Mukul Roy

INTRODUCTION

Radiation therapy is a nascent modality of treatment of cancer which is ever evolving since its inception. Radioactivity as a natural phenomenon was discovered by Henri Becquerel in the year 1895. It was followed by a now famous discovery of radium by Marie and Pierre Curie in the year 1898.Willhelm Roentgen quite accidently discovered X-rays, the mysterious rays which could help to image bones and look inside the body. Biological effects became evident very soon after the discovery of radium and X-rays. They were invented with magical properties of rejuvenation to depilation. Scabies, tinea and tuberculosis were treated with radiation. Serendipity and close observation led to the use of radiation to treat cancer. The early therapeutic applications were based on clinical observation and limitations imposed by technology. Radiation was delivered in multiple fractions as X-ray machines could not deliver erythema dose in one go! Elaborate techniques of radium therapy evolved as external radiation did not penetrate deep enough in the body. Radium-88 was the sole isotope used for brachytherapy till cesium-137 and cobalt-60 were discovered for use. Currently a plethora of radioactive isotopes like iridium-192, palladium-103 and iodine seeds are available for implants. Similarly crackling machines have metamorphosed into highly sophisticated linear accelerators with on-board imaging. However, it was in 1950 that the first telecobalt machine a megavoltage radiation capable of radiating deep-seated tumors was invented. This was a turning point in the history of radiation oncology. Over the last decades, radiation therapy which has evolved on empirical basis has received bench investigations in the realms of radiation biology. Fractionation is not imposed by limitations of technology but a better understanding of tumor cell kinetics, radiation-inflicted injury and repair. Radiation protectors, hypoxic cell sensitizers, hyperthermia, cytotoxic drugs and targeted drugs have been added to potentiate the effects of ionizing radiation. Proton and carbon ion accelerators have become a clinical reality. Particle accelerators have added to the armamentarium of radiation oncologists. This incredible gallop of technology has barely taken a century to evolve. This article will attempt to briefly enunciate various concepts relevant to oncologists and doctors who intend to attend to patients with cancer.

The sole objective of radiation therapy is to deliver therapeutic dose to target volume while sparing normal tissue to the extent possible. The differential delivery of radiation creates a therapeutic ratio which very often is very narrow. In other words the clinician has to be extremely careful in the choice of techniques, fractionation, total dose and any concomitant therapy. Radiation can be delivered from a distance as in teletherapy or from within a cavity as in intracavitary radiation of cervical cancer, or with temporary or permanent implants of radioactive mater. The earlier mentioned is called external-beam radiation therapy (EBRT) and the later as brachytherapy.

External-beam radiation therapy is delivered on telecobalt machines or linear accelerators. Telecobalt machine which was first introduced in 1950 changed the way radiation therapy was practiced. The telecobalt machines house a radioactive material Co-60 of very high specific activity. The natural radioactive decay emits photon of 1.2 MV energy. Photon beams are shaped as square, rectangular or irregular beams and delivered from any coplanar or noncoplanar angles. The divergent beams are similar to those from 4MV linear accelerators in physical distribution. Photons of similar fraction size have similar effects on tumor irrespective of its source, i.e. whether it is sourced from a telecobalt machine or linear accelerator: The fear of nuclear waste and rapid progress in accelerator technology has ensured rapid acceptance of linear accelerators as a crucial component of current departments of radiation oncology.

Linear accelerators produce X-rays of various energies besides electrons. Liner accelerators popularly called linac are versatile and score over telecobalt machines due to the availability of photons with higher depth of penetration and electrons in contrast with limited penetration of depth. Thus both superficial and deep-seated tumor can be treated. Linac-based radiation therapy for cancer therapy began with treatment of the first patient in 1953 in London at Hammersmith hospital with 8 megavolt machine built by Vickers. Later in 1956 Henry Kaplan pioneered linac therapy at Stanford USA. However, it was only in early 1970s that the linacs became robust reliable and routinely used in the clinics of the western world.[1]

Techniques of radiation therapy are largely similar in both telecobalt and linear accelerator; conventional methods rely on square or rectangular shaped beams in a coaxial geometry to treat the target. The lack of beam shaping leads to excessive radiations to normal tissue. The next step in evolution of radiation therapy was cerrobend or custom-based shaping of beams to conform to the tumor geometry. Tumors have no fixed geometry. Thus beam shaping leads to reduced radiation therapy to normal tissue. Inbuilt multi leaves incorporated in the gantry replaced manual blocking of beams. Simultaneous integration of computer aerial tomography in the treatment planning process ensured a giant step forward in three-dimensional conformal radiation. Zelefsky reported the outcome of three-dimensional conformal radiation therapy (3DCRT) in prostate cancer after evaluating a total of 743 patients. He demonstrated the feasibility of dose escalation to 81Gy from 64–68Gy, without a significant addition to bladder or rectal toxicity.[2]

Figures 1A to F demonstrate the effect of various techniques of radiation on normal tissue and conformation index. Intensity-modulated radiation is a particular type of conformal distribution of radiation.

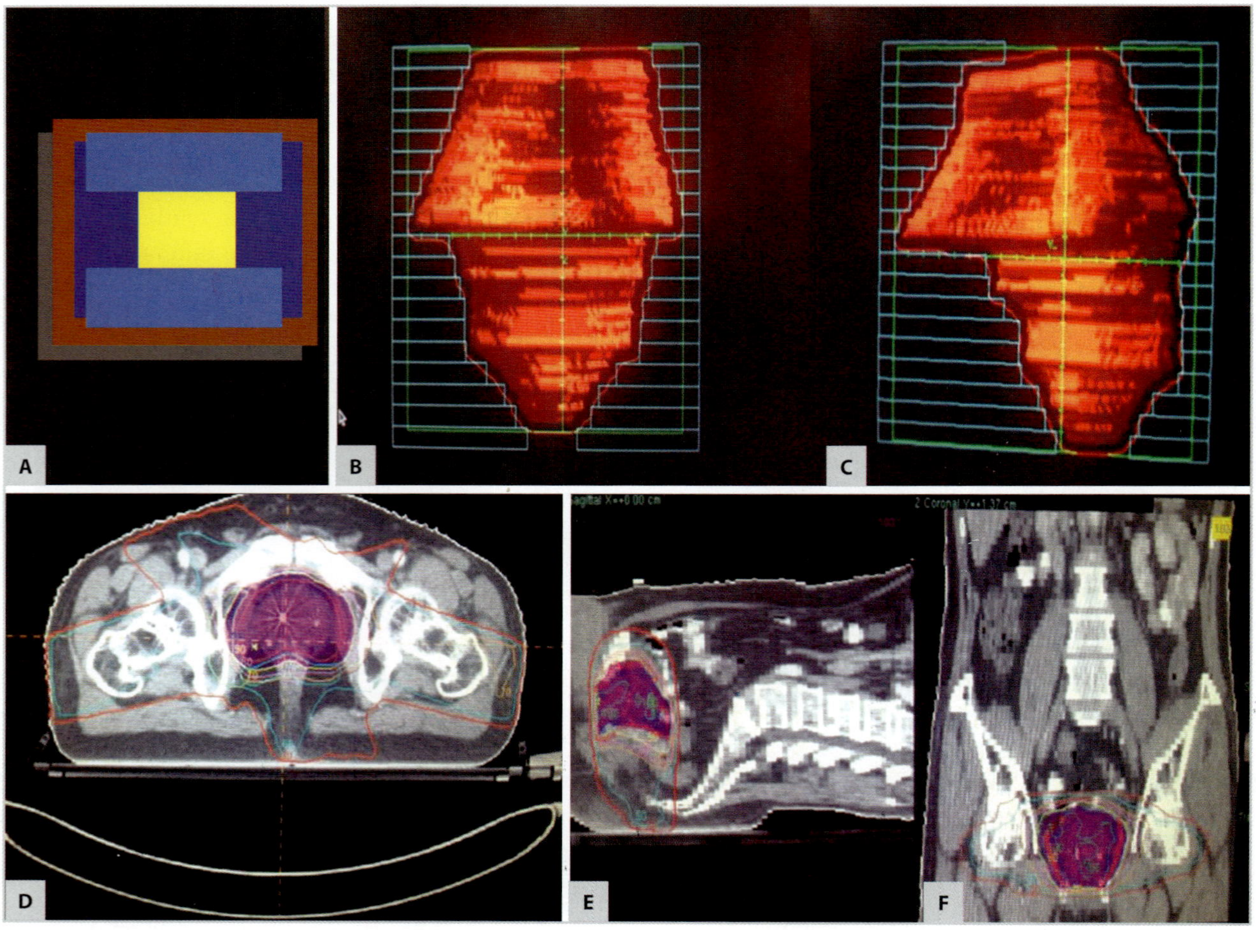

Figs 1A to F: (A) Collimator shaped beam; (B and C) Multi-leaf collimator in three-dimensional radiotherapy (3DRT) for cancer cervix; (D and E) Intensity-modulated radiotherapy (IMRT) in cancer prostate with gold seed implant. 95% Isodose shown in purple color wash; (F) Coronal section—isodose distribution

BIOLOGICAL BASICS OF RADIATION THERAPY

Ionizing radiation randomly interacts with cellular and subcellular targets. The critical target is generally assumed to be deoxyribonucleic acid (DNA), while cellular and nuclear membrane also may be the targets.[3] Radiation induced damage generally manifests as single or double strand breaks in the sugar-phosphate backbone of the DNA molecule. The low linear energy transfer (LET) radiation like electromagnetic radiation act through free radicals while protons impart direct damage. A cascade of molecular events follows cellular damage. Molecular sensors recognize single or double strand break (DSB) of before initiating a repair process. Multiple signaling pathways are involved. The eventual consequence of irradiation of cell depends on defense or sensitivity, innate defense or sensitivity besides quantum and nature of radiation.[4]

Radiation damage to cell is generally manifested as loss of cellular reproductive capacity. That is why rapidly multiplying tumors which undergo reproductive death at each division respond much better than cells with slow proliferation. Cells may also undergo apoptotic death. Repair of DSB's is achieved either with homologous combination repair (HRR) or nonhomologous end joining (NHEJ). HR ensures a faithful repair while NHEJ may not.[5] Cells deficient in repair mechanisms are more sensitive to radiation. That is why a strategy to block *RAD51* gene by using antisense oligonucleotide has shown radiosensitization in glioma cell lines.[6] The biological basis of radiation is built on differential repair kinetics of normal and neoplastic cells, normal tissues repairing faster and more efficiently, intrinsic sensitivity, cytokinetic features of tumor and hypoxia are some other variables which affect the eventual fate of any biological system after having received ionizing radiation (IR).

Regaud in 1927 introduced the idea of fractionation on the basis of experimental observation. Fractionation of the dose ensured sterilization of ram's testis without damaging scrotal skin.[7] Fractionation not only spares normal tissue but also allows for reoxygenation and reassortment of cells, hopefully in more sensitive cell cycle phase like G_1 and M. More recently, it has been found that α/β ratio for prostate cancer cell is between 3 Gy and 3.7 Gy and for rectum is between 4 Gy and 6 Gy. This suggests that a therapeutic ratio may exist in favor of large dose fractions with the obvious potential for shorter overall treatment durations. It improves local tumor control and reduces early and late toxicity, provided appropriate dose constraints for relevant normal tissues are respected. There are economic advantages and patient convenience as well in hypofractionated prostate radiotherapy regimens.

Conventional fractionation which has evolved empirically seems to have achieved optimal results in most cases. Acceleration of dose delivery with altered fractionation and hypofractionation evolved on the basis tumor cytokinetics, better information on delayed changes in normal tissue and of course, tolerance. Mathematical models also have been relied on when designing newer fractionation schedules. Linear Quadric model popularly known as LQ model seems to be fairly robust and reliable in most situations. Controversy exists in totally relying on these models. Similarly, total dose required to annihilate tumor within the range of acceptable therapeutic ratio has evolved empirically. Table 1 shows tumor control probabilities for adenocarcinoma and squamous cell cancer of various sizes. Initial tumor burden, nature of clonogenic cell histology and intrinsic sensitivity determine the total dose required to achieve control or cure. Thus while it may be sufficient to deliver 4,000 cGy in 20 fractions to achieve complete remission in lymphoma, a total dose of 74–80 Gy may be necessary to control adenocarcinoma of prostate. Dose escalation in a clinical situation is limited by normal tissue tolerance. Even the most contemporary technology cannot achieve an ideal therapeutic ratio (Table 2).

TABLE 1: Tumor control probability percentage

Dose	*Histology*	
Dose	Squamous cell carcinoma	Histology adenocarcinoma
5000 cGy over 5 weeks	> 90% subclinical	> 90% subclinical
6000 cGy over 6 weeks	= 90% - T1 lesions of HNSCC = 50% - T3, T4 lesions of HNSCC	
7000 cGy over 7 weeks	= 90% - T2 lesions – HNSCC = 80% - T3, T4 lesions - HNACC	90% clinically possible nodes 2.5–3 cm

Abbreviation: HNSC, head and neck squamous cell carcinoma.

TABLE 2: Fractionation schemes routinely used in the clinic

Fractionation	Schedules
Conventional	180–210 cGy is delivered once a day, 5 days a week
Multiple daily fractions	When 120–150 cGy is delivered at least 6 hours gap, twice a day 5 days a week
Accelerated fractionation	Radiation is delivered twice or thrice a day or higher dose per fraction so that total dose is delivered in a shorter time than conventional radiation
Hypofractionation	Larger dose per fraction delivered less frequently than conventional fractionation
Stereotactic radiation	A very large dose is delivered in short time

TABLE 3: Mechanisms of chemotherapy-induced radiation sensitization

Chemotherapy agent	MOA
Platinum-based compound	Inhibits (a) DNA synthesis (b) Transcription elongation by DNA interstrand cross-links (c) Repair of radiation-induced DNA damage
Taxanes	(a) Arrests cell in G2M phase of cell cycle (b) Induces apoptosis (c) Reoxygenates tumor cells
Topoisomerase I inhibitors	(a) Inhibits repair of radiation-induced DNA strand breaks (b) Redistributes cells to G2 phase of cell cycle (c) Converts radiation-induced SSB's to DSB's
Antimetabolites	(a) Lowers apoptotic threshold (b) Alteration of nucleotide pool (c) Cell cycle redistribution (d) Reoxygenates tumor cells

Abbreviations: SSB, single strand break; DSB, double strand break

Radiotherapy when given in addition to the primary, main or initial treatment is called as adjuvant radiation. An example of adjuvant therapy is the additional treatment usually given after surgery where all detectable disease has been removed, but where there remains a statistical risk of relapse due to occult disease. This is the treatment course commonly employed in head and neck cancers and breast carcinoma where the histopathological features report high risk features like positive surgical margin, lymphovascular invasion, lymphadenopathy with extracapsular extension and perineural invasion. Radiation combined with concurrent chemotherapeutic drugs is used as very popularly treatment of choice in locally advanced head and neck cancers[8] and carcinoma of the nasopharynx.

RATIONALE FOR COMBINATION CHEMORADIOTHERAPY

Radio sensitizer: It improves the probability of local control and in some cases, survival, by aiding the destruction of radio-resistant clones.

Organ-preservation intent: It improves cosmesis and function compared with surgical resection with or without adjuvant treatment.

Chemotherapy: It acts systemically and potentially eradicates distant micrometastases.

The combination of radiation and chemotherapy together was explained by the Steel paradigm[9] which consists of the following:

- Spatial cooperation—radiotherapy acts locoregionally, and chemotherapy acts against distant micrometastases
- Radiation sensitization leads to additive or synergistic effect when given with concurrent chemotherapy (Table 3).

The MACH-NC (meta-analysis of chemotherapy in head and neck cancer) study, which evaluated 63 trials and a total of 10,741 patients, is the largest of the meta-analyses.[10] Individual data rather than literature-based data, with the inclusion of updated data and unpublished trials, were assessed, including individual data updated in 66% of the trials for as long as a median follow-up of 6.8 years. Subcategorization into locoregional treatment with and without concomitant chemotherapy, induction/

adjuvant chemotherapy, and laryngeal preservation with induction chemotherapy, rather than definitive treatment for laryngeal and hypopharyngeal tumors, was reported. No benefit was detected for neoadjuvant or adjuvant chemotherapy, whereas a trend toward a statistically significant benefit (4%) was reported for concurrent or alternating chemoradiation therapy (p = .23).

The most commonly used drug in concurrent setting is cisplatin at a dose of 35–40 mg/m^2 along with hydration. The other compounds are carboplatin, gemcitabine, hydroxyurea, etc.

Many times a lesion may be unresectable or there may be a large tumor burden which makes surgery difficult. In such a scenario, radiation is often delivered first so as to shrink the tumor thereby making the tumor resectable. Neoadjuvant radiation also prevents the microscopic seeding during surgery. This is commonly practiced in locally advanced rectal cancers to convert unresectable disease to a resectable state. It also facilitates sphincter preservation thereby improving the quality of life of such patients.

The literature does justify the use of neoadjuvant chemotherapy in the setting of advanced laryngeal or hypopharyngeal primaries with the dual goals of organ preservation and the treatment of micrometastatic disease. Induction chemotherapy has been considered appropriate in this setting because it does increase laryngeal preservation without compromising overall survival. The landmark Veteran's Affairs Laryngeal Study[11] randomized patients into two arms: induction cisplatin/5-FU for three cycles followed by radiation, or laryngectomy followed by radiation; 332 patients were entered. An evaluation occurred after two cycles of chemotherapy. Patients with a partial response received a third cycle of chemotherapy followed by radiation therapy. Those patients without an initial response to induction chemotherapy received a laryngectomy followed by radiation therapy. Patients with residual disease after the completion of radiation therapy underwent surgical resection. With a median follow-up of 33 months, an estimated 2-year survival rate of 68% in both groups failed to demonstrate a difference in overall survival (p = .9846), although a majority of patients (64%) were able to preserve function of the larynx. Recurrences differed between the two groups, with increased locoregional control (p = .0005) and decreased metastases (p = .016) in the induction chemotherapy group. Given that there was no compromise of overall survival, induction therapy is thought to be feasible in the setting of laryngeal carcinoma to allow organ preservation without compromise of overall survival (Table 4).

Radiation response however can be modified by chemical and physical modalities like hypoxic cell sensitizer, radiation protectors and hyperthermia. Hypoxic cells are 2–3 times more resistant to radiation than oxic cells. Drugs like metronidazole, nimerazole and senazole have been evaluated for oxygen mimetic potentials. Nimerazole and senazole have shown beneficial effects. Yet the clinical use has been disappointing.[12,13]

Amifostine in contrast is a radical scavenger and hydrogen donor. Amifostine which has shown to protect

TABLE 4: Advantages and disadvantages of different chemoradiation sequencing strategies

Strategy	Advantages	Disadvantages
Sequential chemoradiation	• Decrease radiation field size if tumor responds to induction chemotherapy • Optimal systemic therapy • Decreased toxicity	• Prolonged overall treatment time • Local synergy – not utilized
CCRT	• Overall treatment time is less • Radiosenstizing chemotherapeutic agents enhance radiation effects	• Suboptimal systemic therapy • Higher toxicity • Tumor cytoreduction not achieved before starting CCRT
CCRT and adjuvant chemoradiation	• Optimal systemic therapy • Radiosenstizing chemotherapeutic agents enhance radiation effects • Local and metastatic disease control targeted upfront	• Unfavorable toxicity profile • Increased overall treatment time • Compliance for adjuvant chemotherapy is less
Induction chemotherapy and CCRT	• Optimal system therapy • Radiosenstizing chemotherapeutic agents enhance radiation effects	• Higher toxicity • Patient compliance less especially for chemoradiation after induction chemoradiation

Abbreviation: CCRT, cuncurrent chemoradiotherapy

salivary glands and kidney and few other organs could never become a standard of care due to difficulty in daily administration and toxicities. Hyperthermia is another physical modality of treatment which when combined with radiation can increase survival.[14,15] Heating tumor to 42–45°C target hypoxic cells and those cells which are generally resistant to radiation, like S phase of cell cycle. Heating can be achieved by depositing energy with radiofrequency or microwaves. Ultrasound can also be utilized for the same purpose. Hyperthermia with drugs encapsulated in heat sensitive liposomes has yielded excellent results.

BRACHYTHERAPY

Brachytherapy (Greek word brachys, meaning "short-distance"), also known as internal radiotherapy, sealed source radiotherapy, curietherapy or endocurietherapy, is a form of radiotherapy where a radiation source is placed inside or next to the area requiring treatment. The discovery of radium introduced a compact source of unvarying highly penetrating rays, suitable for external or internal application. In 1899, Becqueral had an accidental burn on his skin by carrying a tube of radium in his waist coat pocket. Pierre Curie produced the same effect on his arm skin for confirmation of the same biological effect. This may be considered the beginning of radiation biology. This effect made scientists to think and recognize radium as therapeutic aid in the treatment of disease. In 1901, Danlos and Bloch from St. Louis hospital in Paris treated cutaneous lupus and started the era of brachytherapy. This very early period was followed by the evolutionary period of radium therapy from empiricism or trial and error to the development of an art.

DEVELOPMENT OF NEW RADIONUCLIDES AND RADIATION PHYSICS

Irene and Frederic Joliot Curie discovered man-made radioactivity by bombarding aluminum with alpha particles and obtaining radioactive phosphorus. The first attempt to develop new sources in United States was made by William Myres, who produced Cobalt needles in 1948. Cesium-137 tubes and needles were also produced at around the same time. Ulrich Henschke then introduced in 1965, iridium-192 seeds for removable implants and Au-198 seeds for permanent implants in 1953. Iodine-125 seeds were introduced in 1965 which was found suitable for permanent implant due to its low energy and short half-life. In 1965, Schlea and Stoddard postulated use of californium-252, a neutron emitter for brachytherapy.

Brachytherapy application needed standardization of source strength, the definition and specification of treatment volumes and definition of radiation units. Pierre Curie, a French physicist, suggested to the French doctor Henri-Alexandre Danlos that a radioactive source could be inserted into a tumor. This technique was first applied as a treatment for lupus, but soon after, it was also applied to cancerous tumors. It was found that the radiation caused the tumors to shrink in size. Initially, radium therapy was the province of dermatologists and surgeons. The element was so rare (and expensive) that early practitioners used trivial, ineffective quantities. Initial enthusiasm was replaced by disappointment. But mass exploitation of American (later, African and Canadian) sources of radium ore resulted in the availability of sufficient quantities of the element for practical application. Thereafter progress was rapid, and by 1920 radium therapy had displaced surgery as the preferred treatment for gynecologic malignancy. The past century has witnessed dramatic advances in surgery and pharmacotherapy, but the implantation of radioactive sources has also evolved.

Following these early experiments, interest in brachytherapy grew. Many innovations quickly followed, such as the use of seed therapy for prostate cancer and specialized applicators for cervical cancer. However, the risks of radiation exposure to operators from the manual handling of the radiation sources were soon identified. Consequently the use of brachytherapy declined in the middle of the 20th century. To overcome the problem of unwanted radiation exposure, remote afterloading systems and new radioactive sources were introduced in the 1950s and 1960s. These new systems helped prevent occupational exposure to radiation and made the brachytherapy procedure even safer for patients and operators alike.

In more recent years there has been a "second renaissance" in brachytherapy technological innovations. Three-dimensional (3D) imaging and computerized treatment planning systems and delivery equipment has made brachytherapy a safe and effective treatment for many types of cancer today. Reactor and cyclotron-produced radionuclides, with higher specific activity and lower γ-ray/photon energy, have expanded applicability and patient safety. Computer dosimetry has improved the therapeutic ratio. Remote afterloading has eliminated radiation exposure to personnel. The 21st century is witnessing a renaissance of brachytherapy. History of brachytherapy is given in Tables 5 and 6.

TABLE 5: History of brachytherapy in a nutshell

1896 – Becquerel-Radioactivity	1898 – Madam Curie/Pierre Curie - Radium
1903 – Nobel Prize for Curie's and Becquerel	1903 – First successful case of malignancy basal cell carcinoma of face
1920 – Patterson and Parker tables for radium	1920 – Paris system of IC Rx/Stockholm system
1934 – Manchester system	1953 – Tod and Meredith point A and B defined
1957 – Ir-192 in implants	1965 – Paris system—Interstitial
1960 – Preloaded applicators Stockholm, Paris and Manchester	1960 – Afterloading applicator—Henchke/Fletcher-suit
1962 – First remote after-loading machine	1970 – Co-60 HDR
1985 – HDR Ir-192	2000 – 3D Brachy planning
- CT/MR Compatible applicators	- Inverse planning

Abbreviations: Co, cobalt; CT, computed tomography; HDR, high-dose rate; Ir, iridium

TABLE 6: Radioisotopes used in brachytherapy[16]

Radioisotope	*Energy (MeV)*	*Form*	*Half-life*	*Application*
Radium 226, Ra-222	0.8	Tubes, needles	1620 years	Intracavitatory Historic importance
Cesium-137	0.66	Tubes, needles, seeds	30 years	Intracavitatory, Intersitial
Cobalt-60	1.17, 1.33	Tubes, needles, seeds	5.26 years	Intracavitatory, Interstitial
Iridium-192	0.35	Wires, pellets	74 days	Intracavitatory, Interstitial
Iodine-125	0.035	Seeds	60 days	Interstitial, Permanent
Strontium-90	0.2 β emitter	Plaques	3.4 days	Plaques for ophthalmic use, pituitary tumors
Palladium-103	0.021	seeds	17 days	Permanent interstitial

BRACHYTHERAPY TYPES BASED ON DOSE RATE

Low-dose rate (LDR): This involves implanting radiation sources that emit radiation at a rate of 0.4–2 Gy/h.[17]

Medium-dose rate (MDR): This is characterized by a medium rate of dose delivery, ranging between 2 Gy/h and 12 Gy/h.

High-dose rate (HDR): When the rate of dose delivery exceeds 12 Gy/h.

Pulsed-dose rate (PDR): Pulsed-dose rate brachytherapy involves short pulses of radiation, typically once an hour, to simulate the overall rate and effectiveness of LDR treatment.

TYPES OF BRACHYTHERAPY BASED ON SOURCES PLACED

1. Interstitial: The sources are placed directly in the target tissue of the affected site, such as the prostate or breast[18]
2. Intracavitatory, e.g. cervical cancer
3. Intraluminal, e.g. esophageal cancer
4. Surface: Mould brachytherapy, e.g. skin cancer.

INTENSITY-MODULATED RADIOTHERAPY

Intensity-modulated radiation therapy (IMRT) is the logical evolution of Radiation Therapy, starting from the first fractionated irradiation of patients in a conventional way, evolving into a CRT model, when automatic field sequencing and controlled conformal treatments were developed as a long way to achieve better quality assurance of the radiation therapy process, and finally arriving at modulation of the beam for higher conformality.[19] This evolution can be interpreted as the natural path from one-dimensional treatment to a full 3D treatment process. Conformal radiotherapy started in 1950–60. The main idea was high doses to the tumor and minimum doses to the normal tissues. The purpose was to conform selected isodoses around the tumor and avoid critical structures.

Conformal radiotherapy (CRT) is based on three hypotheses:

- A higher rate of local control to improve the survival rate
- Dose escalation to increase tumor control
- Delivery of higher doses by decreasing the incidence of late effects.

However, there were situations for which 3DCRT could not produce a satisfactory treatment plan because of complex target volume shapes or the close proximity of sensitive normal tissues. This is why IMRT was introduced. Its aim is to overcome the limitations of 3DCRT by adding modulators of beam intensity to beam shaping. IMRT can achieve nearly any dose distributions. IMRT can be used to spare organs-at-risk, for irregular-shaped targets, for treating multiple targets simultaneously. It can be used to enable dose escalation and to treat regions with prior radiation. IMRT is 3D treatment delivery of a 3D plan by modifying the intensity across each beam in complex ways. Intensity modulation uses nonuniform fluence distribution that is modulated by the motion of jaws and leaves. IMRT creates superior dose volume histograms compared to conventional RT. In the dose volume histograms (DVH), the separation between target dose and organ at risk (OAR) doses is greater. In theory, that allows for dose escalation to the target, if necessary. Static IMRT also known as "step and shoot" method is when nothing moves when the beam is on. There are fields with segmentation. In dynamic IMRT, multileaf collimators (MLC) move when the beam is on. There are fields with segmentation plus contribution of the doses between segments.

IMRT modalities based on planning system are:

- Forward planned IMRT
- Aperture-based IMRT
- Inverse planned IMRT
- Monte Carlo based IMRT

Based on delivery systems:

- Multileaf collimators
- Micro-, mini-, virtual-micro MLC
- Tomotherapy devices

Based on treatment techniques:

- Segmented sequential (step and shoot)
- Cinematic sequential (cinematic IMRT)
- Dynamic sequential (sliding window)
- Intensity-modulated arc therapy (IMAT)
- Tomotherapy.

FUTURE OF RADIATION ONCOLOGY

The quest for improving therapeutic ratio continues. Physical optimization of dose distribution of photons seems to have reached a plateau. Particle accelerators like protons and carbon ion are now commercially available. Intensity-modulated radiotherapy with proton can achieve a highly conformal dose distribution while saving normal tissue. However, there is no evidence of protons being superior to photons in improving absolute survival. There is also an attempt to combine newer targeted agents with radiation like bevacizumab, nimotuzumab, sunitinib and cetuximab. Even gold nanoparticles conjugated with receptor-specific ligands are being investigated. Radiation as a modality of treatment can aim to achieve cure, control or palliate.

REFERNECES

1. Thwaites DI, Tuohy JB. Back to the future: the history and development of the clinical linear accelerator. Phys Med Biol. 2006;51:R343-62.
2. Zelefsky MJ, Leibel SA, Gaudin PB, et al. Dose escalation with three-dimensional conformal radiation therapy affects the outcome in prostate cancer. Int J Radiat Oncol Biol Phys. 1998;41(3):491-500.
3. Dizdarogh M. Measurement of radiation induced damage in DNA at the molecular level. Int J Radiat Oncol Biol Phys. 1992;61:175-9.
4. Withers HG. Principle and practice of radiation oncology. In: Perez CA, Brady LW (Eds). Philidelephia (PA): JB Lippincot. 1987; pp. 67-98.
5. Johnson RD, Jasin M. Sister chromatid gene conversion is a prominent double strand break repair pathway in mammalian cells. Embo J. 2000;19:3398-407.
6. Ohinishi J, Jaki T, Hirag Setal. In vitro and in vivo potentiation of radio sensitivity of malignat gliomas by antisense inhibition of the RAD 51 gene. Biochem Biophys Res Commun. 1998;245(2):319-24.
7. Regaud C, Ferronz B. Discordance des effects de rayons X, d'une part dans le testucue, parle fractionment de la dose C R Soc Biol. 1927:97;431-4.
8. Expert Review of Anticancer Therapy, Concurrent Chemotherapy and Radiotherapy for Head and Neck Cancer. 2009;9(3):293-302. doi: 10.1586/14737140.9.3.293.

9. Steel GG, Peckham MJ. Exploitable mechanisms in combined radiotherapy-chemotherapy: The concept of additivity. Int J Radiat Oncol Biol Phys. 1979;5:85-91.

10. Pignon JP, Bourhis J, Domenge C, et al. Chemotherapy added to locoregional treatment for head and neck squamous-cell carcinoma: Three meta-analyses of updated individual data. MACH-NC Collaborative Group. Meta-Analysis of Chemotherapy on Head and Neck Cancer. Lancet. 2000;355:949-55.

11. Induction chemotherapy plus radiation compared with surgery plus radiation in patients with advanced laryngeal cancer. The Department of Veterans Affairs Laryngeal Cancer Study Group. N Engl J Med. 1991;324:1685-90.

12. Huilgol NG, Gupta S, Sridhar CR. Hyperthermia with radiation in the treatment of locally advanced head and neck cancer: a report of randomized trial. J Cancer Res Ther. 2010;6(4):492-6.

13. International Journal of Radiation Oncology Biology Physics, an overview of the initial experience with AK—2123 as a hypoxic cell sensitizer with radiation, in the treatment of advanced head and neck cancers. 1996;34(5):1121-4.

14. Huilgol NG, Gupta S, Sridhar CR. Hyperthermia with radiation in the treatment of locally advanced head and neck cancer: a report of randomized trial. J Cancer Res Ther. 2010;6(4):492-6.

15. van der Zee J, González González D, et al. Comparison of radiotherapy alone with radiotherapy plus hyperthermia in locally advanced pelvic tumours: a prospective, randomised, multicentre trial. Dutch Deep Hyperthermia Group. Lancet. 2000;355:1119-25.

16. Nuclear Wallet Cards 2005. 7th edition. [online] Available from http://www.nndc.bnl.gov/wallet/wc7.html. [Accessed October, 2013].

17. Thomassen B, Das R. The physics and dosimetry of high dose rate brachytherapy. In: Perez and Brady's principles and practice of radiation oncology. 5th edition. Lww. 2008. p. 540-59.

18. Gerbaulet A, Potter R, Mazeron JJ, van Lim Bergen E (Eds). The GEC ESTRO Handbook of Brachytherapy; 2002.

19. Tubiana M, Eschwège F. Conformal radiotherapy and intensity-modulated radiotherapy--clinical data. Acta Oncol. 2000;39(5):555-67.

11 Hormonal Dependence of Malignant Cells

Rajendra Badwe, Sudeep Gupta, Gautam Goyal

INTRODUCTION

Endocrine manipulation of cancer is an excellent example of how the treatment of cancer has evolved over the years utilizing the benefit of evidence based medicine. This intervention has seen progressive evolution from surgical oophorectomy, hypophysectomy to targeted receptor agonists and antagonists and now their usage in rational combinations. Further ahead there will be evaluation of the role of hormonal therapy along with new modules of chemotherapy and targeted therapy. This intervention has also taught us how each step in the search of cure added a small benefit, leading to prolongation of the disease free interval and overall survival.

Tumors of hormone-responsive tissues currently account for greater than 35% of all newly diagnosed cancers in men and nearly 40% of all newly diagnosed cancers in women.[1] The two most common cancers in both men and women, i.e. prostate and breast are under hormonal control. The molecular basis of endogenous hormone levels as an important risk factor for hormone-dependent tumors is also now being appreciated. Although thought to be largely related to environment, it is now increasingly apparent that genetic susceptibility, through germ line polymorphisms in critical genes, plays an important role in production and propagation of cancer.

Since major advancements in the field of hormonal therapies have been in breast and prostate cancers, this chapter will use recurrent examples from these malignancies to illustrate general principles.

HISTORY

In 1896, Beatson[2] was the first to show benefit of hormonal manipulation by surgical oophorectomy in a premenopausal woman with metastatic breast cancer, with temporary regression of disease. Following this discovery, Lathrop and Loeb[3] found that removal of ovaries prevented onset of mammary cancer in a considerable fraction of mice. Lacassagne was the first to show a correlation between development of cancer and hormones, since a steroid with estrogenic activity incited formation of breast cancer.[4]

In prostate cancer, therapy with high-dose estrogens and shortly thereafter castration were introduced successfully by the pioneering work of C Huggins.[5]

In humans, there is a relatively high incidence of cancer involving organs which are under direct endocrine regulation. These are breast, prostate, ovary, uterus and thyroid.

PATHOPHYSIOLOGY

The concept that hormones can influence the development of neoplasia was first developed by Bittner et al. based on experimental studies of estrogens and breast cancer in mice.[6] These observations led to extended studies of the role of hormones in the origin and control of growth. Cancers of the breast, anterior pituitary, adrenal cortex, ovary, endometrium, testis, uterus, lymphoid organs, liver and prostate gland have been induced by alterations in the endocrine environment in experimental animals. There is now also clear evidence that hormones can be carcinogenic in humans.

One of the most interesting developments in the study of neoplasms is the concept of "hormone dependency". Using animal models, Furth[7] postulated a sequence of changes from a normal cell to hyperplasia, to hormone-dependent tumor, to autonomous tumor still responsive to hormones, and finally to fully autonomous neoplasm. The same endocrine alterations necessary for the induction of cancer are also contributory or essential for the continued growth of the neoplasm. The concept of hormone dependence of cancer was soon proved by Huggins and Hodges, who had shown that orchidectomy would induce remissions in men with prostatic cancers.[5]

Principle

In simple words, it is necessary to find a target in the neoplastic cell that is critical for the growth of the tumor and to block that pathway.

There are two principles in the destruction of cancer cells by modification of their endocrine status:

1. Hormone deprivation
2. Hormone interference

The concept of *hormone dependence* and independence came into picture with the help of studies done on prostate cancer. There is a fundamental difference between a normal hormonal target cell and its hormone responsive malignant derivative. In a normal cell of origin, supporting hormones act as catalysts of growth and metabolism, but these compounds are not essential for life of the cell. In contrast, a hormone-dependent cancer cell dies when supporting hormones are blocked or their source is removed. A cancer cell cannot then participate in cellular growth cycles characteristic of the normal cell of origin created by alternately administering and withholding supporting hormone. In many hormone-dependent cancers, like the breast, the prostate and others, the supporting hormones are of cardinal importance in maintaining the life of the malignant cell. This is the principle of cancer control by hormone deprivation or antagonism.

Malignant cells can also be controlled by supplying large amounts of hormones; this is the novel principle of *hormone interference*. Hormone interference causes severe damage or death of cancer through toxicity in the cancer cell while normal cells are relatively undamaged. Not all cancers that regress from hormone deprivation also regress from excessive amounts of the same hormones. An example is the clinical regression of some estrogen receptor (ER) positive breast tumors after administration of high dose estrogen. Thus, breast cancer can regress from either hormone deprivation or hormone interference from excess of hormones. Although the relation of hormones to the origin of these cancers is unknown, the role of hormones in their subsequent growth is of considerable practical importance.

Endocrine therapies are directed at either reducing the synthesis of ligand for the receptor or blocking the receptors present on the tumor cells of hormone-dependent tumors.

The therapies available to block hormone receptor mediated tumor growth are based on two principles:

1. Ligand depletion: Ligand depletion can be achieved surgically by removing the source of hormone production, use of luteinizing hormone releasing hormone (LHRH) analogs leading to decreased production of trophic hormones at pituitary gland or inhibitors of enzymes involved in steroid hormone biosynthesis or by interfering with the feedback mechanisms of sex hormone synthesis at the pituitary/hypothalamic level.
2. Blockade of sex hormone receptor function by use of receptor blockers antihormonal agents.

MOLECULAR EFFECTS OF HORMONAL THERAPIES

Effect on Cell Cycle Regulatory Molecules

Antiestrogens can lead to growth inhibition by arresting the cell cycle in G0/G1 phase.[8,9] Antiestrogenic inhibition of tumor growth in vivo has been reported to result primarily from cell loss that is not cell cycle phase specific.[10] Progression of the cell cycle is governed by the sequential activation of a family of cyclin dependent kinases (CDKs) with the consequent phosphorylation and activation of specific substrates to allow progression through checkpoints in the cell cycle. Since normal physiological regulation of cell cycle progression by extracellular stimuli, including growth factors and steroid hormones, is mediated during G1 phase, the major interactions controlling G1 progression are a central focus to restrict tumor growth.[11-14]

Antiestrogens result in a time dependent decrease in retinoblastoma protein phosphorylation (pRb), thus leading to increased concentrations of hypophosphorylated form, which is growth inhibitory.[15] These early changes in pRb lead to decrease in percentage of S phase cells within several hours. Thus, given the known function of pRb in controlling progression through G1 to S phase, early decreases in the degree of pRb may be central to the inhibition of entry into S phase that is the ultimate consequence of antiestrogen action. Further support for this conclusion is provided by experiments where cells' growth arrested with antiestrogen for 48 hours were "rescued" by addition of estradiol. This resulted in the synchronous entry of cells into S phase within 12 hours, and the proportion of cells in S phase reaching a maximum of 60% at 24 hours.[16,17]

Effect on Cell Cycle Progression

In ER positive breast tumor cells, antiestrogens decrease the rate of thymidine incorporation into the DNA and inhibit the proliferation of cancer cells by acting as growth inhibitory signals. Antiestrogens are predominantly cytostatic in nature rather than cytotoxic and they lead to arrest of cells in the early G1 phase of the cell cycle, with decrease in the relative proportion of tumor cells synthesizing S phase DNA.[8-10] The actively dividing cells are sensitive to antiestrogen mediated growth inhibition. On the other hand, the proportion of dividing cells is decreased in plateau phase of tumor growth, thus rendering them relatively insensitive to antiestrogens. The exact state where cells are arrested, i.e. in G0 or G, does not involve permanent exit from the cell cycle as ligands, such as estrogen (but not other growth factors), can reinitiate the cell cycle. Experiments have shown that reversible inhibition of cell cycle in G0/G1 phase by antiestrogens treated cells can be rescued by use of estrogens, leading to progression of tumor cells into S phase of cell cycle.[18,19]

BREAST CANCER

Estrogens and Breast Tumor

During the evolution of malignant transformation in a cell, the receptors undergo modifications and the cell may retain all or only part of the normal receptor sites. If the receptor is expressed on tumor cell, the growth and function of it is capable of being regulated by the hormonal environment as in normal tissue; however, if the receptor expression is lost or modified due to malignant transformation, the cell is no longer recognized as a target cell by circulating hormones. The absence of specific hormonal receptors on breast tumor tissue indicates hormonal autonomy, thus aiding in selecting breast cancer patients who will benefit from hormonal therapy.

Estrogens act directly to promote growth and differentiation of normal breast tissue. However, estrogen also stimulates the release of prolactin from the pituitary gland, which acts on the breast tissue. Estrogens cannot support breast cancer growth in the absence of a pituitary gland, whereas prolactin can lead to growth of normal breast tissue and tumor, even in the absence of ovaries and adrenals. Estrogens are therefore considered to play only a secondary role in breast tumor growth and regression by some. Another important effect is regression of breast cancer following pharmacologic (high) doses of estrogen. This paradoxical effect of estrogen is due to interference with stimulation of growth by prolactin. This effect can be overcome by increasing the levels of endogenous or exogenous prolactin. Ovaries are the primary site for estrogen secretion, but significant levels of estrogen are also produced by postmenopausal women. The adrenal glands are an important site for steroidogenesis in postmenopausal women. Huggins and Bergenstal found that adrenalectomy, cause regression of metastatic breast and prostate cancer.[20] Hypophysectomy is also effective but is not practiced because of high morbidity and patients are to be maintained on corticosteroids. In fact, high doses of corticosteroids alone are able to control adrenal steroidogenesis. The findings that the steroid androstenedione is converted to estrone in postmenopausal women and that there was significant local production of estrogens by aromatization in peripheral tissue in breast cancer patients, provided a rationale to explain the efficacy of aromatase inhibitors (AI) as therapeutic agents in breast cancer.

Estrogen Receptor

Estrogen receptor manipulation should be considered in light of hormone dependence in breast cancer. When malignant transformation occurs, the cell may retain all or only part of the normal repertoire of receptor sites. If cell retains the receptor sites, its growth and function is potentially capable of being regulated by the hormonal environment as in a normal cell; however, if receptors are lost from the cell as a consequence of malignant transformation, it is no longer recognized as a target by circulating hormones and endocrine control is absent. This could explain why patients fail to respond to endocrine therapy if their tumors lack ER.

Receptor assay at the time of biopsy or surgery can be used to determine whether an endocrine therapy should be a part of the neoadjuvant or adjuvant regimen. One could choose to include pharmacological doses of androgen or estrogen. If the primary tumor or a biopsy of metastatic tissue reveals ER, then an endocrine therapy is must as part of the overall therapeutic schedule.

If estrogen and androgen are essential to cause the growth of breast and prostate cancers, then antagonist drugs that block hormone action would be valuable therapeutic agents. The discovery of antiestrogens was the next step in treatment of hormone-dependent breast tumor.

The use of tamoxifen in breast cancer was the next big step. Jensen proposed the use of ER assay to identify women who are likely to be benefitted by hormonal treatment lead to use of tamoxifen in them.[21] It is now known that tamoxifen is more likely to enhance the survival of women with ER-positive tumors and prevents the development of ER-positive breast cancer. Tamoxifen is not only predominantly used as the first-line therapy in metastatic breast cancer, but it has also been used in adjuvant treatment. In addition to tamoxifen and other nonsteroidal antiestrogens, steroidal antiestrogens have been described that exhibit pure antagonist activity, in contrast to the partial antagonist properties of tamoxifen. Such compounds are potentially more potent than tamoxifen and show efficacy in tumors resistant to tamoxifen. Thus antiestrogens of various structural classes with differing tissue specific estrogen agonist/antagonist properties are established and have an expanding role in the management of breast cancer patients.[22]

Tamoxifen is effective in premenopausal patients despite increases in circulating estrogen due to interruption of the hypothalamic pituitary axis feedback. Decreasing levels of estrogens from the ovary lead to reflex rise in secretion of gonadotropins due to negative feedback loop of the hypothalamic-pituitary axis. AIs are not used in premenopausal women because the powerful action of gonadotropins can reverse ovarian aromatase blockade. Another strategy used in premenopausal women, is to use sustained release preparations of LHRH agonists to cause desensitization of the pituitary gland or to use LHRH antagonist to block gonadotropins release. As a result, the reduction in gonadotropins causes a medical oophorectomy. Combination of LHRH agonist and an antiestrogen effectively decreases the availability of estrogen to the tumor, as with the combination of LHRH agonist and AIs.

Although steroidogenesis in ovary of reproductive age women derives from feedback regulated axes as in the male, the steroid and germ cell production in the female is cyclical. Since estrogen is the major hormone providing negative feedback, inhibition of aromatase (by AIs) will increase LH and follicle stimulating hormone (FSH) production, which increases aromatase expression in an effort to overcome the blockade. Gonadectomy will cause LH and FSH to rise and androgen or estrogen replacement lowers LH but not FSH, since inhibin B remains absent. Similarly, natural menopause occurs when all follicles and thus granulosa cells are depleted, and estradiol production falls while LH and more specifically FSH rise. Long-acting GnRH agonists act by desensitizing the pituitary gonadotropes and suppressing LH (and FSH) and therefore testosterone and estrogen synthesis. Supraphysiologic doses of exogenous androgens and estrogens or progestins also lower LH, testosterone, and estrogen estradiol (E2) production but not FSH and also exert direct hormone actions on the body.

The postmenopausal ovary makes little or no estrogen, and estrogen derived from androgen precursors [dehydroepiandrosterone (DHEAS, AD)] of ovarian and adrenal origin. The aromatase enzyme in postmenopausal women is expressed mainly in adipose tissues, including those of the breast, but also in breast cancers themselves. Since LH and FSH, which are already elevated in postmenopausal women, do not regulate aromatase expression in these tissues, the potent, irreversible AIs used clinically are very effective in suppressing E2 synthesis in postmenopausal women and treating ER-positive breast cancers in these women.

When AIs are administered to premenopausal women, estrogen decreases only transiently, and subsequently a new steady-state is reached. The use of AIs in premenopausal women with ER+ breast cancer would be ineffective, unless combined with therapy to prevent overcoming the blockade. Such treatments might include surgical or chemical oophorectomy and suppression of LH and FSH with high-dose progestins or long-acting GnRH agonists or antagonists. The benefit of "total estrogen blockade" in premenopausal women with ER+ breast cancers using leuprorelin and anastrozole can also be used. Because AI therapy in women who have ceased menses for over 12 months and thus are clinically menopausal effectively suppresses E2 and eliminates most negative feedback on the gonadotropes, LH and FSH might rise even higher. In some women, this gonadotropin surge, which mimics the mid-cycle surge, induces ovulation and/or menses in some women. Often only one cycle is experienced, but this phenomenon, which is rather distressing to patient and doctor alike, also brings into question whether the menopausal status has been correctly assigned. Will such patients still benefit from AI therapy? In general, patients with a single episode of menstrual cycle on an AI can be considered postmenopausal, although serum estradiol measurements before and during AI therapy are required in this setting. As long as serum estradiol remains low, AI therapy remains an option.

Clinical Use in Breast Cancer

Endocrine therapy has been a mainstay for the treatment of breast and prostate cancer for decades, and receptor blockers or enzyme inhibitors are the first-line therapies of metastatic disease in recent years. Treatment strategies to eliminate production of key steroids must consider the optimal targets, alternate pathways that might bypass the blockade, and the endocrine consequences of deranged steroid flux. In many instances, combination therapies with other agents are necessary to prevent side-effects of upstream steroids and/or physiologic adaptations, which might overcome the blockades.

The antiestrogen tamoxifen, is the compound of choice for the treatment of breast cancer and was first described in 1967 by Harper and Walpole.[23] It is a triphenylethylene derivative and is structurally closely related to the well-known nonsteroidal estrogen diethylstilbestrol (DES). The pharmacology of tamoxifen is quite complex. It has partial agonistic activity and has been shown to induce uterine growth. Such compounds are described as "antiestrogens with partial agonistic activity". The balance in the expression of antagonistic and agonistic activity not only depends on the dose applied, but also the target organ looked for.

This residual estrogenic activity, which is associated with a higher incidence in endometrial carcinomas during adjuvant treatment, stimulated the search for antiestrogens with reduced agonistic activity and also increased antagonistic properties, as tamoxifen is not able to inhibit completely either the estrogen-stimulated uterine growth or the growth of breast cancers comparably to ovariectomy. New antiestrogens with improved potency and reduced estrogenic effects are discovered, but none of them have been found to be completely free of estrogenic activity, and the tumor-inhibiting effects in them are no better than those of tamoxifen. "Pure" antiestrogens have been found only recently.

A complete blockade of ER function also be achieved by use of pure antiestrogens. In contrast to AIs, pure antiestrogens are able to block ER activation by ligands other than estradiol and can also interfere with ligand-independent ER activation. In addition to estradiol, progesterone has a strong proliferative effect in breast cancer. Antiprogestins have been tried for clinical breast cancer therapy. The ability of these compounds to induce tumor cell differentiation that leads to apoptosis is unique among all other endocrine therapeutics.

Tamoxifen can lead to remissions in about 30% of the patients (approximately 60% if ER-positive). But in cases of advanced breast cancer, nearly all tumors become resistant to tamoxifen after a median duration of remission of about 18 months.[24] Tamoxifen withdrawal response characterized by partial remission on tamoxifen withdrawal, is seen in 10–30% of tamoxifen treated patients. The likely explanation is that the (partial) agonistic property of tamoxifen becomes a dominant control mechanism during the course of treatment.[25] The mechanism of resistance is due to selection of cells stimulated by tamoxifen, as against the estrogen independent cells. It is suggested that "the cause of resistance lies in the selection of cells that are stimulated by tamoxifen rather than the selection of completely estrogen independent cells".[26] These tamoxifen resistant cells are still responsive to the growth inhibitory action of pure antiestrogens. Upfront use of pure antiestrogens may be superior to tamoxifen in response rate and time to progression. Also they may lead to tumor regression in patients with progression on treatment with tamoxifen.

Further clinical trials must show whether the principle of total ER blockade is superior to other second-line therapies, especially those using AIs. It remains to be elucidated whether the properties of pure antiestrogens not only to block the action of estradiol but also, to prevent ER stimulation by other estrogenic substances (such as adrenal estrogens or phytoestrogens from dietary intake), whether constitutive ER activation without any ligand and activation resulting from the cross-talk with the growth factor signal- transduction cascade will bring a clinical benefit when compared to AIs. Finally, it is beyond question that the existing pure antiestrogens can be improved. The compounds known so far are not orally available and animal experiments reveal that quite high doses are needed to obtain good therapeutic effects. For a broad clinical application presumably a pure antiestrogen with higher efficacy and an easier mode of administration is desirable.

Principles of Hormone Treatment in Breast Cancer

- For a drug to be used, the tumor tissue must have the hormone receptors, whose action is to be modified either with the use of agonists or antagonists. There is no benefit of use of hormonal treatment in receptor negative patients.
- Responsive tumors commonly respond to subsequent hormonal manipulations after response and progression, with a previous hormone therapy.
- Response to hormonal therapy is slow (i.e. it cannot be evaluated for about 6–8 weeks).
- Fast growing tumors and/or visceral involvement respond less well to hormonal treatment.
- All hormonal agents have the potential to cause a "flare" of the disease, an apparent worsening with increased bone pain, hypercalcemia, etc. This is not necessarily an indication to discontinue the drug,

although manifestations (e.g. hypercalcemia) should be corrected. Flare reactions, when they occur, do so within the first few weeks of therapy.

- Withdrawal responses (i.e. response seen when hormone therapy is discontinued) may also be seen in hormonally responsive tumors.
- Hormone therapy has been found to be detrimental when combined with cytotoxic chemotherapy. So, there is no benefit, or even harm of combining cytotoxic chemotherapy with hormonal therapy.
- The combination of two antihormonal drugs has not shown to be superior to single drug, except for the use of hormonal agent with LHRH agonists in premenopausal women.
- Hormonal agents have proven benefit and can be used in neoadjuvant, adjuvant as well as metastatic setting.

Most of the above applies to the use of hormones in advanced breast cancer. Tamoxifen is also used as adjuvant treatment (i.e. to prevent recurrence after primary breast cancer). Today, tamoxifen is the endocrine treatment of choice for all stages of breast cancer in hormone positive premenopausal women in both adjuvant and metastatic disease. It is also approved for the reduction of the incidence of breast cancer in high-risk women.

HORMONES IN PROSTATE CANCER

Androgen receptor (AR) is the key regulator in prostate cancer, and androgen ablation is the treatment of choice for patients of advanced prostate carcinoma. Androgen ablation therapy includes, reduction of serum testosterone levels by orchidectomy, high-dose estrogens or LHRH agonists. A further step is the blockade of the AR function by use of AR antagonists such as cyproterone acetate (CPA) or flutamide.[27] The combination of serum testosterone depletion together with an antiandrogen (referred to as total androgen blockade) has been reported to show a certain benefit.[28]

Testosterone and DHT in Prostate Cancer

Circulating testosterone acts by three potential mechanisms. Binding of testosterone to androgenic receptor lead to androgenic effects in tissues such as spermatic tubules, where it stimulates sperm production. In the prostate, the enzyme 5α-reductase converts testosterone to dihydrotestosterone (DHT), which leads to formation of the prostate and male external genitalia in fetal life, and prostatic hyperplasia in old age. Similarly, aromatase enzyme in mammary tissue metabolizes testosterone to a potent E2. As testosterone and DHT control the growth of prostate cancer, so methods to block testosterone and DHT synthesis and/or action are to be envisioned. Surgical orchidectomy, DES, LHRH agonists, and AR blockers (bicalutamide) are examples of different strategies to block testicular testosterone production or action, and dutasteride inhibits conversion of testosterone to DHT by 5α-reductase enzymes. The problem with AR antagonists is that most are partial agonists or incomplete antagonists, and upregulation of LH and thus testosterone might overcome the blockade. The development of more potent compounds such as abiraterone can solve the problem. In contrast, Gonadal suppression strategies fail to address the abundant DHEAS and DHEA derived from human adrenal gland. Adrenal androgen elimination in castration resistant prostate cancer (CRPC) explains the therapeutic benefit of CYP17A1 inhibitor ketoconazole, thus decreasing the adrenal production of steroids. Similarly dexamethasone and prednisone suppress adrenocorticotropic hormone (ACTH) production and thus adrenal DHEAS production.

The major breakthrough in the field of hormone medicine was the discovery of the fact that pulsatile release of a small peptide, known as LHRH, regulates the secretion of LH and FSH. The findings that the pituitary gland becomes rapidly desensitized by prolonged stimulation with LHRH leading to decreased production of LH and FSH. Sustained release preparations of highly potent LHRH agonist analogs effectively produce a medical oophorectomy and block testicular androgen synthesis in men and ovarian estrogen synthesis in women (Fig. 1). The application of sustained release preparations used to treat premenopausal breast cancer and prostate cancer is now known to be an effective therapy, thereby avoiding surgical procedures and endocrine ablation. Hormones or orchidectomy are generally used in symptomatic metastatic prostate cancer.

The first antiandrogen was steroidal compound CPA. CPA is able to antagonize the testosterone stimulated growth of the normal prostate in the orchidectomized man and also inhibit the growth of prostate tumors. As it also has progestational activity, it interferes with the feedback mechanism and thereby inhibits LH secretion and so lowers testosterone production.[29] On the other hand bicalutamide is a "pure" antiandrogen (nonsteroid), which strongly inhibits testosterone stimulated growth of the prostate, but has inhibitory effects inferior to those of CPA.[30] Bicalutamide also blocks the ARs present in brain, leading to stimulation of LH secretion and

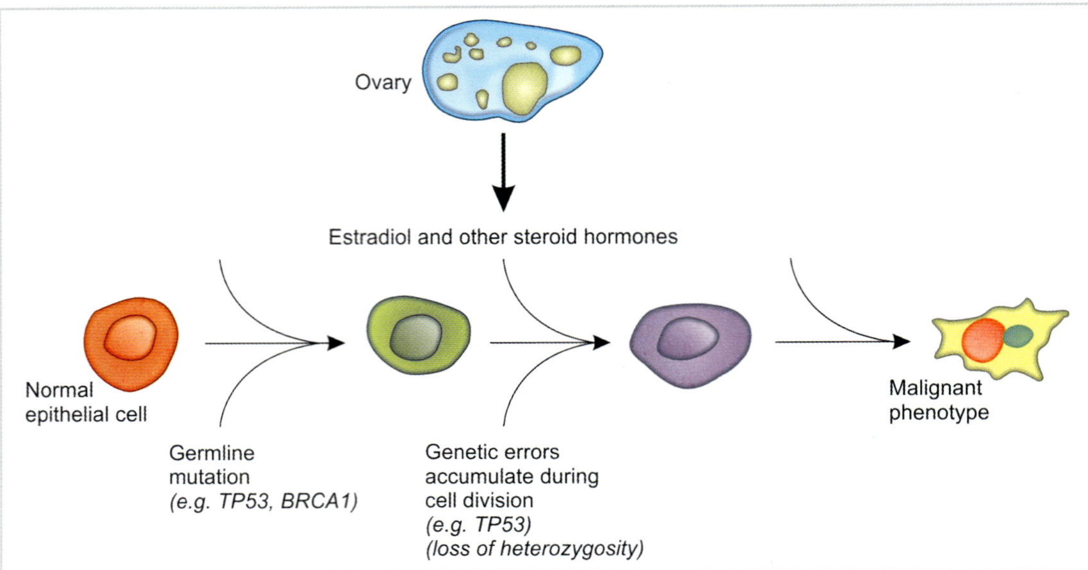

Fig. 1: Pathological basis of hormone induced cancers

increased testosterone levels. Bicalutamide is to be used in the clinic in combination with orchidectomy or LHRH agonists, as the testosterone increasing properties of this antiandrogen are counteracted.[31] In this regards CPA is an ideal antiandrogen, as it only acts at the level of the AR as an antagonist, and also lowers testosterone production.[29]

After the initial response to androgen deprivation, nearly all patients progress within 6–24 months of therapy.[32] In prostate tumors that have progressed on androgen ablation the AR is often overexpressed. It is now clear that most of the relapsed prostatic carcinomas and even the bone metastases of these tumors still contain AR and that these receptor levels even tend to be enhanced.[33] Other mechanism is the presence of mutates AR, which can be activated by adrenal steroids, estrogens, progestins and even antiandrogens. Thus, progression of tumors in the presence of androgen ablation therapies can be due to acquired androgen hypersensitivity or AR activation by ligands other than DHT. The third mechanism may be the acquisition of autocrine pathways such as activation of epidermal, fibroblast growth factor, mTOR or PIK3 pathways. Surgical or medical orchidectomy, prevents the synthesis of testicular androgens, but the synthesis of adrenal androgens that can be peripherally converted to active forms is not affected. The activation of AR by growth factors induces androgen dependent genes and expression of the endogenous PSA gene in cells. So, these AR dependent effects are observed even in the absence of androgens. This ligand-independent AR activation of prostate cancer by growth factors is unlikely to be antagonized by therapies to reduce serum testosterone levels (orchidectomy, LHRH).

Antiandrogen Withdrawal Syndrome

It has been shown that patients with advanced prostate cancer that initially responded following flutamide treatment and underwent tumor progression showed a remission following the withdrawal of the antiandrogens.[34] This paradox shows that the tumor progression might not be caused by an outgrowth of hormone independent tumor cells, but by pathways other than the classical ones and can be stimulated even with antiandrogens. It implies that, even after relapse on androgen ablation therapies, the AR still plays a major role in progression of cancer cells. So AR still remains a target for relapsed prostate cancer.

None of the antiandrogens known so far decrease the levels of their receptor. Antiandrogens that effectively reduce the AR levels, as is the case for the pure antiestrogens and the ER, could be superior blockers of all AR-mediated effects. In tumors where the AR is the key mediator of cell growth, an effective elimination of the AR could be the ideal way to suppress cancer progression. With improved therapeutic modalities a complete blockade of all AR-mediated functions that contribute to tumor cell proliferation should be achieved. Effective blockade of AR activity cannot be achieved by a more complete reduction of serum testosterone levels, and that a compound that directly interacts with the AR may be better. Such an AR blocker is highly effective being able to block the AR even if the cells are androgen hypersensitive.

Endocrine Combination Therapy

As with cytotoxic chemotherapy, the future of hormonal therapy lies in combination of antihormonal agents. In prostate cancer antiandrogens are combined with LHRH agonists or surgical orchidectomy. Although in breast cancer combinations hormonal agents are not routinely used,[35] but presently the combinations of AIs with LHRH agonists in premenopausal women and AIs with fulvestrant in postmenopausal women is being used increasingly. As breast cancers are stimulated by estrogens and progestins, a combination of antiestrogens and antiprogestins is obvious. In one of the studies using an antiprogestin together with an antiestrogen, either tamoxifen or a pure antiestrogen, it was found that the tumor-inhibitory effects of such a combination is superior to those of either therapy alone.[36] But still the regular use of combination of antiestrogen and antiprogestins is not practiced.

Principles of Hormone Treatment in Prostate Cancer

- There is no benefit of checking for hormone receptor expression in prostate cancer as cells have cytoplasmic expression of androgen expression.
- Hormone treatment can be used in neoadjuvant, adjuvant and advanced settings of prostate cancer.
- Blockage of testosterone production (either surgical or medical orchidectomy) is the mainstay of treatment of advanced prostate cancer. All of the further treatment must include the component of orchidectomy. There is no benefit of any treatment in the absence of orchidectomy.
- In contrast to breast cancer, responses to sequential hormonal therapies in prostate cancer are less common.
- As in breast cancer, there is no benefit of combining two hormonal therapies at a single time, except for the use of LHRH to suppress testosterone production along with the androgen blockade.
- Response to hormonal therapy is slow (i.e. for about 6–8 weeks).
- All hormonal agents have the potential to cause a "flare" of the disease, an apparent worsening with increased bone pain, hypercalcemia, etc. Care should be taken while starting treatment in patients with signs of spinal cord compression or urinary tract obstruction. This is not necessarily an indication to discontinue the drug. Flare reactions, when they occur, do so within the first few weeks of therapy.
- Withdrawal responses (i.e. response seen when hormone therapy is discontinued) may also be seen in hormonally responsive tumors.
- Hormone therapy has not shown any benefit when combined with chemotherapy. But, as per the basic principle, medical orchidectomy with LHRH agonist is to be maintained continuously even for the patients on chemotherapy.

Bicalutamide is an antiandrogen that inhibits either androgen uptake into cells or the binding of androgen in the nucleus of target cells. Bicalutamide thus blocks the effects of both testicular and adrenal androgen. It may thus be used in combination with an LHRH agonist to achieve "total androgen blockade". Initial treatment with LHRH agonists results in an increase in gonadotropin secretion. This can cause a "flare", which can be dangerous in patients with impending spinal cord compression or urinary tract obstruction. Bicalutamide is used to block this initial flare. Bicalutamide may also be used alone as hormonal therapy in symptomatic metastatic prostate cancer.

HORMONAL USE IN OTHER TUMORS

As already mentioned, there are a variety of tumors besides breast and prostate cancer expressing steroid hormone receptors. It has been shown for gynecological tumors, i.e. endometrial carcinoma where high-dose progestins are used clinically, whereas use of tamoxifen has been disappointing.[37] Similarly in brain tumors like meningiomas, a large number of progesterone receptors are found.[38] Few small clinical studies have shown that the antiprogestin mifepristone can lead to remissions of these meningiomas. In melanomas, ER has also been demonstrated. A combination of dacarbazine with the antiestrogen tamoxifen proved to cause a longer survival than dacarbazine alone.[39] Hepatocellular carcinoma is predominantly diagnosed in male patients, and use of the antiandrogen CPA has been reported to lead to responses in this tumor type. Other tumors expressing hormone receptors are colorectal carcinomas and carcinomas of the stomach.[40] Such receptors have been detected even in lung cancer. This could open a wide field of preclinical and later clinical research to obtain treatment modalities that do not have the serious side-effects of cytotoxics, especially in an adjuvant setting or in combination with established treatments. Also, the discovery of selective ER modulation with tamoxifen and raloxifene and the demonstration that tamoxifen and raloxifene have estrogen-like effects on bone but antiestrogenic effect on the breast has opened the door to new opportunities for the discovery of novel compounds to treat a number of diseases associated with the menopause such as osteoporosis, coronary heart disease, and breast and endometrial cancers.

NEWER PERSPECTIVES

Recently a number of groups including ours have become interested in innovative use of endocrine and other therapies in the perioperative period. This has been motivated by observations that primary breast cancer surgery during the luteal phase of the menstrual cycle has been shown to result in superior long term outcomes. A randomized trial to test this hypothesis was conducted at Tata Memorial Hospital wherein an injection of progesterone was administered just prior to primary surgery in an attempt to recapitulate the luteal phase.[40] While the result in the total trial population showed no effect of this intervention, an analysis in lymph node positive population showed a significant improvement in both the disease-free and overall survival. A number of other innovative strategies are currently under evaluation at our and other centers.

REFERENCES

1. Jemal A, Bray F, Center MM, et al. Global Cancer Statistics. CA Cancer J Clin. 2011;61:69-90.
2. Beatson GT. On the treatment of inoperable cases of carcinoma of the mamma: Suggestions for a new method of treatment, with illustrative cases. Lancet. 1896;2:10-7, 162-5.
3. Loeb L. Further Investigations on the Origin of Tumors in Mice: VI. Internal Secretion as a Factor in the Origin of Tumors. J Med Res. 1919;40:477-96.
4. Lacassagne A. Compt. rend. Acad. d. sc. 195: 630, 1932.
5. Huggins C, Hodges CV. Studies on prostatic cancer: I. The effect of castration, of estrogen, and of androgen injection on serum phosphatases in metastatic carcinoma of the prostate, 1941. J Urol. 2002;168:9-12.
6. Bittner JJ. Possible Relationship of the estrogenic hormones, genetic susceptibility, and milk influence in the production of mammary cancer in mice. Cancer Res. 1942;2:710-21.
7. Furth J. A meeting of ways in cancer research: thoughts on the evolution and nature of neoplasms. Cancer Res. 1959;19:241-58.
8. Musgrove EA, Wakeling AE, Sutherland RL. Points of action of estrogen antagonists and a calmodulin antagonist within the MCF-7 human breast cancer cell cycle. Cancer Res. 1989;49: 2398-404.
9. Sutherland RL, Reddel RR, Green MD. Effects of oestrogens on cell proliferation and cell cycle kinetics. A hypothesis on the cell cycle effects of antioestrogens. Eur J Cancer Clin Oncol. 1983;19:307-18.
10. Sutherland RL, Hall RE, Taylor IW. Cell proliferation kinetics of MCF-7 human mammary carcinoma cells in culture and effects of tamoxifen on exponentially growing and plateau-phase cells. Cancer Res. 1983;43:3998-4006.
11. Grana X, Reddy EP. Cell cycle control in mammalian cells: role of cyclins, cyclin dependent kinases (CDKs), growth suppressor genes and cyclin-dependent kinase inhibitors (CKIs). Oncogene. 1995;11:211-9.
12. Sherr CJ. Cancer cell cycles. Science. 1996;274:1672-7.
13. Sutherland RL, Prall OW, Watts CK, et al. Estrogen and progestin regulation of cell cycle progression. J Mammary Gland Biol Neoplasia. 1998;3:63-72.
14. Sherr CJ. G1 phase progression: cycling on cue. Cell. 1994;79: 551-5.
15. Riley DJ, Lee EY, Lee WH. The retinoblastoma protein: more than a tumor suppressor. Annu Rev Cell Biol. 1994;10:1-29.
16. Prall OW, Rogan EM, Musgrove EA, et al. c-Myc or cyclin D1 mimics estrogen effects on cyclin E-Cdk2 activation and cell cycle reentry. Mol Cell Biol. 1998;18:4499-508.
17. Prall OW, Sarcevic B, Musgrove EA, et al. Estrogen-induced activation of Cdk4 and Cdk2 during G1-S phase progression is accompanied by increased cyclin D1 expression and decreased cyclin-dependent kinase inhibitor association with cyclin E-Cdk2. J Biol Chem. 1997;272:10882-94.
18. Lippman ME, Bolan G. Oestrogen-responsive human breast cancer in long term tissue culture. Nature. 1975;256:592-3.
19. Lippman M, Bolan G, Huff K. The effects of estrogens and antiestrogens on hormone responsive human breast cancer in long-term tissue culture. Cancer Res. 1976;36:4595-601.
20. Huggins C, Bergenstal DM. Inhibition of human mammary and prostatic cancers by adrenalectomy. Cancer Res. 1952;12: 134-41.
21. Jensen EV, Block GE, Smith S, et al. Estrogen receptors and breast cancer response to adrenalectomy. In: Hall TC (Ed). Prediction of Response in Cancer Therapy. Washington DC: National Cancer Institute Monographs; 1971. pp. 55-70.
22. Jensen EV, Jacobson HI. Basic guides to the mechanism of estrogen action. Recent Prog Horm Res. 1962;18:378-414.
23. Harper MJ, Walpole AL. A new derivative of triphenylethylene: effect on implantation and mode of action in rats. J Reprod Fertil. 1967;13:101-19.
24. DeFriend DJ, Howell A, Nicholson RI, et al. Investigation of a new pure antiestrogen (ICI 182780) in women with primary breast cancer. Cancer Res. 1994;54:408-14.

25. Nicholson RI, Francis AB, McClelland RA, et al. Pure anti-oestrogens (ICI 164384 and ICI 182780) and breast cancer: is the attainment of complete oestrogen withdrawal worthwhile? Endocr Relat Cancer. 1994;1:5-17.

26. Steinberg GD, Isaacs JT. Pharmacological approaches to the management of metastatic prostatic cancer. In: Hickman JA, Tritton TR (Eds). Cancer Chemotherapy. London: Blackwell. 1993; pp 322-43.

27. Labrie F, Bélanger A, Dupont A, et al. Science behind total androgen blockade: from gene to combination therapy. Clin Invest Med. 1993;16:475-92.

28. Patterson JS. Clinical aspects and development of antioestrogen therapy: a review of the endocrine effects of tamoxifen in animals and man. J Endocrinol. 1981;89 Suppl: 67P-75P.

29. Neumann F. Pharmacological basis for clinical use of antiandrogens. J Steroid Biochem. 1983;19:391-402.

30. El Etreby MF, Habenicht UF, Louton T, et al. Effect of cyproterone acetate in comparison to flutamide and megestrol acetate on the ventral prostate, seminal vesicle, and adrenal glands of adult male rats. Prostate. 1987;11:361-75.

31. Tucker H. Non-steroidal anti-androgens in the treatment of prostate cancer. Drug Future. 1990;15:255-65.

32. Crawford ED, Eisenberger MA, McLeod DG, et al. A controlled trial of leuprolide with and without flutamide in prostatic carcinoma. N Engl J Med. 1989;321:419-24.

33. Ruizeveld de Winter JA, Janssen PJ, Sleddens HM, et al. Androgen receptor status in localized and locally progressive hormone refractory human prostate cancer. Am J Pathol. 1994;144:735-46.

34. Scher HI, Kelly WK. Flutamide withdrawal syndrome: its impact on clinical trials in hormone-refractory prostate cancer. J Clin Oncol. 1993;11:1566-72.

35. Muss HB. Endocrine therapy for advanced breast cancer: a review. Breast Cancer Res Treat. 1992;21:15-26.

36. Nishino Y, Schneider MR, Michna H. Enhancement of the antitumor efficacy of the antiprogestin, onapristone, by combination with the antiestrogen, ICI 164384. J Cancer Res Clin Oncol. 1994;120:298-302.

37. Horvath G, Stendahl U, Kalling M, et al. Antiestrogenic treatment of advanced and recurrent carcinoma corpus uteri—a phase II study of toremifene. Anticancer Res. 1990;10:323-5.

38. Huisman TW, Tanghe HL, Koper JW, et al. Progesterone, oestradiol, somatostatin and epidermal growth factor receptors on human meningiomas and their CT characteristics. Eur J Cancer. 1991;27:1453-7.

39. Schneider MR. Hormone antagonists: discovery of steroid hormones for specific cancer therapy. Arch Pharm (Weinheim). 1993;326:769-84.

40. Badwe R, Hawaldar R, Parmar V, et al. Single-injection depot progesterone before surgery and survival in women with operable breast cancer: a randomized controlled trial. J Clin Oncol. 2011;29(21):2845-51.

12 Genetics and Cancer

Rajiv Sarin

GENETICS OF SPORADIC AND HEREDITARY CANCERS

All cancers are biologically a "genetic disease" due to the universal finding of alterations or mutations in genes and/or chromosomes in all types and stages of cancers. Unlike other diseases where the term "genetic" implies a hereditary or congenital condition, for cancer the term "genetic" refers to its molecular pathology and not necessarily its hereditary nature. Any cancer is described as a "hereditary cancer" when it presents as a classical Mendelian inherited disease, as a "familial cancer" when some family history of cancer is present but insufficient to be classified as a Mendelian disorder or as "sporadic cancer" in the absence of any family history of malignancy. The Mendelian inheritance of cancer is generally autosomal dominant, inherited from either maternal or paternal family. Some rare inherited cancer predisposition syndromes are autosomal recessive with both parents being carriers of a recessive mutation.

Hereditary cancers arise from germline mutation in one of the few dozen high penetrance cancer predisposition genes.[1] These germline mutations are usually inherited from either or both parents but sometimes it is a de novo (new) germline mutation that was not present earlier in the family. Germline mutations are present in all the body (somatic) cells of a carrier. Some of the cells in a specific organ of a germline mutation carrier acquire additional genetic alterations and this could trigger the development of cancer. The germline mutations can be passed down to offspring resulting in Mendelian inheritance of cancer. In nonfamilial or sporadic cancers, the genetic alterations occur in a cell (somatic mutation) which becomes cancerous. As somatic mutations are passed down to the daughter somatic cells, but not to the germ cells, the cancer risk is not passed on to the offspring of the patient with sporadic cancer. Depending on their normal role in cell growth and its regulation and how they cause cancer, the cancer-associated genes are classified as "tumor suppressor genes" or "proto-oncogenes".

Over the last few decades, knowledge of specific somatic and germline gene mutations and chromosomal alterations in diverse cancers has helped in molecular subclassification and targeted therapy in few cancers. It has also helped in confirmation of the hereditary nature of some cancers and appropriate genetic counseling for surveillance and cancer prevention in mutation carriers. General principles of the genetic basis of cancer, the tumor suppressor genes and oncogenes will be discussed here with focus on the clinical and laboratory genetics as relevant to hereditary cancers.

BURDEN OF HEREDITARY CANCERS

A series of large epidemiological studies have established that 2–5% of all cancers in the Caucasian population are hereditary. Moreover, 10–20% of cancers are termed familial due to some family history of cancer but not exhibiting classical Mendelian inheritance or syndromic features. In developing countries, hereditary cancers are more likely to be underreported due to lack of awareness as well as specialized cancer genetics services. Many hereditary cancers present without a strong family history or characteristic external phenotypic features and can be diagnosed as hereditary only with detailed clinical genetics assessment and/or genetic testing. Considering a conservative estimate of only 2% cancer cases being hereditary, the total number of new hereditary cancers in India will be 20,000 per year. The number of individuals requiring counseling, clinical and genetic evaluation with or without genetic testing would be several fold higher as all the first degree relatives of persons with hereditary cancer could possibly benefit with such evaluation.[2] There are only a few reports from the developing countries of small cohorts of hereditary cancer families and their mutation spectrum in hereditary breast-ovarian cancer syndrome (HBOC) and hereditary colorectal cancers.[3-14] In the largest Indian cohort of 1,500 families with diverse hereditary cancer syndromes registered at the Tata Memorial Hospital, Mumbai, HBOC and hereditary colorectal cancers are the most common hereditary cancers and account for 60% of all hereditary cancer families (unpublished data). With increasing awareness about the condition among physicians and the public there is increasing referral of such families for evaluation and genetic counseling. The cancer genetics clinic at the Tata Memorial Hospital is presently registering 500 new hereditary cancer families each year (Box 1).

GENETIC MECHANISM OF CANCER DEVELOPMENT: MULTISTEP CARCINOGENESIS AND GENOMIC INSTABILITY

Malignant transformation or carcinogenesis whether occurring spontaneously or due to a known carcinogen, is a long multistep process with three major steps of initiation, promotion and progression. Each stage of malignant transformation has its unique set of cellular dysfunction and genetic alterations. One of the most widely accepted model of multistep carcinogenesis has been propounded by Fearon and Vogelstein.[15] Using the example of colonic carcinoma arising from adenomatous polyps, they proposed that for cancer to develop from a normal cell, it should acquire and accumulate over a period of time deleterious mutations in approximately 5–10 key tumor suppressor genes or oncogenes (Fig. 1).

Through a series of genetic alterations, cancer cells acquire certain traits that are considered as hallmarks of cancer[16] and required for the cancer cell to grow continuously and eventually metastasize. In the "clonal theory" of cancer, a normal cell that has undergone the process of malignant transformation gets selective growth advantage and through clonal expansion develops into a malignant tumor. In its natural history each tumor develops sub-clones with wider molecular and phenotypic heterogeneity.

Most cancers also show various degrees of "genomic instability" which is characterized by chromosomal aberrations, copy number variation, mutations and loss of heterozygozity (LOH) in the tumor. Often, it is difficult to determine if genomic instability is the cause of cancer or the effect of cancer. In certain hereditary cancer syndromes, such as the hereditary nonpolyposis colon cancer (HNPCC), cancer development is driven by the genomic instability due to the underlying inherited defect in deoxyribonucleic acid (DNA) mismatch repair genes.[17] In contrast, genomic instability in sporadic cancer is due

Box 1: High index of suspicion for a cancer being hereditary if one or more feature is present

- History of any cancer in two or more relatives on maternal or paternal side of the family
- Cancer occurring at unusually young age, generally a decade or two before the usual age
- Multifocal or bilateral or multiple primary cancer in an individual
- Cutaneous, ophthalmic, endoscopic or radiological feature of cancer syndrome

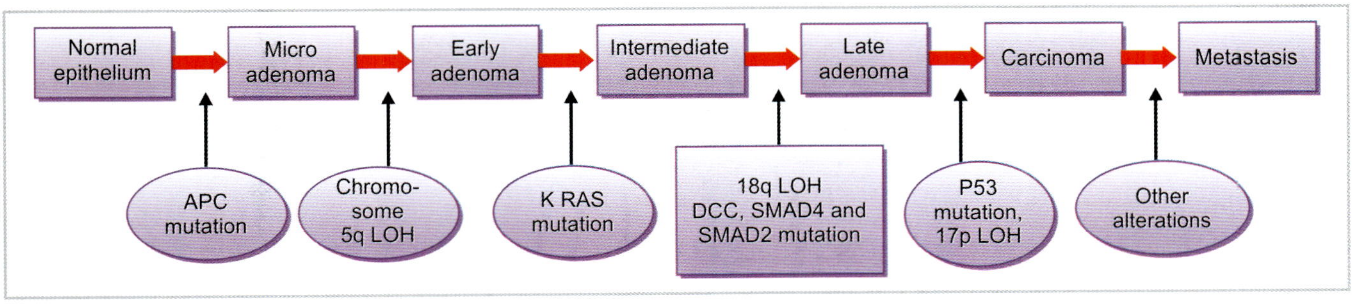

Fig. 1: Stepwise carcinogenesis model for colorectal cancer by Vogelstein

TABLE 1: Tumor suppressor genes and oncogenes

	Proto-oncogenes	*Tumor suppressor genes (TSG)*
Examples	RET, MYC, K-RAS, EGFR	TP53, BRCA1/2, RB, APC, MLH1
Normal cellular function	Oncogenes, which are the activated form of Proto-oncogenes are key cell signaling genes which drive cell division or proliferation under specific physiological and pathological conditions	They control the integrity of cell division and DNA repair or induce programmed cell death when required. Various TSGs control cell cycle progression (RB), apoptosis (TP53) or DNA damage repair (BRCA1 or MLH1)
Effect of mutation on cellular function	Sustained and uncontrolled growth that is a prerequisite for cancer	Inefficient apoptosis, DNA damage repair or cell cycle control promotes cancer development and progression
Type of Mutations and alleles affected for deleterious effect	**Gain-in-Function** mutation in one allele (usually point mutation at specific loci) or gene amplification	**Loss-of-Function** mutation of both alleles (Knudson's two hit model) by chromosomal deletion, frameshift, nonsense or missense mutation
Therapeutic exploitation of mutations	Inhibitors against signaling molecules and growth factors, e.g. imatinib, trastuzumab	Enhanced platinum sensitivity and synthetic lethality with PARP inhibitors for BRCA1 mutations

to accumulation of several gene alterations during the course of malignant transformation and progression.

TUMOR SUPPRESSOR GENES AND ONCOGENES

As their names suggest, these genes when dysfunctional are associated with cancer development and progression. In simple terms, the normal function of tumor suppressor genes (TSGs) is to control the integrity of cell division and DNA repair or induce programmed cell death when required. Similarly, oncogenes, which are the activated form of proto-oncogenes, are cellular growth signals that drive cell division or proliferation (Table 1). Various TSGs control cell cycle progression (e.g. *RB*), apoptosis (e.g. *TP53*) or DNA damage repair (e.g. *BRCA1* or *MLH1*). Various oncogenes regulate signaling pathways of cell proliferation and cell cycle control (e.g. *MYC, RAS, RET* or *EGFR*, etc.). Whereas, genetic alterations (mutations or chromosomal alterations) in oncogenes cause cancer by gain-in-function, TSGs are implicated in cancer due to mutations which cause their loss-of-function. These mutations or chromosomal alterations result in major changes in the length, conformation or interaction of the aberrant protein coded by them which affects its normal activity. These genetic mechanisms are operational in sporadic as well as hereditary cancers. In addition to the background chromosomal alterations observed in cancers in general, the most frequently mutated gene in diverse tumors is *TP53*.[18] Rarely the mutation in *TP53* is inherited as a germline mutation which gives rise to strong inherited predisposition to a range of early onset cancers as part of the Li-Fraumeni syndrome (LFS). The TSGs are also described as "gatekeeper genes" which control critical check points in the cell cycle (*TP53, APC, RB*, etc.) or the "caretaker genes" which maintain genomic integrity through efficient DNA repair (*BRCA1*, nucleotide excision repair and the mismatch repair genes).

Mutations in specific domains of oncogenes or creation of fusion genes by specific translocations of some key genes result in gain of function and constitutive activation of mechanisms controlling cell proliferation. Somatic mutations or overexpression in one or more oncogenes is present in almost all cancers and in some cancers it has prognostic or therapeutic implications. It provides sustained growth stimulus in the primary tumor and metastases. The clinically relevant examples include point mutations in phosphate binding loop of *KRAS* in pancreatic, colon and lung cancer; catalytic kinase domain of *EGFR* in head and neck, lung, and pancreatic cancers; overexpression of *C-ERBB2* in breast cancer and the *BCR-ABL* fusion gene in chronic myeloid leukemia (CML).[1] *RET* is the only example of an oncogene with inheritable germline mutation, which causes the multiple endocrine neoplasia-2 (MEN-2) syndrome.

THE TWO-HIT MODEL OF KNUDSON AND HEREDITARY RETINOBLASTOMA

How the two alleles of tumor suppressor genes are inactivated sequentially in cancer development is best explained by the "two-hit hypothesis" proposed by Knudson in 1971.[19] Though applicable to all tumor suppressor genes, it was first proposed and best exemplified by hereditary and sporadic retinoblastoma. The two-hit model explains that both alleles of a tumor suppressor gene are to be inactivated for tumor development and the characteristic clinical presentation of hereditary cancers at a younger age and with much higher probability of multifocal or bilateral primaries as compared to their sporadic counterparts. If a child is born with the first hit in the form of an inherited germline mutation in the first allele of *RB* gene, this mutation is present in all somatic cells including millions of retinal cells. There is a very high probability that within the first few years of life, the *RB* gene in any one of the retinal cells will acquire a second hit (mutation of the second allele) and triggers the development of hereditary retinoblastoma. This underlying genetic defect predisposes survivors of hereditary retinoblastomas to a high risk of developing sarcomas anywhere in the body—within and outside the field of radiotherapy given for treatment of retinoblastoma.

EPIGENETICS AND CANCER

While it is has been known for long that alteration in the DNA sequence (genetic alterations) are passed down to the daughter cell, only recently it became apparent that certain alteration in the genome or gene expression can also be inherited by the daughter cells even in the absence of any change in the DNA sequence. These are called epigenetic changes. One of the most frequently reported epigenetic change is altered gene expression due to methylation of DNA in the CpG islands (cytosine precedes guanine) of the promoter region of a gene. The epigenetic modification could be through acetylation of the histones that could silence tumor suppressor genes. Epigenetic alteration in cancers is common[20] with several cancers showing genome hypomethylation, especially in the CpG islands of tumor suppressor gene and specific patterns of histone modification. Because of the differential epigenetic changes between the tumor and normal cells and their reversible nature, some epigenetic changes are attractive drug targets. Inhibitors of the histone deacetylase (HDAC) and others are being developed and evaluated in large translational research programs and in clinical trials.[21] Clinical relevance of understanding the epigenetic changes is highlighted by the ability of promoter region methylation of the *MGMT* gene to predict response to temozolomide chemotherapy for glioblastoma.[22]

CLINICAL PRESENTATION AND EVALUATION OF HEREDITARY CANCERS

Almost all cancers have their hereditary counterparts. In general, 2–5% of all cancers are Mendelian hereditary conditions and 10–20% of all cancers are familial with some family history of cancer. The proportion of hereditary cancers varies from less than 1% for some tobacco induced cancers; 5% for breast cancer and colorectal cancer; 10% for ovarian cancer and sarcoma; and 20% for retinoblastoma and some other rare childhood cancers like adrenocortical carcinomas and choroid plexus tumors.[23] In the last 20 years the genetic basis of almost all hereditary cancer syndromes has been established. The underlying germline mutation is in one of the several dozen high penetrance tumor suppressor genes (*RB*, *TP53*, *BRCA1*, *BRCA2*, etc.) or a proto-oncogene (*RET*). In contrast to their sporadic counterparts, hereditary cancers not only tend to occur at younger age, or as bilateral or multifocal cancers, they could also have distinct differences in molecular or pathological features. With the exception of few rare autosomal recessive syndromes, such as xeroderma pigmentosum (XP), ataxia telangiectasia, Bloom syndrome and a few others, vast majority of hereditary cancer syndromes are autosomal dominant and described in Tables 2 and 3.

In many common hereditary cancer syndromes, no "phenotypic features" are clinically evident before the cancer-specific symptoms or signs appear. These include the HBOC, HNPCC, LFS and MEN-2A. However, many cancer predisposition syndromes have characteristic phenotypic features present since birth or appearing later in life but years or decades before the cancer diagnosis (Tables 2 to 4). The most common phenotypic features across diverse syndromes are in the form of benign skin or mucosal pigmentation or lesions characteristic of specific syndromes like neurofibromatosis type 1 (NF1), XP, tuberous sclerosis (TSC), Peutz-Jeghers syndrome (PJS), MEN-2B, etc. In some other syndromes, detailed evaluation with ophthalmoscopy, endoscopy or imaging will show characteristic benign or hamartomatous lesions, polyps or cysts in internal organs or retina as in Von Hippel–Lindau disease (VHL), familial adenomatous polyposis (FAP), TSC, NF1, etc. In syndromes without characteristic external or internal phenotypic features, the diagnosis of a specific hereditary cancer syndrome is based essentially on careful family history for the organ and histology of

TABLE 2: Hereditary cancers affecting breast and gynecological organs

Genetic syndrome; *Gene* (chromosome) **Penetrance** (Lifetime risk of cancer in mutation carriers)	**Clinical presentation and phenotype**	**Screening guidelines for high risk individuals** (Gene mutation carrier; If genetic testing has not been done, all 1st degree relative of a hereditary cancer patient or gene mutation carriers are considered as high risk)
Hereditary breast ovarian cancer (HBOC) syndrome. *BRCA1*(17q); *BRCA2* (13q) Autosomal dominant **Penetrance** Breast cancer (70–80%), Ovarian cancer (30–50%) Male breast cancer, prostate, pancreas, colon, etc. (especially in BRCA2 carriers)	Cancer presents at young age (a decade or two earlier than sporadic cancers). 50% women with breast cancer would develop synchronous or metachronous bilateral breast cancer. Double primaries in breast and ovaries is pathognomonic of HBOC irrespective of family history. BRCA1 associated breast tumors are generally ER, PR and C-ERBB2 negative (Triple –ve) and poorly differentiated	**Breast cancer screening** from 25 years age or 5 years before youngest breast cancer in the family, whichever is earlier • Monthly self-breast examination • 6-monthly clinical breast examination by a trained clinician • Annual mammography and/or breast MRI if dense breasts. **Ovarian cancer screening,** from 30 years age or 5 years before youngest cancer in the family whichever is earlier. Regular screening may be considered if prophylactic salpingo-oophorectomy has not been performed though its utility in detecting early stage cancer not well established. • Annual or more frequent transvaginal sonography (TVS) and CA-125 **Male members of HBOC families** from age 40 years or earlier • Self-breast examination; 6-monthly clinical breast examination • Yearly PSA and digital rectal examination
Li-Fraumeni syndrome (LFS). *TP53*(17p) Autosomal dominant; **Penetrance** Life-time risk of any cancer is >90%. SBBLA- Sarcoma (soft tissue or bone sarcoma); Breast cancer, brain tumors, leukemia, adrenocortical tumors, lung and any other cancer	Presents with childhood or early onset cancers and multiple primary cancers in survivors. Sarcoma before 45 years of age in proband with one 1st degree relative with cancer before 45 years of age and one 1st or 2nd degree relative with cancer before 45 years of age or sarcoma at any age	Comprehensive intensive screening for common LFS cancers can reduce mortality (*Villani A. et al. Lancet Oncol.* 2011;12:559-67) • Breast screening in females as for HBOC • Annual comprehensive physical examination • Annual whole body MRI with brain MRI • USG of abdomen and pelvis 6-monthly • Colonoscopy every 2 to 5 years starting at age 25 or younger. • Blood for CBC, ESR, LDH every 4 months
Cowden syndrome. *PTEN*(10q). Autosomal dominant Breast cancer (30–50%). Bowel cancer (20%), follicular thyroid cancer (5–10%)	Macrocephaly, cobblestone-like papules in gingivobuccal mucosa. Facial trichilemmomas, acral keratosis and gastrointestinal (GI) polyps	Breast cancer screening as for HBOC but may start at later age Annual thyroid USG No other definite screening guidelines but screening for GI and gynecological cancers can be instituted as per personal and family risk
Peutz-Jeghers syndrome (Details under hereditary gastrointestinal cancers)	Hamartomatous lesions, GI cancers and breast cancer	Breast screening as for HBOC Other details under hereditary GI cancers
Hereditary non-polyposis colon cancer (HNPCC) syndrome. (Details under GI cancers)	In addition to GI cancers, endometrial cancer risk 30–60%	Endometrial cancer screening with USG starting at age 40 years or 5 years before earliest endometrial cancer in the family whichever is earlier

cancers occurring in the family, age of onset of cancer and bilateral, or multifocal involvement. Based on phenotypic features and family history whenever a hereditary cancer syndrome is suspected, detailed cancer and syndrome specific clinical, radiological or laboratory investigations are required to uncover associated phenotypic features or clinically silent cancers. In the absence of characteristic features of a particular syndrome or its associated gene mutation, a differential diagnosis of syndromes is made as there is considerable overlap in clinical presentation of diverse syndromes. In all cases, especially in equivocal cases, genetic testing through DNA mutation analysis of the suspected gene(s) is the key to confirm the syndromic diagnosis and in estimating the cancer risk with appropriate genetic counseling for the family.

ASCERTAINING FAMILY HISTORY

The hereditary nature of a cancer is not always apparent. This can be ascertained or suspected only through a detailed family history by a person familiar with the typical and atypical history seen in such families and

TABLE 3: Hereditary cancers affecting gastrointestinal organs

Genetic syndrome; *Gene* (chromosome) **inheritance pattern; Penetrance** (Lifetime risk of cancer in mutation carriers)	**Clinical presentation and phenotype**	**Screening guidelines for high risk individuals** (Gene mutation carrier; If genetic testing has not been done, all 1st degree relative of a hereditary cancer patient or gene mutation carriers are considered as high risk)
Hereditary nonpolyposis colon cancer (HNPCC) syndrome or lynch syndrome Autosomal dominant. Mismatch repair genes ***MSH2***(2p), ***MLH1***(3p), ***MSH6***(2p), ***PMS2***(7p), ***PMS1***(2q) **Penetrance:** All cancers (70–90%) Colorectal (50–75%). Endometrial (30-60%) Less commonly other GI, Pelvi-ureteric or hepatobilliary cancer. Variant of HNPCC with brain tumor is **Turcot's syndrome** and with sebaceous adenoma/carcinoma is **Muir-Torre syndrome**	Up to few dozen polyps in 20–30% cases. Right sided colon cancer in 70% cases and at younger age. Amsterdam - II Criteria for HNPCC • At least 3 relatives with HNPCC related cancer • At least 2 generation affected • At least one is 1st degree relative of other two • At least 1 case < 50 years • FAP is ruled out	Colonoscopy every 1–2 years from age 25 years or earlier and annually from 45 years of age Physical examination including neurological, dermatological and breast examination annually USG and SOS biopsy for endometrial cancer annually Urine analysis annually No consensus on the frequency of screening. More intensive screening in individuals with early onset cancers in the family or personal history of polyps
Familial adenomatous polyposis (FAP) ***APC***(5q) Autosomal dominant Penetrance: Any Cancer - almost 100% Colorectal carcinoma (95%) Desmoid tumor or fibromatosis (50%) Papillary thyroid cancer (15–20%) Infrequently other GI, liver or brain tumors Other benign lesions in 50%	Hundreds to thousands of polyps by 2nd decade leading to cancer by 4th decade. **Attenuated FAP** has fewer (10–100) polyps. **Gardner syndrome:** FAP variant with extracolonic lesions (Dental abnormalities, epidermoid cysts, osteoma, fibroma, CHRPE) or cancers	Prophylactic surgery is not done—annual or more frequent colonoscopy and upper GI endoscopy from late teens depending upon polyp burden and dysplasia. Annual or more frequent endoscopy of rectum after colectomy with ileorectal anastomosis. After ileal pouch —anal anastomosis or ileostomy, endoscopic evaluation of ileal pouch or ileostomy every 1–3 years. For attenuated FAP, prophylactic surgery may be deferred and colonoscopy (with polypectomy) may be done every 1–3 years
Peutz-Jeghers syndrome. *STK11*(19p) Autosomal dominant **Penetrance:** All Cancers (50%) Common cancers include breast, colorectal, pancreatic, endometrial, ovarian and testicular	May present with intussception in childhood due to hamartomatous jejunal / GI polyps. Mucocutaneous melanocytic macules in lips and buccal mucosa (95%). Multiple/atypical naevi	• Breast screening in females as for HBOC • USG of abdomen and pelvis 6-monthly • Upper GI and colonoscopy every 2–3 years from age 25 or younger • Pancreas—MRCP or EUS every 2–3 years from 25 years
Recessive hereditary colon cancer Gene: **MutYH** (1p34). Autosomal recessive	Ten to hundreds of polyps. Features of Gardner's syndrome not seen	• Colonoscopy from 25 years. Frequency 1–3 years as per polyp burden and dysplasia

the clinicopathological features indicative of hereditary variants of diverse cancers. Underreporting of hereditary cancers is a global phenomenon and access to specialized hereditary cancer registries and clinics increases the rate of syndrome identification.[24] It assumes special significance in developing countries with greater constraints for detailed and accurate family history, syndrome specific work-up and poorly developed or nonexistent referral services to specialized cancer genetics clinics.[4] Some oncologists have concerns that genetic testing may increase the distress in the family members[25] and may be influencing referral of high-risk families for genetic counseling and testing.

Underreporting of hereditary cancer is more likely if the leading question is inappropriate. For example, a lady with breast cancer being asked, "Did your sister, mother or aunt had breast cancer?" may fail to identify half of the HBOC families where the index case has paternal inheritance and about a quarter of the families where the other cancers are ovarian, male breast or prostate cancer. Family history of cancer is more likely to be uncovered with a broader question like, "Was anyone in your mother's or father's side of the family ever suspected to have had any type of cancer?" Cancer patients who report any family history of cancer require detailed interview for constructing a pedigree showing the relationship of the cancer affected persons, type of cancers, age at diagnosis, etc.

Many Indian families are unable to reliably report the age and type of cancers that their relatives had in the past and access to their medical records is difficult. Reliable syndromic diagnosis is based on the age at cancer

TABLE 4: **Neurocutaneous and other syndromes with inherited cancers**

Genetic syndrome (Gene; chromosome) penetrance	*Clinical presentation and phenotype*	*Screening guidelines for high risk individiuals*
Neurofibromatosis Type 1-NF1 (*NF1;* 17q) Autosomal dominant. Optic pathway glioma in 15% cases and malignant peripheral nerve sheath tumor–MPNST in 5-15% cases	Skin neurofibromas / Café-au-lait spots in all cases. Axillary freckling and iris Lisch nodules in >90% cases. Plexiform neurofibromas and learning disabilities is seen in a third of children. Optic glioma in 15% and scoliosis in 10% cases	Annual physical, eye and skin examination. Neuroimaging if any relevant symptoms or signs. MRI to rule out MPNST if suspected. Endocrine evaluation if any growth abnormalities
Neurofibromatosis Type 2-NF2 (*NF2*; 22q) Autosomal dominant. B/L vestibular schwannoma in 85%; Schwannoma in 65%; Meningioma in 50%; Other gliomas in 5% cases	Cutaneous stigmata of NF1 generally absent but few (<6) Café-Au-Lait spots in some. Bilateral vestibular schwannomas which present as deafness or other schwannomas are characteristic	Neuroimaging with MRI for vestiblular and spinal schwannomas and meningioma at regular intervals and for any new neurological symptom or sign. Regular audiometric evaluation
Tuberous sclerosis. *TSC1*(9q)**,** *TSC2*(16p) Autosomal dominant. Sub-ependymal giant cell astrocytomas (SEGA) is a characteristic benign tumor of TS Ependymoma and renal cell carcinoma (RCC)	Calcified sub-ependymal nodules and cortical tubers are pathognomonic. Facial angiofibroma (adenoma sebaceum). Characteristic hypopigmented ash leaf spots and shagreen patches. Cardiac rhabdomyoma / renal angiomyolipoma are common. Autism, learning difficulties and epilepsy common	Annual physical examination and clinico-radiological evaluation of organs likey to be involved (brain, kidneys, heart). Sutable interventions may be done to prevent bleeding or renal failure from renal angiomyolipoma
von Hippel Lindau disease-VHL (*VHL*; 3p) Autosomal dominant. Hemangioblastoma (60%); RCC (40%); Pheochromocytoma (15%)	Retinal Angioma are the earliest lesions detected at a mean age of 25 years in 40-70% cases. Multiple renal, liver & pancreatic cysts common. Renal cancer is likely to be bilateral	Annual physical, ophthalmogical, urine cytology and abdominal USG examination
Xeroderma pigmentosum **Nucleotide excision repair genes (XPA, XPB, XPC, ERCC4, ERC5, ERCC6, DDB2 and POLH)** Basal cell carcinoma (BCC), squamous cell carcinoma (SCC) or melanoma in most cases	Extreme UV sensitivity causing keratosis and skin and conjunctival cancers in exposed areas by adulthood. More severe manifestations in tropical countries. BCC most common, followed by SCC and melanoma. Neurological abnormalities common in XP-B, XP-D, and XP-A	Strict compliance to sun avoidance and UV protection rom childhood with regular skin and ophthalmological evaluation to detect and treat cancers early. Baseline neurological evaluation with rehabilitation
Hereditary retinoblastoma – RB (*RB1*; 13q) Autosomal dominant. A third of RB are hereditary. Childhood retinoblastoma (90%) sarcoma in adolescence or adult life (25%)	Presents at younger age bilateral or multifocal involvement. No family history in B/L RB suggest *de novo* germline mutation or incomplete penetrance or spontaneous RB regression in a parent. Sarcoma with or without previous ocular radiotherapy	Monthly retinal examination in 1st year, then quarterly till RB diagnosis, or in its absence up to 5 years of age. Sarcoma risk of sarcoma to be considered
Multiple endocrine neoplasia 2A/2B (MEN2A and MEN2B). ***RET***(10q). Autosomal dominant. Medullary thyroid cancer: (70-100%). Pheochromocytoma (30-50%). Penetrance is influenced by location of mutation in RET gene	**MEN2A:** Family history of MTC/ Pheochromocytoma (PH). Hyperparathyroidism in 20% cases. No external phenotype. **MEN2B:** Aggressive early onset MTC in almost all cases; PH in 50% cases. Tongue and lip neuromas; thickened corneal nerve, marfanoid habitus, intestinal ganglio-neuromatosis. **Familial MTC:** FH of MTC in absence of PH / other features	Prophylactic thyroidectomy in 1st year of life in MEN2B with most aggressive category 'D' RET mutation (M918T/A883F); by 5 years in risk category C (C634); deferred beyond 5 years of age in intermediate – low risk category 'B' / 'A' if annual basal stimulated calcitonin / USG normal
Bloom syndrome. BLM (15q26)**:** Autosomal recessive; Prone for all cancers, particularly AML and multiple primaries. Short, thin individuals with characteristic narrow face, large ears, high pitched voice, telangiectasia and facial butterfly pigmented patch with immunodeficiency and infertility. No screening guidelines		
Fanconi anemia. 14 Genes *(*FANC-A to FANC-O); Autosomal recessive; Bone marrow failure starts in childhood and progresses to malignancy, often AML. Solid tumors also seen; Skin pigmentation; malformation of the heart, kidney, and limbs; endocrinopathy and growth retardation. No definite screening guidelines		

TABLE 5: Cancer types in various hereditary cancer syndrome

Cancer type (Especially at younger age or with family history of same or related cancer)	*Hereditary cancer syndrome*
Breast cancer, GI cancers, Lung cancers	Seen in several hereditary cancer syndromes
Ovarian cancer	Hereditary breast ovarian cancer (*BRCA1/2* gene)
Male breast cancer	
Endometrial cancer	Hereditary Nonpolyposis colon cancer (*MMR* genes)
Retinoblastoma (often bilateral)	Hereditary retinoblastoma (*RB1* gene)
Medullary thyroid cancer	Multiple endocrine neoplasia (MEN) type 2 (*RET* gene)
Pheochromocytoma	
Soft tissue or bone sarcoma	Li-Fraumeni syndrome (*TP53* gene)
Adrenocortical carcinoma	
Choroid plexus tumor	
Optic pathway glioma	Neurofibromatosis Type 1 (*NF1* gene)
Malignant peripheral nerve sheath tumor (MPNST)	Neurofibromatosis Type 2 (*NF2* gene)
Acoustic neuroma (often bilateral)	Von Hippel-Lindau's disease (*VHL* gene)
Cerebellar or spinal hemangioblastoma	Tuberous Sclerosis (*TSC1* and *TSC2* genes)
Subependymal giant cell astrocytoma (SGCA)	Gorlin's syndrome (*PTCH1* gene)
Multiple basal cell carcinoma	

diagnosed and the site and type of cancers in the family. Accurate syndromic diagnosis governs the surveillance advice as well as the genes to be tested in the family. In such situations, careful "verbal autopsy" adapted for Indian social and healthcare set-up can help ascertain the cause of death[26] and cancer type in long dead or distant relatives. Not missing a family history of characteristic phenotypic features or cancers which are typically seen in specific hereditary cancer syndrome (Table 5) is most important. Ovarian cancer is frequently misreported as "abdominal, stomach or uterus cancer" by relatives. Colorectal cancer is also misreported as abdominal or stomach cancer. Careful questioning about recurrent ascites or bloated abdomen with or without cachexia in the last stages is almost pathognomonic of terminal ovarian cancer. Extensive prolonged diarrhea is pathognomonic of end stage metastatic medullary thyroid cancer in MEN type 2 families. Sometimes the broad description of previous treatment helps in making the diagnosis of cancer and its type. Limb amputation in adolescence is indicative of bone or soft tissue sarcoma, colostomy is indicative of colorectal cancer and mastectomy or lumpectomy plus radiotherapy is indicative of breast cancer. There is now increasing use of electronic medical records or databases across hospitals in India. Information about the full name of the deceased patient, year of first visit to the hospital and any other relevant information could facilitate ascertainment of their cancer diagnosis. Release of medical information of deceased patients may require written consent of the next of kin.

GENETIC TESTING, ITS INDICATIONS AND INTERPRETATION

Genetic testing is the process of studying the germline DNA for specific genetic alterations. DNA for genetic testing is extracted from normal cells—usually from lymphocytes in blood or sometimes the buccal cells in buccal scrapings or mouth wash samples. The DNA alterations in the gene of interest is studied by Sanger sequencing on automated capillary DNA sequencing machines. Some genetic alterations like chromosomal alterations require conventional or newer cytogenetic techniques for detection. Large genomic rearrangements (LGR) in the form of deletions or duplication of one or more exons of the gene of interest are not detected by Sanger sequencing and requires special techniques like the multiplex ligation-dependent probe amplification (MLPA). To confirm the hereditary nature and syndromic diagnosis of cancer, a specific gene or genes that are likely to be mutated in the syndrome are tested, e.g. *BRCA1* and *BRCA2* in HBOC or *TP53* in Li-Fraumeni syndrome. Based on the personal and family history of specific cancers, the probability of finding mutation in a gene can be predicted by the use of validated models such as the BRCAPRO or Myriad models for *BRCA1/2* genes in HBOC.[27] Genetic testing is recommended if the probability of finding mutation is predicted to be 10% or more.[28] In a family with a suspected hereditary cancer syndrome, it is preferable to start genetic testing with a person diagnosed with a syndrome-specific cancer (e.g. patient with medullary thyroid cancer in a MEN syndrome family). When DNA sample from a cancer affected person in such a family is not available, unaffected first degree relatives of cancer patients may be subjected to syndrome-specific genetic testing to ascertain their carrier status and risk of developing certain cancers. For example, healthy son of a lady who died of double malignancies of colon cancer and endometrial cancer may be tested for HNPCC syndrome-related mismatch repair (MMR) gene mutations. In such situations when no cancer affected member of the family has been tested earlier and a cancer gene mutation in a family is not known, negative gene test result in a healthy member is not very informative and does not rule out hereditary cancer risk in the family.

The biological effect of an alteration in the DNA sequence of a gene implicated in the cancer syndrome depends on the type of DNA change and its location within the gene. In general, sequence alterations in such genes are pathogenic or disease causing if the protein coded by them is shortened or truncated by frameshift or nonsense mutations. Similarly, mutations in the splice site cause aberrant splicing and are pathogenic. Some missense mutations (substitution of one amino acid by another) could be pathogenic if they occur in specific sites of a proto-oncogene (e.g. *RET, KRAS*) or cause conformational changes in biologically important domains of some tumor suppressor genes such as *TP53*. However, most missense mutations may have little or no biological effect and are classified as single nucleotide polymorphisms (SNP). Similarly, no or very weak biological effect or pathogenicity is expected from change in a nucleotide base which does not change the coded amino acid (synonymous mutation) or it is in the noncoding deep intronic region.

If a small possibility of a false negative or false positive result due to technical or administrative reasons is ruled out, genetic testing to ascertain the genetic basis of a hereditary cancer could have the following four possible results:

1. Detection of a mutation that is already reported in the literature or databases as a pathogenic or deleterious germline mutation. Some mutations in a gene may have never been reported previously but the class of mutation (frameshift or nonsense) is clearly predicted to be deleterious as they result in truncated protein.
2. No mutation or sequence variation is seen in the gene. This could imply:
   a. It is a sporadic cancer, especially if the family history is not strong. Sometimes more than one cancer cases could occur in the family as a chance occurrence.
   b. The genetic alteration is in the form of large genomic rearrangement which will not be detected on Sanger sequencing and may warrant MLPA analysis.
   c. Mutation may be present in some other known or as yet unknown gene. This may warrant examination in some other genes, especially if the family history is very strong. This negative genetic testing by sequencing and MLPA for *BRCA1/2* may be followed by mutation testing for *TP53*, *CHEK2* and some other genes.
3. Detection of a sequence variant which is previously reported as harmless or a polymorphism. Some gene mutations may have never been reported previously but the class of mutation (synonymous mutations or deep intronic mutations) is clearly predicted to be harmless.
4. Detection of a sequence variation of unknown clinical significance. This may be a new or previously reported missense or intronic region mutations that is yet to be but characterized for its pathogenecity.

In addition to technical and interpretative issues, genetic testing has several other Ethical, Legal and Social Implications (ELSI) and is therefore suggested by genetic counselors or attending doctors only when inherited cancer predisposition is suspected and testing is likely to aid in the clinical management for patients or unaffected individuals who may be at a high risk of cancers.[28] The process of pre-test counseling with informed special consent and post-test counseling are integral components of genetic testing. Trained genetic counselors and clinical cancer geneticists are best suited to address the wide range of ethical, psychosocial, technical and medical management issues emanating from genetic testing.

CANCER SCREENING AND PREVENTION IN HIGH-RISK INDIVIDUALS/MUTATION CARRIERS

The main purpose of identifying inherited cancer predisposition and its genetic basis in a family is to safeguard the high-risk individuals in the family by using a proven strategy for cancer prevention or early detection. Appropriate genetic testing can confirm the presence of a deleterious mutation in the index case or proband. Testing for this specific gene mutation can help identify other family members who may have inherited this mutation and benefit from specific screening or preventive measures. However, when genetic testing is not available or the results are noninformative, all first degree relatives of an individual suspected with a specific hereditary cancer syndrome are considered as high risk for developing specific cancers. Such high-risk individuals should be counseled about their cancer risk; symptoms and signs of different cancers; and effective methods for prevention or early detection for common cancers in the suspected hereditary condition. Chemoprevention with tamoxifen and/or oral contraceptives can reduce the risk of some cancers like breast cancer and ovarian cancer respectively in *BRCA1/2* mutation carriers.[28] However, for most cancers, effective primary prevention may require prophylactic surgical removal of thyroid for *RET* mutation,[29] rectum and colon for *APC* mutation[30] and ovaries, tubes and/or breast for *BRCA1/2* mutation carriers.[28] Syndrome-specific screening using imaging, clinical examination and sometimes tumor markers is advised for high-risk individuals tailored for their age and gender as per established guidelines described in Boxes 2 and 3.[4,28,30,31]

Box 2: Recommendations for females from HBOC families or with a *BRCA1/2* mutation[4,28,30]

A. Breast cancer screening starting at the age of 25 years or 5 years before the age of earliest cancer in the family:
   - Monthly breast self-examination
   - Six-monthly clinical breast examination by a trained clinician
   - Annual breast imaging with mammography and/or breast magnetic resonance imaging (MRI) in young women with dense breasts

B. Ovarian cancer screening, starting at the age of 30 years or 5 years before the age of earliest cancer in the family, whichever is earlier. Its utility in detecting early stage ovarian cancer is not well established but baseline and annual screening is advised if prophylactic salpingo-oophorectomy has not been performed

- Annual or more frequent transvaginal sonography (TVS)
- Annual or more frequent CA-125 tumor markers

Box 3: Recommendations for high-risk males from HBOC families

- Monthly breast examination and 6-monthly clinical breast examination from the age of 40 years or earlier depending on family history
- Yearly prostate-specific antigen (PSA) and digital rectal examination from the age of 40 years or earlier

Preventive strategies in high-risk women from HBOC families vary from noninvasive chemoprevention with anti-estrogens to prophylactic bilateral mastectomy with breast reconstruction or prophylactic oophorectomy. Prophylactic oophorectomy reduces the risk of ovarian cancer by almost 99% (rare occurrence of primary peritoneal carcinoma still exists) and also reduces the risk of breast cancer by 50%. While bilateral prophylactic nipple-sparing mastectomy with reconstruction can reduce breast cancer risk by more than 95%, issues regarding breast reconstruction, reoperation rates and the psychosexual aspects of such surgery in healthy young women have to be discussed in detail as the survival benefit of the procedure is yet to be established.[32]

MOLECULAR TAXONOMY OF CANCERS AND ITS CLINICAL RELEVANCE

The present system of clinicopathological classification of diverse tumors was developed in the 20th century and takes into account the natural history of cancers, distinct morphological features of cancer cells, its supporting stroma and immunohistochemical patterns. While the clinicopathological classification of cancer has served well in guiding treatment and predicting prognosis of a group of patients, it is inconsistent in predicting clinical outcome or therapeutic response in individuals or subgroups. Over the last decade, this clinicopathological system has been complemented with molecular taxonomy for some cancers. The molecular taxonomy of cancer is based on newly recognized common pattern of alterations in a set of genes. These alterations are in the form of specific mutations, expression changes or structural chromosomal changes. These molecular patterns are usually discovered through global profiling of gene expression, gene mutations, protein expression and structural rearrangements in a set of clinically and pathologically characterized and annotated tumor samples. Linked with clinical outcome data, molecular taxonomy has been validated in independent cohorts for some cancer types. In a few cancer types or subtypes, molecular taxonomy can complement clinico-pathological classification for more refined diagnosis with better prediction of prognosis or response to specific treatment, especially targeted therapies that are developed against specific genetic alterations. Estrogen and progesterone receptor status in breast cancer is the first and perhaps the best example of clinically relevant molecular taxonomy. Developed in the era of conventional classification, hence not claimed as molecular subclassification, it not only predicts prognosis and response to hormonal therapy but also represents a distinct biological and molecular entity. The other examples of clinically useful molecular or genetic characterization includes N-myc and *HER2/Neu* gene amplification or overexpression predicting prognosis in neuroblastoma and breast cancer respectively, and predicting response of breast cancer to trastuzumab or lapatinib; aid diagnosis and predict response to chemotherapy in oligodendroglioma (1p19q deletion); aid diagnosis for Ewing's sarcoma (EWS-FLI1 translocation) and various hematolymphoid malignancies (cell surface markers and chromosomal translocations); predict response of lymphoma to anti-CD-20 antibody rituximab. The legendary success of imatinib in molecularly characterized CML is the best example of understanding and clinically exploiting the underlying genetic alteration by targeting the *BCR-ABL* fusion gene produced by the t(9;22)(q34.1;q11.2) translocation.

MOLECULAR DIAGNOSTIC TECHNIQUES IN CANCER

The genetic defects in cancer are characterized by sequence changes or mutations in the DNA; numerical or structural aberrations in chromosomes; and overexpression or silencing of genes and their protein products. Advances in more sensitive and high throughput molecular techniques along with better mechanistic understanding of how specific genetic alterations contribute to cancer development and behavior, or its response to specific treatment has helped establish the field of molecular diagnostics. Molecular diagnostic tests are being developed to correlate single or global gene alterations (mutations, chromosomal alterations and expression) with clinically relevant diagnostic, prognostic or predictive abilities.[33] Being increasingly used for specific indications, the cost, time and overall clinical utility of some of these molecular tests is debatable. Some of the important molecular diagnostic techniques used in oncology are outlined below.

Fluorescent In Situ Hybridization

This technique is used for qualitative and quantitative evaluation of chromosomal aberrations in the tumor cells. Using special sample preparation and hybridization methods, fluorescent in situ hybridization (FISH) can be used for cells in mitosis as well as the interphase. Specific fluorescent probes are used, which hybridize with the chromosomal region of interest and then visualized using slide-based systems or flow cytometry systems. In slide-based systems, FISH-stained cells are fixed to a conventional or a confocal fluorescence microscope slide and observed as an image. In the flow systems, FISH-stained cells are prepared in suspension, and the suspension is allowed to flow in a narrow stream across a laser beam wherein the detector records their fluorescent intensities to detect chromosomal changes, if any. Fluorescent in situ hybridization is most commonly used in studying translocations in pediatric tumors and hematolymphoid malignancies and in quantitating overexpression of *HER2/Neu* in breast cancer.

Microsatellite Instability

Microsatellites are tandem repeats (one after another) of one, two or three specific nucleotides anywhere in the DNA. For example, a pentadinucleotide repeat of cytosine and adenine (CA) would consist of five successive CA, i.e. CACACACACA. The mono-, di- and trinucleotide repeats are widely distributed in the genome of all life forms but their exact biological role is not fully understood. When nucleotide sequences are arranged as repetitive bases, they are prone to add or lose one or more repeats during the course of normal DNA replication. As a result, the repetitive sequences exist in many polymorphic forms in a given population. Highly polymorphic repetitive sequences in the form of short tandem repeat (STR) markers are widely used in biomedical research and DNA fingerprinting. Changes in the length of repeat sequences can be detected by capillary electrophoresis of the DNA fragment on automated DNA sequencer. A panel of STR markers studied together would invariably show that two unrelated individuals differ in the length of at least some of the STR markers. However, repeat length of any STR will be same in DNA from different tissues from the same individual and same allele is passed on to the next generation. This forms the basis of human identification and DNA fingerprinting for research and forensics. Due to underlying genetic defect in the DNA mismatch repair (MMR) genes as seen in HNPCC, the normal process of rectifying repeat length errors introduced during DNA replication is hampered. Carriers of germline mutation in the *MMR* genes in HNPCC families show microsatellite instability (MSI) with insertion or deletion of repeats in the DNA of the replicating colonic tumor. This introduces discordance between the repeat lengths of STR markers in the tumor DNA as compared to the normal DNA from lymphocytes of the same patient. For HNPCC, a panel of five microsatellite markers recommended by NCI (Bethesda panel) is used for detection of MSI. If the lengths or number of repeats of two or more microsatellite markers are found to be different between normal and tumor tissue then the tumor is said to be microsatellite unstable or MSI-high. This is indicative of a defective MMR system with a possible mutation in one of genes—*hMLH1*, *hMSH2* or *hMSH6*. The MSI test helps in deciding if *MMR* gene sequencing is warranted and the priority of genes (*MLH1*, *MSH2* or *MSH6*) to be sequenced based on absence of IHC staining of specific MMR proteins.

Gene Expression Profiling

The differential expression of genes in the cancerous cells as compared to the normal cells of the same tissue origin can provide clues about the genes whose overexpression may be driving or sustaining cancer, and genes whose loss of expression may be allowing development and promotion of cancer. Pathway specific or global expression of hundreds to thousands of genes can be studied using microarrays. The probes are attached to a coated matrix which are then hybridized to a test and control sample to read the differences in intensities of hybridized product and thereby the expression. Expression profiling studies have led to molecular classification of breast cancers, lymphomas and other tumors. It allows better understanding of the pathways relevant to development of cancer type and in identifying molecular targets for cancer diagnosis and therapy.

Automated DNA Sequencing

The process includes polymerase chain reaction (PCR) amplification of the coding region of the gene of interest, DNA sequencing to know its nucleotide sequence and biological interpretation of any sequence variation identified. Sequencing of DNA extracted from the normal tissues like blood or buccal cells reveals germline genetic alterations. Sequencing of DNA extracted from the tumor tissue reveals the somatic genetic alteration. For germline genetic analysis, the DNA is generally extracted from 3–6 mL of blood collected in ethylene diamine tetra-acetic acid (EDTA) tubes. Unlike RNA, the DNA is a stable molecule and blood sample for DNA analysis can be transported without cold chain or stored for few days at room temperature or 4°C. However, degraded DNA from autolyzed or poorly processed formalin fixed paraffin embedded tumor tissue may not yield satisfactory sequence information. The Sanger sequencing method for which Frederick Sanger received his 2nd Nobel Prize in 1980 is now automated and is the gold standard for identifying or confirming DNA sequence variation or mutation. This method uses dideoxynucleotides which terminate the chain during in vitro DNA replication. A fragment of the gene to be sequenced is amplified using PCR. The PCR product is cleaned and sequenced using fluorescently labeled nucleotides and their analogs which are incorporated into a newly synthesized strand and detected as they sequentially pass across a laser to give an output of nucleotide sequence. Each nucleotide is assigned a specific color so the result is in the form of a chromatogram. The nucleotide sequence in the sample being analyzed is compared with known reference sequence of normal individuals. As described earlier, the interpretation of this comparison may reveal no sequence change, pathogenic change or mutation, harmless change or polymorphism or a sequence variation of unknown clinical significance.

RECENT ADVANCES AND FUTURE AVENUES

Few decades of basic research in cell and molecular biology of cancer has provided insight in the molecular and genetic basis of cancer and some mechanisms that drive the development and progression of cancer. In the last decade, some of this knowledge has been translated to develop molecular classification of cancer, for identifying individuals at very high risk of developing cancer and in developing drugs against specific targets in the cancer cell. While this has ushered a new era of personalized or molecular medicine in cancer, its overall impact in the clinical management or clinical outcome of common cancers has been very modest till now.[34] Nevertheless, proof of concept has been established with a revolutionary change in the clinical management and outcome for germline mutation carriers of some high penetrance genes like *RET*, *BRCA1*, *MMR*, etc. and for few cancers with specific genetic alterations such as chronic myeloid leukemia, gastrointestinal stromal tumors (GISTs) and molecular variants of some other cancers.

In the last few years, there have been renewed efforts for comprehensive genomic characterization of various cancers using new high throughput technology platforms like the Next Generation Sequencing (NGS). International Cancer Genome Consortium (ICGC), the largest ever-global collaborative project in biomedical research aims to comprehensively characterize the genomic alterations in all the cancer types with public health relevance in different parts of the world. India, one of the seven founding members of the ICGC is characterizing gingivobuccal cancers. It is hoped that ICGC and similar projects would facilitate faster development of new biomarkers, clinically relevant molecular sub-classification of different cancers and identify key driver genes which would serve as targets for new drugs.[35] Such studies are identifying a large number of genetic alterations, many of which were previously not known to be associated with cancers. However, there are several challenges in exploiting the exponentially increasing information on genomic alterations in various cancers and making them clinically relevant. These include reliable and validated bioinformatic analyzes; high throughput functional characterization of new genetic alteration; lack of suitable animal models; redundancy of many newly discovered genetic pathways; time, effort and failures in prospective clinical trials evaluating targeted therapies and new biomarkers.

For hereditary cancers, genetic testing can identify individuals at high risk of developing cancer, but issues of incomplete penetrance (some mutation carriers not developing cancer) and the variable age at cancer diagnosis is a major challenge in genetic counseling. Living in a hereditary cancer family is a complex experience that may affect the cognitive and psychosocial functioning of the individual.[36] There is also a need to generate long-term data on the efficacy of chemoprevention and prophylactic surgeries and understand the psychosocial and quality of life issues surrounding genetic testing in diverse cultural backgrounds.[37] A meta-analysis of controlled trials has shown that appropriate genetic counseling results in improving the cancer risk perception without increasing general anxiety or cancer-specific worry.[38] The benefits of genetic testing may be overemphasized by media frenzy surrounding stories of genetic testing and prophylactic double mastectomy by celebrities like Angelina Jolie. There is also a growing trend of direct-to-consumer predictive genetic testing. While some families would benefit, it may be associated with psychosocial as well as medical issues in healthy individuals who without going through genetic counseling before genetic testing[39] may suddenly find themselves grappling with a complex medical decision based on a test report.

REFERENCES

1. Sarin R. Cancer Genetics. In: Munjal YP (Ed). API Textbook of Medicine, 9th edition;2010.
2. Asian BRCA consortium. In response to "Angelina Jolie's double mastectomy and the question of who owns our genes" (letter to editor). BMJ. 2013;346:f3340.
3. Rajkumar T, Soumittra N, Pandey D, et al. Mutation analysis of hMSH2 and hMLH1 in colorectal cancer patients in India. Genet Test. 2004;8(2):157-62.
4. Kowtal P, Vyas S, Joshi N, et al. Hereditary breast ovarian cancers: genetic testing and its implications. J Obstet Gynecol Ind. 2007;57(4):298-306.
5. Hansa J, Kannan R, Ghosh SK. Screening of 185DelAG, 1014DelGT and 3889DelAG BRCA1 mutations in breast cancer patients from North-East India. Asian Pac J Cancer Prev. 2012;13(11):5871-4.
6. Chakraborty A, Mukhopadhyay A, Bhattacharyya D, et al. Frequency of 5382insC mutation of BRCA1 gene among breast cancer patients: an experience from Eastern India. Fam Cancer. 2013;12(3):489-95.
7. Vaidyanathan K, Lakhotia S, Ravishankar HM, et al. BRCA1 and BRCA2 germline mutation analysis among Indian women from south India: identification of four novel mutations and high-frequency occurrence of 185delAG mutation. J Biosci. 2009;34(3):415-22.
8. Soumittra N, Meenakumari B, Parija T, et al. Molecular genetics analysis of hereditary breast and ovarian cancer patients in India. Hered Cancer Clin Pract. 2009;7(1):13.
9. Vinodkumar B, Syamala V, Abraham EK, et al. Germline BRCA1 mutation and survival analysis in familial breast cancer patients in Kerala; South India. J Exp Clin Cancer Res. 2007;26(3):329-36.
10. Saxena S, Chakraborty A, Kaushal M, et al. Contribution of germline BRCA1 and BRCA2 sequence alterations to breast cancer in Northern India. BMC Med Genet. 2006;7:75.
11. Hedau S, Jain N, Husain SA, et al. Novel germline mutations in breast cancer susceptibility genes BRCA1, BRCA2 and p53 gene in breast cancer patients from India. Breast Cancer Res Treat. 2004;88(2):177-86.
12. Valarmathi MT, Sawhney M, Deo SS, et al. Novel germline mutations in the BRCA1 and BRCA2 genes in Indian breast and breast-ovarian cancer families. Hum Mutat. 2004;23(2):205.
13. Rajkumar T, Soumittra N, Nancy NK, et al. BRCA1, BRCA2 and CHEK2 (1100 del C) germline mutations in hereditary breast and ovarian cancer families in South India. Asian Pac J Cancer Prev. 2003;4(3):203-8.
14. Valarmathi MT, A A, Deo SS, et al. BRCA1 germline mutations in Indian familial breast cancer. Hum Mutat. 2003;21(1):98-9.
15. Fearon ER, Vogelstein B. A genetic model for colorectal tumorigenesis. Cell. 1990;61(5):759-67.
16. Hanahan D, Weinberg RA. Hallmarks of cancer: the next generation. Cell. 2011;144(5): 646-74.
17. Lynch HT, de a Chapelle A. Hereditary colorectal cancer. N Engl J Med. 2003; 348(10):919-32.
18. Nag S, Qin J, Srivenugopal KS, et al. The MDM2-p53 pathway revisited. J Biomed Res. 2013;27(4):254-71.
19. Knudson AG Jr. Mutation and cancer: statistical study of retinoblastoma. Proc Natl Acad Sci USA. 1971;68(4):820-3.
20. Esteller M. Epigenetics in cancer. New Eng J Med. 2008;358(11):1148-59.

21. Zhang L, Lei J, Shan Y, et al. Recent Progress in the Development of Histone Deacetylase Inhibitors as Anti-Cancer Agents. Mini Rev Med Chem. 2013 Oct 25. [Epub ahead of print] [Accessed January,2014].
22. Stupp R, Hegi ME, Mason WP, et al. Effects of radiotherapy with concomitant and adjuvant temozolomide versus radiotherapy alone on survival in glioblastoma in a randomised phase III study: 5-year analysis of the EORTC-NCIC trial. Lancet Oncol. 2009;10(5):459-66.
23. Tabori U, Shlien A, Baskin B, et al. TP53 alterations determine clinical subgroups and survival of patients with choroid plexus tumors. J Clin Oncol. 2010;28(12):1995-2001.
24. Sturgeon D, McCutcheon T, Geiger TM, et al. Increasing Lynch syndrome identification through establishment of a hereditary colorectal cancer registry. Dis Colon Rectum. 2013;56(3):308-14.
25. Van Riel E, Wárlám-Rodenhuis CC, Verhoef S, et al. BRCA testing of breast cancer patients: medical specialists' referral patterns, knowledge and attitudes to genetic testing. Eur J Cancer Care (Engl). 2010;19(3):369-76.
26. Gajalakshmi V, Peto R, Kanaka S, et al. Verbal autopsy of 48000 adult deaths attributable to medical causes in Chennai (formerly Madras), India. BMC Public Health. 2002;2:7.
27. Lindor NM, Lindor RA, Apicella C, et al. Predicting BRCA1 and BRCA2 gene mutation carriers: comparison of LAMBDA, BRCAPRO, Myriad II, and modified Couch models. Fam Cancer. 2007;6(4):473-82.
28. Balmaña J, Díez O, Rubio IT, et al. BRCA in breast cancer: ESMO Clinical Practice Guidelines. Ann Oncol. 2011;22(6):vi31-4.
29. Grubbs EG, Waguespack SG, Rich TA, et al. Do the recent American Thyroid Association (ATA) Guidelines accurately guide the timing of prophylactic thyroidectomy in MEN2A? Surgery. 2010;148(6):1302-9.
30. National Comprehensive Cancer Network. NCCN Guidelines. [online] Available from http://www.nccn.org/professionals/physician_gls/f_guidelines.asp [Accessed January, 2014].
31. National Center for Biotechnology Information. (2014) Online Mendelian Inheritance in Man (OMIM) database. [online] Available from http://www.ncbi.nlm.nih.gov/omim [Accessed January, 2014].
32. Lostumbo L, Carbine NE, Wallace J. Prophylactic mastectomy for the prevention of breast cancer. Cochrane Database Syst Rev. 2010;(11):CD002748.
33. Sarin R, Kowtal P. Inherited predisposition to cancer and issues in genetic testing. Evidence Based Management of Cancer: Guidelines for Molecular Diagnostics in Oncology. Mumbai: Tata Memorial Hospital; 2008. pp. 1-13. ISBN: 978-81-904583-1-3
34. Sarin R. Criteria for deciding cost-effectiveness for expensive new anti-cancer agents. J Cancer Res Ther. 2008;4(1):1-2.
35. International Cancer Genome Consortium, Hudson TJ, Anderson W, et al. International network of cancer genome projects. Nature. 2010;464(7291):993-8.
36. Bakos AD, Hutson SP, Loud JT, et al. BRCA mutation-negative women from hereditary breast and ovarian cancer families: a qualitative study of the BRCA-negative experience. Health Expect. 2008;11(3):220-31.
37. Sarin R. Inheritance of maladies and the gene fairy. J Cancer Res Ther. 2013;9(3):341-2.
38. Braithwaite D, Emery J, Walter F, et al. Psychological impact of genetic counseling for familial cancer: a systematic review and meta-analysis. Fam Cancer. 2006;5(1):61-75.
39. Gray SW, Hornik RC, Schwartz JS, et al. The impact of risk information exposure on women's beliefs about direct-to-consumer genetic testing for BRCA mutations. Clin Genet. 2012;81(1):29-37.

13 Nanotechnology in Cancer Diagnosis and Treatment: A New Frontier

Neil Desai

INTRODUCTION

In recent years, there have been intense efforts focusing on the development of nanotechnology-based diagnostics and therapeutics for a wide variety of diseases, particularly oncology. Nanotechnology relies on the use of nanoscale constructs to provide a new paradigm for a wide range of diagnostic and therapeutic applications. The nanotechnology approach offers numerous potential benefits, including increased sensitivity, enhanced targeting and penetration, personalization of therapies, increased solubility and bioavailability, improved pharmacological, pharmacokinetic and biodistribution profiles, reduced systemic toxicity, and controlled drug release. As a result, nanotechnology-based medical products have increased sensitivity, speed and specificity of diagnostics, and improved clinical efficacy and toxicity profile for therapeutic agents. Ongoing research focuses on multifunctional capabilities to further enhance selectivity and multiplexing in diagnostics, targeting for drug delivery, and overcoming drug resistance. Nanotechnology represents an exciting approach for the development of novel diagnostic and therapeutic tools for the treatment of cancer.

Nanotechnology is the creation of useful materials, devices and systems to manipulate matter at molecular scale in nanometer range, where a nanometer is one billionth of a meter (Fig. 1).[1] Nanotechnology is widely applied to many fields, including electronics, magnetics, optics, information technology, materials development and biomedicine. Due to their small size that is similar to large biomolecules, nanoscale materials and devices can readily interact with biomolecules and translate molecular-based science into clinical advances. During the recent years, there has been tremendous growth in nanotechnology and its application in all areas of medicine. Since most biological processes occur at the nanoscale, the ability of nanotechnology to monitor and manipulate these processes offers invaluable tools for biomedical research and development. In particular, research efforts focusing on nanotechnology-based agents result in significant advances for the diagnosis and treatment of cancer, and hold great potential to revolutionize the field of oncology (Fig. 2).[2]

To date, there is no definitive size range for nanotechnology products. Typically, nanotechnology refers to the manipulation of matter with at least one dimension sized from 1 nm to 100 nm. The Food and Drug Administration of United States considers a product to incorporate nanotechnology if it has at least one dimension in the nanoscale range (approximately 1–100 nm) or exhibits properties or phenomena attributable to its dimension(s) even outside the nanoscale range, up to 1 μm.[3]

Due to high surface to volume ratio, nanomaterials have unique physical and chemical properties that are distinctive from bulk material.[4] There are numerous types of nanomaterials that have seen broad application in oncology and the rank is rapidly increasing. Based on composition, these nanomaterials can generally be classified as organic and inorganic. Organic nanomaterials use organic molecules as building blocks; examples of this group include lipid-based structures such as liposomes, protein-based nanoparticles, dendrimers, carbon nanotubes, silicon-based nanoporous materials, emulsions, and polymer-based nanoparticles. Inorganic nanomaterials use inorganic elements, for example, metals

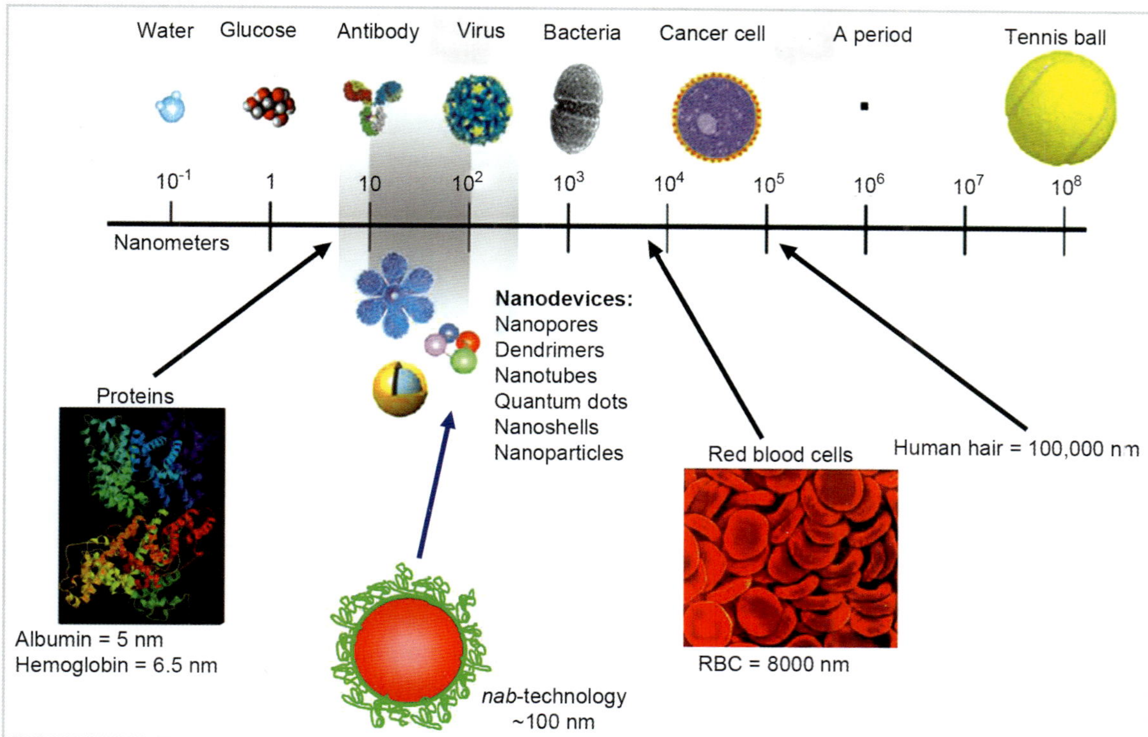

Fig. 1: The size of different objects, biomolecules and nanodevices

Source: Image modified from NCI Alliance for Nanotechnology in Cancer (http://nano.cancer.gov/learn/understanding/) anc McNeil SE. Nanotechnology for the biologist. J Leukoc Biol. 2005;78(3):585-94.[1]

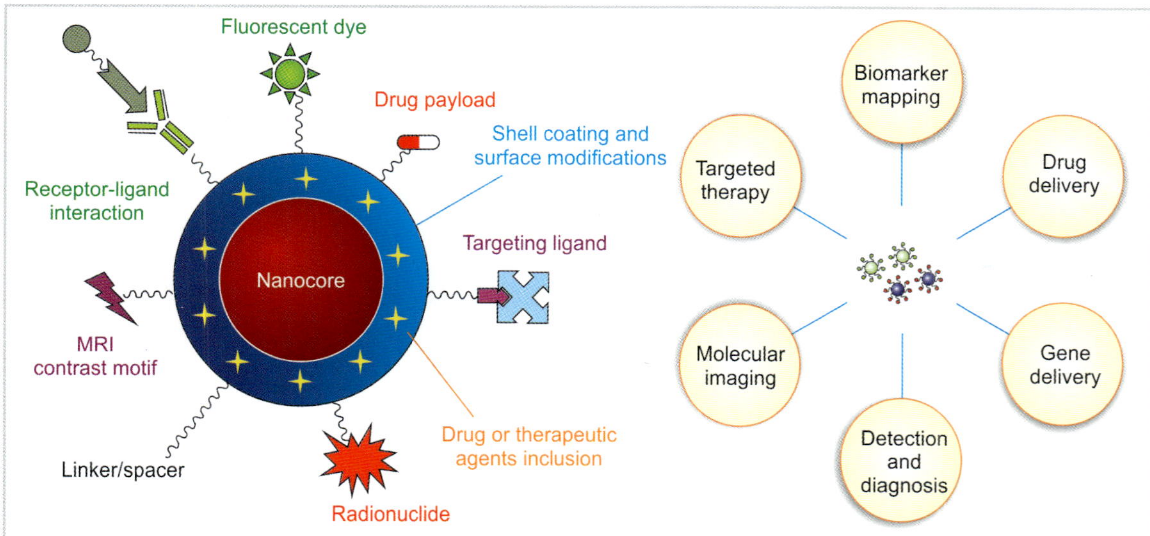

Fig. 2: Scheme of multifunctional nanoparticle for different applications in nanomedicine

Source: Image adapted from Reference 2

as the core; examples of this group include quantum dots, nanoshells, gold nanoparticles and superparamagnetic iron oxide nanoparticles. In addition, nanoconstructs such as nanocantilevers and nanocircuits have been key components of novel devices, providing sensitive detection capabilities at the nanoscale. This review summarizes broad applications of nanotechnology in diagnosis and treatment of cancer.

NANOTECHNOLOGY APPLICATION IN CANCER DIAGNOSIS

The use of nanotechnology in cancer diagnosis can provide major advantages over conventional diagnostic methods, in increased sensitivity, improved accuracy and rapidity of tests. Major advances have been made in recent years in the area of in vitro detection and diagnosis, and tumor imaging in vivo.

Both nanoparticles and nanotechnology-based devices are used in these applications (Figs 3A to D).[5-7] The most commonly used nanoparticles in cancer diagnosis are quantum dots (QDs), nanoshells, and gold nanoparticles. QDs are spherical, fluorescent light-emitting semiconductor nanoparticles with sizes of 2–10 nm. QDs are composed of an inorganic elemental core (e.g. cadmium, technetium, zinc, selenide, mercury, tantalum and indium) with a metal shell.[8] Nanoshells are spherical nanoparticles consisting of a dielectric core (usually silica) surrounded by a thin metal shell (typically gold), with a dimension of approximately 10–300 nm.[9] QDs and nanoshells convert electrical energy into light using plasmon-mediated conversion. Both quantum dots and nanoshells are optically tunable and have emission/absorption properties that range from ultraviolet (UV) to infrared.[10] Gold nanoparticles have vivid optical properties due to localized surface plasmon resonance (LSPR), which confers them with distinctive light scattering and photothermal properties based on their shapes.[11]

A major advantage of QDs and nanoshells over organic fluorophore dyes is that they are several magnitudes more resistant to photobleaching, and can emit narrow emission peaks with minimum overlapping.[10] Multiple QDs excited by a single light source can emit light at different wavelengths, allowing simultaneous measurement of multiple molecular targets labeled with QDs.[12] Relatively larger than quantum dots, nanoshells offer similar imaging properties and applications without the potential heavy metal toxicity. The superior optical properties of these nanoparticles allow for greater sensitivity in signal detection.

Nanotechnology-based devices are also under development for cancer diagnosis. The nanocantilevers (Fig. 3A), which resemble tiny diving boards made of silicon, could be used in high-sensitivity detectors because they vibrate at different frequencies when molecules of the target for detection bind to them. The cantilevers studied in the recent work range in length from a few microns to tens of microns, and are about 20 nanometers thick, which is also roughly the thickness of the antibody coating. Nanocircuits (Fig. 3B) are electrical circuits composed of three different fundamental components, including transistors, interconnections, and architecture, which are fabricated and operate on the nanometer scale. The small circuits can be fitted on a computer chip, allowing faster and more complex functions using less power.

In Vitro Detection and Diagnosis

Tumor biomarkers and circulating tumor cells are useful indicators of the presence of tumors and metastasis. Nanoparticles, such as QDs, nanoshells, gold nanoparticles and magnetic nanoparticles, can be conjugated with antibodies, peptides and other functional moieties. Direct conjugation of targeted antibodies to the surface of nanoparticles preserves high affinity, minimizes nonspecific binding, and can achieve multiplex detection of molecular targets. The bright fluorescence emitted by nanoparticles such as quantum dots and nanoshells enables identification of targets in low levels in cancer cells, resulting in increased sensitivity. Several studies have shown high specificity of QDs for labeling of molecular targets. Because QDs have fluorescent properties and are electron dense, they can be used as probes for light microscopy and simultaneous visualization of multiple subcellular structures by electron microscopy. A QD-based assay has been developed that allows quantitative detection of estrogen receptor, progesterone receptor, and HER2/neu in paraffin-embedded human breast-cancer cells and tumor samples. Simultaneous multiplex detection of six breast-cancer proteins has also been achieved by use of direct conjugation of QDs to an optical detection and spectroscopy. Silica-shell-coated surface enhanced Raman scattering (SERS) nanoshell probes allow spectroscopic labeling of multiple biomarkers in tissue samples. Conjugation of tumor-specific targeting moieties such as HER2/neu antibody to nanoshells allows for targeted imaging in vitro.[10] Raman scattering immunohistochemistry involves staining tissues with biomarker-specific antibodies linked to gold nanoparticles and fluorescent dyes. After the antibody binds to its target, the Raman scattering signal can be detected and visualized by fluorescent microscopy. In summary, use of nanoparticle conjugates and Raman probes offer the possibility of quantifying multiple proteins simultaneously on single tumor sections or small cancer samples; treatment decisions can then be made on the basis of these results.

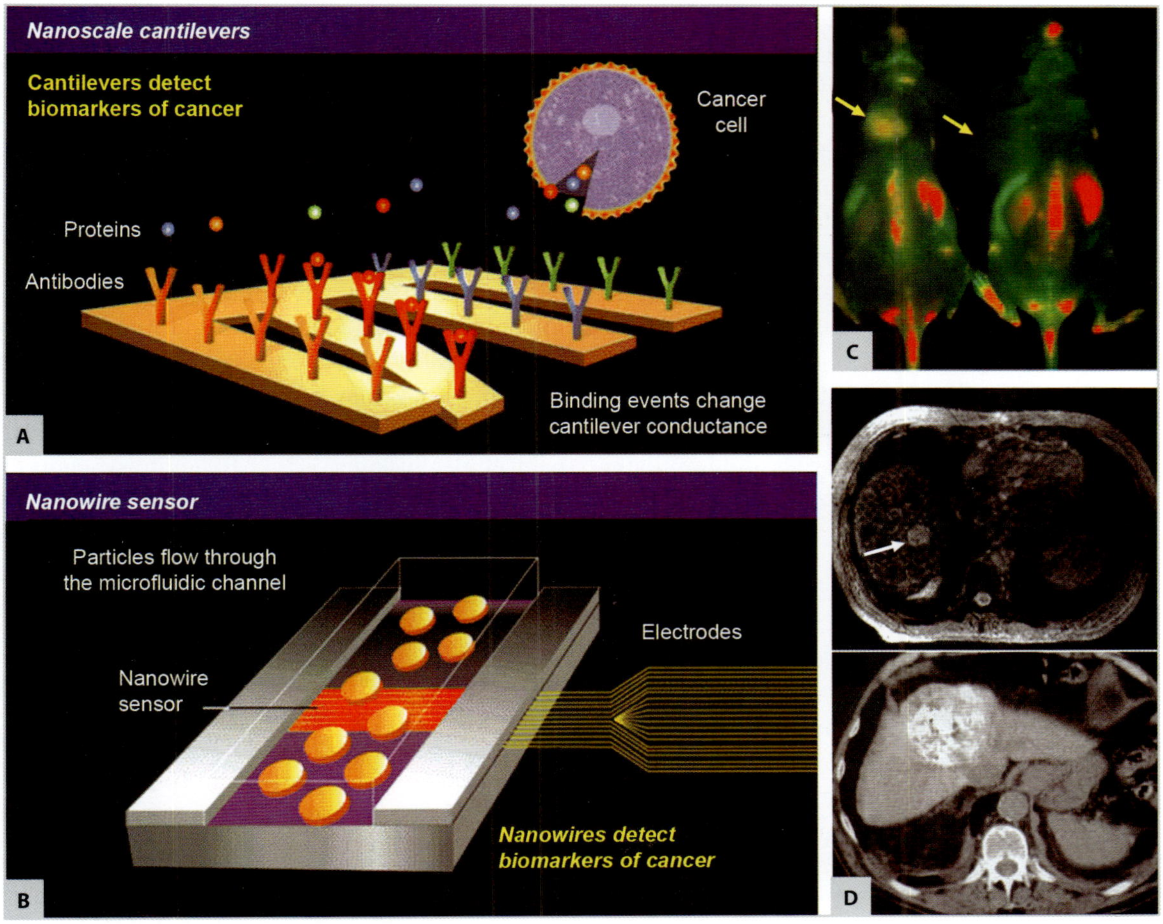

Figs 3A to D: Examples of diagnostic applications of nanotechnology

A. Nanocantilevers: Flexible nanoscale cantilevers coated with antibodies capable of binding specific protein substrates can cetect very low concentrations of cancer biomarker proteins present in patient samples

Source: Image adapted from NCI Alliance for Nanotechnology in Cancer (http://nano.cancer.gov/learn/understanding/nanotech_cantilevers.asp)

B. Nanowires: Nanoscale sensing wires detect molecular particles such as cancer biomarkers flowing through a microfluidic channel

Source: Image adapted from NCI Alliance for Nanotechnology in Cancer (http://nano.cancer.gov/learn/understanding/nanotech_ranowires.asp)

C. Quantum dots: In vivo imaging of U87MG tumor-bearing mice (yellow arrows) at 6 hours post-injection of 200 pmol of RGD-conjugated quantum dots (left) or control quantum dots (right). Improved accumulation is seen for RDG-targeted quantum dots.

Source: Images adapted from Reference 5

D. Superparamagnetic iron oxide nanoparticles (SPION) as MRI contrast agent: MR images of the hepatic dome after injection of ferumoxide iron oxide nanoparticles (top) and conventional gadolinium-based contrast agents (bottom). Note that the liver tissue darkened following injection of iron oxide nanoparticles (top), providing better contrast of the tumor.

Source: Images adapted from References 6 and 7

In addition to the in vitro detection of tumor biomarkers, antibody-conjugated quantum dots were used to detect tumor circulating cells in the peripheral blood of patients with non-small cell lung cancer (NSCLC) for early diagnosis and monitoring of recurrence.[13] Magnetic nanoparticles conjugated with antibodies have also been used to concentrate and detect circulating tumor cells in patient blood samples.

Devices incorporating nanotechnology offer improved detection tools for cancer. Because of the higher sensitivity compared to larger devices, nanocantilevers allow the development of advanced sensors that detect minute quantities of analytes such as rare tumor-specific proteins or nucleotide sequences from patient blood or tissue samples (Fig. 3A). Nanocircuits constructed with nanowires, carbon nanotubes, and QDs can be adapted to monitor biological processes in a true molecular scale, e.g. the measurement of single molecule enzymology with carbon nanocircuits (Fig. 3B). Microfluidic devices offer fast and sensitive detection of analytes with a minimum amount of samples. The detection of tumor biomarkers from patient samples can provide an early diagnosis of tumors before a symptom is manifested or a tumor mass is discovered. It also enables fast genotyping of cancer patients, aiding the selection of the appropriate targeted molecular therapies as the basis for personalized medicine. Overall, nanotechnology allows the development of so-called "lab-on-a-chip" devices, which could make it possible to replace bulky lab equipment with miniature sensors, saving time, energy and materials and improving sensitivity and accuracy.

Tumor Imaging In Vivo

Several types of nanoparticles have seen extensive use for in vivo tumor imaging, including QDs, nanoshells, gold nanoparticles and magnetic nanoparticles. These nanoparticles can be conjugated with specific targeting moieties, including antibodies, oligonucleotides, biotin, streptavidin, or peptides, and have been studied for in vivo imaging applications in oncology. Antibody-conjugated polymeric micelle-coated cadmium selenide/zinc sulfide (CdSe/ZnS) QDs demonstrated efficient targeting and imaging in a human prostate cancer xenograft model,[14] and arginine-glycine-aspartic acid (RGD) peptide-labeled cadmium telluride/zinc sulfide (CdTe/ZnS) QDs could target and image tumor vasculature in vivo (Fig. 3C).[5,15] Peptide-conjugated phospholipid-micelle-encapsulated silicon QDs showed feasibility for in vivo tumor imaging without cellular and tissue toxicities.[16,17] Nanoshells have been used in vivo as a contrast agent for imaging with optical coherence tomography and photoacoustic tomography.[10] Gold nanoparticles conjugated to endothelial growth factor receptor (EGFR) antibodies showed ability to detect precancerous lesions in cervical biopsies.[18]

Magnetic and superparamagnetic nanoparticles have been widely used in cancer diagnosis as MRI contrast agents. Nanoparticles consisting of iron, nickel, cobalt and manganese could exhibit magnetic properties. Due to the thermal fluctuations of magnetic moments that reverse direction, some magnetic nanoparticles, termed as superparamagnetic nanoparticles, display no magnetic behavior in the absence of the magnetic field.[19] Superparamagnetic iron oxide nanoparticle (SPION) is the most commonly used type in biomedical applications, which is typically composed of iron oxide maghemite (γ-Fe_2O_3) and iron oxide core smaller than 15 nm in size. SPIONs have greater magnetic susceptibility than traditional paramagnetic gadolinium-based MRI contrast agents, enabling higher sensitivity and the detection of smaller tumor lesions by SPIONs (Fig. 3D).[6,7] SPIONs approximately 50–100 nm in size show rapid hepatic uptake following intravenous administration and are used to detect liver tumors.[20] In contrast, ultrasmall SPIONs 5–10 nm in size allows uptake in lymph nodes through interstitial lymphatic fluid transport and have been used clinically with high-resolution MRI to detect small lymph node metastases in patients with breast, lung, prostate, endometrial and cervical cancer.[10] Several SPIONs have been clinically approved as MRI contrast agents, including ferumoxides (Feridex IV®, by Berlex Laboratories; and Endorem®, by Guerbet), used for liver and spleen imaging and approved in the United States, Europe and Japan; ferucarbotran (Resovist®, by Bayer Healthcare), used for detecting liver cancer and approved in Europe and Japan; and Lumirem (Gastromark®, by AMAG Pharmaceuticals, Inc.), used for gastrointestinal luminal contrast and approved in the US, Europe and Brazil.[21] Magnetic nanoparticles conjugated with tumor-specific moieties can be further targeted to tumors. Superparamagnetic nanoparticles conjugated with antibodies to HER-2 and luteinizing hormone-releasing hormone (LHRH) were demonstrated to detect breast cancer cells in vivo by MRI.[10,22] Other targeting moieties used with magnetic nanoparticles for MRI include $\alpha v\beta 3$ antagonist for tumor neovasculature imaging,[23] telomerase specific sequence for cancer cell detection,[24] and annexin V for the detection of apoptotic cells.[25]

Other nanoparticle-based MRI contrast agents have also been tested. Dendrimers are repeatedly branched polymeric macromolecules with numerous arms extending from the center that form perfect 3D geometric structures.[26] Dendrimers have also been used as advanced contrast agents in MRI to aid visualization of cancer.[27] Single walled carbon nanotubes (SWNTs) coupled to paramagnetic gadolinium particles can be used as a high-performance MRI contrast agent.[28]

NANOTECHNOLOGY APPLICATION IN CANCER THERAPY

Increasing numbers of nanotechnology-based cancer therapies have been tested and some have been clinically approved. Examples of nanomaterials in therapeutic applications include liposomes, micelles, albumin-based

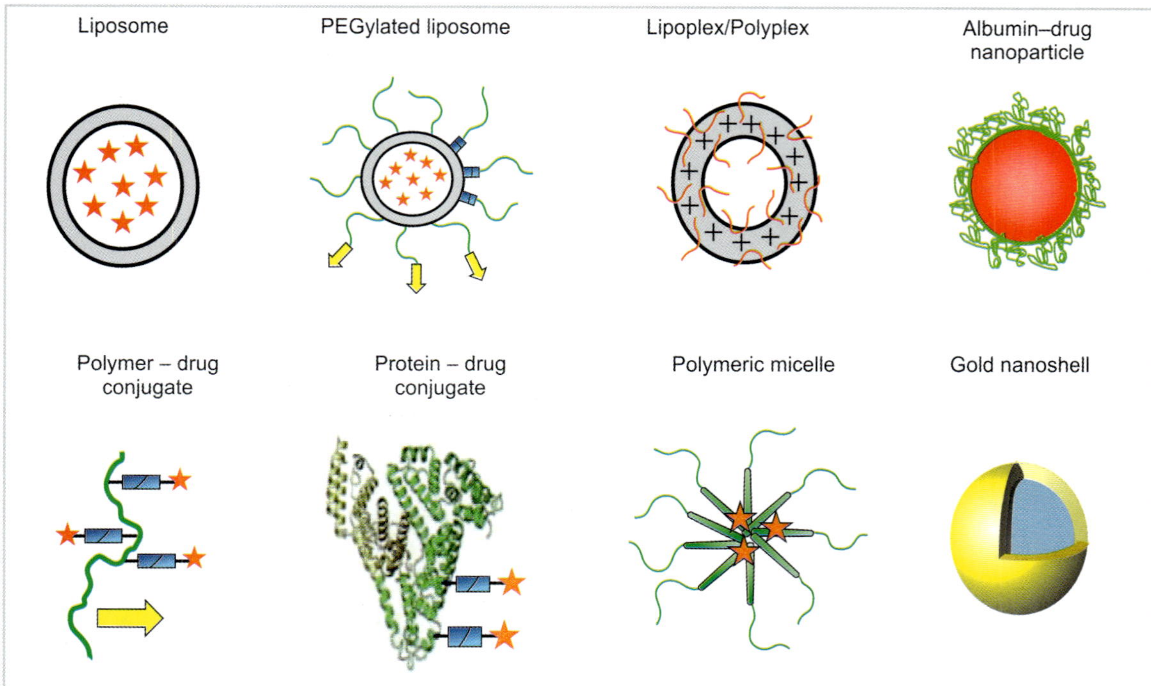

Fig. 4: Examples of nanotechnology-based therapeutic agents in clinical development or commercially available

Source: Image adapted from Reference 29

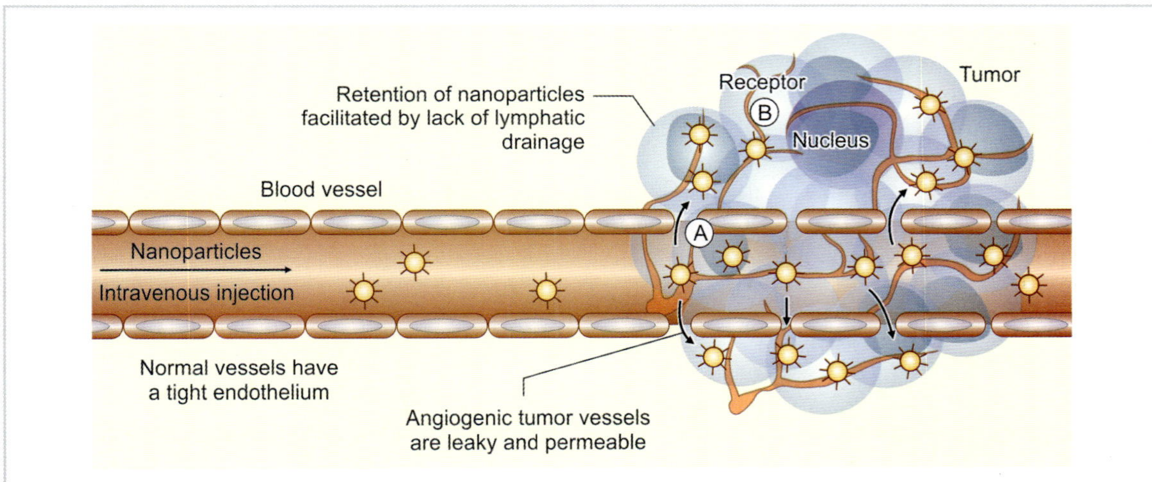

Fig. 5: Enhanced drug delivery to solid tumors with nanoparticles

(A) Passive delivery (EPR). Nanoparticles accumulate in tumors through leaky and permeable tumor vasculature and impaired lymphatic system; (B) EPR+targeted delivery. Nanoparticles with tumor-specific targeting moieties bind to cancer cell receptors resulting in enhanced drug delivery.

Source: Image adapted from Reference 30

nanoparticles, polymer nanoparticles, gold nanoparticles and nanoshells (Fig. 4)[29] Compared with conventional chemotherapies, these nanomedicines possess major advantages in overcoming biological barriers, preferentially targeting tumors, decreasing toxicities and improving clinical efficacy.

The delivery of nanoparticles to tumors can be enhanced by passive targeting and active targeting mechanisms (Fig. 5).[30] For passive targeting, the high permeability of tumor vasculature with fenestrations ranging between 0.2 μm and 1.2 μm and reduced lymphatic drainage lead to enhanced permeability and retention effect (EPR) in the tumor microenvironment and improve the delivery of nanoparticles into tumor.[31,32] The organized structures of nanoparticles allow for active targeting by the incorporation of various tumor-specific targeting moieties, such as ligands for receptors, peptides, proteins, antibodies and nucleotides, to enhance tumor drug delivery and uptake.[33] The unique properties and multicomponent structure of nanoparticles confer them with the ability to overcome layers of biological barriers and preferentially target tumors, which increases efficacy, reduces systemic drug exposures, and decreases side effects.

Delivery of Hydrophobic Drugs

The delivery of hydrophobic drugs typically requires toxic solvents and surfactants such as Cremophor® and Tween®, which impair drug distribution and are associated with severe side effects. The incorporation of hydrophobic drugs into nanoparticle structures eliminates the use of toxic solvents and offers clear advantages over their conventional counterparts by improving solubility, pharmacokinetics, drug release, tissue distribution and toxicity profile.

Liposomes and polymeric micelles are nanoscale vehicles used as drug delivery platforms for both hydrophobic and hydrophilic molecules. Liposomes are self-assembled phospholipid-based vehicles composed of lipid bilayers. Micelles are monolayered colloidal vehicles and smaller in size than liposomes. For hydrophobic chemotherapeutics, liposomes can increase solubility and reduce drug toxicity. Currently, three liposomal formulations of anthracyclines have been clinically approved, including liposomal daunorubicin (DaunoXome®), approved for Kaposi's sarcoma in the US; liposomal doxorubicin (Myocet®), approved for metastatic breast cancer in combination with cyclophosphamide in Europe; and pegylated liposomal doxorubicin (Doxil®/Caelyx®), approved for both Kaposi's sarcoma and refractory ovarian and breast cancer in the US. Despite high antitumor activity, the use of conventional anthracyclines is limited by cardiac toxicity with high cumulative doses.[34] Liposomal anthracycline formulations contain nanoparticles measuring 100 nm in size and were developed to improve the therapeutic index of anthracyclines. In clinical studies, in first-line treatment of patients with metastatic breast cancer, both liposomal doxorubicin and pegylated liposomal doxorubicin demonstrated similar efficacy but significantly lower cardiac toxic effects and less neutropenia compared with conventional doxorubicin.[35,36] While liposomes are relatively stable and biodegradable, conventional "non-stealth" liposomes can be taken up by mononuclear phagocyte system (MPS) and rapidly cleared from circulation, and tend to aggregate. In contrast, pegylated stealth liposomes with an amphipathic polyethylene glycol (PEG) coating can significantly decrease uptake by macrophages and inhibit liposome aggregation, thereby improving stability and extending in vivo circulation half-life.[37-39] However, pegylated liposomal doxorubicin leads to higher concentrations in the skin, resulting in a side effect called palmar plantar erythrodysesthesia (PPE)/hand-foot syndrome,[36] which is not associated with conventional doxorubicin and nonpegylated liposomal doxorubicin.[40]

Liposomes and micelles are also versatile platforms to deliver other hydrophobic small molecule drugs. Studies have investigated the liposomal formulation of the hydrophobic drugs cisplatin, paclitaxel, docetaxel, and curcumin.[41-44] CPX-351 (Cytarabine:Daunorubicin liposome injection, Celator Pharmaceuticals Inc, Ewing, NJ, USA) is currently in a phase 3 clinical trial in patients with untreated high-risk acute myeloid leukemia,[45] and CPX-1 (Irinotecan HCI:Floxuridine liposome injection) has completed a phase 2 clinical trial in patients with colorectal cancer.[46] Liposomes and micelles can be coated with tumor-specific antibodies for tumor targeting. Immunomicelles carrying monoclonal nucleosome (NS)-specific 2C5 antibody (mAb 2C5) and loaded with paclitaxel resulted in an increased drug accumulation in the tumor and greater tumor growth inhibition compared with free paclitaxel or paclitaxel in non-targeted micelles in a preclinical mouse model of Lewis lung carcinoma.[47] Doxorubicin-loaded liposomes carrying mAb 2C5 also showed higher antitumor efficacy compared with nontargeted doxorubicin-loaded liposomes.[48] Liposomes can be synthesized with self-hydrolysable lipids to allow for time-controlled drug release.[49] Liposomes engineered to contain a small amount of air are acoustically active and can be triggered to release loaded drugs by ultrasound.[50]

Albumin is a key plasmic carrier of hydrophobic molecules and is highly accumulated in proliferating tumors.[51,52] Tumor cells use albumin as a major energy and nitrogen source through endocytosis and lysosomal degradation, with the resulting amino acids used in de novo protein synthesis. Expression of mutated *Ras* in tumor cells leads to stimulation of macropinocytosis to import albumin and other extracellular proteins, which provide a source of amino acids required for cancer cell growth, particularly glutamine.[53] Albumin binds to gp60 albumin receptor on endothelial cell surface and activates caveolae-mediated transcytosis across tumor blood vessel endothelium.[54] Albumin can bind to numerous proteins, and the majority of which are extracellular proteins.[55] The first approved protein nanotechnology-based chemotherapeutic, *nab*-paclitaxel (Abraxane®) is a solvent-free 130 nm albumin nanoparticle formulation of paclitaxel. *nab*-Paclitaxel is approved globally for the treatment of metastatic breast cancer and is also recently approved in the US for the first-line treatment of locally advanced or metastatic NSCLC, in combination with carboplatin, in patients who are not candidates for curative surgery or radiation therapy. Conventional formulations of hydrophobic paclitaxel require the solvents Cremophor EL and ethanol, which are associated with significant toxicities including neuropathy and severe hypersensitivity reactions.[56,57] *nab*-Paclitaxel achieved a 50% higher maximum tolerated dose (300 mg/m^2 vs 175 mg/m^2 for solvent-based paclitaxel, every 3 weeks), a shorter infusion time (30 minutes vs 3–24 hours with solvent-based paclitaxel) without the need for premedication to prevent solvent-related hypersensitivity reactions.[58] In a phase 3 study in patients with metastatic breast cancer, *nab*-paclitaxel outperformed solvent-based paclitaxel in terms of antitumor activity, time to progression, and safety profile.[59] In a phase 3 study in patients with advanced NSCLC, *nab*-paclitaxel as first-line therapy was efficacious and resulted in a significantly improved overall response and less neuropathy compared with solvent-based paclitaxel.[60] In a recent phase 3 study, in patients with treatment-naive metastatic pancreatic cancer, the addition of *nab*-paclitaxel to gemcitabine significantly improved overall survival compared with gemcitabine alone.[61] In a phase 3 study in chemotherapy-naïve patients with metastatic melanoma, *nab*-paclitaxel showed a statistically significant improvement in progression-free survival compared with dacarbazine chemotherapy.

Polymeric nanoparticles (PNPs) are highly versatile in targeted delivery of therapeutic agents for cancer. These nanoparticles are often modified with PEG, which inhibits plasma protein binding, reduces uptake by MPS and prolongs systemic circulation.[62] A large number of PNPs carrying anticancer agents have been tested. Poly ethylene glycol-poly (lactic-co-glycolic) acid (PEG-PLGA) nanoparticles carrying recombinant human endostatin (Endostar, Simcere Pharmaceutical Group, Nanjing, China) was approved by the Chinese State Food and Drug Administration, in 2005, for the treatment of NSCLC. Other examples of PNPs include PNP-sirolimus,[63] PLGA-lecithin-PEG nanoparticle with AS1411 antinucleolin aptamers,[64] aptamer-functionalized Pt(IV) prodrug-PLGA-PEG nanoparticle against prostate cancer,[65] aptamer-conjugated PEG-PLGA paclitaxel nanoparticle against glioma,[66] and folic acid–conjugated PEG-PLGA nanoparticles loaded with vincristine sulfate.[67] BIND-014 (BIND Therapeutics, Cambridge, MA, USA), a PNP that targets PSMA and contains docetaxel, is currently in phase 2 clinical trials in patients with NSCLC and prostate cancer.[68] In addition, Aurimune (CytImmune Sciences Inc, Rockville, MD, USA) are colloidal gold nanoparticles with surface binding of tumor necrosis factor (TNF) and PEG-Thiol, which preferentially deliver hydrophobic drugs to cancer sites with minimal accumulation in healthy tissue (Fig. 6A).[69]

Delivery of Nucleic Acids

Nanotechnology is also investigated as a tool for the delivery of macromolecules to cancer sites. Ribonucleic acid (RNA) interference is a naturally occurring endogenous regulatory process where short double-stranded RNA causes sequence-specific post-transcriptional gene silencing. Small interference RNA (siRNA) can be used to directly silence the expression of aberrant proteins implicated in cancer proliferation, representing a promising therapeutic strategy for cancer. However, there remains a major hurdle for the safe and effective delivery of human gene therapy and gene-silencing siRNA, short hairpin RNA (shRNA), and microRNA (miRNA). Due to their high negative charges, large molecular weight and size, and instability, naked nucleic acids undergo rapid enzymatic degradation in human plasma and are also entrapped in organs with mononuclear phagocytic system, particularly liver.[71] Multiple nanoparticle-based deoxyribonucleic acid (DNA) and RNA delivery systems are under development for gene delivery to various human tumors. DNA plasmids can be coupled with cationic and neutral lipids to form lipid-nucleic-acid nanoparticles, which protect DNA molecules from degradation.[72,73] The surface of nanoparticles can be further conjugated with PEG molecules and tumor-specific targeting antibody to increase gene delivery into tumor.[72] DNA plasmids can also be encapsulated in biocompatible poly(D,L-lactide-co-glycolide) polymer-based nanoparticles using a multiple emulsion-solvent evaporation method.[74] The adsorption of siRNA to polyalkylcyano acrylate nanoparticles significantly improved siRNA stability and cellular uptake,[75] and siRNA can be incorporated into noncovalent polyethylenimine-complexed siRNA nanoparticles for in vivo systemic delivery.[76] CALAA-01 (Arrowhead Research Corporation, Pasadena, CA, USA), a polymer nanoparticle consisting of a cyclodextrin-containing polymer, a PEG steric stabilization agent and

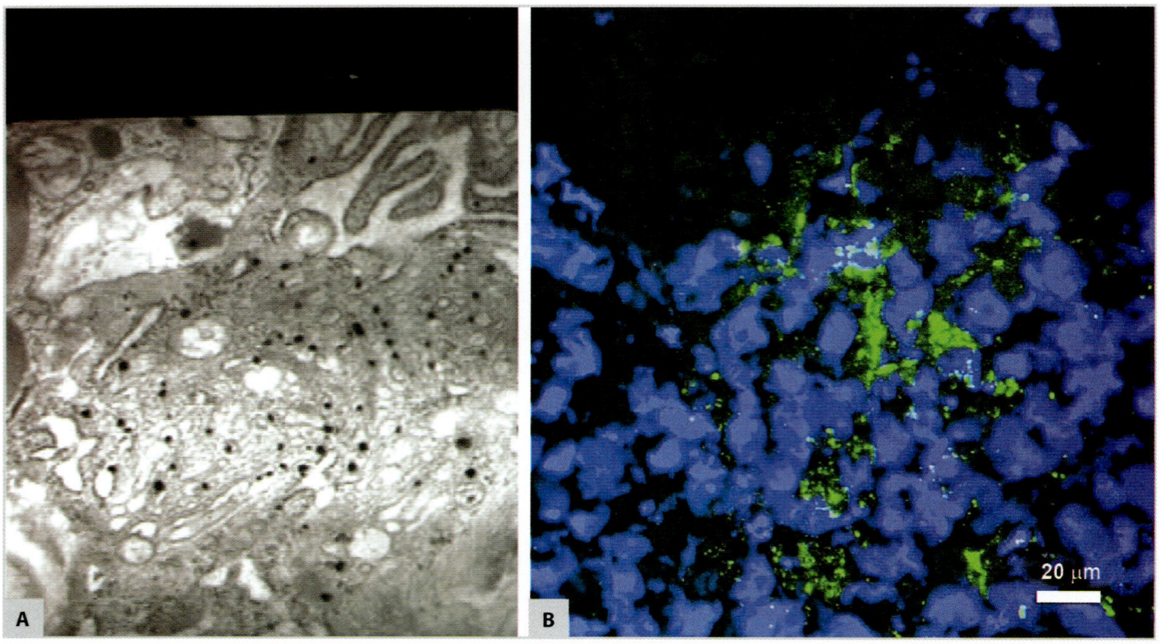

Figs 6A and B: Intracellular accumulation of nanoparticles following in vivo delivery

A. Electron microscopic analysis of tissue biopsies from a cancer patient treated with Aurimune showed accumulation of gold nanoparticles with surface binding of tumor necrosis factor (TNF) and PEG-Thiol in cancer cells.

Source: Image adapted from Reference 69

B. Confocal image showing that nanoparticles (green) of CALAA-01 (cyclodextrin polymer-siRNA nanoparticle with human transferrin) have entered a patient's cancer cells (nucleus=blue) but not the adjacent healthy tissue.

Source: Image adapted from Reference 70 with credit to Jonathan Choi and Jonathan Zuckerman, Caltech.

human transferrin as targeting ligand, and carrying siRNA against the M2 subunit of ribonucleotide reductase is currently in a phase 1 clinical trial in patients with solid tumors (Fig. 6B).[70,77]

Gold nanoparticles can be engineered to release antisense DNA oligonucleotides and cytotoxic agents under photoactivation in conjunction with their photothermal ablation therapeutic activity. For example, Trans-activating transcriptional activator (TAT)-lipid coated 40 nm hollow gold nanoshells could target to tumors and release siRNA following pulse near infrared (NIR) laser induction, providing both temporally and spatially controlled release.[78]

Liposomes can also be loaded with nucleotides to deliver gene therapy and gene silencing agents. In a phase 1 clinical study in patients with breast and ovarian cancer, intracavity injection of *E1A* gene complexed with cationic liposomes demonstrated *E1A* gene expression and accompanied HER2/neu gene downregulation in tumor cells and reduced tumor proliferation.[73] Liposomes modified with TAT peptide containing cationic lipids formed firm noncovalent complexes with DNA and allowed for in vitro and in vivo gene delivery.[79] ALN-VSP (Alnylam Pharmaceuticals, Cambridge, MA, USA) is a lipid nanoparticle delivering siRNAs against kinesin spindle protein (KSP) and vascular endothelial growth factor (VEGF) genes and has been tested in phase 1 clinical trial against liver cancer.[80]

Thermal Ablation Treatment of Cancer

Noninvasive thermal ablation therapy is a promising local treatment option for cancer. Use of nanoparticles can increase targeting accuracy of thermal ablation therapy to tumors and improve therapeutic efficacy. Several nanomaterials have been used for this purpose, including gold nanomaterials, iron nanoparticles, magnetic nanoparticles and carbon nanotubes. Heating of the particles can be induced by magnets, lasers, ultrasound, photodynamic therapy and low-power X-rays. In addition to direct destruction of tumor cells by heat, hyperthermia can also enhance the effects of chemoradiation treatments.[81]

Nanoshells have been used as theranostic agents in vivo in photothermal ablation therapy by acting as photoabsorbers to generate heat and destroy cancer cells when exposed to NIR light.[9,82] For example, AuroShell® particles (Nanospectra Bioscience, Houston, TX, USA) are nanoshells that can thermally destroy cancer tissues using a NIR laser source and are under clinical study for refractory head and neck cancer and metastatic lung cancer.[83]

Gold nanoparticles have many different shapes, including nanospheres, nanorods, nanostars, hollow nanoshells, nanoboxes and nanocages, which allows them to have tunable LSPR peaks in the NIR region and release energy as heat following NIR irradiation.[11] Polydopamine-coated gold nanorods conjugated with EGFR antibody caused selective killing of tumor cells following laser irradiation.[84]

Carbon nanotubes are carbon cylinders composed of benzene rings. Nanotubes with small sizes have been shown to be internalized by cells through endocytosis.[85] Carbon nanotubes can be engineered to target tumor cells by adsorbing different molecules to their surface and used in diagnostic and therapeutic applications. Folic acid conjugated SWNTs can specifically target folate receptor expressing cancer cells, and can be used for photothermal ablation treatment by absorbing NIR light and producing heat.[86]

Theranostic Applications

Multiple functions can be incorporated into nanoparticles to allow for theranostic (combination of therapeutic and diagnostic) platforms and real-time tracking of cancer treatment.[87] For example, blue-emitting zinc oxide (ZnO) QDs were combined with biodegradable chitosan for tumor-targeted drug delivery,[88] and examples of QD nanoparticles carrying chemotherapeutics include QD-aptamer-doxorubicin, folic acid-conjugated carboxymethyl chitosan with QD and fluorouracil (5-FU), and cadmium sulfide (CdS) QD combined with daunorubicin.[89] The conjugation of carbon nanotubes and QDs allows localization of the cancer cells by imaging with QDs, and subsequent cell killing via drug release or thermal treatment.[90] QDs modified with cationic moieties can form nanoplexes with siRNAs, which provides stability, targeting and the ability to trace the siRNA delivery.[89]

Magnetic and superparamagnetic nanoparticles are also desirable theranostic agents for magnetic hyperthermia treatment and as drug or gene delivery platforms, as they can provide monitoring and quantitative determination of biodistribution by MRI, and specific tumor delivery by tumor targeting moieties and/or magnetic field.[19] Magnetic nanoparticles produce heat when exposed to an alternating current (AC) magnetic field, which allows for local magnetic hyperthermia treatment and destruction of cancer cells. Clinical studies have shown that magnetic hyperthermia treatment is feasible and well tolerated.[91,92] Recently approved in Europe, NanoTherm® nanoparticles (MagForce AG, Berlin, Germany) are water soluble superparamagnetic nanoparticles with a size of approximately 15 nm composed of iron oxide core and an aminosilane coating. After direct introduction into the tumor, the nanoparticles are activated by a magnetic field that changes its polarity 100,000 times per second to generate heat for the local treatment of solid tumors.

Several magnetic nanoparticles have undergone both preclinical and clinical studies as drug delivery platforms, including magnetically-guided nanoparticles loaded with epidoxorubicin, mitoxantrone attached to magnetic nanoparticles of ferrofluid (magnetic liquid) and doxorubicin adsorbed to magnetic targeted carriers. In preclinical tumor models, these magnetic nanoparticles produced complete tumor remissions;[93-95] however, in clinical trials these magnetic nanoparticles showed no clinically significant toxicities and successful tumor localization, but had a relatively poor tumor response.[19,94,96,97] Magnetic nanoparticles have also been investigated for the delivery of nucleic acids through magnetofection, which concentrates and transfects cells in the area of a solid tumor using a magnetic field.[98]

SUMMARY AND CONCLUSION

The application of nanotechnology-based diagnostic and therapeutic agents is rapidly growing. However, most of these products are in preclinical and early stage clinical studies, with relatively few receiving clinical approval. Numerous challenges and hurdles exist at different development stages for these agents. The complexity of nanoparticles as multicomponent three-dimensional constructs requires careful design and engineering, detailed analysis and reproducible scale-up and manufacturing process to achieve a consistent product with the intended physicochemical characteristics, biological behaviors, and pharmacological profiles. The safety and efficacy need to be carefully examined in preclinical and clinical studies, particularly in context of the biodistribution, targeting to intended tumor sites, potential toxicity to normal tissues, and immune toxicities. For example, polymer-encapsulated QDs are generally nontoxic to cells and small animals, but their long-term in vivo toxicity and degradation in humans need to be carefully studied. Overall, nanotechnology-based agents may require additional development and regulatory considerations compared with conventional agents.

Even with the above challenges, the applications of nanotechnology in cancer have expanded dramatically during the latest years. This review only provides a glimpse of the fast growing field. Novel agents are constantly invented for diagnostic purpose as imaging tools and contrast agents, and for therapeutic purpose as small molecule drug and macromolecule carriers and as photothermal or magnetic hyperthermal agents. In the near future, nanotechnology-based agents will make strong contributions to personalized medicine based on their ability to target tumor-specific molecules expressed in a particular patient. Multifunctional nanoparticles that can act as theranostic agents will be the trend of new development, with their great advantage in real-time monitoring of drug distribution and clinical efficacy. In conclusion, novel nanotechnology platforms are highly promising to significantly advance cancer imaging and therapeutics and offer great potential to improve clinical outcomes of cancer patients.

ACKNOWLEDGMENT

Dr Shihe Hou's expert editorial and writing assistance of this manuscript is greatly appreciated.

REFERENCES

1. McNeil SE. Nanotechnology for the biologist. J Leukoc Biol. 2005;78(3):585-94.
2. Liu Z, Kiessling F, Gatjens J. Advanced nanomaterials in multimodal imaging: design, functionalization, and biomedical applications. Journal of Nanomaterials. 2010.
3. United States Food and Drug Administration (2011). Draft guidance: considering whether an FDA-regulated product involves the application of nanotechnology.[online] Available from http://www.fda.gov/regulatoryinformation/guidances/ucm257698.htm [Accessed October,2013].
4. Emerich DF, Thanos CG. The pinpoint promise of nanoparticle-based drug delivery and molecular diagnosis. Biomol Eng. 2006;23:171-84.
5. Cai W, Chen X. Preparation of peptide-conjugated quantum dots for tumor vasculature-targeted imaging. Nat Protoc. 2008;3(1):89-96.
6. Hofmann-Amtenbrink M, Hofmann H, Montet X. Superparamagnetic nanoparticles-a tool for early diagnostics. Swiss Med Wkly. 2010;140:w13081.
7. Ramsey D, Geschwind J. Chemoembolization of unresectable hepatocellular carcinoma: a review. Appl Radiol. 2004;33(3).
8. Yezhelyev MV, Gao X, Xing Y, et al. Emerging use of nanoparticles in diagnosis and treatment of breast cancer. Lancet Oncol. 2006;7:657-67.
9. Hirsch, LR, Stafford RJ, Bankson JA, et al. Nanoshell-mediated near-infrared thermal therapy of tumors under magnetic resonance guidance. Proc Natl Acad Sci. USA. 2003;100: 13549-54.
10. Cuenca AG, Jiang H, Hochwald SN, et al. Emerging implications of nanotechnology on cancer diagnostics and therapeutics. Cancer. 2006;107:459-66.
11. Ahmed A, Al Tamimi DM, Isab AA, et al. Histological changes in kidney and liver of rats due to gold (III) compound [Au(en)Cl(2)] Cl. PLoS One. 2012;7:e51889
12. Han M, Gao X, Su JZ, et al. Quantum-dot-tagged microbeads for multiplexed optical coding of biomolecules. Nat Biotechnol. 2001;19:631-5.
13. Wang Y, Zhang Y, Du Z, et al. Detection of micrometastases in lung cancer with magnetic nanoparticles and quantum dots. Int J Nanomedicine. 2012;7:2315-24.
14. Gao X, Cui Y, Levenson RM, et al. In vivo cancer targeting and imaging with semiconductor quantum dots. Nat Biotechnol. 2004;22:969-76.
15. Cai W, Shin DW, Chen K, et al. Peptide-labeled near-infrared quantum dots for imaging tumor vasculature in living subjects. Nano Lett. 2006;6:669-76.
16. Erogbogbo F, Yong KT, Roy I, et al. In vivo targeted cancer imaging, sentinel lymph node mapping and multi-channel imaging with biocompatible silicon nanocrystals. ACS Nano. 2011;5:413-23.
17. Erogbogbo F, Yong KT, Hu R, et al. Biocompatible magneto-fluorescent probes: luminescent silicon quantum dots coupled with superparamagnetic iron(III) oxide. ACS Nano. 2010;4:5131-8.
18. Sokolov K, Follen M, Aaron J, et al. Real-time vital optical imaging of precancer using anti-epidermal growth factor receptor antibodies conjugated to gold nanoparticles. Cancer Res. 2003;63:1999-2004.
19. Prijic S, Sersa G. Magnetic nanoparticles as targeted delivery systems in oncology. Radiology and oncology. 2011;45:1-16.
20. Stark DD, Weissleder R, Elizondo G, et al. Superparamagnetic iron oxide: clinical application as a contrast agent for MR imaging of the liver. Radiology. 1988;168;297-301.
21. Wang Y. Superparamagnetic iron oxide based MRI contrast agents: current status of clinical application. Quant Imaging Med Surg. 2011 1(1):35-40.
22. Artemov D, Mori N, Okollie B, et al. MR molecular imaging of the Her-2/neu receptor in breast cancer cells using targeted iron oxide nanoparticles. Magn Reson Med. 2003;49:403-8.

23. Winter PM, Caruthers SD, Kassner A, et al. Molecular imaging of angiogenesis in nascent Vx-2 rabbit tumors using a novel alpha(nu)beta3-targeted nanoparticle and 1.5 tesla magnetic resonance imaging. Cancer Res. 2003;63:5838-43.
24. Grimm J, Perez JM, Josephson L, et al. Novel nanosensors for rapid analysis of telomerase activity. Cancer Res. 2004;64:639-43.
25. Schellenberger EA, Bogdanov A, Hogemann D, et al. Annexin V-CLIO: a nanoparticle for detecting apoptosis by MRI. Mol Imaging. 2002;1:102-7.
26. Jabir NR, Tabrez S, Ashraf GM, et al. Nanotechnology-based approaches in anticancer research. Int J Nanomedicine. 2012;7:4391-408.
27. Lee CC, MacKay JA, Frechet JM, et al. Designing dendrimers for biological applications. Nat Biotechnol. 2005;23:1517-26.
28. Sitharaman B, Kissell KR, Hartman KB, et al. Superparamagnetic gadonanotubes are high-performance MRI contrast agents. Chem Commun (Camb). 2005;21(31):3915-7.
29. Desai N. Integration of nab-technology into clinical drug development. In: BIschoff J (Ed). Nanotechnologie beim Mammakarzinom-Grundlagen und aktuelle Perspektiven. UNI-MED;2013. pp. 22-31.
30. Desai N. Challenges in development of nanoparticle-based therapeutics. AAPS J. 2012;14:282-95.
31. Dong X, Mumper RJ. Nanomedicinal strategies to treat multidrug-resistant tumors: current progress. Nanomedicine (Lond). 2010;5: 597-615.
32. Greish K. Enhanced permeability and retention of macromolecular drugs in solid tumors: a royal gate for targeted anticancer nanomedicines. J Drug Target. 2007;15:457-64.
33. Lammers T, Hennink WE, Storm G. Tumour-targeted nanomedicines: principles and practice. Br J Cancer. 2008;99:392-7.
34. Chlebowski, RT. Adriamycin (doxorubicin) cardiotoxicity: a review. West J Med 1979;131(5):364-8.
35. Batist G, Ramakrishnan G, Rao CS, et al. Reduced cardiotoxicity and preserved antitumor efficacy of liposome-encapsulated doxorubicin and cyclophosphamide compared with conventional doxorubicin and cyclophosphamide in a randomized, multicenter trial of metastatic breast cancer. J Clin Oncol. 2001;19:1444-54.
36. O'Brien ME, Wigler N, Inbar M, et al. Reduced cardiotoxicity and comparable efficacy in a phase III trial of pegylated liposomal doxorubicin HCl (CAELYX/Doxil) versus conventional doxorubicin for first-line treatment of metastatic breast cancer. Ann Oncol. 2004;15:440-9.
37. Rovira-Bru M, Thompson DH, Szleifer I. Size and structure of spontaneously forming liposomes in lipid/PEG-lipid mixtures. Biophysical journal. 2002;83:2419-39.
38. Allen C, Dos Santos N, Gallagher R, et al. Controlling the physical behavior and biological performance of liposome formulations through use of surface grafted poly(ethylene glycol). Biosci Rep. 2002;22:225-50.
39. Zhu J, Xue J, Guo Z, et al. Vesicle size and stability of biomimetic liposomes from 3'-sulfo-Lewis a (SuLea) containing glycolipids. Colloids Surf B Biointerfaces. 2007;58:242-9.
40. Waterhouse DN, Tardi PG, Mayer LD, et al. A comparison of liposomal formulations of doxorubicin with drug administered in free form: changing toxicity profiles. Drug Saf. 2001;24:903-20.
41. Burger KN, Staffhorst RW, de Vijlder HC, et a . Nanocapsules: lipid-coated aggregates of cisplatin with high cytotoxicity. Nat Med. 2002;8:81-4.
42. Crosasso P, Ceruti M, Brusa P, et al. Preparation, characterization and properties of sterically stabilized paclitaxel-containing liposomes. J Control Release. 2000;63:19-30.
43. Immordino ML, Brusa P, Arpicco S, et al. Preparation, characterization, cytotoxicity and pharmacokinetics of liposomes containing docetaxel. J Control Release. 2003;91:417-29.
44. Thangapazham RL, Puri A, Tele S, et al. Evaluation of a nanotechnology-based carrier for delivery of curcumin in prostate cancer cells. Int J Oncol. 2008;32:1119-23.
45. Bayne WF, Mayer LD, Swenson CE. Pharmacokinetics of CPX-351 (cytarabine/daunorubicin HCl) liposome injection in the mouse. J Pharm Sci. 2009;98:2540-8.
46. Batist G, Gelmon KA, Chi KN, et al. Safety, pharmacokinetics, and efficacy of CPX-1 liposome injection in patients with advanced solid tumors. Clin Cancer Res. 2009;15:692-700.
47. Torchilin VP, Lukyanov AN, Gao Z, et al. Immunomicelles: targeted pharmaceutical carriers for poorly soluble drugs. Proc Natl Acad Sci. USA. 2003;100:6039-44.
48. Lukyanov AN, Elbayoumi TA, Chakilam AR, et al. Tumor-targeted liposomes: doxorubicin-loaded long-circulating liposomes modified with anti-cancer antibody. J Control Release. 2004;100:135-44.
49. Ahmed F, Discher DE. Self-porating polymersomes of PEG-PLA and PEG-PCL: hydrolysis-triggered controlled release vesicles. J Control Release. 2004;96:37-53.
50. Huang SL, MacDonald RC. Acoustically active liposomes for drug encapsulation and ultrasound-triggered release. Biochim Biophys Acta. 2004;1665:134-41.
51. Herve F, Urien S, Albengres E, et al. Drug binding in plasma. A summary of recent trends in the study of drug and hormone binding. Clin Pharmacokinet. 1994;26:44-58.
52. Stehle G, Sinn H, Wunder A, et al. Plasma protein (albumin) catabolism by the tumor itself—implications for tumor metabolism and the genesis of cachexia. Crit Rev Oncol Hematol. 1997;26:77-100.
53. Commisso C, Davidson SM, Soydaner-Azeloglu RG, et al. Macropinocytosis of protein is an amino acid supply route in Ras-transformed cells. Nature. 2013;497:633-7.
54. Schnitzer JE. Caveolae: from basic trafficking mechanisms to targeting transcytosis for tissue-specific drug and gene delivery in vivo. Adv Drug Deliv Rev. 2001;49:265-80.
55. Gundry RL, Fu Q, Jelinek CA, et al. Investigation of an albumin-enriched fraction of human serum and its albuminome. Proteomics. Clinical applications. 2007;1:73-88.
56. Mielke S, Sparreboom A, Mross K. Periphera neuropathy: a persisting challenge in paclitaxel-based regimes. Eur J Cancer. 2006;42:24-30.
57. Irizarry L, Luu T, McKoy J, et al. Cremophor EL-containing paclitaxel-induced anaphylaxis: a call to action. Community Oncology. 2009;6:132-4.

58. Ibrahim NK, Desai N, Legha S, et al. Phase I and pharmacokinetic study of ABI-007, a cremophor-free, protein-stabilized, nanoparticle formulation of paclitaxel. Clin Cancer Res. 2002;8:1038-44.
59. Gradishar WJ, Tjulandin S, Davidson N, et al. Phase III trial of nanoparticle albumin-bound paclitaxel compared with polyethylated castor oil-based paclitaxel in women with breast cancer. J Clin Oncol. 2005;23:7794-803.
60. Socinski MA, Bondarenko I, Karaseva NA, et al. Weekly nab-paclitaxel in combination with carboplatin versus solvent-based paclitaxel plus carboplatin as first-line therapy in patients with advanced non-small-cell lung cancer: final results of a phase III trial. J Clin Oncol. 2012;30:2055-62.
61. Von Hoff DD. Final results of a randomized phase III study of weekly nabpaclitaxel plus gemcitabine versus gemcitabine alone in patients with metastatic adenocarcinoma of the pancreas. In: American Society of Clinical Oncology's (ASCO) 2013 Gastrointestinal Cancers Symposium, San Francisco; 2013.
62. Owens DE, Peppas NA. Opsonization, biodistribution, and pharmacokinetics of polymeric nanoparticles. Int J Pharm. 2006;307:93-102.
63. Woo HN, Chung HK, Ju EJ, et al. Preclinical evaluation of injectable sirolimus formulated with polymeric nanoparticle for cancer therapy. Int J Nanomedicine. 2012;7:2197-208.
64. Aravind A, Jeyamohan P, Nair R, et al. AS1411 aptamer tagged PLGA-lecithin-PEG nanoparticles for tumor cell targeting and drug delivery. Biotechnol Bioeng. 2012;109:2920-31.
65. Dhar S, Gu FX, Langer R, et al. Targeted delivery of cisplatin to prostate cancer cells by aptamer functionalized Pt(IV) prodrug-PLGA-PEG nanoparticles. Proc Natl Acad Sci. USA. 2008;105:17356-61.
66. Guo J, Gao X, Su L, et al. Aptamer-functionalized PEG-PLGA nanoparticles for enhanced anti-glioma drug delivery. Biomaterials. 2011;32:8010-20.
67. Chen J, Li S, Shen Q, et al. Enhanced cellular uptake of folic acid-conjugated PLGA-PEG nanoparticles loaded with vincristine sulfate in human breast cancer. Drug Dev Ind Pharm. 2011;37:1339-46.
68. Hrkach J, Von Hoff D, Ali MM, et al. Preclinical development and clinical translation of a PSMA-targeted docetaxel nanoparticle with a differentiated pharmacological profile. Sci Transl Med. 2012;4(128):128ra139.
69. Libutti SK, Paciotti GF, Byrnes AA, et al. Phase I and pharmacokinetic studies of CYT-6091, a novel PEGylated colloidal gold-rhTNF nanomedicine. Clin Cancer Res. 2010;16:6139-49.
70. Halford B. Tiny Tech To Treat Cancer. C&EN. 2012;90(23):10-5.
71. Wang J, Lu Z, Wientjes MG, et al. Delivery of siRNA therapeutics: barriers and carriers. AAPS J. 2010;12:492-503.
72. Hayes ME, Drummond DC, Kirpotin DB, et al. Genospheres: self-assembling nucleic acid-lipid nanoparticles suitable for targeted gene delivery. Gene Ther. 2006;13;646-51.
73. Hortobagyi GN, Ueno NT, Xia W, et al. Cationic liposome-mediated E1A gene transfer to human breast and ovarian cancer cells and its biologic effects: a phase I clinical trial. J Clin Oncol. 2001;19:3422-33.
74. Prabha S, Labhasetwar V. Nanoparticle-mediated wild-type p53 gene delivery results in sustained antiproliferative activity in breast cancer cells. Mol Pharm. 2004;1:211-9.
75. Schwab G, Chavany C, Duroux I, et al. Antisense oligonucleotides adsorbed to polyalkylcyanoacrylate nanoparticles specifically inhibit mutated Ha-ras-mediated cell proliferation and tumorigenicity in nude mice. Proc Natl Acad Sci USA. 1994;91:10460-4.
76. Urban-Klein B, Werth S, Abuharbeid S, et al. RNAi-mediated gene-targeting through systemic application of polyethylenimine (PEI)-complexed siRNA in vivo. Gene Ther. 2005;12:461-6.
77. Davis ME. The first targeted delivery of siRNA in humans via a self-assembling, cyclodextrin polymer-based nanoparticle: from concept to clinic. Mol Pharm. 2009;6:659-68.
78. Braun GB, Pallaoro A, Wu G, et al. Laser-activated gene silencing via gold nanoshell-siRNA conjugates. ACS Nano. 2009;3(7):2007-15.
79. Torchilin VP, Levchenko TS, Rammohan R, et al. Cell transfection in vitro and in vivo with nontoxic TAT peptide-liposome-DNA complexes. Proc Natl Acad Sci USA. 2003;100:1972-7.
80. Tabernero J, Shapiro GI, Lorusso PM, et al. First-in-humans trial of an RNA interference therapeutic targeting VEGF and KSP in cancer patients with liver involvement. Cancer Discov. 2013;3(4):406-17.
81. Jain KK. Advances in the field of nanooncology. BMC Med. 2010;8:83
82. O'Neal DP, Hirsch LR, Halas NJ, et al. Photo-thermal tumor ablation in mice using near infrared-absorbing nanoparticles. Cancer Lett. 2004;209:171-6.
83. Morton JG, Day ES, Halas NJ, et al. Nanoshells for photothermal cancer therapy. Methods Mol Biol. 2010;624:101-17.
84. Ahmed N, Fessi H, Elaissari A. Theranostic applications of nanoparticles in cancer. Drug Discov Today. 2012;17:928-34.
85. Kam NW, Dai H. Carbon nanotubes as intracellular protein transporters: generality and biological functionality. J Am Chem Soc. 2005;127:6021-6.
86. Kam NW, O'Connell M, Wisdom JA, et al. Carbon nanotubes as multifunctional biological transporters and near-infrared agents for selective cancer cell destruction. Proc Natl Acad Sci. USA. 2005;102:11600-5.
87. Li JM, Wang YY, Zhao MX, et al. Multifunctional QD-based co-delivery of siRNA and doxorubicin to HeLa cells for reversal of multidrug resistance and real-time tracking. Biomaterials. 2012;33:2780-90.
88. Yuan Q, Hein S, Misra RD. New generation of chitosan-encapsulated ZnO quantum dots loaded with drug: synthesis, characterization and in vitro drug delivery response. Acta Biomater. 2010;6:2732-9.
89. Yong KT, Wang Y, Roy I, et al. Preparation of quantum dot/drug nanoparticle formulations for traceable targeted delivery and therapy. Theranostics. 2012;2:681-94.
90. Madani SY, Shabani F, Dwek MV, et al. Conjugation of quantum dots on carbon nanotubes for medical diagnosis and treatment. Int J Nanomedicine. 2013;8:941-50.

91. Johannsen M, Gneveckow U, Eckelt L, et al. Clinical hyperthermia of prostate cancer using magnetic nanoparticles: presentation of a new interstitial technique. Int J Hyperthermia. 2005;21: 637-47.
92. Maier-Hauff K, Rothe R, Scholz R, et al. Intracranial thermotherapy using magnetic nanoparticles combined with external beam radiotherapy: results of a feasibility study on patients with glioblastoma multiforme. J Neurooncol. 2007;81,53-60.
93. Lubbe AS, Bergemann C, Huhnt W, et al. Preclinical experiences with magnetic drug targeting: tolerance and efficacy. Cancer Res. 1996;56:4694-701.
94. Alexiou C, Arnold W, Klein RJ, et al. Locoregional cancer treatment with magnetic drug targeting. Cancer Res. 2000;60:6641-8.
95. Goodwin SC, Bittner CA, Peterson CL, et al. Single-dose toxicity study of hepatic intra-arterial infusion of doxorubicin coupled to a novel magnetically targeted drug carrier. Toxicol Sci. 2001;60:177-83.
96. Lubbe, AS, Bergemann C, Riess H, et al. Clinical experiences with magnetic drug targeting: a phase I study with 4'-epidoxorubicin in 14 patients with advanced solid tumors. Cancer Res. 1996;56:4686-93.
97. Wilson MW, Kerlan RK, Fidelman NA, et al. Hepatocellular carcinoma: regional therapy with a magnetic targeted carrier bound to doxorubicin in a dual MR imaging/ conventional angiography suite--initial experience with four patients. Radiology. 2004;230(1):287-93.
98. Jahnke A, Hirschberger J, Fischer C, et al. Intra-tumcral gene delivery of feIL-2, feIFN-gamma and feGM-CSF using magnetofection as a neoadjuvant treatment option for feline fibrosarcomas: a phase-I study. J Vet Med A Physiol Clin Med 2007;54(10):599-606.

14 Translational Research in Oncology

CS Pramesh, Rajendra Badwe

RESEARCH IN CANCER

Cancer is a major public health problem worldwide, accounting for close to 8 million deaths annually, with more than two thirds of them being in low- and middle income countries.[1,2] It is expected that by the year 2020, the annual global cancer burden will reach 20 million with nearly 10 million deaths. The World Health Organization developed three principles for management of the cancer burden—they estimated that about one third of cancers could be prevented by effective primary prevention methods, another one-third could be detected early by effective screening methods and another third could have improved survival and better quality of life with comprehensive treatment methods.[3] It appears inevitable that a systematic approach to cancer research should embrace basic science, clinical and epidemiological research with multidimensional interaction between them. Cancer is a complex disease with a multitude of changes in several genes—the importance of molecular mechanisms of carcinogenesis from the genome wide level is being increasingly recognized.[4] A number of changes in solitary nucleotide polymorphisms (SNPs) and gene signatures have been identified based on results from the human genome project and genome wide association studies (GWAS).[5] It is important to note that these discoveries were made by combining population data with laboratory in vitro findings to examine the molecular mechanisms of carcinogenesis.[6] There have been tremendous advances in the technology to facilitate cancer research in the past few years, including better understanding of the biology of cancer, comprehensive cancer genome profiling, genetically engineered mouse models, quantitative and qualitative analysis of biospecimens with clinical annotations, nanotechnology and important advances in imaging.[6] Therefore, the past and the present seem poised to launch the future of cancer research into areas never explored before.

A BRIEF HISTORY OF CANCER RESEARCH

Few papers chronicle the history of cancer research as well as DeVita and Rosenberg's manuscript to commemorate the 200th anniversary of the New England Journal of Medicine (NEJM).[7] A summary of their paper is presented in this section of the chapter. Research on cancer started in the 19th century with the discovery of the cellular origins of cancer by Virchow. Subsequent advances in that era include the postulation of the "seed and soil hypothesis" of cancer metastasis by Paget, viral carcinogenesis by Rous and the chromosomal mutational theory by Boveri. Much of the later research on cancer was driven by landmark discoveries in basic research. These included the elegant experiments by Avery in 1944 that showed that the cellular information was transmitted by deoxyribonucleic acid (DNA) and not by proteins, which sequentially led to the discovery of the structure of DNA by Watson and Crick in 1953 and later, the deciphering of the genetic code by Nirenberg and colleagues in 1961. While the results from these important discoveries led to a common dogma that genetic information was transmitted from DNA to ribonucleic acid (RNA) and resulted in protein synthesis, the discovery of reverse transcriptase proved that the converse (transmission of information from RNA to DNA) could also happen. The ability to cleave DNA at specific "restriction sites" paved the way for the molecular biology revolution and the subsequent breakthrough of sequencing of the human genome.

Parallel to these advances in basic cancer research, there were important improvements in treatment of cancer. Surgery, by far the earliest treatment modality for cancer, started from a philosophy of being able to remove organs affected by cancer, "progressed" to the Halstedian principles of radical (and supraradical) surgery and then to a more conservative and rational approach, based on clinical trials. The introduction of cobalt teletherapy in 1950, heralded the era of modern radiation oncology. Subsequent technological advances have enabled radiation oncologists to target the tumor more precisely, sparing adjacent vital structures, thereby reducing morbidity and improving cure rates. Although research in chemotherapy started in the beginning of the 20th century, it was the discovery of the therapeutic benefit of nitrogen mustard (for lymphomas) in 1943, and folate antagonists (for leukemias) in 1948, which gave this research the needed impetus. The results of two landmark studies in breast cancer in the 1970s firmly established the role of chemotherapy in solid tumors and since then, billions of dollars have been pumped in towards discovering newer chemotherapeutic agents. The discovery of imatinib in the early part of the 21st century brought a paradigm shift in the drug discovery process with convincing evidence that specific molecular aberrations could be targeted. The last decade has seen a plethora of new molecules specifically targeting known driver mutations in several cancers. Although research in immunotherapy established the role of interleukin-2 in the treatment of melanoma and renal cell carcinoma, it was the discovery of newer antibodies that has given it an important role in modern cancer therapy. These antibodies, which act by inhibiting the growth factor receptors on the surfaces of cancer cells, now have an established role in the management of lymphomas (rituximab) and melanoma (ipilimumab).

A cursory look at these advances in basic cancer research and improvements in treatment outcomes seems to indicate a disconnect between progress in these important areas of research. However, while this might be true for the greater part of this story, it seems evident that much of the therapeutic innovations in the past two decades have been directly related or based in principle on parallel breakthroughs provided by basic research. In today's age, it would be naive to assume that basic and clinical research follows two parallel tracks, close to each other but never meeting. On the contrary, they should be seen as two tracks moving forward close to each other, with several connections but intermittently indistinguishable from each other to provide important translational research breakthroughs. It therefore becomes crucial for today's oncologist to be aware of the principles and practice of basic, clinical and epidemiological research to be a truly translational researcher.

TRANSLATIONAL RESEARCH

The ultimate goal of translational research is to improve the overall health of the general public through a multidisciplinary integration of basic, clinical and population-based research strategies.[8] The director of the United States office of Scientific Development and Research made a distinction between basic and applied science as follows:[9]

"Basic research is performed without thought of practical ends. It results in general knowledge and an understanding of nature and its laws. This general knowledge provides the means of answering a large number of important practical problems, though it may not give a complete specific answer to any one of them. The function of applied research is to provide such complete answers."

The American Cancer Society defines basic science[10] as "pure science, provides the knowledge and background required for later research into human health problems. In cancer research, this is often lab study in fields like biochemistry, cell biology, or genetics that are not aimed at treating a specific cancer, but may be used later as part of the basis for a treatment." Translational research, on the other hand, is not easily defined—many basic scientists view it as a unidirectional process of using laboratory discoveries to develop diagnostics and therapeutics to be tested in clinical trials; public health researchers, on the other hand, view translational research as a process of developing evidence-based interventions and implementing them in routine clinical practice, thereby ensuring that research knowledge, new diagnostics and therapeutics actually reach the population for whom they are intended and implemented correctly.[11] It has been acknowledged that "translational research means different things to different people but it seems important to almost everyone."[11] Therefore, it becomes important to understand what the term means and the various areas of biomedical research that it represents.

What is Translational Research?

Translational research has been regarded as a "switch" from concept to practice.[6] For most academic researchers, it means the utilization of knowledge from basic science research to develop new treatment options for patients: the classical "bench to bedside" approach. The endpoint of this type of research is to bring a new treatment to clinical use. This enterprise has been described as follows: "effective translation of the new knowledge, mechanisms, and techniques generated by advances in basic science research into new approaches for prevention, diagnosis, and treatment of disease is essential for improving health."[12] From a different (but equally important) perspective, translational research also means transferring the knowledge of new treatments to the actual patients or the population that will benefit from it—the new treatment which is the endpoint of the bench to bedside approach, now becomes the starting point for this type of translational "implementation" research.[11] The Institute of Medicine's Clinical Research Roundtable described two blocks in the translational research enterprise, which are now referred to as T1 and T2 research.[13] The first block or T1 research was described by the roundtable as "the transfer of new understandings of disease mechanisms gained in the laboratory into the development of new methods for diagnosis, therapy, and prevention and their first testing in humans." The T2 block of translational research was described as "the translation of results from clinical studies into everyday clinical practice and health decision making."[13]

Members of the Evaluation Committee of the Association for Clinical Research Training (ACRT) of the National Institute of Health (NIH) developed the following working definition[8] for translational research, which is both comprehensive and operational:

"Translational research fosters the multidirectional integration of basic research, patient-oriented research, and population-based research, with the long-term aim of basic research and patient-oriented research that leads to new or improved scientific understanding or standards of care. T2 research facilitates the movement between patient-oriented research and population-based research that leads to better patient outcomes, the implementation of best practices, and improved health status in communities. T3 research promotes interaction between laboratory-based research and population-based research to stimulate a robust scientific understanding of human health and disease."

Other authors[14] further classify translational research as a continuum from T0 to T4 as follows—T0: description and discovery research; T1: discovery to health applications, including diagnostics and therapeutics; T2: health

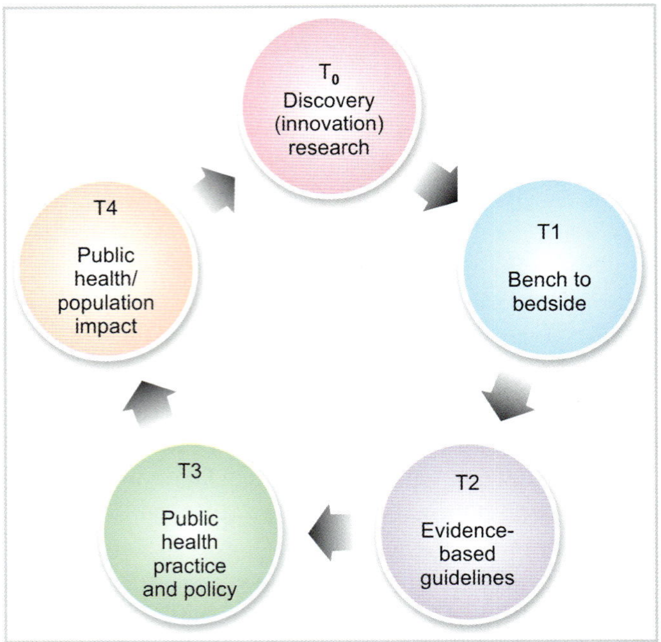

Fig. 1: The multidisciplinary multidirectional interaction between the various forms of translational research

applications to evidence-based guidelines; T3: guidelines to health practice; T4: health practice to population outcomes. Clearly, translational research is much more than the traditionally defined "bench to bedside" research. These definitions of translational research emphasize that it is both multidimensional as well as multidirectional drawing from the lab, the clinic and the community (Fig. 1). In this chapter, subsequent reference will use the ACRT definitions with detailed description of the T1, T2 and T3 phases of translational research.

Need for Translational Research

The benefits of translational research are based on the realization that understanding disease processes is fundamental to providing rational treatment options, that establishing efficacy in a clinical trial precedes universal applicability of new treatment options and that the most efficacious treatment is useless unless it is readily implementable in the community. It is unfortunate that in spite of major advances in our understanding of biology, pathophysiology of disease, molecular mechanisms of health and disease, and high end technologies to study all of these, the translation of this knowledge into improvements in public health has been less than optimal.[15] It is disconcerting that in spite of several decades of knowledge about the contribution of tobacco use, physical inactivity, and poor diet to chronic, noncommunicable diseases like diabetes, cardiac disease and cancer, this has not translated into reductions of the public health burden of these diseases.[16]

Healthcare costs have escalated in the recent past, secondary to improved life expectancy characterized by an aging population, conversion of several acute illnesses to chronic conditions and high costs of conventional cancer treatment.[17] There is an urgent need to identify universally accessible, cost effective treatment options that improve overall cancer outcomes and reduce mortality. Much of the escalated costs of cancer treatment stems from the fact that many patients have to be treated for a few to benefit (most new drugs have shown benefits only to a small percentage of patients treated with it). "Personalized therapy" towards which much of current translational research in cancer is directed, has the potential to be able to identify those who are most likely to benefit, thereby giving a superior therapeutic benefit ratio. Equally importantly, it also has the potential to identify those unlikely to benefit from these treatment options, sparing unnecessary toxicity and reducing treatment costs. While these have obvious advantages in resource-constrained economies, they are important even in highly developed "first-world" countries, which are now increasingly feeling the pinch of high healthcare costs for cancer treatment.

T1 Research—Bench to Bedside (Discovery to Applications) Research

T1 translational research is by far the most understood form of translational research because this has been the traditional definition of the term. It is intuitively appealing that discoveries in the laboratory "translate" into true diagnostic and therapeutic benefits in the clinic—the classical bench to bedside story. Basic research has conventionally focused on mechanisms of disease, trying to understand the pathophysiology from health to disease and the molecular mechanisms underlying them. Some authors[14] have further divided this phase into T0 and T1 research. T0 research is the phase which deals exclusively with "description and discovery" while T1 research deals with translating these discoveries into diagnostic and therapeutic health applications.

There are numerous examples of T1 research fulfilling its potential with the discovery of new treatment options. In cancer, no drug discovery has exemplified the benefits of T1 research as much as the discovery of new targeted agents for several cancers. Identification of the C-KIT pathway led to the discovery of imatinib in chronic myeloid leukemia and gastrointestinal stromal tumors, revolutionizing the treatment of these cancers.[18] The impact of the discovery of the HER-2 pathway and subsequent utilization of trastuzumab in breast cancer is a remarkable example of basic science research translating into real human benefit in a common cancer.[19] Lung cancer treatment has changed dramatically in the past decade—while it was dumped into either non-small cell or small cell lung cancer a decade back, we have strong evidence that not just histology (squamous vs nonsquamous) but also mutation status [epidermal growth factor receptor (EGFR) mutations, EML4-ALK translocations amongst others] are important for prognostication as well as to guide treatment.[20,21] The remarkable breakthroughs with clinical trials of gefitinib and erlotinib in EGFR mutated patients and crizotinib in EML4-ALK translocated patients are striking examples of how basic research has caused paradigm shifts in cancer treatment.

T2 Research—Guidelines to Population (Health Practice)

Type 2 translational research involves research into the systems and processes by which proven, efficacious treatment is adopted and implemented in the community with a view to increasing their population impact. The Society for Prevention Research Type 2 Translational Task Force identified two core challenges[22] for promoting T2 translational research: "(1) building infrastructure and capacity to support systems-oriented scaling up of evidence-based interventions, with well-integrated practice-oriented T2 research and (2) developing an agenda and improving research methods for advancing T2 translation science". In many ways, these are bigger challenges than those facing T1 translational research because the systems and processes are far different and the magnitude of the implementation process far bigger. The decision to accept, adopt and implement an evidence-based intervention in a real-world situation is dependent on time and cost-effective approaches, a strong connect to community needs and an organizational leadership which places emphasis on research-proven interventions and practices.[23] There has been a relative lack of funding for T2 translational (implementation) research compared to T1 (discovery) research. This is unfortunate as many authors feel that more lives would probably be saved by the widespread implementation of existing known efficacious treatment than the discovery of new treatment options. Controversial though, this statement might be, it demonstrates a need for a policy level rethink on priorities for translational research funding.

T2 translational research has had far reaching effects on the population in several areas of healthcare including reducing tobacco, alcohol and drug abuse, physical inactivity, unhealthy eating, teen pregnancy, and several others.[24] However, there are numerous studies which indicate that only a small proportion of the public actually benefit from evidence-based interventions[11,25] and that few public health interventions are actually evidence-based even in the US.[22,26-28] To illustrate this, a recent study showed data suggesting that only 10.2% of acute care hospitals in the US have access to the EGFR mutation test in spite of overwhelming evidence that this was a crucial investigation required to treat advanced lung cancer.[29] It is sobering to realize that the time taken for a clearly effective intervention to be adopted widely in public health can take 17 years or more depending on the intervention.[30] Clearly, there are gaps between proving the efficacy of an intervention and establishing effectiveness in the community. An increased emphasis on implementation research has the potential to save lives, reduce health problems and improve overall quality of life.[22] Importantly, it also has the potential to save money by shifting investments from high-cost, low-efficacy processes to low-cost, high-impact interventions.[31]

The Translation Science to Population Impact (TSci Impact) framework[22] suggests that the two core challenges identified to translational research can be overcome with a conceptual framework of four phases of translation with continuous information feedback loops between them: pre-adoption, adoption, implementation and sustainability. In the pre-adoption phase, the emphasis is on gaining information and knowledge about the new intervention from all stakeholders—the policy makers, the physicians and the general public—and establishing that it is indeed efficacious. Adoption research involves a systematic study of factors which the stakeholders listed above consider would influence the decision to adopt the intervention, including decision making tools. These include research on potential funding for the implementation, attitudes towards the intervention, incentives to ensure adoption by the stakeholders, health economics and organizational readiness for change. Implementation research focuses on research on a broad range of factors affecting implementation of effective interventions in the community. These are aimed at how specific strategies can be used to integrate evidence-based interventions into specific systems and situations, e.g. schools, community centers, etc. These include research on keeping target populations and organizations engaged, estimating how faithful the actual implementation is to the original intervention, methods of integration of the evidence-based intervention into existing systems and the monitoring of the intervention, and the impact on the community. Finally, sustainability research evaluates the long-term adoption and institutionalization of these interventions, and studying how they can be expanded across specific situations and delivery systems. This phase of research would include examining factors contributing to long-term implementation like availability of funding, organizational stability and capability, sustainability of the community teams, and the strength of the policy making process.[22]

T3 Research—Population to Bench

T3 translational research deals with how population research generates hypotheses which can be tested in laboratories and the converse, how laboratory research is used in population-level health interventions.[8] Several examples of T3 translational research exist, including molecular and genetic epidemiology, public health genomics, etc. Newer technologies like next generation sequencing, gene expression profiles and proteomics are being developed with the aim of personalized cancer care with targeted therapy, and discovery of biomarkers for early detection and prognostication.[32] Although a number of these genome-based applications are ready for use in the population, the translation of these discoveries in community practice has been slow.[33,34] It is expected that discoveries in the laboratory that prevent cancer or detect and intervene early in the disease process will have the highest impact in reducing mortality from cancer.[35] Research on genes involved in cancer causation can be used in assessment of lifetime cancer risk, targeted prevention, early detection and manipulation of behavioral and environmental factors to reduce cancer risk, and thereby reduce the cancer burden in the primary healthcare and population settings. Research is already ongoing on the molecular and genetic characterization of tumors, prognostic and predictive biomarkers, and pharmacogenomics to improve the safety and efficacy of cancer therapeutics in the hospital setting.[32]

The Translational Research Team

The single most important factor for the success of a translational research program is the close interaction between the basic scientists, clinical researchers, and the epidemiologists with considerable inputs from biostatistics, bioinformatics, molecular imaging, bioengineering, cell biology, physics, structural chemistry and numerous other specialties. State-of-the-art research in each of these individual disciplines would be meaningless if there is no integrated approach between them. This has probably been the biggest challenge that most institutions have had to face. The lack of a common language between these specialties has led to each of them working in their individual silos, content with advancing their own field without having an impact on human health and disease. Probably the reason for this is the lack of training during each of these career tracks in the other disciplines—the basic scientist rarely has an insight into problems in the clinic or the population, the clinician researcher has no knowledge of the possibilities of basic research or the applicability in the community and the epidemiologist lacks understanding of the processes in basic science or the solutions for clinical problems. This problem is compounded by the physical and cultural separation of these departments in many institutes, thereby limiting opportunities for researchers to network and collaborate on important human health issues. While it may still be a distant dream for a single individual to be able to be an expert in these three widely disparate branches of healthcare, most leaders in translational research have been able to straddle at least two of these disciplines and have a working knowledge of the third.

Training in Translational Research

Currently, there is clear realization that translational research requires formal training to be able to bridge this metaphoric gap between these three important disciplines. A number of structured short- and medium-term training programs are now available for researchers from basic science, clinical research and epidemiology to be able to understand the other fields better. Training in translational research would vary and would need to be customized depending on the trainee's background, expertise, and area of research which they plan to pursue.[8] Common areas of learning would include basic training in study design, biostatistics, bioethics and research integrity, human subject protection, searching for funding sources, writing research proposals, and grant applications. Most importantly, researchers need to be trained on communication and negotiation skills, tact and humility— mandatory traits to thrive in a multidisciplinary collaborative team.[8] Future planning to augment the translational research enterprise should address the basic flaws in training in these three core areas, and attempt to provide physical and cultural proximity to each other. Clearly, an integrated approach between basic, clinical and epidemiology research is crucial for the translational research endeavor to be successful.

Potential of Translational Research

The translational researcher has never had it so good—important technological advances like high throughput DNA sequencing, protein identification, expression arrays, highly sophisticated imaging systems have all combined to provide powerful research tools to answer fundamental biological questions.[17] While these tools have spurred progress in many fields of biomedical research, the impact on newer hypotheses and discoveries in cancer research is particularly exciting. This rapid increase in research technologies, combined with the unprecedented quantum of data available, have encouraged researchers to take multidimensional looks at common but complex diseases and explore new strategies of treatment. This new knowledge gives a unique opportunity to understand disease based on hitherto unknown genomic, proteomic and metabolomic profiles.

The Challenges of Translational Medical Research

Embracing the concept of translational research brings forth several new challenges. Firstly, all stakeholders need to realize that basic, clinical and epidemiological researches need to integrate seamlessly for accelerated progress in cancer research. Policy makers and administrators need to understand that this integration is not just helpful, but is mandatory for any meaningful improvements in cancer outcomes. Traditional (artificial) organizational barriers like departments, specialties, and disciplines need to be broken to create convergence of ideas, problems and solutions.[17] Secondly, researchers from all these fields have to realize that cutting edge research is now a huge team sport. The era of the lone crusading researcher who is able to come up with cataclysmic breakthroughs is over. Researchers who are used to working in isolated silos have to reorient themselves as small (but important) parts of a huge research machine with an intricate network. Newer (and for biomedical research, novel) disciplines like bioinformatics, structural chemists, systems biologists and several others—all have to be integral parts of this team. The true translational research leader has to be able to create common goals from amongst the varied aspirations of the individuals constituting the team. Thirdly, creating and sustaining a critical mass of clinician-scientist-epidemiologist is not easy and requires adequate training and mentoring of researchers as well as protected time away from the increasing pressures of patient care. Finally, access to translational research technologies has to be universal and easy. While there have undoubtedly been important advances in these technologies, these are also expensive, and this could be a difficult problem to overcome especially in developing countries. Considering that knowledge about fundamental biological processes in health and cancer are still not understood well enough to convert this information into more effective treatment and prevention, it is important that current efforts in translational research are sustained and accelerated. With growing awareness amongst policy makers and researchers and an unprecedented increase in research funding for translational research, we are confident that these challenges can be overcome in the near future.

REFERENCES

1. World Health Organization (2010). Burden: mortality, morbidity and risk factors. [online] Available from: http://www.who.int/nmh/publications/ncd_report_chapter1.pdf [Accessed October, 2013].
2. World Health Organization (2010). GLOBOCAN 2008. [online] Available from http://globocan.iarc.fr [Accessed October, 2013].
3. Ngoma T. World Health Organization cancer priorities in developing countries. Ann Oncol. 2006;17(Suppl 8):viii9-14.
4. Stratton MR. Exploring the genomes of cancer cells: progress and promise. Science. 2011;331:1553-8.
5. Broderick P, Wang Y, Vijayakrishnan J, et al. Deciphering the impact of common genetic variation on lung cancer risk: a genome-wide association study. Cancer Res. 2009;69:6633-41.
6. Cao Y, DePinho RA, Ernst M, et al. Cancer research: past, present and future. Nat Rev Cancer. 2011;11:749-54.
7. DeVita VT, Rosenberg SA. Two hundred years of cancer research. N Engl J Med. 2012;366:2207-14.
8. Rubio DM, Schoenbaum EE, Lee LS, et al. Acad Med. 2010;85:470-5.
9. United States Office of Scientific Research and Development, Bush V. In: Bush V (Ed). Science, the endless frontier: a report to the President. Washington, DC: United States Government Printing Office; 1945.
10. American Cancer Society (2013). Cancer glossary. [online] Available from http://www.cancer.org/cancer/cancerglossary/index [Accessed October, 2013].
11. Woolf SH. The meaning of translational research and why it matters. JAMA. 2008;299:211-3.
12. Fontanarosa PB, DeAngelis CD. Basic science and translational research in JAMA. JAMA. 2002;287:1728.
13. Sung NS, Crowley WF, Genel M, et al. Central challenges facing the national clinical research enterprise. JAMA. 2003;289:1278-87.
14. Khoury MJ, Gwinn M, Ioannidis JP. The emergence of translational epidemiology: from scientific discovery to population health impact. Am J Epidemiol. 2010;172:517-24.
15. Zerhouni EA. Space for the cures: science launches a journal dedicated to translational research in biomedicine. Sci Trans Med. 2009;1:1-2.
16. Collins JL, Marks JS, Koplan JP. Chronic disease prevention and control: coming of age at the Centers for Disease Control and Prevention. Prev Chronic Dis. 2010;6:A81.
17. Zerhouni EA. US Biomedical research: basic, translational and clinical sciences. JAMA. 2005;294:1352-8.
18. Druker BJ, Sawyers CL, Kantarjian H, et al. Activity of a specific inhibitor of the BCR-ABL tyrosine kinase in the blast crisis of chronic myeloid leukemia and acute lymphoblastic leukemia with the Philadelphia chromosome. N Engl J Med. 2001;344:1038-42.
19. Slamon DJ, Leyland-Jones B, Shak S, et al. Use of chemotherapy plus a monoclonal antibody against HER2 for metastatic breast cancer that overexpresses HER2. N Engl J Med. 2001;344:783-92.
20. Lynch TJ, Bell DW, Sordella R, et al. Activating mutations in the epidermal growth factor receptor underlying responsiveness of non-small-cell lung cancer to gefitinib. N Engl J Med. 2004;350:2129-39.
21. Kwak EL, Bang YJ, Camidge DR, et al. Anaplastic lymphoma kinase inhibition in non-small-cell lung cancer. N Engl J Med. 2010;363:1693-703.
22. Spoth R, Rohrbach LA, Greenberg M, et al. Society for Prevention Research Type 2 Translational Task Force Members and Contributing Authors. Addressing Core Challenges for the Next Generation of Type 2 Translation Research and Systems: The Translation Science to Population Impact (TSci Impact) Framework. Prev Sci. 2013;14:319-51.
23. Dobbins M, Cockerill R, Barnsley J, et al. Factors of the innovation, organization, environment, and individual that predict the influence five systematic reviews had on public health decisions. Int J Technol Assess Health Care. 2001;17:467-78.
24. National Research Council (US) and Institute of Medicine (US) Committee on the Prevention of Mental Disorders and Substance Abuse Among Children, Youth, and Young Adults: Research Advances and Promising Interventions (2009). In: O'Connell ME, Boat T, Warner KE (Eds). Preventing mental, emotional, and behavioral disorders among young people: progress and possibilities. Washington (DC): National Academies Press; 2009.
25. McGlynn EA, Asch SM, Adams J, et al. The quality of health care delivered to adults in the United States. N Engl J Med. 2003;348:2635-45.
26. Gottfredson GD, Gottfredson DC, Czeh ER, et al. National study of delinquency prevention in schools. [online] Available from: https://www.ncjrs.gov/pdffiles1/nij/grants/194116.pdf [Accessed October, 2013].

27. Ringwalt C, Vincus A, Hanley S, et al. The prevalence of evidence-based drug use prevention curricula in US middle schools in 2005. Prev Sci. 2009;10:33-40.

28. Mendel RA (2000). Less hype, more help: Reducing juvenile crime, what works—and what doesn't. [online] Available from: http://www.aypf.org/publications/mendel/MendelRep.pdf [Accessed October, 2013].

29. Lynch JA, Khoury MJ, Borzecki A, et al. Utilization of epidermal growth factor receptor (EGFR) testing in the United States: a case study of T3 translational research. Genet Med. 2013;15:630-8.

30. Boren SA, Balas EA. Evidence-based quality measurement. J Ambul Care Manage. 1999;22:17-23.

31. Woolf SH. A closer look at the economic argument for disease prevention. JAMA. 2009;301:536-8.

32. Khoury MJ, Clauser SB, Freedman AN, et al. Population sciences, translational research, and the opportunities and challenges for genomics to reduce the burden of cancer in the 21st century. Cancer Epidemiol Biomarkers Prev. 2011;20:2105-14.

33. Gwinn M, Grossniklaus D, Yu W, et al. Horizon scanning for new genomic tests. Genet Med. 2011;13:161-5.

34. Varmus H. Ten years on—the human genome and medicine. New Engl J Med. 2010;362:2028-9.

35. Ogilvie D, Craig P, Griffin S, et al. A translational framework for public health research. BMC Public Health. 2009;9:116.

15

The Impact of Minimally Invasive Surgery in Oncology

Shailesh Puntambekar, Geetanjali Agarwal-Joshi, Saurabh Joshi, Akhil Lawande

"Science progresses more by opposition than appreciation"

"The world hates change, but it is the only thing that has brought progress" (**Charles Kettering**)

INTRODUCTION

Surgical practise has undergone radical changes in the last century. This saw the development of video laparoscopy and robotic surgery. What was considered as a "gold standard" open surgery was suddenly challenged by the development of keyhole "surgery". Keyhole surgery was already existing till 1980 for sterilization and diagnostic purposes, but rapid development and acceptance lead to its use in benign surgeries like appendicectomy and cholecystectomy.[1] The oncosurgeons though, understated the benefits and didn't embrace the technology wholeheartedly, for fear of suboptimal long-term results. A few centers and enthusiastic surgeons started using minimally invasive surgery (MIS) to deal with cancers. Slowly and steadily early reports of MIS in pelvic lymphadenectomy,[2] radical hysterectomy,[3] laparoscopic colorectal surgeries,[4] esophagectomies,[5] lobectomies and radical prostatectomy were published.[6] Almost any abdominal or thoracic procedure can now be dealt with MIS.

Over the last 25 years, there has been a significant technological advancement in the field of laparoscopy. This advancement has led to better visualization, high quality resolution through high-definition camera systems. The visual aids were further aided by better lights like Xenon and light-emitting diode, CO_2 insufflators and gas warming systems. The only energy source available during conventional surgery was electrocautery. There has been a surge in the development of energy sources.

First time in literature a sound energy was designed for cutting and coagulation (Harmonic Ace®). This lead to safety as the maximum temperature generated is 80°C with minimal lateral spread. Since the field of vision is limited in laparoscopy these features are important to avoid damage to the surrounding structures. The smoke generated is much less than the conventional electrocautery and energy is delivered only at the end of the instrument. The other energy sources are vessel sealing instruments like LigaSure™, EnSeal® and tripolar. These devices can seal vessel up to 7 mm and thus obviating the need to apply clips or suture or ligate. This leads to an avascular dissection and avoids frequent change of instruments. Revolution into different types of energy sources leads to their use in open surgery as well, with many surgeons performing Whipple's/hepatectomies and anterior rectal dissection with total mesorectal excision with hand held probes or harmonic scalpels.

Minimally invasive surgery is instrument dependent and hence there has been rapid development of various instruments which is beyond the scope of this communication. Suffice to say that a wide range of high quality instruments are available enabling the surgeon to perform different surgeries in an appropriate and precise way.

Though there were major developments in visual aids, instrumentations and energy sources, the acceptance of laparoscopy has been rather tardy in oncology. The reasons are:

- Depth of perception
- Skill development due to use of straight sticks
- Assistant dependent
- Limited field of vision
- Longer learning curve
- Majority of trained oncosurgeons had their training in pre-laparoscopic era.[7]

This to the development of 3D camera systems and robotic surgery. Robotic surgery was approved by US Food and Drug Administration in 2000 for clinical use. The first robotic procedure performed was robotic prostatectomy. There was an immediate acceptance of this all over USA. The urologist could easily perform this procedure and now the American Urological Association (AUA) recommends this as the procedure of choice for cancer prostate. We will evaluate the comparative data with open and laparoscopic prostatectomies in the subsequent paragraphs. Since 2001, almost all organs have been tackled robotically. The robot probably fills the skill gap needed to do laparoscopic surgery thus making it feasible for an ordinary surgeon to perform complex surgeries. The biggest advantage is the ease of suturing, 3D vision, intuitive movements and easy learning. One need not be a great laparoscopic surgeon to perform robotic surgery. Robotic cancer surgery is now also being applied for superficial organs like thyroid, breast and reconstructive surgery trans-oral robotic surgery (TORS) has also developed for pyriform fossa and other hypopharyngeal lesions.

Oncologic principles such as no touch isolation, en block resection of the primary tumor, tumor free surgical margins have to be followed while doing laparoscopy. The extent of lymph node (LN) dissection and the proximal ligation of vascular pedicles before touching the tumor should also be the same as that in open surgery. The lymph node yield is an independent factor which decides the adequacy of MIS. The specimen should be protected during removal from the wound. This can be achieved by using an endobag. This prevents tumor implantation or port site metastasis. Besides the known benefits of laparoscopic surgery, morbidity and mortality should be either less or comparable to that of open surgery. The disease free survival (DFS) and overall survival (OS) are important end points when treating cancer. Follow-up results in the last two decades has shown that DFS and OS are comparable in laparoscopic or open surgery for colorectal, uterine, gastric and esophageal cancers.

When laparoscopy cannot achieve the same clearance conversion to open surgery is indicated. Conversion to open surgery should not be related to complication but should be a mature decision when an adequate clearance cannot be achieved. Laparoscopic surgery, based on normal interleukin 6 (IL-6) concentrations,[8] maintains immune function within the normal range as opposed to open surgery. Other inflammatory changes are significantly decreased in laparoscopy as well. In an immunocompromized patient, laparoscopy could be an invaluable diagnostic or therapeutic modality.[7,9,10]

LAPAROSCOPY IN ONCOLOGY

Laparoscopy in oncology can be divided basically into four types of procedures: (1) diagnosis; (2) staging; (3) palliative; (4) therapeutic.

Diagnosis and Staging

This can be used for staging of lymphomas, all upper abdominal cancers like stomach, pancreas, liver and gallbladder, ovarian masses. Laparoscopy is now an integral part of perioperative assessment of patients with pancreatic malignancy.[11,12] Unresectability of the tumor can be determined at the time of diagnosis and staging.

Palliative

The main palliative procedures are gastric and biliary bypass. Cuschieri was the first to report a series of biliary bypass,[13] and the first reported laparoscopic gastrojejunostomy was by Wilson and Verma.[14] Palliative internal iliac artery ligation for bleeding, managing adhesive obstruction and nerve blocks for pain relief, (celiac axis block) are often indications where MIS could be considered.

Therapeutic

Besides the known advantages laparoscopic surgery like less perioperative morbidity, decrease hospital stay, less pain and decrease incidence of wound dehiscence, the additional advantages include:

Evidence based surgery

- Less blood loss, less pain and minimal scarring
- Early return of bowel activity
- Immunological response (proposed but not proven)
- Early initiation of adjuvant treatment
- Reduced hospital stay by 2 or 3 days.

Intra-abdominal laparoscopic surgery can be divided into two parts. The line of division lies at the umbilicus. The cancers in the supraumbilical lesion lap is used for staging. Various institutes as MD Anderson Center and Memorial Sloan-Kettering Cancer Center used this for gastric, pancreatic and periampullary cancers before deciding on laparotomy or laparoscopy. As a positron emission tomography or computed tomography scan cannot pick up peritoneal and omental deposits. Laparoscopy can thus avoid major laparotomy in 10–15% of patients. All the supraumbilical cancers are laparoscopy assisted while those below the umbilicus can be laparoscopy-assisted or total laparoscopic procedures. Supraumbilical cancers can have lot of anatomical variations while the pelvis has very little anatomical variations; port positions will therefore remain constant for pelvic tumors; they are in the form of an inverted C (Fig. 1). For supraumbilical tumors the port positions will vary. The pelvic port positions are the same for rectal, bladder and uterine surgery, and this standardization helps to perform surgery with ease. The patient position is always modified Lloyd-Davis irrespective of the site of surgery. This allows the surgeon to move all around the patient thus enabling access to all quadrants. This is the greatest advantage of keyhole or minimal access surgery.

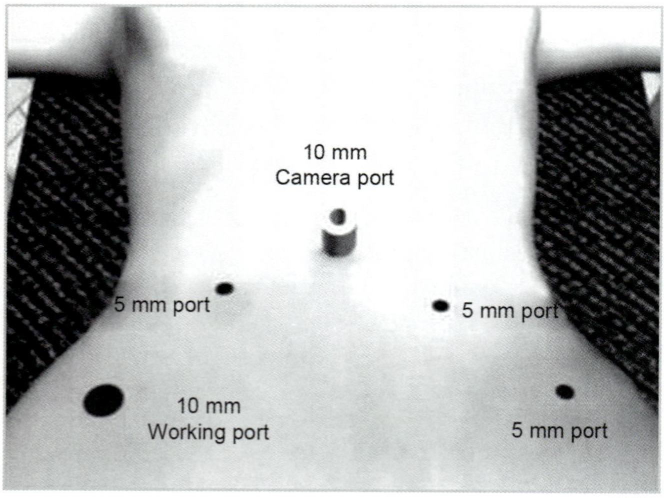

Fig. 1: Port positions

TABLE 1: Comparison between laparoscopic and robotic surgery

	Laparoscopy	*Robotic*
Vision	2D	3D
Depth perception	Poor	Good
Movements	Restricted	Intuitive
Learning curve	Steep	Short
Suturing	Difficult	Easy
Access	All quadrants	One quadrant
Tissue feel	Present	Absent

Robotic ports are unforgiving ports and only one quadrant surgery can be performed in a particular robotic position. For example, cystoprostatectomy can be done, but for urinary diversions the robot has to be re-docked in another position. Except for this disadvantage, robotic surgery has all benefits of minimal access surgery with vision comparable to that of open surgery as illustrated in Table 1.

Robotic surgery is mainly used for complex surgeries, and particularly done where the space is limited as in pelvis or thorax.

Thoracoscopy

In thoracoscopic surgery the biggest advantage of minimal access surgery is visualization, better access and precision in an area where complex anatomy and important structures lie. The biggest advantage is avoidance of a painful thoracotomy, which impacts on lung function and results in low compliance. Esophageal mobilization, lung resection and removal of mediastinal masses are commonly performed oncosurgeries by MIS.

ESOPHAGUS

Minimally access surgery has revolutionized many areas of surgery since its introduction in late 1980s. The common denominator in minimal access surgery is to perform the same operation as in the open approach but through a smaller incision. This reduces the operative trauma without compromising the principles of surgical oncology. Application of laparoscopy in esophagectomy has been slow because of associated complexities, decreased tactile control, possibly increasing the risk of injuring adjacent vital structures, compromised margins, inadequate LN retrieval and tumor dissemination including port site metastasis; however, with the potential to reduce trauma, using MIS may reduce high morbidity and mortality associated with these procedures.[14] The laparoscopic approach also holds the advantage in those cases in which radiological evidence of operability is equivocal, avoiding a major laparotomy and delay in further palliative management.

The various minimally access surgical techniques to esophagectomy use either thoracoscopy or laparoscopy, or a combination of both techniques. Transhiatal approach was initially described by Denk in 1913, and later popularized by Orringer.[15] The side effect of transhiatal approach was blunt mediastinal dissection, resulting in intraoperative bleeding and recurrent laryngeal nerve injury. DePaula et al.[16] were the first to demonstrate the feasibility of laparoscopic transhiatal esophagectomy in a series of 12 patients. Avital et al.[17] published a retrospective analysis of 22 patients undergoing transhiatal esophagectomy (Table 2).

Simon et al.[20] retrospectively analyzed 29 patients and mentioned the advantages of magnified dissection in laparoscopic trans-hiatal esophagectomy (THE), especially of gastroesophageal junction. The pressure of pneumoperitoneum aids the dissection of the esophagus and ensures a wide dissection. Concerns about adequate nodal dissection were raised. Torek[21] performed the first successful transthoracic esophageal resection. Right thoracotomy and abdominal approach was described by Lewis in 1946. Tanner in 1947 described the Ivor-Lewis procedure.[22] In 1998, Luketich[23] and colleagues described the combined thoracoscopic and laparoscopic approach overcoming the disadvantage of laparoscopic transhiatal approach mainly difficulty in mobilizing the middle third esophagus. Smithers et al. (2001) reported their experience with 162 patients who underwent thoracoscopic esophageal mobilization in prone position. Martin et al. (2005) promoted the prone position as the deflated lung lies forward out of the operating field and requires no extra port for a lung retractor (Table 3). Smithers et al. (2001) reported their experience with 162 patients who underwent thoracoscopic transthoracic esophagectomy (TTE) in prone position; the median survival time was 29 months which was similar to the same group's experience with an open Ivor-Lewis technique. Nguyen et al.[19] described a technique similar in principle to the technique described by Swanson and colleagues (2001), which consisted of an initial right thoracotomy for complete dissection of the esophagus followed by a laparotomy for mobilization of the gastric conduit and a cervical anastomosis. Nguyen used thoracoscopy instead of thoracotomy and laparoscopy instead of laparotomy. The advantages of thoracoscopy include improved visualization with better hemostasis, and the ability to evaluate proximal and middle-third tumor for possible extension to other mediastinal structures.

Use of hand-assisted laparoscopic and thoracoscopic surgery in radical esophagectomy with three-field lymphadenectomy for thoracic esophageal cancer was described by Suzuki et al.[24] But thoracoscopic esophagectomy fell into disrepute because of longer operative time, increasing morbidity, hence defying its advantages. Thus the choice for a particular minimally access approach to esophagectomy was based on the location of tumor, its extension and radiological LN enlargement. One of the major and common drawbacks of minimally access esophagectomy was the longer operative

TABLE 2: Laparoscopic transhiatal esophagectomy

Author	*Number of patients*	*Conversion*	*Mean operative time (minute)*	*Mean blood loss (mL)*	*Mortality*	*Morbidity*	*Mean hospital stay*	*Mean no. of LN harvested*
DePaula et al.[16]	12	1 (8.3%)	256	-	0	5	7.6	NA
Swanstrom et al.[18]	9	0	390	290	0	4	6.4	NA
Avital et al.[17]	22	1 (4.5%)	380	220	1 (4.5%)	4	8	14.3
Puntambekar et al.	98	0	155	250	5 (5.5%)	10	8	10

Abbreviations: LN, lymph node; NA, not applicable

TABLE 3: Transthoracic esophagectomy

Author	*Number of patients*	*Conversion*	*Mean operative time (minute)*	*Mean blood loss (mL)*	*Mortality*	*Morbidity*	*Mean hospital stay*	*Mean no of LN harvested*
Martin et al.	36	2	190–360	Upto 1,500	2 (5.5%)	15	8–61	-
Nguyen et al.[19]	46	2	210–520	Upto 1,500	4.3%	12	4–60	10.3
Puntambekar et al.	108	2	180	Upto 500	2 (3.7%)	5	5–20	15

Abbreviations: LN, lymph node

time and need for extensive surgical experience. The learning curve as well as the time taken to complete these procedures can be reduced by standardization of steps and preventing repetition, which is the aim of this atlas. Luketich et al.[23] recently reported the largest series to date of minimally invasive esophagectomies. They reported their experience in 222 patients operated during a 6-year period with a combined laparoscopic and thoracoscopic approach. They reported a 7.5 hours median operative time which decreased to 4.5 hours after the 29th procedure. In a high-volume centre. Selection of laparoscopic THE and TTE, will depend on the location of the tumor and patient status.[25,26] Stomach is the usual conduit. Drainage procedure is generally avoided. Cervical anastomosis is performed in two layers end-to-side hand-sewn.[27]

Operative Technique

1. After induction of general anesthesia, standard intratracheal single lumen intubation follows. Patient is then positioned in prone decubitus position on a standard apparatus in order to support on the head, thorax and pelvis. Abdomen is maintained free for breathing excursions. Position of the arms is very important in order to get abduction of the scapula. The arms are positioned on a support device in flexion of the shoulders and elbows. In this way the area between the spine and the inner edge of the scapula is broadened.
2. Three trocars are placed along the inner edge of the right scapula. The first at the level of the medial lowest point of the scapula, a 10 mm, (can be 5 mm) for the "0" degree thoracoscope. The second, at the level of fourth intercostal space, 10 mm; the third, at the level of eighth intercostal space 5 mm (Fig. 2). The first trocar is introduced open in the thoracic cavity after control by finger palpation that the space is free of adhesions. After introduction of the first trocar a positive insufflation of 7 mm Hg is initiated in order to retract enough the right lung for an adequate visualization of the posterior mediastinum.
3. Inspection is performed of the thoracic cavity and the esophageal area in order to assess if resection is possible. As in conventional surgery, presence of metastases, in the pleura or lung, and local ingrowth of the tumor and fixation will preclude a thoracoscopic resection. Dissection starts anteriorly by cutting the pulmonary ligament, and the anterior pleura along the lung outside the plane of vagus nerve, from the pericardial sac to the hilum of the right lung (right pulmonary vein and right bronchus) up to the azygos vein.
4. Posteriorly, the mediastinal pleura is cut longitudinally at the posterior edge of the esophagus lateral to the esophagus, anterior of the azygos vein from the costophrenic angle to the arch of the azygos vein (Fig. 3).
5. Along the plane of the descending aorta, the esophagus with periesophageal LNs and fat is dissected free, taking care to safe guard the thoracic duct. Vascular branches from the aorta to the esophagus at this level have to be clipped in order to avoid bleeding. The rest of branches are divided by means of a harmonic shears or bipolar coagulation. In this way, the posterior plane of the pericardium, right atrium and contralateral pleura is reached.
6. Furthermore, the azygos vein is dissected free and preserved (Fig. 4).

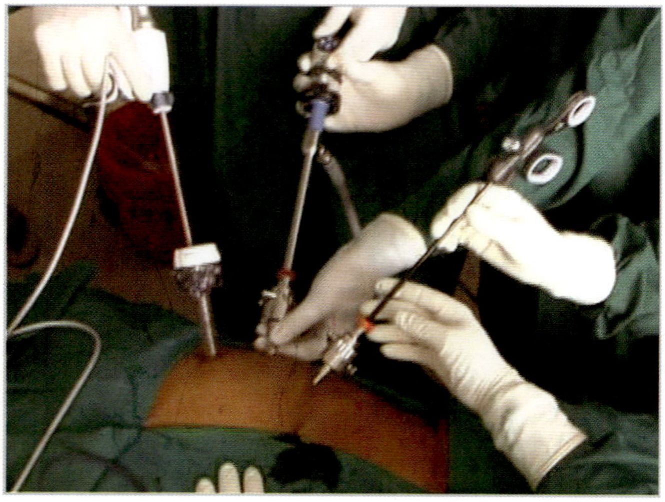

Fig. 2: Surgeon, camera assistant and port position in prone position

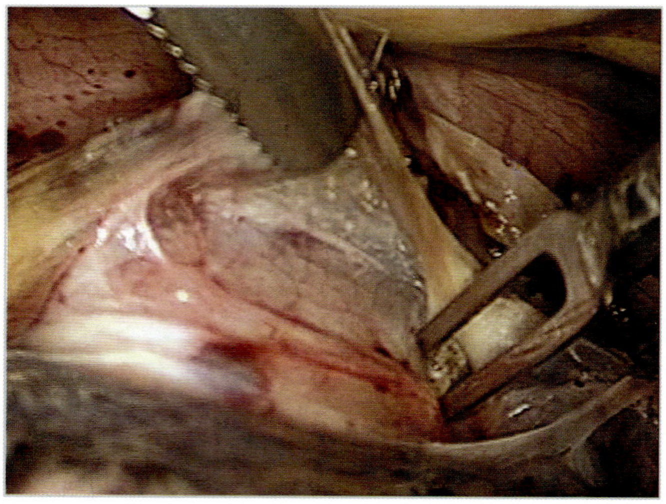

Fig. 3: Pleural cut taken outside the plane of vagus

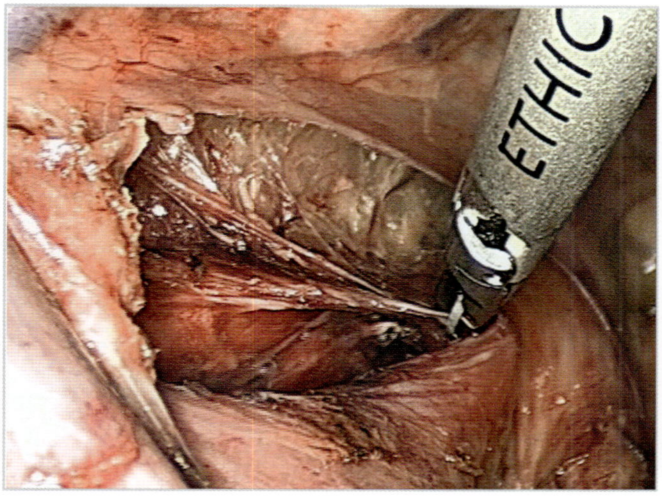

Fig. 4: Supra-azygous mobilization of esophagus

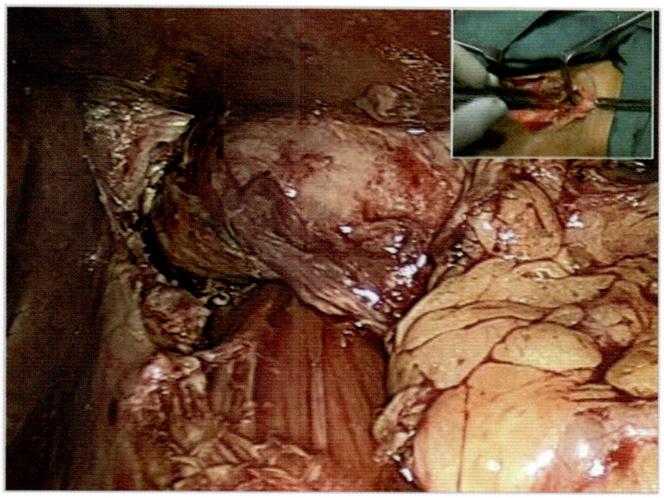

Fig. 5: Gastroesophageal (GE) junction and hiatus after gastric mobilization; inset: simultaneous cervical mobilization of esophagus

7. Dissection proceeds with extensive lymphadenectomy of the right bronchus, carina and left bronchus resection. Lymphadenectomy is "en bloc," hence all the LN remain attached to the specimen.
8. Dissection continues between esophagus and trachea (pars membranacea) in proximal direction, to stop 3 cm from the apex of the thoracic cavity.
9. After hemostasis control, patient is turned and put in supine position and bilateral thoracic drains are kept.
10. Patient is placed supine for the laparoscopic and cervical phase of the operation. Stomach is mobilized completely with preservation of the gastroepiploic vessels and an extensive lymphadenectomy of the celiac trunk is performed. Last part of the laparoscopic approach is the dissection of the hiatal area in which the hiatus is enlarged anteriorly and carefully a communication is made with the thoracic dissected area. At the end of the laparoscopic phase, a second team will approach the esophagus at the cervical area and after division of the esophagus [and attached a nasogastric (NG) tube to the distal part of the divided esophagus] the specimen is retrieved by the abdominal surgeon through a transumbilical incision of 5 cm, protected by a hand assisted device. A 4 cm wide gastric tube is created extracorporeally by means of a 10 cm linear stapler device. No pyloromyotomy or pyloroplasty or Kocher maneuver is performed. After closure of the abdominal wound, insufflation is restarted and under laparoscopic control, the gastric tube, fixed to the NG tube is transhiatal placed into the cervical region. Final situation cervical hand-sewn anastomosis is done in two layers (Fig. 5).

COLON AND RECTAL CANCER

The development of laparoscopy in the treatment of colorectal cancer has been an evolving process since 1990. The MIS approach for malignant colorectal cancers has met with a lot of skepticism till the results of several large randomized controlled trials (RCT) were published in 2002.[28-31] The initial reports were based on retrospective data and these assessed the feasibility, safety and oncological results of laparoscopic surgery. The various trials which gave evidence to laparoscopic colorectal surgery are the Lacy trial from University of Barcelona (Table 4). This trial compares laparoscopy versus open colectomy of right and left colon. Patient with transverse colon carcinoma, obstructive lesion, T4 lesion and prior surgery were excluded.

The laparoscopic colorectal cancer surgical technique can be divided into:

- Hand-assisted laparoscopic surgery
- Single port surgery
- Robotic surgery.

The total laparoscopic procedures are:

- Abdominoperineal resection (APR)
- Right and left hemicolectomy
- Total proctocolectomy.

The only totally laparoscopic procedure is APR. The other procedures are laparoscopic assisted as a small incision is taken to extract the specimen.

Indications for laparoscopic colorectal surgery:

- T1–T3 lesion
- N0 or N1

TABLE 4: **Oncologic outcomes of trials**

Cancer outcomes	*Barcelona (2002)*	*COST (2004)*	*Taiwan (2006)*
	Laparoscopy versus open	Laparoscopy versus open	Laparoscopy versus open
Median	44 months (27–85): 43 months (27–85)	4.4 year overall	40 months (18–27) 23:29
Tumor recurrence Distant Locoregional Peritoneal seeding Port/Incision site	18:28 7:09 7:14 3:5 1:0	76:84 2:1	23:29 1:1
Time to recurrence (months)	15:17		
5 year overall survival (%) I II III	82:74 85:94 75:77 72:45	79:78 84:94 78:81 60:63	
5 year disease free survival (%) I II III	 80% vs 76% 70% vs 45% 	78:80 92:96 82:88 62:60	 80% vs 70% 67% vs 62%
Cancer related survival (%) I II III	91:79 100:99 88:85 84:50		
Adjuvant therapy	68:59	Not significant	All stage III

Abbreviations: COST, clinical outcomes of surgical therapy

TABLE 5: **Large randomized controlled trials comparing laparoscopic and open colon cancer resections: study design and patient demographics**

	Barcelona[28]	*COST*[29]	*COLOR*[30]	*CLASICC*[31]
Accrual years	1993–1998	1994–2001	1997–2003	1996–2002
Study sites	Single center	Multicenter	Multicenter	Multicenter
Surgery	Laparoscopic-assisted	Laparoscopic-assisted	Laparoscopic-assisted	Laparoscopic-assisted
Exclusion criteria	TC, DM, IO, PCS	TC, DM, IO, SMI, IBD, FP, P, OM	TC, SF, DM, IO, PCS, PM, BMI > 30	TC, IO, PM, P
Primary endpoint	Cancer related survival	Time to tumor recurrence	Cancer free survival at 3 years	Margin positivity, operative mortality
Subjects (n)	L: 106 O: 102	L: 435 0: 428	L: 536 O: 546	L: 273 O: 140
Median follow-up	L: 44 O: 43	52.8	Long-term results not yet reported	49.5

Abbreviations: COST, clinical outcomes of surgical therapy; COLOR, colon carcinoma laparoscopic or open resection; CLASICC, conventional versus laparoscopic-assisted surgery in patients with colorectal cancer; TC; DM; IO; PCS; SMI; IBD; FP; P; OM; SF; BMI, body mass index; PM

- No peritoneal deposits
- No distant metastasis
- Medically fit for surgery.

Contraindications for laparoscopic colorectal surgery:

- T4 lesion
- Obstructive disease
- Perforation
- Severe malena
- N2 disease
- Distant metastasis
- Peritoneal deposits
- Ascites.

Technical issues:

- Laparoscopic right hemicolectomy

- Laparoscopic low anterior resection (LAR)
- Laparoscopic APR.

Right Hemicolectomy

Indications

- T1–T3 tumors of the right colon
- Crohn's disease
- Tuberculosis of the ascending colon.

Energy Sources

- Harmonic scalpel
- Bipolar energy
- EnSeal® bipolar source.

Anesthesia

Combination of regional (spinal or epidural) is used along with general anesthesia. The use of regional anesthesia leads to sympathetic blockade. This causes the small bowel to contract and remain on the left side.

Patient Position

The patient is placed in right lateral position. A right side tilt of 45 degrees is given. A bolster is kept on right side.

The camera is placed at the umbilicus or just above the umbilicus depending upon the patient's BMI. An 11 mm working port placed anterior to camera port in mid-clavicular line in the right hypochondrium. A 5 mm port is placed in the same line lower down in the suprapubic region. Thus a triangulation is achieved. Another 5 mm port is placed in the right iliac fossa for the assistant.

Procedure

Step 1: The first step is to do an exploratory laparoscopy and visualize the tumor. The small bowel is then placed in the left iliac fossa and the omentum is placed in the supracolic compartment. This step helps to display the entire colonic mesentery along with the superior mesenteric artery and the vein.

Step 2: The assistant holds the colon at the hepatic flexure and retracts it upward. The patient is then placed in 30 degrees head low position. The entire colonic mesentery is put under stretch. The second position of duodenum is easily visualized beneath the thin mesentery. The best way to open the retroperitoneal is to take a cut at this level and expose the duodenum. Once the cut is taken, CO_2 insufflations opened the space completely. This space is further opened and dissection should continue to expose the Gerota's fascia. This dissection is done by using gauze; this blunt dissection is done very easily staying anterior to duodenum and Gerota's fascia. The plane of dissection should continue till the lateral abdominal wall is reached.

Step 3: The right colic artery is seen due to previous step. The peritoneal space below the artery is also an avascular space and is opened with harmonic scalpel which exposes the retroperitoneal space. This dissection is done from the medial to lateral space. The ureters and the gonadal vessels can be seen at this stage. The plane of dissection should be above this structure and should continue till lateral wall reached. This dissection is also done by pushing gauze in the retroperitoneal space.

Step 4: The right colic artery and vein are then dissected from their origin and all the fibrofatty tissue along with the nodes is dissected (Fig. 6). The ileocolic vessels are clipped at the origin with Hem-o-lok® (TELEFLEX MEDICAL, NC 27709) clip and divided (Fig. 7).

Step 5: Cut pedicle is held by the assistant and the retrocolic dissection completed. At this stage, the hepatic flexure dissected from below the peritoneal attachment at hepatic flexure is cut.

Step 6: The right branch of middle colic along with the vein is seen anterior to head of pancreas. These vessels are carefully dissected and nodes along them are removed. These vessels are then clipped and ligated. The retrocolic space below the cecum and terminal ileum is dissected. This exposes the common iliac vessels.

Step 7: The assistant then pulls transverse colon downward. Supracolic omentum is then separated from hepatic

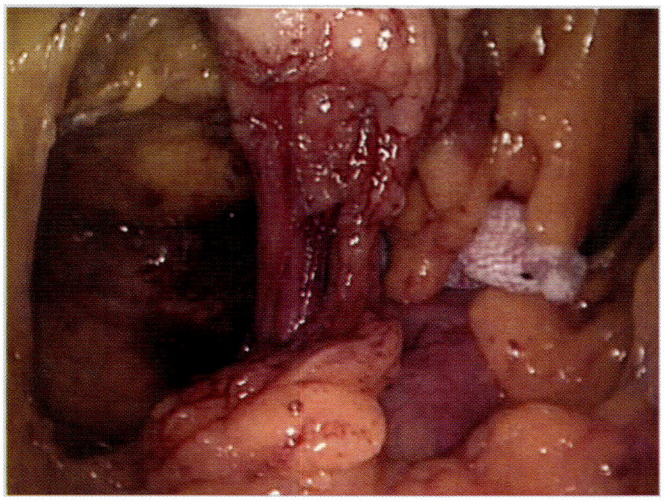

Fig. 6: The opening of the peritoneum below the right colic pedicle

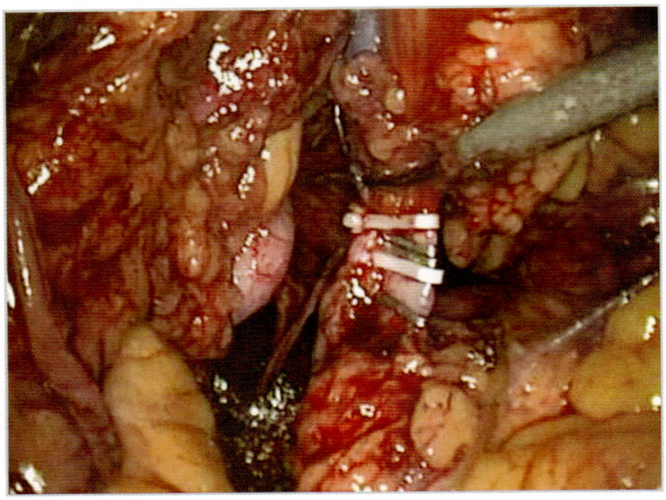

Fig. 7: The ligation of ileocolic vessels

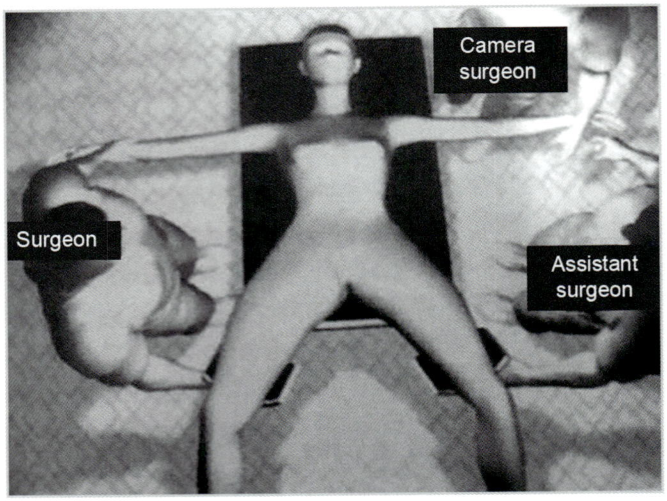

Fig. 8: Surgeon's position on right side and assistant on the left

flexure till the mid transverse colon. The lesser sac entered in supracolic region.

Step 8: The assistant pulls the cecum medially. The lateral peritoneum is cut from cecum till the hepatic flexure. The important step is put the tissue under traction so that dissection can be done in the avascular plane.

Step 9: The entire ascending colon along with the cecum and terminal small bowel is thus freed from all attachments. The resection and anastomosis can be done intracorporeally or extracorporeally. We preferred to do extracorporeal transection. We take a small transverse incision about 5 cm at level of transverse colon. This specimen is delivered after wound protection, and the anastomosis is done manually or with staplers drain placed through the port in the right fossa.

Laparoscopic Low Anterior Resection

Indications

- T1–T3 tumor of lower rectum
- T4 tumors—post-neoadjuvent chemoradiation.

Contraindication

Medically unfit patients

Instruments needed:

- Harmonic scalpel
- Bipolar energy
- EnSeal® bipolar source.

Anesthesia

Combination of regional (spinal or epidural) along with general anesthesia is used to induce the patients. The use of regional anesthesia leads to sympathetic blockade. This causes the small bowel to contract and prevents it from coming into pelvic cavity during the dissection.

The surgeon stands on right side and the assistants are on the left side. The working port is on the right side in the McBurney's point; this position gives a wider range of movements of the right hand.

Patient Position

The patient is placed in modified Lloyd-Devies position. A bolster is placed at the level of anterosuperior iliac spine (Fig. 8). This breaks the pelvis and hence, puts the small intestine in the right iliac fossa.

Port Position

Five ports are placed for all pelvic surgeries. A 10 mm camera port is at the umbilicus. A 10 mm port is placed in the McBurney's point on the right side. A 5 mm port is placed in the pararectal region at the level of umbilicus in midclavicular line. A similar set of two 5 mm ports are placed as a mirror image of the right port on the left side.

Procedure

Step 1: The assistant surgeon holds the sigmoid colon upward and toward the pelvis, thereby, making the inferior mesenteric pedicle prominent.

Step 2: Peritoneal cut lateral to the inferior mesenteric pedicle is taken at the level of sacral promontory. The peritoneal cut is extended cranially and caudally. This opens the retroperitoneal space. The dissection is then carried below the inferior mesenteric pedicle from the medial to the lateral side. This exposes the left ureter and gonadal vessels. The dissection is further carried laterally to expose the psoas muscle.

Step 3: All the fibrofatty tissue along the inferior mesenteric artery and the vein is resected. The artery is thus exposed and separated from the vein. The artery is clipped as closed to its origin and divided. The vein is dissected further cranially till the duodenojejunal flexure is reached. The vein is divided at this level (Fig. 9).

Step 4: The distal cut and of the pedicle is lifted by the assistant's right hand and retracted upward. This opens the presacral area. The CO_2 insufflation assists in opening this space further. At this stage, the autonomic nerves are seen on either side on the posterolateral aspect. The ureters are always lateral to the nerves.

Step 5: The presacral dissection started in the presacral fascia. The plane of dissection is always above the fascia and below the rectal fat. The left hand grasper of the assistant gives upward traction to open the plane further, while the left hand grasper of assistant holds the rectum steady. The harmonic scalpel helps to do a bloodless dissection, this plane called as "holy plane". The dictum is that fat belongs to the rectum and the plane of dissection should be always above the fat. This dissection is done medial to the autonomic nerves. The dissection is carried downward till the distal limit of levator ani reached.

Step 6: Once the posterior dissection is completed, the assistant surgeon's right hand pulls the rectum on the left side. This stretches the peritoneal folds on the right side. The left hand grasper of the assistant surgeon holds the bladder peritoneum in males or uterus in females. This exposes the pouch of Douglas (POD). The surgeon's left hand grasper pushes the rectum further on the left side and the right peritoneal cut is taken to free the rectum completely. The rectum is further pushed to the left and cut is extended up to the levator ani. The plane of dissection is always lateral to the rectal fat and medial to the autonomic nerves (Fig. 10).

Step 7: The POD is entered from the right side. The dissection should be between the two layers of Denonvilliers' fascia. The rectum is pulled in the midline cranially by the assistant surgeon's right hand grasper. The left hand grasper continues to pull the peritoneum or uterus upward. The rectum is dissected of the posterior vaginal wall or the seminal vesicles in the two layers of Denonvilliers' fascia. The plane is above the fat of the rectum anteriorly. The dissection is carried downward till the anorectal junction. The cut from the right side is joined to separate the rectum anteriorly and from the right lateral wall. In 30% of patients, the middle rectal artery can be seen in the lateral pedicle during its dissection. This can be coagulated and cut with the harmonic scalpel.

Step 8: The rectum is then pushed to the left side and the left lateral peritoneal cut is taken. This exposes the left ureter as well as the left autonomic nerve. The dissection is done medial to the nerve and the carried downward to join the peritoneal cut from the right side. The left lateral ligament is coagulated and cut to free the rectum completely. The left levator ani with its covering endopelvic fascia is seen.

Step 9: The rectum, sigmoid colon and the descending colon is separated from the peritoneal fold laterally. The mobilization is continued till the splenic flexure is reached. This is essential to achieve a tension free colorectal or coloanal anastomosis.

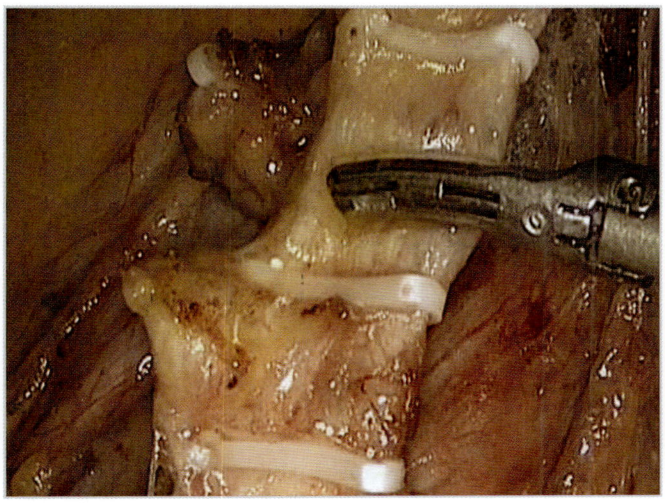

Fig. 9: Ligation of inferior mesenteric pedicles

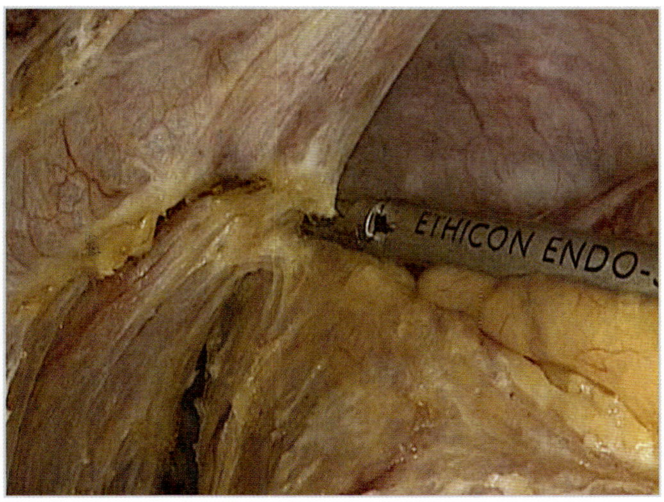

Fig. 10: Lateral mobilization of rectum

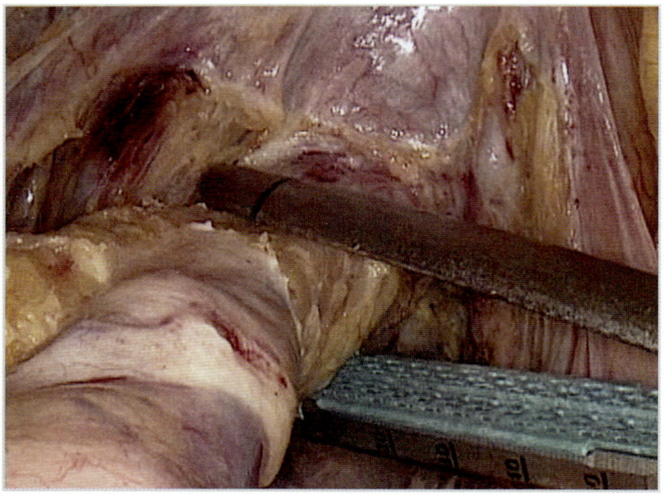

Fig. 11: Division of rectum distal to tumor

Step 10: Once the mobilization is complete a suprapubic 12 mm port is inserted. The distal limit of the tumor is assessed by digital examination and the level of stapling is decided. The stapler is then introduced and the rectum is separated (Fig. 11). The advantage of suprapubic port is in easy stapling of the rectal stump. The advantage is more pronounced in ultralow anterior resections.

Step 11: A small midline or Pfannenstiel incision 5 cm in length is taken. The specimen is delivered using a wound protection. The level of proximal colon transection is decided and colon is transected. The anvil of circular stapler is inserted at this stage. The colon with its anvil is inserted back in the abdomen and the abdomen is closed.

Step 12: The other end of the circular stapler is then inserted per anal through the distal stapled line. The anvil is engaged laparoscopically and the stapler is closed. The stapler is fired. The anastomosis integrity is checked by pushing air from below after filling the pelvis with water. A covering colostomy or an ileostomy may be done as per surgeon's choice. We prefer to do it in ultralow anterior resections. The doughnuts are checked as well as distal margins of resection. A drain is inserted through the left lower port.

- Stretching of the inferior mesenteric pedicle
- The ligation of inferior mesenteric vein at the duodenojejunal flexure and the artery at the origin
- The retraction of cut pedicle upward
- The dissection in the presacral space. The lateral limit on the either side is autonomic nerve
- The dissection in the two layers of Denonvilliers' fascia
- The splenic flexure mobilization
- The insertion of the suprapubic port
- Intracorporeal engagement of the stapler.

Abdominoperineal Resection

Indications

- Low tumors of the rectum
- Anal canal tumor.

The port position, anesthesia, surgeon's position and instruments are the same as in LAR.

Procedure

Step 1 to step 9 are same as in LAR.

Step 10: Once the mobilization of the rectum is completed all around, the dissection should continue further caudally. The levator ani muscles should be defined from all around. If feasible, further caudal dissection engulfing the levator ani muscles can be done. In that case, the perineal dissection is minimized. Anteriorly the dissection can be done till the apex of the prostate is reached.

Step 11: The level of proximal colon transection is decided and the colon is transected. The proximal end is brought out as end colostomy. A small incision at the premarked colostomy site is taken. The rest of the divided rectal specimen is left inside to be delivered perineally.

Step 12: The perineal dissection is done in the same way as is done in open surgery. The specimen is removed and the wound closed primarily keeping a drain.

Important Steps

- Stretching of the inferior mesenteric pedicle
- The ligation of inferior mesenteric vein at the duodenojejunal flexure and the artery at the origin
- The retraction of cut pedicle upward
- The dissection in the presacral space. The lateral limit on the either side is autonomic nerve
- The dissection in the two layers of Denonvilliers' fascia
- The splenic flexure mobilization
- The caudal dissection to expose the levator ani all around
- Division of the colon and bringing the proximal end as colostomy.

HYSTERECTOMY

Uterine malignancies are the second common cause of cancer death in women worldwide. Its incidence appears to have risen in the recent years because of increasing awareness and screening. The gold standard treatment of cervix cancer is radical hysterectomy. Since the first radical hysterectomy performed by Clark in 1895 and the Wertheim's technique of radical hysterectomy in 1898, the radical hysterectomy has evolved into a simpler procedure and the surgical approach has evolved over a period of time into a highly specialized with minimally invasive modality.

The author describes his "Pune technique" of laparoscopic radical hysterectomy with operative steps which are standardized. This makes this technique universally acceptable as it is easily duplicable.

Laparoscopic Radical Hysterectomy

Indications

- Cervical cancers stage 1A2 to stage 2A. Cases of stage 1A1 with a high risk for LN spread are also included in the group
- Endometrial cancer upto stage 2

Preoperative irradiation is not a contraindication for the laparoscopic procedure.

Contraindications

- Tumor size more than 4 cm at largest diameter
- Evidence of peritoneal carcinomatosis or distant metastatic disease
- Evidence of grossly involved LNs.

Procedure

The uterus is hitched in cases of endometrial malignancy. In cases of cervical malignancies a Myoma screw is used and it is introduced from the upper left port and inserted into the fundus for uterine manipulation.

Step 1: Posterior U cut: Uterus is anteverted. The right ureter is identified underneath the peritoneum at the level of sacral promontory. The peritoneum over it is excised with the help of harmonic shears to expose the ureter. This cut is extended down upto the POD keeping the ureters laterally and constantly under vision. The same steps are repeated on the left side and both the peritoneal cuts joined in the POD forming the posterior U cut (Fig. 12).

Step 2: Dissection of rectovaginal space: The peritoneum in the POD is pulled cephalad and with the help of harmonic shears it is incised. The dissection is carried between the two layers of Denonvilliers' fascia. The plane between the fat and the posterior vaginal wall is dissected keeping in mind the dictum "the fat belongs to rectum" (Fig. 13).

Step 3: Dissection of pararectal space: The left ureter is retracted medially and the posterior leaf of broad ligament above the ureter is cut. The cut is extended downward toward the bladder. Ureter forms the medial boundary of the pararectal space and the internal iliac artery forms the lateral boundary. The ureter is retracted medially and the dissection is done parallel to the ureter to open the pararectal space. The uterine artery crosses the pararectal space transversely. The space anterior to the uterine artery and medial to the obliterated hypogastric artery is dissected (Fig. 14). This dissection is continued to the paravesical space upto the levator ani. The uterine vein is seen below the artery. Both the artery and the vein are individually clipped or ligated and then cut. Ureter is retracted medially to expose the uteroscaral and Mackenrodt's ligaments which are seen as a single fan shaped structure (Fig. 15). They are then cut with the harmonic shears in the downward direction toward the levator ani. Same steps repeated on the right side.

Step 4: Anterior U cut: The uterus is retroverted. The peritoneum over the uterovesical fold is cut using the harmonic shears, starting from the round ligament on one side to the other forming the anterior U cut. The fascial plane between the bladder and the uterus is

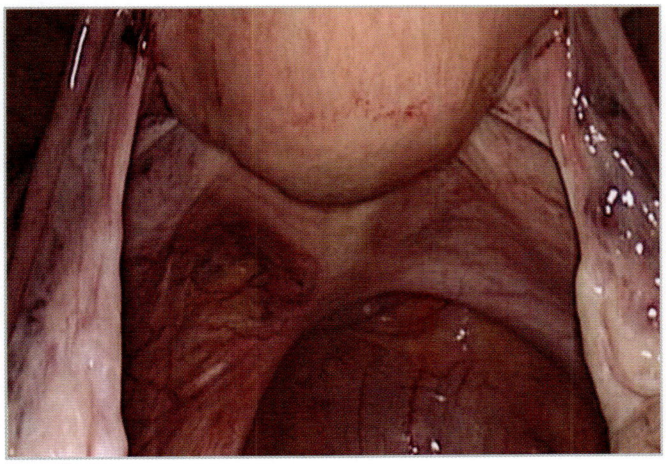

Fig. 12: Posterior U cut

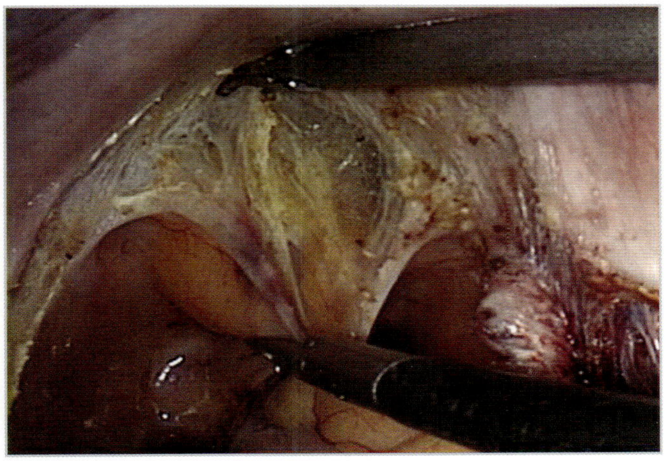

Fig. 13: Dissection in POD. Fat belongs to the rectum, right plane and wrong plane

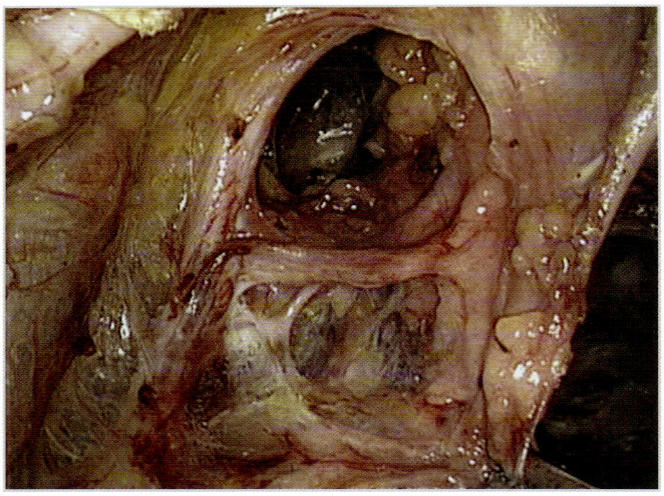

Fig. 14: Left pararectal space. Uterine artery and vein

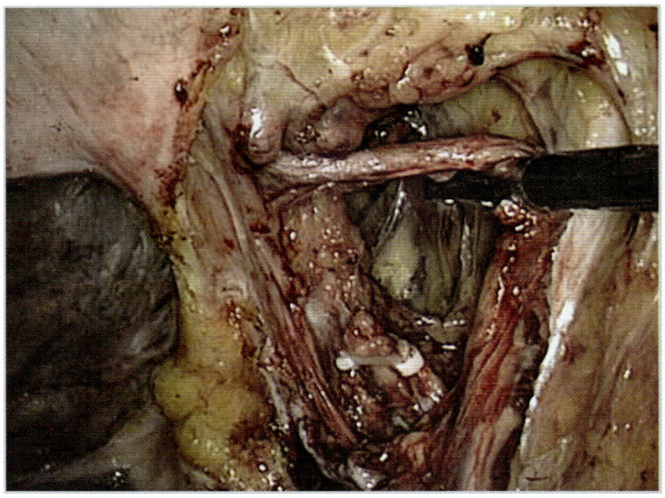

Fig. 15: Right cardinal ligaments seen as single fan shaped structure

developed keeping in mind the dictum "fat belongs to bladder". The peritoneal cut is further extended up to the infundibulopelvic ligaments. A cut is made in the broad ligament and the ureter can now be seen through this broad ligament window.

Step 5: Dissection of ureteric tunnel: The uterus is pulled to the right. The left ureter is traced along its entire course toward the bladder. The bladder peritoneum is held and the bladder is retracted upward. Thus the ureteric tunnel is exposed. This tunnel is dissected with the help of Maryland's forceps (Fig. 16). There are two veins in the roof of the tunnel which can be clipped and then cut. This helps in pushing the ureter further laterally. The ureter can be seen as it enters the bladder at the uterovesical junction. The bladder is pushed further down to achieve a good vaginal cuff, below the growth. The paracolpos is then cut as laterally as possible. These steps ensure that we can obtain maximum amount of paracolpos and the vaginal margin. The same steps are repeated on the right side making the trigonal area visible. Colpotomy is done above this level with the help of harmonic shears. The infundibulopelvic ligaments are then cut and the entire specimen is separated and placed in an endobag.

Step 6: LN dissection: The LN dissection is started at the bifurcation of common iliac artery. The dissection is done with the help of suction cannula as it is relatively atraumatic (Fig. 17). No energy source is used here. All the fibrofatty tissue along the external iliac vein is dissected, sweeping the cannula in a direction parallel to the vessels upto the iliac bone which forms the lateral limit of the dissection. The medial limit is formed by the internal iliac artery, and the lower limit is the obturator nerve. Similar dissection is

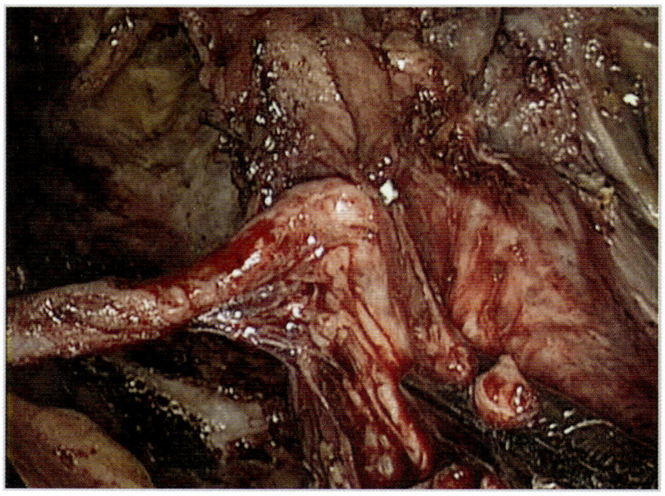

Fig. 16: Left ureteric tunnel dissection

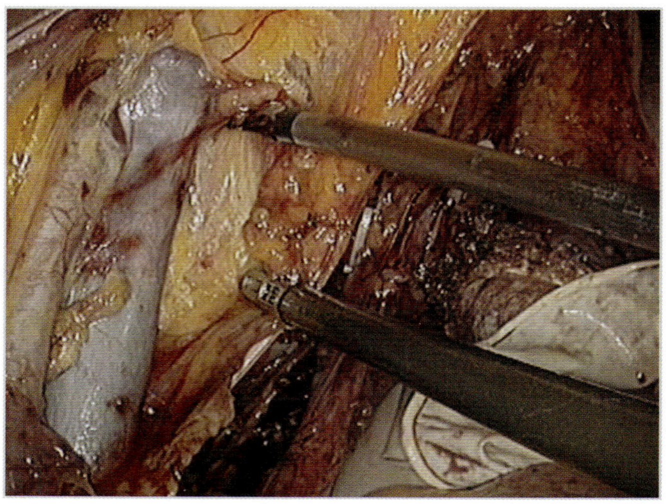

Fig. 17: Left ilio-obturator lymph node dissection

done on both the sides. The entire nodal tissue obtained is put in the endobag.

The endobag is removed vaginally. Hemostasis is achieved. Wound is irrigated with normal saline. Vault is closed with continuous locking intracorporeal suturing with polyglactin 910 2-0, which is introduced through the 10 mm working port. It is not necessary to use any intra-abdominal drain. The ports are removed under vision and the port sites closed. Final appearance of pelvis (Fig. 18).

The Specimen

This technique achieves a Piver type III radical hysterectomy, with a paracervical clearance of more than 3 cm, distal vaginal margin of more than 2.5–3 cm and nodal yield of at least 18–20 nodes.

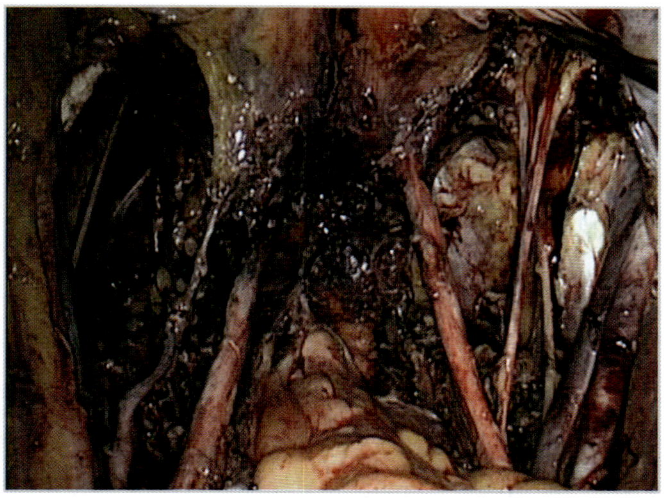

Fig. 18: Road map after completion of dissection

REFERENCES

1. Walker R. The first laparoscopic cholecystectomy. JSLS. 2001;5(1):89-94.
2. Tierney JP, Kusminsky RE, Boland JP, et al. Laparoscopic pelvic lymph node dissection. W V Med J. 1991;87(4):151-2.
3. Nezhat CR, Burrell MO, Nezhat FR, et al. Laparoscopic radical hysterectomy with paraaortic and pelvic node dissection. Am J Obstet Gynecol. 1992;166(3):864-5.
4. Jacobs M, Verdeja JC, Goldstein HS. Minimally invasive colon resection (laparoscopic colectomy). Surg Laparosc Endosc. 1991;1(3):144-50.
5. DePaula AL, Hashiba K, Ferreira EA, et al. Laparoscopic transhiatal esophagectomy with esophagogastroplasty. Surg Laparosc Endosc. 1995;5(1):1-5.
6. Guillonneau B, Vallancien G, et al. Laparoscopic radical prostatectomy: The Montsouris experience. J Urol. 2000;163(2):418-422.
7. Colacchio TA, Yeager MP, Hildebrandt LW. Perioperative immunomodulation in cancer surgery. Am J Surg. 1994;167(1):174-9.
8. Harmon GD, Senagore AJ, Kilbride MJ, et al. Interleukin-6 response to laparoscopic and open colectomy. Dis Colon Rectum. 1994;37(8):754-9.
9. Patel RT, Deen KI, Youngs D, et al. Interleukin 6 is a prognostic indicator of outcome in severe intra-abdominal sepsis. Br J Surg. 1994;81(9):1306-8.
10. Falk PM, Beart RW, Wexner SD, et al. Laparoscopic colectomy: a critical appraisal. Dis Colon Rectum. 1993;36(1):28-34.
11. Hoffman GC, Baker JW, Doxey JB, et al. Minimally invasive surgery for colorectal cancer: Initial follow-up. Ann Surg. 1996; 233(6):790-6.
12. Goh P, Tekant Y, Isaac J, et al. The technique of laparoscopic Billroth II gastrectomy. Surg Laparosc Endosc. 1992;2(3): 258-60.
13. Ballesta-Lopez C, Bastida-Vila X, Catarci M, et al. Laparoscopic Billroth II distal subtotal gastrectomy with gastric stump suspension for gastric malignancies. Am J Surg. 1996;171(2):289-92.
14. Cuschieiri A. Thoracoscopic subtotal esophagetomy. Endosc Surg Allied Technol. 1994;2(1):21-5.
15. Orringer MB, Marshall B, Iannettoni MD. Transhiatal esophagectomy: clinical experience and refinements. Ann Surg. 1999;230(3):392-400.
16. DePaula AL, Hashiba K, Ferreira EA, et al. Transhiatal approach for esophagectomy. In: Toouli J, Gossot D, Hunter JG (Eds). Endosurgery. New York: Churchill Livingstone; 1996. pp. 293-9.
17. Avital S, Zundel N, Szomstein S, et al. Laparoscopic transhiatal esophagectomy for esophageal cancer. Am J Surg. 2005;190(1):69-74.
18. Swanstron LL, Hansen P. Laparoscopic total esophagectomy. Arch Surg. 1997;132(9):943-7.
19. Nguyen NT, Roberts P, Follette DM, et al. Thoracoscopic and laparoscopic esophagectomy for benign and malignant disease: lessons learned from 46 consecutive procedures. J Am Coll Surg. 2003;197(6):902-13.
20. Simon Bann, Moorthy K, Shaul T, et al. Laparoscopic transhiatal surgery of the esophagus. JSLS. 2005;9(4):376-81.
21. Torek F. The first successful case of resection of the esophagus for cancer. JAMA. 1913;60(20):1553.
22. Lewis I. The surgical treatment of carcinoma of the oesophagus with special reference to a new operation for growths of the middle third. Br J Surg. 1946;34:18-31.
23. Luketich JD, Nguyen NT, Schauer PR. Laparoscopic transhiatal esophagectomy for Barret's esophagus with high grade dysplasia. JSLS. 1988;2(1):75-7.
24. Suzuki Y, Urashima M, Ishibashi Y, et al. Hand-assisted laparoscopic and thoracoscopic surgery (HALTS) in radical esophagectomy

with three-field lymphadenectomy for thoracic esophageal cancer. EJSO. 2005;31(10):1166-74.

25. Goldminc M, Maddern G, Le Prise E, et al Oesophagectomy by a transhiatal approach or thoracotomy: A prospective randomized trial. Br J Surg. 1993;80(3):367-70.
26. Pisani P, Parkin DM, Bray F, et al. Estimates of the worldwide mortality from 25 cancers in 1990. Int J Cancer. 1999;83(1):18-29.
27. Putnam JB, Suell DM, McMurtrey MJ, et al. Comparison of three techniques of esophagectomy within a residency training program. Ann Thorac Surg. 1994;57(2):319-25.
28. Lacy AM, Garcia-Valdecacas JC, Delgado S, et al. Laparoscopy-assisted colectomy versus open colectomy for treatment of non-metastatic colon cancer: a randomised trial. Lancet. 2002;359(9325):2224-9.
29. The Clinical Outcomes of Surgical Therapy (COST) Study Group. A comparison of laparoscopically assisted and open colectomy for colon cancer. N Engl J Med. 2004;350(20):2050-9.
30. Hazebroek EJ, COLOR Study Group. COLOR: a randomized clinical trial comparing laparoscopic and open resection for colon cancer. Surg Endosc. 2002;16(6):949-53.
31. Guillou PJ, Quirke P, Thorpe H, et al. Short-term endpoints of conventional versus laparoscopic-assisted surgery in patients with colorectal cancer (MRC CLASICC trial): multicentre, randomised controlled trial. Lancet. 2005;365:1718-26.

16 Toward the Future of Minimal Access Surgery: A Personal Perspective

Tehemton E Udwadia

"The future is not what it is used to be." **(Yogi Bear)**

"The best way to predict the future is to create it." **(Alan Cray)**

INTRODUCTION

The future of minimal access surgery (MAS) is the forward projection of the past and the present. MAS, as we know it today, started in 1985 with a hesitant procedure by a German surgeon Dr Eric Mühe in Böbingen, a town with a few thousand residents, using a 3 cm cannula made out of the tubing of his daughter's bicycle through which, with the aid of a Storz telescope, he performed what he termed the first "closed cholecystectomy". When the German professors of surgery learnt of this heretical surgery by this unknown surgeon, Dr Mühe was chastised and was removed from the German Surgical Society. But Mühe had the courage of his convictions and persevered with the procedure. Sadly, his 98 patients developed common bile duct injury, his peers had him legally prosecuted and Dr Mühe spent the next 5 years in court, litigation and jail.[1,2] In surgery, many truths, sadly, start off as blasphemies.

Yet again, it was in a small town that a French surgeon Dr Philippe Mouret in 1987 performed the first four puncture laparoscopic cholecystectomy as we know it today.[3] Wisely, he did not publicize his procedure, desired to remain in the background, but brought it to the attention of two friends Dr Dubois, Professor of Surgery in Paris and Dr Perissat, Professor of Surgery in Bordeaux, who ratified the procedure. Perissat forcefully presented it on the world stage. To the credit of Dubois and Perrissat, they insisted that credit be given to Philippe Mouret as the originator of laparoscopic cholecystectomy, which rapidly became the "gold standard" for cholecystectomy.[4] This was the genesis of MAS as practised today.

Frowned on and refuted by professors everywhere for the first few years, laparoscopic cholecystectomy was the spring-board for the spread of MAS.[5] Thanks to manufacturer thrust, surgical innovation and patient demand, MAS spread to other organs in the abdomen, and eventuality to be part of surgical procedures in every specialty ranging literally from head to foot. The manifest benefit to the patient are far less pain, less medication, less morbidity, shorter hospitalization, almost no scarring and early return to family and work have ensured that MAS is the surgery of the present moving rapidly to the future. With rapid advances in technology, instrumentation, surgical experience, innovation and outlook, MAS is looking to a future which knows no boundaries and will reach for the stars.

TRAINING

"Build your house on rock, not sand." **(St. Peter)**

More than technology, training is the cornerstone of MAS advance into the future. MAS descended on an unprepared, unsuspecting surgical world like an avalanche, creating a demand for "instant training," totally contrary to the principles of progressive complex training, surgical involvement and operative performance of the hitherto Halstedian method of surgical residency and training over several years. The long, stubborn reluctance of "academic" surgery to accept the validity of MAS perforce mandated the training of MAS surgeons to ad hoc skimpy quick-fix weekend training sessions. The patient generated thirst for surgeons to jump on the MAS bandwagon it was so intense that the education and background of most of the early self-proclaimed MAS surgeons was a weekend course on box trainers and/or pig models.[6] The litany of complications that followed was so horrendous and unending[7] that very soon the realization dawned for the need of a planned, supervised formal MAS training. Sadly, this need is very much prevalent even today, for even today the need to be "with it" promotes several quickfix training programs.[8] For MAS to reach its full potential in the future, it is mandatory that MAS training be accepted as a serious ongoing challenge. MAS training needs to go well beyond skill acquisition to overcome the initial challenges related to loss of depth perception on a flat screen, the fulcrum effect of instruments anchored to the abdominal wall, long instruments with limited grasp which rob the surgeon of his most vital aid—the sense of tactile feedback. It would be unethical and disastrous if this skill acquisition was obtained in the operating room (OR), it needs methods of training which will ensure the patient no harm. There are two areas for this training into the future.

The Residency Program/ Fellowship Courses

In most developed countries, this is the accepted method of gradual education over a few years, which depends heavily on simulator training together with clinical and progressive operative observership, assistance, proctoring, performance, ensuring a safe and competed MAS surgeon. Sadly almost all over the developing world, this ideal training program is at best available to a few centers.

SIMULATOR TRAINING

Outside residency training, this is the platform for the vast majority of surgeons training for MAS all over the developing world.

There are three categories of simulators:

1. Box or mechanical simulators
2. Animal models
3. Virtual reality simulators.

Box Simulators or Mechanical Trainers

Starting from the primitive simulators from the dawn of MAS, box trainers have helped train surgeons from the simplest to complex exercises, and procedures giving requisite manual and visual dexterity (Figs 1 and 2) to the modern advanced technology simulators.[9-12] Apart from being simple, cost-effective and indefinitely reusable box, trainers have established their reliability and validation as competent training modality using various methods of evaluation.[13-15] Being very affordable, trainees can have their own trainers to practise in the office or homes; trainers have today reached a high degree of sophistication for training (Fig. 3). The main disadvantages of these trainers are a lack of tissue feel and feedback, and only a subjective evaluation of progress and improvement.

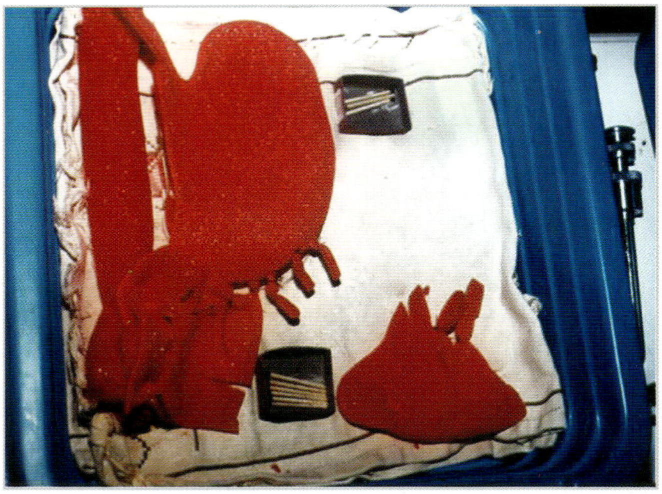

Fig. 1: Earliest primitive box trainer

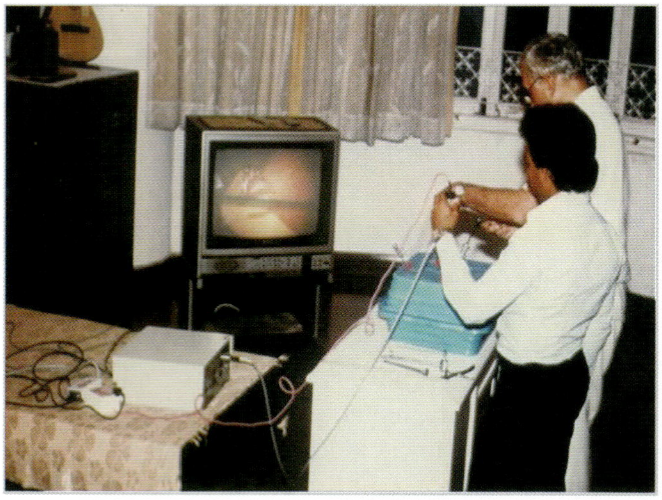

Fig. 2: Early primitive training for minimal access surgery (MAS)

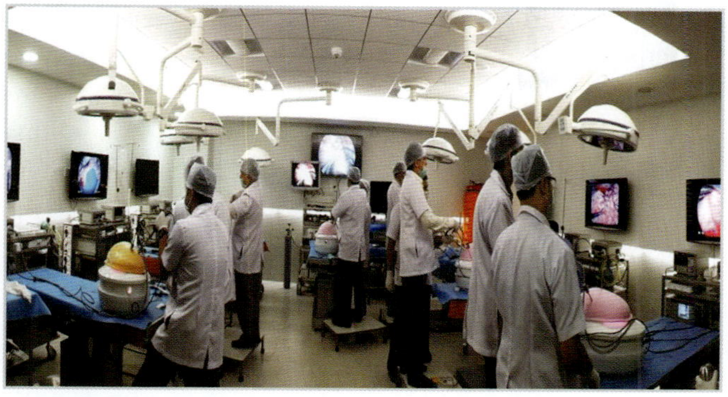

Fig. 3: Minimal access surgery training in a center of excellence

Live Animal Models

While in the early years of MAS training, animal models were frequent training tools for the "crash courses," giving a tissue feel to the training. Worldwide abolition of the use of live animals for experiment and teaching has stopped the use of these simulators.

Virtual Reality

With advances in computer power and technology, virtual simulators are becoming increasingly life-like with some haptic feedback, creation of clinical scenarios as seen at surgery, blood flow, smoke, hemorrhage, bile leak—the works. Of course, all this comes at a very high price.

Comparison of Simulators

Extensive study has concluded that not one method is consistently superior or worse, the tremendously higher cost of virtual reality (VR) simulators does not reflect on improved training end results to the box simulators.[16] One advantage of the VR simulator is that it gives an objective assessment of performance and improvement.

The Actual Reality Trainer

"Actual reality" is the nomenclature I have given to a training modality never before described, created or used for MAS training. This may well be the future of MAS training in developing countries. With ingenuity, improvization, perseverance and passion, a new form of training modality is being perfected at one Center of Excellence for MAS training in Mumbai and is being put to extensive trial. Using conventional economical box trainers, porcine cadavers or blocks of fresh appropriate animal tissue are perfused with blood-like fluid with pulsatile arterial flow of variable speed and pressure created by economical technology.[17] Using identical MAS equipment as used in a modern OR for live surgery, a model is created for repetitive training exercises at very low cost. With the ingenious method of vascularization of specific vessel's[10] for example, hepatic, renal, uterine and mesenteric, can ensure a true-to-life situation for MAS training for cholecystectomy, hepatic resection, donor or partial nephrectomy, myomectomy, hysterectomy, intestinal resection and anastomosis.[18]

TECHNOLOGY

Instrumentation

Three-dimensional technology will certainly be the visual aspect of MAS in the future for it eliminates the serious drawback of 2D vision, thereby approximating MAS to open surgery, improving safety and quality of surgery especially in areas like the pelvis. Camera-chip at the tip of the telescope, flexible tip telescope—the chain of new instrumentation is endless.

Hand instruments are rapidly improving in ergometrics, durability and articulated tip movement to increase range of movement, somewhat replicating the movement of the robotic arm.

Single incision laparoscopic surgery (SILS), where the subumbilical entry area accommodates all ports, is a procedure under evaluation, has necessitated progressive improvization and improvement in instruments to aid overcome the lack of triangulation as is mandated as a safety essential in multiport MAS. SILS enthusiasts have used this method for safe application in a large variety of MAS surgery in general surgery, urology and gynecology.[19] 3 mm instruments should be safer and more appropriate and acceptable as compared to SILS.

Natural Orifice Transluminal Endoscopic Surgery

The desire not to leave the blemish of a single scar on the human body has initiated the somewhat drastic need of entry to the peritoneal cavity for MAS through the vagina, rectum, stomach (all humans do not have a vagina). Despite its enthusiastic proponents, this remains a controversial procedure under trial.[20]

Personally, I would rather have one or even several scars on my skin than a rent in my rectum to do a cholecystectomy or appendectomy!

Robotics

The word 'robot' desived from the Czech word, "robota" means slave labor. Robotics is the current buzzword in MAS.

It would appear tertiary care hospitals would feel deprived and underequipped without one. Two robot instruments, the da Vinci and the Zeus, in current use have an interface for the surgeon, whose hand movement delivers information through computers to robotic arms. The current rush to incorporate, what is still an emerging technology, is driven by market forces, to present a stamp of "excellence and advance" to centers which acquire it. Laparoscopic robotic surgery has advantages over conventional laparoscopic surgery. The rationale of robotic surgery is that it brings laparoscopic surgery closer to the ease and advantages of open surgery and more. It permits 3D vision, incorporates ergometrics and reproduces the versatile (seven) degrees multiple movements of the surgeon's fingers, hand, wrist and forearm, which are severely restricted by the compulsions of conventional laparoscopic surgery. Further, the robot provides a sharp magnified view and eliminates all tremors of the surgeon's hand, ensuring perfect precision in every minute step of the procedure, specifically significant in suturing and anastomosis. Its ultimate utility is in the confined space of the pelvis for radical prostatectomy, or for hysterectomy, lymph node clearance and for cardiac surgery. However, to advocate its indiscriminate use in areas where it has no documented advantage over laparoscopic MAS, in view of the cost of the robot, its maintenance, one-time use of instruments, large size footprint, need for larger OR and fixed operation table position has no rationale whatsoever. There is ample evidence of feasibility of robotic surgery in all MAS procedures, but high quality trials need to be done to determine in which procedures the robot has a distinct advantage and restrict the use of this high technology to those procedures. The jury is still out until long-term follow-up and large volume Randomized Clinical Trial (RCT) reports are available. Longer operative time and unproven outcome data are factors to be taken into account. With greater use and the entry of more manufactures to reduce monopoly of the two current systems, the cost and versatility of robots may improve.

PRAGMATIC EVALUATION

The Surgeon

Training centers for MAS and the trainees so concentrate and emphasize on training on various simulators, each one outdoing the previous simulator to make a life-like scenario of bleeding, smoke, bile-leak that the MAS trainee is mentally programed to feel manual dexterity is all that is required for safe MAS. In today's high-tech and all-for-commerce age, the two other qualities, apart from the hand a surgeon requires—a head and a heart, seem pushed into the background—to the peril of the patient and the profession. The end target of training is not the simulator but an ill, nervous human, who needs professional experience, expertise and kindness. The MAS surgeon, as he progresses, has to face the hype of the media, the push of the manufacturer for their profit, patient demand often misguided by the hypnotic voice of the internet and other influences, professional and monetary. It is for him to evaluate, to separate the grain from the chaff, and, with pragmatic honesty, decide which procedure truly has the patient's interest as the sole criterion.

The Manufacturer

There is no doubt that MAS has reached this degree of advancement, sophistication and safety as a result of the ingenuity, innovation and desire to meet the demands and requirements of the surgeon provided by the endoscope manufacturers. However, it is evident that the manufacturer has to generate maximum profit and the surgeon has to discriminate if a technology newcomer is for the benefit of the manufacturer or the patient.

Minimal Access Surgery in Surgical Oncology

Since its introduction in 1987 and large scale use since 1990, MAS surgeons have extended its indications to oncosurgery. The initial concerns of port site metastasis were unfounded.[21-23] Evidence now supports the use of MAS oncological surgery in many areas.[24-29]

The entry of robotic surgery opens a new field for comparison of results between open surgery, MAS and robotic MAS in oncosurgery. Evidence is growing that in centers of excellence, robotic surgery in specific fields like cancer prostate has an edge over the other procedures.

It must be stressed that comparable long-term results between open and laparoscopic oncosurgery emerge form highly specialized MAS centers and should not be transpolated to the casual MAS surgeon, who would do better justice to the patient by open surgery. "It is ethically wrong to use the patient as a training module".

THE FUTURE

"The only truth in surgery is change"

The future of MAS will be linked with newer technologies and instrumentation which are already under development—articulating hand instruments, breakthrough in optical systems, newer methods of entry like SILS, natural orifice transluminal endoscopic surgery (NOTES), which, at present, are viewed with mental reservation; however, improved technology may perhaps find a place for some enthusiasts in routine surgery.[30,31] Robotic surgery will spread with the entry of newer competitive manufacturers and snowballing technology, the reduced cost, size, increased versatility of robots will ensure their rapidly increasing use, partly manufactures-driven, partly patient-demand driven, partly driven in the interest of patient benefit.

In the distant future, MAS will move into the area of noninvasive surgery. Tissue engineering and stem cell technology will move into organogenesis,[32] with functional development using nanotechnology and adverse tissue culture methodology. Image-guided surgery, the use of the CyberKnife® with a robotic arm and a minute linear accelerator can position the direction of energy to any part of the body from optimal directions. The distant future takes us into the field of nanotechnology which today seems as futuristic and scary as science fiction, but with the exponential growth of the science of nanotechnology, it is predicted to take over surgical procedures as we know today by working at the cellular and molecular level within two to three decades!

These advances, for which society will have to pay for exponentially more, make us appreciate the surgical wisdom of the past. John Hunter in 1762 had predicted "surgery gaining much from the general advance of knowledge might be rendered both knifeless and bloodless". He specifically mentioned "advance in knowledge" (not in surgery) and perhaps 30 years down the line, his prediction will come true after 350 years!

SOCIOECONOMIC REALITY

"Of all forms of inequality, indiscrimination and injustice in healthcare is the most shocking and inhumane."

(Martin Luther King Junior)

As surgeons, we are compelled by the pressure of a sense of duty, pride, patient demand, manufactures push to ensure our equipment and our surgery is as good, if not better, than in any part of the world, which, in our centers of excellence it indeed, is. Observers are awed that just in the city of Delhi, we have more CT scanners, MRI machines and lithotripters than in all Scandinavia put together. We are one of the largest importers of robots. In stark contrast, in the same country, a patient with a strangulated inguinal hernia may not get to see a doctor, leave alone a surgeon. Working in our state of the art hospitals, totally focused on our surgery, equipment, our need (greed) to upgrade it further, we have with determination and studied indifference kept our backs turned to the harsh and sad reality of healthcare in India. After a dozen 5-year plans, the government allocation for healthcare is at best 1% of our gross domestic product (GDP), one-tenth that of China, and less than any of our neighboring countries or several African countries. Our infant and maternal mortality rates are among the highest. One-third of the world's poorest and malnourished children are in India. We accept that 30% of our population is below the poverty line. That, however, is not the bottomline. The poverty line covers the basic necessities of mere existence. With no insurance and meager public health support, if the cost of healthcare is added, the percentage below the poverty line would appreciably increase. Poverty adds greatly to ill health. Surgery is a humanitarian science, so we believe, so we preach.

How much longer can we continue with indifferent tranquility in the face of the injustice of 30% of our population having the ultimate sophistication in healthcare, 70% deprived of basic health amenities.

To add to the irony and injustice it is this deprived 70% that contributes 70% to the national GDP! To me, the true future of MAS lies in bringing the benefits of this advance to all people in all places. Realizing the given economic facts listed above, this would appear to be an impossible, utopian dream and fantasy. As one involved in the spread of laparoscopy and MAS since its very inception in 1972, not only in India, but also in Asia and Africa, I am happy in the knowledge that this dream, hopefully sooner than later, will come true in the developing world. Already the seeds have been sown and have taken root. In the map of India, these dots of seeds are spreading like a measles epidemic. Not only advanced MAS, but also economic innovation toward advanced MAS has emerged from small towns. This is a tribute to the innovation, ingenuity, versatility of the rural surgeons who, working in the backwaters, are the soul, spirit and backbone of Indian surgery, who perforce have to tackle MAS as readily as they, out of necessity, do basic urology, orthopedics, gynecology or oncosurgery.[33]

Each center, where MAS is being done in small towns, India should become a hub from which this surgery will spread. Professors pontificating over weekend courses in small towns cannot help spread MAS as effectively as rural surgeons, who live and work in the ground reality can. The thrust of one Centre of Excellence for MAS training in Mumbai is the training of rural surgeons in MAS and to form on alumni of rural surgeons, who can revert to the Center for help, advice, guidance, intraoperative assistance and proctoring. If we have the will, we shall always find the way. The difficulties in spreading MAS all over the vast country as also over the developing world are truly daunting, and must of necessity go hand in hand with the awareness of spread of public health. The poorest of the poor have as much right to less pain, less medication, less expense, shortened hospitalization and specially for daily wages manual laborers, early return to work and family.[34] The true future of MAS goes way beyond NOTES or robots. As surgeons in a developing country, it is our duty to ensure the universal spread of the benefits of MAS. The possibility of the success of our efforts seems distant, remote for several years. However, the true measure of success is in overcoming the obstacles while trying to succeed.

REFERENCES

1. Muhe E. Die erste Choleyctektomie durch das Laparaskop. Langenbecks Arch Chir. 1986;369:804.
2. Muhe E. The First Laparoscopic Cholecystectomy: Overcoming the Roadblocks on the Road to the Future. Karl Sotrz Lecture in New Technology. Presented at SAGES Annual Meeting; March 26, 1999; San Antonio, Tex.
3. Mouret P. Celioscopic surgery. Evolution or revolution? Chirurgie. 1990;116(10):829-32.
4. Soper NJ, Stockmann PT, Dunnegan DL, et al. Laparoscopic cholecystectomy: the new 'gold standard'? Arch Surg. 1992; 127(8):917-21.
5. Udwadia TE. Laparoscopic Cholecystectomy. Bombay: Oxford University Press; 1991.
6. Soper NJ. Brunt LM, Kerbl K. Laparoscopic general surgery. N Engl J Med. 1994;330(6):409-19.
7. The Southern Surgeons Club. A prospective analysis of 1518 laparoscopic cholecystectomies. N Engl J Med. 1991;324:1073-8.
8. Rogers DA, Elstein AS, Bordage G. Improving continuing medical education for surgical techniques: applying the lessons learned in the first decade of minimal access surgery. Ann Surg. 2001;233(2):159-66.
9. Henriford BT, Backus CL, Mattews BD, et al. Optimal teaching environment for laparoscopic splenectomy. Am J Surg. 2001;181(3):226-30.
10. Derossis AM, Fried GM, Abrahamowicz M, et al. Development of a model for training and evaluation of laparoscopic skills. Am J Surg. 1998;175(6):482-7.
11. Derossis AM, Bothwell J, Sigman HH, et al. The effect of practice on performance in a laparoscopic simulator. Surg Endosc. 1998;12(9):1117-20.
12. Schirmer BD, Edge SB, Dix J, et al. Incorporation of laparoscopy into a surgical endoscopy training program. Am J Surg. 1992;163(1):46-50.
13. Martin JA, Regehr G, Reznick R, et al. Objective structured assessment of technical skill (OSATS) for surgical residents. Br J Surg. 1997:84(2)273-8.
14. Szallay D, MacRae H, Regehr G, et al. Using operative outcome to assess technical skill. Am J Surg. 2000;180(3):234-7.
15. Dhariwal AK, Prabhu RY, Dalvi AN, et al. Effectiveness of box trainers in laparoscopic training. J Minim Access Surg. 2007;3(2):57-63.
16. Sutherland LM, Middleton PF, Anthony A, et al. Surgical simulation: a systematic review. Ann Surg. 2006;243(3): 291-300.
17. Gadgil US. Tissue arterial flow for improved minimal access surgery training (Personal communication). 17-4-13 CEMAST.
18. Gadgil US. Vascularized organ preparation with created pathology for minimal access surgery training (Personal communication). 19-8-13 CEMAST.
19. Bhandarkar D, Mittal G, Shah R, et al. Single-incision laparoscopic cholecystectomy. How do I do it? J Minim Access Surg. 2011;7(1):17-23.
20. Rao GV, Reddy DN, Banerjee R. NOTES: human experience. Gastrointest Endosc Clin N Am. 18(2):361-70.
21. Berends FJ , Kazemier G, Bonjer HJ, et al. Subcutaneous metastases after laparoscopic colectomy. Lancet. 1994;344(8914):58.
22. Hughes ES, McDermott FT, Polglase AL, et al, Tumor recurrence in abdominal scar tissue after large bowel cancer surgery. Dis Colon Rectum. 1933;26(9):571-2.
23. Barbulescu M, Alecu L, Boeți P, et al. Port-site metastases in the laparoscopic surgery for colorectal cancer—still a real concern? Case report and review of the literature. Chirurgia (Bucur). 2012;107(1):103-7.
24. Gemill, EH, McCulloch P. Systematic review of minimally invasive resection of gastro-esophageal cancer. Br J Surg. 2007;94(12):1461-7.
25. Braghetto I, Csendes A, Cardemil G, et al. Open transthoracic or transhiatal esophagectomy versus minimally invasive esophagectomy in terms of morbidity, mortality and survival. Surg Endosc. 2006;20(11):1681-6.
26. Pavlidis TE, Pavlidis ET, Sakantamis AK, et al. The role of laparoscopy in gastric cancer. J Minm Access Surg. 2012;8(2):35-8.
27. Pericleous S, Middleton N, McKay SC, et al. Systematic review and meta-analysis of case-matched studies comparing open and laparoscopic distal pancreatectomy: is it a safe procedure? Pancrease. 2012;41(7):993-1000.

28. Nguyen KT, Geller DA. Outcomes of laparoscopic hepatic resection for colorectal cancer metastases. J Surg Oncol. 2010; 102(8)975-7.

29. Fukunaga Y. Superiority of laparoscopic rectal surgery: Towards a new era. World J Gastrointest Surg. 2011;3(10):142-6.

30. ASGE, SAGES. ASGE/SAGES Working Group on Natural Orifice Translumenal Endoscopic Surgery White Paper October 2005. Gastrointest Endosc. 2006;63(2):199-203.

31. Satava RM. Advanced technologies and the future of medicine and surgery. Yonsei Med J. 2008;49(6):873-8.

32. Davies JA. Welcome to organogenesis. Organogenesis. 2004;1(1):1-2.

33. Udwadia TE. Surgical care for the poor: A personal Indian perspective. Indian J Surg. 2003;65(6):504-9.

34. Udwadia TE. One world, one people, one surgery. Surg Endosc. 2001;15(4):337-43.

17 Oral Premalignant Lesions

Vijay Haribhakti

INTRODUCTION

Oral squamous carcinomas are typically the end results of sustained, persistent and accumulated genetic damage to the oral mucosa by a variety of carcinogens. The major carcinogens include tobacco, alcohol and areca nut; and possibly viruses such as human papillomavirus type 16 (HPV-16). In this multi-step process of carcinogenesis, the mucosa frequently develops morphologic changes that are recognizable clinically, and since these phenotypes predate the manifestation of a carcinoma, they are broadly classified as oral "precancer".

A precancerous lesion is thus an area of morphologically and/or genetically altered tissue that is more likely than normal to develop into a cancer.

The appropriate diagnosis and management of these lesions represent a significant opportunity for prevention of oral cancer. A clear understanding of the range of manifestations and an appreciation of their potential risk is germane to establishing a coherent plan of management in every individual case.

DEFINITIONS AND TERMS

At the very outset, it is important to distinguish between "premalignant lesions" and "premalignant conditions". Lesions are typically "localized" and present as a patch of variable size, while "conditions" are more generalized affectations of the oral mucosa, and may be punctuated with lesions.

Accordingly, premalignant lesions present as a predominantly white patch (leukoplakia) or a beefy red patch (erythroplakia), along with variations.

In contrast, "conditions" present as more widespread mucosal changes, and include submucous fibrosis (SMF) and oral lichen planus (OLP). These conditions must be distinguished from other mucosal alterations, consequent upon a variety of etiologies such as vitamin deficiencies, infections (oral candidiasis), chronic trauma, drugs (e.g. chemotherapy), and radiation therapy.

The hallmark in all cases is epithelial dysplasia, which is the major predictor of malignant transformation.[1]

LEUKOPLAKIA

Oral leukoplakia is defined (WHO, 1978) as "A white patch or plaque that cannot be scraped off and that cannot be characterized clinically or pathologically as any other disease".[2]

By visual inspection, leukoplakias are divided into "homogenous" and "inhomogeneous (speckled)" varieties.

"Homogenous leukoplakia" has a regular, thin, smooth, predominantly uniform white appearance, without erythema or ulceration, and is accompanied by increased keratosis. The risk of malignant transformation is roughly 5%, and hence, the demonstration of severe epithelial dysplasia is uncommon.

"Inhomogeneous leukoplakia" (Figs 1 and 2) has a four to five times higher risk of malignant transformation, and has a mixed white and red (speckled) appearance with an irregular texture. Based on the morphology, the variants include exophytic, papillary and verrucous (or nodular) leukoplakia. An aggressive variant termed as proliferative verrucous leukoplakia (PVL) has a nearly 70% transformation rate. PVL (Fig. 3) often starts as a patch of solitary homogenous leukoplakia that demonstrates only hyperkeratosis without much dysplasia at initial biopsy. However, it recurs and extends relentlessly becoming diffuse, multifocal and hyperkeratotic, with increasing epithelial dysplasia.[3-5]

All cases of inhomogeneous leukoplakia demand biopsy diagnosis to study the degree of epithelial dysplasia and to exclude a carcinoma in situ.

ERYTHROPLAKIA

Erythroplakia (Fig. 4) manifests morphologically as a reddish, velvety patch, often difficult to discern from the surrounding normal mucosa, and is much less common than leukoplakia. These lesions are frequently present in the cheek, floor mouth or soft palate and must be subjected to routine excision biopsy. Majority of them reveal either severe epithelial dysplasia or carcinoma in situ or indeed an invasive carcinoma.

The risk of malignant transformation is high and exceeds 25% in many studies.[6,7]

SUBMUCOUS FIBROSIS (SMF)

This is an extremely common condition in our population and appears to be related to areca nut consumption along with other condiments, presented as a mixture sold under

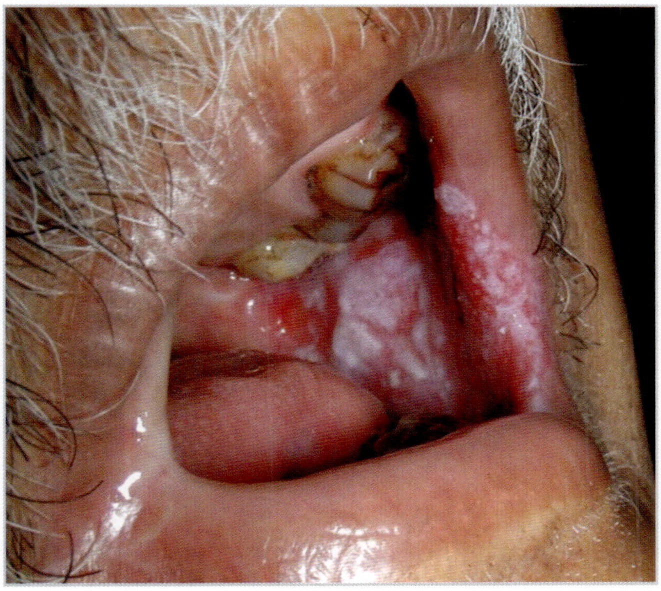

Fig. 1: Speckled leukoplakia

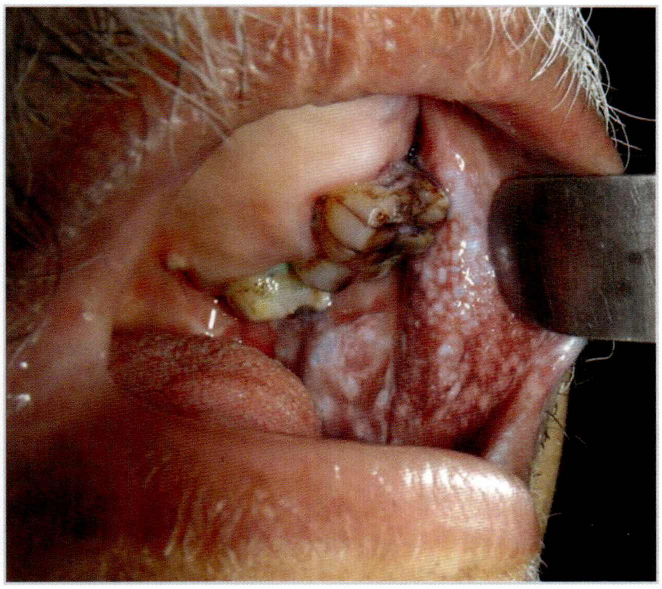

Fig. 2: Supravital staining

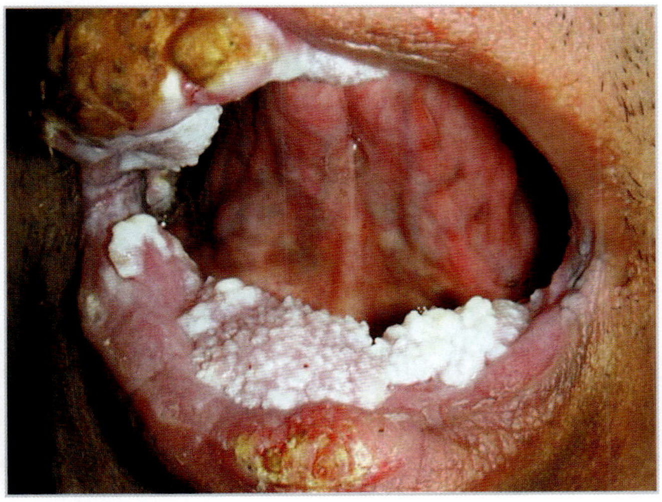

Fig. 3: Complex case—progressive verrucous leukoplakia with verrucous carcinoma

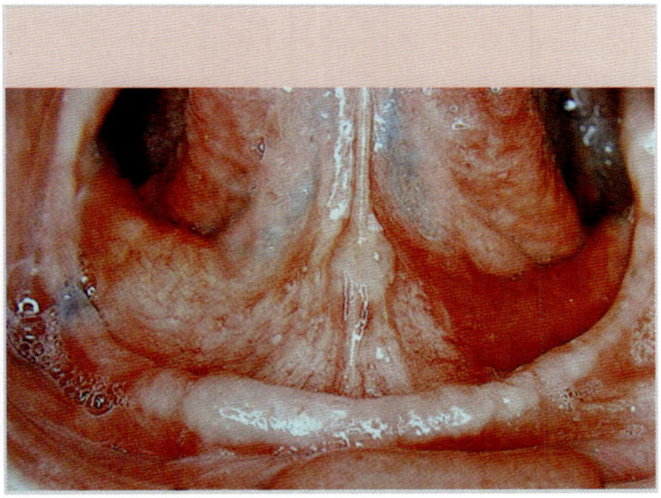

Fig. 4: Erythroplakia involving left floor of the mouth

several brand names such as '*maava*' and '*masala*'. It often starts as subepithelial inflammation manifesting as discomfort and intolerance to spices. The condition progresses relentlessly to SMF and scarring, with mucosal atrophy. The normally pink and pliable mucosa is replaced with a white, inelastic board like lining affecting variable portions of the oral mucosa such as the cheeks, anterior faucial pillars and soft palate. This inexorable progression regularly results in trismus of variable degree, often ending up as complete "lock jaw" with significant functional impairment, affecting food intake, mastication and speech.

Although the precancerous nature of SMF is generally assumed, the malignant transformation rate has been reported as roughly 7%. The major significance of this condition lies in its large prevalence and the significant morbidity it produces. When found as an accompaniment to oral cancer, it renders treatment far more complicated owing to restrictions in mouth opening, friability and poor suture retention. Moreover, the compromised mucosa tolerates radiation poorly, resulting in increasing trismus, poor hygiene, pain and debility.

Even following withdrawal of all etiologic agents, SMF never typically resolves completely to make way for a normal lining. Thus, the management philosophy for this condition has to be long-term and largely involves limiting further progression and countering the morbidity that already exists.

ORAL LICHEN PLANUS (OLP)

This condition of obscure etiology (sometimes reported to be more prevalent with chronic mental stress) is a chronic, inflammatory disease characterized by an autoimmune, T-cell mediated reaction that ultimately results in hyperkeratosis. The incidence is reported to be 1–4% of the general population, and it afflicts the buccal mucosa, tongue, gums and lips.

The common types include "reticular" and "erosive" forms. The reticular variety presents as asymptomatic white lesions in linear or lacy patterns, and represents the commonest form.

Erosive lichen planus presents with erythema and ulceration with white striations at the periphery. This form of OLP is frequently painful, and results in intolerance to spices and severe restrictions in the types and consistencies of food consumed. Relapses and spontaneous remissions are characteristic of this condition.

APPROACH TO A PATIENT (FLOW CHART 1)

A detailed history is first obtained to ascertain the profile of habits in the patient. Of particular significance is the exact type of substance or combinations used and the duration. It is next important to find out if there are any accompanying symptoms, and if so, the duration and impact on food intake and other oral functions.

A very thorough inspection of all mucosal surfaces in the oral space is then carried out systematically to observe the distribution of the lesion or condition.

Digital palpation is necessary to determine the texture of the lesion and to exclude tenderness. If a white patch is present, attempts are made to "scrape it off" with a tongue blade.

Once a provisional diagnosis has been made, further action depends upon the extent of suspicion.

The diagnosis of SMF is quite obvious on inspection and needs no biopsy confirmation. The extent needs to be mapped and documented thoroughly for future comparison, and the extent of mouth opening is assessed by the number of fingers the patient can introduce between the incisors. With restriction, the precise interincisor distance is measured and noted.

The diagnosis of OLP is often not always obvious and needs biopsy confirmation. The author prefers to obtain mucosal tissue biopsy under local anesthesia with a 3 mm dermatologic punch.

With homogenous leukoplakia of a uniform, soft texture, the diagnosis is essentially clinical and does not need biopsy confirmation. Further action depends upon the size, distribution and multiplicity, if any.

Inhomogeneous leukoplakia and erythroplakia invariably need microscopic diagnosis to assess the extent of epithelial dysplasia and to exclude carcinoma in situ. In this situation, supravital staining with toluidine blue (tolonium chloride) can be very helpful. Dysplastic and rapidly multiplying cells that contain higher quantities of DNA and RNA, preferentially take up tolonium chloride. While the sensitivity rates of supravital staining are high, the specificity and positive predictive values are comparatively low. The author frequently employs supravital staining to choose the precise site of biopsy, as also to determine the extent of mucosal resection necessary in an established case. The testing procedure is extremely simple and must be followed accurately.

Flow chart 1: Diagnostic approach—oral lesions

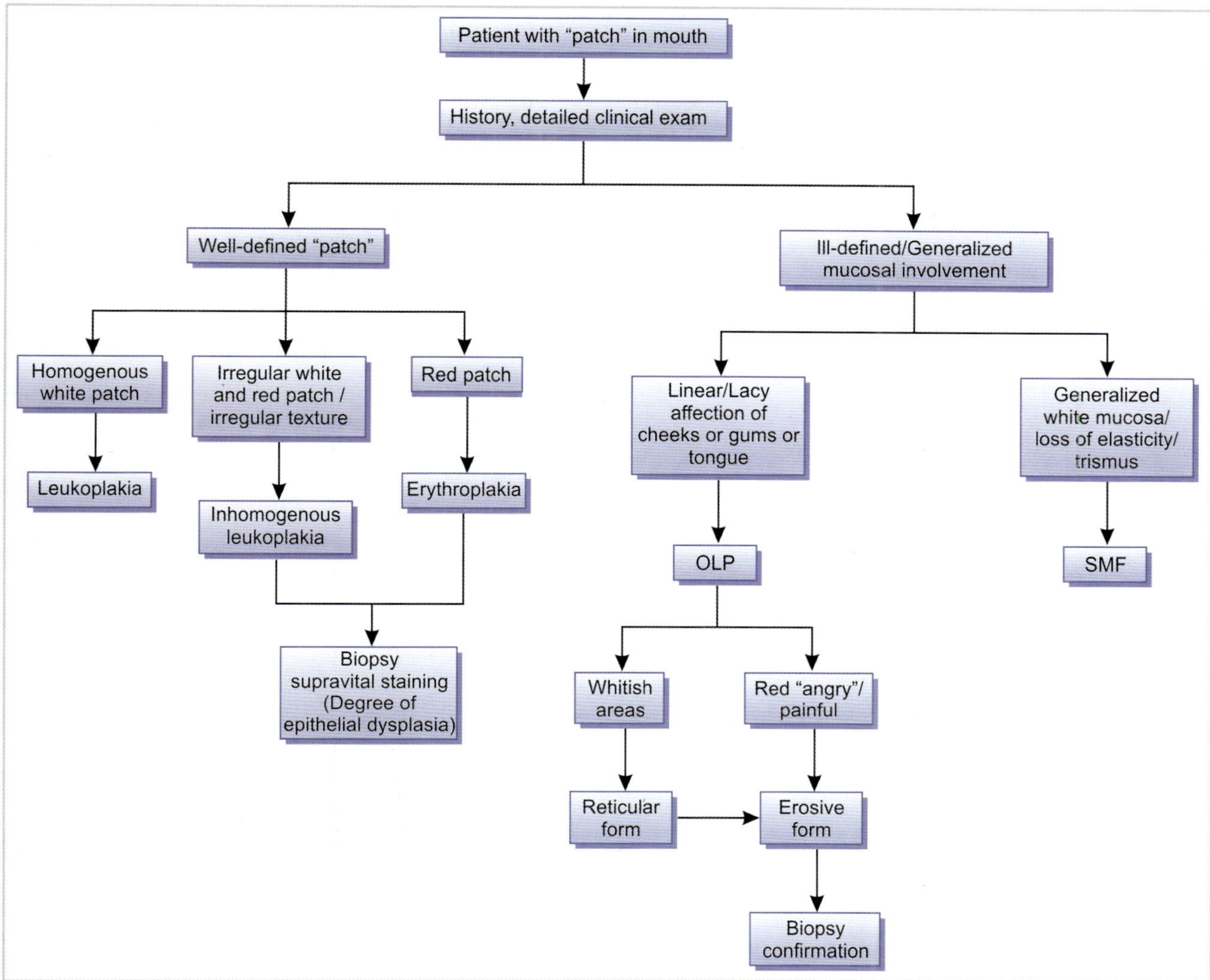

Abbreviations: OLP, oral lichen planus; SMF, submucous fibrosis

The area in question is first dried, either with dry gauze or with dilute acetic acid, keeping the mouth open. Once dried, it is touched with 1% toluidine blue solution using a Q-tip. A generous area over and around the patch is stained and again allowed to stay "dry" for about 30 seconds. Following this, the patient is encouraged to rinse the mouth copiously with plain water. Moist gauze is further used to dab off excess stain, before the area is observed.

A "positive" test is indicated by a deeply staining patch, which stands out against the background of a very lightly stained or unstained surrounding mucosa. If biopsy is planned, a complete excision biopsy of the positively stained area is carried out wherever possible. In the same way, supravital staining is useful to define the limits of excision of a patch, when the patch is located in the midst of abnormal mucosa, e.g. with oral SMF.

BIOPSY INTERPRETATION

The crux of biopsy interpretation is grading the extent of epithelial dysplasia. A set of criteria published by Pindborg et al. is as follows:

- Loss of polarity of basal cells
- Increased nuclear-cytoplasmic ratio
- Drop-shaped rete ridges
- Irregular epithelial stratification
- Increased number of mitotic figures
- Abnormal mitoses
- Cellular and nuclear pleomorphism
- Enlarged, hyperchromatic nuclei
- Loss of intercellular adherence
- Keratinization—single or groups of cells.

Despite apparently objective criteria, the grading of dysplasia into "mild", "moderate" and "severe" categories is essentially subjective. With mild and even moderate dysplasia, the risk of malignant transformation is low at 3–4%. With severe dysplasia, the risk rises to over 40% and is highly significant. In order to address the risks inherent in subjective grading of dysplasia, molecular criteria have been developed and are rapidly evolving. They are as follows:

- DNA aneuploidy
- Loss of heterozygosity
- p53 mutation
- Differentiation markers:
  - Cell surface carbohydrates or keratins.

MANAGEMENT

Despite advances in molecular medicine, current management depends largely upon conventional clinical assessment.

The first question to oneself when a patient presents is: Is this a localized "patch" or a more generalized mucosal "condition"?

Amongst mucosal "conditions," SMF is by far the most important in our population, where chewing habits prevail. Early cases with no significant trismus are managed by strict withdrawal of habits, vitamins and mouth-opening exercises to prevent trismus. Typically, these patients rarely revert to normal, but are able to live largely normal lives without significant handicaps.

Patients with advanced SMF present with thick, board-like mucosa involving cheeks, tonsillar pillars and soft palate, with severe trismus.

Although, management begins conservatively as described above, many patients need surgical correction, with release of trismus, coronoidectomy, medial pterygoid release, and flap replacement. Even following the use of vascularized flaps, mouth-opening exercises have to be continued in order to retain serviceable oral function.

When SMF coexists with oral cancer, it is critically important to recognize that the affected mucosa is brittle, hold sutures poorly, and is quite intolerant to radiation toxicity. Accordingly, tension-free closures must be assured with the use of vascularized flaps, wherever needed. As for radiation, sophisticated planning is advisable, to limit exposure of unafflicted mucosa to the effects of radiation, and to preserve salivary function maximally.

The "management of OLP" usually starts with histologic verification of the clinical diagnosis. The patient is clearly counseled about the remissions and relapses that characterize the condition. For early, minimally symptomatic cases, local steroid gel applications are quite often sufficient. With severe symptoms and major restrictions in spice tolerance and food intake, systemic treatment is required in the form of a "4–6 week course of steroids". Along with this, "vitamins" and local "triamcinolone gels" are helpful. Unconfirmed reports cite persistent mental stress as a possible precipitating factor for relapses, and hence anxiolytics are frequently employed on an empirical basis.

When a patient presents with a "patch", clinical assessment should be able to distinguish between the low-risk "homogenous leukoplakia" and the higher risk "speckled leukoplakia," "erythroplakia" or "nodular leukoplakia". If there is any doubt, supravital staining is employed as described above and an appropriate biopsy performed. In most cases, it is readily possible to discern a definite plane between the mucosa and the underlying muscle, which is preserved intact. With small biopsies and normal surrounding mucosa, primary mucosal closure is recommended for prompt healing.

With larger excisions, it is better to use quilted skin grafts or biologic materials like Kollagen® or AlloDerm®, which permit excellent mucosalization.

In a small number of cases where large patches of homogenous leukoplakia exist and produce persistent concern, limited biopsy is first performed to exclude epithelial dysplasia, following which carbon dioxide laser vaporization may be undertaken.

REFERENCES

1. Reibel J. Prognosis of oral pre-malignant lesions: Significance of clinical, histopathological, and molecular biological characteristics. Crit Rev Oral Biol Med. 2003;14(1):47-62.
2. Neville BW, Day TA. Oral cancer and precancerous lesions. CA Cancer J Clin. 2002;52(4):195-215.
3. Abbey LM, Kaugars GE, Gunsolley JC, et al. Intraexaminer reliability in the diagnosis of oral epithelial dysplasia. Oral Surg Oral Med, Oral Pathol, Oral Radiol Endod. 1995;80(2):188-91.
4. Allen CM. Evidence-based medicine and the clinical practice of oral maxillofacial pathology. Oral Surg, Oral Med, Oral Pathol, Oral Radiol Endod. 1997;84(3):277.
5. Califano J, van der Riet P, Westra W, et al. Genetic progression model for head and neck cancer: Implications for field cancerization. Cancer Res. 1996;56(11):2488-92.
6. Gupta PC, Mehta FS, Daftary DK, et al. Incidence rates of oral cancer and natural history of oral precancerous lesions in a 10-year follow-up study of Indian villagers. Community Dent Oral Epidemiol. 1980;8(6):283-333.
7. Gupta PC, Bhonsle RB, Murthy PR, et al. An epidemiologic assessment of cancer risk in oral precancerous lesions in India with special reference to nodular leukoplakia. Cancer. 1989;63(11):2247-52.

18 Oral Cancers

Vijay Haribhakti

INTRODUCTION

Oral cancer is the sixth most common cancer worldwide and even more important when looked at in the context of India. Among all male cancers, head and neck cancers are most common and among these, oral cancers rank highest in incidence. In the female population too, they are highly significant and come next only to the most prevalent sites, namely cervix and breast. These cancers are intimately related to the prevalence of habits that include tobacco chewing and smoking, alcohol, areca nut, and a variety of other substances packaged together as "*maava*," "*paan masala*," etc. These substances have toxic effects on the oral mucosa and produce a variety of changes, the most common being leukoplakia and submucous fibrosis. These have been dealt with at length in a separate chapter. By far, the most common type of cancer encountered is squamous cell carcinoma, originating from the stratified squamous epithelium that lines the mouth. These account for over 94% of all cases. Other less frequent neoplastic lesions include tumors of minor salivary origin, mucosal melanomas, jaw tumors and sarcomas. The discussion that follows relates essentially to squamous carcinomas, although the fundamentals remain similar with different histologies.

ANATOMICAL BOUNDARIES AND SUBSITES

The oral cavity comprises a number of anatomically distinct subsites, each with unique biological and clinical significance. Cancers originating in individual subsites often exhibit distinct patterns of local extension and spread that must be clearly appreciated.

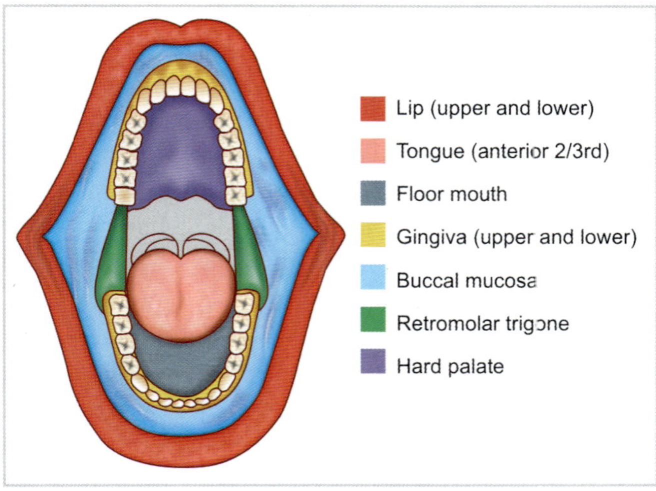

Fig. 1: Oral cavity, subsites

Figure 1 depicts the various subsites within the oral cavity and their approximate boundaries.

GENERAL FEATURES

The vast majority of oral squamous carcinomas manifest as ulcerated lesions, which refuse to heal spontaneously, despite conventional measures. Less frequently, endophytic lesions present with submucosal thickening and induration with relatively small overlying ulceration. Entirely submucosal lesions are more likely to represent tumors originating from minor salivary glands. As lesions evolve, they grow in diameter and depth, encroach upon surrounding anatomical structures, and invade deeper structures such as vessels, nerves, muscles and bone. Once a cancer extends to critical areas such as the masticator space, it has access to anatomical structures that could create pathways for aggressive and lethal extension. Apart from local extension, these cancers frequently exhibit lymph nodal metastases, which in most untreated cases follow predictable patterns of spread. With advancing stage and invasion, they also have the capacity to metastasize to distant sites. The most important sites for systemic spread include the lungs and skeletal system. The presence of lymphovascular emboli is thus an adverse prognostic indicator, as is perineural invasion. Size, thickness and depth of invasion are all important predictors of local aggressiveness and metastatic potential. The stage classification of oral cancers is essentially size-based, and this is a definite limitation which has been addressed in recent updates, which include criteria for invasiveness. Table 1 represents the currently accepted classification system for oral cancers.

A complete clinical evaluation of any lesion must therefore include detailed bimanual palpation to gauge thickness and infiltration of underlying tissues, and anatomical imaging [computed tomography/magnetic resonance imaging (CT/MRI)] to distinguish superficial, proliferative lesions from endophytic, infiltrative and destructive lesions.

In assigning a clinical "T" stage, it is important to measure not only the visually obvious greatest dimension of the lesion, but also to estimate the dimension of the submucosal component by palpation, and the extent of deep invasion by clinical and radiologic signs. Failure to do this often results in fallacious understaging and incorrect treatment planning.

Thorough assessment of large, locally advanced lesions also includes a check for signs of advanced, "inoperable" disease such as induration, erythema and edema of large areas of overlying skin, or evidence of dermal lymphatic permeation with manifestations like cutaneous thickening, edema and *peau d' orange* of the skin of the neck, or deep extension to surgically forbidden areas. It is also important to keep in mind some vital truths like the population of capillary lymphatics in the area of disease, and the inherently greater proclivity for lymphatic spread in areas such as the tongue and floor mouth. Following complete local examination of the primary, the neck is carefully palpated for evidence of nodal metastasis. Majority of patients with oral cancer have variable degrees of secondary infection and consequent reactive nodal enlargement. The presence of firm-to-hard enlarged nodes, especially if accompanied by impaired mobility, is highly suspicious of metastasis. In all cases, the neck is clinically staged, the stage classification being dependent upon size, laterality and multiplicity (Table 2). Based on patterns of cervical node metastasis, the Memorial Hospital group introduced the concept of neck levels, in order to represent the stations most at risk for a given primary cancer. For oral cancers, levels I, II and III are important and must be cleared during a staging neck dissection for a clinically N0 neck at risk. Ultrasound, CT and MRI are important imaging modalities to ascertain the status of the neck.

Enlarged, spherical, hypoechoic nodes with displacement or loss of fatty hilum are highly suspicious findings on ultrasound. On the CT, enlarged nodes (short

TABLE 1: T-staging for tumors of the lip and oral cavity

TX	Primary tumor cannot be assessed
T0	No evidence of primary tumor
Tis	Carcinoma in situ
T1	Tumor 2 cm or less in greatest dimension
T2	Tumor more than 2 cm, but not more than 4 cm in greatest dimension
T3	Tumor more than 4 cm in greatest dimension
T4a Lip	Tumor invades through cortical bone, inferior alveolar nerve, floor of mouth or skin of face
Oral cavity	Tumor invades through cortical bone, into deep extrinsic muscle of tongue (genioglossus, hyoglossus, palatoglossus and styloglossus), maxillary sinus or skin of face
T4b	Tumor involves masticator space, pterygoid plates, or skull base and/or encases internal carotid artery

TABLE 2: N-staging for all head and neck sites except thyroid

Nx	Regional lymph nodes cannot be assessed
N0	No regional lymph node metastasis
N1	Metastasis in a single ipsilateral lymph node, 3 cm or less in greatest dimension
N2	Metastasis in a single ipsilateral lymph node, more than 3 cm but not more than 6 cm in greatest dimension; or in multiple ipsilateral lymph nodes, none more than 6 cm in greatest dimension; or in bilateral or contralateral lymph nodes, none more than 6 cm in greatest dimension
N2a	Metastasis in a single ipsilateral lymph node more than 3 cm, but not more than 6 cm in greatest dimension
N2b	Metastasis in multiple ipsilateral lymph nodes, none more than 6 cm in greatest dimension
N2c	Metastasis in bilateral or contralateral lymph nodes, none more than 6 cm in greatest dimension
N3	Metastasis in a lymph more than 6 cm in greatest dimension

axis > 1 cm) with central necrosis are significant findings, while on the MRI, the demonstration of extranodal extension is a nearly diagnostic finding. The surest way to establish presence of metastatic disease is by fine needle aspiration biopsy with ultrasonography assistance, as needed. In this context, it is important to mention that the practice of incision or excision biopsies for suspicious nodal metastasis is both unnecessary and potentially damaging. An incorrectly placed incision can prove problematic for neck dissection later. The availability of positron emission tomography-computed tomography (PET-CT) imaging has made a significant contribution to the evaluation and management of the metastatic neck. In patients with high T-stage disease and short, thick necks that vitiate reliable clinical examination, the PET-CT is immensely useful, especially when there is an assumed risk of bilateral spread. It is also extremely useful for the monitoring of metastatic nodes that have been treated with chemoradiation alone.

Following thorough clinical, radiological and histological diagnosis, a treatment plan is made, based upon the clinical tumor, TNM stage.

In general, early cancers (stage I and II) are treated with a single modality, while more advanced cancers (stages III and IV) demand combination treatments for effective control.

APPROACH TO TREATMENT

For the oral cavity, surgery remains the primary treatment modality, and the most fundamental treatment is a wide surgical resection with clear margins. All refinements and advances relate to the manner in which this fundamental treatment is delivered with minimal morbidity and maximal efficacy. Most significantly, today there is improved clarity about the determinants of function and esthetics, and the means available for effective preservation and restoration of both.

SURGICAL APPROACHES

Surgical approaches to oral cancers depend upon a variety of factors, chief amongst them being the location and extent of the primary lesion. The other vital factors include the extent of mouth opening and the quality and pliability of the oral mucosa. Apart from primary lip lesions that are immediately accessible, other lesions are tackled by one of the following three approaches:

Peroral (Figs 2 to 5)

In which the lesion is directly approached through the open mouth without any facial incisions. This approach is excellent for early lesions of the anterior cheek and tongue, and selected lesions of the gums and anterior floor mouth. Submucous fibrosis and trismus severely limit this approach. Posterior extension of the primary lesion restricts access by peroral approaches and must be dealt with appropriately

Cheek Flap (Figs 6 to 8)

Through an anterior median lip-split, a cheek flap is raised to provide access to the lesion. In rare instances, access may be gained by a commissure split. In the standard median

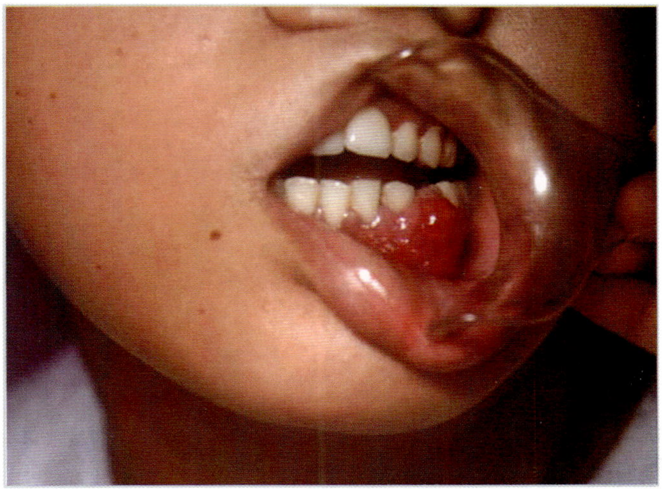

Fig. 2: Carcinosarcoma involving the anterior lower gum with minimal cortical erosion

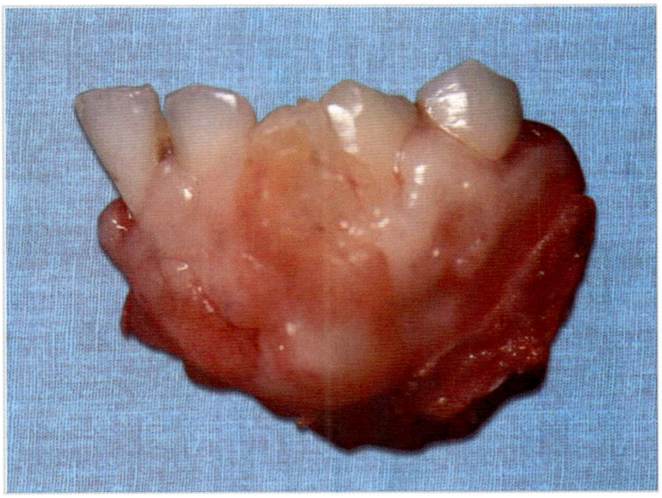

Fig. 3: Peroral resectiion (with clear margins)

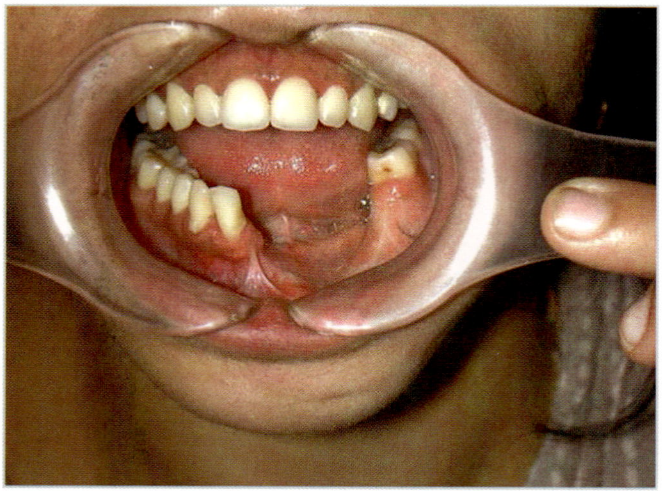

Fig. 4: Primary mucosal reapproximation

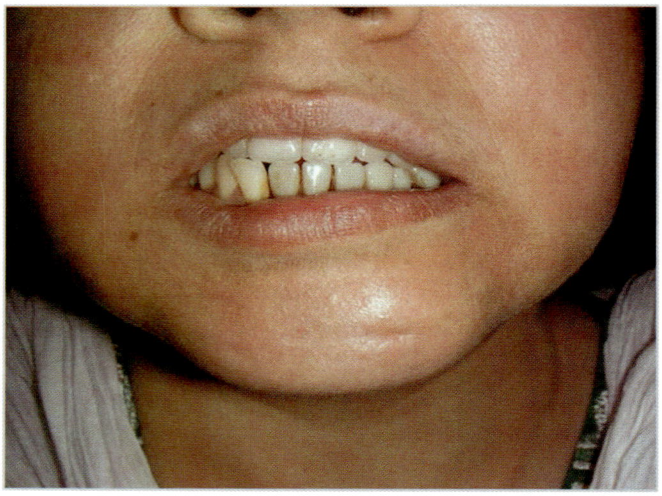

Fig. 5: Final long-term result—dental rehabilitation

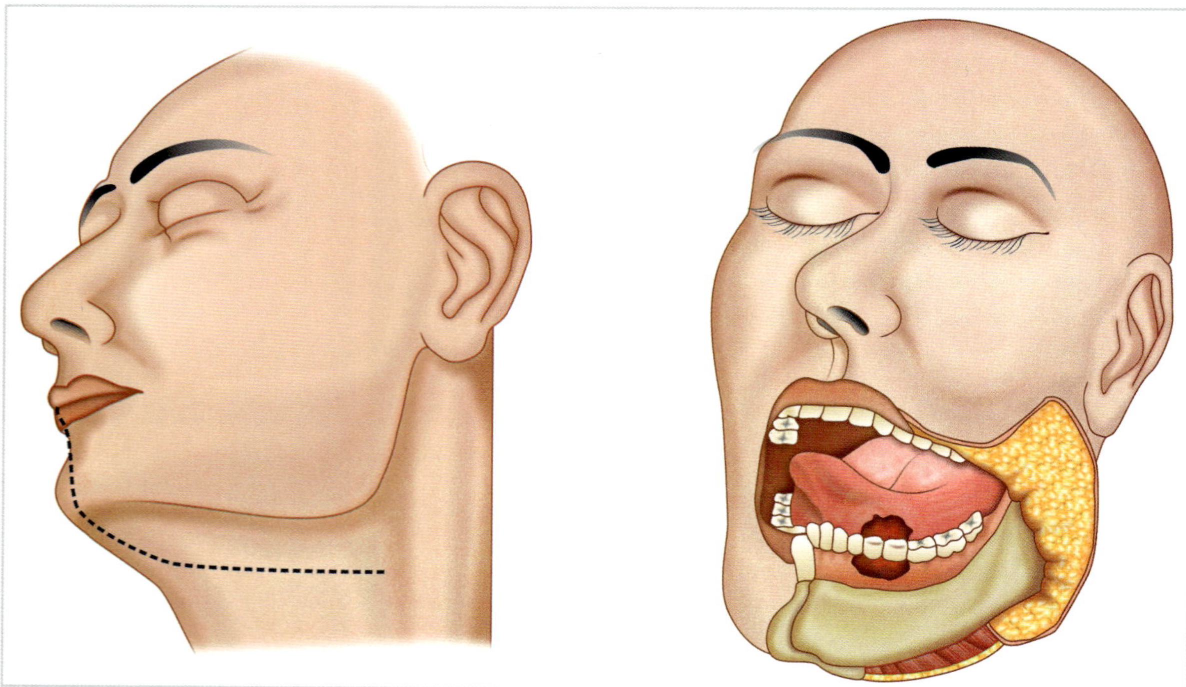

Fig. 6: Lip split with cheek flap

lip-split (Fig. 7), the midline must be accurately marked, preoperatively. In order to restore perfect apposition, it is the author's preference to mark a notch at the white line of the lip, and small "Zs" at the sublabial crease, submental crease and one in between (Fig. 8).

Visor Flap (Fig. 9)

In this approach, the lip split is avoided, and access is gained to the anterior mandible and associated areas, as demonstrated. This concept is useful in selected situations and must be carefully planned.

Managing the Mandible

The mandible is frequently encroached or invaded by the lesion in question, or is in the way, impeding access to a posterior primary site in the tongue base or oropharynx. A clear approach to its management is germane. Whenever a primary lesion originating in the cheek, gum or tongue grows and abuts the mandible, or even produces minimal cortical erosion, it is not necessary to remove a segment of bone, except in instances of advanced disease, where radiologically uninvolved bone is surrounded by tumor. In all other cases, a "rim (marginal) mandibulectomy" is

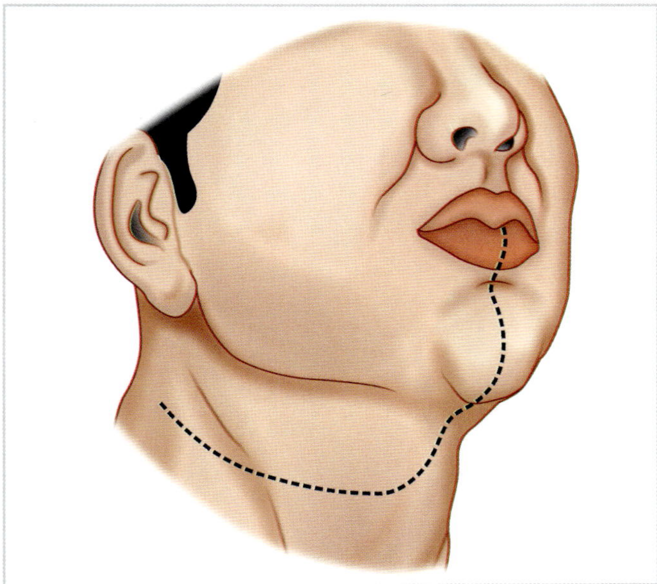

Fig. 7: Standard median lip split incision

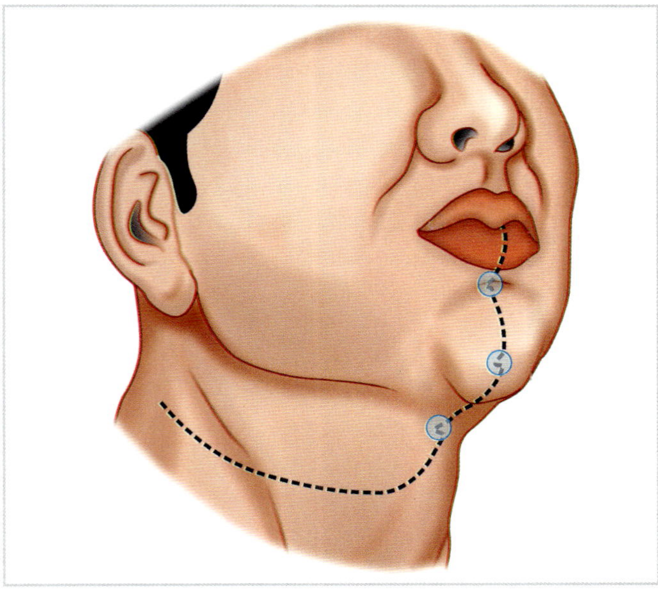

Fig. 8: Modified median lip split with Z's

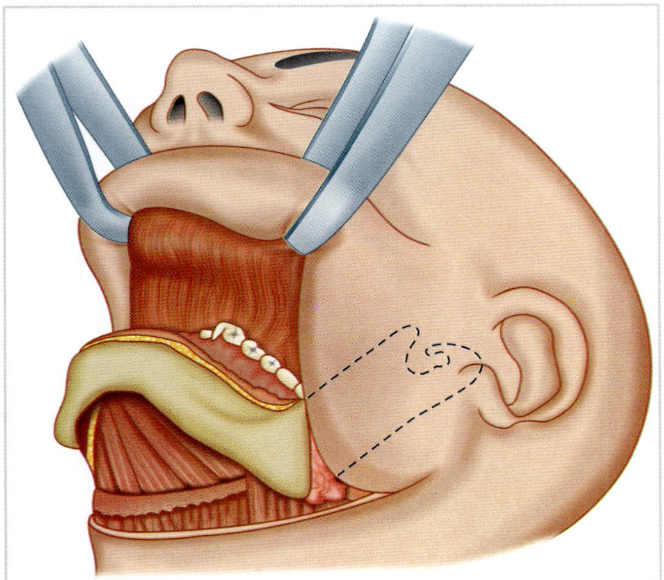

Fig. 9: Visor flap—submandibular incision with access to the anterior mandible

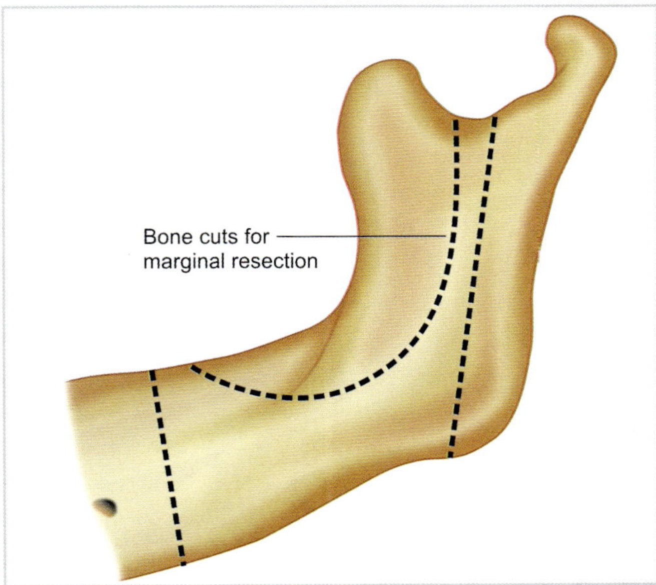

Fig. 10: Bone cuts for segmental or marginal mandibulectomy

undertaken, in which anatomical continuity of the bone is retained by preserving at least a centimeter of bony height and designing a cut that accomplishes a wide three-dimensional resection of the primary, without any compromise to oncologic safety (Fig. 10). When designing a cut for marginal resection for a cancer originating in the tongue and/or floor of mouth, a "lingual cortex" resection may be planned. In the majority of patients; however, a horizontal rim resection is the requirement. Figure 11 demonstrates the correct principles for carrying out a biomechanically sound rim resection.

When the mandible is invaded, an appropriately designed segmental resection is undertaken to achieve clear bony margins. The common designs of mandibular cuts are shown in Figure 10, and are possible to follow in the majority.

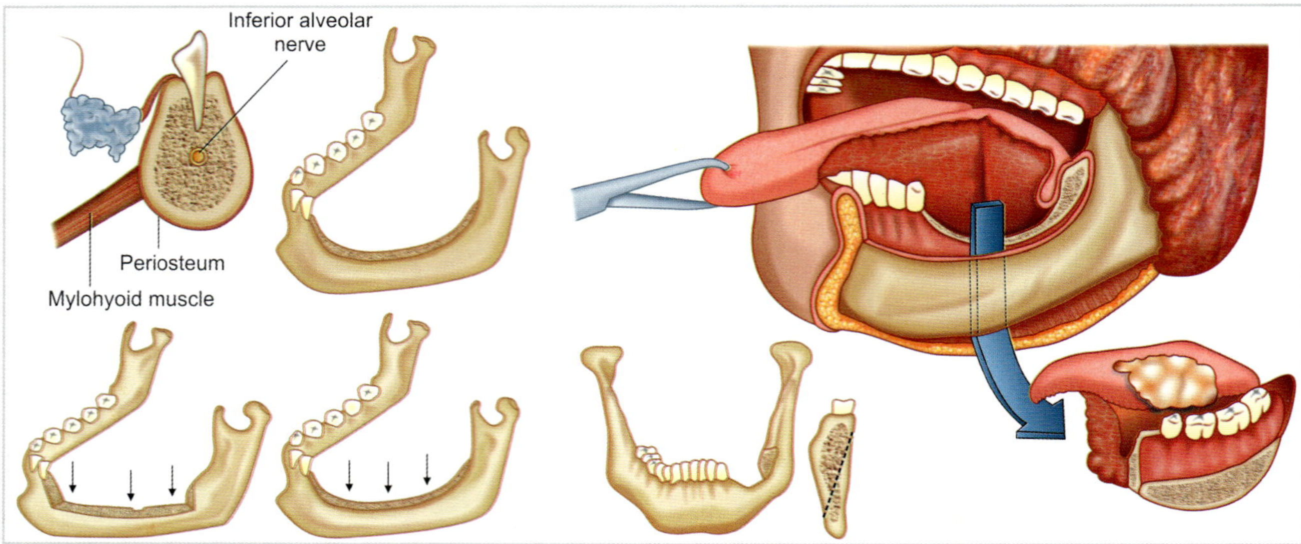

Fig. 11: Marginal mandibulectomy—rationale and design

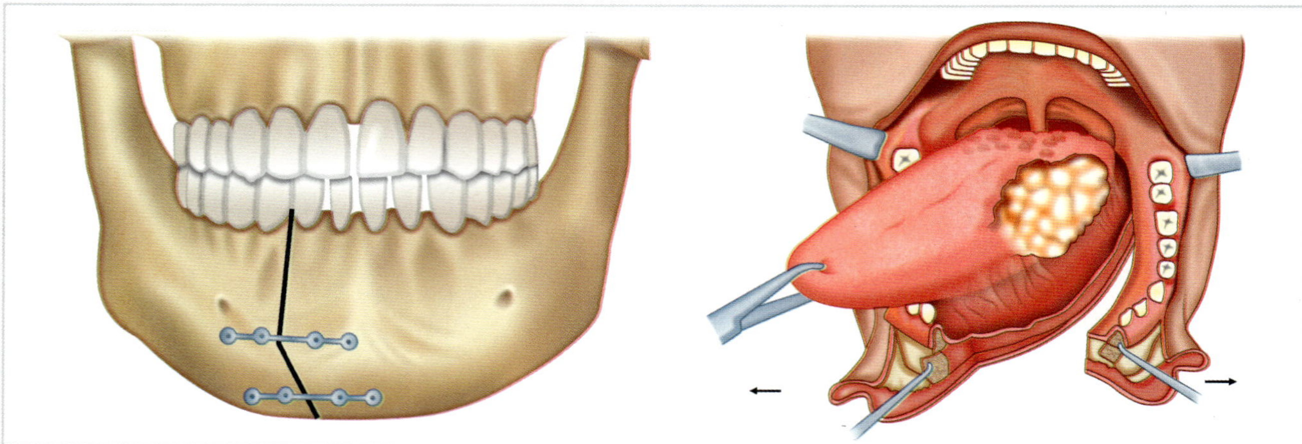

Fig. 12: Paramedian mandibulotomy—posterior lesion of the tongue and oropharynx

When planning the cuts for a segmental resection, it is crucial to estimate the extent of marrow involvement and to ascertain if the inferior dental canal is invaded and the nerve thickened. The earlier "standard" practice of "hemimandibulectomy" with disarticulation at the temporomandibular (TM) joint has very little to recommend it. If a high resolution computed tomography (HRCT) of the mandible reveals erosion into the marrow spaces, it is best to get a correlative MRI scan to study the extent of marrow invasion and the characteristics of the nerve. Based on clinical and radiologic information, the extent of mandibulectomy is always planned in advance, since frozen section information on bone margins is not a possibility. While it is unwise and functionally detrimental to sacrifice unnecessary lengths of bone, it must be borne in mind that clear bony margins are absolutely essential. Positive bone margins raise the risks of failure immensely and are unacceptable.

For approach to the posterior tongue and oropharynx, a paramedian mandibulotomy approach is employed as shown in Figure 12. This design of mandibulotomy is biomechanically more stable and easier to replate than the median mandibulotomy, which is now almost given up in most centers. With these generalizations in mind, it is possible to proceed with subsite-specific considerations.

THE LIPS

The lips are highly specialized musculoelastic "curtains" which separate the moist interior of the mouth from the dry exterior. The vermillion forms a distinctive border that gives the lips their unique esthetic significance. The prime function of the lips is oral competence, which derives from their sphincter-like function. The lower lip acts like a dam and has pronounced functional value, while the upper lip acts like a curtain and has marked esthetic significance. Squamous carcinomas most frequently present on the free margin of the lower lip. Extension in a lateral direction takes them towards the commissures, while deep extension results in invasion of the orbicularis muscle, buccal mucosa, and finally mandibular bone. The commissures and varying portions of the lips can get secondarily involved with cancers originating in the buccal mucosa.

With increasing stage, lymphatic spread occurs predictably to the cervical nodes, level I being the first station. With central lesions, bilateral spread is known. The submental triangle contains tiny nodes that must be assiduously cleared in all cases of primary lower lip cancer. With large central tumors, bilateral supraomohyoid neck dissection must be performed, sparing the external jugular vein on at least one side.

In general, early T1 and T2 lesions are treated with surgical resection with clear margins along with neck dissection, as indicated. As stage advances, surgical resection is followed by adjuvant radiation or chemoradiation.

Lip reconstruction clearly begins with a well-planned surgical resection. The essential aims are restoration of oral competence, commissure diameter, symmetry and circumferential vermillion. As lip tissue is highly specialized, in general, "lip for lip" reconstructions are advisable, keeping in mind the aims just mentioned. The most common techniques employed are the V-Y excision and closure, the Abbe-Estlander flap and the Karapandzic technique (Figs 13 and 14).

When excision involves more than 40% of lip substance, it is best to bring in a thin, fasciocutaneous flap.

While the radial forearm flap with a palmaris longus tendon sling is the most preferred option, the anterolateral thigh flap can be employed in individuals with large requirements and with thin, pliable skin over the thigh.

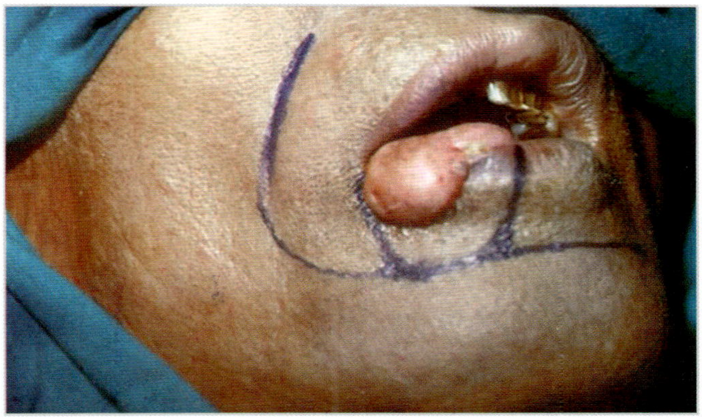

Fig. 13: Squamous carcinoma lower lip

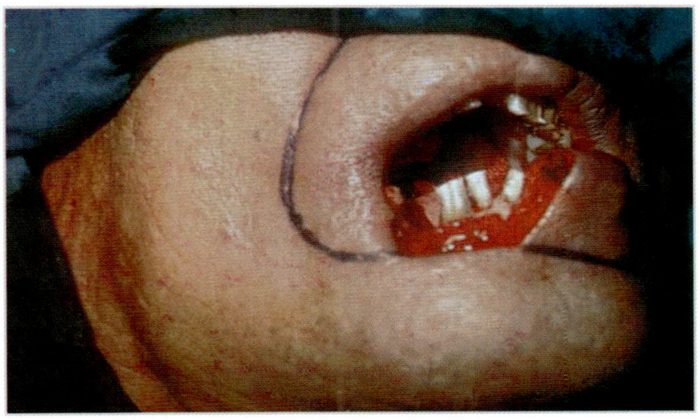

Fig. 14: Karapandzic technique: Loss of commissure plus 30% lower lip

CHEEK AND GUM

The cheeks are multilayered musculoelastic "walls" on either side of the jaws that merge seamlessly into the lips in front, the upper gum above, the lower gum below and the retromolar trigone behind. The mucosal lining in the normal mouth is pink and pliable, and is pierced by the opening of the Stensen's duct, near the second upper molar on either side. Beneath the mucosa (in successive outward planes) lie the submucosal glands, the buccinator muscles, nerves and vessels, subcutaneous fat and skin. The muscles of facial expression traverse in a plane just deep to the neurovascular plane and attach themselves to the modiolus on either side.

Cancers that originate in the central portion of the cheek mucosa extend craniad and caudald up to the respective upper and lower gingivobuccal sulci, anteriorly toward the commissure and lips, and posteriorly toward the retromolar trigone. Posterior spread beyond the pterygomandibular raphe gives tumor cells free access to the contents of the masticator space. The medial pterygoid muscle gets infiltrated early and can lead to trismus. Progressive outward and upward spread from the masticator space involves the masseter muscles, the temporalis and finally the infratemporal fossa. Progressive inward and caudal spread beyond the retromolar trigone results in disease extension to the floor of mouth, and finally the tongue medially, and the tonsillar pillar and palate above. Extension into the masticator space also gives the tumor free access to spread along branches of the mandibular division of the trigeminal nerve.

When tumors demonstrate cranio-caudal spread and are inseparable from bone, it becomes important to exclude cortical erosion by CT imaging. When marrow invasion is suspected, it is best demonstrated by MRI imaging. Soft tissue extension is not so clearly delineated on CT imaging and is facilitated by the "puffed cheek" technique to offer air contrast. With marked posterior extension, it is helpful to get MRI imaging done to study muscle invasion and neurovascular invasion. Thickening of nerves and widening of bony foramina through which the nerves traverse indicate neural invasion. Lymphatic spread of cheek and gum primaries increases with increasing stage and tumor thickness, and occurs in a systematic level-wise spread to the cervical nodes, level I being the first station of spread.

The approach to primary cheek and gum cancers is as follows: For early T1 and T2 lesions, wide surgical resection with clear margins and an appropriate neck dissection is needed. If adverse factors (thick T3/T4 lesion, tumor, invasive margins and nodal spread) are present, radiation is added; chemoradiation being reserved for very high-risk factors like extranodal spread, perineural extension and lymphovascular emboli.

It is very important to have a plan of reconstruction ready in all cases. The major aims of reconstruction are to restore a good, pliable lining capable of withstanding radiation, if indicated. Failure to achieve this can result in fibrous healing and trismus, which is extremely difficult to reverse. In the presence of submucous fibrosis and an unhealthy, nonpliable surrounding mucosa, some form of reconstruction is frequently necessary.

For small defects that can be closed by primary mucosal approximation, either directly or with mobilization, primary closure is best.

For moderate sized, superficial defects with an "adequate" surrounding mucosa, where the floor of the defect has a layer of muscle, reconstruction is possible to accomplish by using a split skin graft, or a full-thickness graft, or even a biological material like Kollagen®.

With deeper, larger, defects and with fibrotic surrounding mucosa, some form of vascularized reconstruction is optimal. The alternatives are numerous and include local, regional or distant tissues.

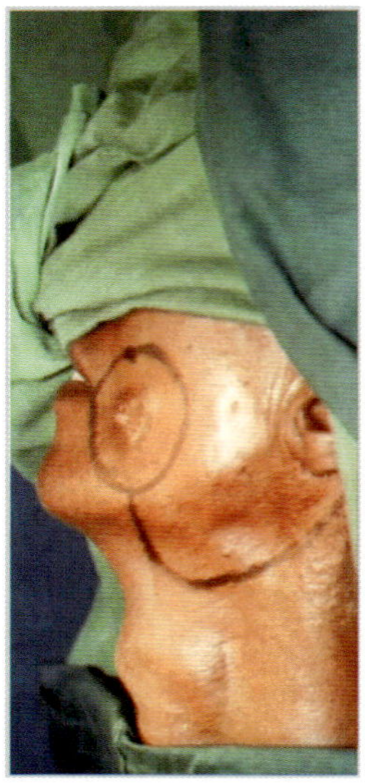

Fig. 15: Composite left cheek-mandible defect

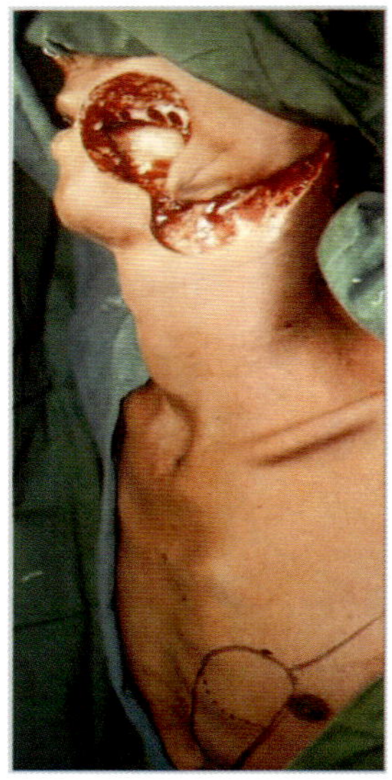

Fig. 16: Reconstruction by bipaddled pectoralis major flap

The "local" options include suctorial fat pad grafts and masseter flaps. The regional options include the temporoparietal fascia, the temporalis muscle, the submental flap and the platysma flap.

With large surface area or large volume defects with exposed bone, it is optimal to bring in a fasciocutaneous free flap such as the free "radial forearm flap" or the "anterolateral thigh flap".

Alternatively, the "pectoralis major" flap may be employed in very thin individuals with a thin layer of subcutaneous fat (Figs 15 to 18).

THE MANDIBLE

The mandible is frequently involved by lesions originating in neighboring subsites such as the cheeks, floor mouth and tongue, or by direct downward spread of primary lower gum cancers. The mechanisms of extension and spread were studied by McGregor and MacDonald and related to the state of dentition of the mandible. In the dentate adult human mandible, involvement begins with cortical erosions on the occlusal surface by the sides of the teeth, in the region of the periodontal membrane. Progressive downward spread involves the marrow spaces of the mandible from where, further extension takes two routes; one, along a broad front, anteriorly or posteriorly within the marrow space of the mandible and once the inferior dental canal is involved, spread can happen along

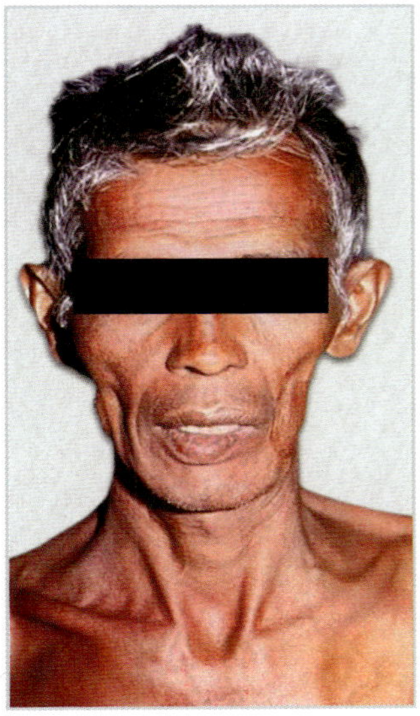

Fig. 17: Final result—front face

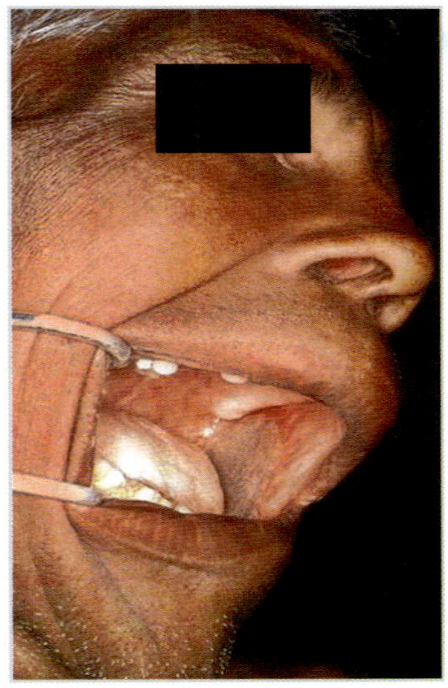

Fig. 18: Final result—mouth opening

the perineurium of the inferior dental nerve, ascending up along the trajectory of V3 to the skull base.

When planning mandibular resection, these patterns have to be borne in mind in order to achieve an oncologically sound resection without sacrificing needlessly large segments of the mandible. Once marrow invasion has occurred, MRI scanning is important to assess the extent and help decide the limits of segmental re-section necessary. While it is important to conserve healthy, uninvolved mandibular bone, it is equally important to recognize that a positive bone margin is dangerous and portends treatment failure. If despite all efforts at imaging and planning, there is a positive bone margin, reexcision must be advocated.

Once segmental resection is performed, some form of reconstruction becomes necessary. All defects involving the central arch segment of the mandible demand reconstruction by vascularized bone.

With posterior segmental defects that completely spare the arch, the type of reconstruction chosen depends upon the extent of bone resected, magnitude and complexity of the associated soft tissue and lining defect, the state of the oral mucosa, presence of trismus, and the philosophy and training of the surgeon. With very substantial soft tissue defects and very little healthy bone available for plate anchorage, it is often pragmatic to restore the soft tissue defect effectively with a soft tissue flap with sufficient skin and bulk.

In all cases, it is essential to restore the normal occlusal relationships of the mandibular remnant, so as to permit mastication to the best extent possible. In patients with severe trismus (due to fibrotic oral mucosa) who need postoperative radiation, it is often advantageous to avoid bony reconstruction, except with defects involving the anterior arch segment.

At the same time, one must recognize that limited defects of the ascending ramus alone, without reconstruction, leave long segments of "unsupported" mandible with resulting cantilevering, malocclusion and functional disability. In summary, it is critically important to decide beforehand:

- If segmental resection is necessary, what is the extent?
- What is the status of the remaining oral mucosa?
- What is the extent of the associated soft tissue defect?
- Is the central arch intact?
- What would be the functional or esthetic consequences of the resection?
- What would be the most optimal plan of reconstruction, keeping in mind the need for further treatment?

The reconstructive options should necessarily include healthy, vascularized, cortical bone suitable for future osseointegration. In most instances, the fibula provides the required bone and soft tissues, and has become the current "workhorse" for mandibular reconstruction (Figs 19 to 25).

The rib as part of the pectoralis major flap was used many years ago for relatively short, straight segmental losses. However, the undependable vascularity made frequent extrusions common, and the futility of a weak, poorly vascularized length of bone was recognized.

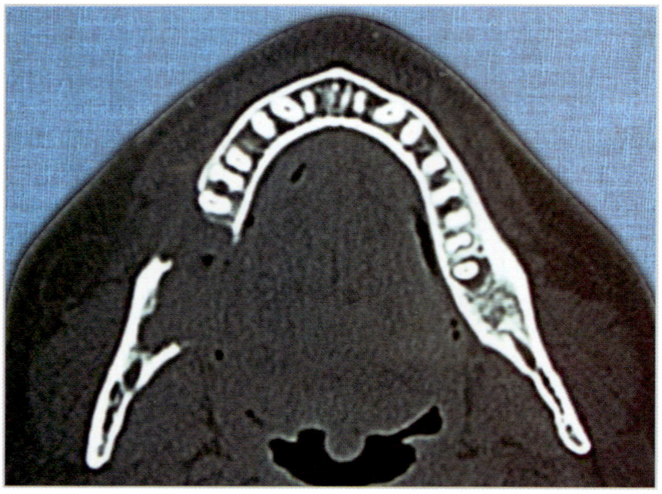

Fig. 19: Squamous carcinoma invading molar area of mandible

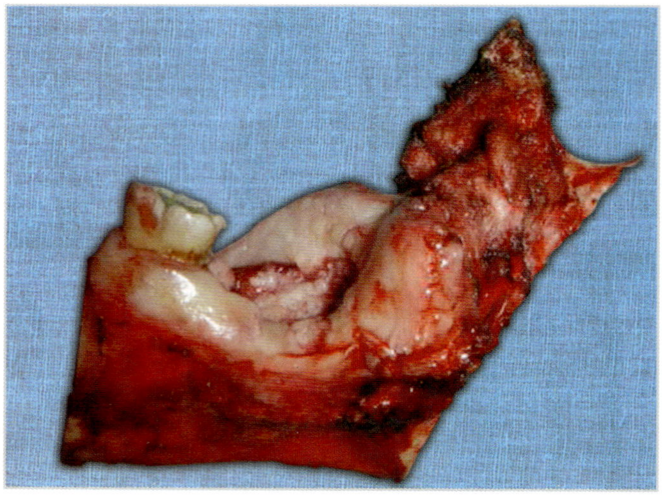

Fig. 20: Segmental resection with clear margins

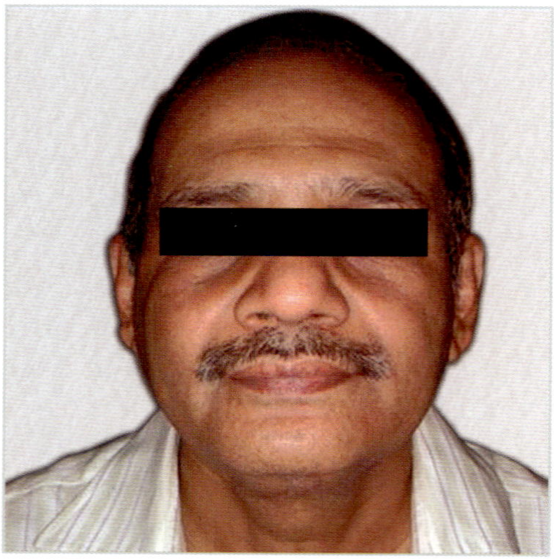

Fig. 21: Final result—fibula graft, front face

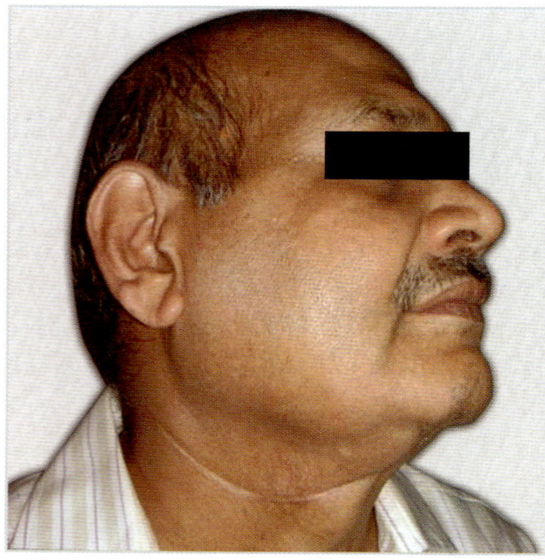

Fig. 22: Final result—fibula graft, profile

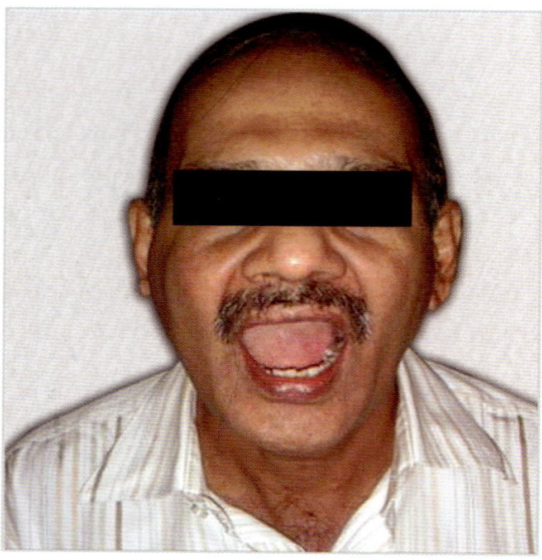

Fig. 23: Final result—fibula graft, open mouth

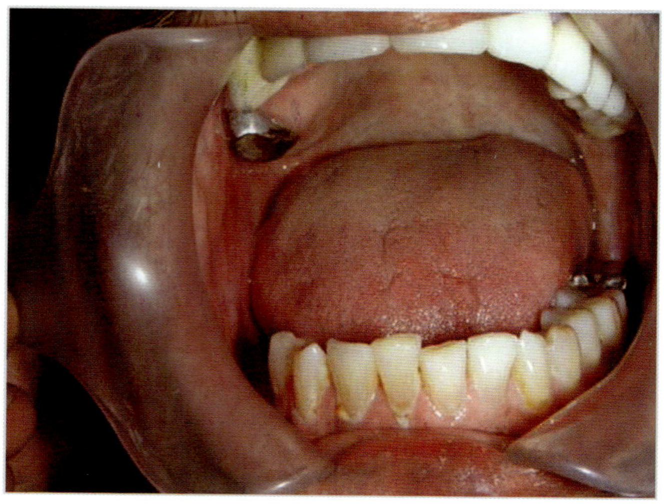

Fig. 24: Final result—intraoral view

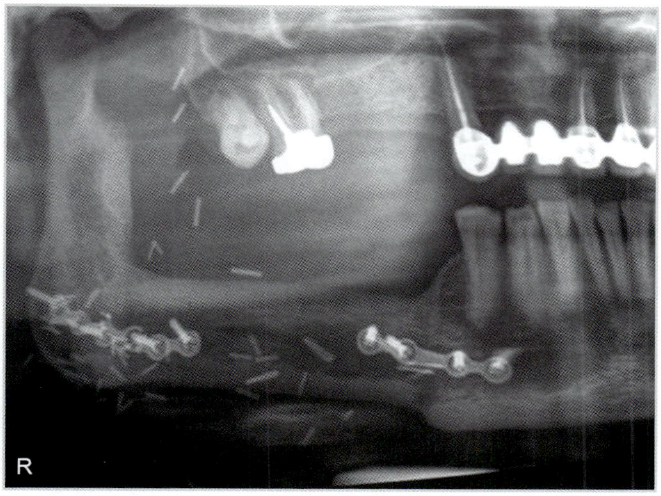

Fig. 25: Orthopantomograph (OPG) at 8 weeks

The vascularized iliac crest was far more frequently used earlier. However, the relatively short pedicle, the bulky soft tissue cuff required for including skin, and poor donor-site qualities, rendered it as a less-favored approach.

RETROMOLAR TRIGONE

This is a critically important location within the oral cavity for a variety of reasons. Situated just behind the last molar tooth, it is comprised of a band of "attached mucosa" overlying the area of the coronoid process origin, and extends up to the retromaxillary area. The integrity of this mucosa is essential to preserve mouth opening. It merges anterolaterally with the cheek mucosa and posteromedially with the tonsillar pillar and glosso-tonsillar sulcus. This area is profusely bathed with capillary lymphatics and has a significant proclivity for lymphatic spread. In its immediate neighborhood is the pterygomandibular raphe, a condensed band of fibrous tissue that extends from the posterior end of the mylohyoid line below to the tubercle of the medial pterygoid plate above. Tumors involving the retromolar area primarily or secondarily have access to several avenues of spread. Deep and downward extension involves the mandible, upward and lateral extension creates access to the contents of the masticator space (containing the muscles of mastication, lingual and inferior dental nerves), medial extension creates access to the floor mouth, tongue and glossotonsillar sulcus below and the tonsillar fossa and soft palate above. Trismus is common with involvement of this area, and is frequently due to invasion of the medial pterygoid muscle. CT imaging of this area is often vitiated by the presence of dental amalgam, and thus, MRI evaluation is important to study soft tissue extension, masticatory muscles, and neurovascular involvement. It is relevant to note that cortical erosion makes it a T4a primary, while invasion of masticatory muscles and neurovascular structure makes it a T4b primary.

Whenever excision of an oral primary cancer entails resection of the retromolar area, some form of reconstruction is required. This is particularly true for lesions originating posteriorly in the upper alveolus or maxilla. Failure to provide adequate reconstruction invariably results in trismus and disability. In general, split skin grafts do not help.

Vascularized thin skin (fasciocutaneous free flaps) or mobilized mucosa is to be preferred, not only for their pliability, but also for their ability to withstand adjuvant radiotherapy.

FLOOR OF MOUTH/TONGUE

The tongue occupies a position of unrivalled functional importance in the oral cavity, and the floor of mouth provides the necessary platform for lingual function. The tongue is crucial for all vital functions of the mouth, i.e. food intake, mastication, deglutition and speech. It is structurally composed of a large number of intrinsic and extrinsic muscles, which make possible its complex movements and alterations in shape and substance. The protrusible tip has critical importance and is intimately related to the articulation of consonant sounds and the movement of food and saliva within the mouth by its sweeping function. The submucosa contains numerous minor salivary glands, largely in the posterior portion. Capillary lymphatics abound within the tongue and floor mouth area, rendering lymphatic invasion common and frequent.

In order to preserve its complex array of functions, it is crucial to avoid tethering of the tongue and to ensure that there is "adequate" substance, especially in its posterior portion, which is responsible for the first phase of deglutition. The oral tongue is the anterior two-third of the organ, located anterior to the circumvallate papillae, and majority of lesions here present along the lateral borders. A tumor typically originating along the lateral border exhibits progressive mucosal spread anteroposteriorly toward the tip in front, or the tongue base behind; or along the undersurface of the tongue, making its way to the floor mouth, and hence, to the mandibular gingiva and bone. Deep extension involves the intrinsic and the extrinsic muscles, and progressively the neurovascular bundle comprising the lingual and hypoglossal nerves and the lingual artery. While the stage classification of tongue cancer is based on size, "T4" is indicative of an infiltrative tumor involving the intrinsic muscles, the neurovascular bundle or mandibular bone.

Clinical examination of a primary tongue lesion necessarily includes visual assessment of forward protrusion of the tongue tip. Ankyloglossia is a grave sign that indicates an advanced T4 lesion invading musculature. Deviation of the tip toward the side of the lesion indicates possible hypoglossal nerve involvement with unopposed action of contralateral extrinsic muscles. Deep palpation and palpation under anesthesia are also critically important to evaluate the extent of muscle invasion. Given the very high proclivity for lymphatic extension, the neck must be carefully assessed, clinically as well as radiologically. While anterior lesions tend to spread first to level I, more posterior lesions tend to go directly to the subdigastric nodes (level II). Skip metastases are known with tongue and floor of mouth primaries. Thus, a staging neck dissection for the N0 neck in patients with a primary tongue or floor of mouth cancer includes levels I–IV. Imaging for tongue and floor mouth primaries includes assessment of the primary site and neck. While CT scanning is preferred for nodal assessment, it is the author's preference to rely on MRI as a regular routine, for accurate assessment of the deep lingual musculature and the neurovascular bundle.

The treatment of T1 and T2 primary cancer of the oral tongue and floor of mouth includes wide surgical resection for the primary lesion together with an appropriate neck dissection. For lesions presenting along the lateral border, the most optimal plan of excision, typically is a laterally-based wedge, which lends itself to good primary closure with excellent function (Fig. 26).

The approach to resection depends on the location and size of the primary. For large, deeply invasive lesions located more posteriorly, a paramedian mandibulotomy is often needed to secure adequate access for a sound, three-dimensional resection.

Reconstruction following excision is aimed at restoring a tongue with maximal functional capability. In order to achieve this, tethering is to be avoided, so as to permit excellent tip function. In general, any loss of substance beyond 30% is an indication for some form of tissue replacement. Primary closure must be carried out in layers to achieve approximation of the divided musculature prior to mucosal closure. In some cases, owing to asymmetrically large losses of mucosa, primary closure could lead to tethering, and thus, skin grafts may be employed to retain optimal functionality. For a significant defect, such as hemiglossectomy, a thin, fasciocutaneous free flap is the method of choice for an optimal reconstruction. The radial forearm flap, hitherto considered the standard of care, is increasingly being replaced by the anterolateral thigh flap in individuals where thin, pliable skin is available. For large volume defects and total glossectomy defects, the anterolateral thigh flap is the current choice. In patients where a hemiglossectomy defect is coupled with a segmental mandibulectomy, bony reconstruction is optimal and the fibular osteocutaneous flap provides all the necessary tissue for an effective reconstruction.

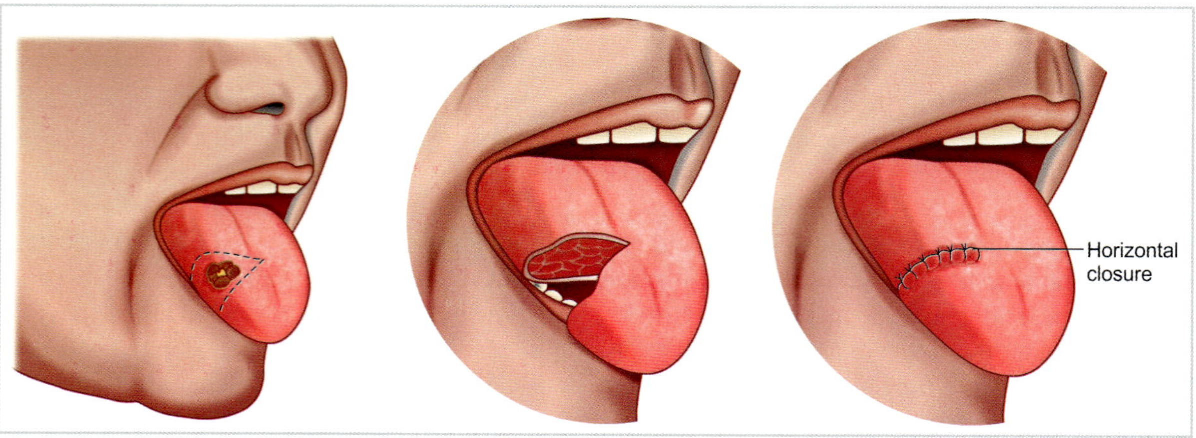

Fig. 26: Lesion at the lateral border oral tongue—wedge excision with primary closure

RADIOTHERAPY

Radiotherapy is the other definitive treatment modality for oral cancer, and can be employed as the only treatment for early disease, where surgery is either not possible for any reason or associated with needless morbidity. For advanced cancers, it is typically brought in after complete surgical resection, and results in improved local and regional control. In carefully selected cases, concomitant chemotherapy is added to further improve local and systemic control.

CHEMOTHERAPY

Chemotherapy has no role in the management of early oral cancer. For advanced cancer, it can be employed in a variety of situations. In far advanced cancers which are primarily inoperable or unresectable, chemotherapy is often employed to "downstage" disease before definitive treatment is introduced. It is also combined with radiotherapy in the presence of definitive criteria such as extracapsular spread with nodal metastasis, very thick, infiltrative primary tumors, lymphovascular embolization, and perineural extension.

BIBLIOGRAPHY

1. Jerjes W, Upile T, Petrie A, et al. Clinicopathological parameters, recurrence, locoregional and distant metastasis in 115 T1-T2 oral squamous cell carcinoma patients. Head and Neck Oncol. 2010;2:9.
2. Ow TJ, Myers JN. Current management of advanced resectable oral cavity squamous cell carcinoma. Clin Exp Otorhinolaryngol. 2011;4(1):1-10.
3. Patel SG, Shah JP. TNM staging of cancers of the head and neck: Striving for uniformity among diversity. CA Cancer J Clin. 2005;55(4);242-58.
4. Rana M, Iqbal A, Warriach R, et al. Modern surgical management of tongue carcinoma: A clinical retrospective research over a 12 years period. Head Neck Oncol. 2011;3:43.
5. Trotta BM, Pease CS, Rasamny JJ, et al. Oral cavity and oropharyngeal squamous cell cancer: Key imaging findings for staging and treatment planning. Radiographics. 2011;31(2): 339-54.
6. Vijayakumar M, Burrah R, Sabitha KS, et al. To operate or not to operate N0 neck in early cancer of the tongue? A prospective study. Indian J Surg Oncol. 2011;2(3):172-5.
7. Zhang H, Dziegielewski P, Biron VL, et al. Survival outcome of patients with advanced oral cavity squamous cell carcinoma treated with multimodal therapy: A multi-institutional analysis. J Otolaryngol Head and Neck Surg. 2013;42:30.

19 Cancer of the Larynx

Vijay Haribhakti

INTRODUCTION

The larynx occupies a position of unrivalled importance in the head and neck region. Apart from phonation, which is the prime modality of communication, the larynx guards the respiratory organs by its vital sphincteric function during the act of deglutition. Situated as it is upon the trachea, the larynx maintains the patency of the airway during respiration. With its crucial role in three fundamental functions, i.e. respiration, deglutition and phonation, the intact larynx has always been regarded as a functioning marvel that should naturally elicit every attempt at preservation (Fig. 1).

The approach to laryngeal cancers has undergone complete metamorphosis since the advent of organ salvage protocols, aimed at offering the best possibilities of control, keeping in mind the dual objectives of cure and organ preservation.

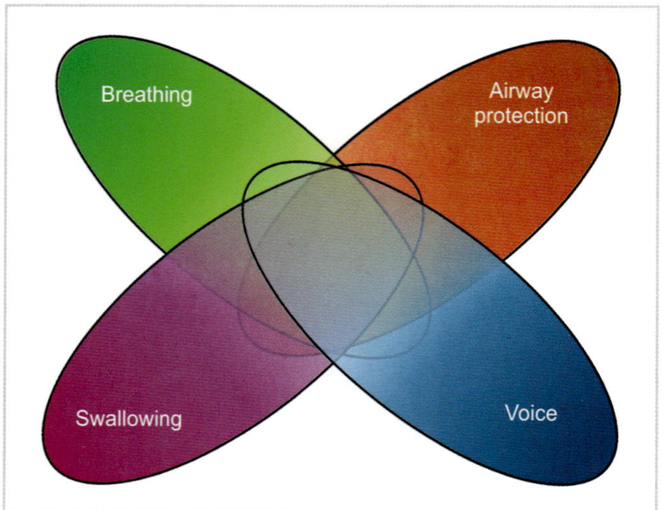

Fig. 1: Functional role of the larynx

Surgical Anatomy of the Larynx

The anatomy of the larynx has to be understood not only in terms of an intricate interplay of cartilages, ligaments, muscles and membranes; but also in terms of the pathways of spread to tumors originating within. In this connection, it is important to comprehend the laryngeal spaces and their boundaries, which explain the mechanisms by which tumors spread within and outside the larynx.

The larynx is divided based on anatomic and embryologic lines:

The "supraglottic larynx" is composed of the epiglottis, aryepiglottic folds and ventricular folds. The "glottis" consists of the two vocal cords, and the anterior and posterior commissures. The junction between the two portions passes through the saccule of the larynx, which represents not only a lymphatic watershed, but also a significant barrier to spread of tumors downward from the supraglottis or conversely upward from the glottis. The biological behavior, patterns of extension and lymphatic spread of tumors originating in these two regions are likewise different. The "subglottis" includes the remaining portion of the larynx up to the inferior border of the cricoid cartilage.

The laryngeal space is divided into three:

1. The "vestibule" is the upper chamber of the laryngeal cavity between the laryngeal inlet and the vestibular folds which enclose the vestibular ligament and associated soft tissues.

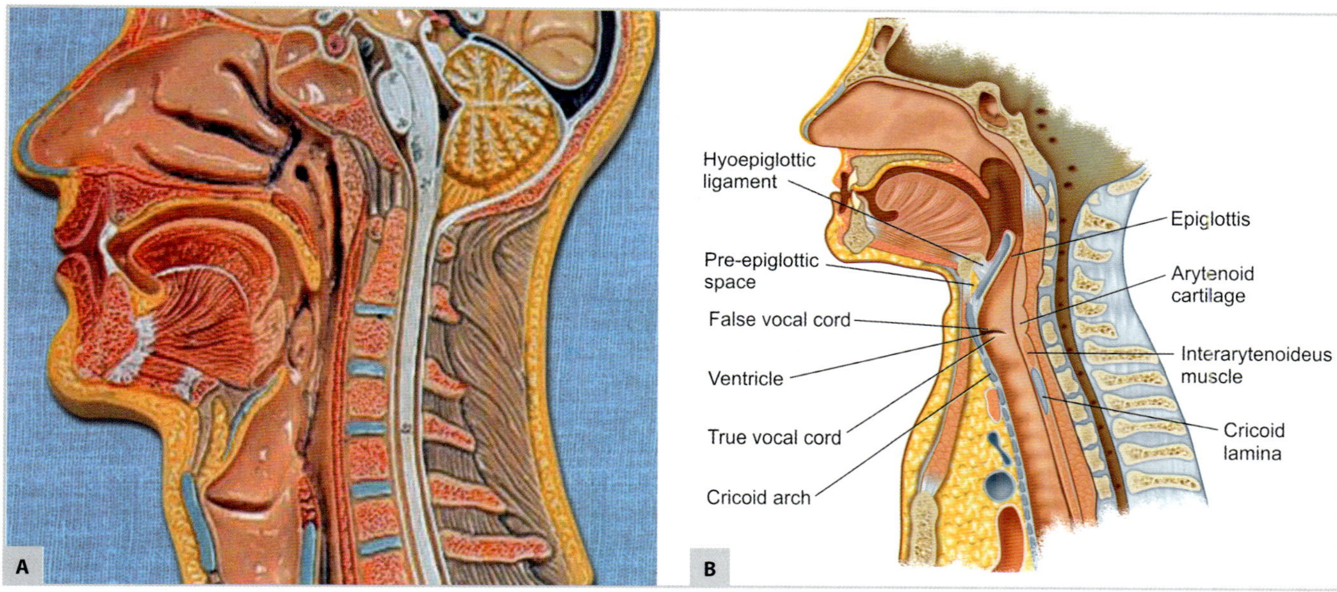

Figs 2A and B: Sagittal anatomy of the larynx

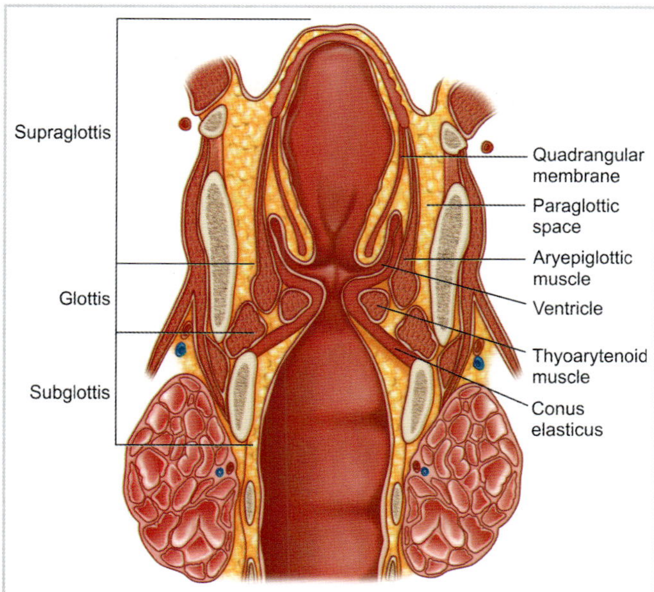

Fig. 3: Surgical coronal anatomy of the larynx

2. The "saccule" (middle part of the laryngeal cavity) is very thin and is between the vestibular folds above and the vocal folds below.
3. The "infraglottis" is the most inferior chamber of the laryngeal cavity and is between the vocal folds (which enclose the vocal ligament and related soft tissues) and the inferior opening of the larynx into the trachea (Figs 2 and 3).

It is important to note that tumors originating in the epiglottis have direct access through fenestrations in the cartilage to the space in front, known as the pre-epiglottic space. This space is bounded by the thyrohyoid membrane anteriorly, the vallecula superiorly, the epiglottis posteriorly and the hyoid inferiorly; and is commonly involved by local spread of supraglottic tumors. Once this space is involved the tumor is staged directly as 'T3'. Tumors involving this area can then spread into the soft tissues of the neck via the rents in the thyrohyoid membrane or inferiorly via the paraglottic space, bounded internally by the quadrangular membrane, and externally by the thyroid cartilage (Fig. 3).

Cancers of the larynx can be classified as advanced stage III or IV either by virtue of locally advanced primary tumors or by the presence of regional lymph node metastasis and are described in terms of their location, number and size. The location of the lymph nodes is described by 'levels' in the neck, the most important ones being II, III and IV (Fig. 4).

DIAGNOSIS

If the tumor originates on the vocal cords or in the glottic region of the larynx, the first warning sign includes hoarseness or change in the quality of voice. With advancing tumors of the glottis, there could be compromise in the airway and consequent stridor. Tumors originating in the supraglottic portion of the larynx remain undetected for long periods of time until they produce odynophagia, halitosis or otalgia. Certain tumors of the supraglottis develop a characteristic change in the quality of speech, known as the "hot potato speech". As these tumors advance and spread across the spaces of the larynx, hoarseness may develop as a late symptom. Not surprisingly, ominous symptoms such as hemoptysis, dysphagia, airway compromise and neck mass are common only in advanced disease.

The most important method of clinical diagnosis of the larynx is with an indirect laryngoscopy (IDL) mirror, which offers an excellent panorama of the inlet of the larynx, vocal cords, vestibular folds as well as the surrounding regions of the supraglottic larynx. This is a simple and vital examination which can either be carried out with a simple IDL mirror, a 90° Hopkins telescope, or with a flexible fiberoptic nasolaryngoscope. In the course of this examination careful note is made of the presence of any tumor, the exact extent of which is documented on a diagram, as also the mobility of the vocal cords. This is important and dictates the staging of any cancer. Careful clinical examination of the neck gives vital information about neck node involvement.

Once a clinical diagnosis of laryngeal cancer is made, it is necessary to obtain sound radiological imaging to ascertain the depth of tumor invasion, the involvement of the laryngeal spaces, i.e. the pre-epiglottic and paraglottic spaces, and also to study the presence of cartilaginous invasion and extralaryngeal spread. Clinically, extralaryngeal spread is possible to diagnose by the absence of what is known as the thyrovertebral crackle. This is a rattling sensation and sound that is produced as the larynx is moved to and fro against the spine posteriorly. Another sign of an advanced cancer is widening of the thyroid cartilage.

Radiological assessment of the larynx is best carried out by means of a high resolution computed tomography (CT) of the larynx.[1] The high resolution CT gives excellent and reliable information about the presence of tumor, the extent of involvement superiorly, inferiorly and the depth of involvement into the paraglottic and pre-epiglottic spaces. It adds critically important information about involvement of laryngeal framework, evidenced by rarefaction or actual destruction of the cartilages of the larynx, most frequently the thyroid cartilage. It gives information about extralaryngeal spread into the soft tissues of the neck, and the presence of lymph node metastasis, commonly to the jugular chain. The most important signs of lymph node metastasis are spherical nodes greater than 1 cm in maximum dimension, with a classical sign of central necrosis.

After imaging of the larynx, the next step is a direct laryngoscopic examination under general anesthesia. This is carried out with a rigid speculum, which is moved around to inspect the laryngeal inlet, surrounding pharynx and finally the laryngeal interior. The entire area of disease is carefully mapped, the adequacy of the airway noted, and at the time of reversal, vocal cord mobility is studied. A biopsy is mandatory to confirm the presence of cancer. For early and small tumors involving only the vocal cords, it is preferable to perform a microlaryngoscopy in order to carefully assess the extent of tumor, and to study supra and infraglottic extension. Once a through clinical, radiological and endoscopic assessment of the patient is complete, the disease is clinically staged and the therapeutic approach planned.

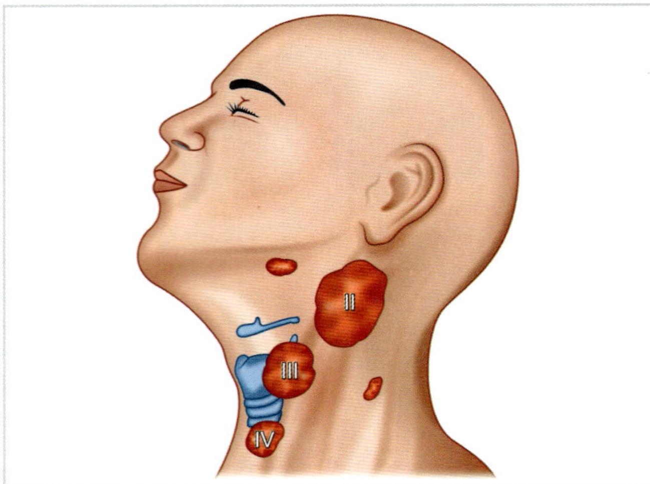

Fig. 4: Lymphatic spread of laryngeal cancer [Level II (sub-diagastric), Level III (mid jugular), Level IV (larger jugular)]

STAGING OF CANCER OF THE LARYNX[2-4]

The Tumor-Node-Metastasis (TNM) system of staging is universally accepted for classification of laryngeal cancer, and is dependent upon surface extent, vocal cord mobility and invasiveness into either the spaces of the larynx or the laryngeal framework. Despite deficiencies in the staging system and considerable variability within a given stage, this classification constitutes a uniform, acceptable language of communication and for expression of treatment results (Table 1).

MANAGEMENT OF LARYNGEAL CANCER

General Principles

T1 and T2 cancers of the larynx whether glottic or supraglottic, are to be managed differently from advanced

TABLE 1: Tumor-node-metastasis (TNM) classification

Primary tumor (T)	
TX	Primary tumor cannot be assessed
T0	No evidence of primary tumor
Tis	Carcinoma in situ
Supraglottis	
T1	Tumor limited to one subsite of supraglottis with normal vocal cord mobility
T2	Tumor invades mucosa of more than one adjacent subsite of supraglottis or glottis (e.g. mucosa of base of tongue, vallecula and medial wall of pyriform sinus) without fixation of the larynx
T3	Tumor limited to larynx with vocal cord fixation and/or invades any of the following: postcricoid area, preepiglottic space, paraglottic space and/or inner cortex of thyroid cartilage
T4a	Moderately advanced local disease
	Tumor invades through the thyroid cartilage and/or invades tissues beyond the larynx (e.g. trachea, soft tissues of neck including deep extrinsic muscle of the tongue, strap muscles, thyroid, or esophagus)
T4b	Very advanced local disease
	Tumor invades prevertebral space, encases carotid artery or invades mediastinal structures
Glottis	
T1	Tumor limited to the vocal cord(s) (may involve anterior or posterior commissure) with normal mobility
T1a	Tumor limited to one vocal cord
T1b	Tumor involves both vocal cords
T2	Tumor extends to supraglottis and/or subglottis and/or with impaired vocal cord mobility
T3	Tumor limited to the larynx with vocal cord fixation and/or invasion of paraglottic space and/or inner cortex of the thyroid cartilage
T4a	Moderately advanced local disease
	Tumor invades through the outer cortex of the thyroid cartilage and/or invades tissues beyond the larynx (e.g. trachea, soft tissues of neck including deep extrinsic muscle of the tongue, strap muscles, thyroid or esophagus)
T4b	Very advanced local disease
	Tumor invades prevertebral space, encases carotid artery or invades mediastinal structures
Subglottis	
T1	Tumor limited to the subglottis
T2	Tumor extends to vocal cord(s) with normal or impaired mobility
T3	Tumor limited to larynx with vocal cord fixation
T4a	Moderately advanced local disease
	Tumor invades cricoid or thyroid cartilage and/or invades tissues beyond the larynx (e.g. trachea, soft tissues of neck including deep extrinsic muscles of the tongue, strap muscles, thyroid or esophagus)
T4b	Very advanced local disease
	Tumor invades prevertebral space, encases carotid artery or invades mediastinal structures
Regional lymph nodes	
NX	Regional lymph nodes cannot be assessed
N0	No regional lymph node metastasis
N1	Metastasis in a single ipsilateral lymph node, ≤ 3 cm in greatest dimension
N2	Metastasis in a single ipsilateral lymph node, >3 cm but ≤ 6 cm in greatest dimension
	Metastases in multiple ipsilateral lymph nodes, none > 6 cm in greatest dimension
	Metastases in bilateral or contralateral lymph nodes, none > 6 cm in greatest dimension
N2a	Metastasis in a single ipsilateral lymph node, > 3 cm but ≤ 6 cm in greatest dimension
N2b	Metastases in multiple ipsilateral lymph nodes, none > 6 cm in greatest dimension
N2c	Metastases in bilateral or contralateral lymph nodes, none > 6 cm in greatest dimension
N3	Metastasis in a lymph node, > 6 cm in greatest dimension
Distant metastasis (M)	
M0	No distant metastasis
M1	Distant metastasis

cancers of the larynx. Subglottic cancers are uncommon and almost uniformly require total laryngectomy. The management of cancers of the larynx has undergone major changes in the recent past.

For early T1 and T2 primaries of the glottis or supraglottis, the most important fact to bear in mind is that they should be treated by a single modality.[5,6] The single modality of treatment chosen depends upon factors related to the tumor, factors related to the patient and factors related to the treating physician. For example, a small T1 tumor of the midportion of the vocal cord is equally and effectively treated by either a transoral laser microsurgical resection or with radiotherapy. The most important thing to recognize is that laser microsurgery achieves excellent control in a single stage treatment with no adverse effects of radiotherapy, which can be kept in reserve for early T1 cancer of the glottis or even of the supraglottis, transoral laser microsurgery is a good treatment to follow provided that the treating surgeon has requisite experience with laser microsurgery.[7-10]

If the extent of tumor is greater and involves both cords as in T1b cancer of the glottis, it is best treated with radiotherapy in order to avoid excessive cord resection, or raw areas at the anterior commissure that could result in synechiae. Patient factors to be borne in the mind are the occupation, respiratory reserve and undoubtedly the patient's fundamental desire. For those early tumors that can be equally effectively treated by surgery or by radiotherapy, it is important to assess whether there is any advantage in terms of quality of voice by either of the treatments. If there is excessive resection of vocal cord substance or the possibility of complications due to bilateral resection, the patient should be appropriately counseled and offered radiotherapy instead of transoral laser microsurgery. Bulky T2 lesions do not give equally good results by both methods and are better treated by radiotherapy with added chemotherapy. The practice of "debulking" a large T2 lesion with laser resection and following it up with radiation is not recommended. Neoadjuvant chemotherapy could be considered in bulky lesions.

Until recently, T2 glottic lesions were frequently treated with vertical partial laryngectomy; and T1, T2 and even selected T3 supraglottic lesions were treated with supraglottic partial laryngectomy. With the advent of laser microsurgery on the one hand and chemoradiation protocols on the other, these procedures are rarely offered today as primary treatment.

The management of advanced stage III and IV cancer of the larynx is now dictated largely by the extent of tumor involvement.[11,12] Today only patients who have gross laryngeal framework invasion should have primary surgery in the form of total laryngectomy. Patients who have T3 and early T4 lesions without gross involvement of the laryngeal skeleton may be offered a combination of chemotherapy and radiotherapy.[13-15] Numerous studies have looked at the optimal sequence of treatment, either neoadjuvant chemotherapy in the form of a two- or three-drug regimen followed by radiotherapy or concomitant chemoradiotherapy, or sequential chemoradiotherapy for very bulky disease. The Radiation Therapy Oncology Group (RTOG) 91-11 trial has established beyond doubt that concomitant chemoradiotherapy offers significant advantages over radiotherapy alone for T3 and selected T4 primaries. For these cancers of the larynx, currently, concomitant chemoradiotherapy is considered the standard of care. Good supportive and symptomatic care is vital as therapy reactions and toxicity can be considerable.

Management of Relapse and Treatment Failure[16,17]

For patients who present with post-treatment relapses, treatment offered depends upon the extent of disease and the possibility of offering function-preserving surgery. For those who have unilateral glottic recurrences, it may be possible to offer vertical partial laryngectomy or laser microsurgery depending upon the situation. For supraglottic failures, a salvage supraglottic laryngectomy is possible. However, this should be very carefully offered only to those patients who are young and have an excellent respiratory reserve. Typically, supraglottic laryngectomy following previous radiotherapy results in significant aspiration and is not a procedure to be advised in patients who have been smokers and have a compromised respiratory reserve. A procedure that may be advocated following failed radiotherapy for glottic cancer is the supracricoid laryngectomy with cricohyoidoepiglottopexy. This is an operation that can be offered for salvage in place of total laryngectomy in patients who have disease restricted to the region of the thyroid cartilage. It is important to realize that involvement of the cricoid cartilage negates the possibility of supracricoid laryngectomy.

Total laryngectomy carried out after failed radiation or chemoradiation has a much higher risk of complications such as wound dehiscence, leaks and fistula. Thus, it is currently advised that all patients who have salvage

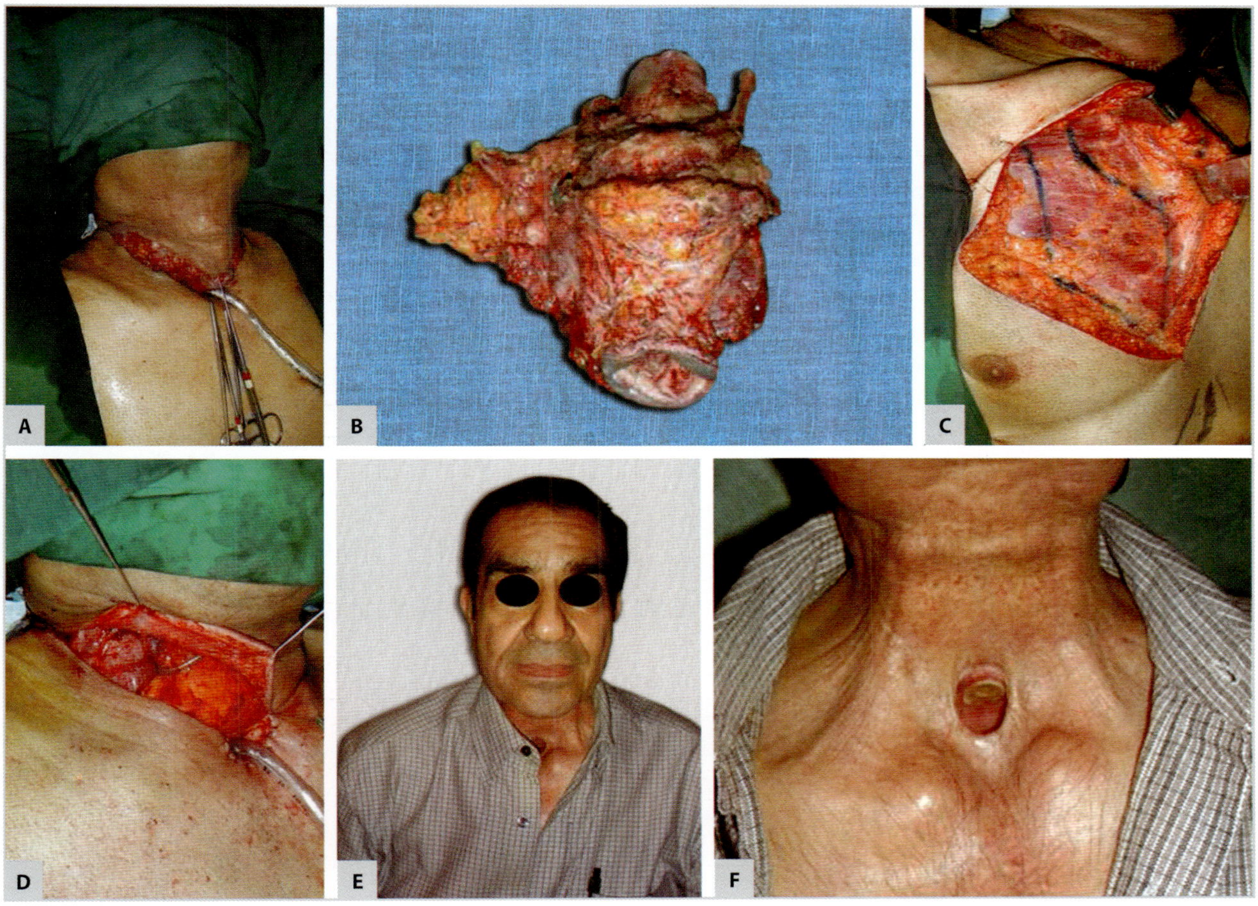

Figs 5A to F: The management principles followed for a patient who failed chemoradiation for a T3 supraglottic cancer and required emergency tracheostomy elsewhere. (A) Severely devitalized skin, induration around the tracheostomy; (B) Total laryngectomy specimen; (C) Design of the pectoralis major myofascial flap; (D) Tension-free skin closure; (E) Final result after 3 weeks; (F) TEP prosthesis in place

laryngectomy, even those where primary closure can be achieved, should receive a pectoralis muscle flap to cover the pharyngeal closure in order to minimize the incidence of leaks and fistulae (Figs 5A to F). Few important points to be borne in mind for salvage laryngectomy are as under:

- The incision for neck dissection and mobilization should as far as possible be separate from the stoma in order to protect it from leaks
- Closure of the pharynx should be easy and tension-free. Adequacy of pharyngeal circumference may be assessed by ability to achieve closure over a 32 Fr tube
- If there is any reduction in the diameter of the pharynx, it is important to undertake augmentation pharyngoplasty by means of a thin vascularized flap. In thin male individuals, the pectoralis major musculocutaneous flap may be used; but in individuals with a large panniculus of subcutaneous fat, it is preferable to use a microvascular radial forearm flap or anterolateral thigh (ALT) flap.

KEY POINTS: Management of Early Stage I and II Cancer of the Larynx

- For early laryngeal cancer, both definitive radiation therapy and larynx conservation surgery (either transoral laser surgery or open partial laryngectomy) generally offer equivalent tumor control and survival. The treatment chosen should be the one that maximizes both survival and functional outcome, i.e. voice production, swallowing and airway protection
- For many patients with early staged cancer of the supraglottis and glottis, laryngeal radiotherapy is recommended rather than surgery because of better functional outcomes. One has to realize, however, that early cancers like those of the midcord in the glottic larynx or small tumors of the epiglottis or the supraglottis can be equally well-managed by transoral laser surgery in which clear margins can be achieved.

Patients who have larger extent of tumor involvement, e.g. invasion of the anterior commissure in glottic cancers or of large portions of the supraglottic larynx, it is preferred to advise radiotherapy. In those patients with stage II cancers who have minimum restriction in cord mobility chemotherapy may be added to optimize the effects of radiotherapy

- For patients with early stage cancer of the subglottic larynx, although total laryngectomy is generally recommended, partial laryngectomy may be offered in conjunction with thyroidectomy and bilateral paratracheal node clearance for those patients where it is applicable. An alternative today is intensity-modulated radiation therapy (IMRT) with the low neck and the upper mediastinum included in the treatment fields
- For early staged supraglottic cancer, bilateral elective neck treatment is recommended for tumors involving midlines structures. The choice of elective bilateral neck dissection versus comprehensive neck radiotherapy depends on the treatment approach for the primary tumor. Patients with early stage glottic cancer with a clinically negative neck can be managed with observation alone for the neck rather than elective neck dissection
- For patients who are treated with primary surgery, postoperative radiotherapy is recommended only in those patients with positive resection margins, lymphovascular embolization, perineural invasion or pathologically positive lymph nodes in the selective neck dissection. Postoperative concurrent chemoradiation is preferable for patients who have positive lymph node metastasis with extracapsular extension
- The major psychological issue that patients experience with total laryngectomy is the permanent stoma. Loss of voice can be rehabilitated effectively.

Management of Stage III and Stage IV Cancer of the Larynx[18-20]

- Prior to a definitive treatment plan, all patients with stage III and IV cancers of the larynx must ideally be seen in a multidisciplinary tumor board experienced in the treatment of head and neck cancer. The selection of a particular treatment approach depends upon the tumor extent and location, patient specific factors such as age, performance status, comorbidities, psychosocial support, physician expertise and the availability of comprehensive rehabilitation possibilities. For most patients with good performance status and with locally advanced stage III or IV cancer, functional organ preservation strategy rather than surgical resection is recommended. Organ sparing approaches may permit larynx preservation, but do not provide survival advantage compared to total laryngectomy. The nonsurgical modalities of treatment include concurrent chemoradiotherapy, induction chemotherapy followed by radiotherapy alone and sequential chemoradiotherapy. Concurrent chemoradiotherapy may be preferable for patients with N0, N1 and N2 presentations while induction chemotherapy may offer advantages for patients with relative higher risk of distant metastasis. Sequential therapy may be particularly useful in patients with large and bulky primary T3 and T4 tumors and/or advanced nodal disease.
- Partial laryngectomy and minimally invasive surgery may be options for carefully selected patients especially those in whom there are relative small primary tumors combined with more extensive neck disease. Postoperative radiotherapy is generally recommended in such patients. Patients who may not be candidates for an organ preservation approach include those patients with tumors that have destroyed both vocal cords, which leave the prospects of retaining adequate laryngeal function very remote. It is likewise for elderly patients with whom the toxicity associated with chemoradiotherapy or full-dose radiotherapy alone is problematic and in those patients with extensive cartilage destruction from the primary tumor.
- Management of the neck is complex and depends upon disease extent, the treatment modality used to treat the primary tumor and the response to therapy.
- For patients who are not candidates for a functional organ preserving approach, total laryngectomy is a potential alternative. Definitive radiotherapy alone may be used as a functional organ preserving approach for laryngeal cancer patients who are not fit candidates for chemotherapy, although there is a higher risk of recurrence, treatment failure and a need for salvage total laryngectomy.
- Adequate post-treatment surveillance and long-term follow-up are crucial to ensure adequate voice rehabilitation and to monitor disease recurrence or a second primary recurrence.

REFERENCES

1. Mancuso AA, Mukherji SK, Schmalfuss I, et al. Preradiotherapy computed tomography as a predictor of local control in supraglottic carcinoma. J Clin Oncol. 1999;17(2):631-7.
2. Thabet HM, Sessions DG, Gado MH, et al. Comparison of clinical evaluation and computed tomographic diagnostic accuracy for tumors of the larynx and hypopharynx. Laryngoscope. 1996;106 (5 Pt 1):589-94.
3. Edge SB, Byrd DR, Compton CC, et al. (Eds). AJCC Cancer Staging Manual, 7th edition. New York: Springer; 2010. pp. 57-67.
4. O'Sullivan B, Shah J. New TNM staging criteria for head and neck tumors. Semin Surg Oncol. 2003;21(1):30-42.
5. Dinshaw KA, Sharma V. Radiation therapy in early glottic carcinoma: significance of prognostic factors and dose fractionation. Indian J Cancer. 1990;27(3):143-53.
6. Mendenhall WM, Amdur RJ, Morris CG, et al. T1-T2N0 squamous cell carcinoma of the glottic larynx treated with radiation therapy. J Clin Oncol. 2001;19(20):4029-36.
7. Steiner W. Results of curative laser microsurgery of laryngeal carcinomas. Am J Otolaryngol. 1993;14(2):116-21.
8. Steiner W, Ambrosch P, Rodel RM, et al. Impact of anterior commissure involvement on local control of early glottic carcinoma treated by laser microresection. Laryngoscope. 2004;114(8):1485-91.
9. Ambrosch P, Kron M, Steiner W. Carbon dioxide laser microsurgery for early supraglottic carcinoma. Ann Otol Rhinol Laryngol. 1998;107(8):680-8.
10. Peretti G, Piazza C, Bolzoni A, et al. Analysis of recurrences in 322 Tis, T1, or T2 glottic carcinomas treated by carbon dioxide laser. Ann Otol Rhinol Laryngol. 2004;113(11):853-8.
11. Hinerman RW, Mendenhall WM, Amdur RJ, et al. Carcinoma of the supraglottic larynx: treatment results with radiotherapy alone or with planned neck dissection. Head Neck. 2002;24(5):456-67.
12. Induction chemotherapy plus radiation compared with surgery plus radiation in patients with advanced laryngeal cancer. The Department of Veterans Affairs Laryngeal Cancer Study Group. N Engl J Med. 1991;324(24):1685-90.
13. Parsons JT, Mendenhall WM, Stringer SP, et al. Salvage surgery following radiation failure in squamous cell carcinoma of the supraglottic larynx. Int J Radiat Oncol Biol Phys. 1995;32(3): 605-9.
14. Forastiere AA, Goepfert H, Maor M, et al. Concurrent chemotherapy and radiotherapy for organ preservation in advanced laryngeal cancer. N Engl J Med. 2003;349(22):2091-8.
15. Bhalavat RL, Fakih AR, Mistry RC, et al. Radical radiation vs surgery plus postoperative radiation in advanced (resectable) supraglottic larynx and pyriform sinus cancers: a prospective randomized study. Eur J Surg Oncol. 2003;29(9):750-6.
16. Weber RS, Berkey BA, Forastiere A, et al: Outcome of salvage total laryngectomy following organ preservation therapy: the Radiation Therapy Oncology Group trial 91-11. Arch Otolaryngol Head Neck Surg. 2003;129(1):44-9.
17. Laccourreye O, Brasnu D, Biacabe B, et al: Neo-adjuvant chemotherapy and supracricoid partial laryngectomy with cricohyoidopexy for advanced endolaryngeal carcinoma classified as T3-T4: 5-year oncologic results. Head Neck. 1998;20(7):595-9.
18. McConnel FM, Mendelsohn MS, Logemann JA. Manofluorography of deglutition after supraglottic laryngectomy. Head Neck Surg. 1987;9(3):142-50.
19. McNeil BJ, Weichselbaum R, Pauker SG. Speech and survival: tradeoffs between quality and quantity of life in laryngeal cancer. N Engl J Med. 1981;305(17):982-7.
20. de Graeff A, de Leeuw RJ, Ros WJ, et al. A prospective study on quality of life of laryngeal cancer patients treated with radiotherapy. Head Neck. 1999;21(4):291-6.

20 Cancer of the Pharynx

Vijay Haribhakti

SURGICAL ANATOMY

The pharynx is a musculofascial "half cylinder" that links the oral and nasal cavities in the head to the larynx and esophagus in the neck, and extends from the skull base above to the esophageal opening below. From above downward, the pharynx is subdivided into three anatomical regions:

1. The Nasopharynx
2. The Oropharynx (OP)
3. The Hypopharynx.

The nomenclature of each is derived from the area that the pharynx is posterior to. Thus, the nasopharynx is behind the nasal space and is bordered anteriorly by the posterior nasal choanae. The OP on the other hand lies behind the oral cavity and is bordered anteriorly by the posterior one-third of the tongue, while the laryngopharynx (hypopharynx) is behind the larynx (Figs 1A and B).

Structurally, the pharynx consists of five layers from inside out, i.e. the mucosa, submucosa, pharyngobasilar fascia, muscular layer and the buccopharyngeal fascia. The mucous membrane consists of columnar epithelium, which is ciliated in some areas. The submucosa contains many small veins forming a venous plexus, and also contains mucous and minor salivary glands and lymphoid tissue. A very important fact is that it is very rich in capillary lymphatics, and therefore, tumors arising in the pharynx exhibit pronounced tendency to lymphatic spread. The pharyngobasilar fascia is attached above to the base of the skull and fills the gap between the constrictor muscles within the pharynx. The muscular layer consists basically of three circumferential muscles that are arranged in overlapping fashion from below upward. Accordingly, the inferior constrictor is the muscle found in the region of the hypopharynx, above is the middle constrictor and right above is the superior constrictor muscle. Finally, the buccopharyngeal fascia forms the outer layer of the pharynx. It is continuous with the visceral fascia of the esophagus and acts as the anterior boundary of the retropharyngeal space.

GENERAL FEATURES

While each region of the pharynx gives origin to tumors with very distinct biological patterns of spread, a few generalizations apply:

- Tumors originating in the pharynx in general have a very conspicuous tendency for submucosal spread. Accordingly, foci of tumor can extend for considerable distances away from the index tumor
- Most tumors arising in the pharynx have a moderate to high histologic grade, which imparts not only a significant potential for local extension and spread, but also a high responsiveness to chemotherapy and radiotherapy
- Capillary lymphatics abound in this region, giving rise to a high incidence of lymphatic metastasis
- Due to contiguity of the component regions and lymphatic crossover beyond the midline, lymphatic spread frequently occurs bilaterally
- Owing to a high proclivity for lymphatic spread, small primaries can often give rise to bulky nodal metastasis. It is for this reason that "unknown primaries" are frequently located in one of the regions of the pharynx, and manifest clinically as nodal masses with no clinically demonstrable primary cancer

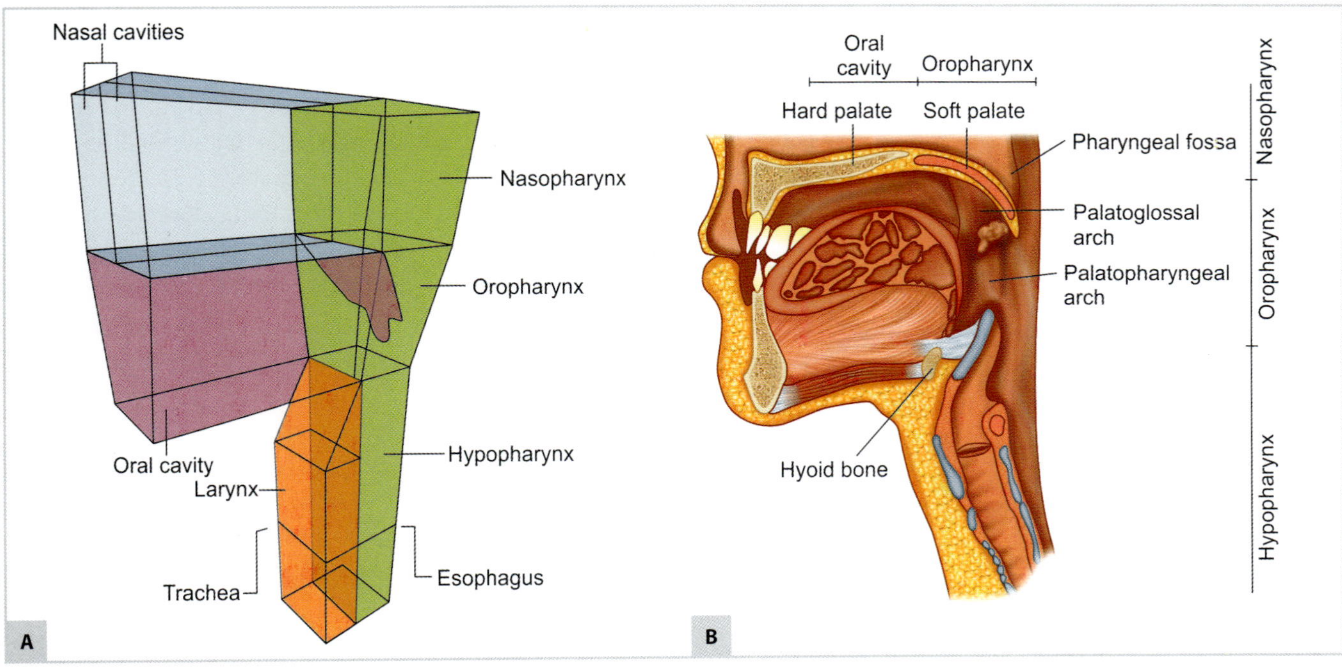

Figs 1A and B: Schematic anatomy of the pharynx

- Given their complex anatomical location, often in close proximity with functionally vital organs such as the tongue and larynx, and their inherent responsiveness to chemotherapy and radiation, majority of pharyngeal cancers are treated primarily by nonsurgical modalities.

THE NASOPHARYNX (FIG. 2)

The most common tumor to affect the nasopharynx is squamous cell carcinoma. Three basic histologies are encountered here: Type 1 is described as the standard keratinizing squamous cell carcinoma, type 2 is the non-keratinizing squamous carcinoma and type 3, which is very common, is the undifferentiated carcinoma. The term lymphoepithelioma is often used to describe epithelial carcinomas with a rich infiltrate of benign lymphocytes.

The etiology of nasopharynx cancer is multifactorial with genetic, viral, dietary and environmental influences playing a possible role. A genetic predisposition has not been explicitly demonstrated, but data from China shows common human leukocyte antigen patterns among some patients with nasopharyngeal cancer. The Epstein-Barr virus has been closely associated with cancers of the nasopharynx. Cigarette smoking and alcohol also appear to be risk factors for this cancer.

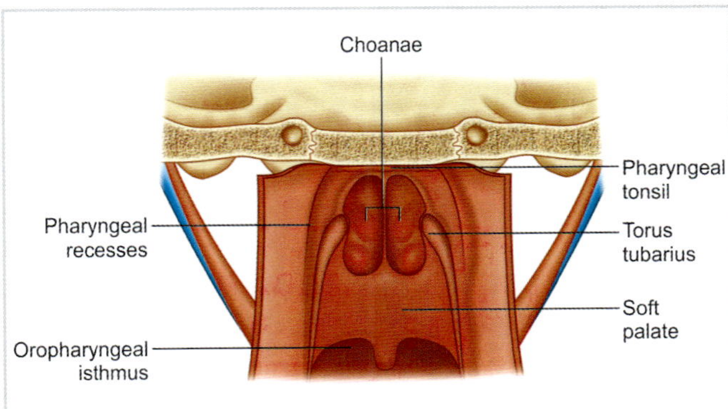

Fig. 2: The nasopharynx

Surgical Anatomy of the Nasopharynx

The nasopharynx is a hollow passage, lined by mucosa and serves to connect the nasal cavity with the OP. It is bounded anteriorly by the posterior nasal choanae and the nasal septum. The floor is formed by the superior surface of the soft palate and is in communication with the OP at the level of the uvula. The posterior wall of the nasopharynx lies anterior to the first two cervical vertebrae, the prevertebral and buccopharyngeal fascia. The roof is formed by the basisphenoid and basiocciput of the skull base. The lateral walls lie medial to the maxillopharyngeal space, pterygoid plates and parapharyngeal space. The pharyngotympanic tube orifices enter the nasopharynx through the lateral walls and each is surrounded by a cartilaginous protuberance, called torus tubarius. A recess behind and below the torus tubarius known as the fossa of Rosenmüller is the most common site of nasopharyngeal cancers.

Cancers of the nasopharynx exhibit multiple routes of local spread, and they may extend into the nasal cavity, OP, parapharyngeal space and the skull base. The sphenoid sinus is more commonly invaded than the other sinuses. The orbit, cervical vertebrae and pterygoid structures may be involved in advanced disease. Invasion of the clivus can occur with advanced tumors. These tumors may extend across the foramen lacerum, ovale or spinosum or to the cavernous sinus, potentially involving the cranial nerves II–VI. The nasopharynx has a very rich lymphatic network with multiple pathways for drainage. The first echelon lymph nodes are in the retropharyngeal space and are named as the nodes of Rouvière. Further caudad spread then happens systematically to the nodes in the upper posterior triangles (level IIb) and to the jugular chain of nodes. It is important to note that nearly 85% of all patients with a primary nasopharyngeal cancer present with a lymph nodal mass in the neck and 50% have bilateral spread.

Clinical Features

The presenting symptoms include most commonly a neck mass, which is a metastatic nodal mass, epistaxis, nasal obstruction, change in voice quality, pain, otalgia, decreased hearing or cranial neuropathies. The diagnosis of nasopharyngeal cancer is made by a combination of clinical and radiological assessment. Clinical assessment includes a detailed head, face and neck examination, palpation of the neck for metastatic nodes and anterior rhinoscopy to study the nasal space. An endoscopic examination of the nasopharynx is routinely performed by means of a 30° rigid telescope or a fiberoptic nasolaryngoscope, introduced through the nostrils. As mentioned earlier, the most common site of origin is the fossa of Rosenmüller. A guided biopsy is typically obtained under endoscopic control for a clear histologic diagnosis, following which, imaging is carried out with a contrast-enhanced computed tomography (CECT) scan. For soft tissue detail, magnetic resonance imaging (MRI) assessment is extremely useful. Following detailed clinical endoscopic and radiologic assessment, the patient is staged by the TNM classification (Table 1).

Goals of Treatment

Goals of treatment of cancers of the nasopharynx include local as well as systemic control. Given the remote anatomical location of the nasopharynx, surgical approach is formidable, and not generally practised. Radiotherapy is the foundation for curative treatment. Chemotherapy has an important role as well in the management of cancers of nasopharynx and is utilized in three ways:

1. Neoadjuvant chemotherapy in clinically high staged disease, to reduce tumor burden before starting off with radiotherapy
2. Concomitant chemoradiotherapy in which radiotherapy is accompanied by weekly injections of chemotherapy
3. Sequential treatment in which neoadjuvant chemotherapy is followed with chemoradiation in place of radiation alone.

The third option is utilized in patients with bulky nodes and very bulky primary tumors. In general, tumors of the nasopharynx, especially undifferentiated carcinomas are extremely sensitive to both chemotherapy and radiation, and show a very impressive response.

In those patients who have residual disease following radical treatment, salvage procedures are carried out. Salvage for nasopharyngeal primaries is in the form of surgical resection. Open surgical resection today is carried out by an approach called the maxillary swing, which

TABLE 1: The tumor-node-metastasis (TNM) classification of cancers of the nasopharynx

Nasopharynx	
T1	Tumor confined to the nasopharynx
T2	Tumor extends to soft tissues
T2a	Tumor extends to the oropharynx and/or nasal cavity without parapharyngeal extension*
T2b	Any tumor with parapharyngeal extension*
T3	Tumor involves bony structures and/or paranasal sinuses
T4	Tumor with intracranial extension and/or involvement of cranial nerves, infratemporal fossa, hypopharynx, orbit or masticator space
The "N" and "M" classification is common to all other head and neck sites.	

*Note: Parapharyngeal extension denotes posterolateral infiltration of tumor beyond the pharyngobasilar fascia

was described and detailed by William Wei from Hong Kong. In this approach, the entire maxilla stays attached to the skin and is swung outward, providing exposure to the nasopharynx for appropriate resection. This is not commonly practised.

More recently, endoscopic procedures have started becoming increasingly popular and endoscopic nasopharyngeal resection is a possible way of approaching residual nasopharyngeal cancer in patients who do not have very large or bulky tumors. Endoscopic nasopharyngectomy can also be used for patients who manifest other tumor types such as minor salivary tumors. Radical radiotherapy to a dose of 65–75 Gy is typically needed to treat a patient effectively with nasopharyngeal cancer. Given its close proximity to important anatomical entities such as the spinal cord and even brain stem, and the need to cover both sides of the neck, nasopharyngeal cancer is optimally treated by an intensity-modulated radiation therapy (IMRT) plan.

The details of chemotherapy are similar to that employed in other head and neck sites. Accordingly, if neoadjuvant chemotherapy is planned, a three-drug regimen that incorporates docetaxel, cisplatin and fluorouracil (TPF) is considered standard. For concomitant regimens, single drug cisplatin is the standard of care. It can either be employed on a weekly regimen at 50 mg/m^2; or at a dose of 100 mg/m^2 on days 1, 21 and 42.

Results of Treatment[1]

An analysis of results of treatment for nasopharyngeal carcinoma demonstrated that median 5-year disease-free survival rates were 40% for patients who had radiotherapy alone and 60% for those who had chemoradiation (P = 0.002).

THE OROPHARYNX (FIG. 3)

Introduction

The commonest tumor type arising in the OP is squamous cell carcinoma, and oropharyngeal cancers have recently attracted considerable attention and interest for a variety of reasons:

- The human papilloma virus-16 (HPV-16) is now an established factor in the etiology of these cancers in a significant proportion of patients[2]
- There is convincing retrospective evidence implicating HPV as a cause for subsequent malignancies in pediatric and young adult (PAYA) cancer survivors
- HPV-mediated cancers in general have improved responses to treatment and survival when compared with non-HPV cancers
- Most investigators agree that patients with HPV-mediated cancers represent an improved prognostic group, a fact that may influence treatment policies in the future

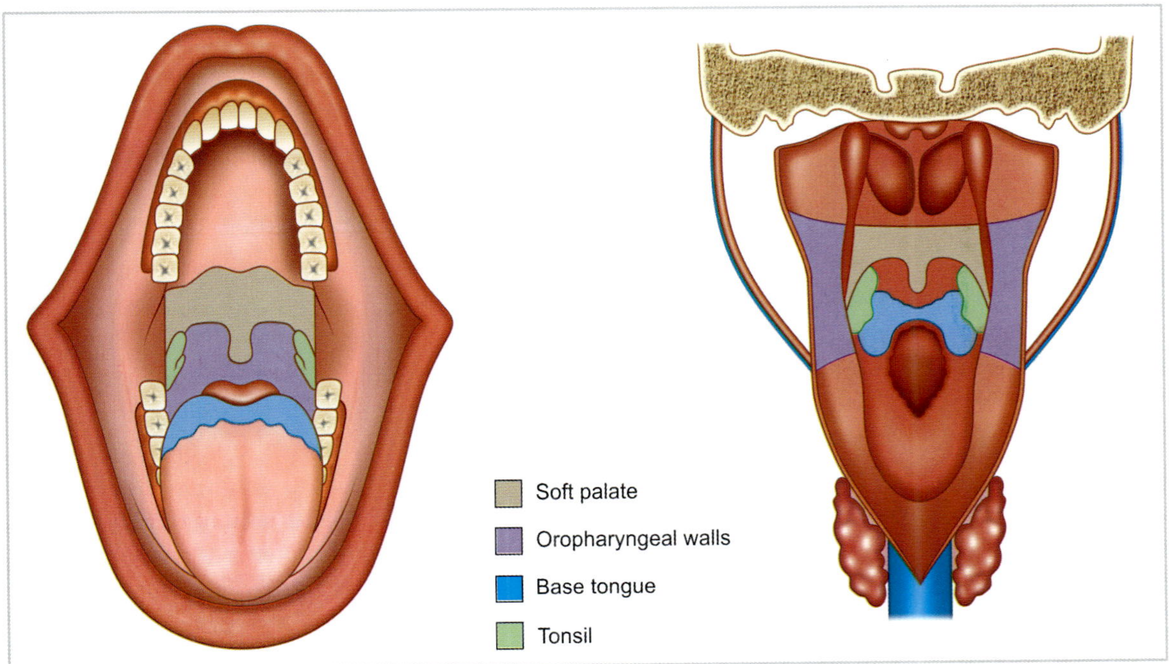

Fig. 3: Anatomic areas within the oropharynx—base tongue, tonsils, tonsillar pillars, soft palate and oropharyngeal walls

- Bonner's study demonstrated improved control rates and survival by the addition of cetuximab to radiotherapy, and subgroup analysis showed that HPV-mediated oropharyngeal cancers did significantly better[3]
- Although traditionally reserved for salvage only, primary surgery for oropharyngeal cancers has been investigated in a number of centers in the context of transoral robotic surgery (TORS).[4]

Surgical Anatomy of the Oropharynx

The oropharynx is literally at the crossroads of the respiratory and food passages, and thus cancers originating here have major implications for the most basic functions of respiration, deglutition and speech. The anatomical components of the oropharynx include the "palatine arch" comprising of the soft palate, faucial arches and palatine tonsils, the base tongue, and the lateral and posterior walls, from the plane of the soft palate above to the hyoid below.

Clinical Features

While early and superficial lesions produce hardly any symptoms, advanced lesions become symptomatic with odynophagia (painful swallowing), dysphagia, referred otalgia and altered speech (hot potato speech). With secondary sepsis that most often supervenes with advanced lesions, there is often severe referred pain, dysphagia and halitosis.

Staging[5] (Table 2)

TABLE 2: Tumor-node-metastasis (TNM) classification

Oropharynx	
TX	Primary tumor cannot be assessed
T0	No evidence of primary tumor
Tis	Carcinoma in situ
T1	Tumor ≤ 2 cm in greatest dimension
T2	Tumor > 2 cm but ≤ 4 cm in greatest dimension
T3	Tumor > 4 cm in greatest dimension or extension to lingual surface of epiglottis
T4a	Moderately advanced local disease. Tumor invades the larynx, extrinsic muscle of tongue, medial pterygoid, hard palate or mandible
T4b	Very advanced local disease. Tumor invades lateral pterygoid muscle, pterygoid plates, lateral nasopharynx, skull base or encases carotid artery
The "N" and "M" classification is common to all other head and neck sites.	

Management

The management of oropharyngeal cancers is subsite and stage dependent. For early T1 and T2 squamous cancers, transoral surgical resection wherever possible is recommended. The exact details of the technique employed, whether conventional, with long diathermy tips or laser microsurgery, or TORS would depend significantly upon the training and experience of the treating surgeon, and patient factors such as the presence of trismus. The neck is treated independently based on clinical and radiologic findings. For the N0 neck, appropriate selective neck dissection for staging should incorporate levels II, III and IV. Open surgery for lateral oropharyngeal lesions frequently needs paramedian mandibulotomy (Fig. 4). When surgery is note feasible or desirable for any reason, radical radiotherapy is administered with curative intent.

For advanced stage III and IV cancers, radiotherapy and chemotherapy are both needed and are combined in much the same way as they are for nasopharyngeal primaries.[6,7] In all these cases, surgery is typically reserved for salvage and involves massive resection and reconstruction. In order to achieve adequate access, the approach to the mandible needs to be carefully decided. Whereas the paramedian mandibulotomy provides adequate access to the base tongue, it cannot be employed in cases where the disease process courses laterally and posterosuperiorly to the glossotonsillar sulcus, pillars and tonsils. In these cases, limited segmental mandibulectomy is essential to achieve adequate three-dimensional clearance. Furthermore, in those patients in whom serious risks of aspiration exist, a total laryngectomy is frequently necessary for physiologic reasons.

Representative Case

The approach noted above is exemplified by a 45-year-old male who presented with an advanced T4 squamous carcinoma involving the vallecula, base tongue and supraglottic larynx. MRI scan revealed a massive tumor involving the oropharynx and supraglottic larynx, sparing the neurovascular bundle of the tongue on both sides. Using a median labiomandibulotomy approach, the anterior tongue was split in the midline to approach the massive primary tumor, which was possible to resect with widely clear margins, incorporating a total laryngectomy and a primary tracheoesophageal puncture (Figs 5A to D).

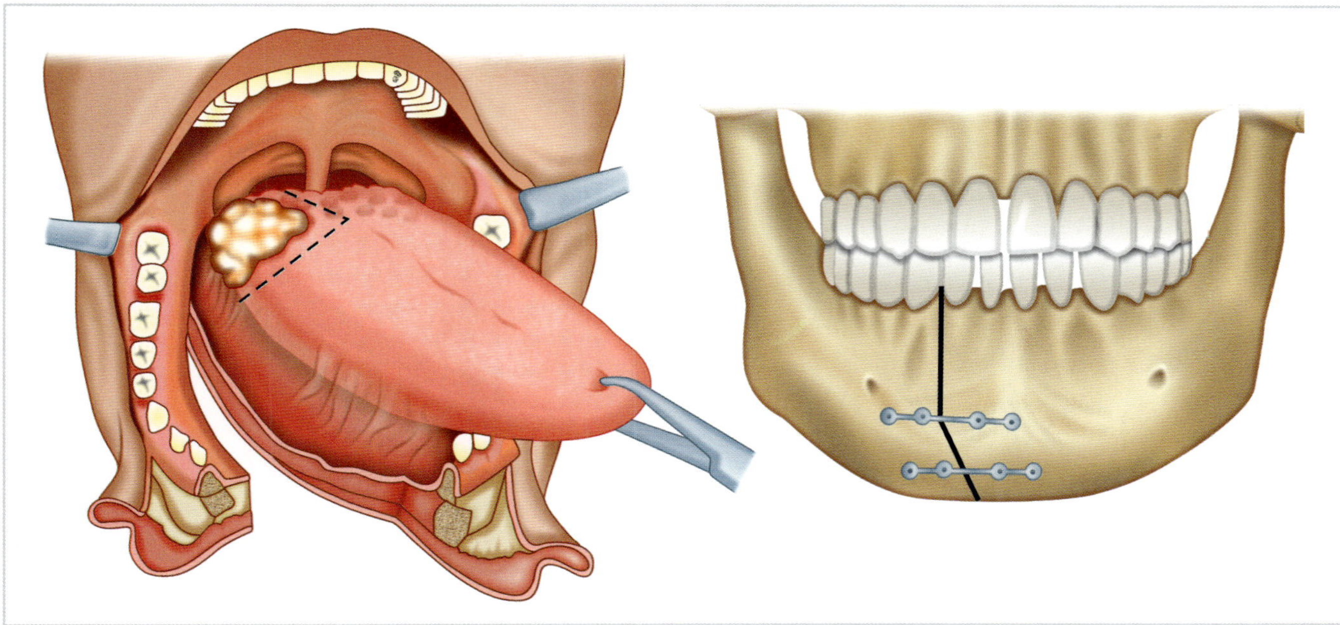

Fig. 4: Paramedian mandibulotomy approach for lateral base tongue tumors

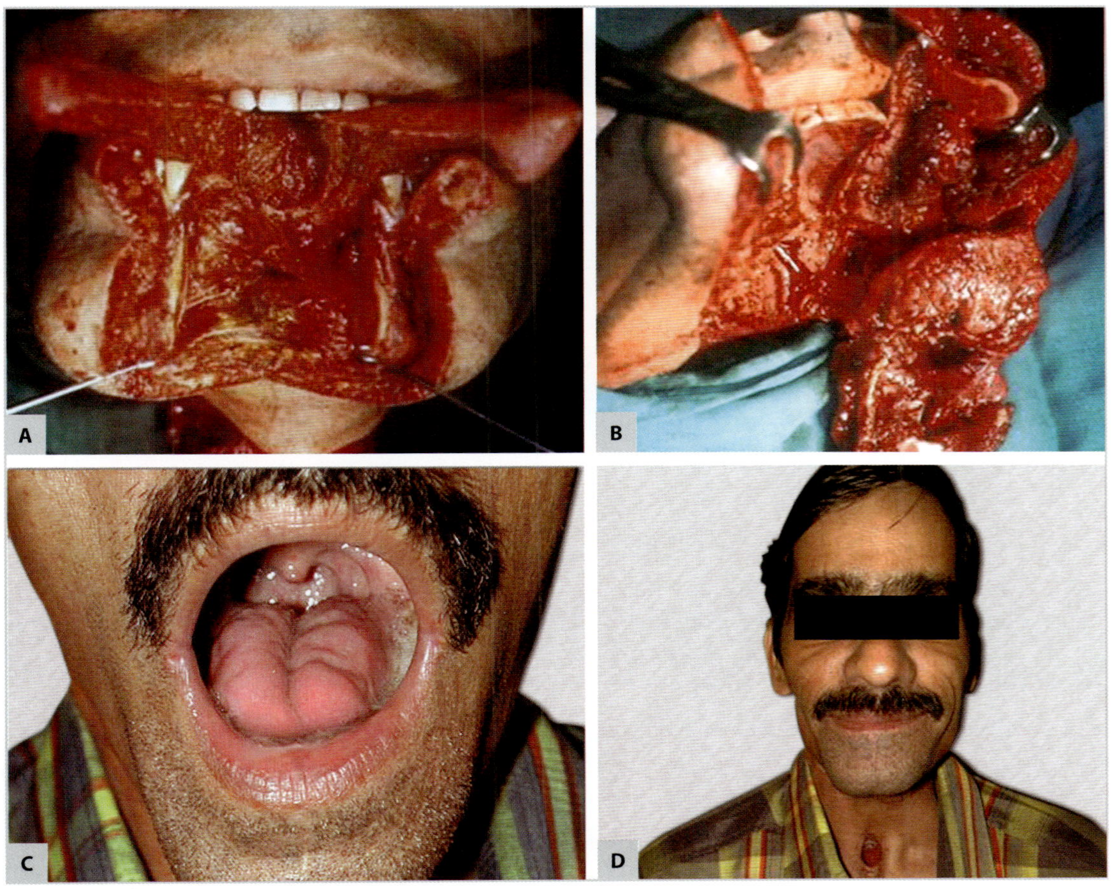

Figs 5A to D: (A and B) Intraoperative photographs demonstrating the approach and specimen delivery; (C and D) Final postoperative result—followed by adjuvant chemoradiation

THE HYPOPHARYNX AND CERVICAL ESOPHAGUS (FIG. 6)

Introduction

Cancers of the hypopharynx are among the most common cancers affecting the pharynx in many parts of the world. In India, hypopharyngeal cancer is the most common among all pharyngeal cancers, and it is also extremely high in incidence in other countries such as France and Spain. The major cause of hypopharyngeal cancer appears to be tobacco addiction along with alcohol. A number of other factors such as genetics have been implicated, but are not proven. The significance of cancers of this region lies in the fact that they are in direct proximity with the larynx, and therefore, their growth and progression produces functional effects in this area, causing major symptoms such as hoarseness, dysphagia and finally aspiration. The major problem with this site is the fact that early cancers remain almost completely silent, and when they manifest with major symptoms, they are typically far advanced and beyond conservative methods of treatment. The cervical esophagus extends from the C6 level up to the thoracic inlet, and is the least frequent site for esophageal cancer (the highest being the lower third). The importance of the cervical esophagus is two-fold: Primary cancers originating here pose a formidable proposition for surgical resection owing to their proximity with the cricopharynx and the consequent difficulty in obtaining an adequate cranial margin. Conversely, cancers originating in the postcricoid area frequently extend downward into the cervical esophagus, rendering it often difficult to obtain a suitable distal margin of resection, necessitating complete laryngopharyngoesophagectomy.

Surgical Anatomy of the Hypopharynx

The hypopharynx (also known as the laryngopharynx) extends from the lower margin of the oropharynx, which is approximately at the level of the tip of the epiglottis or the horizontal plane of the vallecula and extends down until the esophageal opening, at the level C6. The anatomical components of the hypopharynx include the pharyngeal walls, i.e. the posterior pharyngeal wall and the lateral pharyngeal walls, which continue anteriorly into a pair of pyriform sinuses that flank the larynx and continue behind the larynx as the postcricoid area (Fig. 6). The area between the postcricoid mucosa and the cervical esophagus is

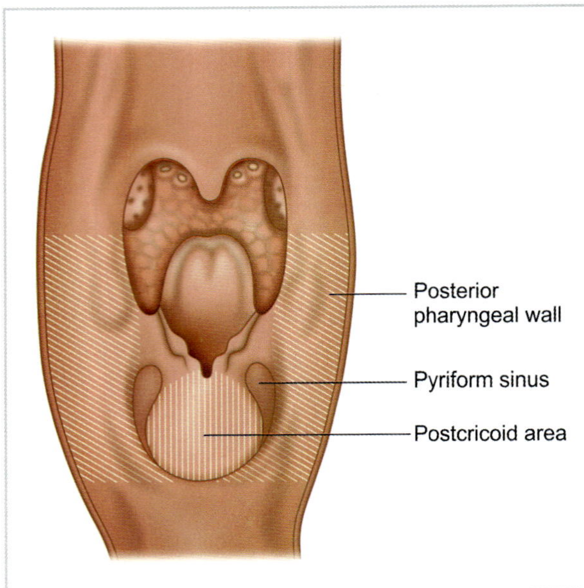

Fig. 6: Anatomical regions in the hypopharynx—pyriform sinus, postcricoid pharynx and pharyngeal walls

perhaps the narrowest area in the entire gastrointestinal (GI) tract.

The surgically important feature of this region is its layered anatomy, which consists of a stratified squamous lining, a submucosa, a muscular layer and a fascial layer. The muscular layer consists of the inferior constrictor, which surrounds almost the lower two-third the hypopharynx, above which is the middle constrictor in the upper most part of the hypopharynx. At the lowest part of the hypopharynx, the inferior constrictor fibers are condensed into a somewhat circular band of fibers, known as the cricopharyngeus, which marks the opening into the cervical esophagus. Between the cricopharyngeus and the thyropharyngeus portions of the inferior constrictor muscle is an area of weakness known as the Killian's dehiscence, and it is from this area that pharyngeal mucosal pouches develop. Outside the muscular layer is the layer of buccopharyngeal fascia, which is continuous with the visceral fascia of the esophagus.

The submucosa of the hypopharynx has a very large population of capillary lymphatics, which makes this an area of easy lymphatic extension. It is also known that tumors originating in this area can manifest significant extent of submucosal spread, and can be found at fairly significant distances away from the primary index tumor. The lymphatics from the hypopharynx course toward the jugular chain of nodes, the most important stations being level II, III and IV. The important mechanism of contiguous extension of tumors originating in the hypopharynx is in a medial and anterior direction, invading the larynx, the thyroid cartilage and finally the ipsilateral lobe of the thyroid gland. When these tumors spread posteriorly and laterally, they can get into the soft tissues of the neck and cause a loss of the thyrovertebral crackle. Downward spread happens into the cervical esophagus. The lymphatics from here gain access to the paratracheal or paraesophageal nodes in the central compartment of the neck (level VI) as well as superior mediastinal nodes (level VII).

Epidemiology, Incidence and Classification of Hypopharyngeal Cancers

The incidence of these cancers is significantly higher in males than in females, and there is significant geographical division in incidence, being highest in countries such as France, Spain and India, and relatively lower in the US and other west European nations. In the hypopharynx, the most common and most important subsite is the pyriform sinus. In certain parts of India, cancers of the postcricoid region are frequent, and are often associated with long-standing anemia, known as the Plummer-Vinson syndrome. The most common histologic type of cancer is the squamous cell carcinoma, and most cancers in this region are of high grade (grade 3–4), in contradistinction to the glottic larynx where most tumors are grade 1 and 2. The significance of this is in their biologic potential for spread and in their responsiveness to chemotherapy and radiation.

Clinical Features

The most common symptoms associated with cancers of the hypopharynx involve a vague feeling of sore throat, a feeling of something "stuck inside the throat," dysphagia, painful swallowing or odynophagia, and very frequently, referred otalgia. As tumors advance and involve the larynx, they may produce vocal cord fixity and manifest as hoarseness, alteration in speech and finally, in far advanced cases, dyspnea and stridor. Since dysphagia is a very important symptom of hypopharyngeal cancer, most significantly in postcricoid cancer where the pharynx is narrowest, it is often found that patients by the time they present for treatment have lost significant weight. Approximately, one-fourth of the patients present with a mass in the neck, with no symptoms referable to the primary. When detailed head and neck examination is performed, a lesion is found in the ipsilateral hypopharynx. One of the nodal groups involved in these cancers is the retropharyngeal group and large retropharyngeal nodes do often present with a syndrome of pain that consists of characteristic occipital pain and pain in the nape of the neck that radiates up to a point behind the eye.

Physical Findings

The most important part of clinical examination is indirect laryngoscopy (IDL) that is performed either with an IDL mirror or with a 90° Hopkin's telescope. Tumors of the pyriform sinus and postcricoid area may be obscured by the presence of significant pooling of saliva, which is seen very often with obstructing lesions of this area. The patient is encouraged to sip a little water to clear out the pharynx before examination is undertaken. At this point of time, it is important to note the pattern of swallowing. If while drinking water, the patient immediately gets into a spell of coughing, it indicates overspill into the larynx and therefore advanced disease, producing fixity of the larynx and aspiration. With large, advanced tumors, we often notice significant swelling in the neck, in the area of the thyroid, and unless a careful examination is carried out, these cancers can sometimes masquerade as a large tumor involving the ipsilateral lobe of the thyroid gland. Widening of the thyroid cartilage and loss of thyrovertebral crackle are other clinical signs of advanced disease.

Following detailed local examination, the neck is palpated for metastatic disease before further investigations are carried out. An important radiological investigation for cancers of this region is the standard barium swallow with air contrast in order to delineate the exact site of obstruction and the extent and the length of obstruction. A contrast enhanced computed tomography (CECT) scan is also critically important to delineate the extent of the tumor, invasion of the larynx, involvement of the laryngeal spaces and invasion of the laryngeal framework and cervical soft tissues. A careful note is also made of the jugular nodes on both sides of the neck. The most important procedure to be carried out in order to accurately stage the disease and map disease extent is direct laryngoscopy, which is carried out under general anesthesia. In those patients who have significant stridor, this may be a somewhat risky examination as the tumor is large and may obstruct the laryngeal opening, rendering intubation very difficult. If the airway is adequately patent, it is preferable to intubate the patient and do a careful examination of both pyriform sinuses and the entire area to map the total tumor extent. A biopsy specimen is obtained at the same time in order to grade the tumor and take a decision regarding further treatment.

TABLE 3: Tumor-node-metastasis (TNM) classification of cancers of the hypopharynx

TX	Primary tumor cannot be assessed
T0	No evidence of primary tumor
Tis	Carcinoma in situ
Hypopharynx	
T1	Tumor limited to one subsite of hypopharynx and/or ≤ 2 cm in greatest dimension
T2	Tumor invades > 1 subsite of hypopharynx or an adjacent site, or measures > 2 cm but not > 4 cm in greatest dimension without fixation of hemilarynx
T3	Tumor > 4 cm in greatest dimension or with fixation of hemilarynx or extension to esophagus
T4a	Moderately advanced local disease
	Tumor invades thyroid/cricoid cartilage, hyoid bone, thyroid gland or central compartment soft tissue[b]
T4b	Very advanced local disease
	Tumor invades prevertebral fascia, encases carotid artery, or involves mediastinal structures

The "N" and "M" classification is common to all other head and neck sites.

Staging of Cancers of the Hypopharynx and Cervical Esophagus

The TNM classification system is most regularly employed, and the classification depends upon the areas of involvement and vocal cord fixity. The most recent updated classification is presented in the Table 3.

Management of Tumors of the Hypopharynx[8]

Early Cancer

In general, it is desirable to treat early staged T1 and T2 cancers with a single modality. With involvement of the cervical lymph nodes, however, the management approach has to be altered to address the nodes. With an N0 neck and an early staged (T1, T2) primary, trans-oral laser microsurgery may be used for suitably located primary lesions, provided that the surgeon has considerable experience with the technique, and it is possible to obtain clear margins. If a staging neck dissection is deemed necessary, an ipsilateral selective neck dissection is performed, incorporating levels II, III and IV. An alternative approach to T1/T2, N0 disease would be radical radiotherapy, with inclusion of the neck in the radiation portals.

For clinically manifest neck disease, the treatment necessarily incorporates surgery, radiation or a combination, together with chemotherapy for selected indications. As a general thumb rule, significant nodal disease does not respond to a single modality, and needs a combination of treatments. Thus, if an early, "radiocurable" primary coexists with significant nodal disease, it is best to treat with upfront concomitant chemoradiation, with surgery reserved for management of residual neck disease. Surgery for the neck may be in the form of a planned, completion neck dissection, or following demonstrable disease in a follow-up investigation such as positron emission tomography-computed tomography. Any open, larynx preserving surgery for T1/T2 primaries is necessarily accompanied by selective staging neck dissection.

Advanced Disease

With advanced T3 and selected T4 primary cancers of the hypopharynx, organ saving protocols are the standard of care unless contraindications exist in a given case. For patients with well-lateralized T3 cancers with fixity of the hemilarynx, it is best to treat with concomitant chemoradiation and follow this up with neck dissection, as necessary. In patients with T3 primary pyriform sinus cancers who cannot receive chemoradiation for any reason, a possible alternative is primary radical surgery with a near-total laryngectomy. This procedure, described originally by Bruce Pearson, has gained considerable popularity in the Indian subcontinent, where advanced pyriform sinus cancers are extremely common. This procedure requires most of one cord, one arytenoid and a hemicricoid to be preserved, with an intact recurrent laryngeal nerve to innervate the voice shunt created. If the interarytenoid mucosa is involved, this procedure cannot be offered. Although this procedure does result in a permanent anterior wall tracheostoma, there is no need for voice prosthesis and the quality of speech is excellent. The key to success with this procedure is creation of an optimal shunt that permits excellent speech and is yet 100% competent. If aspiration occurs due to a suboptimal voice shunt, revision total laryngectomy is essential. With very bulky, high-volume disease or with very bulky nodes, sequential therapy may be carried out in the form of neoadjuvant three-drug chemotherapy (TPF); to be followed with concomitant platinum-based chemotherapy and radiation. In all these treatments one has to remember that dysphagia becomes a very important problem during and after treatment, and therefore these patients need nutritional appliances such as a percutaneous endoscopic gastrostomy or a nasogastric tube.

Patients with deeply infiltrating, circumferential lesions originating in the postcricoid area are at a high risk of developing permanent pharyngeal strictures, and are thus better suited for primary radical surgery in the form of circumferential laryngopharyngectomy. Patients who manifest obvious destruction of the laryngeal framework are also poor candidates for nonsurgical treatment, and should go for primary radical surgery, i.e. laryngopharyngectomy. Primary surgery for advanced cancers of the hypopharynx almost always involves laryngopharyngectomy, the extent of pharyngectomy depending on the extent of involved pharyngeal mucosa. With primary cancers of the pyriform sinus, it is frequently possible to save the mucosa of the contralateral pyriform sinus area and the posterior pharyngeal wall, whereas with tumors originating in the postcricoid region, it is almost always necessary to perform a circumferential laryngopharyngectomy.

Reconstruction

Surgery for cancers of the hypopharynx poses a major reconstructive challenge. The most important goals of reconstruction are:

- Restoration of prompt and effective swallowing
- Freedom from leaks, fistulae and strictures
- Effective rehabilitation of speech.

In order to assure this, it is important that the reconstructed pharynx should be adequate, a simple test being the ability to achieve a tension free closure over a 32 Fr tube. If this is not possible, it is best to perform an augmentation pharyngoplasty, employing a fasciocutaneous flap in most cases. In very thin male individuals, it may be appropriate to use a pectoralis major myocutaneous flap. For circumferential pharyngeal defects, the method of reconstruction selected depends upon the

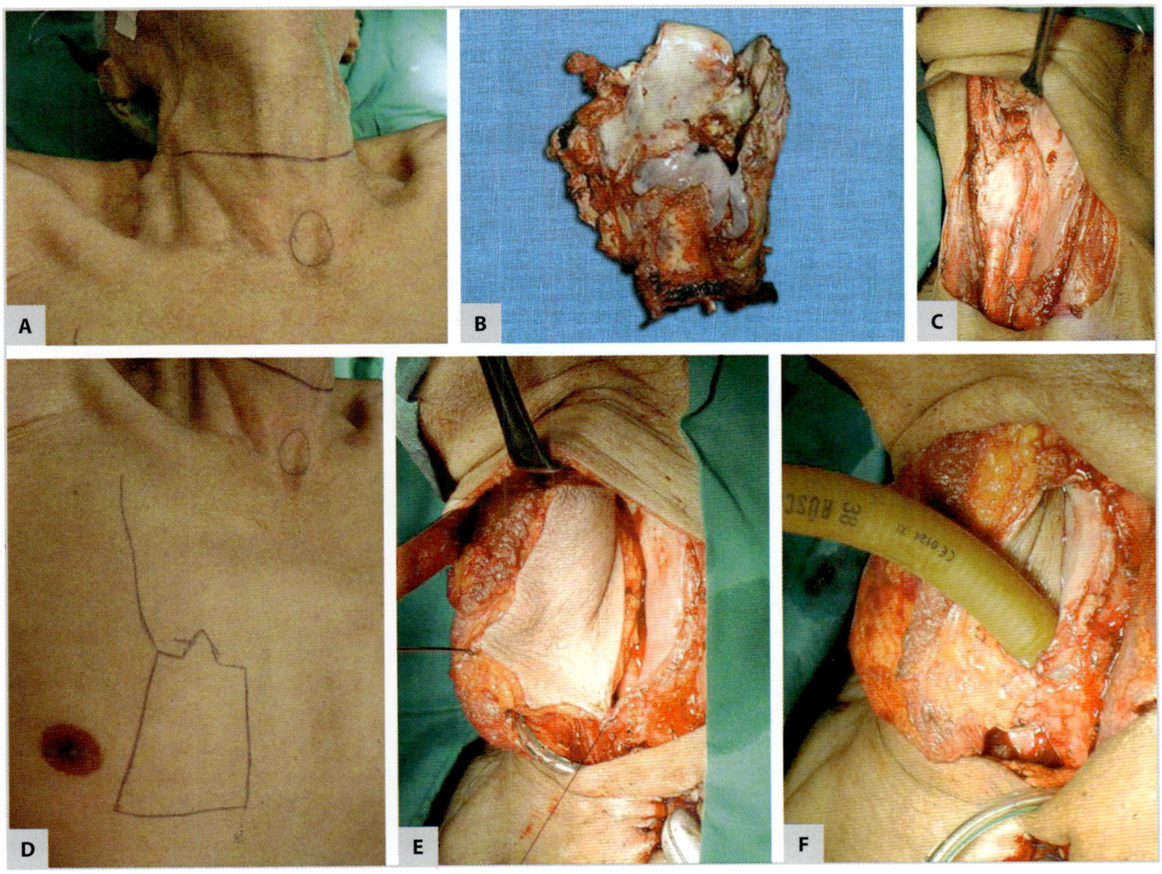

Figs 7A to F: (A) Incision plan; (B) Laryngopharyngectomy specimen; (C) Defect; (D) Flap design; (E and F) Patch pharyngoplasty with adequate luminal diameter

inferior extent of the defect. If the defect is above the thoracic inlet, reconstruction can be performed either with a free jejunal graft or with a tubed fasciocutaneous flap such as the free radial forearm flap or the anterolateral thigh flap. In all cases where there is an adequate party wall, it is best to introduce a voice prosthesis at the time of primary surgery, since most patients with an augmented pharynx develop excellent tracheoesophageal puncture speech. In patients who need a free jejunal graft, the quality of speech rehabilitation with the voice prosthesis is distinctly inferior as the voice has a very moist quality. In patients where the disease is extending down into the cervical esophagus and below the thoracic inlet, it is best to perform a circumferential laryngopharyngoesophagectomy with gastric transposition. In the current scenario, gastric mobilization can be performed laparoscopically, and the stomach pulled up into the neck across the posterior mediastinum, the fundus being anastomosed to the base tongue area.

Representative Cases

1. A lean, elderly male following total laryngectomy with subtotal pharyngectomy, reconstructed with a pectoralis major myocutaneous flap (patch pharyngoplasty) (Figs 7A to F).
2. A 55-year-old male with a postradiation failure for a large postcricoid cancer—total laryngopharyngectomy was performed, with a circumferential defectm reconstructed with a jejunal graft (Figs 8A to D).

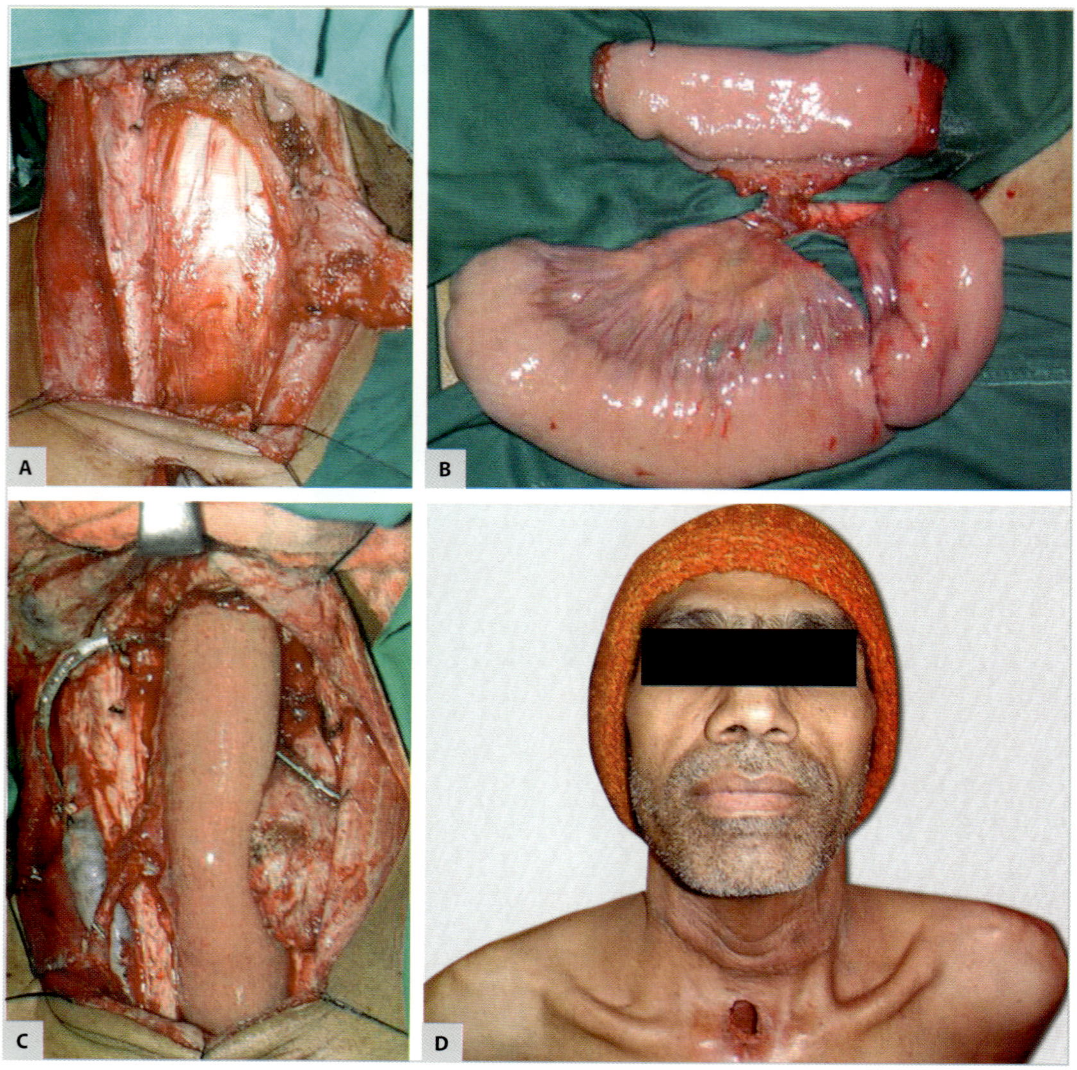

Figs 8A to D: (A) Defect; (B) Segment of jejunum; (C) Vascular anastomosis complete, jejunum in place; (D) Final result—excellent swallowing

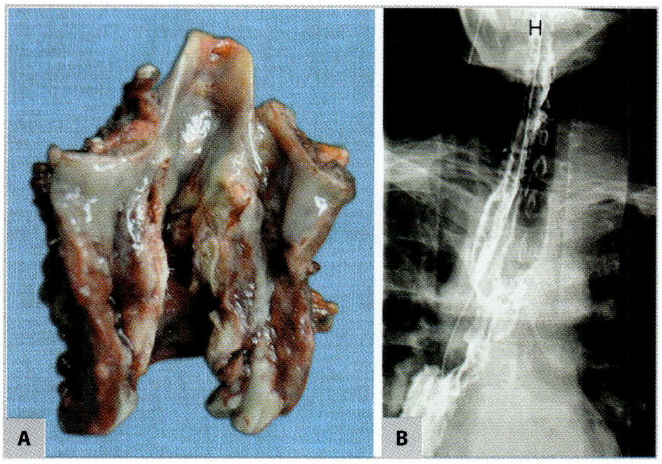

Figs 9A and B: (A) Specimen—total laryngopharyngectomy; (B) Gastric pull-up

3. A 55-year-old male with advanced postradiation failed cancer of the larynx—total laryngopharyngectomy was performed, with gastric pull-up (Figs 9A and B).

Results of Treatment

Results of treatment of the cancers of the hypopharynx depend significantly on the initial stage at presentation. Early stage patients without extensive nodal disease in general do well with radiotherapy alone. With advanced disease, the results depend upon the tumor volume, cartilage invasion and extent of nodal involvement. Typically, large nodes and extracapsular spread have an adverse prognosis and these patients often manifest with secondary tumors and with distant metastatic spread.

REFERENCES

1. Venkitaraman R, Ramanan SG, Vasanthan A, et al. Results of combined modality treatment for nasopharyngeal cancer. J Cancer Res Ther. 2009;5(2):102-6.
2. Ojha RP, Tota JE, Offutt-Powell TN, et al. Human papillomavirus-associated subsequent malignancies among long-term survivors of pediatric and young adult. PLos One. 2013; 8(8):e70349.
3. Bonner JA, Harari PM, Giralt J, et al. Cetuximab prolongs survival in patients with locoregionally advanced squamous cell carcinoma of head and neck: A phase III study of high dose radiotherapy with or without cetuximab. J Clin Oncol. 2004;22(14):5507.
4. Moore EJ, Olsen SM, Laborde RR, et al. Long-term functional and oncologic results of transoral robotic surgery for oropharyngeal squamous cell carcinoma. Mayo Clin Proc. 2012;87(3):219-25.
5. Tauzin M, Rabalais A, Hagan JL, et al. PET-CT staging of the neck in cancers of the oropharynx. Patterns of regional and retropharyngeal nodal metastasis. World J Surg Oncol. 2010;8:70.
6. Cooper JS, Pajak TF, Forastiere AA, et al. Postoperative concurrent radiotherapy and chemotherapy for high-risk squamous-cell carcinoma of the head and neck. N Engl J Med. 2004;350(19):1937-44.
7. Garden AS, Kies MS, Morrison WH, et al. Outcomes and patterns of care of patients with locally advanced oropharyngeal carcinoma treated in the early 21st century. Radiat Oncol. 2013;8:21.
8. Laccourreye O, Veivers D, Hans S, et al. Chemotherapy alone with curative intent in patients with invasive squamous cell carcinoma of the pharyngolarynx classified as T1-T4N0M0 complete clinical responders. Cancer. 2001;92(6):1504-11.

21 Salivary Gland Tumors

Vijay Haribhakti

INTRODUCTION

Neoplasms originating in the salivary glands are an uncommon and a highly heterogeneous group. They can originate from either major salivary glands which are the paired parotid, submandibular and sublingual glands or the minor salivary glands (MSG), which are largely mucous producing glands, scattered across a very large area of the head and neck, e.g. hard palate, soft palate, base tongue and lip. As a general rule of thumb, most tumors originating in the major salivary glands are benign while most tumors originating in the MSGs are malignant.[1] More than 75–80% of all tumors originating in the parotid glands are benign, in the submandibular gland the percentages are roughly 60% (benign) and 40% (malignant); whereas in MSGs, majority of the tumors are malignant (Fig. 1). Salivary tumors, especially the malignant ones, exhibit a marked variability of histology, grade and biological behavior. The most important fact about salivary tumors is that they are essentially surgical problems. Surgery has been and will remain the mainstay of treatment, as majority of these tumors are resistant to radiotherapy as well as chemotherapy.

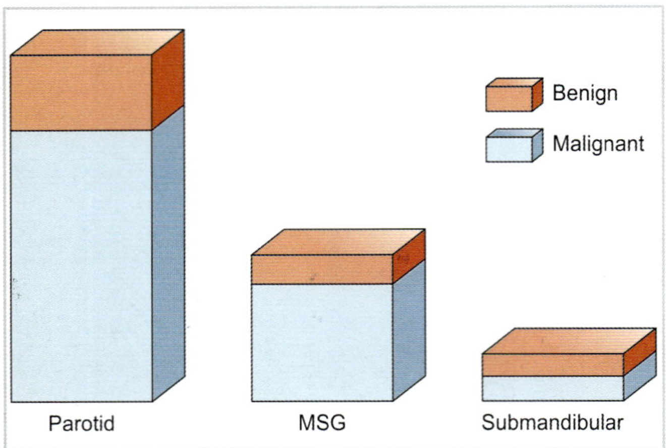

Fig. 1: Salivary tumors—distribution

SURGICAL ANATOMY

The parotid gland overlies the angle of the mandible and is closely related to the cartilage of the external auditory canal posteriorly, the zygomatic process superiorly and the parapharyngeal space in its deep extent. The sternomastoid muscle and the posterior belly of the digastric muscle are related inferiorly to the parotid gland. The facial nerve exists the skull base at the stylomastoid foramen and runs through the substance of the parotid gland, splitting into its major branches in the process (Fig. 2). Although the exact pattern of arborization of the nerve is quite variable, the plane of the facial nerve is critically important and it divides the gland into its superficial and deep lobes. The deep lobes constitute only 20% of the total parotid substance and lie deep to the nerve (Figs 3 and 4).

The submandibular salivary gland (Fig. 5) abuts the body of the mandible superolaterally, related to hypoglossal nerves in the depth, mylohyoid muscle anteriorly and the tail of the parotid gland posteriorly. The marginal mandibular branch of the facial nerve runs along the lateral surface of the gland just deep to the platysma.

The MSGs are small predominant mucous secreting glands located beneath the mucosa of the upper aerodigestive track. These are found in highest concentration in the palate, nasal cavity and oral cavity.

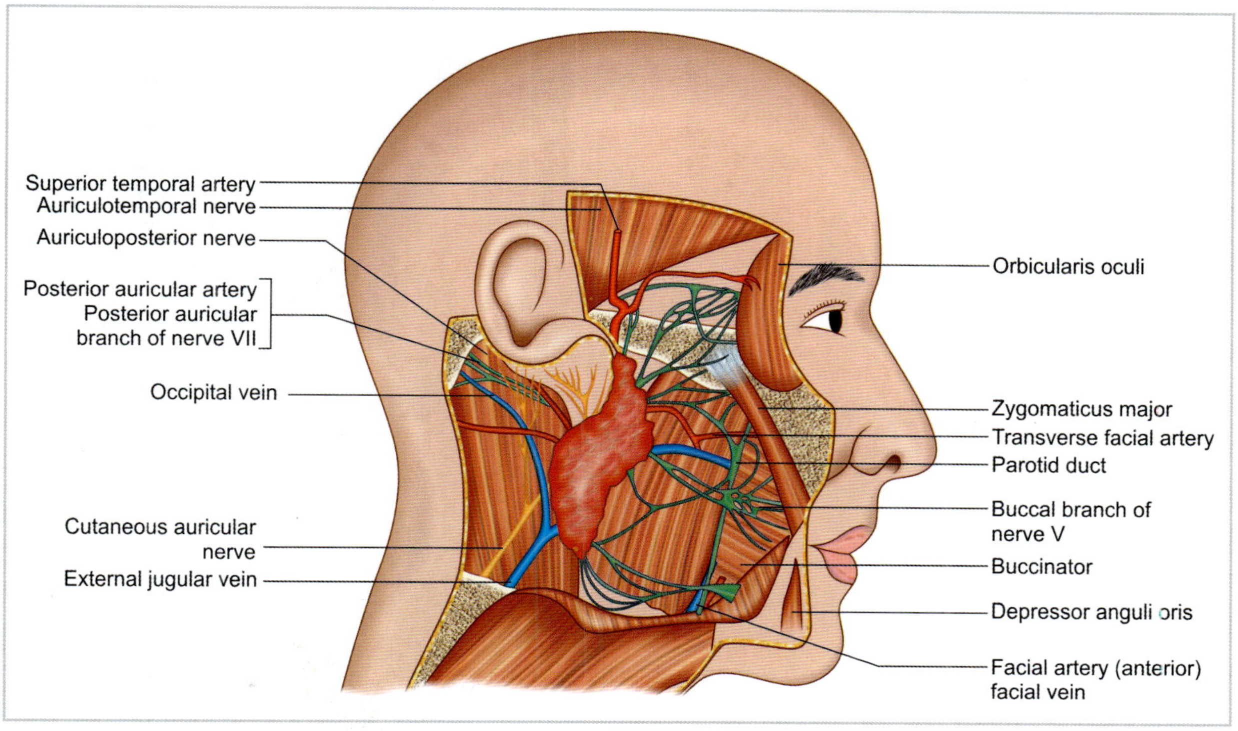

Fig. 2: Parotid gland

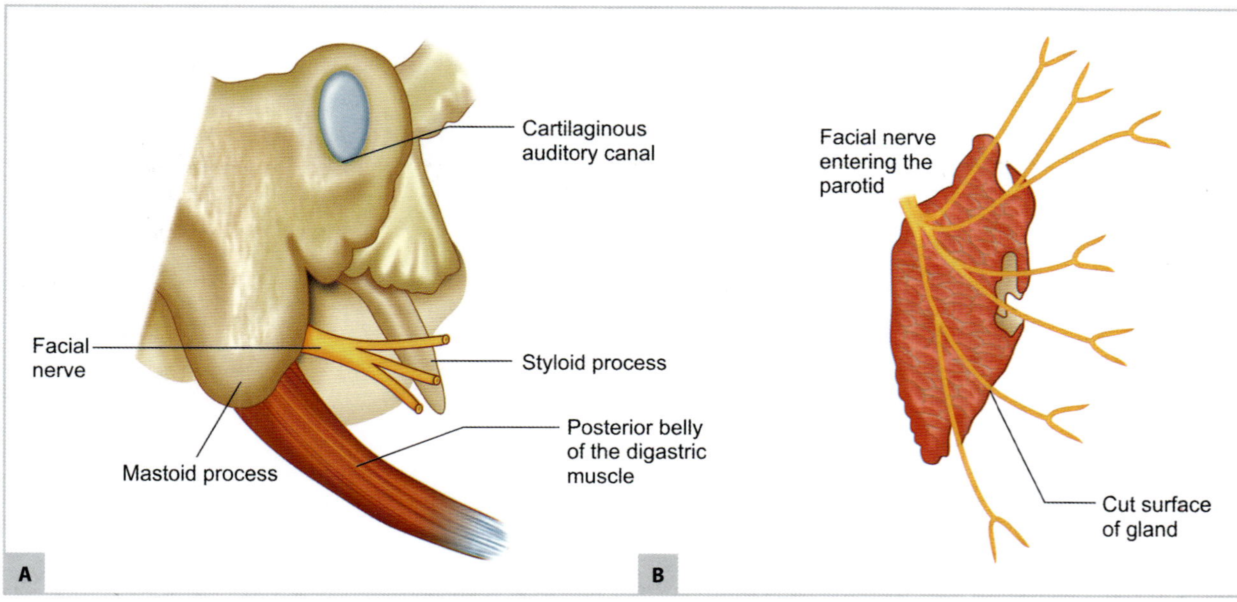

Figs 3A and B: The extracranial course of the facial nerve

CLINICAL FEATURES AND DIAGNOSIS

In majority of patients, salivary tumors present as a painless mass involving the affected gland. There are certain signs that indicate the possibility of malignancy and they are as follows:

- Facial nerve paresis or paralysis
- Presence of significant lymph node enlargement
- Fixity to adjacent anatomical structures
- Ulceration
- Pain
- Rapid growth of the mass.

For neoplasms originating in the MSGs, the presenting signs and symptoms vary according to the location, nature

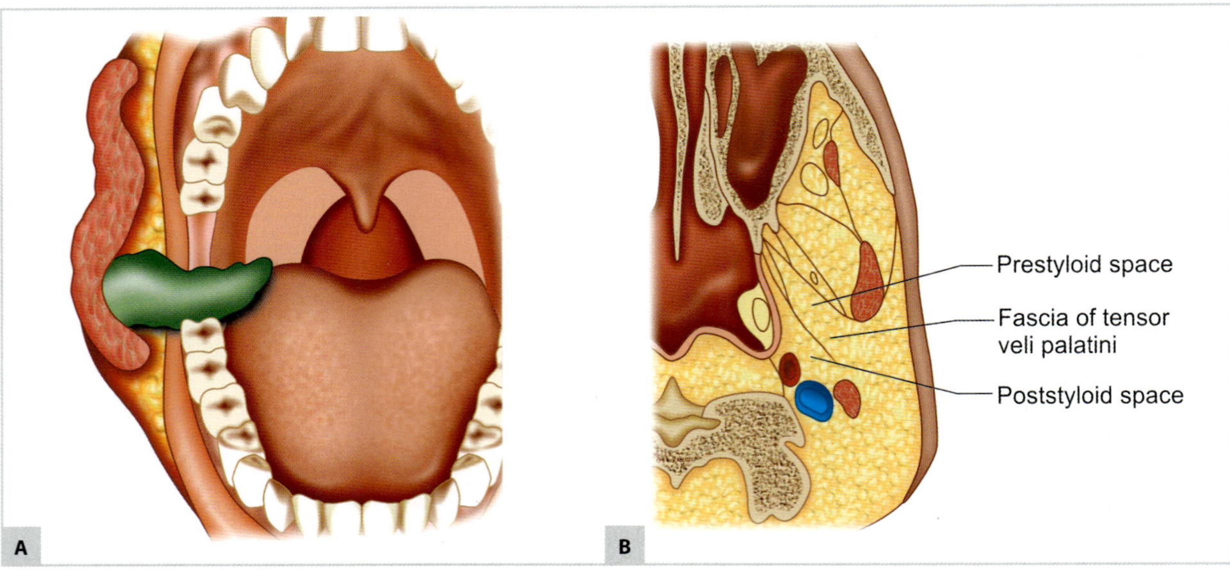

Figs 4A and B: The deep lobe and extension into parapharyngeal space

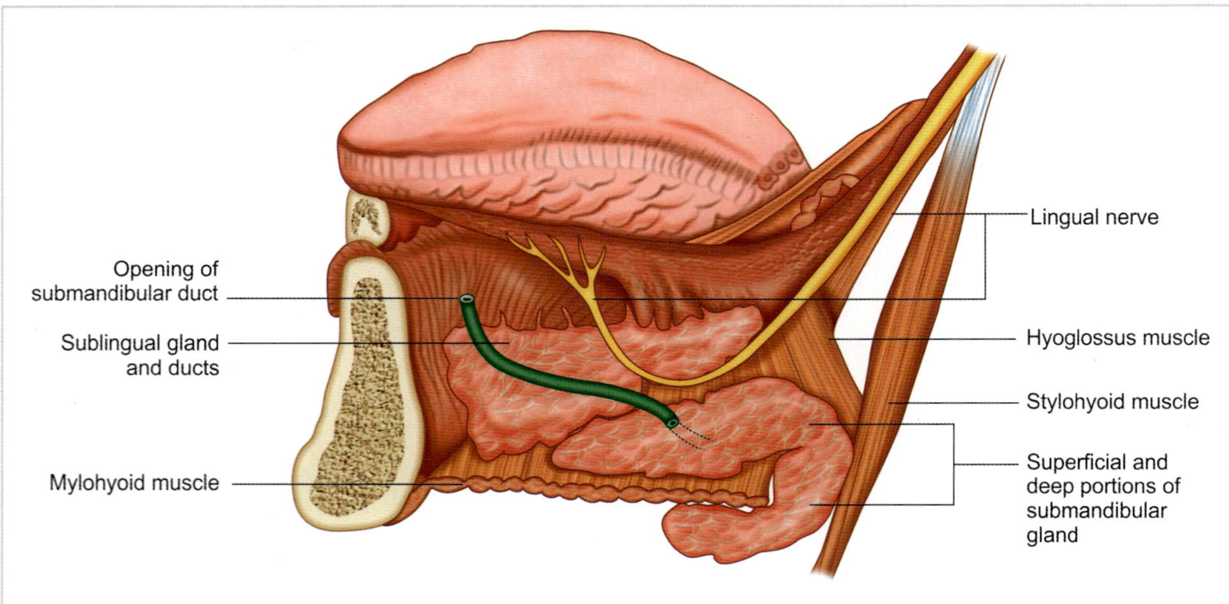

Fig. 5: Submandibular and sublingual glands

and size. Adenoid cystic carcinomas often do not declare themselves at the primary site and may be picked up in the course of a search for the primary with detectable lung metastases. Fine needle aspiration biopsy is a useful way to achieve a cellular diagnosis, especially in a suspected malignant lesion. The findings are of use mainly for counseling the patient in case malignant cells are found. The decision regarding the exact nature of treatment is not based so much on fine needle biopsy because any salivary mass requires surgery. If, however, fine needle biopsy suggests a malignant lesion, and the location is such that it could be in the course of the facial nerve or one of its branches, it helps in preoperative counseling of the patient about the possibility of nerve sacrifice. The other important role of the fine needle biopsy is to distinguish between salivary and nonsalivary tissues, e.g. lymph nodes in the region of the parotid tail masquerading a neoplasm. The imaging for salivary tumors can either be non-anatomical or anatomical. The most important non-anatomical imaging is the ultrasound[2-4] and it answers some very definite questions. It tells us if the mass in question is salivary or extra-salivary and whether it is cystic or solid, and from the pattern of blood supply and the margins, gives us some idea of the nature of the mass.

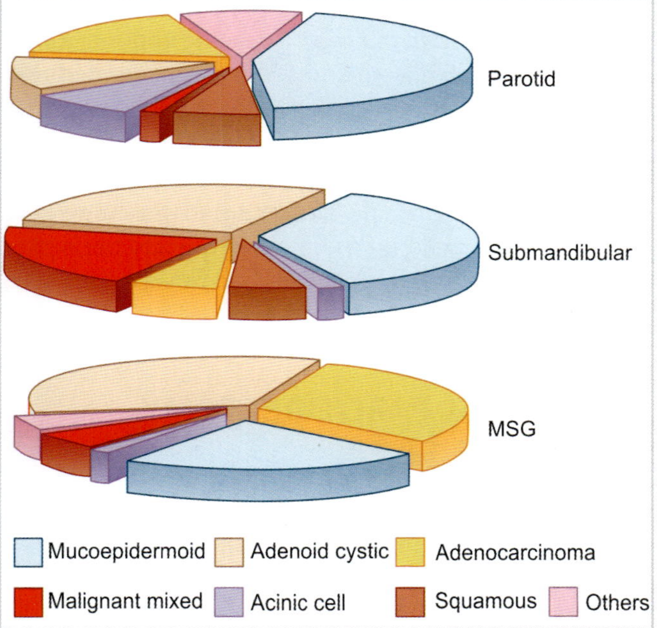

Fig. 6: Most important histologic variants of malignant salivary gland tumors

The anatomical imaging modalities used can be either computed tomography (CT) or magnetic resonance imaging (MRI) scanning. CT scanning is a very adequate way to map out the extent of any salivary neoplasm. However in those patients, where it is essential to study the relationship of a tumor with the nerves, e.g. the trunk of the facial nerve in a parotid mass, MRI scanning is preferred and gives us reliable information about whether the nerve is infiltrated and if so to what extent.

CLASSIFICATION OF SALIVARY TUMORS

Salivary tumors can be either benign or malignant. Among benign tumors, the most common is the pleomorphic adenoma. The other common benign tumors are monomorphic adenoma and Warthin's tumor. Malignant tumors originating from salivary glands can be of various histologies and the most important ones are as shown in Figure 6.[5-7]

MUCOEPIDERMOID CARCINOMA

In mucoepidermoid carcinoma, there are basically three types of cells: (1) mucous secreting cells; (2) epidermal cells; and (3) intermediate cells. The most important factor in classification of mucoepidermoid carcinoma is the histological grade, which can either be well-differentiated grade I, which infiltrates locally and very rarely metastasizes, grade II or moderately differentiated with a high tendency to recur but with rare incidence of metastasis, and finally grade III or poorly differentiated which has a high rate of local recurrence as well as distant metastasis. Thus, the histological grade is critically important with mucoepidermoid cancers.

ADENOID CYSTIC CARCINOMA

"Adenoid cystic carcinoma" or "cylindroma" is one of the most important malignant tumors originating from the salivary tissues and comprises 4–15% of all cancers of salivary glands and 25–31% of all malignant neoplasms of MSGs. The subclassification of adenoid cystic carcinoma[8,9] is based on structure and accordingly three histologic patterns are recognized: (1) tubular; (2) cribriform; and (3) solid. Majority of specimens contain mixed histological patterns. The tubular formation type is the least malignant, while the solid type is most malignant. Survival statistics are very adversely affected by the presence of a solid type adenoid cystic carcinoma. The most important histologic detail to be noted in adenoid cystic carcinoma is the presence of perineural spread. Demonstration of perineural spread is vitally important for adenoid cystic carcinoma and indicates the need for follow-up radiotherapy. Lymph node metastasis, too, have a worse prognosis. Distant metastases adversely affect the overall outcome, although quiescent pulmonary metastases are known to go on for years.

ADENOCARCINOMA

Adenocarcinomas of salivary origin are an important group and present in major as well as MSGs. Tumor grade is important and surgery is the mainstay of treatment.

OTHERS

The other type is acinic cell carcinoma. This is regarded as a low-grade malignancy due to its relatively favorable biological behavior. The next is the malignant mixed tumor (MMT), which account for approximately 3–12% of all cancers of salivary glands. The development of carcinoma in a preexisting benign mixed tumor that is "carcinoma ex-pleomorphic adenoma" occurs in approximate 3–4% of all benign mixed tumors. The risk of developing malignancy increases with increasing duration after the patient first notices the mass, being about 1.5% up to 5 years but as high as 9.5% after more than 15 years. The other important histology is undifferentiated carcinoma of salivary origin, a highly aggressive neoplasm with a very rapid growth rate and a very poor prognosis. Other types are squamous cell carcinoma of salivary tissues and duct carcinomas, both aggressive neoplasms with a very poor long-term outlook. Malignant lymphoma can also involve the salivary glands either as part of a systematic process or as a sole manifestation of the disease. Uncommonly, metastases may be found to salivary glands and this must be borne to mind.

The factors that influence survival in a case of malignant salivary cancer are the following:

- Facial nerve paralysis: Adversely affects the long-term outlook
- Pain: The significance of pain in salivary gland cancer is unclear. Pain as a presenting symptom has been reported in 12–24% of patients with these cancers, and it was found that the 5-year survival of those patients who presented with pain was just 33% as opposed to overall 5-year survival of 66%
- T stage and location of the tumor: A high T stage and certain locations of the cancer affect the prognosis in many cases
- Lymph node metastasis: The presence of lymph node metastasis adversely affects the prognosis in all malignant tumors
- Detailed histopathology: Accurate tumor histological analysis is important in the satisfactory management of the cancer and in prognostication. Low-grade cancers including mucoepidermoid carcinoma and acinic cell carcinoma have a predictably good prognosis. High-grade cancers including "solid" adenoid cystic, squamous cell carcinoma, salivary duct carcinoma, adenocarcinoma, mucoepidermoid carcinoma, MMT and undifferentiated carcinoma have a worse prognosis than low-grade cancers
- Presence of distant metastasis is a predictor of poor prognosis
- Recurrence: The overall recurrence rate of malignant salivary tumors is high, and is between 27% and 38%. Recurrence adversely affects the prognosis.

TREATMENT GOALS AND ALTERNATIVES

The goals of treatment of salivary cancer include cure, while decreasing the treatment morbidity. Surgical resection has long been the mainstay of treatment of salivary tumors and of salivary cancer, radiotherapy being important in an adjuvant setting, while chemotherapy has a limited role. Surgery consists typically of a wide three-dimensional resection with clear margins for the primary, together with an appropriate neck dissection when indicated. Since the parotid gland is by far the most affected site, superficial parotidectomy would be the most frequently performed operation for salivary tumors, followed by submandibular gland resection.

SUPERFICIAL PAROTIDECTOMY—TECHNIQUE

1. Preauricular skin crease incision curving under lobule and continuing into upper neck crease/submandibular crease
2. Extra-platysmal flaps, anterior flap upto anterior border of parotid, and posterior flap upto cartilaginous canal
3. Fascia over sternomastoid muscle incised and parotid tail separated
4. Great auricular nerve identified and anterior division divided in most cases
5. Posterior belly of digastric exposed
6. Superficial lobe separated from auditory canal and retracted forward
7. Dissection continued along superior border of posterior belly of digastric toward tympanomastoid sulcus
8. Main trunk of facial nerve exposed by careful separation of salivary tissues
9. Facial nerve identified at a point where the tip of the mastoid, cartilaginous canal and posterior digastric belly meet
10. Dissection continued until the periphery of the gland
11. Meticulous dissection proceeds along each of the branch of the facial nerve
12. Stensen's duct identified if possible, divided and ligated
13. Hemostasis and closure without suction drains.

MANAGEMENT OF THE NECK

Those patients that initially present with obvious nodal involvement require a therapeutic neck dissection. In all patients where tumors originate in the parotid gland, the most important stations of spread are level II, IIB, III, IV and V. For submandibular salivary glands it is level I to level IV. In those patients who have multiple nodal metastases, it is best to perform a comprehensive neck dissection.

ISSUES IN SALIVARY GLAND SURGERY

The Facial Nerve

In patients with preoperative normal facial nerve function, every effort must be made to demonstrate and preserve the nerve with all its branches. In benign tumors (very large tumors or recurrent, multifocal tumors), the nerve or its branches are frequently entwined with the tumor and must be carefully dissected and preserved. In these situations, radiotherapy may become necessary to address potential spillage. With malignant tumors, the approach to the nerve depends principally on the preoperative function status and the extent of nerve involvement. In majority of cases with proven malignancy, preoperative MRI scanning is carried out to study the relationship of the nerve with the tumor and to study the morphology of the nerve. If thickening is demonstrable, the proximal extent of thickening is noted. If it is possible to demonstrate thickening above the level of the stylomastoid foramen, it is necessary to trace the nerve all the way up.

In a patient undergoing surgery for a malignant tumor, and with normal preoperative facial nerve function, following are important considerations:

- Is the nerve "normal looking," or is it thickened/ inflamed/invaded?
- Is the nerve compressed by the tumor or is it passing through it?
- Is it possible to achieve clear margins at all areas except that related to the nerve?
- If a functioning nerve appears to be directly invaded, it may be sacrificed and a clear nerve margin must idealy be achieved. This is especially true for adenoid cystic carcinomas, where the nerve may be involved for considerable distances proximal to the tumor
- If it is a normal looking nerve, one has to ask if the area around the nerve is the only area that precludes a complete wide excision. If yes, the nerve may be sacrificed in the interest of oncologic safety
- If the tumor extent is such that close or unclear margins are present at many areas, it may be justifiable to spare the nerve by dissecting close to it and securing complete tumor resection nonetheless
- In patients who present with nerve paralysis, it is necessary to sacrifice the nerve in most cases.

Nonsurgical Treatment

In a minority of patients who have large, unresectable neoplasms and who are in need of palliation, external radiotherapy may be used. Particle irradiation (either with fast neutrons or protons) is especially useful for salivary tumors.

Rehabilitation and Quality of Life

In those patients in whom facial nerve sacrifice is required variety of methods exists to rehabilitate function. At the time of surgery, cable grafts may be used to restore function to the extent possible. In later cases with severe disabilities due to facial nerve paralysis a variety of techniques such as microneural reconstruction with the hypoglossal are performed in order to restore animation of the face. Other techniques that can be used are the static and dynamic slings. It is also now possible to perform reanimation surgery with the use of microvascular, microneural free muscle transfer, in which a muscle such as serratus anterior or pectoralis minor or gracilis is transferred along with the nerve to provide animation of the paralyzed face.

REFERENCES

1. To VS, Chan JY, Tsang RK, et al. Review of salivary gland neoplasms. ISRN Otolaryngol. 2012:872982.
2. Huang YT, Jung SM, Ko SF, et al. Diagnostic efficacy of ultrasonography-guided fine needle aspiration biopsy in evaluating salivary gland malignancy. Chang Gung Med J. 2012;35(1):62-9.
3. El-Khateeb SM, Abou-Khalaf AE, Farid MM, et al. A prospective study of three diagnostic sonographic methods in differentiation between benign and malignant salivary gland tumours. Dentomaxillofac Radiol. 2011;40(8):476-85.
4. Javadi M, Asghari A, Hassannia F. Value of fine-needle aspiration cytology in the evaluation of parotid tumors. Indian J Otolaryngol Head Neck Surg. 2012;64(3):257-60.
5. Bussu F, Parrilla C, Rizzo D, et al. Clinical approach and treatment of benign and malignant parotid masses, personal experience. Acta Otorhinolaryngol Ital. 2011;31(3):135-43.
6. Mukherji S, Sheth S. Warthin's tumor of bilateral parotid glands: A case report. J Maxillofac Oral Surg. 2012;11(4):483-6.
7. Carlson J, Licitra L, Locati L, et al. Salivary gland cancer: an update on present and emerging therapies. Am Soc Clin Oncol Educ Book. 2013;33:257-63.
8. Ellington CL, Goodman M, Kono SA, et al. Adenoid cystic carcinoma of the head and neck: Incidence and survival trends based on 1973-2007 Surveillance, Epidemiology, and End Results data. Cancer. 2012;118(18):4444-51. Erratum in: Cancer. 2012;118(21):5448-9.
9. Bhayani MK, Yener M, El-Naggar A, et al. Prognosis and risk factors for early-stage adenoid cystic carcinoma of the major salivary glands. Cancer. 2012;118(11):2872-8.

22 Carcinoma of the Thyroid

Praful Desai, Sarabjeet Kaur Arneja

INTRODUCTION

Cancer of the thyroid is uncommon and constitutes less than 2–3% of all cancers. Among malignancies of endocrine glands thyroid cancer is the most common. Increasing incidence is noted in recent years. It is much more frequent in women to the extent of 75%. Recent data in 2010 from the US reported 44,670 patients with thyroid cancer.[1] In most well-differentiated papillary and follicular types of thyroid cancer the survival rates are high, 90–95%, except in the anaplastic type which is rapidly fatal. The papillary form which is most common constitutes nearly 80% of all thyroid malignancies. Majority are well-differentiated, though mixed pathologic variants are known. The second most common is the follicular type (10%).[1] Five percent of these are the Hürthle cell type which tend to be multicentric and do not concentrate radioactive iodine. Lymph node metastasis and recurrences are common.

Medullary cancer of the thyroid forms about 5% of all thyroid cancers and is a distinct clinicopathologic entity first described by Hazard[2] in 1950. It is often a part of a hereditary syndrome associated with multiple endocrine neoplasia (MEN) 2A or 2B.[3] It is known to arise from hyperplasia of the C-cells in the upper pole of the gland. Lymphomas, Hodgkin's disease, metastatic spread into the thyroid gland (because of its vascularity) and rarely a squamous carcinoma of the thyroid are also known. The other rarer type of pathologic variant is the non-Hodgkin B-cell type and the mucosa-associated lymphoid tissue (MALT) type lymphoma. For all neoplasia of endocrine glands inclusive of thyroid cancers, a good team effort among surgeons, physicians, pathologists and endocrinologists is mandatory for satisfactory therapy outcomes.

ETIOLOGY

Radiation therapy to the mediastinum, chest or neck at an early age is an important factor for the development of papillary carcinoma in younger women. Genetic and familial predispositions are important factors in etiology. Increase in the incidence of thyroid cancer after the Chernobyl and Hiroshima disasters are well-documented and show radiation sensitivity of the thyroid gland. Familial medullary cancer of the thyroid and the more common papillary carcinoma are sometimes preceded by several mutational events, BRAF and RAS mutations, interaction and chromosomal rearrangements.[2] It is the complex interaction of such external and body's own internal genetic changes[4] that initiates the process of carcinogenesis. p53 mutations are described in anaplastic cancers of the thyroid.

PATHOLOGY

Based on cellular differentiation, thyroid neoplasms are divided into tumors exhibiting follicular differentiation and those exhibiting C-cell differentiation; the former comprise more than 95% of the tumors.

Tumors Exhibiting Follicular Differentiation: Specific Types

Follicular Adenoma and Carcinoma

Follicular adenoma is defined as a benign tumor of follicular cell differentiation that is grossly and microscopically completely encapsulated and lacks: evidence of capsular and/or vascular invasion and nuclear features of papillary carcinoma (Fig. 1A). They are almost always solitary;

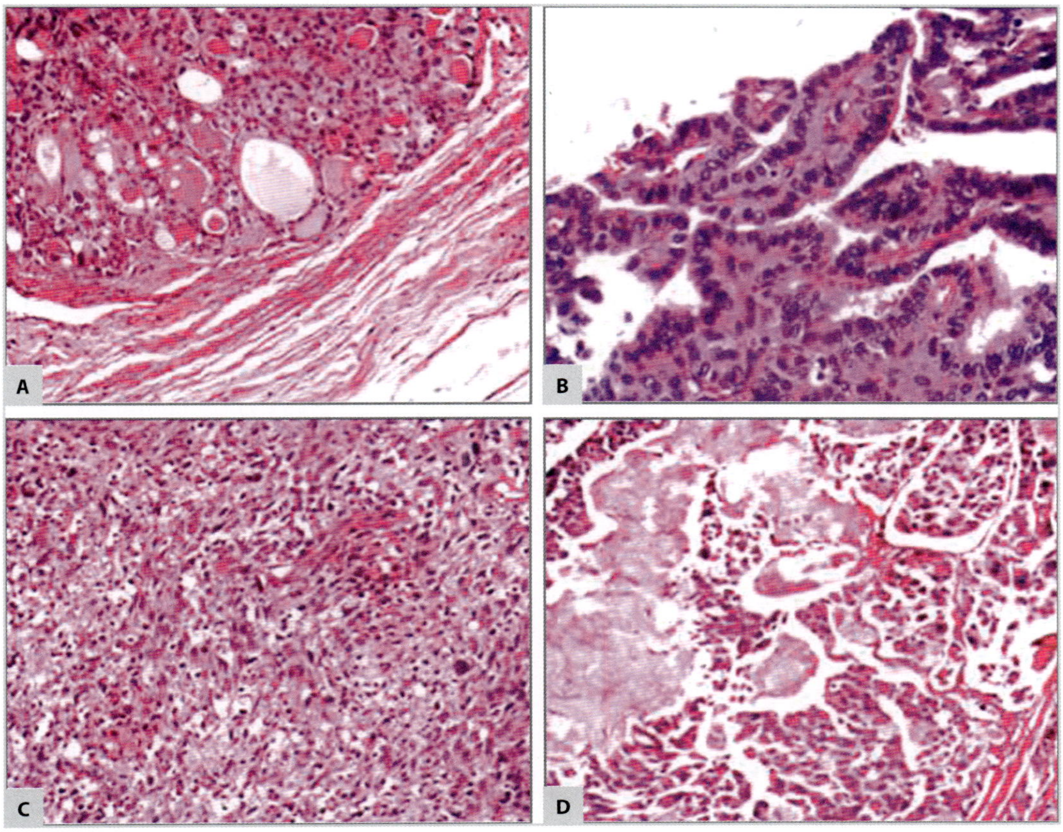

Figs 1A to D: (A) Follicular adenoma, encapsulated tumor with cells in follicular pattern. Cells lack nuclear features of papillary carcinoma; (B) Papillary carcinoma, papillae with characteristic nuclear features; (C) Anaplastic carcinoma, cells in sarcomatoid pattern; (D) Medullary carcinoma, cells in nests separated by hyaline pink material

the architectural and cytological features are different from that of the surrounding normal compressed thyroid gland. A variety of patterns may be seen, normofollicular, macrofollicular, microfollicular and trabecular or solid. The so-called Hürthle cell (oncocytic) neoplasms are variants of follicular adenoma that characteristically contain abundant eosinophilic cytoplasm imparting an oncocytic appearance.[5]

Diagnosis of malignancy in follicular adenomas is dependent on demonstration of blood vessel and/or capsular invasion. Invasion of the capsule must be full thickness for it to qualify as capsular invasion.[6] The vessels showing invasion should be of venous caliber, located within or immediately outside the capsule and contain tumor cells adherent to the wall and protruding into the lumen, being covered by endothelial cells on its free surface.

Papillary Carcinoma

The typical papillary carcinoma contains numerous papillae that are usually complex, branching, with a central fibrovascular core lined by cells with characteristic nuclear features (Fig. 1B):

- Ground glass (optically clear) nuclei with nuclear overlapping
- Nuclear pseudoinclusions
- Nuclear grooves.

Undifferentiated (Anaplastic) Carcinoma

The term undifferentiated or anaplastic carcinoma is used for those tumors, first, that do not make follicles, papillae or trabeculae, but still retain an epithelial appearance, and second that are composed of cells with sarcomatoid appearance and tumor giant cells (Fig. 1C).

Tumors Exhibiting C-Cell Differentiation

Medullary carcinoma is a distinctive type of malignant thyroid tumor composed of C-cells (parafollicular cells).[2] Microscopically, the classic presentation is that of solid proliferation of round to polygonal cells, separated by a vascular stroma and amyloid (Fig. 1D). The latter is seen as extracellular hyaline eosinophilic material that is positive for Congo red stain and shows apple green birefringence under polarized microscopy. The pattern of tumor growth can be trabecular, follicular, solid or pseudopapillary. The amyloid deposition may be abundant, scanty or completely absent. Immunohistochemically, the tumor cells are reactive for pan-neuroendocrine markers such as chromogranin, synaptophysin and the product of C-cells, calcitonin.

STAGING (TABLE 1)

TABLE 1: American Joint Committee on Cancer/Tumor-Node-Metastasis (AJCC/TNM) system

Stage I — T_1 up to 2 cm (limited to thyroid)
Stage II — T_2— 2–4 cm
Stage III — T_3— > 4 cm (minimal extrathyroid extension)
T_4— infiltration into surrounding structures
T_5— encasement of vessels, prevertebral fascia
N_1— regional metastatic nodes N_{1b}— Contralateral or bilateral nodes
Stage $IV_{A, B, C}$— Any T with N_{1b}

CLINICAL FEATURES AND INVESTIGATIONS

Most common thyroid cancers present as a solitary asymptomatic nodule in the gland of a few months duration; occasionally, presence of a node in the lower or mid neck may be the only presenting symptom or sign. A rapidly growing and painful thyroid nodule is often the result of a recent hemorrhage in a benign colloid nodule. A long standing cancerous nodule will grow in size, very gradually. In later stages, the disease may present with obstructive symptoms like dysphagia, mild to moderate difficulty in breathing or hoarseness of voice if the recurrent laryngeal nerve (RLN) is infiltrated by the disease; rarely, the nodule (benign or malignant) may extend into the superior mediastinum through the narrow confines of the thoracic inlet. Symptoms may then increase, particularly cough and a mild stridor depending on the size of the mediastinal extension. This is a common clinical presentation of an advanced papillary or follicular carcinoma. Advanced lesions may present with lymph node metastasis in the neck. Anaplastic cancers often present with a hard plaque or a fixed mass in the thyroid region; often the mass is tethered with restricted mobility and hoarseness due to RLN paresis or palsy. Lymph node metastases are common and often infiltrate to encase the carotid vessels in later stages.

Routine investigations include blood chemistry, thyroid function tests, liver and kidney profiles including serum thyroglobulin. Thyroglobulin (TG) is produced by some forms of differential thyroid cancers and its estimation is of value in the follow up to monitor any residual thyroid tissue or local or distant metastasis. In some ways, but not in all cases it could be considered as a tumor marker. Ultrasound studies of the neck will give extremely useful information about the size, vascularity and multicentricity of the nodules (if any). A multinodular lesion is often benign. Ultrasound study of the neck is a very useful guide for a fine needle aspiration biopsy of the suspect nodule. Nuclear studies and isotope scanning of the neck will give vital information about the type of nodule—"hot or cold" and helps in clinical decisions. A computed tomography (CT) scan of the neck and chest will delineate mediastinal extension. A plain X-ray of the neck (anteroposterior and lateral) will delineate the position of the trachea in large tumors.

FINE NEEDLE ASPIRATION CYTOLOGY

Fine needle aspiration cytology (FNAC) is a simple and very often the most informative diagnostic procedure for a thyroid lesion. A 23 gauge needle should be used to avoid a hemorrhagic aspirate, as lesions are often vascular. A recent painful nodule with hemorrhage, often benign, will almost completely resolve after aspiration. Most of the times, FNAC will give sufficient histologic data for treatment planning in nearly 85–90% of patients. False negative is generally unknown, less than 5% in experienced hands.

TREATMENT

Surgery remains the therapy of choice for malignant lesions of the thyroid. In many patients, a long standing asymptomatic small incidental benign nodule, careful observation suffices as these nodules remain indolent and have a very slow growth. A solitary nodule in a young woman or at any age, however, should be carefully investigated and should be proved to be benign before deciding against surgical excision. Increase in size and cosmesis are other indications for a surgical excision even for a benign nodule. Thyroid suppression for benign nodules is worthwhile as nearly 25% of the benign nodules may regress or remain stable in size for years. Unnecessary surgery for a small benign nodule should be

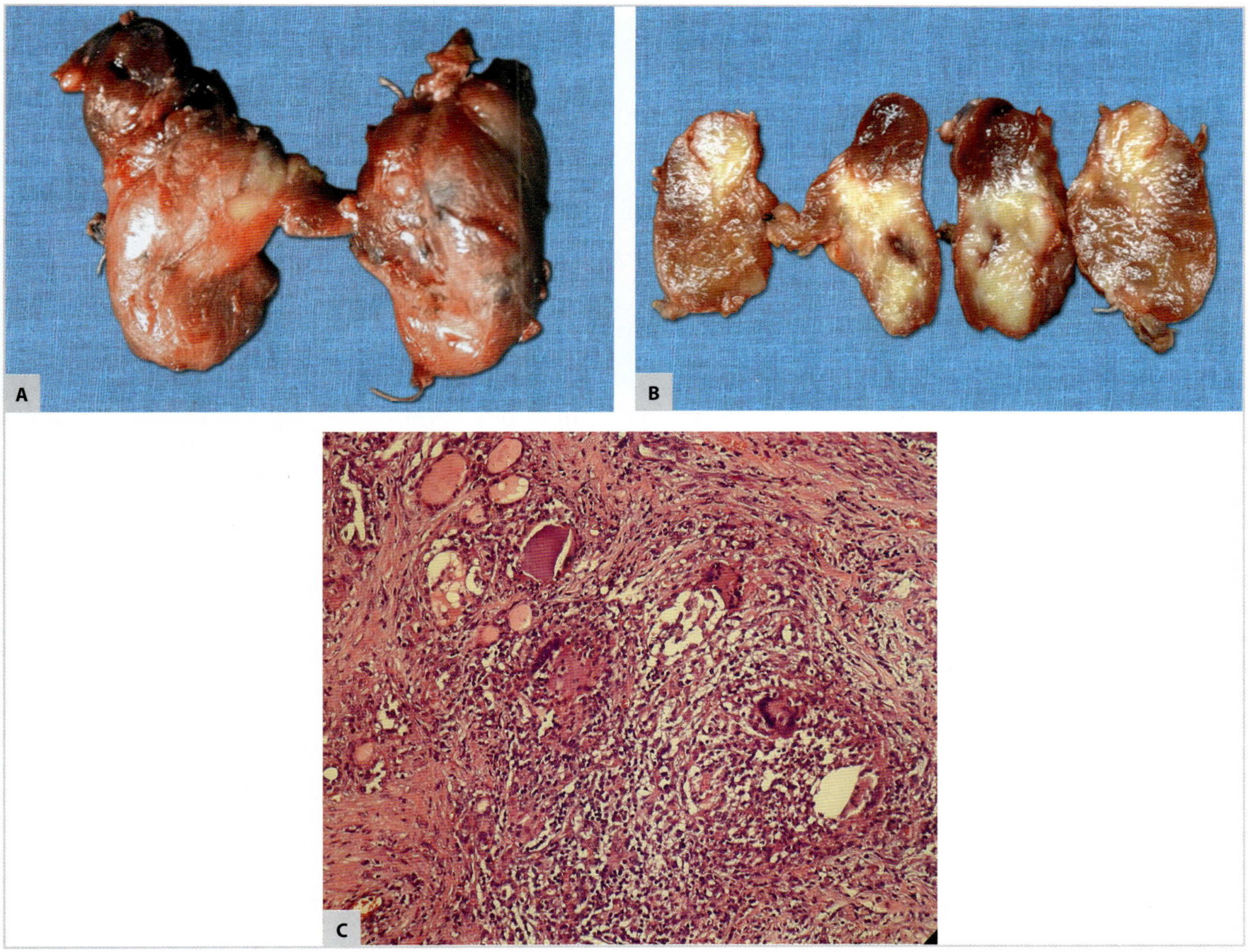

Figs 2A to C: (A) Specimen of total thyroidectomy—suspected of a follicular lesion on fine needle aspiration cytology (FNAC); (B) Cut sections of the specimen showing a homogenous firm lesion; (C) Final histologic diagnosis—granulomatous thyroiditis—groups of follicles disrupted by lymphohistiocytic and neutrophilic infiltrate and multinucleate histiocytic giant cells, one containing engulfed colloid

avoided as unforeseen morbidity due to RLN palsy and cosmetic issues may arise. For papillary and follicular cancers surgery is the treatment of choice. Majority of the times a total thyroidectomy is indicated.[7,8] In rare clinical situations, through FNAC reveals a carcinoma the final histopathological diagnosis can be at variance. A total thyroidectomy often becomes mendatory. Two patients had to undergo total thyroidectomy for an unusual pathology like granulomatous thyroiditis and amyloid infiltration of the total thyroid in a patient of Addison's disease with autoimmune status (Figs 2 and 3). However, debates will continue for a small localized lesion in either lobe or isthmus. Small lesions less than 2 cm without capsular invasion and devoid of macroscopic multicentricity can be considered for a unilateral lobectomy with isthmectomy. A subtotal or near total thyroidectomy leaving behind strips of thyroid tissue safeguarding the RLN and parathyroid glands is indicated for a larger lesion. The final decision is best left to an experienced thyroid surgeon. Strong reason to avoid a total thyroidectomy is because of almost equivalent long-term survivals for as long as 15–20 years (95%) after a subtotal or near total thyroidectomy.

"Medullary carcinoma" has distinctive features as regards its management. When localized within the gland the survival rate at 10 years is high, around 90%, which drops to 20% when it has metastasized to lymph nodes or elsewhere. Increased serum calcitonin and carcinoembryonic antigen (CEA) are important markers for medullary thyroid cancer. Lymph node metastases are frequent. It is known to be associated with pheochromocytoma and investigation to exclude this possibility is important. Long-term 5-year survivals are reported. Medullary cancers of the thyroid may be sporadic or familial and genetic transmission is often due to inherited Mendelian

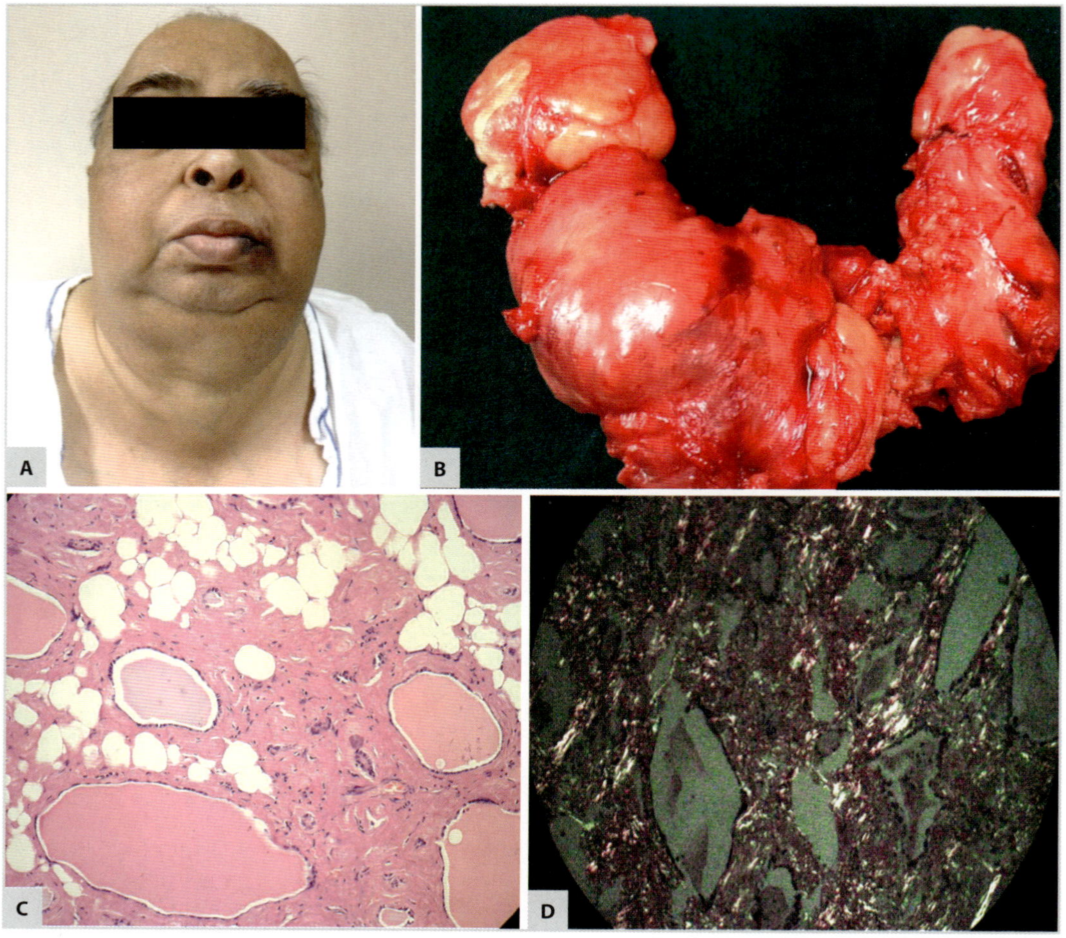

Figs 3A to D: (A, B) 55 years old male with steroid facies (Addison's disease) and a large bilateral goitorous thyroid FNAC indicated lipomatosis. Exclusion of papillary carcinoma (presence of nuclear grooves in FNAC) was suggested. Total thyroidectomy was indicated for mild dysphagia, hoarseness and stridor on recumbency; (C) Colloid containing thyroid follicles surrounded by acellular, homogenous, eosinophilic material (amyloid). Groups of fat cells are also identified (H&E x400); (D) Congo red stain: Amyloid deposits show apple green birefringence on polarisation (400X)

autosomal dominance (MEN-2A).[9] Presence of primary hyperparathyroidism should be excluded. Bilaterality and multicentric nature of the lesion needs to be carefully evaluated before a total thyroidectomy. Medullary carcinoma associated with MEN-2 syndrome is generally more aggressive. Calcitonin estimation is important in follow-up. Rising calcitonin levels in asymptomatic patients often pose difficult decisions in management. Local recurrence, nodal and distant metastases are the main causes of elevated calcitonin levels. Tisell, et al.[10] reports super radical neck dissections going for 10–12 hours of a seemingly normal neck removing 40–60 nodes. Calcitonin levels often drop indicating microscopic nodal involvement responsible for high calcitonin levels in asymptomatic patients. This is debatable as careful observation of asymptomatic patients is a possible alternative despite very high calcitonin levels. Rising calcitonin levels will mandate appropriate investigation to exclude distant metastasis.

MANAGEMENT OF NECK NODES

Lymph node clearance in thyroid cancer needs a special mention. A radical neck dissection is very rarely needed, except in a very advanced primary lesion with heavy nodal burden. Infiltration of the vessels (internal jugular vein, carotid artery) is extremely rare. The nodes are softish, easily removable by gentle finger and sharp dissection. "Berry picking" is a common word used for nodal dissections and indicates the ease with which the nodes can be dissected. Central compartments (Fig. 4) and the superior mediastinum should be carefully searched for presence of nodes.

A preoperative CT scan generally gives sufficient information about the superior mediastinum. A sternal or mediastinal split is very rarely necessary as even a few rare plunging (into the superior mediastinum) thyroid lesions

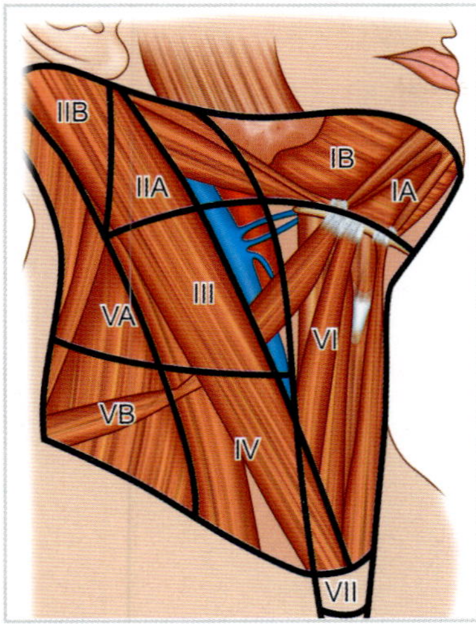

Fig. 4: Different neck compartments

(benign or malignant) can be easily and deftly removed by dissection in the correct intracapsular dissection plane. Palpation and clearance of the nodes on both sides is mandatory if the lesion is bilobar or has crossed the isthmus. Careful palpation of level III is also necessary to avoid leaving behind small involved nodes. Level I and II are very rarely involved except when a large nodal mass is present clinically. The lower posterior triangles (level V A,B) should be carefully palpated and dissected in presence of nodes. The best way to avoid inadvertent parathyroid removal is to work in the intracapsular plane and push the fascial capsule away which will dislodge the parathyroid out of harm. Prophylactic neck dissections are not generally indicated in thyroid malignancies.

A locally aggressive tumor may infiltrate the pretracheal fascia and rarely the tracheal cartilage. A limited involvement of the cartilage of two or three rings of the trachea can be safely excised with a tracheal repair by 3-0 Vicryl® sutures. Occasionally, scraping away of the pretracheal fascial layer will facilitate complete removal. Adequate mobilization of the trachea from the mediastinum and a laryngeal drop will safely ensure a tension-free tracheal anastomosis after excision of three to four tracheal rings. This is important as complete excision of the disease can result in a long-term local control.

ADJUVANT RADIOACTIVE IODINE

Adjuvant radioactive iodine (RA ^{131}I) is generally indicated only after a total thyroidectomy. For lesions, less than 2 cm without capsular invasion and devoid of lymph node involvement particularly at a young age, RA ^{131}I could be avoided after appropriate surgery. The long-term effects of RA ^{131}I therapy are distressing; constant dryness due to lack of saliva and xerostomia of the eyes are difficult to manage in later stages of life. These are easily avoidable in early thyroid cancer management. Postoperative radiotherapy to the neck is necessary in advanced anaplastic cancers or when non-resectable disease is left behind in the operative area. Suppressive hormonal therapy for thyroid-stimulating hormone (TSH) suppression (thyroxine) is the standard (2 μg/kg/day) therapy after surgery and RA ^{131}I treatment. Medullary and anaplastic cancers show no uptake of RA ^{131}I.

LOBECTOMY VERSUS TOTAL THYROIDECTOMY IN THYROID CANCERS

The controversy will continue with relevant data presented for either approach. The strongest argument for a conservative approach (wide lobectomy with isthmectomy) for a small, less than 2 cm differentiated low-risk (papillary or follicular type) thyroid carcinoma shows data of 20-year survival rates in 99% of patients and disease-free survival rates in more than 95% of patients in a recent evaluation of National Cancer Data Base (NCDB) 1985–1998.[1] Modest decrease in local recurrences and increased survival benefit for thyroid cancers of more than 1 cm after total thyroidectomy and a low incidence of RLN palsy and parathyroid injury (2%) is an argument for a total thyroidectomy.

SOLITARY THYROID NODULE — MANAGEMENT ALGORITHM

A good history and clinical examination must precede investigations. A very short history (of days) of pain and sudden enlargement often indicates a recent hemorrhage in a preexistent nodule which needs aspiration and cytologic evaluation. Most of these are benign.

The most common clinical presentation of thyroid cancers is almost always with an asymptomatic solitary nodule localized in a lobe or a solitary lymph node in the neck with an occult primary. A careful evaluation of a solitary thyroid nodule is therefore imperative for appropriate management. The adjoining algorithm (Flow chart 1) is a practical approach modified from the American Thyroid Association guidelines.[11]

Flow chart 1: Solitary thyroid nodule — management algorithm

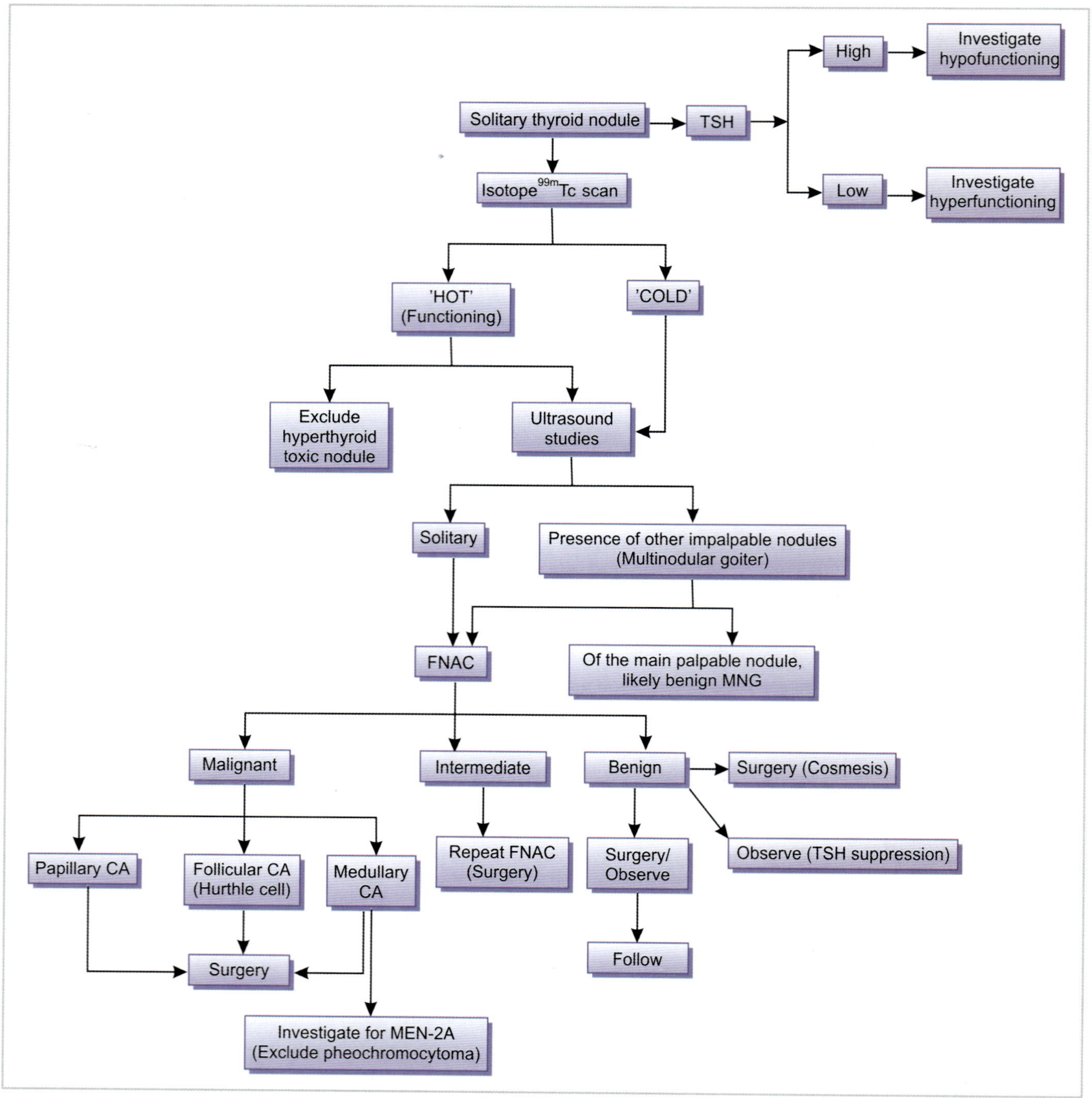

Abbreviations: TSH, thyroid-stimulating hormone; FNAC, fine needle aspiration cytology; MNG, multinodular goiter; CA, carcinoma; MEN-2A, multiple endocrine neoplasia type 2A

REFERENCES

1. Thomas RM, Habra MA, Perrier ND, et al. Well-differentiated carcinoma of the thyroid and neoplasms of the parathyroid glands. In: MD Anderson Surgical Oncology Handbook, 5th edition. Philadelphia: Lippincott Williams and Wilkins; 2011. pp. 550-87.
2. Hazard J, Hawk W, Crile G. Medullary (solid) carcinoma of the thyroid—a clinicopathologic entity. J Clin Endocrinol Metab. 1959;19:152.
3. Qucyle FJ, Moley JF. Medullary thyroid carcinoma: including MEN 2A and MEN 2B syndromes. J Surg Oncol. 2005;89(3):122-9.
4. Learoyd DL, Messina M, Zedenius J, et al. Molecular genetics of thyroid tumors and surgical decision-making. World J Surg. 2000;24(8):922-33.
5. Zampi G, Carcangiu ML, Rosai J. Thyroid tumor pathology. Proceedings of an international workshop, San Miniato, Italy, October 1984. Semin Diagn Pathol. 1985;2(2):87-146.
6. Heffess CS, Thompson LD. Minimally invasive follicular thyroid carcinoma. Endocr Pathol. 2001;12(4):417-22.
7. Billimoria KY, Bentrem DJ, Ko CY, et al. Extent of surgery affects survival of papillary thyroid cancer. Ann Surg. 2007;246(3): 375-81.
8. Chen H, Udelsman R. Papillary thyroid carcinoma: justification for total thyroidectomy and management of lymph node metastases. Surg Oncol Clin N Am. 1998;7(4):645-63.
9. Mulligan LM, Kwok JB, Healey CS, et al. Germ-line mutation of the RET proto-oncogene in multiple endocrine neoplasia type 2A. Nature. 1993;363(6428):458-60.
10. Tisell LE, Hansson G, Jansson S, et al. Reoperation in treatment of asymptomatic metastasizing medullary thyroid carcinoma. Surgery. 1986;99(1):60-6.
11. American Thyroid Association (ATA) Guidelines Taskforce on Thyroid Nodules and Differentiated Thyroid Cancer, Cooper DS, Doherty GM, et al. Revised American Thyroid Association management guideline for patients with thyroid nodules and differentiated thyroid cancers. Thyroid. 2009;19(11): 1167-214.

23 Parathyroid Tumors

Praful Desai

INTRODUCTION

Though parathyroid tumors are rare, it is one of the more common endocrine neoplasms. As a consequence of high calcium and parathormone levels in parathyroid lesions, symptoms of hyperparathyroidism are often the presenting clinical features of a parathyroid adenoma in 80–85% of patients. Carcinoma of the parathyroid is uncommon and forms less than 10% of all parathyroid tumors. Hyperplasia of the parathyroid glands is another cause of primary hyperparathyroidism in about 10% of patients. Secondary hyperparathyroidism, in about 10% of patients is often associated with renal dysfunction which can lead to renal failure. Multiple endocrine neoplasia (MEN 1 and MEN 2A) is an inherited familial cancer syndrome often associated with tumors of the parathyroid glands.[1]

National Cancer Data Base[2] records nearly 100,000 new patients of primary hyperparathyroidism yearly in the USA. Parathyroid carcinomas form only 0.005% of all cancers.[2] Chronic hypercalcemia leading to renal failure often develop secondary hyperparathyroidism leading to cancer of the parathyroid glands. Rarely head and neck radiotherapy can trigger a parathyroid malignancy. The increase in number of parathyroid tumors in the atomic bomb survivors is well-documented.[3] Parathyroid tumors often form a component of MENs (MEN 1) in more than 90% and MEN 2A in around 25%.[4,5] Symptoms of primary hyperparathyroidism needs to be carefully investigated for exclusion of pancreatic and gastric tumors, carcinoids of the small gut and a parathyroid lesion. Usual symptoms of primary hyperparathyroidism are myopathies, asthma, osteoporosis, renal calculi or calcinosis; however, occasionally primary hyperparathyroidism may be asymptomatic. A parathyroid adenoma or carcinoma can also present without any components of MEN 1 or MEN 2A/2B. The latter is often associated with medullary cancer of the thyroid in almost all cases which are bilateral, multicentric and secrete calcitonin and carcinoembryonic antigen. A pheochromocytoma is also known to occur in this complex neoplastic endocrine pathology.

Clinical Features/Investigations/ Management

It is extremely rare to be able to palpate a parathyroid adenoma. Most often symptoms of anorexia, nausea, polyuria, weakness and fatigue are major components particularly when primary hyperparathyroidism (PHPT) is present. Unrecognized PHPT can lead to secondary hyperparathyroidism with chronic hypercalcemia and renal failure. A parathyroid carcinoma, untreated, can also result in end-stage renal disease.[6] Previous history of renal calculi, spontaneous fractures due to osteoporosis and bony pains may be the presenting symptoms (Figs 1A and B). This symptom syndrome should lead toward a clinical suspicion and appropriate biochemical investigations of serum parathormone, calcium, phosphorus and alkaline phosphatase levels should be obtained. An ultrasound and a computed tomography (CT) scan of the neck and mediastinum will help to locate the lesion, if present (Fig. 2). A sestamibi scan (nuclear medicine) can help to localize a parathyroid lesion, particularly if minimally invasive surgery is contemplated. It is rarely used with the availability of modern imaging techniques. Once identified, the presence of a parathyroid lesion should lead to further investigations. Associated MEN 1-2A syndrome by an abdominal CT scan will be determined by the presence of a gastrointestinal tract

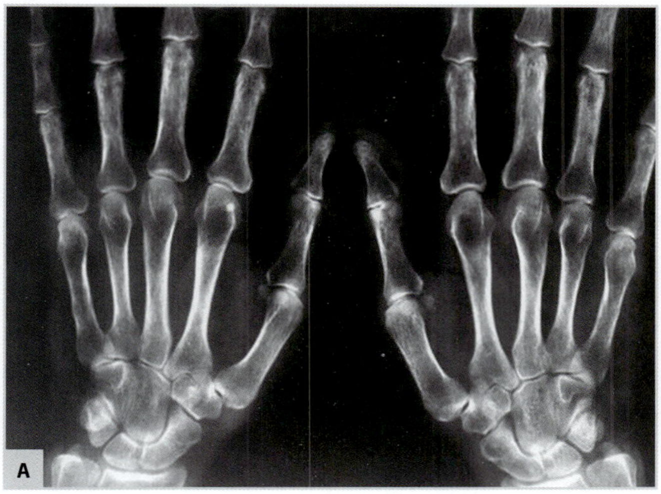

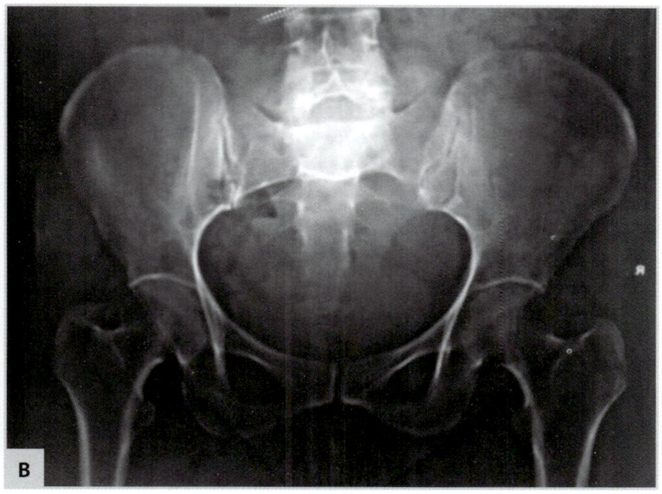

Figs 1A and B: X-rays of both hands and pelvis showing significant generalized osteoporosis

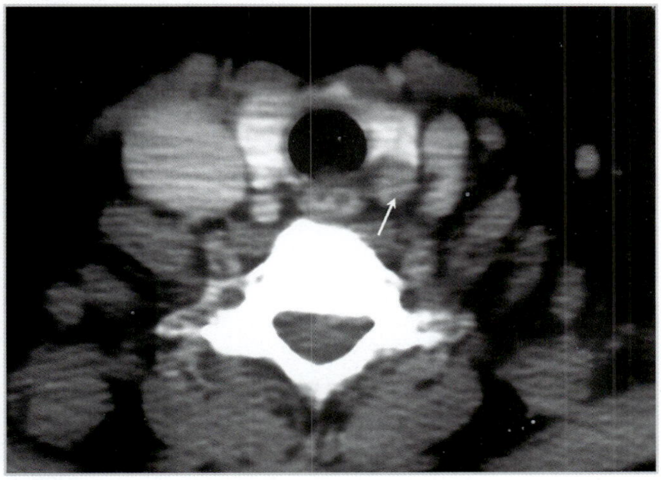

Fig. 2: Computed tomography (CT) scan image clearly defines the rounded shadow of the left inferior parathyroid lesion, inferior to the left lobe of the thyroid

lesion, a pheochromocytoma, gastrinoma, carcinoid or pancreatic neuroendocrine lesions.

The therapy of choice for a parathyroid lesion is a surgical excision. Careful exposure of other parathyroid glands and digital exploration of the superior mediastinum is mandatory (Figs 3A and B). In the presence of a large adenoma, the other parathyroids tend to be functionally suboptimal and sometimes difficult to locate. A thorough and careful exploration is mandatory to avoid a reoperation for a missed adenoma. Superior mediastinum is a rare site for a parathyroid lesion and a CT scan of the mediastinum will help to delineate it. Cancer of the parathyroid glands are rare but can present with a firm to hard neck mass, with fixity or even palpable neck node metastasis. In an advanced lesion, there could be fixity, invasion of vessels, recurrent laryngeal nerve palsy and rarely even infiltration of the trachea and/or esophagus.

The therapy of choice is always a surgical excision with radicality as feasible and indicated. The prognosis remains poor in an advanced lesion which can metastasize and disseminate like any malignancy. Even in a localized lobar carcinoma a total thyroidectomy is indicated if histology shows a carcinoma. Radiotherapy for a locally advanced nonresectable lesion may produce some palliation and chemotherapy with cyclophosphamide, methotrexate and adriamycin have been used with minor responses. A high index of suspicion should be exercised and a firm hard mass should arouse a doubt of a carcinoma. Effective surgical excision may result in survival rates of 13–78% at 10 years.[2] Local recurrence of 25–80% at 5 years are reported in various series.[2]

Hypercalcemic Crisis

Serum calcium levels higher than 15–17 mg/mL can produce a metabolic crisis and is known in parathyroid carcinoma or a long standing large benign adenoma. Extreme weakness, fatigue, polyuria and severe anorexia or nausea are common symptoms—occasionally acute pancreatitis is reported. This can also occur in the setting of associated MEN 1 type of syndrome.[7] Urgent management with hydration, diuretics (Lasix®), steroids and calcitonin are indicated. Intravenous octreotide and zoledronate may be added to reduce and control hypercalcemia. Hypocalcemia can occur postoperatively after excision of a parathyroid adenoma and intraoperative and postoperative calcium support is needed for a variable period of time till the normal parathyroids take over the function.

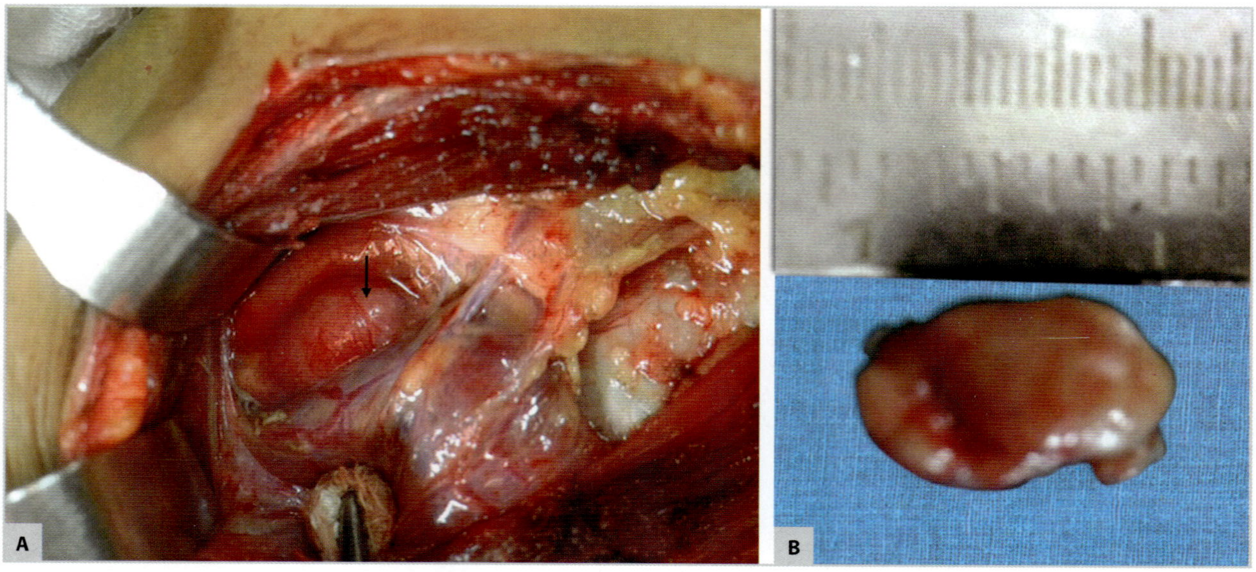

Figs 3A and B: (A) The parathyroid adenoma of the left inferior gland in this case, positioned posterior to the left thyroid lobe, which is mobilized and retracted anteriorly. The lesion abuts the left common carotid artery; (B) Operative specimen

REFERENCES

1. Westin G, Bjorklund P, Akerstrom G, et al. Molecular genetics of parathyroid disease. World J Surg. 2009;33(11):2224-33.
2. Rahbari R, Kebebew E. Parathyroid tumors. In: Devita VT, Lawrence TS, Rosenberg SA (Eds). Cancer, 9th edition. Philadelphia: Lippincott Williams & Wilkins; 2012. p. 1473.
3. Takeichi N, Dohi K, Ito H, et al. Parathyroid tumors in atomic bomb survivors in Hiroshima: a review. J Radiat Res. 1991;32(Suppl):189-92.
4. Fernandez-Ranvier GG, Khareafshar E, Tacha D, et al. Defining a molecular phenotype for benign and malignant parathyroid tumors. Cancer. 2009;115(2):334-44.
5. Abdelgadir AM, Untch BR, Olson JA. Parathyroid carcinoma: current understanding and new insights into gene expression and intraoperative parathyroid hormone kinetics. Oncologist. 2010;15(1):61-72.
6. Kamayama K, Takami H. DNA cytofluorometric analysis using HP/DAPI double staining of parathyroid carcinoma arising in a patient with chronic renal failure and secondary hyperparathyroidism. Oncol Rep. 1999;6(6):1345-7.
7. Dionisi S, Minisola S, Pepe J, et al. Concurrent parathyroid adenomas and carcinomas in the setting of MEN type 1: presentation as hypercalcemic crisis. Mayo Clin Proc. 2002;77(8):866-9.

24 The Metastatic Neck

Vijay Haribhakti

INTRODUCTION

The significance of cervical node metastasis has been recognized since long, and it has been classically said that the mere presence of cervical metastasis reduces survivals by half. The optimal approach and management of the neck, whether "at risk" or clinically positive, is thus absolutely fundamental to the effective management of head and neck cancer. With the exception of differentiated thyroid cancer, in which the presence of lymph node metastasis does not influence ultimate prognosis significantly, for all other histological subtypes the presence and the extent of metastatic disease impacts disease control and survival in a very significant way. Although this section specifically deals with metastatic squamous carcinoma, the conclusions are valid for all other subtypes.

ANATOMY OF THE FASCIA AND SPACES OF THE NECK

In order to understand the phenomenon of cervical metastasis and neck dissections that are employed to treat them, it is important to have a working knowledge of the fascia and spaces of the neck.

The deep fascia of the neck can be discussed under three main headings:

1. The superficial
2. The middle
3. The deep layers.

The superficial or investing layer of the deep cervical fascia originates in the posterior midline at the ligamentum nuchae and runs forward on either side like a muff around the neck and splits to enclose the sternocleidomastoid (SCM) muscles. Hence, the extent of the fascia in the anterolateral neck is from the anterior border of the trapezius muscle coming along the clavicle right up to the suprasternal notch below, and the lower border of the mandible above. The middle layer of the cervical fascia is the visceral layer that encloses the larynx, the esophagus and the thyroid gland. The third is the prevertebral layer of the fascia, which lies over the prevertebral muscles, and is penetrated by the roots of the brachial plexus as they emerge and course downward toward the upper limb.

TRIANGLES OF THE NECK

The neck is divided into a number of triangles by the manner in which certain muscles transverse the neck. The anterior triangle of the neck, which is bounded anteriorly by the midline, superiorly by the inferior border of the mandible and posterolaterally by the SCM muscle, consists of two triangles, divided by the superior belly of the omohyoid muscle. Above the superior belly of the omohyoid, the area is divided into two: the submandibular triangle, which is bounded inferiorly by the digastric muscle, and the carotid triangle between the digastric and the omohyoid. In front, under the chin and between the anterior bellies of the digastric muscles is the submental triangle. The SCM muscle is an important landmark in the neck and the upper part of it encloses an important space known as the submuscular recess, which is the space deep to the SCM muscles and bounded medially by the spinal accessory nerve (SAN). The splenius capitis muscle forms the floor of the recess, and it is an important station for nodal metastasis (level IIb). In general, metastatic disease in the neck follows an organized, predictable pattern of spread from above downward.

NECK LEVELS

Neck levels based on analysis of patterns of spread, the group at the Memorial Sloan Kettering Cancer Center, New York, developed the concept of neck levels. These levels are as follows:

Level I include nodes that are located above the digastric muscle. Level I is again subdivided as level 1A which is the submental triangle and level 1B which is the submandibular triangle. The nodes along the internal jugular veins are classified into three groups: (1) the upper; (2) mid; and (3) lower jugular nodes. The upper jugular nodes are a cluster just beneath the digastric muscle and therefore known as the subdigastric nodes. This is **level IIA**, which is the most important first station of spread for primaries originating in the oral cavity, larynx and pharynx. Below this at the level where the omohyoid crosses the SCM muscles is **level III**, which is the mid jugular nodes and all the way down in the neck along the jugular vein is **level IV**, which is the lower jugular node.

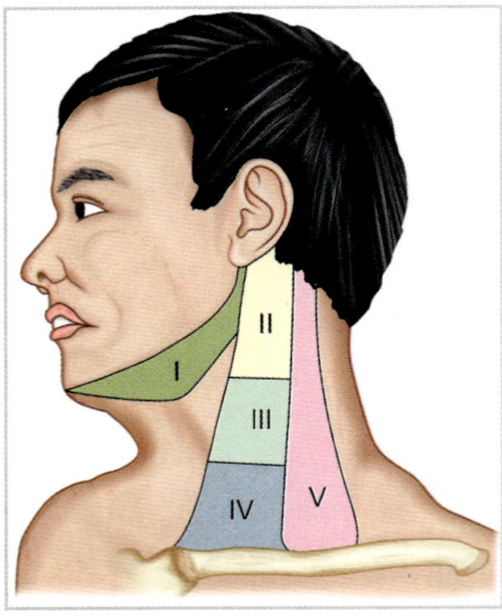

Fig. 1: Neck levels

Level II is subdivided into level IIA and IIB. Level IIA is the group of nodes anterior to the SAN while level IIB are the nodes behind it. This by some is considered to be the uppermost part of the **posterior triangle**, which is designated as **level V**. The nodes that are found in the **central compartment** of the neck between the carotid sheath structures and the viscera are the paratracheal and paraesophageal nodes, also known as **level VI nodes**. Further lower level nodes in the **superior mediastinum** are designated as **level VII**. The concept of levels has brought about complete standardization to the nomenclature of metastatic patterns in the neck.

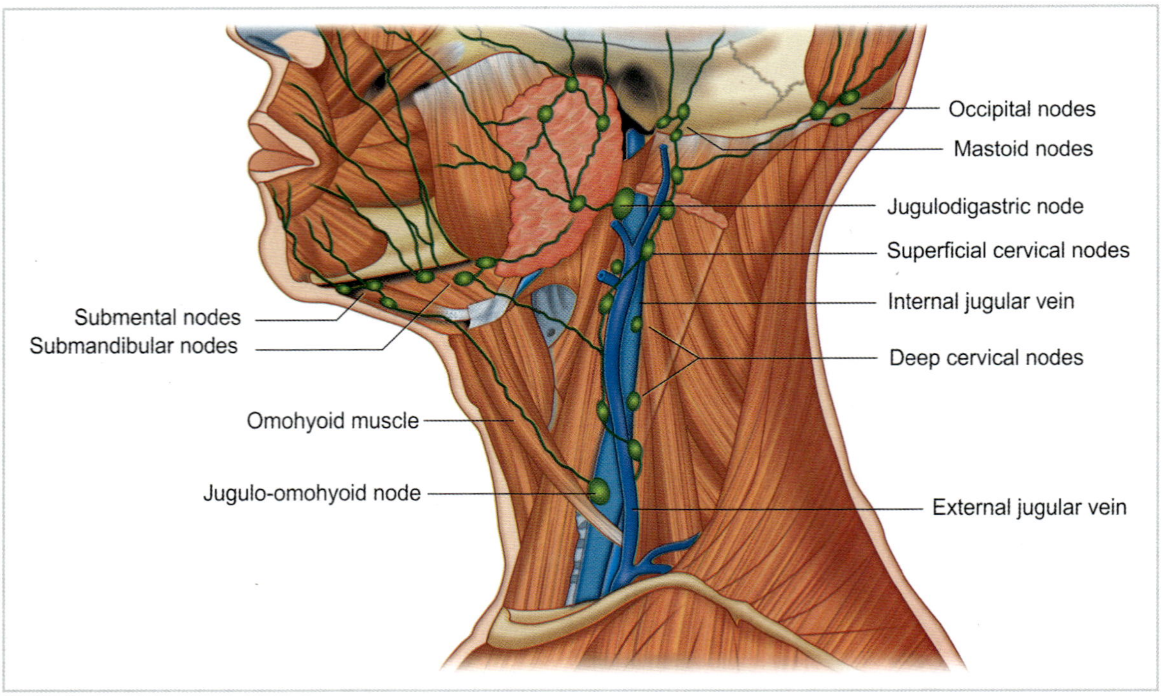

Fig. 2: Important nodal groups

DETERMINANTS OF NODAL METASTASIS

The presence of nodal metastasis is influenced by a variety of factors, of which the site of the primary is highly significant, as there are certain sites which are far more prone to metastatic spread than others. Those areas poor in capillary lymphatics have a low tendency to metastatic spread while those that are richly bathed in capillary lymphatics have much higher proclivity. For example, the free margins of the vocal cord have a practically zero possibility, with hardly 1% incidence of nodal metastasis for an early tumor. On the other hand, for a nasopharyngeal primary the incidence of nodal metastasis is about 80%. In the oral cavity when it concerns the cheek, the more posterior the growth, the more is the propensity for metastatic spread. The tongue by and large is very rich in lymphatics and very prone to metastatic spread. As one moves back from the tip of the tongue to the base, the extent of metastatic spread increases dramatically. The floor of the mouth is also an area highly prone to metastatic spread. In the larynx, while primary glottic cancers hardly ever spread to the nodes, supraglottic cancers spread freely to the nodes, central lesions invading the preepiglottic space manifesting bilateral spread. All subsites in the pharynx, whether nasopharynx, oropharynx or hypopharynx, have a high proclivity for metastatic spread.

Tumor cells that metastasize invade deep down across the basement membrane, then invade into the capillary lymphatics, and through capillary lymphatics are either transmitted down along lymphatic chains to the draining lymph nodes or into the blood stream from which they can again get trapped by lymph nodes. Each node has a hilum through which vessels enter and exit. One of the major hallmarks of metastatic presence in the nodes is an alteration in hilar characteristics of a node. If the hilum is displaced, it is an abnormal finding; and if it is completely destroyed it is almost certain that the node is metastatic. Another important feature of the metastatic nodes is the presence of central necrosis. The T stage of the primary is the next important determinant. More importantly, it is the thickness of the primary and the depth of invasion, which are linked to the risk of metastasis.

CLINICAL FEATURES

The detection of metastatic nodes first requires a thorough clinical examination. Clinical examination of the neck first involves inspection, which reveals only those nodes that are grossly enlarged and frequently invaded. Palpation is important and should be carried out with the anterior muscles of the neck relaxed by flexing the patient's neck gently forward, with the examiner standing behind the patient. With this, all areas of the neck are carefully palpated keeping in mind the presence, size, consistency, multiplicity and mobility of nodes. In general, nodes that are firm to hard are more likely to contain metastasis.

The ultrasound[1] is a useful and important modality for detection of nodal metastasis. The size of the node, characteristics of its hilum, the presence of central necrosis and the overall architecture is noted. Importantly ultrasound permits guided fine needle biopsy, which is simple and accurate method of diagnosing nodal metastasis. Open biopsy for diagnosis of metastatic disease is best avoided. The anatomical imaging modalities for the neck include computed tomography (CT) and magnetic resonance imaging (MRI). A size greater than 1–1.5 cm, spherical shape and central necrosis are highly suspect for metastatic disease. Presence of extracapsular spread is often possible to demonstrate on a MRI. The other method today is the positron emission tomography-computed tomography (PET-CT) scan. The presence of nodes with the above characteristics, with significant standardized uptake value is an indication of metastatic disease. False negative results due to inflammatory nodes are not uncommon. Only histology gives the final answer.

STAGING (TABLE 1)

TABLE 1: Staging of the neck is based upon size, laterality and multiplicity

NX	Regional lymph nodes cannot be assessed
N0	There is no regional node metastasis
N1	Metastasis is in a single ipsilateral lymph node, 3 cm or less in greatest dimension
N2	Metastasis is in a single ipsilateral lymph node, more than 3 cm but not more than 6 cm in greatest dimension; or metastasis is in multiple ipsilateral lymph nodes, none more than 6 cm in greatest dimension; or metastasis is in bilateral or contralateral lymph nodes, none greater than 6 cm in greatest dimension
N2a	Metastasis is in a single ipsilateral lymph node, more than 3 cm but not more than 6 cm in greatest dimension
N2b	Metastasis is in multiple ipsilateral lymph nodes, none more than 6 cm in greatest dimension
N2c	Metastasis is in a bilateral or contralateral lymph node, none more than 6 cm in greatest dimension
N3	Metastasis is in a lymph node, more than 6 cm in greatest dimension

The most important prognostic indicators in a neck dissection are as follows:[2-4]

- Nodal size
- Number of nodes
- Extracapsular spread
- Levels involved
- Lymphovascular emboli (LVE).

MANAGEMENT OF THE METASTATIC NECK

Appropriate management of the metastatic neck is crucially important for many reasons. Information regarding nodal status is the single most significant prognostic determinant for any disease and guides vital decisions concerning adjuvant therapy. Furthermore, control of neck disease is vital, as uncontrolled disease heralds distant spread, local recurrence and compromises survivorship. Surgical management of the neck involves planning of an appropriate neck dissection, based on the clinical staging of the neck. Neck dissections today are classified as either comprehensive, which include all levels (I-V) or selective, in which selected levels are dissected. In a clinically negative (N0) neck, the dissection is probably prophylactic and essentially for staging, while in a clinically positive (N+) neck, the dissection is therapeutic.

The N0 Neck

It is important to decide whether to perform a prophylactic neck dissection or a sentinel node biopsy, or to carefully follow-up the patient. The decision to do a prophylactic neck dissection depends on the site and the stage of the primary lesion and the assumed risk of metastatic spread. When approach to a primary lesion requires the elevation of a cheek flap involving exposure of the neck, a prophylactic neck dissection is worthwhile. At the present time, routine sentinel node biopsy is not considered a standard of care, and must be performed within the context of a clinical trial. The type of prophylactic neck dissection performed for a given primary depends upon the site and to a lesser extent, the stage of the primary cancer. For the N0 neck from oral primaries the levels to be addressed are I, II and III, with the exception of the oral tongue, where high staged and thick primary tumors require level IV to be included in dissection. Accordingly, the most common prophylactic neck dissection for oral primaries (level I–III) is the supraomohyoid neck dissection, with level IV being included in selected cases. For the larynx and the pharynx and other midline sites, levels II, III and IV have to be addressed. Additionally, level VI is included in a number of cases. For tumors originating in the eyelids, facial skin and parotid gland, it is important to clear the pre and periparotid nodes, the level IIb nodes and the posterior triangle nodes as well.

The N1 Neck

In the presence of a single involved node it is necessary to perform a selective neck dissection encompassing levels I–IV for oral cavity primaries, or levels II–VI for midline primaries.

The N2 Neck

For the N2 neck, it is generally advisable to perform a comprehensive neck dissection incorporating all nodal groups at risk. With bilateral metastatic nodes, bilateral dissections are necessary, sparing at least one internal jugular vein. An ipsilateral comprehensive and contralateral selective neck dissection may also be possible in individually selected cases.

The N3 Neck

In the presence of massive neck disease, it is important to establish the anatomical relationship of the mass with the carotid artery. In cases where the common carotid is not encased, surgical resection remains the initial treatment of choice. With common carotid encasement, concomitant chemoradiation or sequential therapy (neoadjuvant chemotherapy followed by chemoradiation), followed by surgery are the alternatives. Carotid artery resection and grafting for metastatic squamous carcinoma is generally inadvisable and hardly ever performed. In previously untreated patients, it may be possible to resect almost all disease, leaving a minimal plaque of disease on the carotid wall, tagged with radiopaque clips. This area is frequently covered with a small muscle flap and subjected to postoperative chemoradiation.

NOMENCLATURE OF NECK DISSECTIONS

The classical radical neck dissection (RND), incorporates levels I to V and sacrifices three important structures, namely the sternomastoid muscle (SCM), internal jugular vein (IJV), and spinal accessory nerve (SAN). Currently, any neck dissection that incorporates levels I to V is termed a 'comprehensive' neck dissection, or modified radical neck dissection (MRND). The three types of MRND are named according to the structures preserved: In MRND 1, only the SAN is preserved. In MRND 2, the SAN and IJV are preserved. In MRND 3 (functional neck dissection, FND, described by Bocca of Italy), all three structures are preserved.

Selective Neck Dissections

The nomenclature of selective neck dissections is based upon the levels dissected. They are as follows:

- Supraomohyoid dissection (I, II, III)
- Lateral neck dissection (II, III, IV)
- Anterolateral neck dissection (I–IV)
- Posterolateral neck dissection (II–V).

THE SURGICAL PATHOLOGY REPORT

A complete surgical pathology report of the neck should include information on the number of metastatic nodes involved from those dissected, the levels and the presence of capsular invasion and perinodal infiltration and extracapsular spread.[5]

Extent of involvement varies tremendously in spectrum from micrometastasis on the one hand, in which only a single 2 mm focus or just free tumor cells may be detected, to complete effacement of nodal architecture. Beyond micrometastasis is minimal disease, where there is tumor without involvement of the capsule. The next stage and most important prognostically is the presence of extracapsular spread. The presence of extracapsular spread is a vital prognostic indicator and is a reflection of the need for aggressive treatment in the form of chemoradiation.[6-9]

CONCLUSION

The management of the metastatic neck is one of the most important aspects in the care of a head and neck patient. Frequent morbidity and mortality results from metastatic disease in the neck despite the control of the primary lesion. Every positive neck, therefore, must be adequately addressed. If the primary modality of treatment is surgery, an appropriate neck dissection must be performed. After completion of the primary mode of treatment (radiotherapy and/or chemotherapy), it is necessary to watch the patient carefully and if indicated to either do a planned neck dissection following completion of initial treatment, or to follow the patient clinically and with PET-CT if needed to decide whether or not a neck dissection is mandated. The N0 neck is managed either by a "wait and watch" conservative approach when the assumed risk of spread is very low. With increasing risk or when the neck is anyway opened in order to approach the primary, an appropriate selective neck dissection is performed.

REFERENCES

1. Sureshkannan P; Vijayprabhu, John R. Role of ultrasound in detection of metastatic neck nodes in patients with oral cancer. Indian J Dent Res. 2011;22(3):419-23.
2. Köhler HF, Kowalski LP. Prognostic impact of the level of neck metastasis in oral cancer patients. Braz J Otorhinolaryngol. 2012;78(6):15-20.
3. Amar A, Chedid HM, Rapoport A, et al. Prognostic significance of the number of lymph nodes in elective neck dissection for tongue and mouth floor cancers. Braz J Otorhinolaryngol. 2012;78(2):22-6.
4. Park SM, Lee DJ, Chung EJ, et al. Conversion from selective to comprehensive neck dissection: is it necessary for occult nodal metastasis? 5-year observational study. Clin Exp Otorhinolaryngol. 2013;6(2):94-8.
5. Wan XC, Egloff AM, Johnson J. Histological assessment of cervical lymph node identifies patients with head and neck squamous cell carcinoma (HNSCC): who would benefit from chemoradiation after surgery? Laryngoscope. 2012;122(12):2712-22.
6. Pendleton KP, Grandis JR. Cisplatin-based chemotherapy options for recurrent and/or metastatic squamous cell cancer of the head and neck. Clin Med Insights Ther. 2013;2013(5).
7. Specenier P, Vermorken JB. Cetuximab: its unique place in head and neck cancer treatment. Biologics. 2013;7:77-90.
8. Rangaraju RR, Sharma JB, Dewan AK, et al. Palliative weekly chemotherapy along with cetuximab in recurrent and metastatic head and neck cancers: a retrospective analysis. Indian J Cancer. 2012;49(1):1-5.
9. Pergolizzi S, Santacaterina A, Adamo B, et al. Induction chemotherapy with paclitaxel and cisplatin to concurrent radiotherapy and weekly paclitaxel in the treatment of loco-regionally advanced, stage IV (M0), head and neck squamous cell carcinoma. Mature results of a prospective study. Radiat Oncol. 2011;6:162.

25 The Role of Diagnostic and Therapeutic Endoscopy in Digestive Tract Malignancies

Samir Parikh

INTRODUCTION

Digestive tract cancers (DC) are a major cause of morbidity and mortality worldwide. Its prevalence is likely to rise due to rising longevity, increasing incidence of obesity and higher consumption of alcohol or smoking. The annual incidence of highly lethal cancers like pancreas equals its annual death rates. At present the cure rates of DC are poor due to the delay in diagnosis, inadequate visual inspection, errors of interpretation, lesion subtlety, inaccurate staging, nonavailability of technology or expertise, high cost of therapy, poor awareness and socioeconomic constraints.

Endoscopy has taken center stage in the diagnosis/therapy of various DC as it allows visualization and targeted biopsy under direct vision. Newer endoscopic techniques of chromoendoscopy (CE) and narrow band imaging (NBI) help to identify premalignant and early lesions. Development of video capsule endoscopy (VCE) or enteroscopy and cholangioscopy techniques now allow visualization of small bowel and bile duct respectively. Endoscopic ultrasonography (EUS) accurately evaluates locoregional stage of DC to offer algorithm-based individualized treatment. Endoscopic ultrasonography-guided fine needle aspiration biopsy (FNAB) improves diagnostic accuracy especially in resectable pancreatic head lesions. Endoscopic ultrasonography is complementary to computed tomography-positron emission tomography/magnetic resonance imaging (CT-PET/MRI) in overall staging of DC. A diagnostic laparoscopy for T3-T4 stomach/colon cancer can detect peritoneal disease and avoid morbidity of unnecessary exploration.

Endoscopic therapy of premalignant lesions prevents development of DC. Endoscopic polypectomy and radio-frequency ablation (RFA) of Barrett's esophagus (BE) play an important role in prevention of colorectal cancer (CRC) and adenocarcinoma of esophagus (ACE) respectively. Endoscopic mucosal resection (EMR) and endoscopic submucosal dissection (ESD) can cure early mucosal luminal DC with organ preservation and lower morbidity compared to surgical resection. Advances in individual skills, better optics and instrumentation have allowed current generation oncosurgeons to use laparoscopy in select cases for resection of DC. In the years ahead natural orifice transluminal endoscopic surgery (NOTES) may evolve. Transanal resection of rectosigmoid cancer is an exciting development. Endoscopic closure of a postoperative leak, application of hemoclips for anastomotic bleeds and balloon dilation of postresection or radiotherapy strictures is considered standard of care in most centers. Endoscopy plays an important role in annual postoperative surveillance for luminal DC. Placing endoluminal stents to bypass an obstruction in advanced DC allows palliation with least morbidity, lower cost and lesser hospital stay. Endoscopic ultrasonography-guided celiac plexus neurolysis (CPN) is a simple technique to palliate pain in terminally ill patients.

Endoscopy, therefore, plays an important role in diagnosis, treatment, prevention and palliation of DC. Improved cure or care in DC is possible with emphasis on early diagnosis, accurate staging, stage based individualized treatment, health awareness and regular follow-ups. Future guidelines for the treatment of premalignant conditions, endoscopic resection of early cancers, use of laparoscopic resections/NOTES, follow-up timings after neoadjuvant chemoradiotherapy need to be standardized and should be sensitive to healthcare resources.

PREMALIGNANT/DYSPLASTIC LESIONS OF DIGESTIVE TRACT

Majority of DC arise from the mucosa. Endoscopic serial evaluations have allowed clinicians to understand the progression of mucosal inflammation to various grades of dysplasia to the development of mucosal cancers. Routine white light endoscopy (WLE) fails to differentiate areas of inflammation from dysplasia and has a miss rate of about 30% to detect intramucosal cancers.[1] High definition endoscopes, newer endoscopic techniques of CE/NBI improve sensitivity and specificity of detecting dysplasia by allowing targeted biopsy.[2-6]

Barrett's esophagus is a metaplastic columnar lined mucosa containing goblet cells most often seen in patients with reflux esophagitis. Relative risk of developing ACE in BE is 30 to 125 times compared to the control population.[7] White light endoscopy is usually sufficient to suspect BE (Fig. 1A). Current recommendations of taking four quadrant biopsies every 1–2 cm in BE is labor intensive, suboptimal and technically difficult.[8] Chromoendoscopy using Lugol's iodine as a staining agent is practised since the last four decades in countries like China with high prevalence of squamous cell carcinoma of esophagus (SCC). Lugol's iodine reacts with glycogen present in mature squamous cell and gives it a "silk crape" appearance. Unstained portion of esophageal mucosa have high chance of high-grade dysplasia (HGD) or carcinoma in situ.[9] Observing a pink color in unstained portion 3 minutes after Lugol's iodine enhances the sensitivity, specificity and positive predictive value to detect HGD/SCC.[2] Loss of mucosal regularity; dilated, elongated and tortuous capillaries on NBI suggest presence of HGD/SCC.[3] An important caveat in the screening programs is to recruit high-risk individuals with premalignant/dysplastic lesions. Both CE and NBI enhance mucosal viewing by increasing contrast. Both techniques are safe, easily available, need experience and allow targeted biopsy in segments of BE to detect dysplasia/carcinoma in situ (Figs 1B and C).[10,11] Recent techniques of confocal laser endomicroscopy (CLE) enhance detection rates of dysplasia/malignancy in BE.[12-14] Narrow band imaging and CLE can detect post-treatment BE/BE with dysplasia.[15,16]

Helicobacter pylori (*H. pylori*) associated chronic gastritis leads to the development of intestinal metaplasia (IM). Intestinal metaplasia is a metaplastic precancerous transformation of gastric mucosa. Type III IM which has brush border, cellular disarray and abundant sulfomucin is premalignant. Presence of diffuse IM carries higher risk for developing adenocarcinoma of stomach (ACS). Detection of IM on WLE is extremely difficult. Narrow band imaging of gastric mucosa is helpful in detecting IM. A light blue crest sign on NBI is highly sensitive to detect IM.[17] Irregular or absent microvascular architecture together with irregular or absent microsurface structures on NBI magnifying endoscopy has high sensitivity to detect mucosal cancers in intestinal metaplastic tissue.[18] Methylene blue stains only dysplastic tissue and is not absorbed by normal gastric mucosa. Chromoendoscopy using methylene blue stain can allow endoscopist to biopsy areas of dysplasia. The degree of heterogenous uptake of the dye directly relates to the degree of dysplasia.[19]

Adenomatous polyp with dysplasia is a premalignant lesion of the colon. White light endoscopy often fails to detect small, sessile serrated polyps in the right colon. High definition WLE, cap-assisted colonoscopy, wide angle colonoscopes, fuse endoscopes and third eye retroscopes have reduced miss rates of polyps in ascending colon.[20-23] Current recommendations for surveillance colonoscopy in patients with ulcerative colitis suggest multiple random biopsies every 10–15 cm distance. This method is labor intensive, time consuming and difficult.

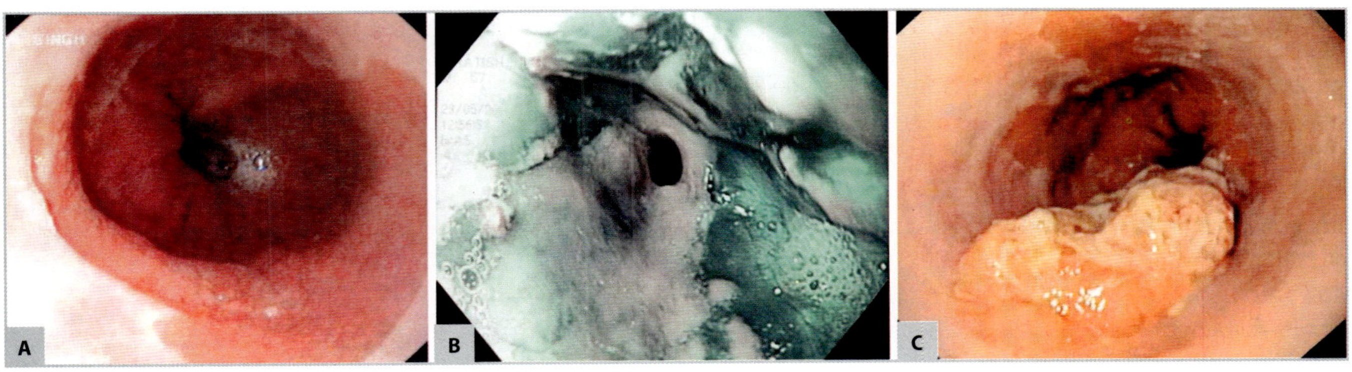

Figs 1A to C: (A) White light endoscopy showing pink mucosa above the Z-line (Barrett's esophagus); (B) Narrow band imaging (NBI) image showing ulcerated dysplastic Barrett's mucosa with stricture; (C) Barrett's mucosa with polypoidal ulcerated adenocarcinoma

Pit pattern type	Characteristics
I	Roundish pits
II	Stellar or papillary pits
III S	Small roundish or tubular pits (smaller than type I pits)
III L	Large roundish or tubular pits (larger than type I pits)
IV	Branch-like or gyrus-like pits
V	Nonstructured pits

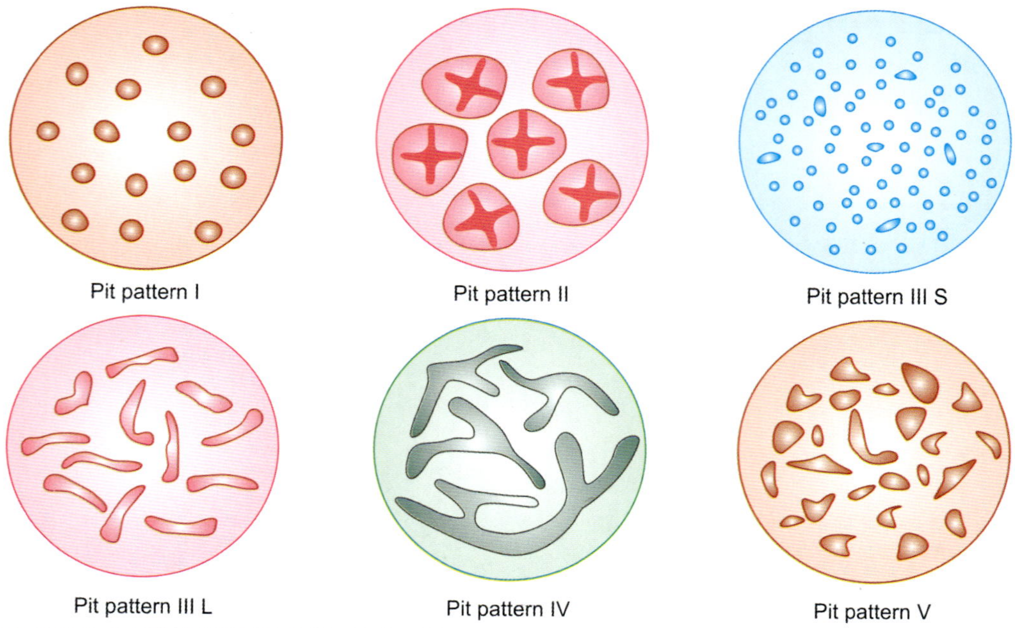

Fig. 2: Kudo's pit pattern

Use of methylene blue stain and CLE in such situation is extremely useful to detect areas of dysplasia whereas NBI is not effective in detection of dysplasia in patients with colitis.[24-26] White light endoscopy fails to differentiate non-neoplastic polyps from neoplastic polyps.[27] Narrow band imaging helps differentiate benign from malignant polyps allowing a recent concept of resect and discard benign polyps without its histological evaluation.[28-30] Narrow band imaging magnifying endoscopy can characterize pit pattern. Kudo's pit pattern (Fig. 2) helps to differentiate non-neoplastic polyp (type I and II) from neoplastic polyps (type III, IV and V)[31] (Fig. 3). Thus, advances in endoscope, endoscopic techniques and improved optical imaging may reduce interval colon cancers in patients on surveillance. Identifying premalignant lesions, dysplasia and intramucosal cancers at an earlier stage will be of immense benefit.

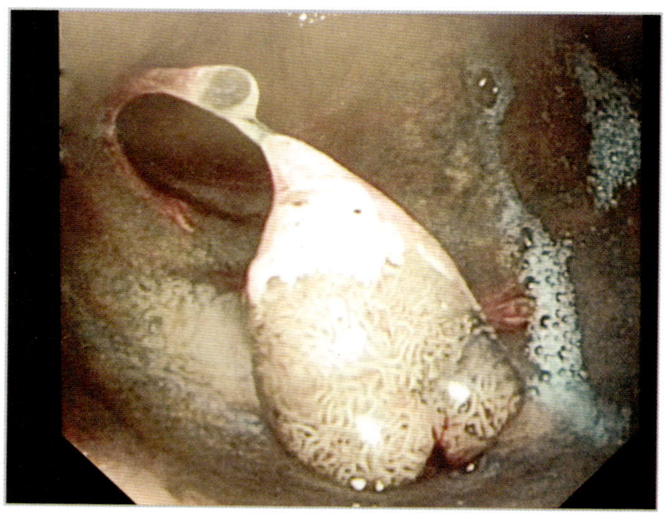

Fig. 3: Narrow band imaging (NBI) image showing Kudo's IIIL pattern, malignant adenomatous polyp

TABLE 1: Various premalignant conditions of digestive tract

Premalignant conditions	
Esophagus	Squamous cell cancer • SCC of aerodigestive tract • Plummer-Vinson syndrome • Zenker's diverticulum • Corrosive/radiation stricture • Primary achalasia cardia Adenocarcinoma • Reflux esophagitis • Barrett's mucosa•
Stomach	Adenocarcinoma • Multifocal atrophic gastritis • Type III intestinal metaplasia • Adenomatous polyp • Fundic polyp > 1 cm in FAP • Gastrojejunostomy for gastric ulcer. • Menetrier's disease • *H. pylori* gastritis (MALT)
Gall bladder and bile duct	Adenocarcinoma • Stones > 1 cm • Anomalous union of pancreaticobiliary ductal system • Adenomyomatosis • Porcelain gall bladder (type II and III)•+ • Primary sclerosing cholangitis • Adenomatous polyps (> 1 cm, rapidly growing)•+ • Caroli's disease, choledochal cyst+ • Hepatolithiasis+
Ampulla	Adenocarcinoma • Ampullary adenoma in FAP•+ • Gardner's syndrome•+
Pancreas	Adenocarcinoma • Hereditary pancreatitis• • Chronic pancreatitis
Colon	Adenocarcinoma • Adenomatous polyps• • Long standing ulcerative pancolitis•

• Surveillance recommended
+ Treatment at diagnosis recommended
•+ Surveillance and treatment recommended
(*Abbreviations:* SCC, squamous cell carcinoma; FAP, familial adenomatous polyposis; MALT, mucosa-associated lymphoid tissue)

Various premalignant conditions of digestive tract are mentioned in Table 1.

The usual sequence of events for development of mucosal cancers is demonstrated in Flow chart 1.

Flow chart 1: Usual sequence of events for development of mucosal cancers

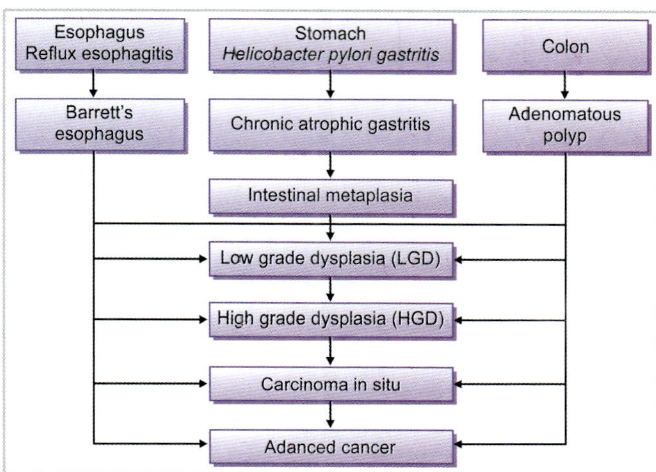

Despite the ability of newer technology to identify dysplasia on endoscopy (virtual histology) the gold standard for its confirmation remains histology. During surveillance the interval between endoscopies depend on the stage of sequence identified on histology. Endoscopic biopsies are performed every 3–5 years if no dysplasia identified, 1–2 yearly if LGD and 6 monthly if HGD is detected in patients with premalignant conditions of DC. Patients with dysplasia may be treated with ablative/endoscopic resection whereas those with carcinoma in situ require EMR/ESD. Just as anti *H. pylori* medical treatment prevents gastric cancers, hepatitis B vaccine prevents hepatocellular cancers, endoscopic detection and treatment of premalignant/early dysplastic tissue can prevent DC.

DIAGNOSIS AND STAGING OF DIGESTIVE CANCERS

Esophagus

Squamous cell carcinoma and ACE account for 95% of esophageal malignant tumors. Short duration, progressive dysphagia in an elderly patient is a common form of presentation. An early stage esophageal cancer appears on endoscopy as superficial plaque, nodule or small ulcer. They are better characterized by CE/NBI which often guides biopsy. A tumor above the submucosa on EUS can be treated by EMR/ESD. About 75% of patients present at an advanced stage with an ulcerated mass, circumferential involvement, a stricture or a tracheoesophageal fistula. Exact location (cervical vs mid esophageal vs lower third), length of the lesion (< 5 cm vs > 5 cm), type (circumferential vs. eccentric), morphology (proliferative vs stricturous) and presence of a fistula have to be recorded as it has direct implications on therapy. Multiple biopsies (about 7) gives least sampling error.[32] Cytology is useful in patients with malignant tight strictures.[32] Once the diagnosis is established EUS is used for locoregional staging and integrated CT-PET for distant disease.[33,34] Endoscopic ultrasonography is more reliable in diagnosing celiac lymph node involvement.[33] A malignant node appears round, hypoechoic, more than 1 cm in size with clear margins. Fine-needle aspiration cytology/fine-needle aspiration biopsy (FNAC/FNAB) is required only in a doubtful node not fulfilling all the above criteria. Patients undergoing PET-CT and EUS both have better outcomes compared to those in whom a single modality is used.[35] Some centers perform bronchoscopy for tumors above carina and laparoscopy for lower third tumors to accurately stage them.[36,37] Both integrated PET-CT and EUS have low sensitivity and specificity to detect residual tumors after neoadjuvant chemoradiotherapy.[38] Reduction in cross sectional volume by 50% on EUS, negative biopsy on esophagoscopy and negative FNAB of lymph node on EUS suggests a good response, high resection rates and better survival post-neoadjuvant chemoradiotherapy.[39,40]

Stomach

Most gastric cancers are diagnosed at a stage where curative resection is not possible (Fig. 4). Anemia,

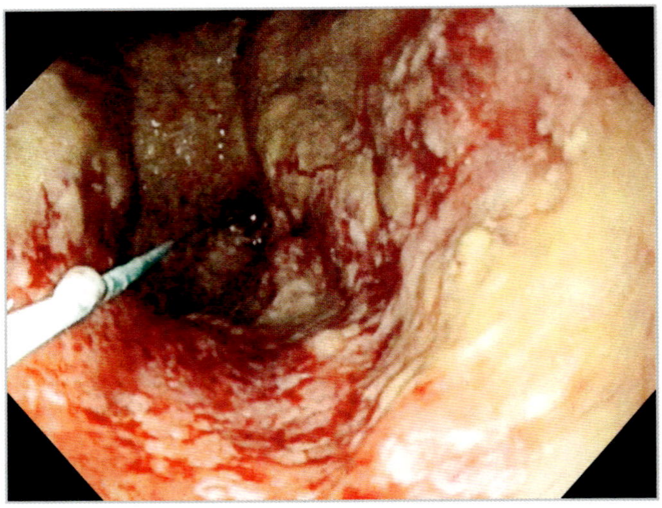

Fig. 4: Diffuse gastric body and antral adenocarcinoma

anorexia, weight loss and vomiting are usual presenting symptoms. All gastric ulcers unlike duodenal ulcers must be biopsied. Even if biopsy from a gastric ulcer is negative a repeat endoscopy after 8 weeks of proton pump inhibitor therapy demonstrating complete healing is the surest way to demonstrate absence of malignancy. Patients with linitis plastica may need well/bite biopsies or even snaring of mucosa to demonstrate malignancy. An early stage intramucosal cancer confirmed on EUS can be treated by EMR/ESD. Integrated PET-CT is accurate to identify nodes and distant metastasis but is ineffective in detecting peritoneal disease.[41] Diagnostic laparoscopy is ideal for diagnosis of peritoneal disease in patients with T3/T4 stage disease.[42]

Small Bowel

Small bowel tumors contribute only 2% of DC despite accounting for 75% of its length and 90% of its mucosa. Common form of presentation include obscure gastrointestinal bleed, anemia, intestinal obstruction, weight loss and intussusception.[43,44] Delay in diagnosis (average about 8 months) and metastasis at the time of detection (about 50%) is related to poor diagnostic yield on CT/MRI/barium studies.[45,46] Neuroendocrine tumors (~ 36%), adenocarcinoma (~ 31%), lymphoma (~ 19%) and gastrointestinal stromal tumors (GISTs ~ 10%) constitute majority of all small bowel tumors.[47] Most adenocarcinoma and Indian lymphomas are proximally located whereas neuroendocrine tumors and western lymphomas are distal. Video capsule endoscopy (VCE) and enteroscopic viewing of small bowel is now performed in most centers as its sensitivity and specificity is higher compared to CT/MRI enteroclysis. Video capsule endoscopy images can

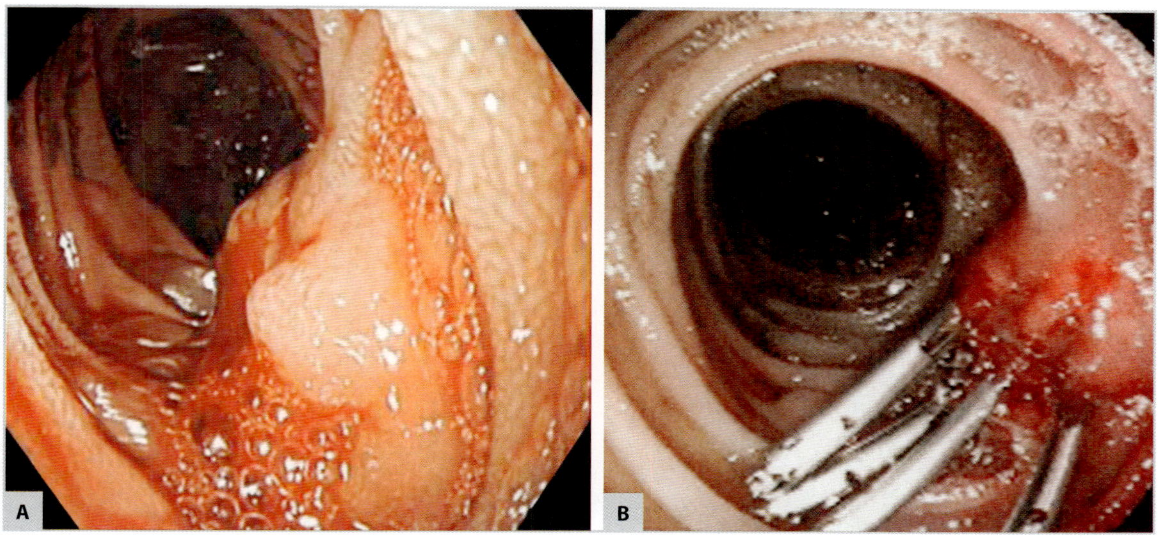

Figs 5A and B: (A) Jejunal ulcerated leiomyoma with bleed; (B) Hemoclips applied, hemostasis achieved

be manipulated to achieve virtual chromoendoscopy to enhance detection or characterization of mucosal lesions.[48] On VCE presence of bleeding, mucosal disruption, mucosal irregularity, polypoidal appearance, change of color are considered major criteria and delayed passage, white villi, invagination are considered as minor criteria to detect malignant tumors.[49] Video capsule endoscopy can miss upto one-third of tumors and ampulla of Vater is seen in only 10%.[50,51] Retention of capsule (> 2 weeks), obstruction (in 24 hours) and inability to take biopsy or offer any therapy are limiting factors of VCE. Currently, patency capsule (dissolves in 40 hours) is under evaluation in patients with suspected malignant stricture.[52] Video capsule endoscopy is recommended every 2–3 yearly in patients with Peutz-Jeghers syndrome and familial adenomatous polyposis (FAP) to detect development of cancer. Patients with lesions within two-thirds of small bowel capsule transit time (in 6 hours) can have tissue diagnosis/polypectomy with per-oral enteroscopes (single balloon/double balloon/spiral) (Figs 5A and B).[53,54] Polypectomy compared to polyp biopsy is the most reliable method to prove or exclude malignancy in a polyp. Cost of equipment, time taken to perform procedure, need for anesthesia and a long learning curve are current problems with the use of the enteroscopes. Perforation and pancreatitis occur in less than 5% patients undergoing enteroscopy.[53]

Colorectal

Colorectal cancer surveillance and screening has marginally reduced the mortality related to colorectal cancer (CRC). Most CRC present as endoluminal masses with ulcerated, necrotic and friable mucosa. Circumferential involvement correlates with "apple-core" appearance on barium/CT imaging and often presents as intestinal obstruction. In patients with Lynch syndrome, synchronous lesions are often identified necessitating complete colonoscopic evaluation. Flat nongranular lesions in right colon are the most common cause of a missed CRC. Effective bowel preparation, detailed evaluation, examination on withdrawal, longer inspection time and high performance skill is required to reduce miss rates. If an EMR/ESD is performed for intramucosal cancer and its adequacy is in doubt proximal segment must be tattooed to help surgeon identify the location. Complete removal of the polyp is the best way to avoid sampling error of biopsies (Figs 6A and B). If a polyp can be lifted by injecting at its base (lift sign) it is unlikely to have submucosal disease. For pedunculated polyps a part of polyp stalk must be sent for histological evaluation. Endoscopic ultrasonography is superior to CT/MRI for locoregional staging of rectal cancers.[55] Endoscopic ultrasonography alters treatment protocol in about 30% patients with rectal cancers.[56] All pararectal lymph nodes are pathological as healthy individuals have no pararectal nodes. Endoscopic ultrasonography is superior to CT/MRI to detect recurrences.[57] Post-surgery/chemoradiotherapy EUS is performed 3 monthly for first 2 years and then 6 monthly in rectal cancers.[57]

Pancreaticobiliary

Ultrasonography is a sensitive method to diagnose malignant biliary obstruction. Computed tomography/magnetic resonance imaging are more sensitive and specific to identify the site and cause of obstructive

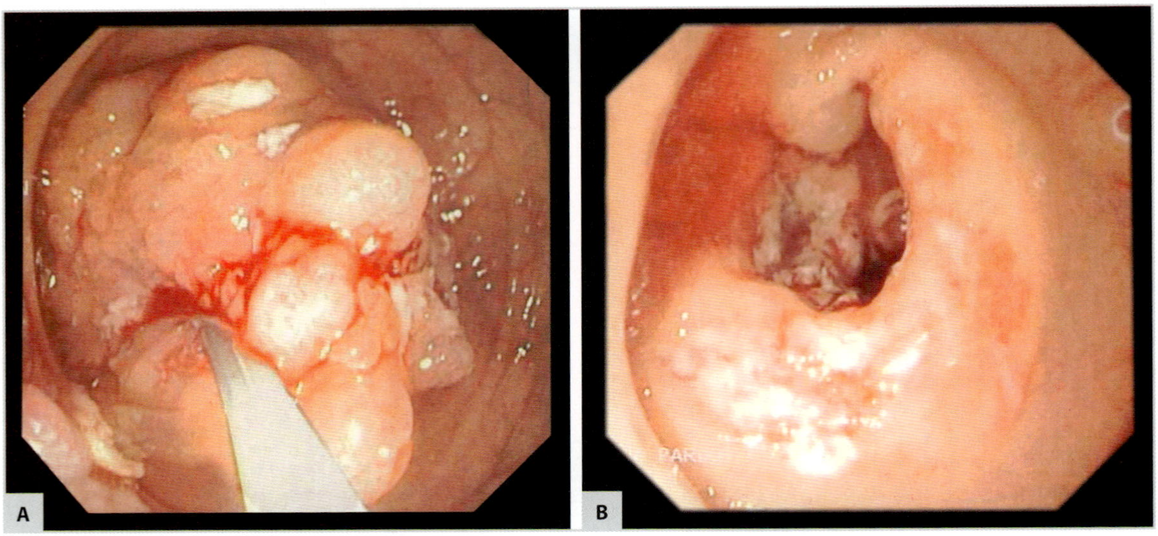

Figs 6A and B: (A) Large rectal villous adenoma, with low-grade dysplasia; (B) Piece meal polypectomy done

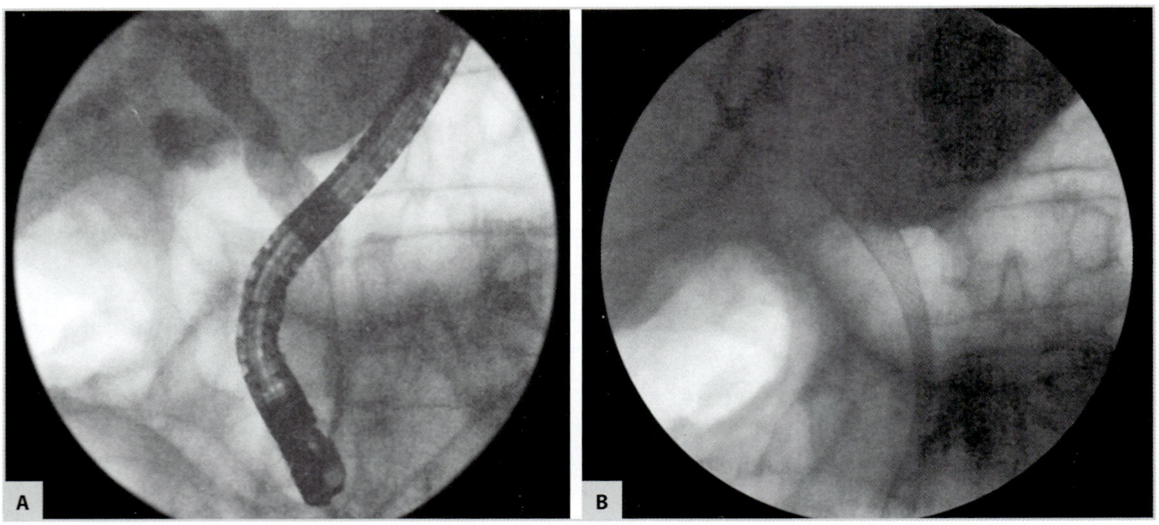

Figs 7A and B: (A) Infradeodenal common bile duct (CBD) stricture, secondary to inoperable carcinoma head pancreas; (B) Self-expandable metal stent placed to alleviate jaundice

jaundice. Endoscopic ultrasonography-guided FNAB is often performed in operable cases of carcinoma of the head of pancreas to confirm the diagnosis. Linear EUS with thin needle (25G) is used to make 6–8 passes under electronic Doppler scan (to avoid bleed) and assessed on site by the cytopathologist.[58] The risk of track seedling using EUS is irrelevant in operable cases as the track falls in resected specimen. All patients post EUS FNAB for carcinoma head pancreas are observed for one day and given antibiotics. Endoscopic ultrasonography-guided FNAB is superior to CT/MRI for large nonfunctional and small functional neuroendocrine tumors of pancreas.[59] Presence of pancreatitis and stent in bile duct interfere with EUS evaluation. For patients with inoperable carcinoma of the head of pancreas presenting with obstructive jaundice, bile duct cytology is sensitive in about 50–60% of cases.[60] Long brush, repeated passage and postdilatation cytology may yield marginally higher detection rates. Malignant biliary strictures are usually short, irregular and bleed on performing cytology during cholangiography. Malignant head mass usually produces a double duct sign on common channel injection of contrast during endoscopic retrograde cholangiopancreatography (ERCP) (Figs 7A and B). For patients with cholangiocarcinoma of the lower end a forceps biopsy using cholangioscope is highly sensitive but difficult to perform.[61] Intraductal ultrasonography (IDUS) performed over the guidewire is easy, rapid and accurate method to diagnose malignant nature of bile duct stricture.[62] It is most useful for hilar cholangiocarcinoma. A malignant stricture on IDUS shows: (a) disruption of normal three layers of bile duct; (b) hypoechoic infiltrating mass with irregular margins; (c) heterogenous echo poor areas invading surrounding tissue; and (d) size greater than 10 mm with asymmetry.[62,63] Intraductal ultrasonography also helps identify longitudinal spread, portal vein and right hepatic artery involvement in hilar cholangiocarcinoma.[64] Confocal laser endomicroscopy with ERCP is highly sensitive and specific in evaluation of indeterminate bile duct stricture.[65]

Ampulla of Vater

Ampullary tumors are uncommon tumors often identified in a patient with obstructive jaundice or as a routine evaluation for FAP (Fig. 8). Ampullary adenoma needs to be differentiated from ampullary adenocarcinoma. If a standard gastroscopic biopsy is inconclusive, EUS must be performed. Patients with IDUS showing no intraductal infiltration or ulcer above the roof of the papilla and absence of a node can be treated by endoscopic ampullectomy.[66]

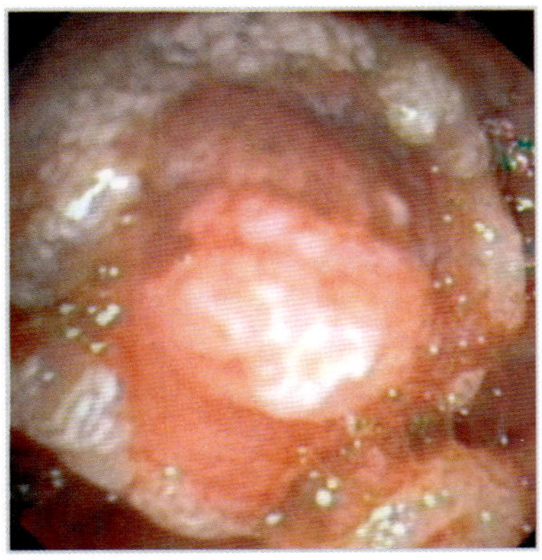

Fig. 8: Large ulcerated ampullary adenocarcinoma with intraductal extension

Gastrointestinal Stromal Tumors

Gastrointestinal stromal tumors (GISTs) are most often located in the stomach and proximal small intestine. Both GISTs and leiomyomas appear as a submucosal mass with smooth margins, normal overlying mucosa with a bulge in the lumen on endoscopic evaluation. They are often detected by chance but may present with gastrointestinal bleed (Figs 9A and B). Standard endoscopic biopsy is neither useful nor recommended. Endoscopic ultrasonography can accurately detect the type of GIST from its layer of origin. A tumor size less than 30 mm, homogenous echo pattern, maintained tissue planes, absence of cystic changes and absence of lymph nodes are good predictors of its benign lesion.[67] Endoscopic ultrasonography-guided FNAB is indicated: (a) when in doubt; or (b) large inoperable GISTs essentially before starting Imatinib.[68] Symptomatic GIST, size greater than 2 cm, malignant on imaging/biopsy needs to be resected.

Gastrointestinal Lymphoma

The gastrointestinal (GI) tract is the predominant site of extranodal lymphoma. Secondary involvement of GI tract in non-Hodgkin's lymphoma is commoner than primary GI tract lymphoma. In about 70% patients, stomach is involved. Endoscopic evaluation may suggest an area of erythema, nodularity, benign looking ulcer, thickening of folds or punched out volcano-like ulcer. Multiple biopsies with well technique (biopsy from same spot) or snare

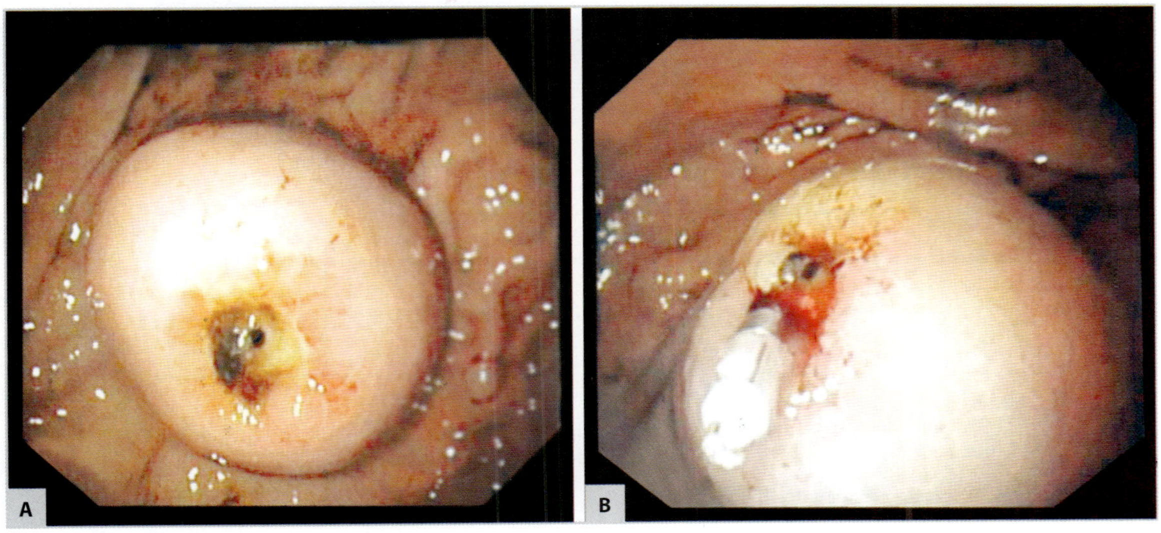

Figs 9A and B: (A) Large gastrointestinal stromal tumor (GIST) located in gastric fundus with central ulcer and bleed; (B) Single hemoclip applied, hemostasis achieved

biopsy is often necessary to diagnose gastric lymphoma. An early stage mucosa-associated lymphoid tissue (MALT) lymphoma without nodes can be treated successfully with anti-*H. pylori* treatment.

Diagnostic Staging Laparoscopy

Diagnostic staging laparoscopy (DSL) is performed in DC patients to assess feasibility of a curative resection. Diagnostic staging laparoscopy is indicated for: (a) esophageal cancer at the cardia;[69] (b) gastric cancer;[70] (c) pancreatic cancer of body/tail;[71] (d) proximal bile duct cancer;[72] and (e) gall bladder cancer[73] when CT/MRI/EUS show a lesion with a possibility of a curative resection. Diagnostic staging laparoscopy should be performed prior to neoadjuvant chemoradiotherapy and prior to resection of liver metastasis from CRC. Its role of staging lymphoma is decreasing. Diagnostic staging laparoscopy aims to identify peritoneal, serosal, omental spread of the disease and prevent negative exploration reducing operative morbidity.

ENDOSCOPIC TREATMENT

Barrett's Esophagus

Patients with dysplastic BE and intramucosal cancer can be treated endoscopically.[73,74] In a few specialized centers endoscopic resections are performed for tumors in superficial submucosa without nodal disease.[75] At present, BE without dysplasia need not be treated by endoscopic method. Dysplastic BE can be treated by EMR and/or ablative treatment whereas BE with mucosal cancer need EMR/ESD. Ablative forms of treatment include radiofrequency, halo system and photodynamic therapy. For circumferential ablation radiofrequency ablation is preferred whereas halo system is preferred for left over BE. For noncircumferential BE, EMR can also be used. Endoscopic resections have distinct advantages; (a) post resection tissue availability for histological evaluation; (b) high success of completely removing the tissue; and (c) lower risk of buried BE which has subsequent risk of cancer.[76] Limitations of endoscopic resection include: (a) about 70% circumferential clearance achieved each time to reduce the risk of subsequent stricture formation; (b) long learning curve; and (c) risk of perforation. Current practice of endoscopic treatment for circumferential dysplastic BE includes endoscopic resection followed by ablation of left over mucosa.[77-79] Endoscopic treatment for BE with intramucosal cancer is indicated when: (a) cancer is limited to mucosa; (b) tumor is well differentiated; (c) size less than 2 cm for macroscopic type I, IIa, IIb; and (d) size less than 1 cm for macroscopic type Ic (Fig. 10). Endoscopic treatment is insufficient if resected tissue has lymphovascular invasion.[74] Risk of recurrent tumor is higher when: (a) Barrett's esophagus is long segment

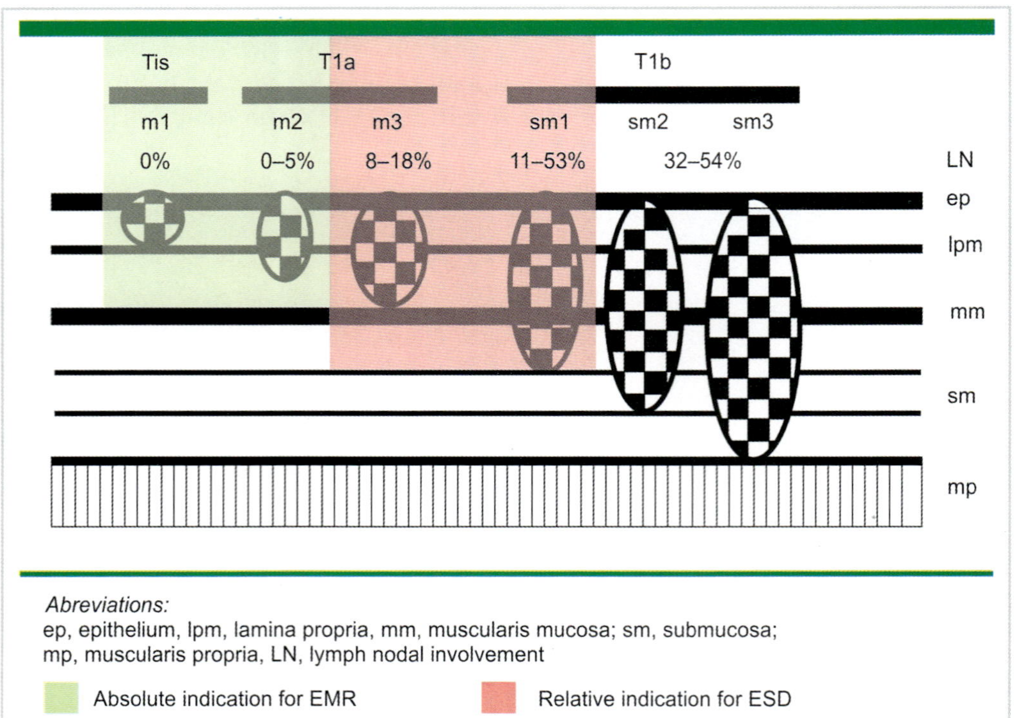

Fig. 10: Subclassification of the depth of superficial esophageal cancer

(> 3 cm); (b) time taken for completing treatment is greater than 10 months; (c) piecemeal resection is done; (d) neoplasia is multifocal; and (e) ablative therapy is not offered after ER.[78] Endoscopic treatment is comparable to surgery with a 5-year cancer free survival with lower morbidity.[79] However, beyond 5 years cancer develops in 12% of patients treated endoscopically suggesting need for a close follow-up.[80]

ENDOSCOPIC RESECTION

Superficial Esophageal Cancer

The risk of lymph node involvement directly correlates with the depth of submucosal invasion. Endoscopic resection (ER) is recommended in high volume centers with good skills in superficial esophageal cancers with no evidence of lymph nodal disease. Though NBI technique helps to identify disease early and EUS can accurately predict the depth of mucosal disease, endoscopically resected specimen is the most reliable method for identifying histopathological type, depth of invasion and lymphovascular involvement. En block resection of the lesion with clear margins (akin to surgical specimen) is the key to reduce recurrences and achieve cure. Subclassification of intramucosal cancer, risk of lymph nodal involvement and indications for endoscopic therapy are based on its depth[81,82] (Fig. 10). Endoscopic description of mucosal cancer is best described as per Paris classification (Fig. 11).[83,84] Various methods of EMR are shown in Figures 12 to 14. Appropriate injection to lift the lesion is the key. Most commonly used solution is a mixture of 1:20,000 adrenaline with sodium hyaluronate. Various steps of ESD are demonstrated in Figure 15.

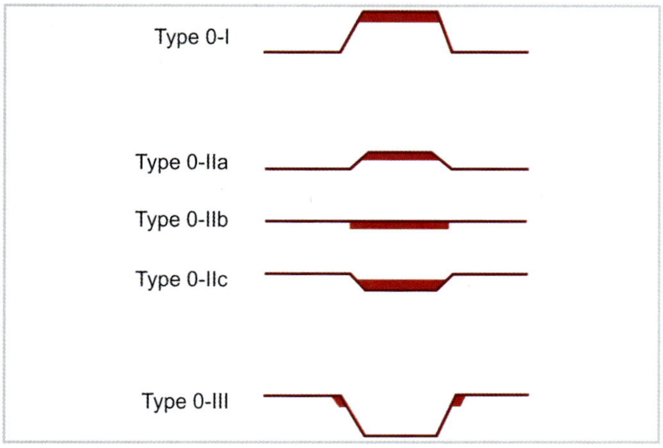

Fig. 11: Paris classification

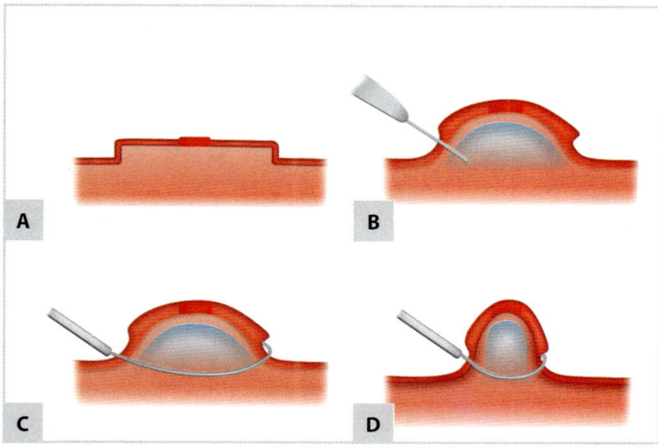

Figs 12A to D: Endoscopic mucosal resection (EMR) technique (injection + snaring)

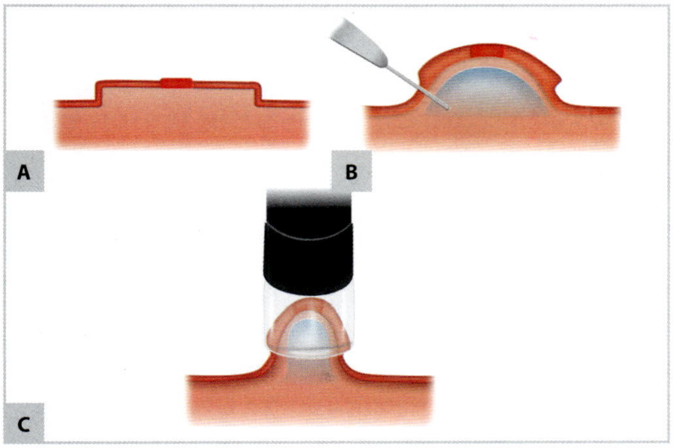

Figs 13A to C: Endoscopic mucosal resection (EMR) technique (injection + hood application)

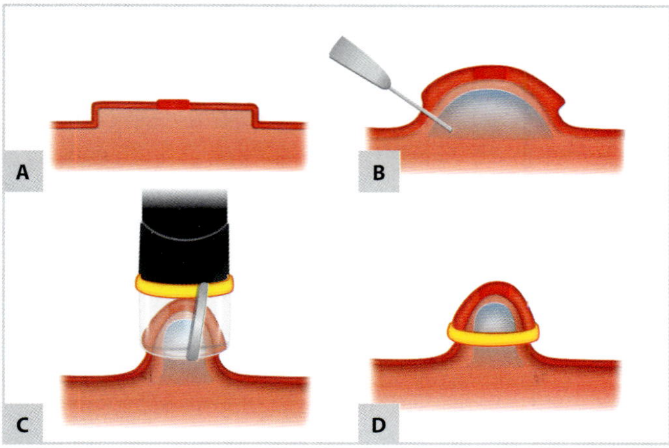

Figs 14A to D: Endoscopic mucosal resection (EMR) technique (injection + band application)

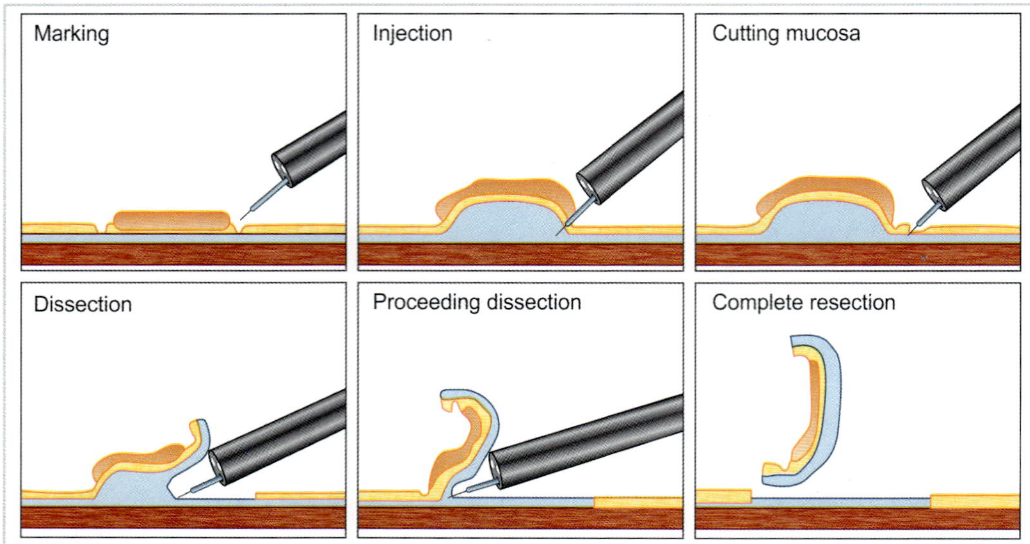

Fig. 15: Steps of endoscopic submucosal dissection (ESD)

En block resections are possible in more than 95% patients and complete resection in more than 85% patients.[85] Risk of perforation is 3–4% and bleeding occurs rarely. Extensive circumferential resections are associated with stricture formation in 15–18% and recurrence/distant metastasis occur in less than 2% patients.[85] Resected specimen must be stretched, pinned at corners and sent for histological evaluation with mucosa down. Both lateral and vertical margins should be tumor free. Regular endoscopic follow-up is a must. Surgery should be offered if margins are unclear or disease recurs. High skills, adequate instrumentation, detailed understanding, intensive learning, thorough knowledge of indications and regular follow-up will enhance the outcome of ER.

Early Gastric Cancer

Early gastric cancer (EGC) is a mucosal or submucosal (T_1 cancer) with or without lymph node disease. Endoscopic treatment can be offered only in patients with no lymph nodal disease. All patients with early gastric cancers must be macroscopically assessed as per Paris classification.[83,84] Lateral extension, site of tumor, type of tumor, depth and lymph nodal disease must be well documented by endoscopy, EUS and histology before deciding on ER. According to Japanese gastric cancer association guidelines, endoscopic resection is indicated in well-differentiated elevated lesions less than 2 cm in size (type 0-I, 0-IIa), less than 1 cm in size flat/depressed (type 0-IIb, 0-IIc) and type IIb-c lesions without ulceration.[86] The extended criteria for endoscopic resection were based on rate of lymph nodal disease about 2.7% with mucosal and about 18% with submucosal extension.[87] They are: (a) well differentiated, type 0-I, less than 3 cm in size with or without ulceration; (b) well differentiated, type IIa of any size without ulceration; (c) well differentiated, type IIb (submucosal depth < 500 μm), less than 3 cm in size; and (d) poorly differentiated, type Ia, less than 2 cm in size.[86] Endoscopic submucosal dissection compared to EMR is better as it is associated with higher rates of en block resection, complete/curative resection and has lower rates of recurrences.[88] Endoscopic submucosal dissection is however associated with higher risk of perforation, bleeding and has longer learning curve compared to EMR.[89]

Early Colon Cancer

Intraepithelial cancers and early mucosal cancers can be treated by EMR/ESD. Detailed evaluation of lesion as per Paris classification, size, circumferential extent and site need to be recorded. A lesion upto 20 mm size can be resected from cecum as it is thin walled whereas in rectum lesion upto 30 mm can be resected safely as rectum is thick walled (Fig. 16). Endoscopic mucosal resection or endoscopic submucosal dissection techniques remain the same. Tattooing with carbon is necessary if a resection is incomplete to help surgeon resect involved area. Endoscopic resection can be achieved in more than 90% of patients with early colon cancer (ECC) with 6–10% risk of complications.[89,90] Perforation during ER should be identified during ER so it can be closed using hemoclips.[91] Early bleeding is prevented by adrenaline used in injection to lift the lesion, however delayed bleeding remains a risk factor.

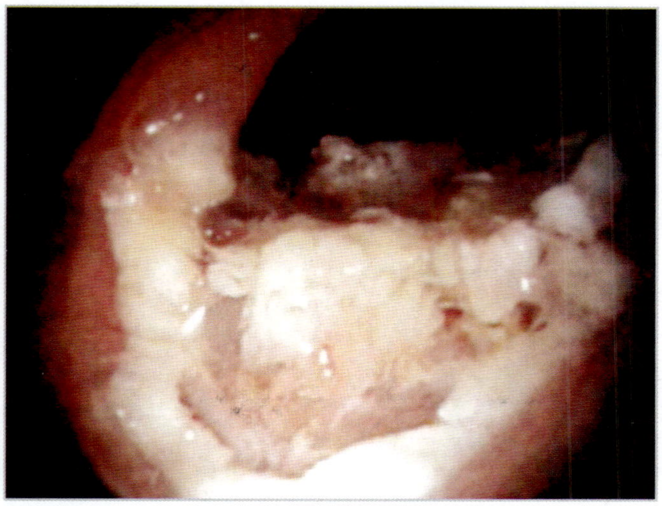

Fig. 16: Postcolonic endoscopic submucosal dissection (ESD) for intramucosal cancer

Ampullary Adenoma

Ampullary adenoma/carcinoma are rare.[92] Patients with FAP have a very high risk to develop ampullary cancer.[93] Transduodenal ampullectomy have high recurrence rates and pancreaticoduodenectomy have considerable morbidity/mortality.[94,95] Endoscopic treatment is recommended for all ampullary adenomas of size less than 5 cm, no ulcer or friability, no firmness on biopsy, positive lift sign and negative intraductal growth or lymph nodal disease on EUS. Removal of an entire adenoma is the only method to rule out malignancy as the false-negative rates even after 6–8 transduodenal endoscopic biopsies are 14–42%.[93,96] Endoscopic sphincterectomy for bile duct and pancreatic duct is followed by prophylactic stenting of pancreatic duct with 3Fr plastic stent. Post-injection adenoma is lifted and en block resection is carried out with a snare. If cancer is detected, the patient undergoes pancreaticoduodenectomy. Bleeding, pancreatitis, cholangitis and duodenal perforations are known complications.[97] Endoscopic ampullectomy should be performed by experts in high volume centers as endoscopically it is considered as a high-risk procedure.[98]

Anticoagulation/antiplatelet drugs must be stopped for 5–7 days prior to ER and restarted 48 hours after completing ER. Patients need to be hospitalized for 24 hours and most centers give single dose antibiotics. Patients with esophageal/gastric ER are given proton pump inhibitors for 6–8 weeks to allow post ER ulcers to heal. Follow-up endoscopy with biopsy is required for patients with intramucosal cancer undergoing ER every 6 monthly for first year and then yearly for at least 5 years.

Based on histology and follow-up, ER are classified as piece meal, en block, curative or complete curative with the latter having the best outcome. Piecemeal removal means endoscopic removal of lesions in multiple pieces. En block resection means removal of lesion in one piece. Curative resection means en block resection with clear vertical and lateral margins. Complete curative resection means no disease after curative resection on check endoscopy with biopsy at 6 months.

LAPAROSCOPIC SURGERY

Laparoscopic surgery is considered as a minimally invasive surgery as it avoids large abdominal wall incision, is associated with less postoperative pain, lower consumption of pain-killers and early postoperative recovery. Depth of vision and better illumination has allowed lap-oncosurgeons to carry out cancer surgery in select patients where it is safe and oncologically sound. For lower third esophageal cancer and gastric cancer several authors in small numbers have demonstrated lesser morbidity and shorter hospital stay with laparoscopic surgery.[99,100] Laparoscopic resection of pancreatic malignancy is not reported feasible, safe or potentially beneficial for patients.[101] Laparoscopic curative resection of early gall bladder cancer is considered a poor indication.[102] Laparoscopic-assisted colectomy and resection of small liver malignant lesions are increasingly performed as it is safe and oncologically sound.[103] Some of the oncologic surgeries are laparoscopic assisted. The delivery of a large specimen will need a small incision occasionally. Increased time of surgery, higher cost, need for trained surgeons and higher rate of conversion are current limitations. In selected elderly patients and an early lesion it appears to be a better form of approach compared to open surgery. For local resection of gastrointestinal stromal tumor, debulking of tumors and minor resections after positive margins with endoscopic procedures, laparoscopic surgery is indicated.

NATURAL ORIFICE TRANSLUMINAL ENDOSCOPIC SURGERY

Natural orifice transluminal endoscopic surgery (NOTES) is a rapidly evolving gastrointestinal intervention wherein peritoneum is approached by an endoscopic access in an organ to perform various therapeutic surgeries. The common routes are transgastric, transanal, transvaginal and transcystic. Absence of abdominal incision; lower incidence of hernia, pain, ileus, adhesions; safety in obese patients; lower hospital and overall cost are distinct advantages.[104] Uncontrolled peritoneal insufflations, bacterial peritonitis, inability to handle major complications, steep learning curve and need for specialized instruments are current limitations of NOTES.[105] After considerable animal experience, transanal rectosigmoidectomy with total mesorectal excision is feasible and oncologically safe opinion.[106,107]

ENDOSCOPIC PALLIATIVE TREATMENT

Esophageal Cancer

Endoscopic palliative treatment for dysphagia is recommended for patients with: (a) locally unresectable tumor; (b) tracheoesophageal fistula; (c) medically poor risk for surgical palliation; (d) refusal and intolerant to chemoradiotherapy; (e) history of aspiration pneumonia; and (f) recurrence after surgery. There are several endoscopic approaches to palliate dysphagia:

- Mechanical
  - Dilation
  - Dilation with stent placement
  - Stent placement with brachytherapy
- Ablative
  - Alcohol intratumoral injection
  - Laser therapy
  - Argon plasma coagulation
  - Cryospray ablation
  - Photodynamic therapy.

Of all the above methods, the best form of palliation is placement of a self-expandable partially covered metal stent (Figs 17A and B).[108] Ideal length of the stent is tumor length plus 4–6 cm (2–3 cm above and below the tumor). They can be placed without dilating malignant stricture thus reducing the risk of perforation. They cover tracheoesophageal fistula reducing the risk of aspiration. Stents are easy to deploy, need little expertise, relieve dysphagia rapidly, remain patent over 3–6 months and are chemoradio compliant. Patient is hospitalized for about 24 hours. Tumor ingrowth/overgrowth, mucosal hyperplasia, migration and its cost are major drawbacks. Stent placement is not recommended if tumor is within 1–2 cm of the cricopharynx and is associated often with reflux when they cross cardia. Tumor ingrowth/overgrowth are treated with placement of another longer stent whereas mucosal hyperplasia is treated with ablative treatment (Figs 18A and B). Most often a single stent palliates dysphagia in more than 90% patients till they survive.

Gastric Cancer

Endoscopic palliative treatment is indicated in patients with advanced gastric cancer with gastric outlet obstruction and are: (a) unfit for palliative resection/gastrojejunostomy; (b) intolerant or refusal for chemoradiotherapy; and (c) have postoperative recurrence. Placement of enteral partially covered self-expandable metal stent is relatively easy, patient friendly method of alleviating outlet obstruction. Enteral stents are not as effective as esophageal stents due to axis shift across the pylorus.

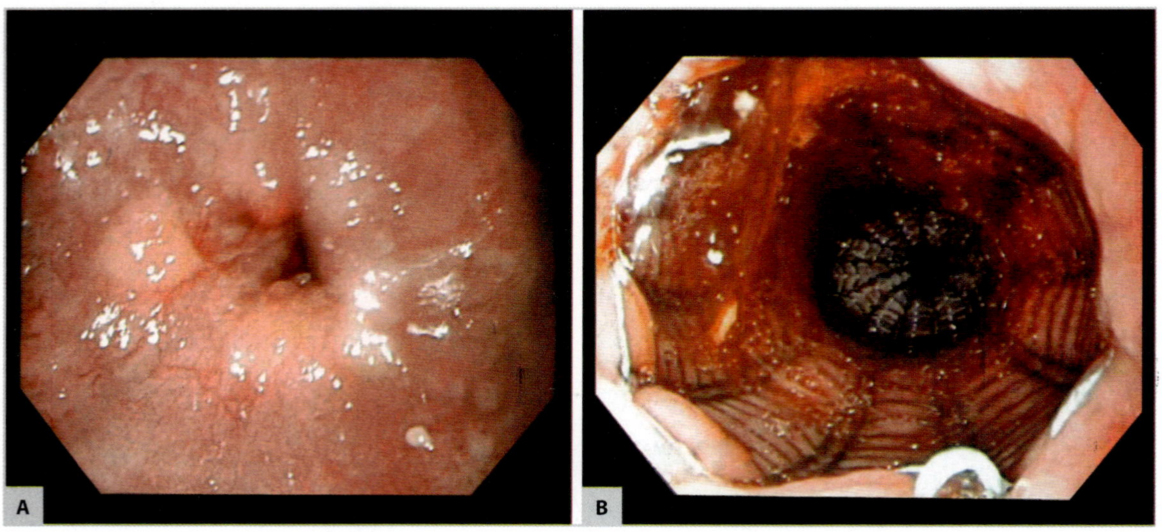

Figs 17A and B: (A) Inoperable midesophageal malignant stricture; (B) Self-expandable metal stent (SEM) placed to relieve dysphagia

Patients with enteral stents have to eat diet low in fiber, eat more often and report in case of recurrence of symptoms early.

Malignant Colorectal Obstruction

Enteral stents are placed in patients with malignant colorectal obstruction who have partial obstruction and are unfit for surgery. In an emergency situation it can avoid colostomy. Placement of enteral stent is cost-effective, associated with low morbidity/mortality compared to emergency stoma followed by resection.[109] Post stenting colon can be prepared to perform colonoscopy and evaluate rest of the colon for synchronous lesions.[110] Often, multiple stents have to be placed to cover tumor adequately.[111] Placement of stent is successful in 92% (46–100%), median patency rates are 106 days (68–288 days), re-intervention are required in 20%, stent migration rates are 11% (0–50%), perforations occur in 45% (0–83%) and re-obstruction in 12% (1–92%).[112] Colonic stent placement in large volume centers with an experienced endoscopist is effective, safe and simple. Delayed perforation is a risk in patients receiving bevacizumab.[113]

Pancreaticobiliary Cancer

At the time of presentation less than 15% of pancreatic and gallbladder cancers are operable.[114] Even after resection 5-year survival rates are poor.[114] The goal of palliative endoscopic therapy is to relieve symptoms of itching/jaundice, improve quality of life, reduce need for recurrent hospitalization with least morbidity of intervention.[115] In patients with inoperable pancreatic head mass, gall bladder cancer and cholangiocarcinoma endoscopic palliation is superior to surgical palliation.[116] Uncovered self-expandable metal biliary stents with post-deployment diameter of 10 mm are preferred over plastic stents with a diameter of 10F (about 2.3 mm) when expected patient survival is greater than 6 months.[117] Plastic stents should be avoided in hilar cholangiocarcinoma as it may interfere with drainage of various segmental branches leading to cholangitis. In a failed cannulation of papilla, EUS-guided guidewire cannulation is preferred over a percutaneous route.[118] About 15–20% of patients with voluminous head cancers can present with gastroduodenal outlet obstruction (GOO). In those with GOO and obstructive jaundice, a biliary stent is placed percutaneously followed by placement of an enteral stent. Patients with resectable hilar cholangiocarcinoma often need stenting of uninvolved segment preoperatively to reduce jaundice. In unresectable hilar cholangiocarcinoma at least 30% of liver volume should be drained. Brachytherapy and photodynamic ablations are only practised in the Western world (Figs 19A and B).

Intractable Pain

Persistent pain is a debilitating symptom of patients with inoperable carcinoma of the pancreas. Endoscopic ultrasonography-guided celiac plexus block (CPB) or celiac plexus neurolysis (CPN) reduces pain, need for morphine use and improves quality of life in about 70–80%

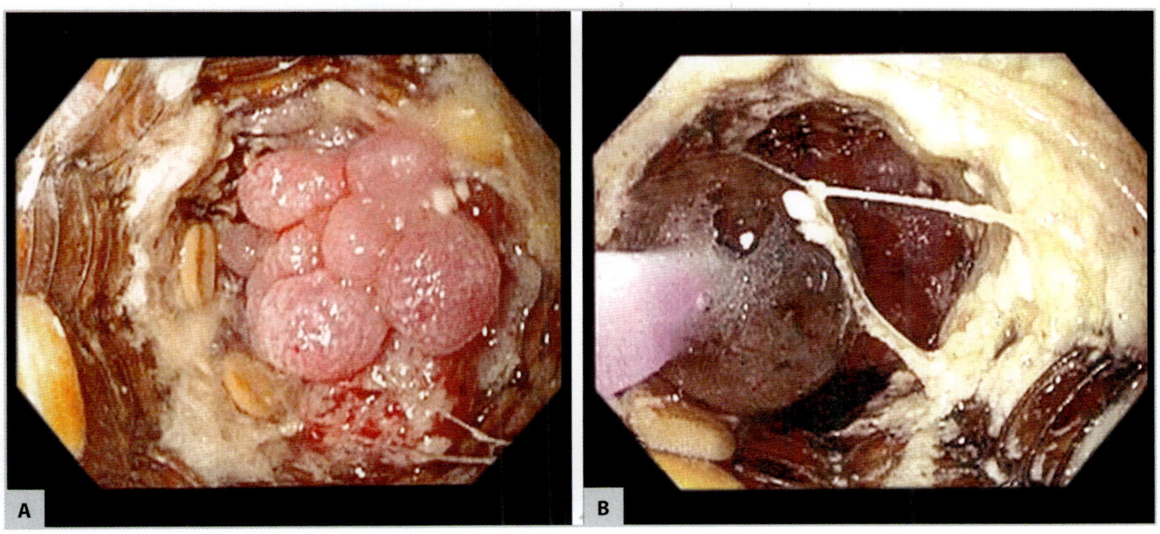

Figs 18A and B: (A) Mucosal hyperplasia at the lower end of self-expandable metal stent (SEM) in esophagus; (B) Balloon dilation followed by ablation was performed

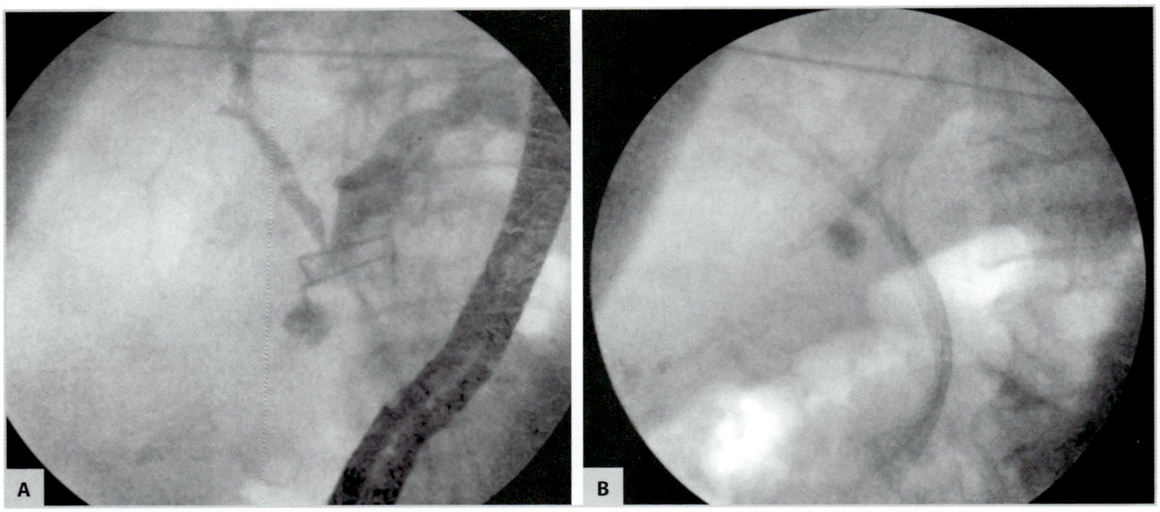

Figs 19A and B: (A) Inoperable hilar cholangiocarcinoma; (B) Two self-expandable metal stent (SEMs) placed, one each in right and left hepatic duct

patients for an average duration of 10 weeks.[114] Alcohol is injected on either side of aorta at the take off point of celiac artery in CPN and an anesthetic agent is used in CPB using 20 gauge needle under EUS guidance. Trans EUS CPN is currently considered as the standard of care for pain palliation of pancreatic cancer predominantly of body and tail.[115]

ENDOSCOPIC TREATMENT OF POSTOPERATIVE/POSTRADIOTHERAPY COMPLICATIONS

Anastomotic bleed occurs in less than 10% of patients undergoing resection. Early bleed (<5 days) in postoperative period is best treated by conservative/radiological methods. Beyond 5–7 days gentle endoscopy (less air insufflation) can be carried out. Injection 1:20,000 adrenaline and application of hemoclips is preferred over thermal therapy which may produce ulcer. Postoperative strictures are most often ischemic in nature. They can be dilated by controlled radial expansion (CRE) balloon through the scope under vision. Often dilation is done sequentially from smaller to larger size balloons. Dilation of anastomotic strictures is rewarding (Figs 20A and B). Post radiotherapy strictures often present late and respond poorly to dilation. Occasionally for a resistant stricture (> 5 dilations)/complex stricture (long >3 cm) a retrievable self-expandable plastic/metal stent is placed under endoscopic guidance. Stent is usually removed after 8–12 weeks (Figs 21A and B). Treatment of postoperative leak is an endoscopic challenge. Application of hemoclips for small defects and placing covered self-expandable metal/plastic stents for larger defects have produced mediocre results.

Endoscopy has become an integral part of surveillance, diagnosis, prevention, treatment of early cancer and palliation of DC. Newer investigational modalities like CLE, endocystoscopy, autofluorescence endoscopy, optical coherence tomography and molecular imaging need to be evaluated in clinical trials.[119,120] Careful endoscopy using newer imaging will allow diagnosis of DC at a stage when it is curable. Stage based individualized treatment of DC is now a reality. Endoscopic R_0 resections for early mucosal cancer has reduced morbidity associated with surgical resections of the past. Placement of enteral stents is an excellent palliative measure for relieving obstruction/jaundice in advanced DC. Laparoscopic approach is increasingly used in select cancers reducing postoperative pain and hospital stay. Natural orifice transluminal endoscopic surgery is making inroads for rectosigmoid cancers.

Newer development, magnification endoscopy and use of specialized accessories however come at a cost. In developing countries like India judicious use of health care resources is a must. Randomized trials need to be planned not just for the effectiveness of a therapy but also to take into consideration health economics. We need better methods to evaluate outcomes of neoadjuvant chemoradiotherapy. Regular follow-ups, health education, multidisciplinary approach and team work will improve care and cure rates of DC.

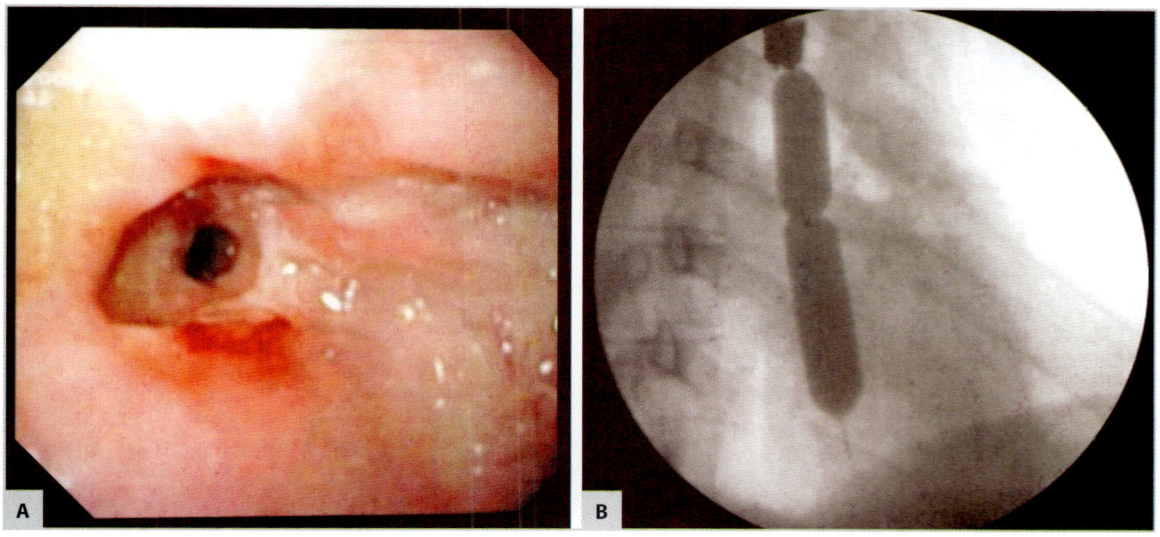

Figs 20A and B: (A) Anastomotic stricture at esophagogastric junction; (B) Dilation done with controlled radial expansion (CRE) balloon

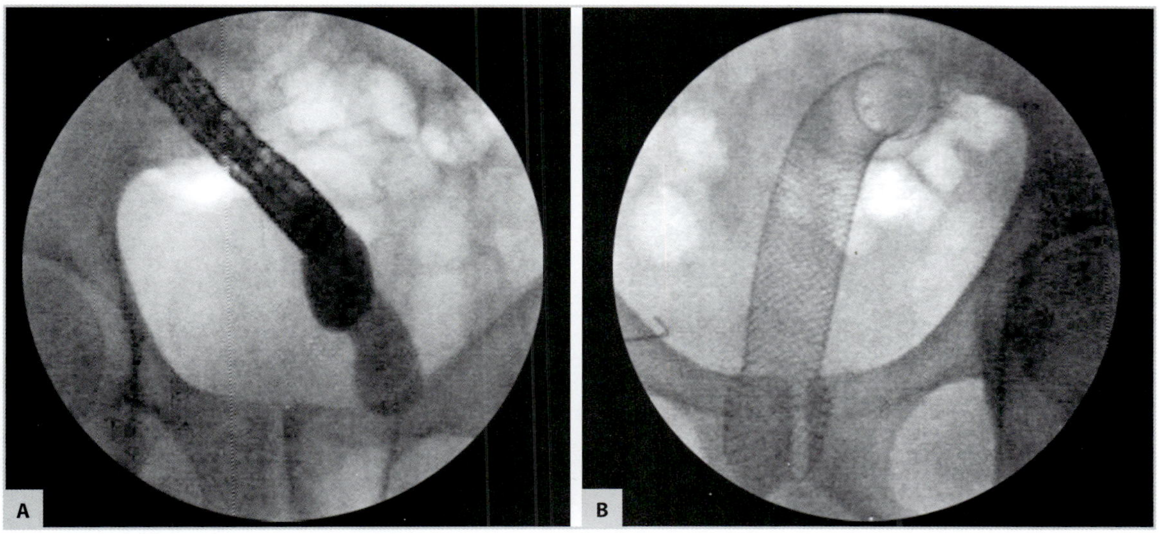

Figs 21A and B: (A) Post-radiotherapy complex rectosigmoid resistant stricture, balloon dilation done; (B) Fully covered retrievable enteral stent placed for 12 weeks

REFERENCES

1. Dawsey SM, Wang GQ, Weinstein WM, et al. Squamous dysplasia and early esophageal cancer in the Linxian region of China: distinctive endoscopic lesions. Gastroenterology. 1993;105(5):1333-40.
2. Shimizu Y, Omori T, Yokoyama A, et al. Endoscopic diagnosis of early squamous neoplasia of the esophagus with iodine staining: high-grade intraepithelial neoplasia turns pink within a few minutes. J Gastroentero Hepatol. 2008;23(4):546-50.
3. Ishihara R, Inoue T, Uedo N, et al. Significance of each narrow-band imaging finding in diagnosing squamous mucosal high-grade neoplasia of the esophagus. J Gastroenterol Hepatol. 2010;25(8):1410-5.
4. Subramanian V, Mannath J, Hawkey CJ, et al. High definition colonoscopy vs. standard video endoscopy for the detection of colonic polyps: a meta-analysis. Endoscopy. 2011;43(6):499-505.
5. Repici A, Di Stefano AF, Radicioni MM, et al. Methylene blue MMX tablets for chromoendoscopy. Safety, tolerability and bioavailability in healthy volunteers. Contemp Clin Trials. 2012;33(2):260-7.
6. Wu L, Li P, Wu J, et al. The diagnostic accuracy of chromoendoscopy for dysplasia in ulcerative colitis: meta-analysis of six randomized controlled trials. Colorectal Dis. 2012;14(4):416-20.
7. Stein HJ, Siewert JR. Barrett's esophagus: pathogenesis, epidemiology, functional abnormalities, malignant degeneration and surgical management. Dysphagia. 1993;8(3):276-88.

8. Falk GW, Rice TW, Goldblum JR, et al. Jumbo biopsy forceps protocol still misses unsuspected cancer in Barrett's esophagus with high-grade dysplasia. Gastrointest Endosc. 1999;49(2):170-6.
9. Mori M, Adachi Y, Matsushima T, et al. Lugol staining pattern and histology of esophageal lesions. Am J Gastroenterol. 1993;88(5):701-5.
10. Sharma P, Hawes RH, Bansal A, et al. Standard endoscopy with random biopsies versus narrow band imaging targeted biopsies in Barrett's oesophagus: a prospective, international, randomised controlled trial. Gut. 2013;62(1):15-21.
11. Silva FB, Dinis-Ribeiro M, Vieth M, et al. Endoscopic assessment and grading of Barrett's esophagus using magnification endoscopy and narrow-band imaging: accuracy and interobserver agreement of different classification systems. Gastrointest Endosc. 2011;73(1):7-14.
12. Sharma P, Meining AR, Coron E, et al. Real-time increased detection of neoplastic tissue in Barrett's esophagus with probe-based confocal laser endomicroscopy: final results of an international, multicenter, prospective, randomized, controlled trial. Gastrointest Endosc. 2011 74(3):465-72.
13. Bertani H, Frazzoni M, Dabizzi E, et al. Improved detection of incident dysplasia by probe-based confocal laser endomicroscopy in a Barrett's esophagus surveillance program. Dig Dis Sci. 2013;58(1):188-93.
14. Canto MI, Anandasabapathy A, Brugge WR, et al. In vivo endoscope-based confocal laser endomicroscopy improves detection of unlocalized Barrett's esophagus-related neoplasia over high resolution white light endoscopy: an international multicenter randomized controlled trial. Gastrointest Endosc. 2012;75(4 Suppl):AB174.
15. Wallace MB, Crook JE, Saunders M, et al. Multicenter, randomized, controlled trial of confocal laser endomicroscopy assessment of residual metaplasia after mucosal ablation or resection of GI neoplasia in Barrett's esophagus. Gastrointest Endosc. 2012;76(3):539-47.
16. Kosaka R, Tanaka K, Tano S, et al. Magnifying endoscopy for diagnosis of residual/local recurrent gastric neoplasms after previous endoscopic treatment. Surg Endosc. 2012;26(8):2299-305.
17. Uedo N, Ishihara R, Iishi H, et al. A new method of diagnosing gastric intestinal metaplasia: narrow band imaging with magnifying endoscopy. Endoscopy. 2006;38(8):819-24.
18. Yoshida T, Kawachi H, Sasajima K, et al. The clinical meaning of a nonstructural pattern in early gastric cancer on magnifying endoscopy. Gastrointest Endosc. 2005;62(1):48-54.
19. Areia M, Amaro P, Dinis-Ribeiro M, et al. External validation of a classification for methylene blue magnification chromoendoscopy in premalignant gastric lesions. Gastrointest Endosc. 2008;67(7):1011-8.
20. Rex DK, Chadalawada V, Helper DJ. Wide angle colonoscopy with a prototype instrument: impact on miss rates and efficiency as determined by back-to-back colonoscopies. Am J Gastroenterol. 2003;98(9):2000-5.
21. Matsushita M, Hajiro K, Okazaki K, et al. Efficacy of total colonoscopy with a transparent cap in comparison with colonoscopy without the cap. Endoscopy. 1998;30(5):444-7.
22. Waye JD, Heigh RI, Fleischer DE, et al. A retrograde-viewing device improves detection of adenomas in the colon: a prospective efficacy evaluation (with videos). Gastrointest Endosc. 2010;71(3):551-6.
23. Pasha SF, Leighton JA, Das A, et al. Comparison of the yield and miss rate of narrow band imaging and white light endoscopy in patients undergoing screening or surveillance colonoscopy: a meta-analysis. Am J Gastroenterol. 2012;107(3):363-70.
24. Buchner AM. Does the dye-based chromoendoscopy improve dysplasia detection in patients undergoing surveillance colonoscopy for long-term ulcerative colitis? Am J Gastroenterol. 2010;105:$S_1$571.
25. Rispo A, Castiglione F, Staibano S, et al. Diagnostic accuracy of confocal laser endomicroscopy in diagnosing dysplasia in patients affected by long-standing ulcerative colitis. World J Gastrointest Endosc. 2012;4(9):414-20.
26. Ignjatovic A, East JE, Subramanian V, et al. Narrow band imaging for detection of dysplasia in colitis: a randomized controlled trial. Am J Gastroenterol. 2012;107(6):885-90.
27. Baxter NN, Goldwasser MA, Paszat LF, et al. Association of colonoscopy and death from colorectal cancer. Ann Intern Med. 2009;150(1):1-8.
28. Dinesen L, Chua TJ, Kaffes AJ. Meta-analysis of narrow band imaging versus conventional colonoscopy for adenoma detection. Gastrointest Endosc. 2012;75(3):604-11.
29. Paggi S, Rondonotti E, Amato A, et al. Resect and discard strategy in clinical practice: a prospective cohort study. Endoscopy. 2012;44(10):899-904.
30. Hewett DG, Huffman ME, Rex DK. Leaving distal colorectal hyperplastic polyps in place can be achieved with high accuracy by using narrow band imaging: an observational study. Gastrointest Endosc. 2012;76(2):374-80.
31. Kudo S, Tamura S, Nakajima T, et al. Diagnosis of colorectal tumorous lesions by magnifying endoscopy. Gastrointest Endosc. 1996;44(1):8-14.
32. Graham DY, Schwartz JT, Cain GD, et al. Prospective evaluation of biopsy number in the diagnosis of esophageal and gastric carcinoma. Gastroenterology. 1982;82(2):228-31.
33. Rösch T. Endosonographic staging of esophageal cancer: a review of literature results. Gastrointest Endosc Clin N Am. 1995;5(3):537-47.
34. Bruzzi JF, Truong MT, Macapinlac H, et al. Integrated CT-PET imaging of esophageal cancer: unexpected and unusual distribution of distant organ metastasis. Curr Probl Diagn Radiol. 2007;36:21-9.
35. van Westreenem HL, Heeren PA, van Dullemen HM, et al. Positron emission tomography with F-18-fluorodeoxyglucose in a combined staging strategy of esophageal cancer prevents unnecessary surgical explorations. J Gastrointest Surg. 2005;9(1):54-61.
36. Riedel M, Hauck RW, Stein HJ, et al. Preoperative bronchoscopic assessment of airway invasion by esophageal cancer: a prospective study. Chest. 1998;113:687-95.
37. Kaushik N, Khalid A, Brody D, et al. Endoscopic ultrasound compared with laparoscopy for staging esophageal cancer. Ann Thorac Surg. 2007;83:2000-2.

38. Zuccaro G, Rice TW, Goldblum J, et al. Endoscopic ultrasound cannot determine suitability for esophagectomy after aggressive chemoradiotherapy for esophageal cancer. Am J Gastroenterol. 1999;94:906-12.
39. Chak A, Canto MI, Cooper GS, et al. Endosonographic assessment of multimodality therapy predicts survival of esophageal carcinoma patients. Cancer. 2000;88:1788-95.
40. Agarwal B, Swisher S, Ajani J, et al. Endoscopic ultrasound after preoperative chemoradiation can help identify patients who benefit maximally after surgical esophageal resection. Am J Gastroenterol. 2004;99:1258-66.
41. Yoshioka T, Yamaguchi K, Kubota K, et al. Evaluation of 18F-FDG PET in patients with advanced, metastatic, or recurrent gastric cancer. J Nucl Med. 2003;44:690-9.
42. Leake PA, Cardoso R, Seevaratnam R, et al. A systematic review of the accuracy and indications for diagnostic laparoscopy prior to curative-intent resection of gastric cancer. Gastric Cancer. 2012;15 suppl 1:S38-47.
43. DiSario JA, Burt RW, Vargas H, et al. Small bowel cancer: epidemiological and clinical characteristics from a population-based registry. Am J Gastroenterol. 1994;89:699-701.
44. Sjöblom SM. Clinical presentation and prognosis of gastrointestinal carcinoid tumours. Scand J Gastroenterol. 1998; 23:779-87.
45. Ciresi DL, Scholten DJ. The continuing clinical dilemma of primary tumors of the small intestine. Am Surg. 1995;61:698-702.
46. Maglinte DD, O'Connor K, Bessette J, et al. The role of the physician in the late diagnosis of primary malignant tumors of the small intestine. Am J Gastroenterol. 1991;86:304-8.
47. Gustafsson BI, Siddique L, Chan A, et al. Uncommon cancers of the small intestine, appendix and colon: an analysis of SEER 1973-2004 and current diagnosis and therapy. Int J Oncol. 2008;33:1121-31.
48. Duque G, Almeida N, Figuiredo P, et al. Virtual chromoendoscopy can be a useful software tool in capsule endoscopy. Rev Esp Enferm Dig. 2012;104(5):231-6.
49. Mergener K, Ponchon T, Gralnek I, et al. Literature review and recommendations for clinical application of small-bowel capsule endoscopy based on a panel discussion by international experts. Consensus statements for small bowel capsule endoscopy, 2006/2007. Endoscopy. 2007;39(10):895-909.
50. Urbain D, De Looze D, Demedts I, et al. Video capsule endoscopy in small bowel malignancy: a multicenter Belgian study. Endoscopy. 2006;38(4):408-11.
51. Clarke JO, Giday SA, Magno P, et al. How good is capsule endoscopy for detection of periampullary lesions? Results of a tertiary referral center. Gastrointest Endosc. 2008;68(2):267-72.
52. Spada C, Spera G, Riccioni M, et al. A novel diagnostic tool for detecting functional patency of the small bowel: the given patency capsule. Endoscopy. 2005;37(9):793-800.
53. Mensink PB, Haringsma J, Kucharzik T, et al. Complications of double balloon enteroscopy: a multicenter survey. Endoscopy. 2007;39(7):613-5.
54. May A, Nachbar L, Pohl J, et al. Endoscopic interventions in the small bowel using double balloon enteroscopy: feasibility and limitations. Am J Gastroenterol. 2007;102:527-35.
55. Kwok H, Bissett IP, Hill GL. Preoperative staging of rectal cancer. Int J Colorectal Dis. 2000;15:9-20.
56. Harewood GC, Wiersema MJ, Nelson H, et al. A prospective, blinded assessment of the impact of preoperative staging on the management of rectal cancer. Gastroenterology. 2002;123:24-32.
57. Lohnert MS, Doniec JM, Henne-Bruns D. Effectiveness of endoluminal sonography in the identification of occult local rectal cancer recurrences. Dis Colon Rectum. 2000;43:483-91.
58. Harewood GC, Wiersema MJ. A cost analysis of endoscopic ultrasound in the evaluation of pancreatic head adenocarcinoma. Am J Gastroenterol. 2001;96:2651-6.
59. De Angelis C, Carucci P, Repici A, et al. Endosonography in decision making and management of gastrointestinal endocrine tumors. Eur J Ultrasound. 1999;10:139-50.
60. Monsfield JC, Griffin SM, Wadehra V, et al. A prospective evaluation of cytology from biliary structures. Gut. 1997; 40: 671-7
61. Tamada K, Ueno N, Tomiyama T, et al. Characterization of biliary strictures using intraductal ultrasonography: comparison with percutaneous cholangioscopic biopsy. Gastrointest Endosc. 1998;47:341-9.
62. Vazquez-Sequeiros E, Baron TH, Clain JE, et al. Evaluation of indeterminate bile duct strictures by intraductal US. Gastrointest Endosc. 2002;56:372-9.
63. Tamada K, Tomiyama T, Wada S, et al. Endoscopic transpapillary bile duct biopsy with the combination of intraductal ultrasonography in the diagnosis of biliary strictures. Gut. 2002;50:326-31.
64. Tamada K, Nagai H, Yasuda Y, et al. Transpapillary intraductal US prior to biliary drainage in the assessment of longitudinal spread of extrahepatic bile duct carcinoma. Gastrointest Endosc. 2001;53:300-7.
65. Meining A, Chen YK, Pleskow D, et al. Direct visualization of indeterminate pancreaticobiliary strictures with probe based confocal laser endomicroscopy: a multicenter experience. Gastrointest Endosc. 2011;74(5):961-8.
66. Napolean B, Saurin JC, Scoazec JY, et al. Do endoscopic ultrasound and intraductal ultrasonography allow to orientate the treatment of ampullary tumour? Endoscopy. 2001;33:A2770.
67. Palazzo L, Landi B, Cellier C, et al. Endosonographic features predictive of benign and malignant gastrointestinal stromal cell tumours. Gut. 2000;46:88-92.
68. Watson RR, Binmoeller KF, Hamerski CM, et al. Yield and performance characteristics of endoscopic ultrasound-guided fine needle aspiration for diagnosing upper GI tract stromal tumors. Dig Dis Sci. 2011;56:1757-62.
69. de Graaf GW, Ayantunde AA, Parsons SL, et al. The role of staging laparoscopy in oesophagogastric cancers. Eur J Surg Oncol. 2007;33:988-92.
70. Muntean V, Mihailov A, Iancu C, et al. Staging laparoscopy in gastric cancer. Accuracy and impact on therapy. J Gastrointestin Liver Dis. 2009;18:189-95.

71. Stetanidis D, Grove KD, Schwesinger WH, et al. The current role of staging laparoscopy for adenocarcinoma of the pancreas: a review. Ann Oncol. 2006;17:189-99.
72. Guidelines of Diagnostic laparoscopy. Society of American Gastrointestinal and Endoscopic Surgeons. Practice/Clinical guidelines; 2011.
73. Fleisher DE, Overholt BF, Sharma VK, et al. Endoscopic radiofrequency ablation for Barrett's esophagus: 5-year durability outcomes from a prospective multicenter trial. Gastrointest Endosc. 2010:71:AB117-8.
74. Ell C, May A, Pech O, et al. Curative endoscopic resection of early esophageal adenocarcinomas (Barrett's Cancer). Gastrointest Endosc. 2007;65:3.
75. Manner H, May A, Pech O, et al. Early Barrett's adenocarcinoma with "low-risk" submucosal invasion: long-term results of endoscopic resection with curative intent. Am J Gastroenterol. 2008;103:2589-97.
76. Mino-Kenudson M, Ban S, Ohana M, et al. Buried dysplasia and early adenocarcinoma arising in Barrett's esophagus after porfimer-photodynamic therapy. Am J Surg Pathol. 2007;31: 403-9.
77. Gondrie JJ, Pouw RE, Sondermeijer CM, et al. Effective treatment of early Barrett's neoplasia with stepwise circumferential and focal ablation using the HALO system. Endoscopy. 2008;40:370-9.
78. Pech O, Behrens A, May A, et al. Long-term results and risk factor analysis for recurrence after curative endoscopic therapy in 349 patients with high-grade intraepithelial neoplasia and mucosal adenocarcinoma in Barrett's oesophagus. Gut. 2008;57:1200-6.
79. Pouw RE, Wirths K, Eisendrath P, et al. Efficacy of radiofrequency ablation combined with endoscopic resection for Barrett's esophagus with early neoplasia. Clin Gastroenterol Hepatol. 2010;8:23-9.
80. Prasad GA, Wu TT, Wigle DA, et al. Endoscopic and surgical treatment of mucosal (T1a) esophageal adenocarcinoma in Barrett's esophagus. Gastroenterology. 2009;137:815-23.
81. Oyama T, Miyala Y, Shimaya S, et al. Diagnosis and long term results and prognosis of M_3 and SM_1 esophageal cancer. Lymph node metastasis of M_3, SM_1 esophageal cancer. Stomach Intest. 2002;37:71.
82. Guidelines for the treatment of esophageal cancer. The Japan Esophageal Society, 2007.
83. The Paris endoscopic classification of superficial neoplastic lesions: esophagus, stomach and colon: November 30 to December 1, 2002. Gastrointest Endosc. 2003;58:S3-43.
84. Endoscopic Classification Review Group. Update on the Paris classification of superficial neoplastic lesions in the digestive tract. Endoscopy. 2005;37:570-8.
85. Ono S, Fujishiro M, Niimi K, et al. Long-term outcomes of endoscopic submucosal dissection for superficial esophageal squamous cell neoplasms. Gastrointest Endosc. 2009;70:860-6.
86. Japanese Gastric Cancer Association. JGCA gastric cancer treatment guideline, 2004.
87. Gotoda T, Yanagisawa A, Sasako M, et al. Incidence of lymph node metastasis from early gastric cancer: estimation with a large number of cases at two large centers. Gastric Cancer. 2000;3:219-25.
88. Oka S, Tanaka S, Kaneko I, et al. Advantage of endoscopic submucosal dissection compared with EMR for early gastric cancer. Gastrointest Endosc. 2006;64:877-83.
89. ASGE Technology Committee, Kantsevoy SV, Adler DG, Conway JD, et al. Technology status evaluation report: endoscopic mucosal resection and endoscopic submucosal dissection. Gastrointest Endosc. 2008;68:11-8.
90. Moss A, Bourke MJ, William SJ, et al. Predictors of therapeutic success for endoscopic resection (EMR) of laterally spreading tumors (LSTs) and large sessile colonic polyps: results of prospective multicenter Australian Colonic EMR (ACE) study. Gastrointest Endosc. 2010;71:AB111.
91. Swan MP, Bourke MJ, Moss A, et al. The target sign: an endoscopic marker for the resection of the muscularis propria and potential perforation during colonic endoscopic mucosal resection. Gastrointest Endosc. 2011;73:79-85.
92. Pandolfi M, Martino M, Gabbrielli A. Endoscopic treatment of ampullary adenomas. JOP. 2008;9:1-8.
93. Heinrich S, Clavien PA. Ampullary cancer. Curr Opin Gastroenterol. 2010;26:280-5.
94. de Castro SM, van Heek NT, Kuhlmann KF, et al. Surgical management of neoplasms of the ampulla of Vater: local resection or pancreaticoduodenectomy and prognostic factors for survival. Surgery. 2004;136:994-1002.
95. Farnell MB, Sakorafas GH, Sarr MG, et al. Villous tumors of the duodenum: reappraisal of local vs extended resection. J Gastrointest Surg. 2000;4:13-21.
96. Bohnacker S, Soehendra N, Maguchi H, et al. Endoscopic resection of benign tumors of the papilla of Vater. Endoscopy. 2006;38:521-5.
97. Norton ID, Gostout CJ, Baron TH, et al. Safety and outcome of endoscopic snare excision of the major duodenal papilla. Gastrointest Endosc. 2002;56:239-43.
98. Hernandez LV, Catalano MF. Endoscopic papillectomy. Curr Opin Gastroenterol. 2008;24:617-22.
99. Avital S, Zundel N, Szomstein S, et al. Laparoscopic transhiatal esophagectomy for esophageal cancer. Am J Surg. 2005;190:69-74.
100. Carboni F, Lepiane P, Santoro R, et al. Laparoscopic surgery for gastric cancer: preliminary experience. Gastric Cancer. 2005;8:75-7.
101. Croce E, Olmi S, Bertolini A, et al. Laparoscopic surgery of pancreatic cancer: state of the art. Hepatogastroenterology. 2005;52(66):1889-94.
102. Cho JY, Han HS, Yoon YS, et al. Laparoscopic approach for suspected early stage gallbladder carcinoma. Arch Surg. 2010;145(2):128-33.
103. Bianchi PP, Rosati R, Bona S, et al. Laparoscopic surgery in rectal cancer: a prospective analysis of patient survival and outcomes. Dis Colon Rectum. 2007;50(12):2047-53.
104. Swain P. A justification for NOTES--natural orifice transluminal endosurgery. Gastrointest Endosc. 2007;65:514-6.
105. Chukwumah C, Zorron R, Marks JM, et al. Current status of natural orifice transluminal endoscopic surgery (NOTES). Curr Probl Surg. 2010;47:630-68.

106. Lacy AM, Adelsdorfer C. Totally transrectal endoscopic total mesorectal excision (TME). Colorectal Dis. 2011;13 suppl 7:43-6.
107. Velthuis S, van den Boezem PB, van der Peet DL, et al. Feasibility study of transanal total mesorectal excision. Br J Surg. 2013;100(6):828-31.
108. ASGE Standards of Practice Committee, Evans JA, Early DS, et al. The role of endoscopy in the assessment and treatment of esophageal cancer. Gastrointest Endosc. 2013;77:328-34.
109. Targownik LE, Spiegel BM, Sack J, et al. Colonic stent vs. emergency surgery for management of acute left sided malignant colonic obstruction: a decision analysis. Gastrointest Endosc. 2004;60:865-74.
110. Baron TH, Dean PA, Yates MR, et al. Expandable metal stents for the treatment of colonic obstruction: techniques and outcomes. Gastrointest Endosc. 1998;47:277-86.
111. Baron TH, Rey JF, Spinelli P. Expandable metals stent placement for malignant colorectal obstruction. Endoscopy. 2002;34:823-30.
112. Watt AM, Faraghar IG, Griffin TT, et al. Self-expanding metallic stents for relieving malignant colorectal obstruction: a systemic review. Ann Surg. 2007;246:24-30.
113. Small AJ, Coelho-Prabhu N, Baron TH, et al. Endoscopic placement of self expandable metal stents for malignant colonic obstruction: long-term outcomes and complication factors. Gastrointest Endosc. 2010;71:560-72.
114. Kaufman M, Singh G, Das S, et al. Efficacy of endoscopic ultrasound guided celiac plexus block and celiac plexus neurolysis for managing abdominal pain associated with chronic pancreatitis and pancreatic cancer. J Clin Gastroenterol. 2010;44:127-34.
115. Catalano M, Ahmed U, Chauhan S. Celiac plexus neurolysis (CPN) in the treatment of refractory pain of pancreatic cancer: site specific response to therapy. Gastrointest Endosc. 2005;1:AB273.
116. Smith AC, Dowsett JF, Russell RC, et al. Randomised trial of endoscopic stenting versus surgical bypass in malignant low bile duct obstruction. Lancet. 1994;344:1655-60.
117. Moss AC, Morris E, Layden J, et al. Do the benefits of metal stents justify the costs? A systematic review and meta-analysis of trials comparing endoscopic stents for malignant biliary obstruction. Eur J Gastroenterol Hepatol. 2007;19:1119.
118. Giovannini M, Moutardier V, Pesenti C, et al. Endoscopic ultrasound-guided bilioduodenal anastomosis: a new technique for biliary drainage. Endoscopy. 2001;33:898-900.
119. Tsai TH, Zhou C, Tao YK, et al. Structural markers observed with endoscopic 3-dimensional optical coherence tomography correlating with Barrett's esophagus radiofrequency ablation treatment response. Gastrointest Endosc. 2012;76(6):1104.
120. Li Z, Zuo XL, Li CQ, et al. In vivo molecular imaging of gastric cancer by targeting MG7 antigen with confocal laser endomicroscopy. Endoscopy. 2013;45(2):79-85.

26 Cancer of the Esophagus

Praful Desai, Ganesh Balasubramaniam

INTRODUCTION

Esophageal cancer is the eighth most common cancer worldwide, with 481,000 new cases (3.8% of the total) estimated in 2008, and the sixth most common cause of death from cancer with 406,000 deaths (5.4% of the total).[1] These figures encompass both adenocarcinoma and squamous cell carcinoma (SCC) types. More than 80% of the cases and deaths occur in developing countries. Esophageal cancer is a relatively rare form of cancer, but some world areas have a markedly higher incidence than others: China, Iceland, India, Japan and UK appear to have a higher incidence, as well as the region around the Caspian Sea. In India the incidence rates vary across the country. High incidence of cancer of esophagus has been reported from Caspian littoral of Iran, Central and East Asia and certain areas of China.[2] In India, there are an estimated 29,000 new esophageal cancer cases and 26,000 deaths as per the GLOBOCAN estimates.[1] The age-adjusted incidence rates vary across India from $3.8/10^5$ in Barshi to $30.4/10^5$ in Aizawl among males and from $2.2/10^5$ in Barshi to $11.9/10^5$ in Dibrugarh among females (Figs 1A and B).[3]

In India, esophageal cancer is the most common malignancy involving the gastrointestinal tract in Karnataka, Tamil Nadu, Kerala and Assam.[4] In Kashmir, esophageal cancer is extremely common. There is scarcity of epidemiological studies in this malignancy.[5] Esophageal cancer has a peculiar geographical distribution and shows marked differences in incidence within a particular geographical region. Rao, et al.[6] (1996) reviewed the Indian studies on esophageal cancer and discussed in

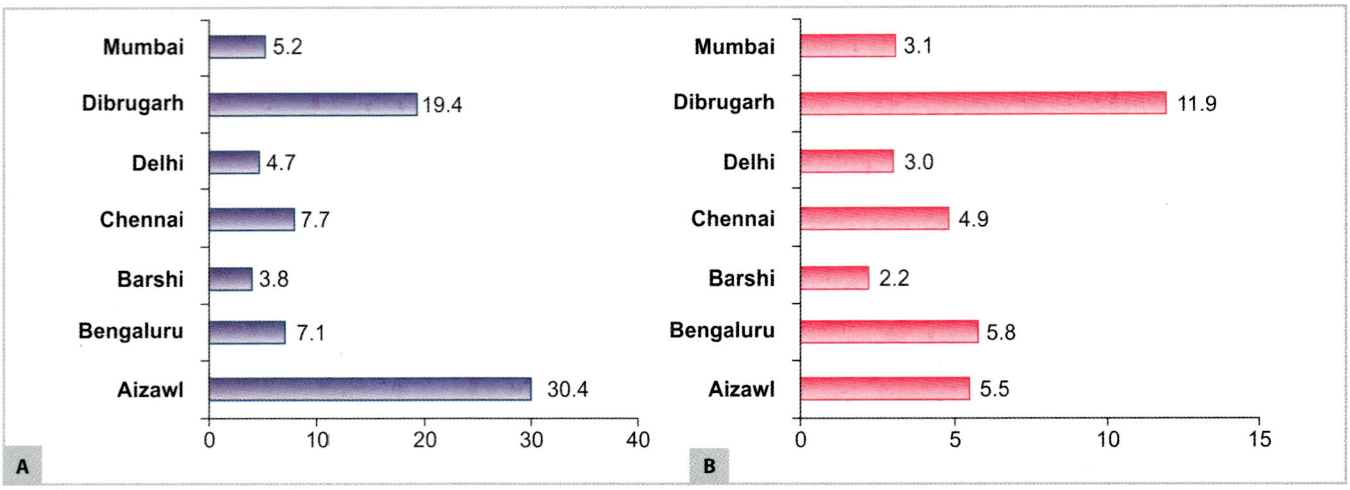

Figs 1A and B: (A) Age-adjusted incidence rates in males—India; (B) Age-adjusted incidence rates in females—India

detail aspects on incidence, mortality and risk factors. Presently, as there seems little prospect of early detection of this cancer, an understanding of the etiological factors may suggest opportunities for its primary prevention.

ASSOCIATED FACTORS

There are several risk factors that are associated with esophageal cancer. The chance of getting esophageal cancer is low at younger ages and increases with the age. Less than 15% of cases are found in people younger than age 55; also men have three-fold higher rates than women.[1] People with gastroesophageal reflux disease (GERD) of a long duration are at higher risk for esophageal cancer; GERD can cause Barrett's esophagus. This can progress to epithelial metaplasia, dysplasia and subsequent carcinoma over a period of years (> 10 years). Though screening for early diagnosis of esophageal cancer is an impractical proposition in India or elsewhere, a selective screening approach could be considered in the endemic regions of India (Kashmir, Assam and Northeast India) in a population with tobacco habits and symptoms of acidity or reflux regurgitation. Endoscopy and contrast studies may be worthwhile in this group and early diagnosis is feasible. Dysphagia is a late symptom and this effort may be worthwhile for a potentially lethal disease which is generally diagnosed late. Early diagnosis of stomach cancer in Japan is a classic example of screening producing huge benefits for a potentially serious disease.

The use of tobacco products like cigarette or cigar or smokeless tobacco like chewing tobacco are known to increase the risk for esophageal cancer. There are many studies from India as well from other parts globally which has demonstrated this association.[7] Alcohol increases the risk for esophageal cancer and is known to affect the squamous cell type more than the adenocarcinoma of the esophagus[8] among others. The combined habit of smoking and alcohol increases significantly the risk for esophageal cancer. "Diet" high in fruits and vegetables are known to reduce the risk whereas meat eaters are prone to higher risk for esophageal cancer. There are studies from India and Western countries as well; fruits and vegetables provide a number of vitamins and minerals that may help prevent cancer.[9] Red meat, lamb and boiled meat were directly associated with the risk of esophageal SCC, whereas total white meat, poultry, fish and liver were mainly protective against this malignancy.[10]

People who are overweight or obese have a higher chance of getting adenocarcinoma of the esophagus. This is in part explained by the fact that people who are obese are more likely to have esophageal reflux. Besides these there are other risk factors such as achalasia cardia, tylosis and injury to the esophagus (lye, a chemical found in strong industrial and household cleaners).

The current knowledge of risk factors will prove to be beneficial in understanding the disease thereby providing leads for prevention, through screening or primary prevention.

PRETHERAPY WORK-UP AND INVESTIGATION

Apart from the routine laboratory investigations, a profile of hepatorenal and cardiopulmonary function studies would be mandatory if surgical resection is a consideration. Contrast studies, endoscopy and biopsy are mandatory; a CT scan study of the chest and abdomen are essential for assessing the total profile of a given tumor. Endoscopic ultrasound for T-N status is optional and not done routinely at all centers. Operability is based on many different criteria. A T_3N_{1-2} lesion diagnosed on endoscopic ultrasound is not necessarily a contraindication for surgery as other clinical and investigational criteria need to be evaluated before treatment decisions are made in a given clinical setting.

A positron emission tomography-computed tomography (PET-CT) evaluation is again optional. False positive results are not uncommon, since reactive or inflammatory or tubercular nodes often give false positive results. The benefit of identifying distant metastatic lesions exists; however, this must be histologically proven before accepting the M stage. The true value of this expensive investigation is debatable and will depend on the clinician. Assessment of treatment response by PET-CT after chemoradiotherapy is also optional as simpler methods can also indicate response. Though surgical approach is steadfast and generally accepted when the disease is localized within the esophagus, the following considerations are vital for a final therapeutic decision. Complementary and combination therapy with surgery, radiotherapy and chemotherapy as and when indicated should be the rule and a team approach is mandatory before a final treatment decision.

SURGICAL APPROACH

TABLE 1: Standard surgical approaches

	Site of lesion	*Surgical approaches*
Adenocarcinoma	Cardioesophageal junction, lower esophagus, cardia	Left thoracoabdominal Ivor-Lewis/Tanner (TTE) Transhiatal (THE)
Squamous carcinoma		
Squamous carcinoma	Middle one-third lesion	Three-stage total esophagectomy (TTE) Transhiatal esophagectomy (THE)
Adenocarcinoma (rare)		
Squamous carcinoma	Cervical	Poor candidates for surgery Chemotherapy/radiotherapy/stenting, etc. are better options
Squamous carcinoma	Supra-aortic	
Squamous carcinoma	Thoracic inlet	

Abbreviations: TTE, transthoracic esophagectomy; THE, transhiatal esophagectomy

LOCALIZED (LOCOREGIONAL) ESOPHAGEAL CANCER

Though surgical excision remains the therapy of choice in this clinical setting, a number of trials have indicated a better disease-free and 5-year survival by combining neoadjuvant chemoradiotherapy [three cycles cisplatin/fluorouracil (5-FU)/paclitaxel and 45 Gy radiation therapy][11,12] followed by a surgical resection, 3–4 weeks later. This is not universally accepted as neoadjuvant chemoradiotherapy can produce postoperative complications including cardiopulmonary and problems with anastomotic healing; particularly so if, radical chemoradiotherapy has been used. Combination therapy is indicated if the lesion, though resectable, is locoregionally advanced. Surgical results of lesions of the supraaortic region and thoracic inlet are unsatisfactory and are better treated by definitive chemoradiotherapy, with surgery only as a salvage option. Indeed, any lesion with a length greater than 6 cm is best managed by neoadjuvant chemoradiotherapy. It is then assessed for a surgical resection or definitive chemoradiotherapy, if the response is satisfactory with a significant regression of the lesion and complete relief of dysphagia.

The debate about the types of surgical procedures and the views regarding two- or three-field nodal dissection will continue; however, certain surgical principles have remain steadfast.

- A good proximal margin of 5 cm or more in the surgical specimen (Fig. 2)
- Nodal dissection of two-field [adequate regional dissection (ARL)] is an accepted standard. This includes (a) celiac and left gastric; (b) gastric lesser curvature and (c) mediastinal, hilar region (Figs 3A to C)

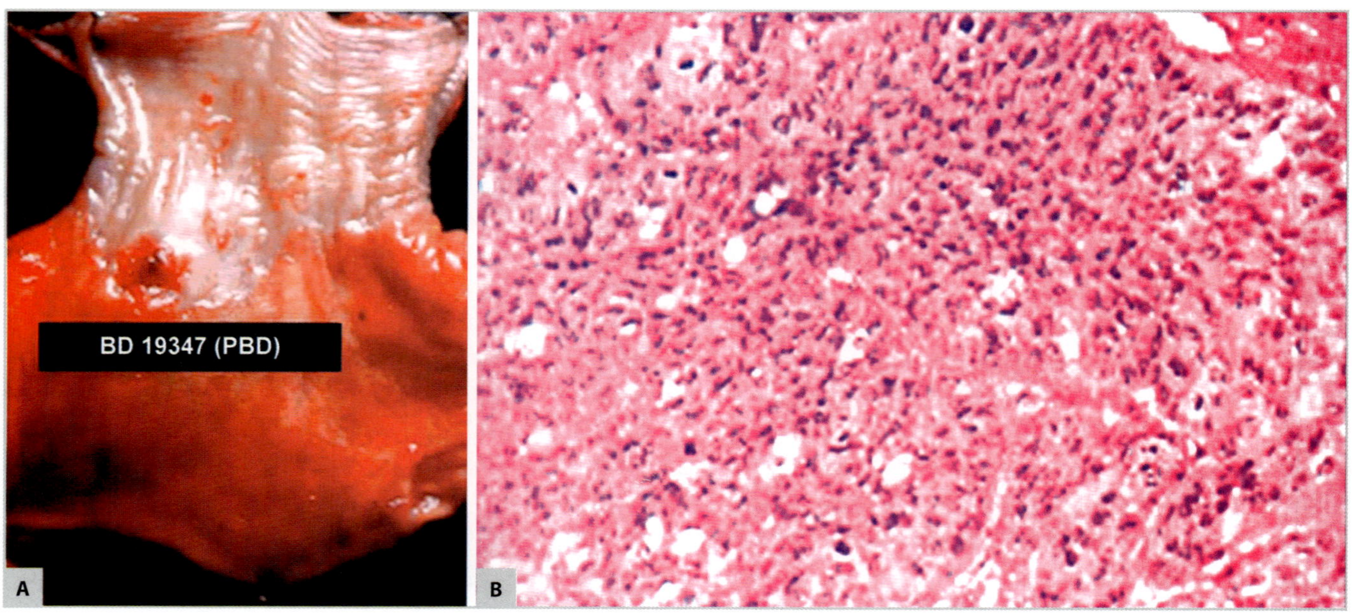

Figs 2A and B: (A) Early cardioesophageal lesion—resected specimen via left thoracoabdominal approach. Good proximal margin greater than 5 cm. Margins shrink in vitro; (B) Operative specimen of resection and histology. Extremely active tumor

- A three-field dissection (including low cervical) would be a natural consequence of a total esophagectomy, where a right thoracotomy is a part of the procedure in a three-stage procedure (abdomen, right chest and neck)
- For lesions of the lower one-third and cardia, a left thoracoabdominal approach is generally a very adequate procedure and a total esophagectomy is not always necessary (Figs 4A to C) (Table 1)
- An Ivor-Lewis approach with a high right intrathoracic anastomosis is a very satisfactory procedure with a mortality rate of less than 5% in high volume hospitals and surgeons. This procedure is being increasingly practised now even by those earlier performing total esophagectomy (Fig. 5)
- For lesions of the middle one-third extending proximally, a total esophagectomy with a three-field dissection becomes mandatory with a cervical anastomosis; the surgical approach could be transhiatal or transthoracic. The three-field nodal dissection carries with it an increased risk and incidence of recurrent laryngeal nerve injury and pulmonary morbidities. Proponents of three-field nodal dissection claim some improvement in results, not generally duplicated.[13-15]

It is worthwhile to note that the THE evolved in the 1980s, primarily to avoid the serious complications of

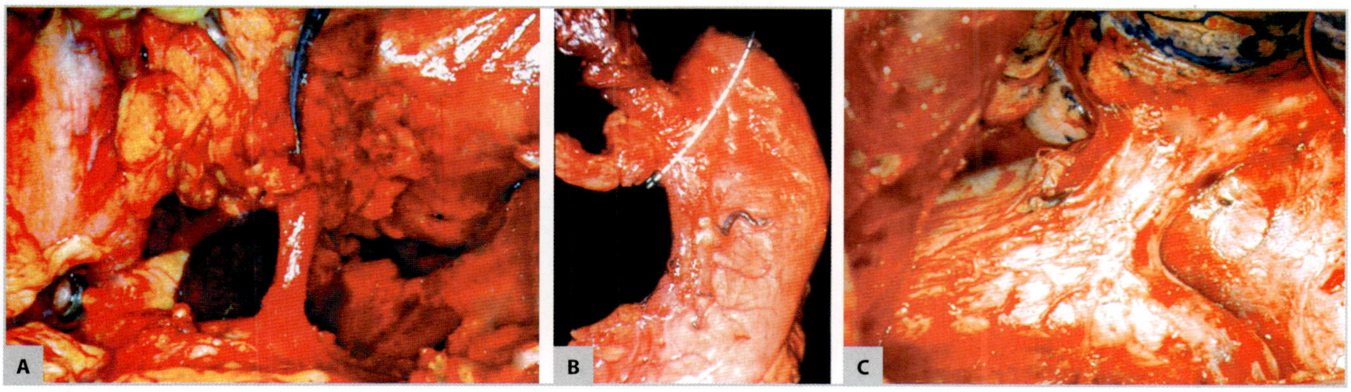

Figs 3A to C: (A) Celiac axis nodal clearance; the left gastric artery is cleared of nodes and fatty tissue, and should be ligated at the upper border of the pancreas; (B) Clearance of nodes from lesser curvature of the stomach; (C) Subcarinal nodal clearance in the right chest, the right and left bronchus, and subcarinal area is clearly visible (two-field dissection) (ARL)

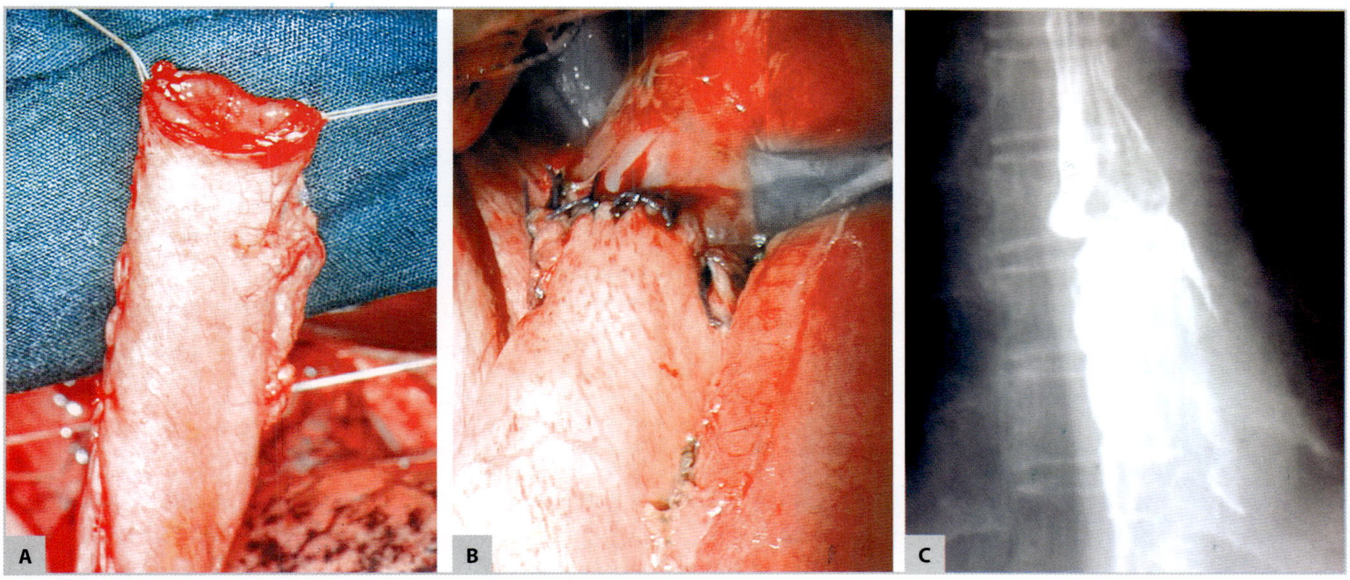

Figs 4A to C: (A) Gastric tube conduit prepared for the anastomosis; (B) Hand-sewn left sided esophagogastric anastomosis for a lesion in the lower one-third of the esophagus. Anastomosis just below the aortic arch. Descending thoracic aorta is clearly visible next to the stomach tube; (C) Contrast study 6 months later of the same patient showing a smooth passage with a wide anastomosis (above the left inferior pulmonary vein). Left sided thoracic—abdominal approach for cancer at the cardia

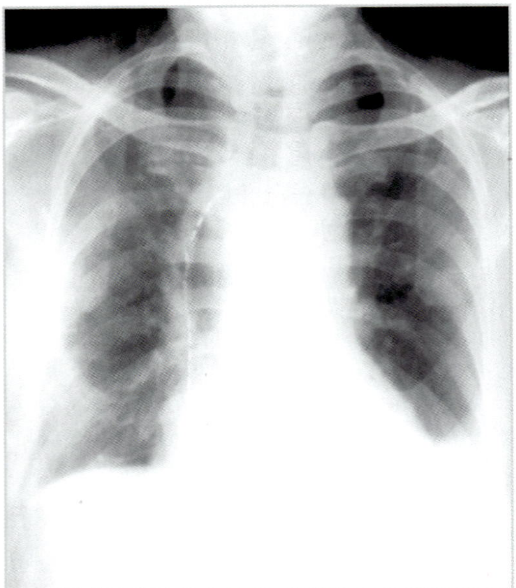

Fig. 5: The stomach conduit is seen lying snugly in the mediastinum with the anastomosis above the arch of aorta high (Ivor-Lewis) in the right chest

an anastomotic disruption in the right or left chest. With increasing experience over the years the leakage rate is now less than 5% (even 2% in high volume hospitals and surgeons) and with aggressive management of an anastomotic disruption, most patients are salvaged from this dreaded complication. Many authors prefer a total esophagectomy even for a lesion of the lower one-third and cardia via a transhiatal (TH) approach. This will depend on the comfort zone of the surgeon. THE would be preferable for a patient with a low cardiopulmonary reserve.

Transthoracic and Transhiatal Esophagectomy and Open/Minimally Invasive/Robotic Esophagectomy

Arguments and debates will continue over these issues as it has happened ever since TH approach and the minimally invasive surgery (MIS) began to be performed more frequently. It is now beyond any doubt, based on many well-studied randomized trials that the results are nearly equivalent in experienced hands, vis-à-vis node retrieval, complications and long-term results. There is also little doubt that every single case of resectable esophageal cancer need not undergo a total esophagectomy as lesions of the lower reaches of the esophagus and cardia can be easily and effectively handled by a subtotal esophagectomy (Ivor-Lewis or left thoracoabdominal approach). It may be of interest to note the very recent publication of Leuketich, et al.[16] of 1,000 MIS (with cervical anastomosis) in which there is now a shift toward a subtotal (Ivor-Lewis) type of esophagectomy with a right intrathoracic anastomosis. More importantly, it is the comfort zone of the operating surgeon, open or MIS or robotic, which is more important rather than any major differences in the procedure. Less pain, less complications and an earlier hospital discharge of 2–3 days are usually mentioned with MIS/robotic surgery. The overall complications, the node retrievals, the disease-free survival (DFS) and overall survival (OS) are almost comparable. The learning curve of all the three techniques is long and difficult. An experienced open surgeon can master the other techniques expeditiously; the reverse is probably not true.[17-20]

NODAL DISSECTION (TWO-FIELD/THREE-FIELD)

Adequate Regional Dissection (ARL)

The three-field dissection for a lesion high in the middle one-third will be a natural consequence of a total esophagectomy. The profuse lymphatic drainage of an organ extending over three anatomic regions is a major issue in the surgical treatment of esophageal cancer. It is true that in advanced esophageal cancer (T3N2) lymph nodes away from the site may be involved (e.g. cervical nodes) from a lower esophageal cancer (8–10%); however, these are hardly the cases that one would plan for a surgical therapy. It is, therefore, unjustifiable and is not a strong enough reason to subject 90% of patients to a total esophagectomy and a three-field dissection, which is compatible with greater morbidity and complication. Even the long-term survival results are not significantly superior in comparison with an ARL and a two-field dissection; (coeliac, gastric, mediastinal and hilar)[21] (Figs 6 to 8).

A right-sided intrathoracic esophagogastrostomy (Ivor-Lewis) anastomosis and a left-sided subaortic anastomosis will ensure a good proximal margin of at least 5 cm or more for most lesions of the CO junction, cardia and lower middle third esophageal cancers.

Quantum of Node Retrieval

An average retrieval of 15 nodes is considered adequate surgery and conveys a good dissection. Recent reports indicate that quantum of node retrieval is very comparable with either [transthoracic (TT) or TH] approaches whereas some indicate that TT node retrieval is greater. This is indeed a theoretical debate and generally does not impact on ultimate control or cure rates. Clearance of 15

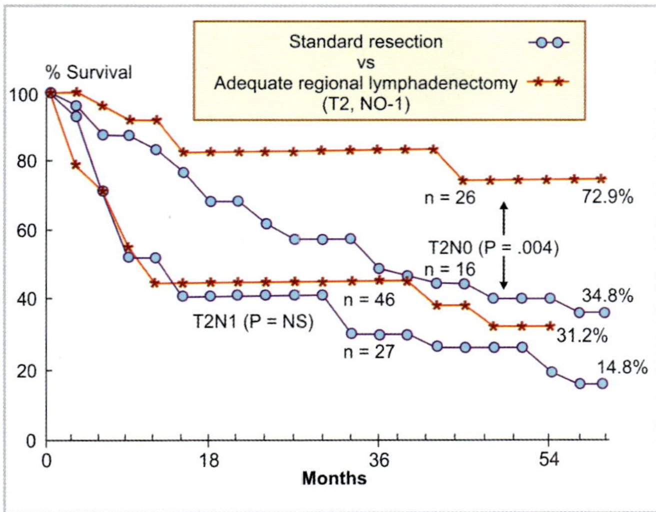

Fig. 6: The standard resection versus adequate regional (ARL) lymphadenectomy (T2, NO-1)[21]

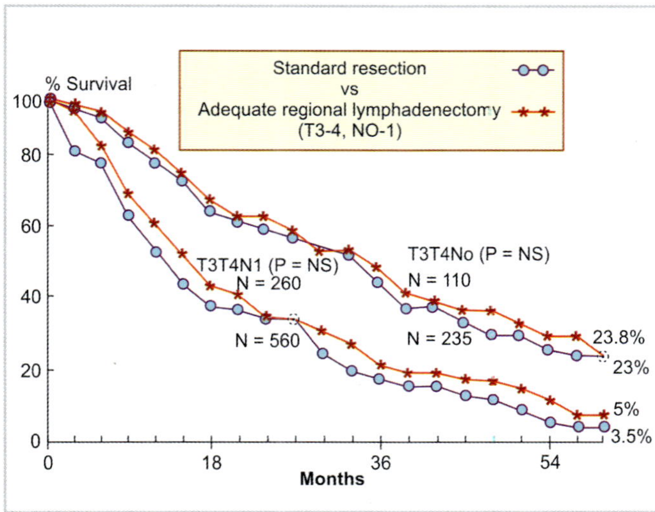

Fig. 7: The standard resection versus adequate regional (ARL) lymphadenectomy (T3–4, NO-1)[21]

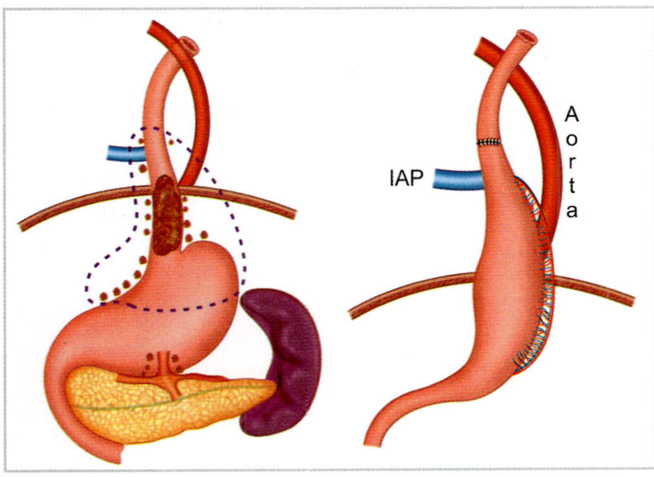

Fig. 8: The extent of resection and nodal clearance for a lesion in the lower esophagus and cardia. The left esophagogastric anastomosis is well above the inferior pulmonary vein (IPV) about 3–4 cm below the aortic arch. Via left thoracoabdominal approach

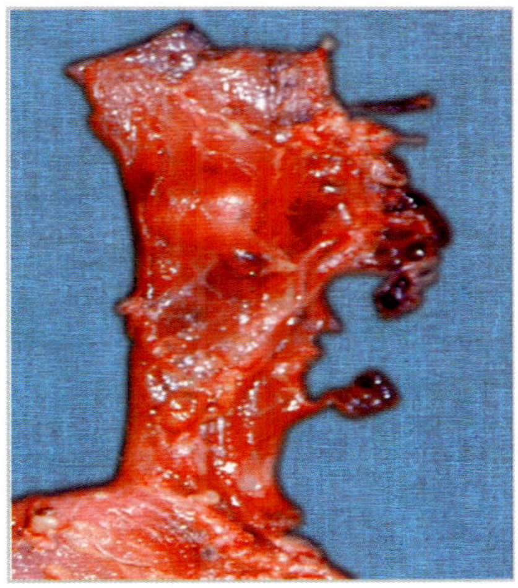

Fig. 9: Specimen of esophagectomy with two-field dissection (Ivor-Lewis)

metastatic nodes or more, generally does not improve survival rates as prognosis is inversely proportional to the number of involved nodes (Fig. 9).

Recent studies regarding the impact of high volume surgeon and high volume institutions, for very major surgeries like esophagectomy, pancreatectomy and liver resections, etc. have been studied extensively by many authors.[22] There is little doubt that the survival rates for such technically demanding procedures are better and complications and morbidities are lower with high-volume surgeons working in a high-volume tertiary institution. Centralization of such difficult surgical procedures, therefore, needs to be seriously considered.

Anastomotic Breakdowns

The bane of esophageal surgery is the serious complication due to an anastomotic leakage. It is now conclusively shown that high-volume surgeons and hospitals[22] consistently report leakage rates of less than 5% and mortality rates of 2–4% at many centers. Cervical anastomosis disrupts more often (15%) than intrathoracic (5%) and can result in significant morbidity; mediastinitis, strictures, repeated dilatations and a poor quality of life are commonly seen. The genesis of TH total esophagectomy was based on the reasons to avoid an intrathoracic anastomosis leakage and the consequent serious surgical complications. With experience in most centers, this complication is now rare and managed efficiently as mortality due to this reason is now quite uncommon and less than 5%.

Prevention and Management of Anastomotic Leaks

The leakage rate either with hand-sewn or staplers are comparable, though strictures are probably more common with staplers than hand-sewn absorbable sutures. The fundamentals of a safe anastomosis lie in vascular cut ends of esophagus and the stomach, and tension free loose anastomosis. The simpler the anastomosis the greater the chances of safe healing; whether interrupted or continuous, a 3-0 Vicryl™ suture is the safest material to use. It is not the number of stitches which holds or heals the anastomosis. It is the vascularity and tension free anastomosis which has the maximum chance of primary healing. Despite all the precautions and experiences that one brings to bear in esophageal surgery, the surgeon has to contend and deal with the problem of anastomotic breakdowns. The incidence is reported from 5 to 30% or as low as 2% or even 0% in experienced hands; generally speaking, the incidence is inversely proportional to the experience of the operating surgeon. Currently, in most centers of excellence, dehiscence rate of around 5% seems acceptable and is compatible with good esophageal surgery; what is more important is early diagnosis and effective management of the leak because most of these patients are salvageable.

TYPE OF ANASTOMOTIC DISRUPTIONS

Type I—Major

Usually occurs between the 4th and the 7th postoperative day. The patient rapidly deteriorates with a breakdown of cardiopulmonary function with signs and symptoms of bronchospasm, shock, collapse and dyspnea; X-ray studies may reveal pneumothorax or collapse of the lung with pleural fluid; thoracic drain may not show increase in drainage as the infected discharges are often loculated in the mediastinum, interlobar fissure and phrenicocostal sinuses.

Immediate management will require urgent resuscitative measures, a thoracotomy for rapid evacuation of infected material from the chest with appropriate drains; ensure expansion of the lung, adequate antibiotic therapy, restoration of a normovolemic state and ventilatory support as indicated. It is futile to reanastomose disrupted necrotic ends unless the disruption is minimal. A very major total disruption will require an end-cervical esophagostomy and a feeding jejunostomy or gastrostomy. The stomach tube may have to be disengaged and brought out as a gastrostomy; such severe disruptions are now rarely seen with increasing experience in esophageal surgery. Appropriate total parenteral nutrition and caloric intake are most important. A feeding jejunostomy at the end of primary resection is not always mandatory, though some surgeons prefer it as a choice for postoperative feeding. A fatality is always at hand if such aggressive management is not instituted as an emergency measure in very major, near total breakdown of the anastomosis. In experienced hands such major breakdowns are extremely rare.

Type II—Moderate

This is the more common type of dehiscence and occurs during the same postoperative period (between 4 and 8 days). Stomach end necrosis is the more common site; occasionally, the sutured lesser curvature of the gastric conduit gives way. Rarely, there can be a complete failure to heal at the anastomotic site. The symptoms which should arouse suspicion to achieve an early diagnosis of this complication are those of a less than smooth postoperative progress, viz. a moderate spike in temperature, mild bronchospasm, mild dyspnea for no apparent reason and tachycardia. Generally the cardiovascular profile is stable, though the leukocyte count shows an upward trend and the chest X-ray shows patches of pneumonitis and air or fluid collection which is not over a large area. The thoracic drain may or may not show increase in the exudates and auscultation of the lungs will reveal diminished air entry, crepitations or clinical evidence of a collapse. It is imperative that at the earliest evidence of clinical suspicion and presence of signs mentioned above, attempts must be made to prove or disprove a suture line dehiscence. The most efficient way to do this is to aspirate chest fluid if any and oral contrast study to see the security of the anastomosis. There may be a 25–30% escape of the contrast in the pleural cavity and nearly 70% may still be passing normally through the anastomosis into the stomach.

Rapid decisions have to be made regarding management approach vis-à-vis a thoracotomy or an intensive conservative approach. Generally, if a good lung expansion is ensured, the stomach segment is well-decompressed, nutrition is effectively maintained by a jejunostomy or parenteral hyperalimentation and the patient does not show any evidence of septicemia, nearly all patients can be salvaged by a conservative approach. The breakdown will heal in about 10–14 days during which the patient needs to be supported with appropriate and adequate antibiotics, physiotherapy, etc. Generally, ventilator supports are not indicated in this group of patients unless the pO_2, pCO_2 levels continue to be abnormal. The chest picture will rapidly improve, pyrexia will settle and the overall clinical condition will steadily get better. A repeat Conray™ study can be done after 2 weeks and if the anastomosis has healed, oral intake can be gradually started. In some patients (25–30%) in this group, if the condition worsens within 24–48 hours after diagnosis, thoracotomy to efficiently drain infected or loculated pockets may become necessary. The cardinal principles in the management of anastomotic breakdown, therefore, are:

- Rapid evacuation and drainage of infected effluents in the chest or abdominal cavity when indicated
- Nutritional support through a jejunostomy and/or parenteral hyperalimentation
- Adequate and efficient antibiotic therapy
- Thorough lung expansion
- Supportive therapy with proteins, vitamins, whole blood, albumin, etc.
- Physiotherapy

Type III—Minor (Contrast Study—Radiologic Leak)

Most of these are asymptomatic and only rarely require active treatment. These are diagnosed incidentally, when a thin contrast medium (Conray™) is given before starting oral feeds. A thin streak of outpouching or a linear streak in the mediastinum is the most common finding; often, these streaks empty out into the anastomotic area and into the stomach. Patients are generally asymptomatic. Very occasionally, a mild bronchospasm may occur which will rapidly subside with bronchodilators. The reason for this kind of "radiologic outpouching" is the slightly asymmetric apposition between esophagus and the substituted segments (stomach or colon). No active therapy is needed and the patients may be kept off feeds for 2 or 3 days when these minor outpouching seals off.

CHEMORADIOTHERAPY AS DEFINITIVE TREATMENT

More reports[23,24] now indicate this as a therapy of choice to avoid the severity, morbidity and complications of esophageal surgery even in resectable lesions of the esophagus. For locally advanced lesions, this approach often provides good palliation and occasionally a long-term survival (Figs 10A to D). Selection of patients for this mode of therapeutic approach is therefore important. Generally our experience shows that proliferative, noninfiltrating type of lesions respond very adequately whereas strictured, obstructive and cicatrizing type of lesions responds poorly to chemoradiotherapy. In a study, nearly 70% respond adequately to consider chemoradiotherapy as a primary definitive treatment for this type of lesions. Further studies are needed to appropriately select patients for chemoradiotherapy as a definitive primary treatment for esophageal cancers.

PALLIATION

The most distressing symptom of the disease is dysphagia. In many of the terminally advanced patients relief of dysphagia is a major concern. Palliative chemoradiotherapy and surgical resections have already been discussed. A major source of relief for dysphagia is the expandable metal stents which could be carefully traversed through the stenosed diseased area. Blockage due to food debris, overgrowth of cancer and dislocation of stents are known complications (Fig. 11). This should be considered only when surgery, chemoradiotherapy have been ruled out.

CHEMOTHERAPY

Squamous cell carcinoma of the esophagus and the rarer adenocarcinoma are significantly responsive to chemotherapy. Cisplatin based chemotherapy with 5-FU and occasionally taxanes elicit partial response and occasionally complete pathologic responses (15–20%) particularly in proliferative noninfiltrating lesions.

Chemotherapy is usually considered in the following clinical settings:

- As a definitive therapy: Along with radiotherapy in advanced esophageal cancers which are beyond the ambit of surgical resection. In postcricoid, thoracic inlet and supraaortic regions, surgical results are poor and chemoradiotherapy is often used concurrently or sequentially with equivalent results of surgery with little morbidity
- Neoadjuvant (upfront) chemotherapy or Chemoradiotherapy together are often used to downstage the disease. Generally a response assessment is made 2 weeks after completion of three cycles and 40 Gy of radiotherapy to consider the possibility of a surgical resection, clinically and by imaging studies. Heavy doses of radiation, more than 50 Gy and more than three cycles of chemotherapy can result in severe postoperative morbidities and complication with increased

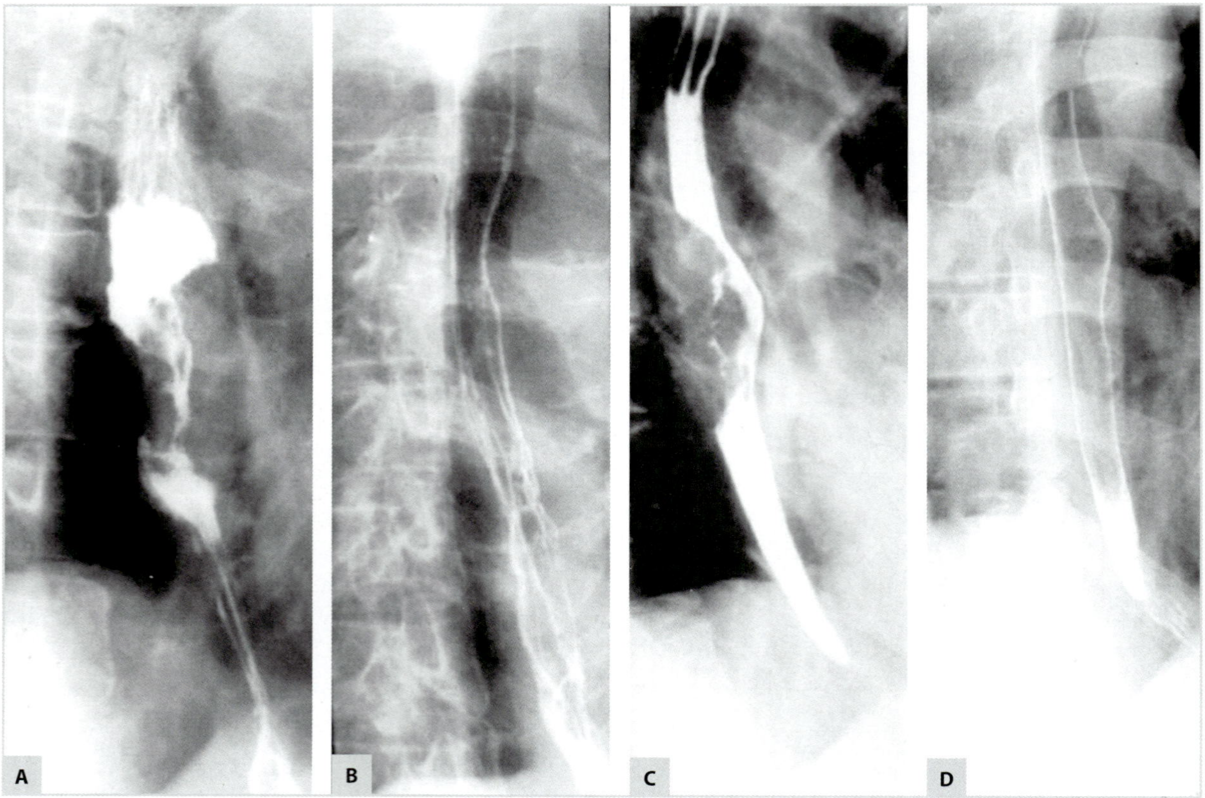

Figs 10A to D: Two different patients with locally advanced lesions of the middle esophagus showing very satisfactory responses with chemoradiotherapy. Prolonged palliation extending from 8 months to 4 years. Predominantly proliferative lesions

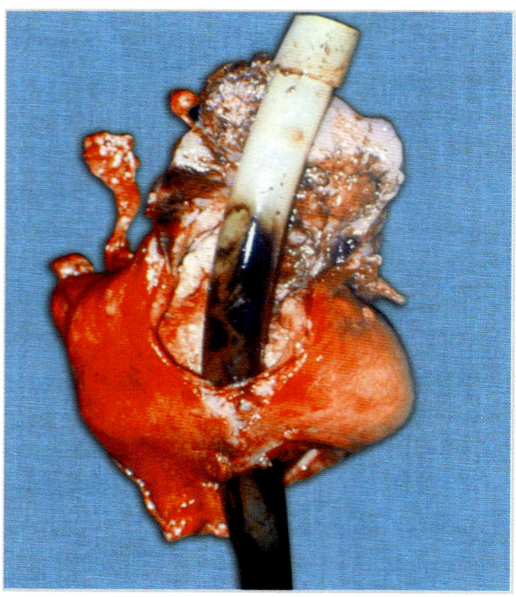

Fig. 11: Resected specimen of the esophagus with an in situ stent. A proper assessment of resectability of the lesion is mandatory before stenting. Complications due to stents are not uncommon

anastomotic leaks. A few trials have shown positive results [Medical Research Council (MRC) trial][11]

- Adjuvant (postoperative) chemoradiotherapy: After major resectional surgery, adjuvant chemotherapy or radiotherapy is poorly tolerated and no documented data are at hand of any significant improvement of either DFS or OS. Chemotherapy, therefore, is best used in an upfront neoadjuvant setting.

Studies about chemotherapy sensitivity to a given lesion have been published without any definitive result; overall, however, the proliferative, noninfiltrating (even bulky size) type of lesions respond much better (including complete pathologic responses) than the obstructive, infiltrative and stenosing (stricture type) types of esophageal cancers. Surgery in this group should therefore be considered per primam (Figs 12A to D) (Table 2).

TABLE 2: Chemotherapy or radiotherapy response in cancer esophagus

Type of lesion		*Responses*			*%*
	N	*CR*	*PR*	*NR*	
Ulcerative—stenotic infiltrative	65	0	10	55	15
Proliferative	101	20	54	27	73* (CR/PR)
Ulceroproliferative	34	0	15	19	44
	200				

*p ≤ 02

Abbreviations: CR, complete remission; PR, partial remission; NR, no response

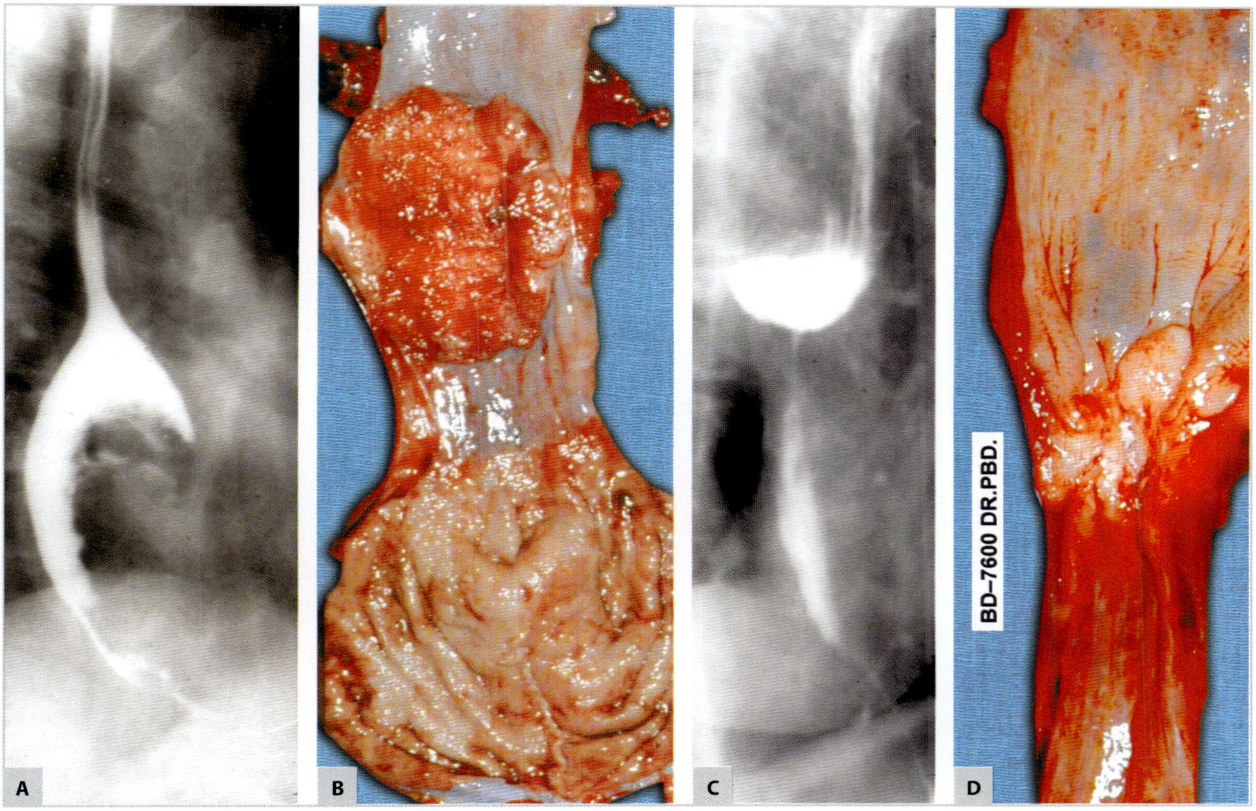

Figs 12A to D: (A and B) Esophagograms and specimens of a predominantly proliferative lesion and obstructive, cicatrizing lesion; (C and D) The former responds very effectively with neoadjuvant chemotherapy unlike obstructing lesions which respond properly

TRACHEOESOPHAGEAL FISTULA

This is a potentially dangerous and lethal complication of locally advanced esophageal cancers. Very rarely in neglected cases patients may initially present with complaints of persistent cough (saliva aspiration) and obvious inability to swallow, fever, aspiration pneumonia and weight loss are constant features. Majority of tracheoesophageal fistulae occurs in the upper thoracic region or occasionally in the middle third. Only palliation is feasible.

- Expandable metal stents can occasionally block a small tracheoesophageal fistula temporarily; larger tracheoesophageal fistulae are difficult to palliate. If the patient's general condition is good and investigations reveal localized disease in a short segment, attempts can be made toward aggressive palliation by improving nutrition by:
  - A feeding gastrostomy or jejunostomy and re-evaluation after 3–4 weeks
  - End-cervical esophagectomy with closure of the distal end in the neck to prevent aspiration pneumonias and hectic fever
- Chemotherapy: Two to three cycles (cisplatin based) could be administered during this phase as occasionally in around 10% the fistula may close if there is disease response. Rarely, due to necrosis, fistula can worsen
- Radiation therapy is contraindicated in presence of a TE fistula due to the danger of worsening the fistula due to radiation necrosis
- If the general condition improves and in the event of a good response, attempts to do a colonic bypass (retrosternal) by a cervical esophagocolostomy and cologastrostomy is a theoretical possibility. These are severe procedures and are compatible with morbidity and mortality. However, in very rare suitable clinical setting, this procedure can be considered. No attempt should be made to do esophagectomy.

At the most palliation can last 6–8 months. Untreated, most patients will succumb in 2–3 months. A considered decision after a detailed discussion with the patient and relatives is imperative. Best supportive care is an alternative with poor outcomes in this very distressing complication of neglected esophageal cancer.

REFERENCES

1. Ferlay J, Shin HR, Bray F, et al. (2010) GLOBOCAN 2008: Cancer Incidence and Mortality Worldwide: IARC CancerBase No. 10. [online]. Available from http://www.iarc.fr/en/publications/eresources/cancerbases/ [Accessed January, 2014].
2. Kamangar F, Malekzadeh R, Dawsey SM, et al. Esophageal cancer in Northeastern Iran: a review. Arch Iran Med. 2007;10(1):70-82.
3. National Cancer Registry Programme, Indian Council of Medical Research. Two year Report of the Population Based Cancer Registries, 2006-2008. National Cancer Registry Programme, 2009, Bangalore, India.
4. Chitra S, Ashok L, Anand L, et al. Risk factors for esophageal cancer in Coimbatore; southern India: a hospital-based care control study. Indian J Gastroenterol. 2004;23(1):19-21.
5. Khan NA, Lone MM, Fir Afroz, et al. Clinico-pathological profile of carcinoma oesophagus and esophago-gastric junction in Kashmir. JK Practitioner. 2004;11:182-5.
6. Rao DN, Desai PB, Ganesh B. Epidemiological observations on cancer of the oesophagus—a review of Indian studies. Indian J Cancer. 1996;33(2):55-75.
7. Ganesh B, Talole SD, Dikshit R. Tobacco, alcohol and tea drinking as risk factors for esophageal cancer: A case-control study from Mumbai, India. Cancer Epidemiol. 2009;33(6):431-4.
8. Sharma MK, Gour N, Pandey A, et al. Epidemiological study of risk factors for oral, laryngeal and esophageal cancers at a tertiary care hospital in India. Asian Pac J Cancer Prev. 2011;12(5):1215-8.
9. Pohl H, Wrobel K, Bojarski C, et al. Risk factors in the development of esophageal adenocarcinoma. Am J Gastroenterol. 2013;108(2):200-7.
10. De Stefani E, Deneo-Pellegrini H, Ronco AL, et al. Meat consumption, cooking methods, mutagens, and risk of squamous cell carcinoma of the esophagus: a case-control study in Uruguay. Nutr Cancer. 2012;64(2):294-9.
11. Medical Research Council Oesophageal Cancer Working Group. Surgical resection with or without preoperative chemotherapy in oesophageal cancer. A randomised controlled trial. Lancet. 2002;359(9319):1727-33.
12. Lerut T, Moons J, Coosemans W, et al. Multidisciplinary treatment of advanced cancer of the esophagus and gastroesophageal junction: a European center's approach. Surg Oncol Clin N Am. 2008;17(3):485-502.
13. Akiyama H, Tsurumaru M, Udagawa H, et al. Radical lymph node dissection for cancer of the thoracic esophagus. Ann Surg. 1994;220(3):364-72.
14. Nishimaki T, Suzuki T, Kanda T, et al. Extended radical esophagectomy for superficially invasive carcinoma of the esophagus. Surgery. 1999;125(2):142-7.
15. Hulscher JB, van Sandick JW, de Boer AG, et al. Extended transthoracic resection compared with limited transhiatal resection for adenocarcinoma of esophagus. N Engl J Med. 2002;347(21):1662-9.
16. Leuketich JD, Pennathur A, Awais O, et al. Outcomes after minimally invasive esophagectomy: review of over 1000 patients. Ann Surgery. 2012;256(1):95-103.
17. Rindani et al. Data from meta-analysis 5483 patients 1986-1996.
18. Connors RC, Reuben BC, Neumayer LA, et al. Comparing outcomes after transthoracic and transhiatal esophagectomy: a 5-year prospective cohort of 17,395 patients. J Am Coll Surg. 2007;205(6):735-40.
19. Stiles BM, Mirza F, Coppolino A, et al. Clinical T2-T3N0M0 esophageal cancer: the risk of node positive disease. Ann Thorac Surg. 2011;92(2):491-6.
20. Orringer MB, Marshall B, Chang AC, et al. Two thousand transhiatal esophagectomies: changing trends, lessons learned. Ann Surg. 2007;246(3):363-72.
21. Desai P, Deshpande R, et al. Adequate regional lymphadenectomy in cancer of the esophagus. Dis Esophagus. 1992;5:99-105.
22. Birkmeyer JD, Siewers AE, Finlayson EV, et al. Hospital volume and surgical mortality in United States. N Engl J Med. 2002;346(15):1128-37.
23. Arnott SJ, Duncan W, Gignoux M, et al. Preoperative radiotherapy for esophageal cancer. Cochrane Database Syst Rev. 2005;19(4):CD001799.
24. Roth J, Pass H, et al. Randomised clinical trial of pre-postoperative adjunct chemotherapy with cisplatin and bleomycin for ca esophagus. J Thorac Cardiovasc Surg. 1998;96:242-8.

27 Carcinoma Stomach

Praful Desai, Bhavna Parikh, Nagraj G Huilgol, Ganesh Balasubramaniam

INTRODUCTION

Despite a reasonably significant knowledge of etiology, modern investigations and imaging capabilities, cancer of the stomach is diagnosed late the world over, except in Japan and some Southeast Asian countries where screening is routine for this disease owing to its high prevalence. The prognosis, even after appropriate therapy is dismal with a 5-year survival rate of less than 25% globally, in contrast to those in Japan where 5-year disease free survival (DFS) is reported to be greater than 70% and reaching even more than 90% where mucosal or submucosal cancers (stage I) are routinely diagnosed by screening and treated with appropriate therapy. Overall, however, the incidence is showing a decline due to proper management of increasing reflux disease and control of *H. pylori* infections.[1]

EPIDEMIOLOGY

The global burden of cancer, as per the recent GLOBOCAN estimates,[2] is approximately 12.6 million new cancer cases and 7.6 million cancer deaths each year. Gastric cancer is the fourth leading site of cancer in the world; there are nearly 1 million new cancers and 0.7 million cancer deaths due to gastric cancer. Gastric cancer is now more common in Asia than in US or Europe. Until the 1980s, gastric cancer was the most common type of cancer in the world. Since then, the rates have fallen in all developed countries and overall rates are now about 15% lower than in 1985. Forty-two percent of cases occur in China alone. Gastric cancer is the second most common cause of death due to malignancy accounting for 736,000 deaths, 9.7% of the total. High-risk areas are China, Japan, Eastern Europe, Central and South America. Low-risk areas are Southeast Asia, Northern and Eastern Africa, USA, Australia and New Zealand.[3-5]

Historically, the rates of gastric cancer were remarkably high in the more developed countries, but the rates have considerably reduced in many of these countries recently. The morbidity and mortality due to gastric cancer indicates a downward trend in most countries world-wide. The decline initially began in countries with low gastric cancer incidence such as the US.[6] Decline in countries with high incidence like Japan was slower.[7] Part of the decline may be due to the recognition of certain risk factors such as *Helicobacter pylori* and other dietary and environmental risks.[8] Gastric cancer is the fifth leading site of cancer among all sites in males and seventh among females in India; however, there are variations in the occurrence of gastric cancer within India. The incidence rates of gastric cancer in India is very low compared to Western countries and the number of new gastric cancers is about 34,000 with a male predominance ratio of 1:2. It is estimated that by the year 2020, there would be approximately 50,000 new gastric cancers annually.

The incidence of gastric cancer has been higher in southern India, viz. Chennai;[9] however, recent data shows that the incidence rates are highest in the Northeastern region [National Cancer Registry Program (NCRP), 2009]. As per the latest reports available from the NCRP (2009), gastric cancer incidence rate in males was 11.75 in Chennai and 9.5 in Bengaluru while among females it was 6.01 and 5.60 in Chennai and Bengaluru respectively. In Mumbai, the rates are as low as 4.9 per 100,000; in Bengaluru, it is the leading site of cancer among males while in Chennai, it is the second leading site of cancer. The population-based survival studies, another indicator of health infrastructure and success of treatment, indicate that despite improvement in treatment modalities, prognosis from stomach cancer remains poor. The 5-year survival rate for stomach cancer is approximately 20%. Survival rates are higher in countries which have screening programs that lead to early detection and where distal cancer (which has a better prognosis) predominates. The 5-year relative survival for stomach cancer in India from 1992 to 1994 was observed to be 6% mainly because of late presentation. Over the years, 1982–2005, the incidence of gastric cancer has remained more or less stable (though there are variations in some years), both in Chennai and in Bengaluru, while in Mumbai, it has shown a decline from 7.1 to 4.9 per 100,000 during the same period.[10]

In a recent study from India to determine the association of *H. pylori* infection, dietary items and habits in population where consumption of smoked and salted meat is not high, reported similar *H. pylori* status between gastric cancer patients and controls and concluded that high intake of carbohydrates, low intake of vegetables and fruits, habits like smoking, tobacco chewing and alcohol intake were more frequent in patients with gastric cancer than among controls. It may be noted that though there are several studies conducted in India over the last decade, they failed to confirm the association between *H. pylori* infection and gastric cancer mainly because of high prevalence of *H. pylori* infection in Indian population, inadequate sample size, power of the study and failure to adjust for other confounding variables. Probably, studies with adequate power and addressing the issue of interaction between *H. pylori* and other lifestyle-related factors and dietary variables will provide a lead to understand the etiology of gastric cancer in India in relation to *H. pylori* infection.[11]

DIET

Diet plays a major role in gastric carcinogenesis. Gastric cancer rates have declined over the years. Researchers all over the world have tried to explore to ascertain the reasons for the decline. It is known that diet is one of the important factors associated with gastric cancer, besides other factors of concern. Strong evidence has been provided that high consumption of fresh fruit and raw vegetables and a high intake of antioxidants vitamins (such as A and C) appears to lower the risk of stomach cancer. Pickled food, high rice intake, spicy food, excess chilly consumption, consumption of high-temperature foods smoked dried salted meat, use of soda and consumption of dried salted fish have emerged as significant dietary risk factors in various parts of India. These practises are prevalent in Southern and Eastern states of India where a higher frequency of gastric cancer is also observed.

TOBACCO

Role of tobacco in gastric cancer has been studied by many across the world. Trédaniel et al. (1997)[12] conducted a review and meta-analysis of 40 studies that provide a quantitative estimate of the association between tobacco smoking and gastric cancer risk. The results suggest a relative risk of 1.6 in smokers compared to non-smokers. Smoking tobacco has been found to be an independent risk factor for stomach cancer. Current smokers were found to be at a higher risk as compared to non-smokers and ex-smokers. A significantly increased risk was observed with increased smoking in a South Indian study. Increased risk was also observed among the tobacco chewers. The risk showed an increasing trend with increase in frequency and amount of tobacco use and decreasing trend with the number of years since the practise of consuming tobacco was discontinued. Tobacco use in any form (chewing, smoking and drinking) was observed to increase the risk of stomach cancer in Mizoram, a Northeastern state of India.

ALCOHOL

A study from China suggested alcohol consumption (every drinker) showed an enhanced significant risk for gastric cancer after adjustment for smoking and other confounders. In a study conducted in Mumbai, alcohol intake did not emerge as a risk factor for gastric cancer. In the Indian context, due to social stigma, it is difficult to measure the alcohol intake of an individual. Reviews of alcohol and gastric cancer have consistently rejected an association. However, a specific association with cancers of the gastric cardia has been suggested by studies in USA, Italy and Spain.[13]

OBESITY

In a meta-analysis of Cohort studies from China, the combined results of this meta-analysis, however, indicated that overweight and obesity are associated with an increased risk of gastric cancer. The strength of the association also increases with increasing body mass index.

ETHNICITY

There are a host of other factors as socioeconomic status, geography, previous stomach surgery, Ménétrier's disease (hypertrophic gastropathy), pernicious anemia, type A blood, inherited cancer syndromes, hereditary diffuse gastric cancer (HDGC), hereditary nonpolyposis colorectal cancer, familial adenomatous polyposis, BRCA1 and BRCA2, some types of stomach polyps, certain occupations and immune deficiency, are associated in many different ways in the etiology of gastric cancer.[14]

GENETICS

Strong genetic mutations and familial transmission of the disease is well-documented. The biological genesis of most cancers depends on the cascade of molecular events leading to the development and progression of the disease and gastric cancer is no exception. Vascular endothelial growth factor (VEGF) is a major factor in angiogenesis in many cancers including stomach cancer. E-cadherin is an important self-adhesive factor. CDH1 gene encodes E-cadherin and mutation of the former and loss of expression of the latter is a key player in the development of familial gastric cancer. HDGC represents a minority of gastric cancer cases. It is appropriate for relatives with a strong family history of diffuse gastric cancer to have CDH1 gene mutation testing after the age of 25 years. It was hypothesized that prophylactic total gastrectomy should be offered to such CDH1 mutation carriers in the famiy.[15] Stomach cancer families are known; the most famous and historical is that of Napoleon Bonaparte. Rarely, precursor polyps, villous adenomas, as a part of diffuse intestinal polyposis syndrome (Peutz-Jeghers syndrome) have been known occasionally to lead to stomach cancer. Avoidance of causative factors, early surveillance and treatment of upper gastrointestinal symptoms in appropriate family members and screening in endemic areas are therefore of great significance in a major preventive and therapeutic effort against this difficult cancer.

PATHOLOGY

Most (95%) lesions are adenocarcinomas and often classified as "intestinal type" (well to moderately differentiated) and "diffuse type" (poorly differentiated—signet ring type). The anaplastic—*linitis plastica* type of lesions (leather bottle stomach) are aggressive and involve the whole stomach in its later stages. Consequent to the increasing incidence of gastroesophageal reflux disease (GERD) there is an increasing incidence of proximal (gastric cardia) and gastroesophageal (GE) junction cancers which form nearly 50% of all gastric cancers. The distal (noncardia) antral cancers are often a consequence of *H. pylori* infections and are decreasing in incidence because of effective management of *H. pylori* infection. Untreated, *H. pylori* induced gastritis and ulcerated lesions progress to intestinal metaplasia, dysplasia and finally to cancer. These are generally intestinal type as aforementioned, well-differentiated and have a better prognosis than the diffuse type. Rarely, lymphomas, gastrointestinal stromal tumors and neuroendocrine lesions can arise in the stomach, which form less than 5% of all gastric cancers.

Symptomatology/Diagnosis/ Investigations

At best, early symptoms are generally vague and neglected by the patient. They are usually passed off as indigestion, acidity, fullness after a meal or a vague upper abdominal discomfort. A lesion at the cardia may initially cause dysphagia. An obstructive lesion in the antrum and pyloric region will produce obstructive symptoms with persisted vomiting. Rarely hematemesis may occure due to a large ulcerative or polypoidal fundal or body lesion (Figs 1A to C). Chronic anemia may result as a consequence leading malena. Persistence of such symptoms coupled with a family history or otherwise should lead to an appropriate investigation. Anorexia, loss of weight and a palpable mass are indicative of an advanced disease when only palliation can be offered. In a disease where 50% will die in the first year after diagnosis, the importance of prevention and early diagnosis cannot be overemphasized.

Important symptoms should, therefore, be promptly investigated by a good routine clinical examination of the abdomen, neck and per rectal examination; lab studies, tumor marker studies of CEA/CA 19-9 are worthwhile; endoscopy with a biopsy is vital and imaging by a computed tomography (CT) scan are necessary for a baseline study. A positron emission computed tomography (PET-CT) is optional, but may be indicated in an advanced clinical setting when neoadjuvant chemotherapy or radiotherapy is often used. Assessment of response after two to three cycles is useful in planning further therapy, regarding exploration for a resection. It is estimated that the therapeutic approach may change in about 20% of patients with a PET-CT which may help avoid an unnecessary exploration. The importance of laparoscopic staging before exploration has received much attention and in

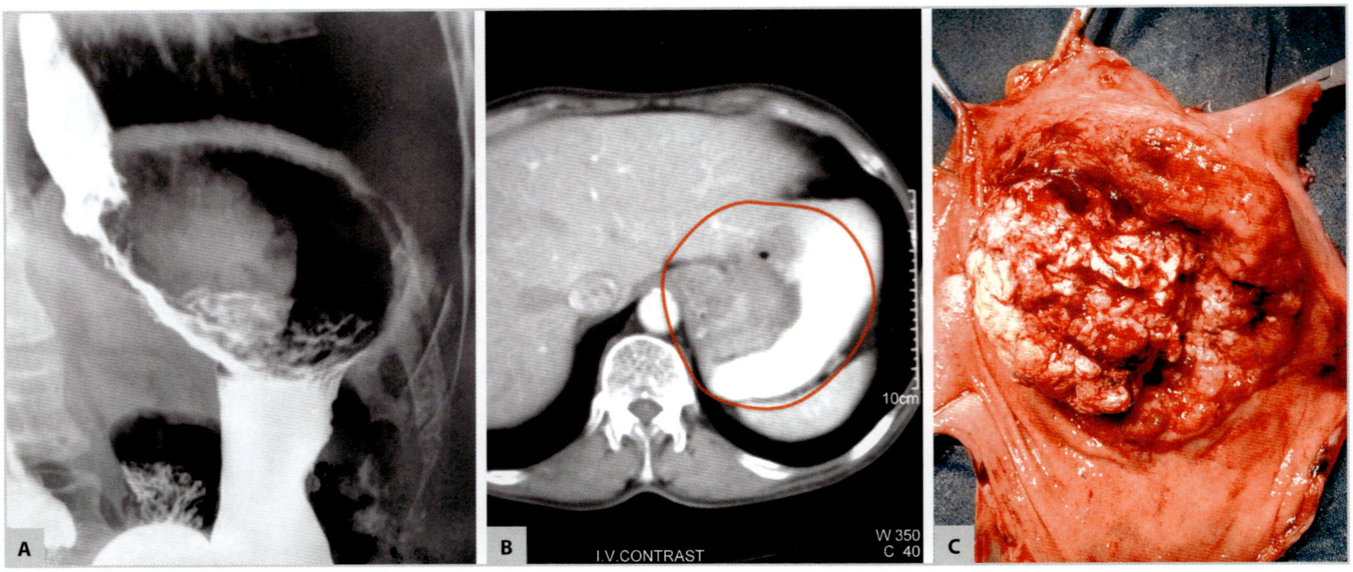

Figs 1A to C: (A and B) Barium study and CT scan reveals a large mass in the fundal region excised by radical proximal gastrectomy; (C) Operative specimen. Most stomach cancers are diagnosed late

a suspected advanced disease (peritoneal or omental seedlings) it is a useful procedure and may help change the therapeutic approach. Endoscopic ultrasound studies are optional and not always indicated and depend on an individual or institution protocol. Most patients, more than 70% present late and only palliative forms of therapy will be possible.

Treatment

The current standard of care in the therapy of all malignant solid tumors is a complementary approach of surgery, chemotherapy and radiotherapy appropriately used in neoadjuvant, adjuvant or sequential approach. There is little doubt that this approach has increased, (based on evidence) the DFS, overall survival (OS) and cure rates in varying degrees for most solid tumors and stomach cancer is no exception. A team approach for initial therapy planning is, therefore, imperative and mandatory. Very early lesions, diagnosed mainly during a screening trial are limited to the mucosa (T_1) and can be dealt endoscopically by endoscopic mucosal resection. This is frequent in the Japanese literature due to their large screening program. Since most stomach cancers are advanced at presentation, initial assessment and decision whether to treat with an intention to cure or palliation is therefore vital.

Surgery (Table 1 and Fig. 2)

There is little doubt that in a localized disease where the surgeon, after appropriate assessment (based

TABLE 1: Surgical approaches depend on the site and extent of disease

	Site	*Procedure*
a	Predominantly fundal growth → cardioesophageal	Distal esophagectomy with proximal gastrectomy
b	Predominantly antral growth	Radical distal gastrectomy
c	Mid body	Variable, depending on the site of lesion (> 5 cm margin)
d	Diffuse/Linitis plastica	Total gastrectomy with 4–5 cm of lower esophagus

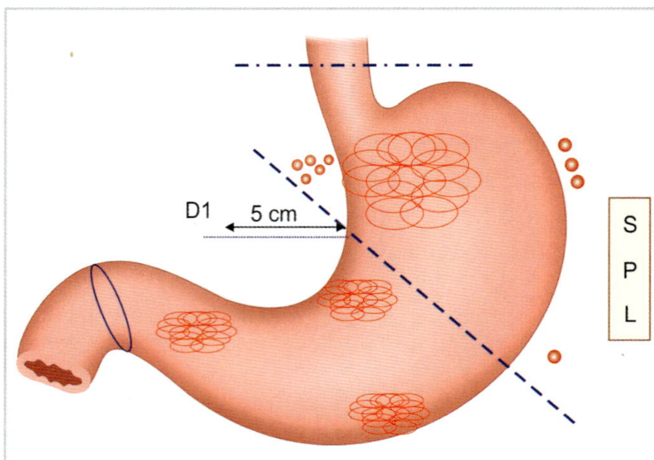

Fig. 2: Usual sites of primary lesion: cardioesophageal junction, fundus, lesser and greater curvature (body) and distal (antral). D1 dissection entails clearance of nodes and lesions 5–7 cm beyond the disease

on investigations), can achieve a good macroscopic clearance, "surgery" will remain the therapy of choice. This will include a distal radical gastrectomy for lesions of the antrum and distal body; and a radical proximal gastrectomy for lesions of the cardia, fundus and proximal body. Total gastrectomy with a lower esophageal stump of 5 cm is the therapy of choice of an organ localized anaplastic cancer of the stomach, (linitis plastica). Lesions localized distally and proximally do not merit a total gastrectomy if an adequate free margin of 5–7 cm is available, as most patients succumb to distant (liver) metastasis. Recurrent anastomotic recurrences are known if adequate free margins have not been achieved at surgery.

Lymph Node Dissection (Fig. 3 and Table 2)

The debate about D_1, D_2 and D_3 dissection will continue though various studies have now proven [Medical Research Council (MRC)/Dutch trials] that D_1 dissection (5 cm beyond the lesion) and D_2 dissection (including hepatic, celiac, complete perigastric and gastrosplenic areas) are sufficient (depending on the size, extent and the site of the primary lesion). The D_3 variant involving splenectomy distal pancreatectomy, paraaortic dissection, etc. are neither justified nor proven to be beneficial; there

TABLE 2: Nodal dissection

Dissection	*Procedure*
D_1	Standard: greater + lesser omentum 5 cm either side of tumor Left gastric group of nodes—up to the origin of the left gastric artery at the level of the upper border of the pancreas
D_2	D_1 + splenic, celiac, pancreatic, hepatic, para-aortic, superior and inferior pancreatic nodes
D_3	D_2 + splenectomy, distal pancreatectomy, para-aortic dissection

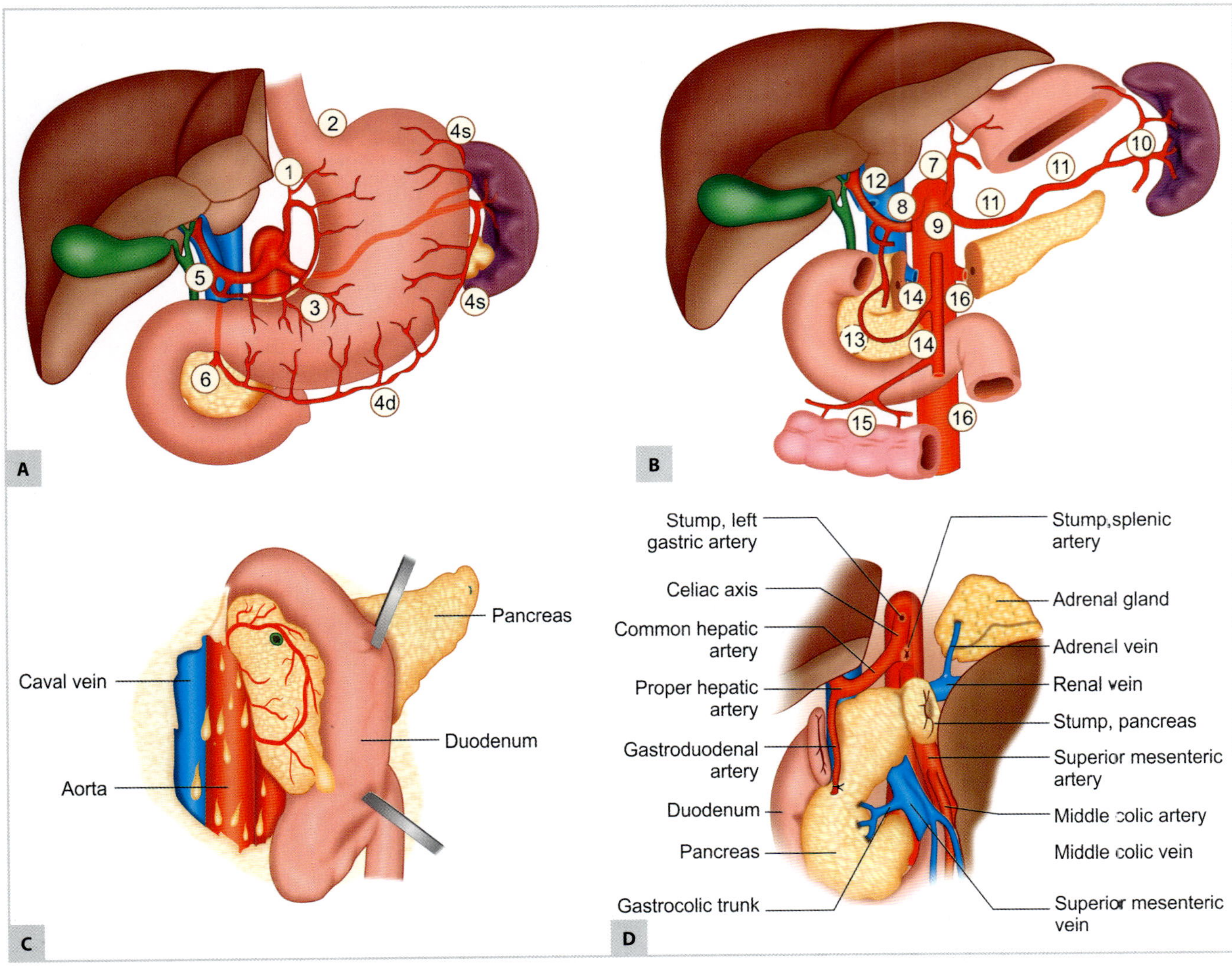

Figs 3A to D: (A and B) Lymphatic drainage of the stomach; (C and D) Completion of extensine D_3 dissection–rarely performed

TABLE 3: Medical Research Council (MRC)/Dutch trials—D_1D_2 dissection[19,20]

	British trial (MRC) %		Dutch trial %	
	D_1	D_2	D_1	D_2
Mortality	6	13	4	10
Morbidity	28	46	25	43
5-year survival	35	33	45	47

TABLE 4: N stage based on the extent of nodal involvement

Stage	Procedure	Number of nodes
N_1	Perigastric within 5 cm	one to five nodes
N_2	Coeliac, splenic, hepatic	6–15 nodes
N_3	Pancreatic, Para-aortic	> 15 nodes

is no significant difference in survival between D_1 and D_2 dissections on the contrary, morbidity, mortality or long-term complications completely negates the benefit of D_3 dissections and even in some cases of D_2 dissection (Tables 3 and 4). Individual surgical decisions are often necessary at surgery regarding inclusion of the D_2 dissection.[16-18] For advanced obstructive lesions, bypass surgery (gastrojejunostomy) is often indicated when noninvasive methods are contraindicated.

The surgical approach to stomach cancer should be decided on the findings at exploration. In a resectable lesion ($T_{2,3}N_{0,1}$) an adequate clearance of the primary and nodes is generally feasible and a R_0 (complete resection) resection should be the aim; if the nodal burden is high a D_2 node dissection is performed. No significant benefit accrues from even a D_2 dissection when more than 10 nodes are involved; however, combination therapy (chemotherapy and surgery) may add an incremental benefit on DFS of a few months or a year in some cases (Fig. 4). Results are poor when a R_1 (residual microscopic disease) or R_2 (residual macroscopic disease) dissection is forced because of advanced disease (Fig. 5).

Peritoneal Carcinomatosis in Stomach Cancer

Generally a late disease, few patients present with diffuse celomic spread. Palliative chemotherapy and supportive care is the usual approach. Hyperthermic intraperitoneal chemotherapy after debulking is practised in secondary or tertiary centers. Complication and morbidity are significant and overall results do not merit it as an acceptable form of therapy except in tertiary centers within the ambit of a clinical trial. The same treatment scenario applies to peritoneal carcinomatosis in colorectal and ovarian cancers, though the results reported in this group show a 5 years control from 10 to 15%. Better outcomes are reported in ovarian carcinomatosis.

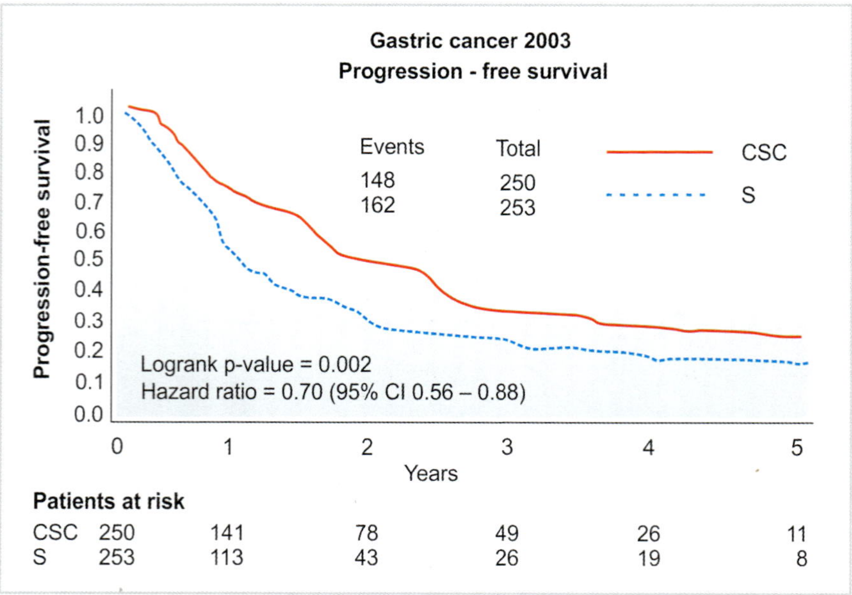

Fig. 4: Results with surgery (S) alone and combination therapy—chemotherapy-surgery-chemotherapy (CSC)

[*Courtesy:* Persiani R, D'Ugo D, Rausei S, et al. Prognostic indicators in locally advanced gastric cancer (LAGC) treated with preoperative chemotherapy and D2-gastrectomy. J Surg Oncol. 2005;89(4):227-36]

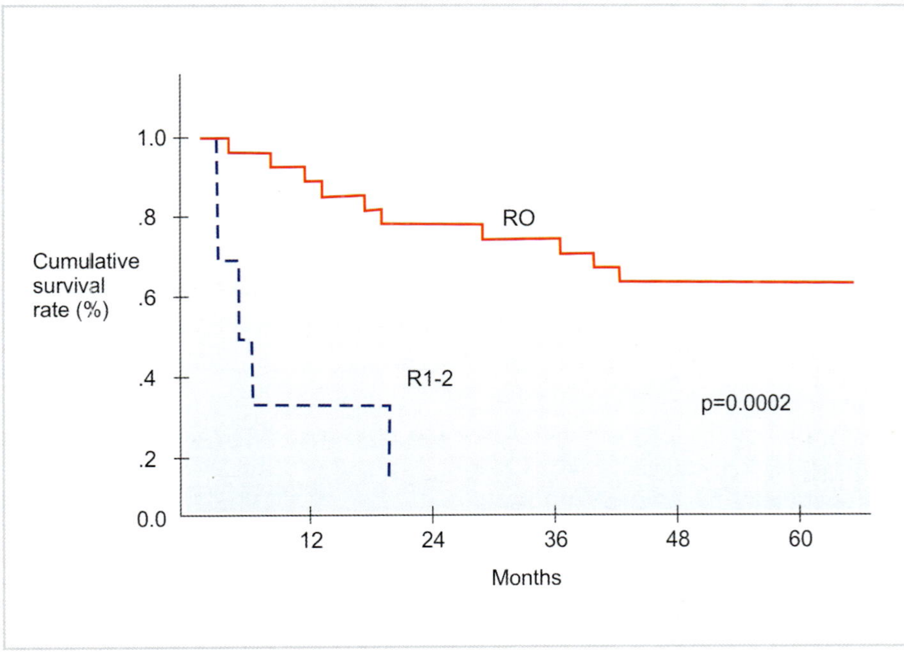

Fig. 5: Cumulative survival in locally advanced gastric cancer (LAGC) after preoperative chemotherapy: effect of R category

[*Courtesy:* Persiani R, D'Ugo D, Rausei S, et al. Prognostic indicators in locally advanced gastric cancer (LAGC) treated with preoperative chemotherapy and D2-gastrectomy. J Surg Oncol. 2005;89(4):227-36]

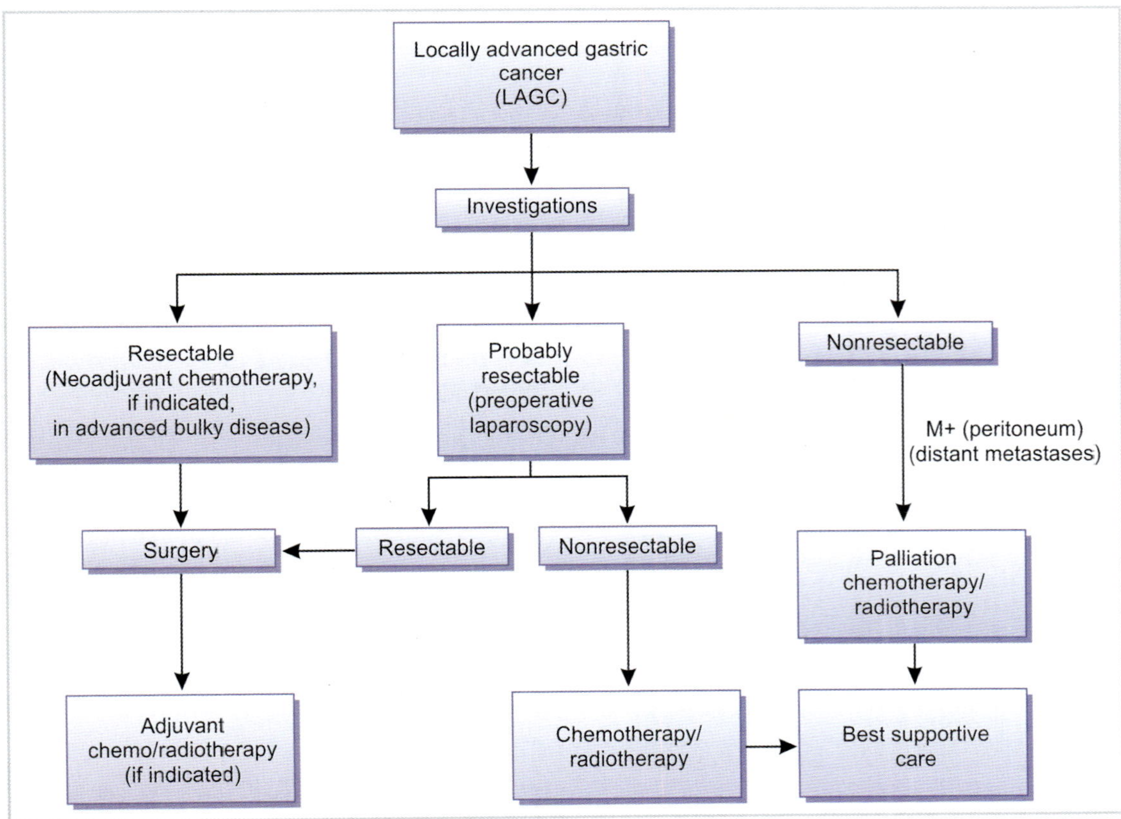

Combination Therapy for Carcinoma Stomach (Chemoradiotherapy/ Biological Therapy)

Evidence-based data prove the efficacy, though only incremental, of chemoradiotherapy. It is appropriate that a locoregionally advanced lesion should be down staged by a neoadjuvant chemotherapy approach which generally consists of two or three cycles of chemotherapy either with or without concurrent radiotherapy (up to 45 Gy).[21] Imaging (PET-CT) methods can assess response of the primary and nodal disease 2 weeks after cessation of neoadjuvant therapies to decide whether surgical approach should be exercised. This decision vests on the clinical setting and investigations. A very significant response (subjective and objective) may be an indication to continue chemotherapy or radiotherapy as a definitive therapy. A surgical approach to resect the primary lesion often results in maximum palliation which can prevent pain, bleeding and obstruction due to the primary lesion. A team approach with a surgical lead would be worthwhile.

Targeted (Biological) Therapy

Beyond morphology, genetic molecular studies of every cancer yields an increasing understanding about the progression of cancer from its inception to growth, due to proliferation (epidermal growth factor) and subsequent metastasis due to angiogenesis (VEGF).[22] Monoclonal antibodies like bevacizumab (Avastin®), trastuzumab (Herceptin®) are now used in clinical practise targeted to cell growth, proliferation and prevention of metastasis due to angiogenesis (VEGF) (Fig. 6). Herceptin® (trastuzumab) and Avastin® have been used along with chemotherapy as an adjuvant after definitive surgery. No robust or clear data is yet on hand regarding its impact on DFS or OS except in breast and colon cancers. Cetuximab is often used in stomach and head and neck cancers with varying results. Clearly, the toxicity, morbidity and host factors need to be weighed carefully against the advantages of a few incremental survivals of few months. The years ahead will clarify whether targeted biological therapy will stand the test of time. The role of EGFR and VEGF are being increasingly researched upon. Though breast, ovarian and colonic cancers respond favorably to biological targeted therapy (Herceptin®-Avastin®) the same is not of equivalent efficacy in stomach cancer.

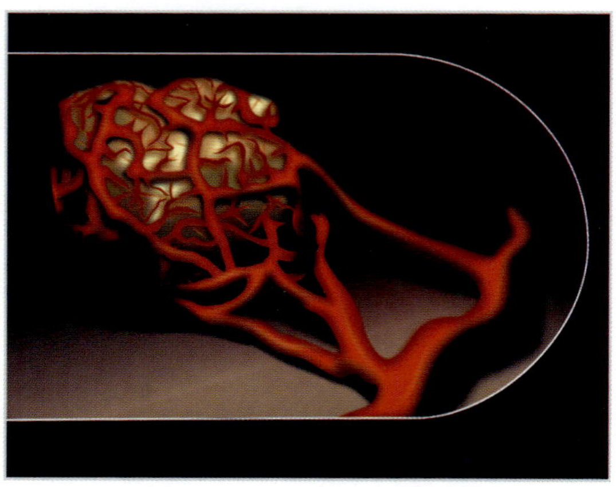

Fig. 6: Anti-angiogenesis therapy aims to control hematogenous metastasis

Recurrent Metastatic Disease

This is a frequent occurrence. When metastatic disease is disseminated majority of patients will require only palliative chemotherapy. Radiotherapy along with Zometa® (bisphosphonates) has to be considered in presence of skeletal metastasis. Metastasis occurring in a single site after a long latent period (2 years or more), which can be surgically resected without morbidity, is known to provide effective palliation with a significant remission period.

Chemotherapy

Surgery is the mainstay of treatment for cancer of stomach. However, microscopic disease in spite of a R_0 resection is responsible for regional as well as distant metastasis. Systemic treatment in neoadjuvant, adjuvant and metastatic setting is an important treatment modality for this disease based on a given clinical scenario.

Adjuvant Chemotherapy

There have been various clinical trials to study role of adjuvant chemotherapy in operated cases of stomach cancer. Majority of trials had small number of patients and could not show significant advantage over surgery alone. Earle and Maroun[23] included the only non-Asian trials and found to have absolute risk reduction of 4% with chemotherapy. Panzini et al.[24] included 17 studies. They reported a hazard ratio of 0.83 in favor of chemotherapy. Though most of the meta-analysis did not include individual patient data, it indicates modest benefit for systemic postoperative therapy.

Perioperative (Neoadjuvant) Chemotherapy

In view of many patients presenting with locally advanced disease where a R_0 dissection cannot be achieved, preoperative chemotherapy is advised. Goals of neoadjuvant therapy are to downstage the disease and to kill microscopic cells. Many phase II studies involving the use of injection cisplatin and injection fluorouracil (5FU) preoperatively demonstrated good objective responses. Assessing the response after neoadjuvant chemotherapy is a challenging task. Recently, PET-CT scan is used to assess the response (Figs 7A and B). It is found to be useful based on the standardized uptake value measure. All gastric tumors, however, may not be fluorodeoxyglucose (FDG) avid. The landmark "Medical Research Council Adjuvant Gastric Infusional Chemotherapy (MAGIC)" trial was reported by Dr David Cunningham[25] after a well-designed phase III trial. This trial included patients with gastric cancer, cardioesophageal junction tumors and lower esophageal adenocarcinomas. Patients receive "epirubicin, cyclophosphamide, 5FU (ECF)" regimen in neoadjuvant and adjuvant fashion. There was no increase in surgical mortality and morbidity. There was an improved R_0 resection. At a median follow-up of 4 years, there was a significant improvement in DFS and OS.

Role of Adjuvant Chemoradiation

There have been various clinical trials on adjuvant chemoradiation. These studies have mainly used 5FU based regimens. One of the landmark trials was "Intergroup 0116" trial.[20] This involved giving 5FU with leucovorin regimen followed by concurrent chemoradiation (45 Gy) and then further two cycles of 5FU with leucovorin. The results including OS, DFS and locoregional control favored adjuvant chemoradiation.

Treatment of Advanced (Stage IV) Disease

This is an incurable stage of the disease. Patients often present with a large mass, supraclavicular nodes in the neck and ascites. These are very advanced cases and may not even merit chemotherapy in this clinical setting. The role of chemotherapy was studied against best supportive care due to potential toxicities of chemotherapy drugs. It was concluded that patients with good performance status should be offered chemotherapy as it has a modest but real benefit in survival. There are many chemotherapeutic drugs used as a single agent treatment like 5FU, capecitabine, tegafur, anthracyclines, cisplatin, taxanes and irinotecan. These have shown response rates of approximately 17–49%. Hence, a combination chemotherapy is recommended to improve results. A combination of injection cisplatin and injection 5FU is one of the most widely accepted regimens. This combination has consistently produced similar results in various trials. The response rates have varied between 20% and 41% and median DFS between 3.7 months and 7.3 months in various trials. Two-year survival was 10–15%. This combination has been compared with various other combinations, e.g. (a) 5FU, adriamycin, methotrexate (FAMTX), (b) etoposide, 5FU and leucovorin. These have not shown any additional benefit. Van Custen, et al. reported a study TAX 325 in 2006.[26] This study compared docetaxel, cisplatin and 5FU (DCF) combination with only cisplatin, 5FU (CF). DCF showed better time to progression and 2-year survival rates. Toxicity increased in DCF arm (hematological

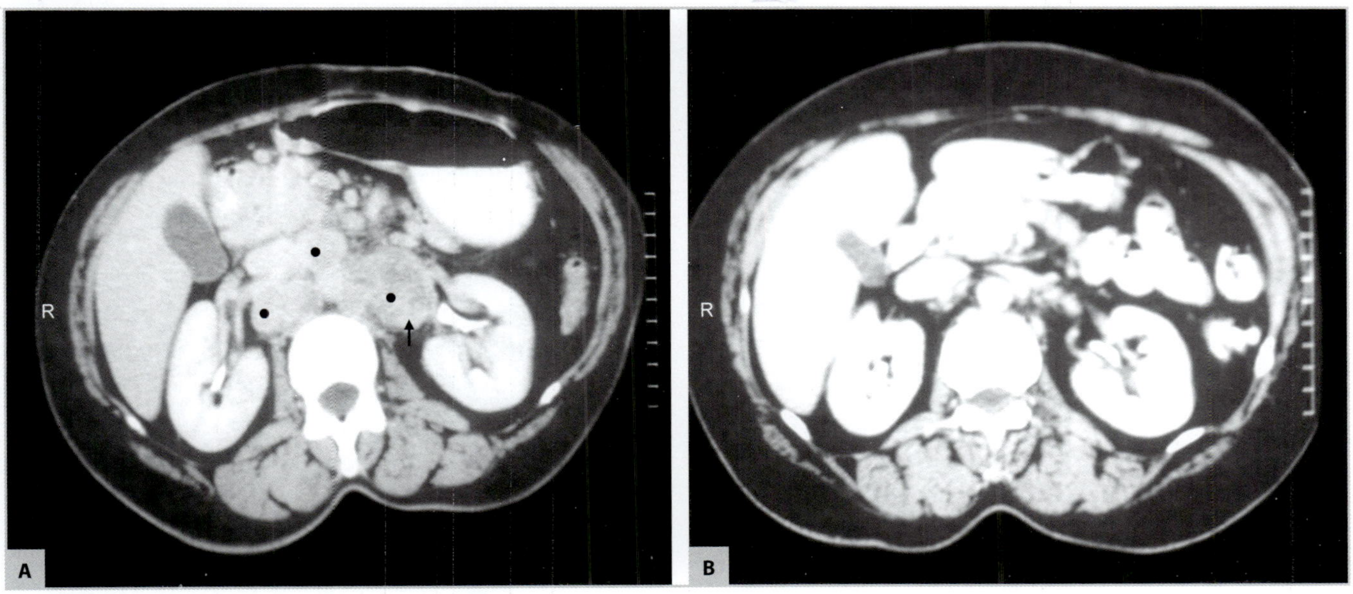

Figs 7A and B: (A) Computed tomography scan showing large metastatic nodes in the para-aortic region in a patient with cancer of the fundus of the stomach; (B) Postchemotherapy showing complete response to neoadjuvant chemotherapy. Patient ultimately underwent a surgical resection, survival 11 months before disseminated liver metastases developed and non-hematological) but treatment related mortality was similar in both the arms. Hence, DCF is a preferable regimen in a patient with good performance status. "ECF" regimen consisting of epirubicin, cisplatin and 5FU is another well-studied regimen. It has shown good survival data (14% at 2 years) with manageable toxicity. Other less commonly used combinations like leucovorin, 5FU, irinotecan (FOLFIRI), irinotecan with cisplatin have been used. FOLFIRI has been found to be non-inferior to CF. Oxaliplatin based regimens [folinic acid, 5FU, oxaliplatin (FOLFOX)] have been studied. Peripheral neuropathy was the dose limiting toxicity. The overall response rate was 50% and median OS of 10–12 months. Another landmark study was REAL-2.[27] This trial was primarily designed to know the exact role of oxaliplatin and capecitabine in the management of stomach cancer. It was a four-arm study:

1. Arm A: ECF
2. Arm B: EOX—epirubicine, oxaliplatin, 5FU
3. Arm C: ECX—epirubicine, cisplatin, capecitabine
4. Arm D: EOX—epirubicine, oxaliplatin, capecitabine

The trial was well-balanced with 250 patients in each arm. There was no difference in median OS between various arms. The 1-year survival was also similar. The conclusion was that oxaliplatin could be substituted for cisplatin and capecitabine for 5FU. This is useful for patients with renal dysfunction, cardiac dysfunction or difficult intravenous access (for continuous infusion of 5FU).

Role of Targeted Therapy in Metastatic Cancer of Stomach

Trastuzumab (HERCEPTIN)

This is a monoclonal antibody to HER2/neu. This is indicated if the tumor tissue is expressing HER2/neu + 3 on immunohistochemistry or by fluorescence in situ hybridization technique. About 15–20% of stomach cancers can have expression of HER2/neu. Trastuzumab has been combined with chemotherapy in the dose of 8 mg/kg as a loading dose and 6 mg/kg every 3 weeks. Trastuzumab can be continued as a maintenance therapy after chemotherapy is over. Cardiac function needs to be monitored with trastuzumab.

Bevacizumab

This is an antiangiogenic agent which can be combined with chemotherapy. It can be given intravenous 15 mg/kg every 3 weeks.[28] It can lead to thromboembolic phenomenon, bleeding, and GI perforations. Hence, patients on bevacizumab require close monitoring.

Commonly Used Regimens (Table 5)

TABLE 5: Commonly used regimens

Regimen	*Dose*
ECF	Day 1: epirubicin 50 mg/m^2 IV bolus + cisplatin 60 mg/m^2 IV Day 1–21: 5FU 200 mg/m^2 IV continuous infusion over 24 hours daily Repeat cycle every 3 weeks for three cycles preoperatively and three cycles postoperatively
CF	Day 1 and 29: cisplatin 75–100 mg/m^2 IV Day 1–4 and 29–32: 5FU 750–1,000 mg/m^2 IV continuous infusion over 24 hours
DCF	Day 1: docetaxel 75 mg/m^2 IV + cisplatin 75 mg/m^2 IV Day 1–5: 5FU 750 mg/m^2/day IV. Repeat cycle every 3 weeks Or Day 1: docetaxel 75 mg/m^2 IV + cisplatin 75 mg/m^2 IV. Day 1–5: 5FU 1,000 mg/m^2 IV continuous infusion over 24 hours, daily Repeat cycle every 4 weeks

Abbreviations: ECF, epirubicin, cisplatin, 5FU; 5FU-fluorouracil; IV, intravenous; CF, cisplatin, 5FU; DCF, docetaxel, cisplatin, 5FU

Radiotherapy

Role of radiotherapy as the sole treatment in gastric cancer is limited to palliation. Hematemesis and obstruction due to locally advanced gastric cancer can be effectively palliated by radiating to the dose of 4,000–5,000 cGy in 4–5 weeks. Simple parallel opposed fields may be all that is necessary to achieve effective palliation. The median survival improved to 36 months from 27 months when patients received chemotherapy and radiation therapy as compared to observation alone. Three-year recurrence free interval increased from 31 to 48% in patient who received chemoradiation. Similarly, preoperative radiation can downstage stage I and IV gastric cancer to pave way for increased resectability. Zhang et al.[29] have reported 5- and 10-years survival rates of 30% versus 20%, and 20% and 13% for preoperative radiation therapy versus surgery alone. In this study radiotherapy was prescribed to partial stomach fields and regional nodes were not necessarily included. A dose of 4,000 cGy was delivered in 4 weeks on a high energy accelerator.

Preoperative chemoradiation is another approach which has shown effectiveness in increasing resectability rates, DFS and OS. Continuous infusion of 5FU (15 mg for 1 kg) on day 1–6 and cisplatin 75 mg/m^2 on day 7 for two cycles repeated twice was administered to patients of locally advanced esophagus (65%) or gastric cardia (35%).

Simultaneous radiation therapy was started on the day 1 of the first cycle of chemotherapy. A total dose of 4,000 cGy was delivered on high energy accelerator. No difference in operative morbidity was evident in those who received chemoradiation and those who did not. Those who received preoperative chemoradiation lived substantially longer 37% versus 7% at 3 years.[30]

Adenocarcinoma of the stomach is fairly radio responsive. Hence, 30 Gy in 10 fractions is adequate for palliation while 40–50 Gy is effective in pre or postoperative radiation alone or in conjunction with chemotherapy. Techniques of radiation can vary from simple parallel opposed fields on a megavoltage beam to intensity modulated radiation. Target volume depends on the extent of the disease and nature of resection. Regional nodes are included along with tumor bed for radiation following surgery.

Acute side effects include fatigue, nausea, vomiting, weight loss, bowel motility disorder, gastritis or ulceration and radiation dermatitis. Most of these sequels can be medically managed. Late sequel are permanent changes in bowel habits, small bowel obstruction, hepatic or renal dysfunction and myelopathy. A close attention to radiation techniques can minimize the chances or severity of late sequel. Hypofractionated radiation is not recommended except in a palliative setting.

REFERENCES

1. Gajalakshmi CK, Shanta V. Lifestyle and risk of stomach cancer: A hospital-based case-control study. Int J Epidemiol. 1996;25(6):1146-53.
2. Ferlay J, Shin HR, Bray F, et al. (2010). GLOBOCAN 2008. Cancer Incidence and Mortality Worldwide: IARC CancerBase No. 10. [online] Available from http://www.iarc.fr/en/publications/eresources/cancerbases/ [Accessed January, 2014].
3. Parkin DM, Bray F, Ferlay J, et al. Global cancer statistics, 2002. CA Cancer J Clin. 2005;55(2):74-108.
4. Parkin DM. International variation. Oncogene. 2004;23(38):6329-40.
5. Parkin DM, Whelan SL, Ferlay J. et al. (2005) Cancer Incidence in Five Continents Volumes I to VIII. [online] Available from http://www.iacr.com.fr/statist.htm [Accessed January, 2014].
6. Haenszel W. Variation in incidence of and mortality from stomach cancer, with particular reference to the United States. J Natl Cancer Inst. 1958;21(2):213-62.
7. Hirayama T. Epidemiology of cancer of the stomach with special reference to its recent decrease in Japan. Cancer Res. 1975;35(11 Pt 2):3460-3.
8. Laroiya I, Pankaja SS, Mittal S, et al. A study of ***Helicobacter pylori*** infection, dietary pattern and habits with gastric cancer in South India. Asia Pacific J Tropical Dis. 2012;2(1):24-6.
9. Mathew A, Gangadharan P, Varghese C, et al. Diet and stomach cancer: A case-control study in South India. Eur J Cancer Prev. 2000;9(2):89-97.
10. Rao DN, Ganesh B, Dinshaw KA, et al. A case-control study of stomach cancer in Mumbai, India. Int J Cancer. 2002;99(5):727-31.
11. Trédaniel J, Boffetta P, Buiatti E, et al. Tobacco smoking and gastric cancer: review and meta-analysis. Int J Cancer. 1997;72(4):565-73.
12. International Agency for Research on Cancer. (1988). IARC monographs on the evaluation of carcinogenic risks to humans, Volume 44, Alcohol Drinking. [online] Available from http://monographs.iarc.fr/ENG/Monographs/vol44/volume44.pdf [Accessed January, 2014].
13. Verma Y, Pradhan PK, Gurung N, et al. Population-based cancer incidence in Sikkim, India: report on ethnic variation. Br J Cancer. 2012;106(5):962-5.
14. Russel MC, Hsu C, Mansfield PF, et al. In: Feig BW, Ching CD (Eds). Primary gastric malignancies. The MD Anderson Surgical Oncology Handbook. Philadelphia: Lippincott Williams & Wilkins; 2011. pp. 270-321.
15. Dixon M, Seevaratnam R, Wirtzfeld D, et al. A RAND/UCLA appropriateness study of the management of familial gastric cancer. Ann Surg Oncol. 2013;20(2):533-41.
16. Bonenkemp JJ; Hermans J, Sasako M, et al. Extended lymph-node dissection for gastric cancer. N Engl J Med. 1999;340(12):908-14.
17. Bonenkemp SS, Songun I, Hermans J, et al. Randomised comparison of morbidity after D1 and D2 dissection for gastric cancer in 996 Dutch patients. Lancet. 1995;345(8952):745-8.
18. Cuschieri A, Weeden S, Fielding J, et al. Patient survival after D1, D2 resections for gastric cancer: long-term results of the MRC randomized surgical trial. Surgical Co-operative Group. Br J Cancer. 1999;79(9-10):1522-30.
19. Songun I, Putter H, Kranenbarg EM, et al. Surgical treatment of gastric cancer: 15-year follow-up results of randomised nationwide Dutch D1D2 trial. Lancet Oncol. 2010;11(5):439-49.
20. Cuschieri A, Fayers P, Fielding J, et al. Postoperative morbidity and mortality after D1 and D2 resections for gastric cancer: preliminary results of the MRC randomised controlled surgical trial. The Surgical Cooperative Group. Lancet. 1996;347(9007):995-9.
21. Mcdonald SS, Smalley S, Benedetti J, et al. Chemoradiotherapy after surgery compared with surgery alone for adenocarcinoma of stomach or gastroesophageal junction. N Eng J Med. 2001;345(10):725-30.
22. Folkman J. What is the evidence that the tumors are angiogenesis dependent? J Nat Cancer Inst. 1990;82(1):4-6.
23. Earle CC, Maroun JA. Adjuvant chemotherapy after curative resection for gastric cancer in non-Asian patients: revisiting a meta-analysis of randomized trials. Eur J Cancer. 1999;35(7):1059-64.

24. Panzini I, Gianni L, Fattori PP, et al. Adjuvant chemotherapy in gastric cancer: a meta-analysis of randomized trials and a comparison with previous meta-analyses. Tumori. 2002;88(1):21-7.

25. Cunningham D, Allum WH, Stenning SP, et al. Perioperative chemotherapy versus surgery alone for resectable gastroesophageal cancer. N Eng J Med. 2006;355(1):11-20.

26. Van Custem E, Moiseyenko VM, Tjulandin S, et al. Phase III study of docetaxel and cisplatin plus fluorouracil compared with cisplatin and fluorouracil as first-line therapy for advanced gastric cancer: a report of the V325 study group. J Clin Oncol. 2006;24(31):4991-7.

27. Cunningham D, Rao S, Sterling N, et al. Randomized multicenter phase III study comparing capecitabine with fluouracil and oxaliplatin with cisplatin in patients with advanced oesophago–gastric cancer: the REAL 2 trial. J Clin Oncol. 2006;24:1825.

28. Pisters Peter, Kelsen DP, Tepper JE. Cancer of stomach. Cancer: Principles and Practice of Oncology, 8th edition. Philadelphia: Lippincott Williams & Wilkins; 2008. p. 1043.

29. Zhang ZX, Gu XZ, Yin WB, et al. Randomized clinical trial on the combination of preoperative irradiation and surgery in the treatment of adenocarcinoma of gastric cardia (AGC)—report on 370 patients. Int J Radiat Biol Phys. 1998;42(5):929-34.

30. Walsh TN, Noonan N, Hollywood D, et al. A comparison of multimodality therapy and surgery for esophageal adenocarcinoma. N Eng J Med. 1996;335(7):4662-467.

28 Tumors of the Small Bowel

Ratna Parikh, Praful Desai

INTRODUCTION

Primary malignant lesions of the small bowel are very rare and forms only 1% of gastrointestinal (GI) tract cancers. Reasons have been postulated to explain this low incidence.[1] Secretions of the small bowel are nonacidic and hence less irritating to the mucosa. The rapid transit of the intestinal contents through the small gut and the absence of anaerobic bacteria, which converts bile acids into carcinogens, is probably the reason for the rarity of small bowel cancers. Excess of lymphoid tissue may be of some significance as a protective factor and the presence of enzyme benzopyrene hydroxylase may be responsible for detoxification of carcinogens.

Small bowel lesions may be primary or metastatic in origin. Commonly occurring tumors are presented in Table 1.

ETIOLOGY

Bile acids are considered carcinogenic, particularly after cholecystectomy,[3] due to increased exposure of the mucosa to bile. Bile stasis due to obstruction or a blind loop syndrome leads to bacterial overgrowth and could be a causative factor. Gastrointestinal dysfunction can disrupt normal physiology and has a possible tumorigenic effect. Other contributory factors are familial polyposis, adult celiac sprue, Peutz-Jeghers syndrome, Gardner's syndrome, Crohn's disease and Von Recklinghausen's neurofibromatosis.

TABLE 1: Commonly occurring tumors of the small bowel[2]

Primary	*Secondary (metastatic from)*
Lymphomas (7.3%)	Colon
Stromal tumor (8.4%)	Ovary
Adenocarcinoma (36.9%)	Lung
Carcinoid (37.4%)	Melanoma

CLINICAL PRESENTATION

The early symptoms of small intestine cancer tend to be vague, which often delays the diagnosis. The most common presentation is a chronic dull or colicky abdominal pain which occurs in majority of patients. Acute or subacute bowel obstruction, gastrointestinal hemorrhage (occult), weight loss, malnourishment, recurrent bowel perforation and occasionally a palpable abdominal mass are other presenting features.

DIAGNOSTIC WORK-UP

Apart from routine clinical and laboratory investigations, fecal occult blood, urinary 5-HIAA (5-hydroxyindoleacetic acid) to rule out a carcinoid, upper gastrointestinal endoscopy, contrast imaging study, small bowel enema, video capsule endoscopy, and a computed tomography (CT) scan will detect lesions in 97% patients. Occasionally, intraoperative endoscopy may help in diagnosis though it is not a routine study.

CARCINOID TUMORS

Carcinoid neoplasms are neuroendocrine tumors arising from the amine precursor uptake and decarboxylation

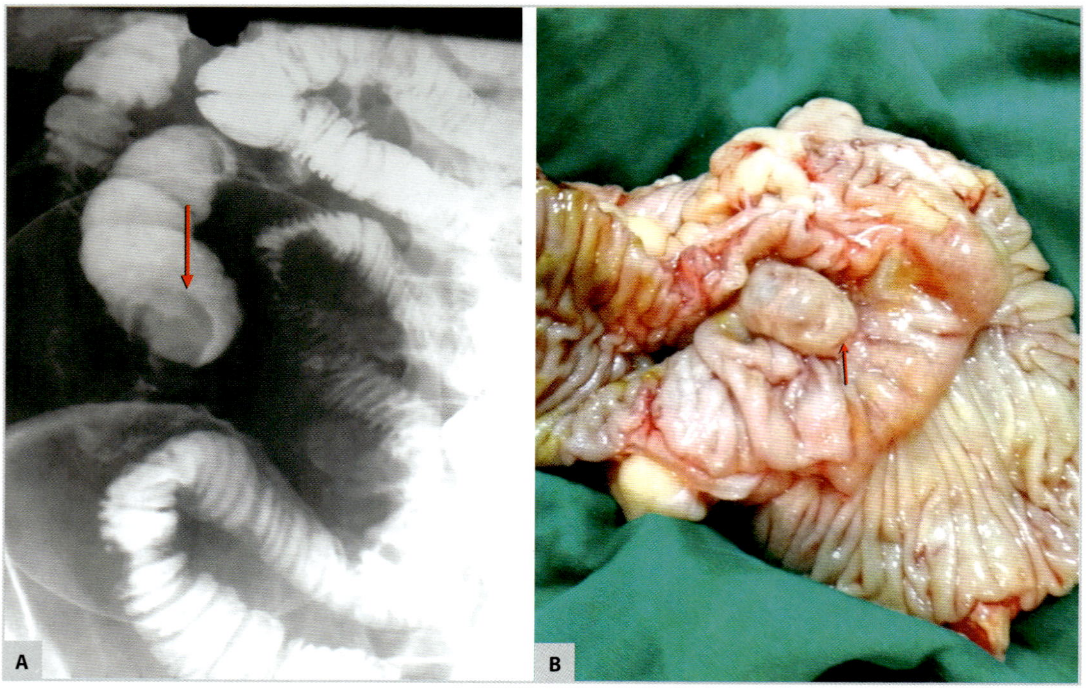

Figs 1A and B: (A) Small bowel enema of a patient with a carcinoid lesion in the ileocecal region, three other small synchronous lesions were found in the ileum intraoperatively when the small bowel was explored. These lesions were not seen on radiography; (B) Resected specimen of the ileocecal carcinoid

(APUD) cells of the intestine. These are generally slow growing and 44% of all gastrointestinal carcinoids, originate in the small intestine.[4] Most of them are in the ileum and less commonly in the jejunum (Figs 1A and B). It usually occurs in the elderly around the sixth decade. The diagnosis of an intestinal carcinoid is often delayed. They may be diagnosed incidentally at surgery for other abdominal disorders. Recurrent abdominal pain and subacute/chronic recurring intestinal obstruction are common symptoms. Rarely a gastrointestinal bleed may occur. Carcinoid syndromes occur in 20%[5] of patients characterized by flushing, wheezing, sweating and diarrhea.

Gastrointestinal carcinoid tumor cells produce hormonally active polypeptides and amines. Serotonin is secreted in urine after metabolism as 5-HIAA. The hormones secreted are kinin, histamines and prostaglandins. Secretory products such as chromogranin are diagnostic of a functional or a nonfunctional tumor. Localization of carcinoids can be accomplished by 111-indium (90% sensitivity) or a metaiodobenzylguanidine (MIBG) scintigraphy. This surveys the whole body and detects small primary or metastatic lesions. Scintigraphy can be combined with positron emission CT to increase sensitivity and define any systemic spread (Fig. 2).

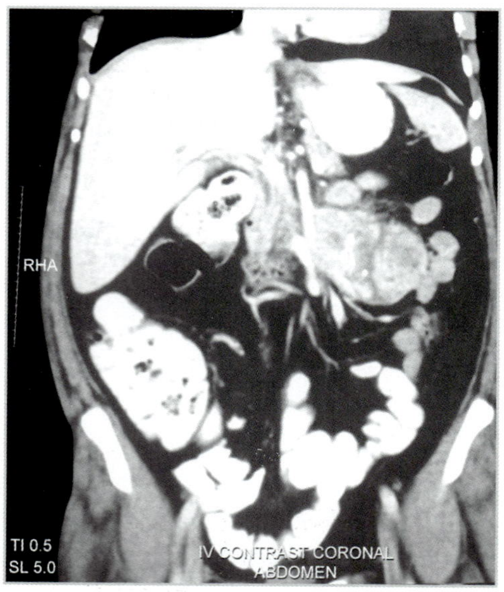

Fig. 2: Neuroendocrine tumor of the jejunum. Patient presented with episodes of subacute intestinal obstruction. Intraoperatively, there was a large mass arising from the jejunum and extending into the mesentery encasing the superior mesenteric vessels

TREATMENT

The therapy of choice is an adequate surgical excision, with nodal extension when feasible. Small bowel carcinoids are multicentric in 20–40% of patients. Ileal carcinoids commonly metastasize even when small; carcinoids in the midgut (jejunum, ileum and appendix) produce symptoms of hormone excess when bulky or metastatic. The stress of surgery, anesthesia and/or chemotherapy can precipitate a carcinoid crisis; octreotide (somatostatin analog) should therefore be given preoperatively to patients with a metastatic carcinoid. A wide resection with the adjacent mesentery and lymph nodes is a standard therapy. Occasionally, a local excision of a small carcinoid is feasible. Intraoperatively, a complete examination of the small bowel is mandatory as multicentricity is known. As these lesions are generally slow growing, even in the presence of metastases a wide excision is justified. For appendiceal carcinoids, less than 1.5 cm in size, an appendicectomy is adequate unless the base is involved. A right hemicolectomy is indicated for lesions near the base and larger than 1.5 cm. Duodenal carcinoids account for 4% of all gastrointestinal carcinoids. Most are located in the periampullary region. They can present with icterus, obstruction, abdominal pain or gastrointestinal bleeding. Zollinger-Ellison syndrome can occur in 10% of patients. A local excision or a pancreaticoduodenectomy is indicated depending on the size and site of the lesion.

Patients with a symptomatic carcinoid syndrome can be treated medically. Somatostatin analogs are known to improve symptoms. A number of studies[6] have shown that octreotide can significantly slow down tumor growth in more than 50% patients and causes regression in 10–20% patients. Interferon-alpha has been advocated in the therapy of carcinoid tumors with symptomatic relief in 75% patients and tumor response in 10% of patients.[7,8] A number of chemotherapeutic agents have shown a response rate ≤ 20%.[9] Similarly, external beam radiation has a limited benefit in treating carcinoid tumor.[10]

The prognosis with small bowel carcinoids is better than other gastrointestinal tract lesions. Localized disease with a complete resection has a 100% five-year survival rate; this drops to 68% in a patient even with resection of a metastatic lesion. Unresectable disease has a 38% five-year survival rate.[6]

Adenocarcinoma

Adenocarcinomas of the small intestine are found mainly in the duodenum (65% periampullary). Predisposing cause for small bowel adenocarcinoma are inherited germ line mutations—*K-ras* gene found in 14–53% of small intestine adenocarcinoma and chronic inflammatory diseases. Familial adenomatous polyposis (FAP) and hereditary nonpolyposis colorectal carcinoma (HNPCC) have a 100 fold higher risk of small bowel adenocarcinoma.[11] Newer data suggest patients with Peutz-Jeghers syndrome are 18 times more likely to develop small bowel malignancy.[12] Crohn's disease and celiac disease are other predisposing factors[13] for small bowel cancers. Clinical presentation is a gastrointestinal bleed or chronic anemia. Gastric outlet obstruction results with a large intraluminal mass. Seventy to eighty percent are resectable and the 5-year survival rate is around 20–30%. Surgical treatment is resection of the primary lesion and associated lymph nodes. For a duodenal adenocarcinoma a wide local excision or a pancreaticoduodenectomy is performed depending upon the size and location of the lesion. For advanced small intestinal adenocarcinoma chemotherapy consisting of 5-fluorouracil (5-FU), oxaliplatin, leucovorin and irinotecan are used as indicated. Adjuvant chemoradiation may produce some benefit. Intraoperative radiation therapy by an electron beam or external radiation for a positive resection margin or an unresectable disease is often considered for achieving palliation. Adenocarcinomas of small intestine are generally radioresistant.

Sarcoma

Small bowel sarcomas account for 10% of small bowel cancers. Leiomyosarcoma and gastrointestinal stromal tumors (GISTs) account for 75% of small intestinal sarcomas. The less common tumors are fibrosarcoma, liposarcoma and angiosarcoma. Sarcomas are slow growing and are frequently found in the jejunum and ileum. They locally invade surrounding tissues and may metastasize to the lung, liver and bones. Clinical presentation is usually abdominal pain, a mass or bleeding. Intestinal obstruction may be rare as they tend to be extramural. Surgical resection is the treatment modality; however, often they are unresectable. Chemoradiation has a limited role for small bowel sarcomas.

Lymphoma

Lymphomas of the small bowel may be primary or as a part of a systemic disease. The stomach is the most common site for primary lymphoma followed by the small intestine. Lymphomas in the small intestine occur in the distribution of lymphoid follicles which explains its greater prevalence in the ileum. The B-cell and T-cell lymphomas are the usual variants. Most T-cell lymphomas are likely to be ulcerated plaques or strictures in the proximal small bowel. B-cell lymphomas tend to be annular or polyploidal masses in the distal and terminal ileum.[14,15]

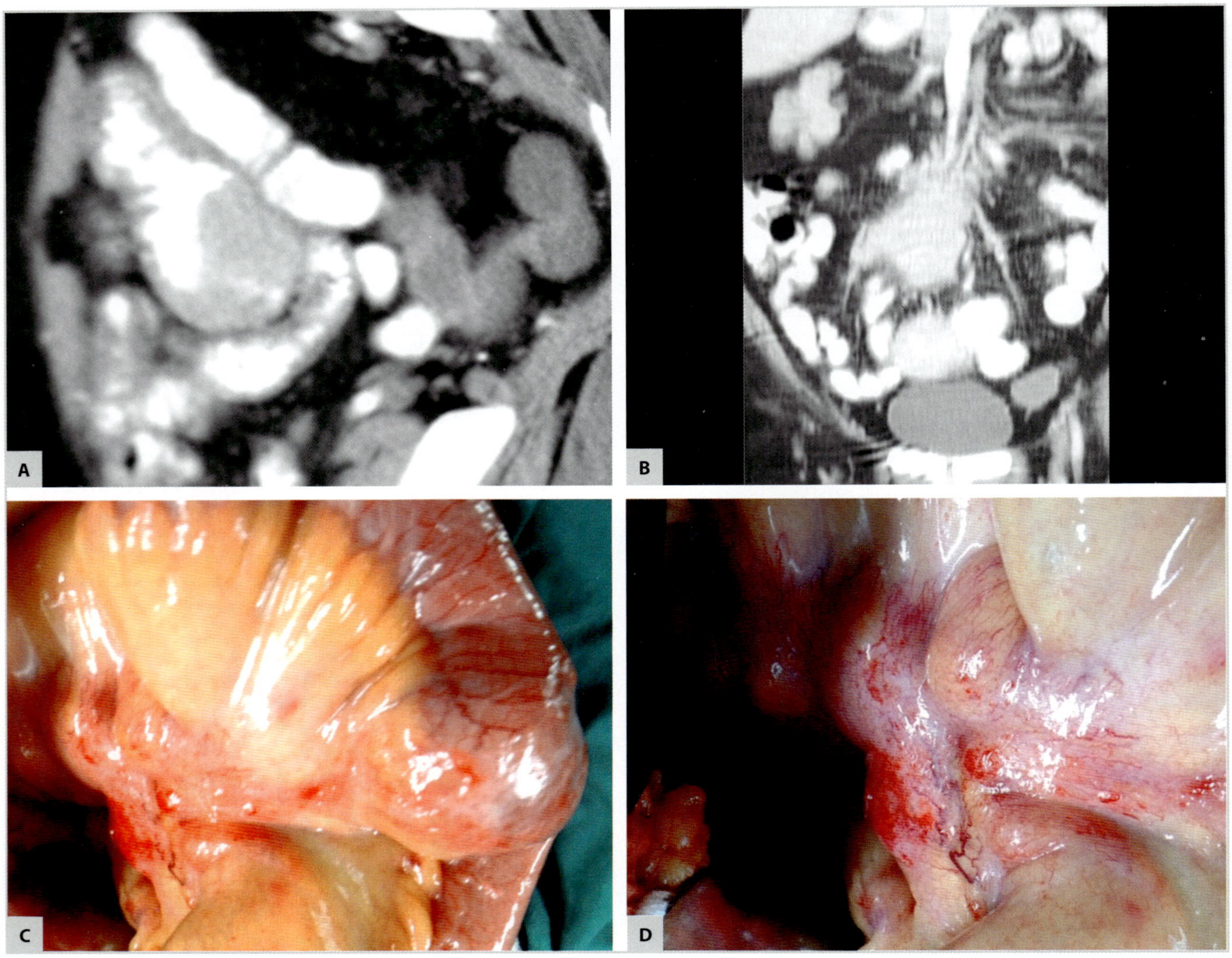

Figs 3A to D: (A and B) Computed tomography (CT) scan showing primary lymphoma with nodal mass in the ileum and encasement of mesenteric vessels; (C and D) Intraoperative photographs of the same patient showing the lesion (resected) and mesenteric lymph nodes (treated with chemotherapy)

A bulky small bowel lesion favors the diagnosis of a lymphoma. Imaging studies show a thickened segment or a mass with or without mesenteric adenopathy (Figs 3A to D). Surgical intervention is indicated, if the diagnosis is in doubt or if there are complications (obstruction, bleeding or perforation). Adjacent lymph nodes can be removed if feasible, along with the primary. Adjuvant chemotherapy is exhibited after histologic diagnosis. The CHOP therapy (cyclophosphamide, doxorubicin, vincristine and prednisone) is the standard protocol even after complete resection (R_0) or if there is residual disease (R_1-R_2). Radiation therapy is reserved for treatment of initially bulky tumors, residual recurrent disease, nodal metastases or positive resection margins. Radiotherapy can rarely produce significant morbidity (necrosis, bleeding and bowel perforation). Survival data show that low grade B-cell lymphoma has the best outcome and T-cell lymphoma the worst, due to resistance to chemotherapy. Five-year survival of patients with small bowel lymphoma ranges from 50% to 70%.[16–18]

Metastatic

Metastasis to the small bowel and the mesentery is commonly seen from cancer of the ovary, colon, lung, breast as a part of diffuse abdominal carcinomatosis. This is usually hematogenous and/or lymphatic dissemination. This may produce small bowel obstruction or perforation and appropriate surgical therapy is needed. Therapy for the primary lesion should be considered on its merits.

REFERENCES

1. Lowenfels AB. Why are small-bowel tumours so rare? Lancet. 1973;1:24-6.
2. Billimoria KY, Bentrem DJ, Wayne JD, et al. Small bowel cancer in the United States: changes in epidemiology, treatment and survival over the last 20 years. Ann Surg. 2009;249(1):63-71.
3. Lagergren J, Ye W, Ekbom A. Intestinal cancer after cholecystectomy: is bile involved in carcinogenesis? Gastroenterology. 2001;121:542-7.
4. Modlin IM, Lye KD, Kidd M. A 5-decade analysis of 13,715 carcinoid tumors. Cancer. 2003;97:934-59.
5. Akerström G, Hellman P, Hessman O, et al. Management of midgut carcinoids. J Surg Oncol. 2005;89:161-9.
6. Feig B, Ching CD. Small bowel malignancies and carcinoid tumours. The MD Anderson Surgical Oncology Handbook, 5th edition. Lippincott, Williams & Wilkins. pp.323-46.
7. Modlin IM, Latich I, Kidd M, et al. Therapeutic options for gastrointestinal carcinoids. Clin Gastroenterol Hepatol. 2006;4:526-47.
8. Kölby L, Persson G, Franzén S, et al. Randomized clinical trials of the effect of interferon-alpha on survival in patients with disseminated midgut carcinoid tumours. Er J Surg. 2003;90:687-93.
9. Rougier P, Mitry E. Chemotherapy in the treatment of neuro-endocrine malignant tumors. Digestion. 2000;62 Suppl 1:73-8.
10. Schupak KD, Wallner KE. The role of radiation therapy in the treatment of locally unresectable or metastatic carcinoid tumors. Int J Radiat Oncol B ol Phys. 1991;20:489-95.
11. Rodriguez-Bigas MA, Vasen HF, Lynch HT, et al. Characteristics of small bowel carcinoma in hereditary nonpolyposis colorectal carcinoma. International Collaborative Group on HNPCC. Cancer. 1998;83:240-4.
12. Giardiello FM, Welsh SB, Hamilton SR, et al. Increased risk of cancer in the Peutz-Jeghers syndrome. N Eng J Med. 1987;316:1511-4.
13. Senay E, Sachar DB, Keohane M, et al. Small bowel carcinoma in Crohn's disease. Distinguishing features and risk factors. Cancer. 1989;63:360-3.
14. Domizio P, Owen RA, Shepherd NA, et al. Primary lymphoma of the small intestine. A clinicopathological study of 119 cases. Am J Surg Pathol. 1993;17(5):429-42.
15. Ruskoné-Fourmestraux A, Aegerter P, Delmer A, et al. Primary digestive tract lymphoma: a prospective multicentric study of 91 patients. Gastroenterology. 1993;105(6):1662-71.
16. Daum S, Ullrich R, Heise W, et al. Intestinal non-Hodgkin's lymphoma: a multicenter prospective clinical study from the German Study Group on Intestinal non-Hodgkin's Lymphoma. J Clin Oncol. 2003;21(14):2740-6.
17. Radaszkiewicz T, Dragosics B, Bauer P. Gastrointestinal malignant lymphomas of the mucosa-associated lymphoid tissue: factors relevant to prognosis. Gastroenterology. 1992;102:1628-38.
18. Silberman H, Silberman A. Principles and Practice of Surgical Oncology. Lippincott, Williams and Wilkins. Small Bowel tumours, 44;812-27.

29 Cancer of Colon, Rectum and Anal Canal

Praful Desai, Sarabjeet Kaur Arneja, Bhavna Parikh

CARCINOMA OF THE COLON

INTRODUCTION

There is a fair amount of commonality between colon and rectal cancers in its etiology, clinical presentation, approach to diagnosis and management. Specific differences will be alluded to in a separate section on rectal cancers.

Colorectal cancer (CRC) is the third most frequent cancer in males after lung and prostate cancers. The incidence worldwide is declining due to early diagnosis, a direct consequence of routine fecal occult blood test (FOBT), appropriate management of inflammatory bowel disease, chronic ulcerative colitis and endoscopic management of polyps and adenomas of the colorectum. It is largely a disease of our habits and lifestyle; a predominantly exclusive non-vegetarian diet high in red meat, high cholesterol content with a low fiber component. Lesions mentioned above are often precursors of cancer. Diet rich in vegetables, fruits, antioxidant vitamins are reported to be protective but are devoid of any robust evidence. Age adjusted incidence rates of cancer colon and rectum show geographic variations in metropolitan cities and rural areas in India (Figs 1A and B).

A genetic background in the first-degree relatives particularly of colon cancers, hereditary syndromes of familial adenomatous polyposis (FAP), hereditary nonpolyposis colon cancer (HNPCC)—also known as Lynch syndrome with autosomal dominant inheritance and chronic ulcerative colitis require careful familial surveillance. Histologic diagnosis of polyps and adenomas can lead to early diagnosis and effective therapy. Treated early, both colon and rectal cancer has a satisfying 5-year control rate of greater than 65–70%.

PATHOLOGY

Adenomas

All adenomas by definition consist of dysplastic epithelium. Adenomas may harbor an intramucosal carcinoma or invasive carcinoma. The risk of malignant transformation is dependent on size of polyp and adenoma type, tubular versus villous.[1] If more than 75% of the epithelium demonstrates tubular or villous architecture, they are labeled as tubular or villous adenoma respectively.[2] The lesions that fall in between are labeled as tubulovillous adenomas.

Tubular Adenomas

Grossly they may be pendunculated/stalked or sessile. They tend to be rounded with a relatively smooth surface. Microscopically they show proliferation of glands and tubules lined by adenomatous epithelium (Fig. 2).

Villous Adenomas

The lesion shows similar adenomatous lining; however, the overall growth pattern or configuration is composed of villous projections (Fig. 3). The criteria of dysplasia are defined as per the World Health Organization (WHO) system[3] into low grade and high grade. All adenomas by definition carry low-grade dysplasia. This term is equated with adenomatous change. High-grade dysplasia encompasses carcinoma in situ and includes both

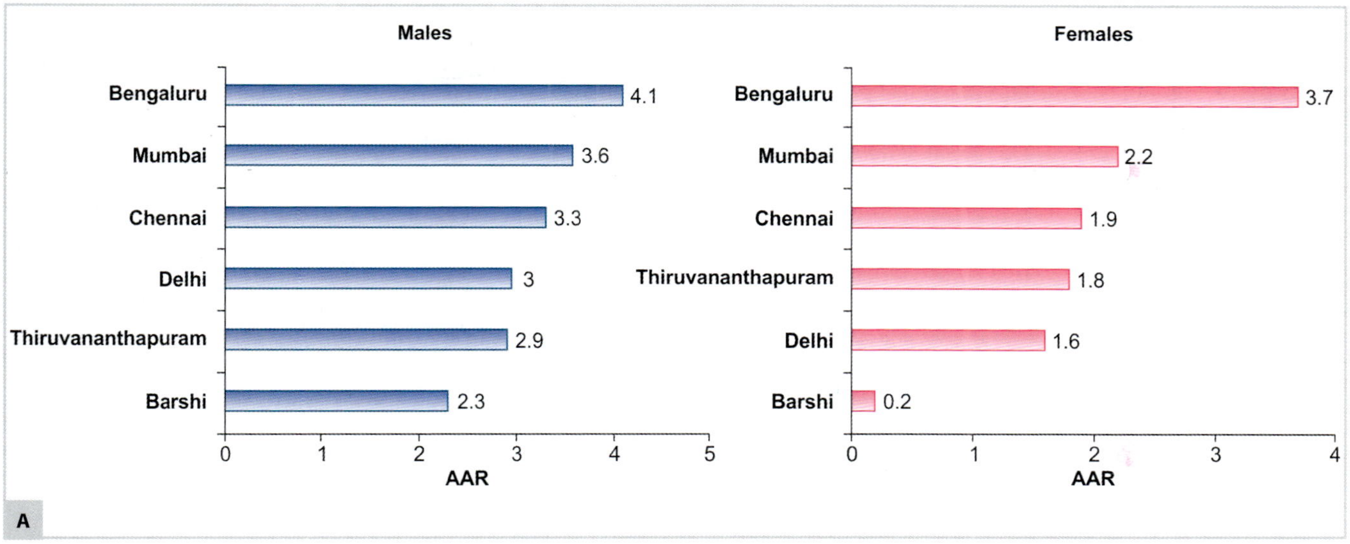

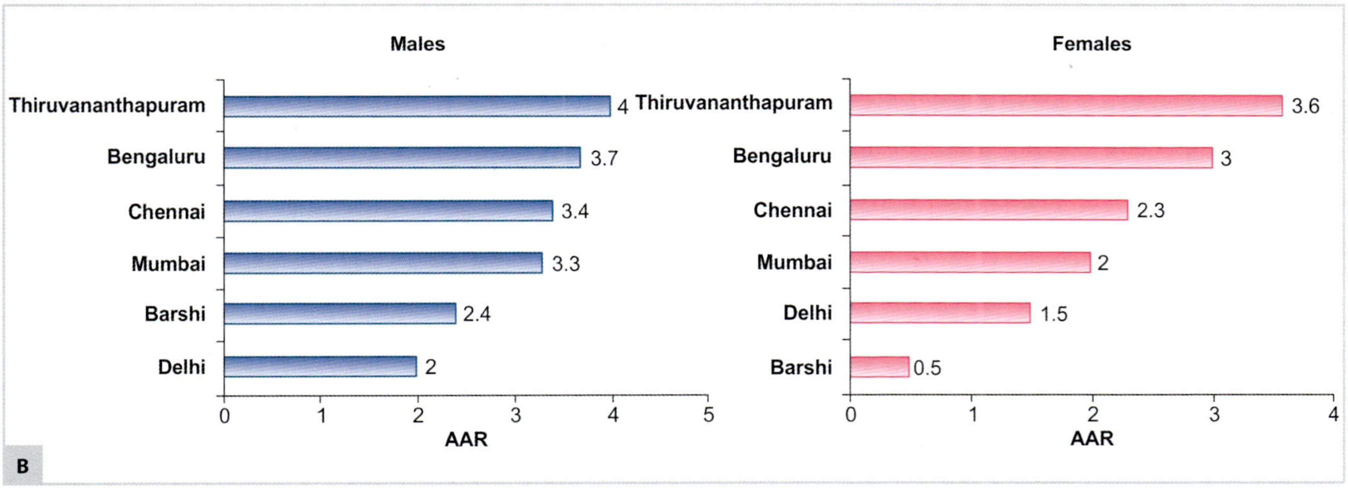

Figs 1A and B: (A) Age-adjusted rate (AAR) per 100,000 population India—cancer colon; (B) AAR per 100,000 population India—cancer rectum shows geographic variations in metropolitan cities and rural areas.
(*Sources:* National Cancer Registry Program Report 2006-2008)

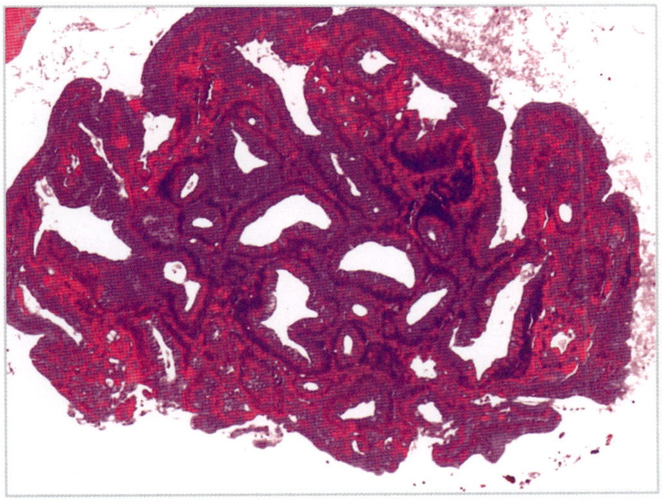

Fig. 2: Microscopic appearance of tubular adenoma composed of tubular glands

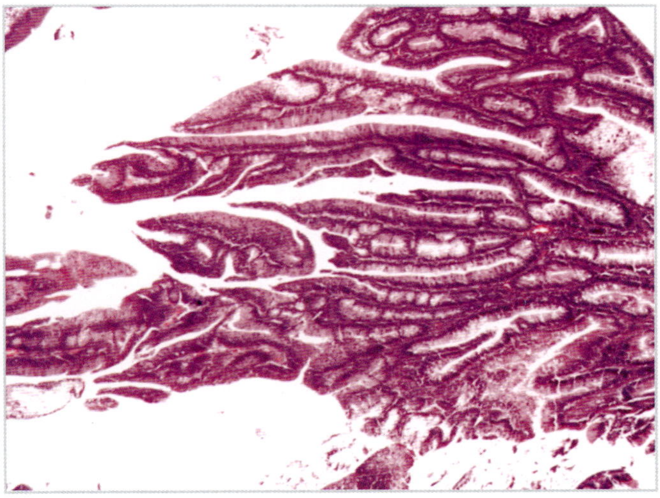

Fig. 3: Microscopic appearance of villous adenoma composed of villiform structures

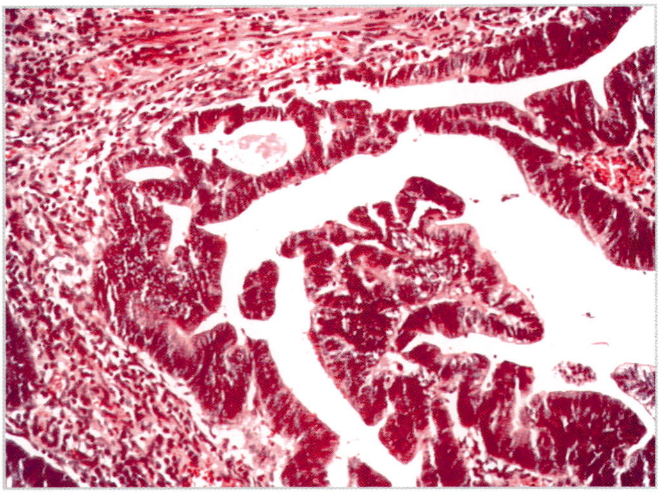

Fig. 4: Adenomatous polyp with high-grade dysplasia. Cribriform pattern with high-grade cytologic atypia

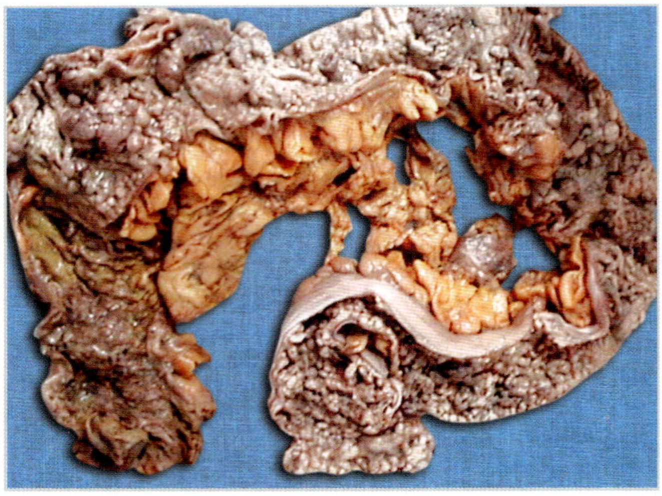

Fig. 5: Gross appearance of familial adenomatous polyposis. The entire large bowel is carpeted by hundreds and thousands of polyps

architectural and cytologic changes. Architecturally the crypts in high-grade dysplasia show irregular branching, confluence of glands and cribriform pattern. Cytologically the nuclei are enlarged hyperchromatic and show loss of stratification (Fig. 4).

Adenocarcinoma

Macroscopically CRCs can be polypoid-fungating or ulcerative-infiltrating lesions. On cut section grayish-white tumor tissue is seen replacing the bowel wall. Microscopically they may be classified as well differentiated, moderately differentiated or poorly differentiated.

Other Microscopic Types[3]

- Mucinous carcinoma
- Signet ring carcinoma
- Small cell carcinoma (oat cell cancer)
- Adenosquamous carcinoma
- Squamous cell carcinoma
- Undifferentiated (medullary) carcinoma.

Familial Forms of Large Bowel Cancer

Familial Adenomatous Polyposis

It is an autosomal dominant disorder[4,5] in which hundreds or thousands of adenomatous polyps carpet the large bowel. The microscopic appearance of polyps is no different from sporadically occurring adenomatous polyps. The genetic defect is in the adenomatous polyposis coli (APC) gene located on chromosome 5q21.[6,7] The tumors occurring in this background manifest much earlier, usually in the second decade of life. Molecular techniques can be used to diagnose this disorder presymptomatically by determining the germline mutation in relevant genes (Fig. 5).

Hereditary Nonpolyposis Colorectal Cancer

This is due to germline mutation in one of the DNA mismatch repair genes, MLH1, MSH2, MSH6 and PMS2 that results in microsatellite instability (MSI).[8-10] This imparts 50% risk of developing large bowel cancer in a first-degree relative of an affected patient.

Neuroendocrine Tumors

Macroscopically they may appear as polypoid to plaque like lesions, usually nonulcerated. Microscopically they appear as patterned tumors composed of small uniform cells disposed in nests, trabeculae or festoons. Immunohistochemically they stain for pan-neuroendocrine markers (chromogranin, synaptophysin or neuron-specific enolase).

Gastrointestinal Stromal and Smooth Muscle Tumors

These are biologically and morphologically similar to their gastric and small intestinal counterparts referred to elsewhere.

DIAGNOSIS/INVESTIGATIONS

The initial symptoms are often vague and transitory. Gastrointestinal (GI) dysfunction symptoms like abdominal pain after oral intake, heaviness, change in bowel habits, alternating diarrhea and constipation, weakness, unexplained anemia and loss of weight are usual symptoms in the initial stages. A simple FOBT points towards a colonic or rectal pathology. A palpable mass in the ascending, transverse, descending colon or sigmoid region is indicative of a lesion which has invaded the serosa. Rarely a patient may present with a palpable liver and/or ascites indicative of a diffuse spread in the liver and peritoneal cavity (omentum, parities, miliary seedlings). In this clinical setting, abdominal paracentesis to study the presence of malignant cells is a routine to confirm diffuse peritoneal spread. In a suspected advanced lesion, a laparoscopy would be advisable before a final decision to explore for even a palliative resection.

Routine investigations will include a complete colonoscopy and a biopsy. Imaging studies are the next logical step to detect the site, extent and spread of the disease (Fig. 6). A positron emission tomography-computed tomography (PET-CT), though not mandatory, is often performed. False negatives in the form of reactive nodes in the abdomen and chest are not uncommon with a PET study and should be viewed in totality with the clinical scenario. Therapeutic decisions should not be changed unless a histology is available of a reportedly PET scan-positive metastatic distant spread. Routine blood chemistry, cardiopulmonary and hepatorenal function studies are mandatory before treatment planning. Special attention should be given to protein levels, particularly the albumin level (above 3 g) which is a prerequisite before planning surgery in CRCs. Tumor markers carcinoembryonic antigen (CEA) and carbohydrate antigen 19.9 (CA 19.9) is worthwhile as a baseline parameter in all colorectal cancers.

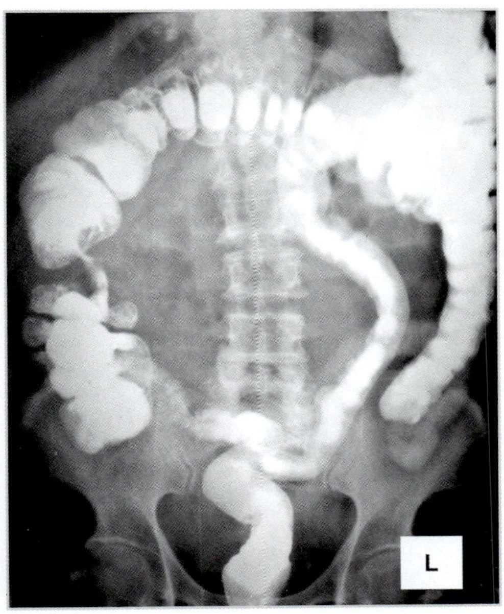

Fig. 6: Barium study of a patient with a lesion in the ascending colon

STAGING

Historically, the Dukes' (A, B, C) classification was generally adopted; however, currently the tumor-node-metastasis (TNM) classification is the one commonly accepted as it helps in planning therapy based on TNM staging. The T classification ranges from T_{is} (carcinoma in situ) to $T4_{a,b}$ when the lesion invades other organs or penetrates the visceral peritoneum. The N stage is based on number of nodes retrieved at surgery and ranges from N1 (1–3 positive nodes) and $N2_{a,b}$ (4–7 nodes). M refers to distant metastasis with $M1_{a,b}$ as referral to one or more organ involvement or peritoneal infiltration (Table 1).

TABLE 1: TNM classification of CRCs

T-Staging	
T_{1s}	Carcinoma in situ. Invasion of lamina propria
T_1	Submucosal invasion
T_2	Muscularis mucosa
T_3	Upto subserosa, pericolic or perirectal invasion
T_4	• Upto serosa • Invasion of other organs or structures
N-Staging	
N_1	• 1 node involvement • 2 to 3 nodes involvement • Mesenteric involvement
N_2	More than 4 nodes • Upto 6 nodes • More than 7 nodes
M-Staging	
M_1	• One organ involvement • Two or more organs involvement
Stage	
I	$T_1 T_2$
IIA	T_3
IIB	T_{4a}
IIC	T_{4b}
IIIA	$T_{1.2} N_1$
IIIB	$T_{3.4} N_{2a}$
IIIC	$T_{4a.b} N2_{a.b}$
IVA	Any T Any N M_{1a}
IVB	Any T Any N M_{1b}
Duke Staging (CRC)	
A	Mucosal involvement
B	Invasion muscularis propria
C	Upto serosa. Lymph nodes and adjacent organs
D	Distant metastasis

This extensive TNM staging is recent and clarifies further the simple and practical old DUKE's classification (A to D) for colo-rectal cancers. Beyond a point, exhaustive classification like the TNM (in CRC) can only be of prognostic value without any therapeutic impact. The historic Duke's classification is still useful in planning adjunctive therapy, e.g. Duke's stage C will require adjunctive chemotherapy.

TREATMENT PLANNING

For a localized lesion, the therapy of choice remains a standard resection of a right, a transverse and a left hemicolectomy or a sigmoidectomy depending on the site of the lesion. A transverse colectomy (Fig. 7) will require a good mobilization of the hepatic and splenic flexure for a loose tension-free and vascular anastomosis; similarly, resection of a sigmoid cancer will require mobilization of the splenic flexure to ensure a tension-free colorectal anastomosis in the pelvis or at the pelvic brim. Ligation of the inferior mesenteric artery and vein at its origin may become necessary to ensure a tension-free anastomosis; in such a situation, the marginal artery will be the sole supply to the colonic end. In patients with diabetes and hypertension, ligation of the inferior mesenteric artery at its origin can lead to anastomotic dehiscence. If possible, ligation at its origin should be avoided as the nodes around the pedicle can be easily dissected without ligation at its origin.

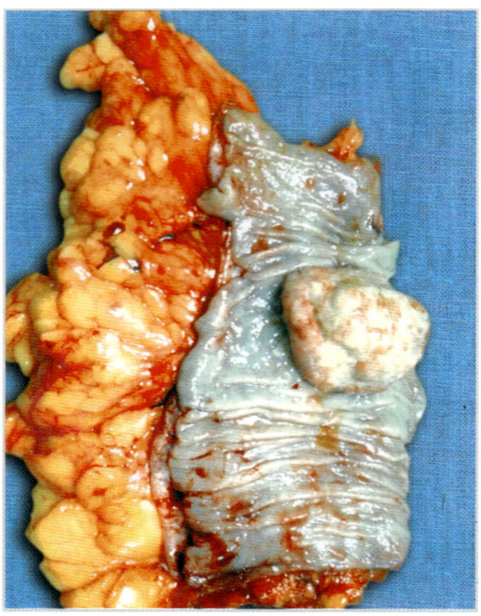

Fig. 7: Specimen of a polypoidal lesion in the transverse colon

Total colectomy will be necessary in rare instance of multiple colonic cancers (5–8%) and an ileorectal anastomosis will be in order. Patients with chronic ulcerative colitis, FAP and HNPCC will likewise require a total colectomy with ileorectal anastomosis or rarely a total proctocolectomy with a permanent ileostomy if the rectal stump is heavily involved. In patients with minor or moderate involvement of the rectum, the stump could be carefully surveyed every 6 months by a careful sigmoidoscopy. Rarely, in order to avoid an ileostomy, intraperitoneal ileal pouch and ileoanal anastomosis[11] have occasionally been performed with varying results impacting on the quality of life by incontinence, continual diarrhea and impotence. Nearly 10% of patients or more may have to convert to a permanent ileostomy. A well-executed colostomy after an abdominoperineal resection (APR) can often permit a better quality of life than ileoanal anastomosis. The question of proximal diversion after surgery will depend upon the adequacy and the confidence of the surgeon about the state of the anastomosis. A temporary transverse colostomy or an ileostomy will safeguard against sepsis due to an anastomotic breakdown, particularly in cases where the surgeon is concerned about the vascular adequacy of the anastomosis.

A locally aggressive colonic lesion is apt to involve the abdominal wall or the peritoneum. Infiltration of adjoining organs like the bladder (sigmoid carcinoma), a segment of the small bowel, part of the stomach wall (transverse colon) or rarely even the head of the pancreas (ascending colon lesion). If the disease can be efficiently resected with safety, sacrifice of the involved organs is not a contraindication. Long-term control rates have been reported. A colo-Whipple resection is also within the ambit of an experienced oncologic surgeon which can result in a good control of the disease. In an obstructed colonic lesion, a proximal diversion is advisable prior to a planned standard surgical procedure after 2–3 weeks. Retrieval of around 15 lymph nodes is considered adequate surgery by either open method or minimally invasive surgery (MIS). This is proven by number of randomized trials like the Clinical Outcomes of Surgical Therapy Study Group (COST)[12], the Conventional versus Laparoscopic-Assisted Surgery in Colorectal Cancer (CLASICC),[13] etc. with equivalent long-term results.[14,15] It is therefore a closed chapter about discussing the method of surgery. It depends on the comfort zone of the surgeon. Increasingly larger number of patients now undergo laparoscopic colectomy.

Minimally invasive surgery, robotic surgery and the "open" approach have their advocates. Number of trials—COST[12], CLASICC[13], Colon Cancer Laparoscopic or Open Resection (COLOR) Study[16] have proved the adequacy and equivalency in terms of node retrieval (up to 15 nodes) and even long-term results at 3 years and 5 years. Colonic resection with MIS is now increasingly practiced at most places. The advantage of less pain and shortened hospitalization by 2 or 3 days and earlier GI tract recovery are reported advantages. Case selection is imperative and patients with a large body mass, and difficult, infiltrating larger tumors are best resected by an open approach. The comfort zone of the surgeon and his expertize in MIS and robotic procedures will be the final call vis-a-vis the surgical approach.

COMPLICATIONS OF COLONIC SURGERY

By far and large appropriately conducted surgery for colon cancer in a properly selected patient should be devoid of any major complication which endangers life, except in the rare event of a cardiopulmonary or a cerebral event. By far the commonest complication is an anastomotic disruption, the incidence of which is less than 5% in experienced hands. The "adage", "even the best looking anastomosis can leak" is indeed a truism. Attention to preoperative nutrition, protein values, electrolytes, etc. and most importantly a safe technique (hand sutured or stapled) are important preoperative and operative steps. Anastomotic breakdowns are either minor or major. With appropriate drainages (placed at completion of surgery) most minor leakages heal within 5–7 days; major breakdown may require an urgent fecal diversion in the form of an ileostomy or a transverse colostomy depending upon the site of anastomosis. Adequate total parenteral nutrition and controlling sepsis with antibiotics are important steps which will heal majority of leaks in 2–3 weeks. A re-exploration is a distinctly rare event and needs to be considered with appropriate drainages in the event of diffuse peritonitis. Overall mortality after colonic resection is less than 2–3%.

NEOADJUVANT CHEMOTHERAPY IN COLONIC CANCERS

A colonic cancer confined to the organ without local infiltration and excessive nodal burden (as determined by imaging studies, CT scan) should be generally resected without any upfront neoadjuvant chemotherapy (NACT). Postoperative (adjunctive) chemotherapy should be considered if indicated after detailed histopathology; however, a large T4 resectable lesion with excessive nodal burden or synchronous liver metastasis should be excised after standard three or four cycles of NACT. This often effectively downstages the disease and may even permit a R_0 (no residual disease) resection of the primary lesion 3 weeks after the completion of NACT.

CARCINOMA OF THE RECTUM

INTRODUCTION

Despite many seeming similarities in CRCs in clinical presentation and diagnostic approach, rectal cancer management requires a distinctly different approach; the narrow confines of the pelvic anatomy, the lack of a serosa in its middle and lower segments, the importance of the anal sphincter preservation, when indicated, and the response to chemoradiotherapy of rectal lesions are all special issues which play a major role in the successful management of rectal cancer. The concept of trans-mesoretal excision (TME) proposed by Heald et al.[17,18] has significantly changed the surgical technique and approach to rectal cancer management and has significantly reduced local pelvic and recurrence rates after surgery.

Two studies, Stockholm[19,20] and rectal study group have clearly indicated, based on documented evidence that high volume therapeutic team (surgeons, chemotherapist and radiotherapist) and high volume institutions make a significant difference in the results and outcomes of rectal cancer management. It is therefore obvious that though CRCs are often treated in a similar fashion important and significant insights are needed for appropriate management of rectal cancers.

ETIOLOGY

Generally the same causative factors (mainly dietetic) are operative in rectal cancers. Polyps, adenomatous lesions, involvement of the rectum in chronic ulcerative colitis with colonic cancer are important etiological factors. Rarely, nonhealing chronic high fistula-in-anorectal region could induce a malignant lesion in the rectum. The adenoma-hyperplasia-carcinoma sequence of a colonic polyp also holds true for a rectal polyp.

CLINICAL PRESENTATION AND INVESTIGATIONS

By far the most frequent symptom is rectal bleeding which is usually fresh, before, during or after defecation. A sense of incomplete evacuation is an extremely common symptom because of partial blockage of the rectal lumen depending on the size and volume of the lesion. Mild to moderate degree of lower abdominal or rectal discomfort or pain may be associated with above symptoms. Clinical examination generally reveals a normal abdomen.

Digital Per-Rectal Examination

By far the most important clinical assessment of a rectal lesion can be obtained by a digital evaluation of the rectum in experienced hands. The size of the lesion, its morphologic character (polypoidal noninfiltrative or ulcerative and infiltrating), the amount of circumferential involvement, infiltration of the rectal wall and proximity or infiltration of the prostate gland and the degree of luminal obstruction can be efficiently gauged by a careful rectal examination. The distance from the anal verge, the possibility of sphincter preservation surgery (in the event of surgical approach) and the amount of pararectal tethering signifying involvement of the rectal wall can all be efficiently estimated and helps in planning of therapy (NACT-radiotherapy/chemotherapy, surgery). Further investigations like sigmoido-colonoscopy, rectal biopsy and a transrectal ultrasound (TRUS) (Fig. 10) study will be helpful to complete the data necessary for proper assessment, staging and treatment planning. A CT, PET/CT and/or magnetic resonance imaging (MRI) scans will complete the list of pretreatment assessment before the final therapeutic approach for rectal cancer can be planned.

The forgotten art of clinical examination is a victim of the plethora of investigations that we have at our command. It is indeed necessary to use modern investigations prudently and intelligently. It is unwise to use them just because they are at hand. A PET/CT is probably more useful to assess recurrences post-therapy in a asymptomatic patient with a rising tumor marker. The presence of reactive and inflammatory nodes often gives a false-negative result on the PET scan. A good routine CT of the chest and abdomen or an MRI is enough routine investigation. A TRUS often gives an accurate assessment of the rectal wall involvement and the presence of pararectal lymph nodes (false-negative known) for clinical staging. A study of tumor markers CEA/CA 19.9, very often conveys the tumor burden, though nearly 35% of colorectal lesions will show normal values. Very high CEA greater than 100 IU/mL generally indicates celomic or metastatic spread to the liver. A high value is extremely useful as a monitor in post-therapy evaluations.

FUNDAMENTAL PRINCIPLES OF THERAPY

Majority of patients (> 60%) present late with a large tumor T3 with N1 or N2 disease. Clinical staging even with appropriate imaging investigations has its limitations and in colorectal lesions; the nodal status cannot be totally relied upon, as inflammatory and reactive nodes vitiate the clinical assessment; however, a good per-rectal digital examination often gives a fairly accurate assessment of the state of resectability of the primary lesion in the rectum.

Preoperative Downstaging of Rectal Cancer—the Need for Neoadjuvant Chemoradiotherapy

Rectal cancers are chemo- and radiosensitive. Large data base clearly show that downstaging of the lesion almost always occurs. The decision to give neoadjuvant chemoradiotherapy (NACRT) should be made jointly by the team of surgeon, chemotherapist and radiation oncologist. Three to four cycles of chemotherapy and 40 Gys of radiotherapy is the usual combination. Occasionally concurrent chemoradiotherapy may produce severe symptoms and radiotherapy or chemotherapy can be used as a single-agent neoadjuvant therapy. The disadvantage of sequential chemoradiotherapy is time consuming and surgery could be delayed by 2.5–3 months. Assessment of response should be evaluated 3 weeks after completion and an appropriate surgical procedure should then be planned about a week after the assessment. Complete clinical response after chemoradiotherapy is around 15–20% of patients so treated. A pathologic complete response in the resected specimen occurs in around 8–10%.[21,22] Initial surgery may be forced in presence of an obstructed lesion (stenting or transverse colostomy) or severe bleeding which can be controlled with radiotherapy. The selective use of NACRT for patients with rectal cancer who achieve a complete clinical response appears to achieve similar oncologic outcomes for patients who have achieved a pathologic complete response after NACRT and rectal resection, while conferring the advantage of avoiding the morbidity of rectal resection.[23] Definitive

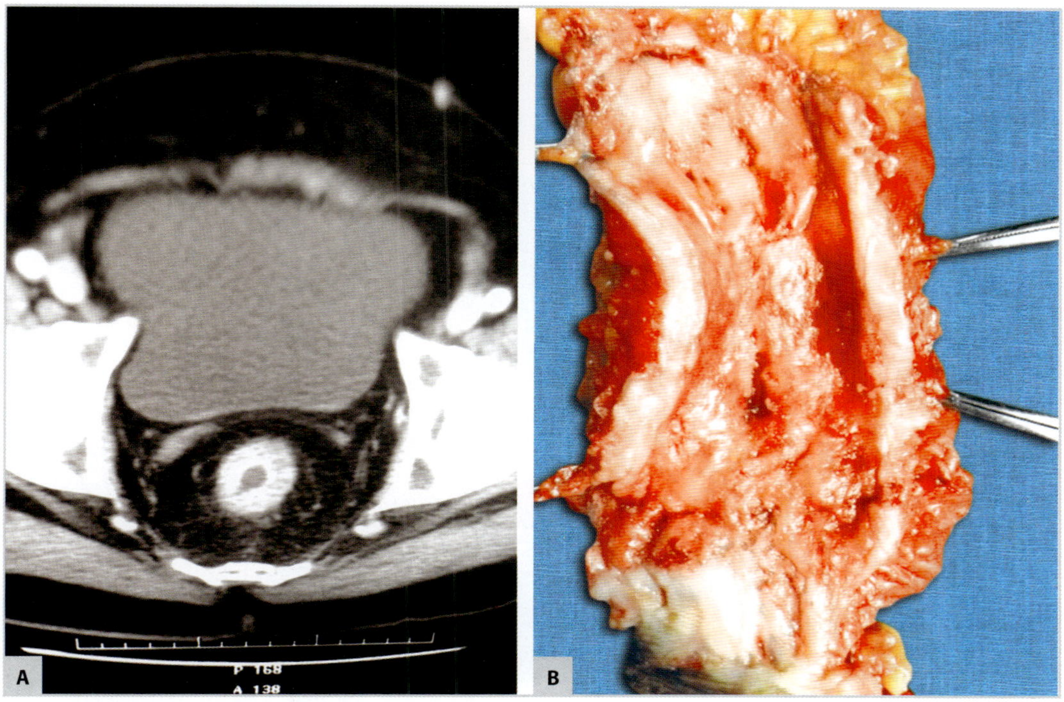

Figs 8A and B: (A) Computed tomography (CT) scan study of a lesion in the lower rectum postchemoradiotherapy; (B) Specimen at surgery 6 weeks later showing extreme thickening of the rectal wall and a necrotic ulcerating lesion. Dissection in the low pelvis becomes difficult after chemoradiotherapy because of pelvic fibrosis

chemoradiotherapy as a primary therapy for rectal cancers is receiving increasing attention in order to salvage the rectum (Figs 8A and B).

Surgery

A provisional initial assessment needs to be made about the inevitability of an APR (very low lesions within 5 cm of the anal verge) or the feasibility of a sphincter-saving procedure—either a colorectal or coloanal anastomosis.[24] Stretching or pushing the limits to perform a sphincter-saving procedure is an unwise surgical decision as the lower the anastomosis, greater are the chances of anastomotic disruption, strictures, local recurrences, incontinence, continual diarrhea and often sexual issues of impotence and retrograde ejaculation. Even bladder dysfunction is frequent (Figs 9 to 11).

A well-executed end colostomy offers a better quality of life after the initial (negative) impact of a colostomy which slowly and steadily wanes. However, appropriately indicated low sphincter-saving anterior resection has a satisfying outcome as the postoperative problems of frequent diarrhea resolves within 6–8 months as the storage capacity of the pouch or the rectum improves. The need for a covering ileostomy or a transverse colostomy depends on the surgeon's decision regarding the state of anastomosis; it is mandatory in very low colorectal or coloanal anastomosis as leakages are common (more than 10%). With a safe and very vascular colorectal anastomosis diversion could be avoided as per the discretion of the surgeon.

Hand-Sewn and Stapler Anastomosis

There is no major or significant difference in the outcome between the two methods. The choice depends on the comfort zone of the surgeon. Many conventional surgeons still use 2-0, 3-0 vicryl sutures for hand-sewn anastomosis. Unabsorbable staplers may cause marginally high strictures, particularly in anastomosis which are of smaller circumference like esophageal anastomosis. Stapler anastomosis are time saving. Good primary healing of the anastomosis depends not on staplers or hand-sewn methods, but on good vascular ends which are tension-free.

The Concept of Total Mesorectal Excision in Rectal Surgery and Circumferential Margins

One of the major issues in the therapy of mid and lower one-third cancers of the rectum is the frequency of local recurrence in the pelvis after surgery, even after NACRT. The incidence varies from 8% to 43%,[25] as per literature review.

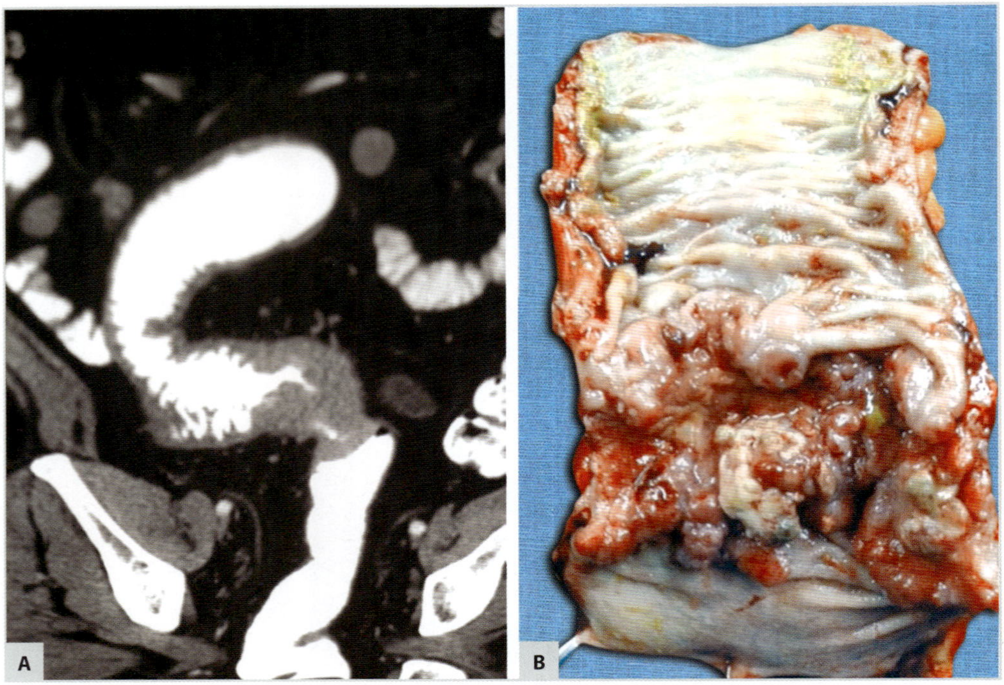

Figs 9A and B: Computed tomography (CT) contrast study of a sigmoid carcinoma and the operative specimen. A low anterior sphincter-saving procedure with a good 4 cm distal-free margin

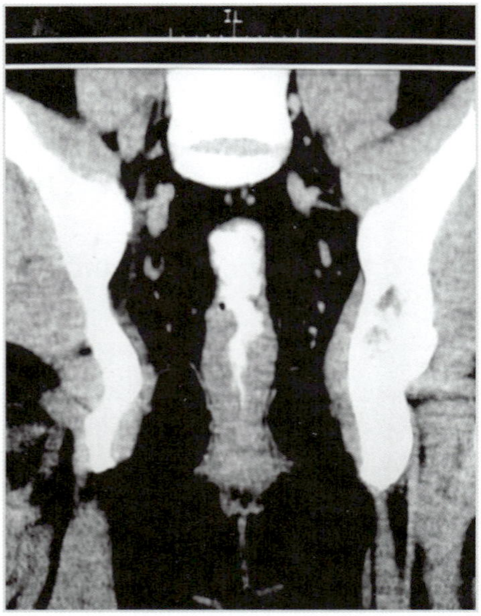

Fig. 10: Carcinoma rectum in a 25-year-old person with extreme narrowing and cicatrization of the rectum with circumferential involvement all around

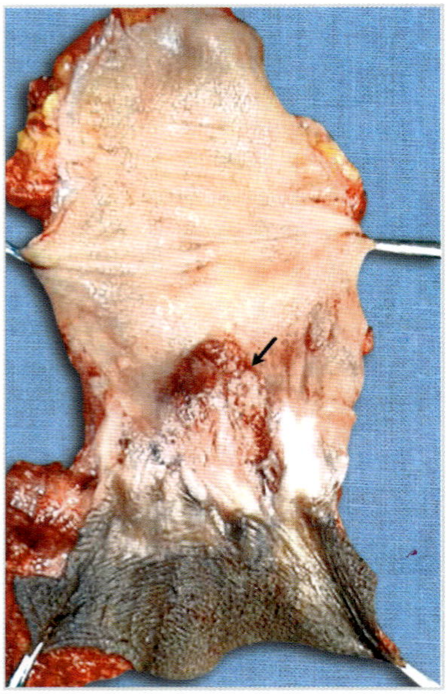

Fig. 11: Adenosquamous carcinoma at the anorectal junction, operative specimen

Recurrences usually occur in the pelvis and pararectal space, mainly in the lymph nodes and soft tissues—despite adjuvant radiotherapy. In a seminal and probably a practice changing contribution by Heald et al.[17,18] pointed out the importance of the mesorectum as encasing a large number of pararectal lymph nodes. He showed the very significant reduction in local recurrences[26] by a proper surgical excision alone which includes the mesorectum. In narrow confines of the pelvis, the technique of TME needs to be observed and mastered. It has a significant learning curve. He also pointed out about the importance of circumferential margins as of equal or greater importance than the distal margin. While a 2–2.5 cm distal margin clearance is acceptable, the circumferential margin clearance should be around 5 cm from the depth of the center of the cancer in the rectum.[27-30] The concept of TME and its approach and circumferential margins are shown in Figures 12 and 13.

An appropriate surgical technique with TME and postoperative radiotherapy in T2N1 or larger lesions will significantly reduce local recurrences in the pelvis

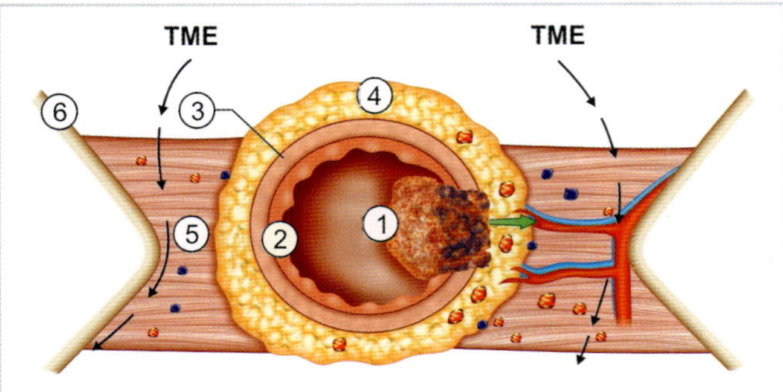

Fig. 12: The concept of total mesorectal excision (TME) and circumferential margins in surgery for rectal cancer

1. Tumor invading the muscle layer and into the perirectal fat (4) and nodes in the pelvic space (5); 2. Submucosa; 3. Muscle layer; 4. Perirectal tissue–must be included in the specimen; 5. Pelvic or pararectal space tissues has been metastatic lymph nodes which must be removed by a transmesorectal excision (TME) can depicted by arrows. Leaving behind the nodes is a major cause for pelvic recurrences after surgery for rectal cancer; 6. Pelvic wall

and perineum after rectal cancer surgery (Table 2). This technique should be meticulously followed in lower, middle and upper one-third rectal cancers (5 cm, 6–10 cm and 11–15 cm) from the anal verge respectively.

Minimally Invasive (Laparoscopic), Robotic and Open Surgery for Cancer Rectum

Minimally invasive (Lap + Robotic) and open surgery debates will continue. There is enough evidence for equivalence in colonic surgery as regards node retrieval and long-term results. Rectal surgery—APR; high and low anterior resections and coloanal anastomosis are recent inclusions and current data point towards equivalence though robust evidence in not yet at hand.

The negative spin off from MIS and robotic surgery show an increased incidence of autonomic nerve damage leading to impotence (nervi erigentes)[31] anastomotic leakages and increased local recurrences. Covering ileostomy for a year or more is mandatory after low pelvic anastomosis. Patients with a large body mass index (BMI) and difficult, large and adherent tumors are best tackled by open surgery. Conversion to open surgery is reported in 5–8% with greater complications and hence appropriate case selection is of vital importance.

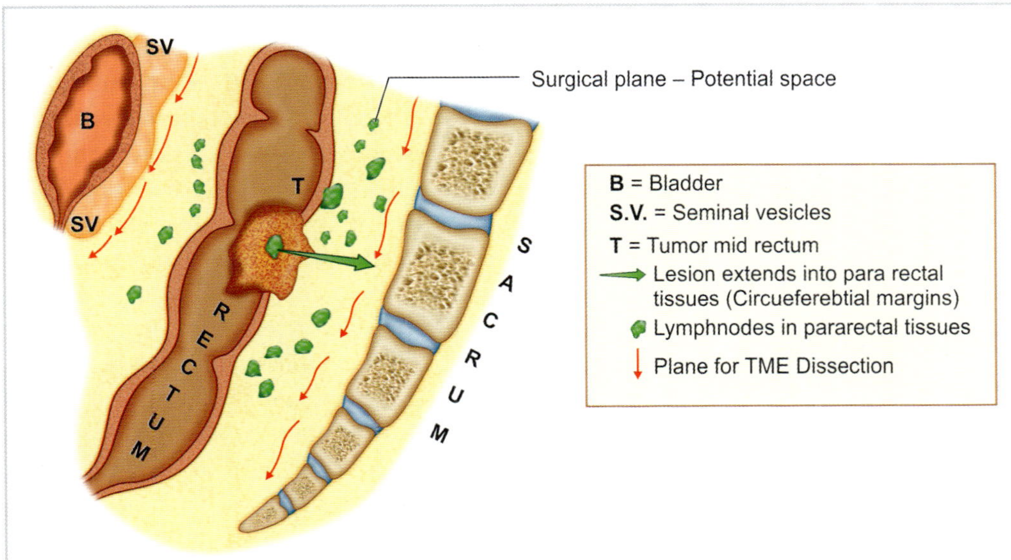

Fig. 13: Surgica approach for trans-mesorectal excision (TME) and obtaining a good circumferential margin for surgery in rectal cancer. A major factor in reducing pelvic recurrences after surgery for rectal cancer

(Significant numbers of pararectal nodes are embedded within the mesorectal mesentery. The mesorectum therefore needs to be excised with the rectum for retrieval of pararectal nodes. Figure 13 shows the plane of dissection behind the seminal vesicles and prostate anteriorly and in the avascular presacral fascia posteriorly. The lateral dissection in the pelvis is limited by the pelvic wall; however, ligation of middle and lower rectal vessels near the pelvic wall w ll ensure removal of all nodes draining the mid and lower rectum which will significantly reduce local pelvic recurrences. Metastatic nodes will require adjunctive pelvic radiotherapy.)

TABLE 2: Local recurrence of rectal cancers

Literature review	4–55%
Adjuvant radiotherapy	13–35%
Adjuvant chemotherapy + radiotherapy	8–15%
Optimized surgery alone	4%

Source: O'Higgins N. J Surg Oncol. 2004;87(3):109-15.

Table 2 emphasizes the importance of adequate surgery for rectal cancers in reducing pelvic recurrences.

Selection of Surgical Approach for Mid-lower Rectal Cancers

Patients for sphincter saving procedures should be carefully selected for either open or MIS procedures. Large lesions > 6 cm, which are often adherent are best approached by open surgery. Attempt with MIS or robotic surgery can lead to increase in local recurrences and often anastomotic disruptions. The lower the anatomosis (< 5 cm from the dentate line) the leaks are higher, and margin positivity is frequent. Conversion to open surgery is needed more frequently.

Polyps—Adenomas

Endoscopic management is generally the therapy of choice. A pedunculated polyp is easily managed by endoscopic excision—the base of the pedicle requires histologic assessment. A sessile narrow-based lesion can also be effectively managed by the endoscopist with a careful excision. A tethered or a firm base should be carefully and superficially excised as the chance of a perforation exists. The histology should subsequently decide the further course of action.

Obstructive Rectal Cancers

In less than 10% of CRCs (particularly the left colon, sigmoid and rectum), patients may present with signs of subacute or acute bowel obstruction. Diversion colostomy at an appropriate level has been the conventional approach followed by resection of the lesion after 2 or 3 weeks. Recent experiences with metallic stenting will avoid a colostomy though blockage and dislodgment of the stent is known and may require a re-evaluation.

Transanal Endoscopic Microsurgery

Transanal endoscopic microsurgery (TEM) of the early lesions of mid and lower rectum (T1N0) and anal canal is a feasible procedure which avoids a laparotomy.[32] Special facilities and instrumentation are needed. No long-term results are yet available and the inability to reach the mesorectum (nodes) is a disadvantage. The presence of nodal metastasis in T1 lesions is reported to be around 10%.

Adjuvant Radiotherapy

Adjuvant radiotherapy to the pelvis is often indicated, particularly in locally advanced lesions with multiple nodal involvement. Postoperative recurrences in the pelvis and perineum are very common after surgery for a T3N2 lesion of the rectum and postoperative radiotherapy therefore is mandatory. The concept of TME has dramatically diminished local recurrences in the pelvis, and appropriate surgical technique needs to be carefully observed, learnt and executed. Adjuvant chemotherapy is often exhibited along with radiotherapy.

Extrahepatic and Liver Metastasis in Colorectal Cancers

Currently an aggressive approach is the standard of care in metastatic disease in CRC. Localized resectable extrahepatic disease, hilar node metastasis, locoregional recurrences are no longer considered formal contraindications to surgery.[33] A major practice changing paradigm shift has however steadily evolved in the surgical management of liver metastasis over the last decade and is now firmly established as the therapy of choice and standard of care. Cautious surgical therapy toward either a synchronous or metachronous liver metastasis has now become the sine qua non for surgery of metastatic liver lesions.[34] The first resection of a metastatic liver lesion in colon cancer was performed in 1943.[35] This significant change has happened because of more efficient chemotherapy drugs resulting in downstaging of the primary disease and liver metastasis. Increasing experience in limited and even major hepatic resections now has acceptable morbidity and mortality. With large volume institutions and surgeons, the mortality is well below 5% and the 5 and 10 years survival rates range from 50% to 25% respectively[32,36,37] when liver metastases are aggressively managed.

Each clinical setting of a patient of CRC with liver metastasis therefore needs to be individualized before deciding upon the surgical approach. The following principles need to be generally followed:

1. Neoadjuvant chemotherapy is indicated when there are multiple metastasis in either lobe or two to three in either lobes—this helps to determine the chemosensitivity of the drug in a given patient

2. If the metastatic lesion is solitary and superficial, synchronous resection with the primary resection is feasible
3. It is generally inadvisable to simultaneously resect a major colonic or rectal lesion with multiple segments or even a large single segment hepatic resection
4. Major multiple segmental resections are best undertaken electively after NACT (four to six cycles) and resection of the primary lesion
5. Even in presence of liver metastasis, initial resection of the primary colorectal lesion is indicated if there is significant pain, obstructive symptoms and/or significant bleeding from the primary tumor
6. Even major left or right hepatectomy can be considered, particularly if the primary disease has remained controlled for at least 2–3 years. The prognosis is better if there is a long and significant latent period between the treatment of the primary lesion and the metastatic event
7. A joint multidisciplinary team of surgeons and chemotherapists should best decide the issues and therapy approach in a given case of CRC with liver metastasis.

The surgical approach of simultaneously handling an infected colonic lesion and a highly vascular organ like liver is best avoided. When a major resection is required neoadjuvant chemotherapy can significantly reduce the size and number of metastatic lesions in the liver and subsequent surgery for liver metastatic lesion is generally much safer with minimum morbidity (Fig. 14).

Peritoneal Carcinomatosis—Hyperthermic Intraperitoneal Chemotherapy (HIPEC)

Cancers of the GI tract from stomach to rectum are eminently treatable when diagnosed in stage I to stage III. This has been possible because of effective chemotherapy and good supportive care. Even in stage IV, with liver metastasis, appropriate combination therapy (chemotherapy, surgery) results in a significant 3 years and 5 years survival. A major problem, however, is when a patient with CRC present initially or late in the course of disease with extensive peritoneal involvement and carcinomatosis involving the omentum, the peritoneal surfaces, ascites and miliary carcinomatosis.[38]

Up until now, there was no significant proactive therapy approach for a patient with this clinical setting except best supportive care. A seminal therapeutic contribution is from Sugarbaker[39] who considered extensive cytoreductive surgery (CRS) followed immediately by HIPEC (44°C), before abdominal closure. Perioperative or early postoperative chemotherapy (POC) was another similar approach.

Phase II and III trials showed some minor to moderate improvement in survival for a few months. The morbidity, significant mortality and the long learning curve[40,41] for this procedure have been a major deterrent for a wider and general acceptance of this procedure. The CRS often involves multiple organ and bowel resections (6–8 hours) with omentectomy and peritonectomy resulting in a high rate of complications, sepsis and morbidity.[42-45] There are no randomized trials between best supportive care and HIPEC due to paucity of numbers. These procedures should not be performed beyond the ambit of a tertiary care center except in a clinical trial scenario. Disseminated peritoneal surface malignancies still remain an unsolved therapeutic issue and the only way out is to diagnose GI tract cancers early and effective treatment in stages II and III.

Systemic Therapy for Colorectal Cancer

Systemic therapy for CRC has evolved rapidly in the last decade. Five fluorouracil (5-FU) has been the backbone of systemic therapy for these cancers. Various combinations have been tried with 5-FU to increase or modify its effect,

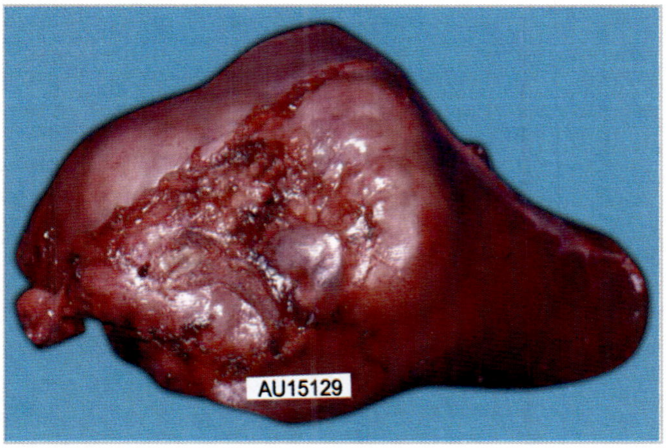

Fig. 14: Right hepatectomy specimen of a large metastatic lesion from the colon 3 years after the primary surgery. Patient survived 3½ years posthepatectomy

e.g. levamisole, leucovorin (LV), interferon, etc. Out of all these agents, LV has been accepted widely as a synergistic agent with 5-FU.

Systemic therapy in patients with CRCs is indicated in various clinical situations.

- Adjuvant therapy (colon)
- Metastatic setting
- Neoadjuvant therapy for rectal cancers.

Adjuvant Therapy

This is indicated in all stage III colorectal tumors. National Surgical Adjuvant Breast and Bowel Project (NSABP) C-03 was the landmark trial comparing 5-FU + LV arm versus MOF (methyl-CCNU, Oncovin, 5-FU) arm in Dukes stage "B" and "C" colon cancer. The overall survival at 3 years was 84% versus 77% in these arms respectively. This led to exclusion of MOF completely from the management of CRC and established 5-FU/LV as a standard arm.[46] Further development of adjuvant treatment involved adding injection oxaliplatin and/or injection irinotecan. One landmark trial is "MOSAIC" trial.[47] This was a randomized trial with infusion 5-FU/LV biweekly with and without oxaliplatin. With the median follow-up of 38 months, 3-year DFS was 72% for FOLFOX versus 66% for LV5FU2. Stage III patients benefited more than stage II in this study. Hence, oxaliplatin is established as the standard of care for adjuvant treatment of CRC. Regarding irinotecan, initial studies compared it with bolus 5-FU/LV versus irinotecan paired with either bolus 5-FU/LV (IFL). IFL arm showed inferior results.[48] There are other trials which used infusion 5-FU/LV with or without irinotecan (FOLFIRI). ACCORD II trial randomized 400 patients[49] and PETACC trial randomized 3,278 patients.[50] This agent did not show any benefit versus infusion 5-FU/LV. Hence, irinotecan has no role in adjuvant treatment of CRC.

Role of Oral Chemotherapy in Adjuvant Setting

Oral chemotherapy agents, viz capecitabine and tegafur have been studied in adjuvant setting. These agents are equivalent to only bolus 5-FU/LV regimens. Since bolus 5-FU/LV is used quite rarely in adjuvant setting, their use in this setting is much less. In an era of oxaliplatin-based chemotherapy for adjuvant treatment, these oral agents can be considered only when one wants to consider giving only 5-FU/LV bolus therapy. This can be for patients with stage II, and those who are reluctant for infusion 5-FU/LV therapy. The oral chemotherapy drugs do not have any role in treatment of stage III patients.

In stage II disease, benefit of adjuvant chemotherapy is questionable. In patients with high-risk stage II with evidence of: (1) obstruction or perforation, (2) poorly differentiated cancer, (3) preoperated elevated CEA, (4) high S phase fraction and (5) T4 tumors may behave like stage III tumors biologically and hence adjuvant chemotherapy is justified. For stage II patients, paraffin block can be studied for high-frequency MSI (MSI-H) phenotype.[46] Patients with MSI-H phenotype will not benefit from 5-FU based therapy. Hence, these high-risk stage II patients should not be subjected to chemotherapy.

Metastatic Setting

Patients may present with synchronous metastatic disease or develop metastases at a later stage (metachronous). While assessing patients with synchronous metastatic disease, it is important to set the goal at the outset while deciding whether the lesion is potentially resectable. The surgical approach in a patient with synchronous metastasis will depend on the clinical setting of a given case. If there is multicentric diffuse metastasis, primary chemotherapy is mandatory. Severe symptoms due to primary lesion (obstruction, pain) will mandate early resection. If the metastasis in the liver is superficial, solitary and resectable, surgery can be done concurrently. The authors favor only resection of primary lesion so that opportunity to see and evaluate the response to chemotherapy in liver metastasis exists. The preferred regimens will be FOLFOX. Targeted therapy may be considered if eligible. In disseminated unresectable stage IV disease, systemic therapy (chemotherapy and/or targeted therapy) is the only therapeutic approach. If these patients have been treated with oxaliplatin-based regimens earlier, irinotecan-based regimens like FOLFIRI can be considered.

Oral Chemotherapy

Capecitabine: This is a prodrug of 5-FU and gets converted to 5-FU in vivo. It is found to be useful for liver metastasis due to its high concentration in the liver. It has its peculiar side effects of hand-foot syndrome, mucositis and GI toxicity. The bioavailability and metabolism are unpredictable and require close monitoring and dose adjustment. This drug is contraindicated in patients with renal dysfunction as it is metabolized by renal route.

Tegafur-uracil with oral leucovorin: This is also a prodrug of 5-FU and needs to be given along with oral LV. It has minimum incidence of hand-foot syndrome, mucositis and GI toxicity. It is a well-tolerated drug for second-line therapy.

Targeted Therapy

Role of targeted therapy in management of colorectal cancer

Targeted therapy is a new therapeutic modality which can be considered in a setting of metastatic CRC (Fig. 15). It has no role in an adjuvant setting. The understanding of various pathways at cellular levels for carcinogenesis and its progression has led to development of targeted therapy. Five agents in this category (Table 3) are in clinical use of which only two agents are approved in India, viz. cetuximab and bevacizumab.

Eligibility criteria for using anti-EGFR drugs

The paraffin block tissue should be studied for KRAS mutation expression. If there is no mutation, i.e. KRAS wild-type, then only anti-EGFR drugs are indicated.[51] In presence of KRAS mutation, the tumor is nonresponsive and these agents are contraindicated. The side effects include occasional hypersensitivity reaction, acneiform rash and diarrhea.

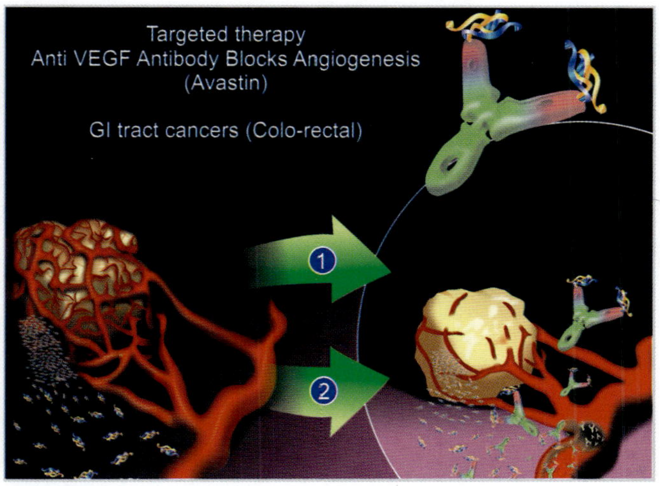

Fig. 15: Targeted therapy

Dose of cetuximab

Loading dose of 400 mg/m^2 followed by 250 mg/m^2 intravenous (IV) every week along with chemotherapy. Recently biweekly infusion is also considered to increase patient's compliance so that cetuximab can be combined with biweekly chemotherapy protocols (FOLFOX/FOLFIRI).

Role of anti-VEGF agents: Angiogenesis is one of the most important mechanisms of carcinogenesis. Intravenous bevacizumab is the first agent in this class. It can be used as a first-line or second-line metastatic setting therapy. It produces modest response as a single agent and is more effective when combined with chemotherapy.[52] It should not be combined with anti-EGFR agents.

Newer targeted agents: In antiangiogenesis group, there are promising new agents, e.g. regorafenib, aflibercept, axitinib. These are not in yet common use in India.

In the anti-EGFR agent group, panitumumab is the relatively new agent which is currently used with a modest response.

Neoadjuvant Chemotherapy

Concurrent chemotherapy with radiation (5-FU or capecitabine) followed by surgery is commonly used in locally advanced rectal cancers. This will downstage the disease and may enable sphincter-saving surgery. After a definitive surgery, principles of adjuvant treatment are same as those for colon cancer.

Protocols

Protocols have been shown in Flow chart 1 and Table 4.

TABLE 3: Five agents in targeted therapy

Class of drug	*Target*	*Drug*
MAB (monoclonal antibody)	EGFR1	Cetuximab (approved)
MAB	EGFR 1	Panitumumab
MAB	VEGF	Bevacizumab (approved)
Small molecule	VEGFR-TIG 2	Regorafenib
MAB	VEGF-A and VEGF-B	Aflibercept

Abbreviations: MAB, monoclonal antibody; EGFR, epidermal growth factor receptor; VEGF, vascular endothelial growth factor; VEGFR, VEGF receptor.

TABLE 4: Protocols of chemotherapy

FOLFOX	Oxaliplatin 85 mg/m^2 IV infusion day 1 Leucovorin 200 mg/m^2 IV infusion 2 hours day 1 + 2 5-FU 400 mg/m^2 IV bolus over 2–4 minutes day 1 followed by 5-FU 600 mg/m^2 IV infusion over 22 hours day 1 + 2
FOLFIRI	Irinotecan 180 mg/m^2 IV over 90 minutes concurrently with folinic acid 400 mg/m^2 IV over 2 hours followed by 5-FU 400 mg/m^2 IV bolus then 5-FU 2,400 mg/m^2 IV over 44 hours repeated every 2 weeks
CAPOX	Oxaliplatin 130 mg/m^2 IV infusion day 1 Capecitabine 1,000 mg/m^2 twice daily PO day 1–14 every 3 weeks for 6 cycles

Abbreviations: FOLFOX, 5-FU, oxaliplatin, leucovorin; FOLFIRI, 5-FU, irinotecan, leucovorin, oxaliplatin; CAPOX, capacitabine, oxaliplatin

Flow chart 1: Therapy algorithm of colorectal cancer

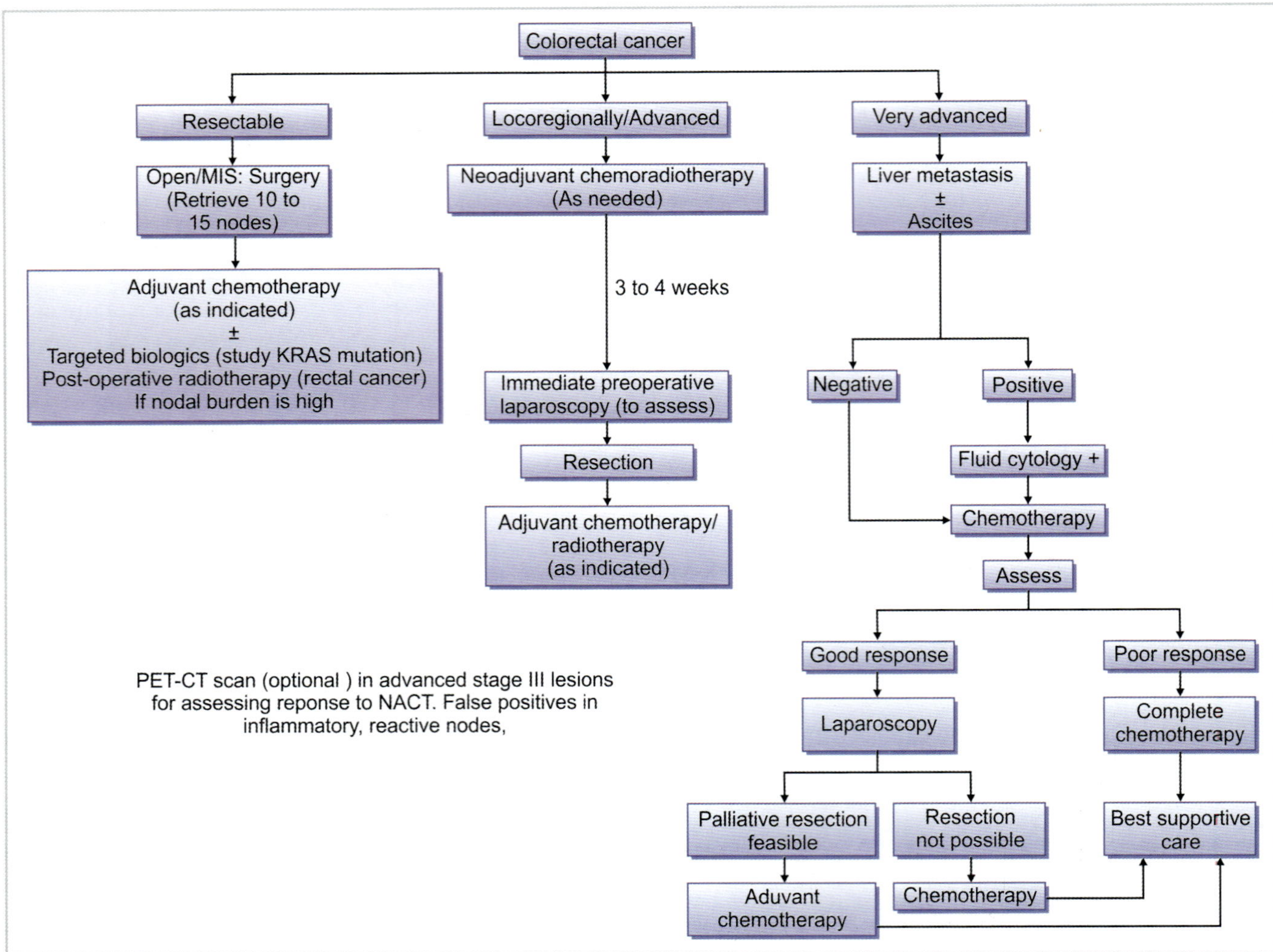

CANCERS OF THE ANAL CANAL

INTRODUCTION AND ETIOLOGY

The anal canal extends from the anal verge to about 1.5 cm up to dentate line and is lined by squamous epithelium. All lesions are squamous cell cancers. Rarely melanoma of the anal canal and rectum are reported. Important etiological factors are sexually transmitted disease (STD), human immunodeficiency virus (HIV) and human papillomavirus (HPV)-related infections. This group has a higher incidence in homosexuals and individuals with habits which promote anal canal cancers. It is rare in women but not unknown. There is a 40–95% association with HPV DNA.[53] Age adjusted rate of anal canal are shown in Figure 16.

DIAGNOSIS AND PRETHERAPY WORKUP

The clinical features are ulcerating lesions in the anal canal which often spills over to the anal verge and occasionally on to the perianal skin. Generally painful at presentation, they are often misdiagnosed as fissures. A nonhealing ulcerative lesion should be biopsied. Inguinal node metastasis is common in large ulcerated lesion and a fine-needle aspiration cytology (FNAC) is easily obtained. A CT scan evaluation will reveal the status of pelvic nodes. A good digital per anal-rectal examination, and if necessary examination under anesthesia to avoid pain should be performed. The degree of its extent into the anal canal, its infiltrative nature and extension into the soft tissues should be properly assessed.

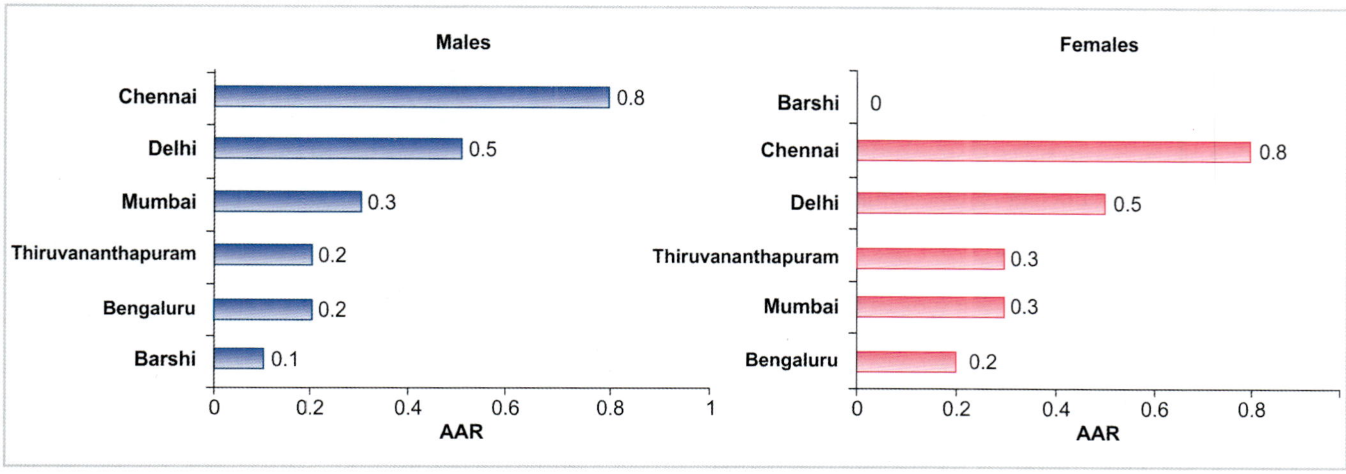

Fig. 16: Age-adjusted rate (AAR) per 100,000 population India—cancer anal canal

PATHOLOGY

Condyloma and Other Human Papillomavirus-related Lesions

In the anal region, HPV is associated with a variety of benign and malignant proliferative lesions, of which condyloma acuminatum is the most common.[54,55] Approximately 7–20% of anal condylomas show dysplasia on microscopic examination.[56,57] The HPV types most commonly encountered are 6, 11, 16 and 18, but 31, 35 and 39 have also been found.[57] The high-risk HPV infection-associated lesions often show overexpression of p16 (a tumor suppressor gene product) and a high Ki-67 (MIB-1) index.[58,59]

Anal Intraepithelial Neoplasia

Anal intraepithelial neoplasia (AIN) is the term used for the lesions traditionally designated as dysplasia, Bowen disease or in situ squamous carcinoma (CIS).[60] Using criteria similar to lesions in the cervix, AIN lesions are divided into three grades (AIN 1, AIN 2, AIN 3) or mild, moderate or severe dysplasia.[3]

Squamous Cell Carcinoma

Grossly most anal carcinoma arises near the pectinate line and grows either upward into the rectum and surrounding tissues or outward to the perianal tissues.[61] Traditionally, these tumors are classified as squamous cell carcinomas.[62] However, two distinct types of squamous carcinoma have been proposed (1) squamous cell carcinoma, analogous to the one seen on skin (2) cloacogenic (transitional, basaloid) carcinoma, believed to be originating from the transitional epithelium of this region and simulating light microscopic features of this zone.[63]

Adenocarcinoma

Most adenocarcinomas found in the anal canal represent downward extension of rectal adenocarcinoma or arise in colorectal type mucosa that is present above the dentate line. Macroscopically and microscopically, they are similar to colorectal type adenocarcinoma, and except for their low location do not represent a special entity.

Malignant Melanoma

Malignant melanomas are relatively rarer tumors, and account for 1–3% of all anal canal tumors.[64,65] Grossly they appear as single or multiple polypoid smooth surfaced masses. Due to their polypoid appearance they are often misdiagnosed as a thrombosed hemorrhoid.[66] Their morphologic and immunohistochemical profile is similar to those of melanomas at other sites.[67]

TREATMENT

The therapy of choice is chemoradiotherapy[68] and the standard drugs used are cisplatin, 5-FU and mitomycin-C in various combinations. Concurrent or sequential administration of chemoradiotherapy should be planned based on patient's general condition and his tolerance capacity. Most lesions respond satisfactorily and can be kept under observation. Total therapeutic response will occur only 8–10 weeks after completion of chemoradiotherapy.

Inguinal and pelvic node metastasis should be managed by either a superficial or a radical node dissection as needed. Thirty to fifty percent of patients will have positive nodes in larger lesions. A complete clinical and pathologic response is known and digital examination of the site of the lesion will show a depressed scar like fibrous tissue. No biopsies need to be performed during follow-up unless recurrence of a painful ulcer becomes symptomatic due to pain or bleeding. Occasionally a covering left ileal colostomy needs to be performed if, during therapy, symptoms of pain, bleeding and obstipation are severe. In the event of a recurrence of disease or poor response to chemoradiation, an APR with a permanent left colostomy will become mandatory.

REFERENCES

1. Konishi F, Morson BC. Pathology of colorectal adenomas: a colonoscopic survey. J Clin Pathol. 1982;35:830-41.
2. Reissenweber N, Gualco G, Ardao G, et al. The interrelationship between tubular and papillary sectors of tubulo-villous colorectal adenomas: comparative morphometric analysis and evaluation of cell proliferation. Hum Pathol. 1998;29:431-7.
3. Hamilton SR, Vogelstein B, Kudo S, et al. Carcinoma of the colon and rectum. In: Hamilton SR, Aaltonen LA (Eds). Pathology and Genetics of Tumours of the Digestive System (World Health Organization Classification of Tumours). Lyon, France: IARC Press; 2000. pp. 105-19.
4. Rustgi AK. Hereditary gastrointestinal polyposis and nonpolyposis syndromes. N Engl J Med. 1994;331:1694-702.
5. Sachatello CR. Familial polyposis of the colon. A four-decade follow-up. Cancer. 1971;28:581-7.
6. Bodmer WF, Bailey CJ, Bodmer J, et al. Localization of the gene for familial adenomatous polyposis on chromosome 5. Nature. 1987;328:614-6.
7. Leppert M, Dobbs M, Scambler P, et al. The gene for familial polyposis coli maps to the long arm of chromosome 5. Science. 1987;238:1411-3.
8. Jass JR. Diagnosis of hereditary non-polyposis colorectal cancer. Histopathology. 1998;32:491-7.
9. Lynch HT, de la Chapelle A. Hereditary colorectal cancer. N Engl J Med. 2003;348:919-32.
10. Lynch HT, Kimberling W, Albano WA, et al. Hereditary nonpolyposis colorectal cancer (Lynch syndromes I and II). I. Clinical description of resource. Cancer. 1985;56:934-8.
11. Fazio VW, Kiran RP, Remzi FH, et al. Ileal pouch anal anastomosis: analysis of outcome and quality of life in 3707 patients. Ann Surg. 2013;257:679-85.
12. Clinical Outcomes of Surgical Therapy Study Group. A comparison of laparoscopically assisted and open colectomy for colon cancer. N Engl J Med. 2004;350:2050-9.
13. Guillou PJ, Quirke P, Thorpe H, et al. Short-term endpoints of conventional versus laparoscopic-assisted surgery in patients with colorectal cancer (MRC CLASICC trial): multicentre, randomised controlled trial. Lancet. 2005;365:1718-26.
14. Fleshman J, Sargent DJ, Green E, et al. Laparoscopic colectomy for cancer is not inferior to open surgery based on 5-year data from the COST Study Group trial. Ann Surg. 2007;246(4): 655-62.
15. Jayne DG, Thorpe HC, Copeland J, et al. Five-year follow-up of the Medical Research Council CLASICC trial of laparoscopic-assisted versus open surgery for colorectal cancer. Br J Surg. 2010;97:1638-45.
16. Veldkamp R, Kuhry E, Hop WC, et al. Laparoscopic surgery versus open surgery for colon cancer: short-term outcomes of a randomised trial. Lancet Oncol. 2005;6:477-84.
17. Heald RJ, Husband EM, Ryall RD. The mesorectum in rectal cancer surgery—the clue to pelvic recurrence? Br J Surg. 1982;69:613-6.
18. Heald RJ, Ryall RD. Recurrence and survival after total mesorectal excision for rectal cancer. Lancet. 1986;1(8496):1479-82.
19. Preoperative short-term radiation therapy in operable rectal carcinoma. A prospective randomized trial. Stockholm Rectal Cancer Study Group. Cancer. 1990;66:49-55.
20. Randomized study on preoperative radiotherapy in rectal carcinoma. Stockholm Colorectal Cancer Study Group. Ann Surg Oncol. 1996;3:423-30.
21. Smith JD, Ruby JA, Goodman KA, et al. Nonoperative management of rectal cancer with complete clinical response after neoadjuvant therapy. Ann Surg. 2012;256:965-72.
22. Habr-Gama A, Perez RO, Nadalin W, et al. Operative versus nonoperative treatment for stage 0 distal rectal cancer following chemoradiation therapy: long-term results. Ann Surg. 2004;240:711-7.
23. Habr-Gava A, Perez RO, Proscurshim I, et al. Pattern of failure and survival for nonoperative treatment of stage c0 distal rectal cancer following neoadjuvant chemoradiation therapy. J Gastrointest Surg. 2006;10:1319-28.
24. Steele GD, Herndon JE, Bleday R, et al. Sphincter-sparing treatment for distal rectal adenocarcinoma. Ann Surg Oncol. 1999;6(5):433-41.
25. Scott N, Jackson P, al-Jaberi T, et al. Total mesorectal excision and local recurrence: a study of tumour spread in the mesorectum distal to rectal cancer. Br J Surg. 1995;82(8):1031-3.
26. Quirke P, Durdey P, Dixon MF, et al. Local recurrence of rectal adenocarcinoma due to inadequate surgical resection. Histopathologic study of lateral tumour spread and surgical excision. Lancet. 1986;2:996-9.
27. Adam IJ, Mohamdee MO, Martin IG, et al. Role of circumferential margin involvement in the local recurrence of rectal cancer. Lancet. 1994;344:707-11.
28. Nagtegaal ID, Quirke P. What is the role for the circumferential margin in modern treatment of rectal cancer? J Clin Oncol. 2008;26:303-12.

29. Birbeck KF, Macklin CP, Tiffin NJ, et al. Rates of circumferential resection margin involvement vary between surgeons and predict outcomes in rectal cancer surgery. Ann Surg. 2002;235:449-57.
30. Trakarnsanga A, Gonen M, Shia J, et al. What is the significance of the circumferential margin in locally advanced rectal cancer after neoadjuvant chemoradiotherapy? Ann Surg Oncol. 2013;20:1179-84.
31. Luca F, Valvo M, Ghezzi TL, et al. Impact of robotic surgery on sexual and urinary functions after fully robotic nerve-sparing total mesorectal excision for rectal cancer. Ann Surg. 2013;257:672-8.
32. Collinson R, Mortensen N. TEMS for tumours of the rectum. In: Johnson CD, Taylor I (Eds). Recent Advances in Surgery 31. London: Royal Society of Medicine Press; 2008. pp. 141-54.
33. Elias D, Liberale G, Vernerey D, et al. Hepatic and extrahepatic colorectal metastases: when resectable, their localization does not matter, but their total number has a prognostic effect. Ann Surg Oncol. 2005;12:900-9.
34. Poston GJ, Adam R, Alberts S, et al. OncoSurge: a strategy for improving resectability with curative intent in metastatic colorectal cancer. J Clin Oncol. 2005;23:7125-34.
35. Poston GJ. Standing on the shoulders of giants. Eur J Surg Oncol. 2008;34:253-5.
36. Figueras J, Valls C, Rafecas A, et al. Resection rate and effect of postoperative chemotherapy on survival after surgery for colorectal liver metastases. Br J Surg. 2001;88:980-5.
37. Choti MA, Sitzmann JV, Tiburi MF, et al. Trends in long-term survival following liver resection for hepatic colorectal metastases. Ann Surg. 2002;235:759-66.
38. Verwaal VJ, Bruin S, Boot H, et al. Eight-year follow-up of randomized trial: cytoreduction and hyperthermic intraperitoneal chemotherapy versus systemic chemotherapy in patients with peritoneal carcinomatosis of colorectal cancer. Ann Surg Oncol. 2008;15:2426-32.
39. Sugarbaker PH, Graves T, DeBruijn EA, et al. Early postoperative intraperitoneal chemotherapy as an adjuvant therapy to surgery for peritoneal carcinomatosis from gastrointestinal cancer: pharmacological studies. Cancer Res. 1990;50:5790-4.
40. Smeenk RM, Verwaal VJ, Zoetmulder FA. Learning curve of combined modality treatment in peritoneal surface disease. Br J Surg. 2007;94:1408-14.
41. Mohamed F, Moran BJ. Morbidity and mortality with cytoreductive surgery and intraperitoneal chemotherapy: the importance of a learning curve. Cancer J. 2009;15:196-9.
42. Votanopoulos KI, Swett K, Blackham AU, et al. Cytoreductive surgery with hyperthermic intraperitoneal chemotherapy in peritoneal carcinomatosis from rectal cancer. Ann Surg Oncol. 2013;20:1088-92.
43. Hill AR, McQuellon RP, Russell GB, et al. Survival and quality of life following cytoreductive surgery plus hyperthermic intraperitoneal chemotherapy for peritoneal carcinomatosis of colonic origin. Ann Surg Oncol. 2011;18:3673-9.
44. Franko J, Gusani NJ, Holtzman MP, et al. Multivisceral resection does not affect morbidity and survival after cytoreductive surgery and chemoperfusion for carcinomatosis from colorectal cancer. Ann Surg Oncol. 2008;15:3065-72.
45. Wagner PL, Austin F, Maduekwe U, et al. Extensive cytoreductive surgery for appendiceal carcinomatosis: morbidity, mortality, and survival. Ann Surg Oncol. 2013;20:1056-62.
46. Ribic CM, Sargent DJ, Moore MJ, et al. Tumor microsatellite-instability status as a predictor of benefit from fluorouracil-based adjuvant chemotherapy for colon cancer. N Engl J Med. 2003;349(3):247-57.
47. André T, Boni C, Mounedji-Boudiaf L, et al. Oxaliplatin, fluorouracil, and leucovorin as adjuvant treatment for colon cancer. N Engl J Med. 2004;350(23):2343-51.
48. Sargent DJ, Niedzwiecki D, O'Connell MJ, et al. Recommendation for caution with irinotecan, fluorouracil, and leucovorin for colorectal cancer. N Engl J Med. 2001;345(2):144-5.
49. Ychou M, Raoul J, Douillard JY, et al. A phase II randomised trial of LV5FU2 + irinotecan versus LV5FU2 alone in adjuvant high-risk colon cancer (FNCLCC Accord02/FFCD9802). Ann Oncol. 2009;20:674-80.
50. Van Cutsem E, Labianca R, Hossfeld D, et al. Randomized phase III trial comparing infused irinotecan/5-fluorouracil (5-FU)/folinic acid (IF) versus 5-FU/FA (F) in stage III colon cancer patients (PETACC 3). 2005 ASCO Annual Meeting Proceedings. J Clin Oncol. 2005;23:16s.
51. Karapetis CS, Khambata-Ford S, Jonker DJ, et al. K-ras mutations and benefit from cetuximab in advanced colorectal cancer. N Engl J Med. 2008;359(17):1757-65.
52. Saltz LB, Clarke S, Diaz-Rubio E, et al. Bevacizumab in combination with oxaliplatin-based chemotherapy as first-line therapy in metastatic colorectal cancer: a randomized phase III study. J Clin Oncol. 2008;26(12):2013-9.
53. Feig BW, Ching DC (Eds). The MD Anderson Surgical Oncology Handbook, 5th edition. Philadelphia, PA: Lippincott Williams and Wilkins; 2011.
54. Noffsinger A, Witte D, Fenoglio-Preiser CM. The relationship of human papillomaviruses to anorectal neoplasia. Cancer. 1992;70:1276-87.
55. Palefsky JM. Human papillomavirus-associated anogenital neoplasia and other solid tumors in human immunodeficiency virus-infected individuals. Curr Opin Oncol. 1991;3:881-5.
56. Law CL, Qassim M, Thompson CH, et al. Factors associated with clinical and sub-clinical anal human papillomavirus infection in homosexual men. Genitourin Med. 1991;67:92-8.
57. Puy-Montbrun T, Denis J, Ganansia R, et al. Anorectal lesions in human immunodeficiency virus-infected patients. Int J Colorectal Dis. 1992;7:26-30.
58. Lu DW, El-Mofty SK, Wang HL. Expression of p16, Rb, and p53 proteins in squamous cell carcinomas of the anorectal region harboring human papillomavirus DNA. Mod Pathol. 2003;16:692-9.

59. Samama B, Lipsker D, Boehm N. p16 expression in relation to human papillomavirus in anogenital lesions. Hum Pathol. 2006;37:513-9.
60. Strauss RJ, Fazio VW. Bowen's disease of the anal and perianal area. A report and analysis of twelve cases. Am J Surg. 1979;137:231-4.
61. Fenger C. Anal canal tumors and their precursors. Pathol Annu. 1988;23(Pt 1):45-66.
62. Dillard BM, Spratt JS, Ackerman LV, et al. Epidermoid cancer of anal margin and canal. Review of 79 cases. Arch Surg. 1963;16:772-7.
63. Gillespie JJ, MacKay B. Histogenesis of cloacogenic carcinoma. Fine structure of anal transitional epithelium and cloacogenic carcinoma. Hum Pathol. 1978;9:579-87.
64. Morson BC, Volkstädt H. Malignant melanoma of the anal canal. J Clin Pathol. 1963;16:126-32.
65. Klas JV, Rothenberger DA, Wong WD, et al. Malignant tumors of the anal canal: the spectrum of disease, treatment, and outcomes. Cancer. 1999;85:1686-93.
66. Winburn GB. Anal carcinoma or "just hemorrhoids"? Am Surg. 2001;67:1048-58.
67. Angeras U, Jönsson N, Jönsson PE. Primary anorectal malignant melanoma. J Surg Oncol. 1983;22:261-4.
68. Nigro ND, Vaitkevicius VK, Considine B. Combined therapy for cancer of the anal canal: a preliminary report. Dis Colon Rectum. 1974;17:354-6.

30 Pseudomyxoma Peritonei

Ratna Parikh, Praful Desai, Sarabjeet Kaur Arneja

INTRODUCTION

The first case of pseudomyxoma peritonei (PMP) was described by Rokitansky in 1842. However, the terminology was given by Werth in 1884; he associated it with a mucinous ovarian tumor. Frankel in 1901 co-related this term with the cyst of the appendix.[1] Pseudomyxoma peritonei is a rare condition with overall incidence of 1–2 per million per year. Seventy-five percent are women between the age of 45–75 years.[2] Long et al. reported a 45% five-year survival rate and a 40% ten-year survival rate.[3]

PATHOLOGY

Pseudomyxoma peritonei is a clinical term characterized by mucin in the abdominal or peritoneal cavity.[4] Epithelial tumor cells are identifiable microscopically within the abundant lakes of mucin, implying that mucinous deposits are not acellular purely mucinous material. Primary lesion in most cases is mucinous neoplasm of the appendix.[5] Grossly, the lesion is seen as multiple gelatinous nodules on peritoneal surfaces of intra-abdominal organs. Microscopically, the bulk of the lesion is composed of lakes of extracellular mucin accompanied by strips and nests of well-differentiated mucin-producing adenocarcinoma cells.[6] The implants are typically noninvasive, paucicellular and exhibit low-grade cytologic atypia. High-grade atypia or invasion indicates peritoneal carcinomatosis rather than pseudomyxoma peritonei (Figs 1A and B).[7]

Pseudomyxoma peritonei (jelly-belly) is a slow growing cancer which usually begins in the appendix. Occasionally the ovary, bowel or bladder may be the trigger sites. The tumor within the appendix produces a jelly-like substance, mucin. As a result the appendix swells up and the tumor breaks through the wall and tumor cells spread into the peritoneal cavity. These cells produce mucin or gelatinous substance which fills the peritoneal cavity.[8] Due to gravity, the pouch of Douglas, the right retrohepatic space and the left abdominal paracolic gutter fills with a mucoid tumor mass. Due to constant bowel mobility the mucinous lesions do not deposit on the bowel or its mesentery. Untreated the mucinous tumor will eventually compress vital structures. Pseudomyxoma peritonei does not spread by hematogenous or lymphatic pathways (Figs 2A to C).[9]

DIAGNOSIS

Pseudomyxoma peritonei lesions are usually difficult to diagnose and has a long latent period before it becomes symptomatic. Patients may present with vague abdominal or pelvic pain, distention, unexplained weight gain, change in bowel habits, infertility in women or symptoms of appendicitis. Computed tomography and/or MRI scan is usually adequate to make a diagnosis (Figs 3A and B). Tumor markers like carcinoembryonic antigen (CEA), CA 125 and CA 19-9 may be useful. Occasionally, PMP is detected on laparoscopy performed for infertility or during surgery for appendicitis.

TREATMENT

Cytoreductive Surgery and Hyperthermic Intraperitoneal Chemotherapy

Cytoreductive surgery involves removal of most of the visible lesions by peritonectomy (stripping of the involved peritoneum) and resection of involved organs

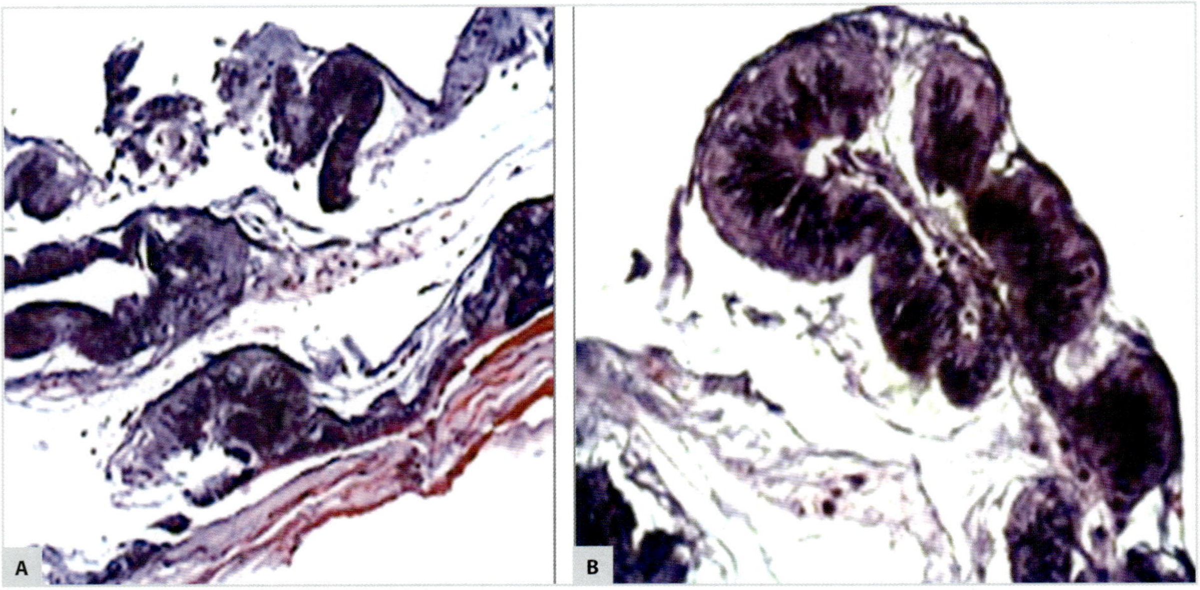

Figs 1A and B: (A) H&E staining, 20x magnification. Strips of well-differentiated mucinous neoplasm floating in large extracellular lakes of mucin; (B) H&E staining, 40x magnification. High-power view of the neoplastic epithelium. The cells exhibit low-grade nuclear atypia

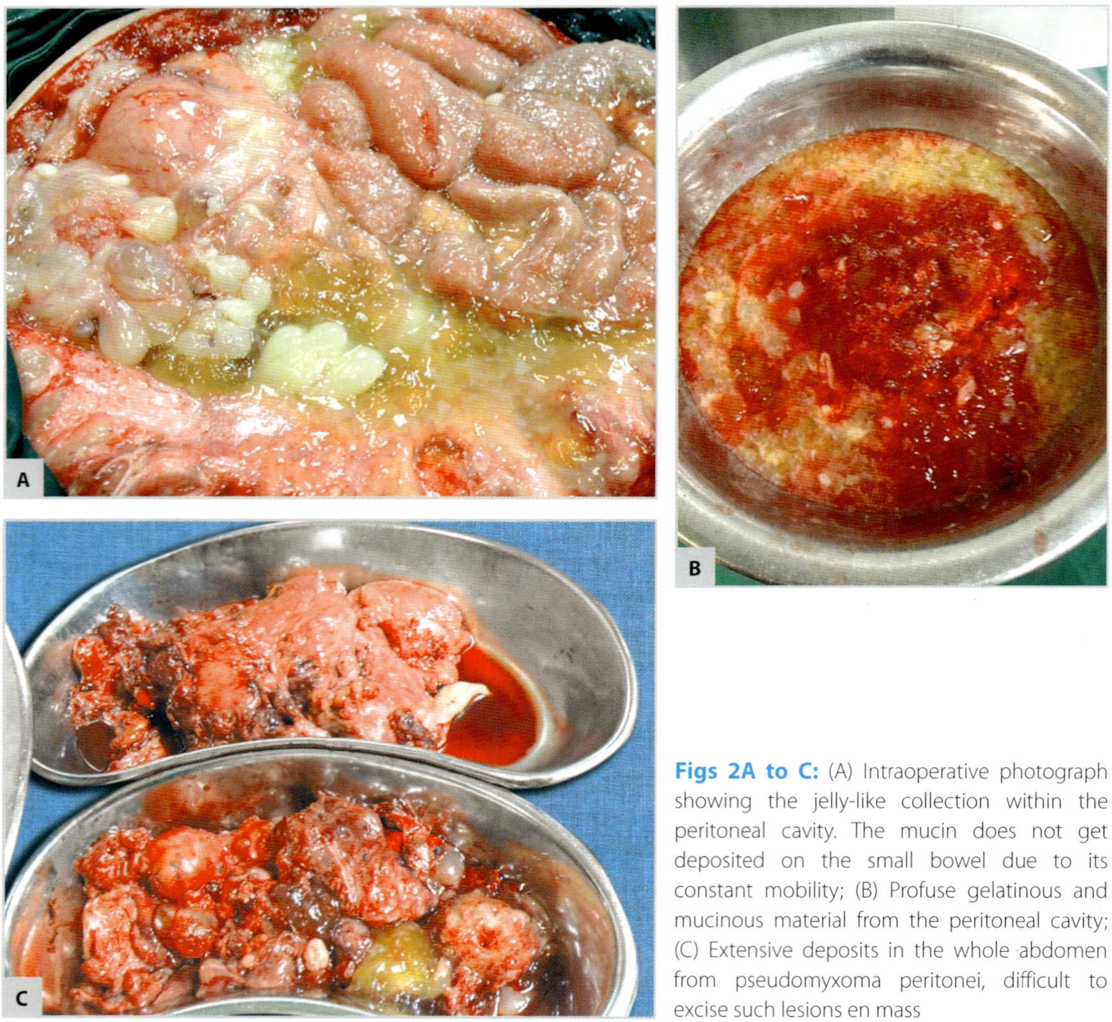

Figs 2A to C: (A) Intraoperative photograph showing the jelly-like collection within the peritoneal cavity. The mucin does not get deposited on the small bowel due to its constant mobility; (B) Profuse gelatinous and mucinous material from the peritoneal cavity; (C) Extensive deposits in the whole abdomen from pseudomyxoma peritonei, difficult to excise such lesions en mass

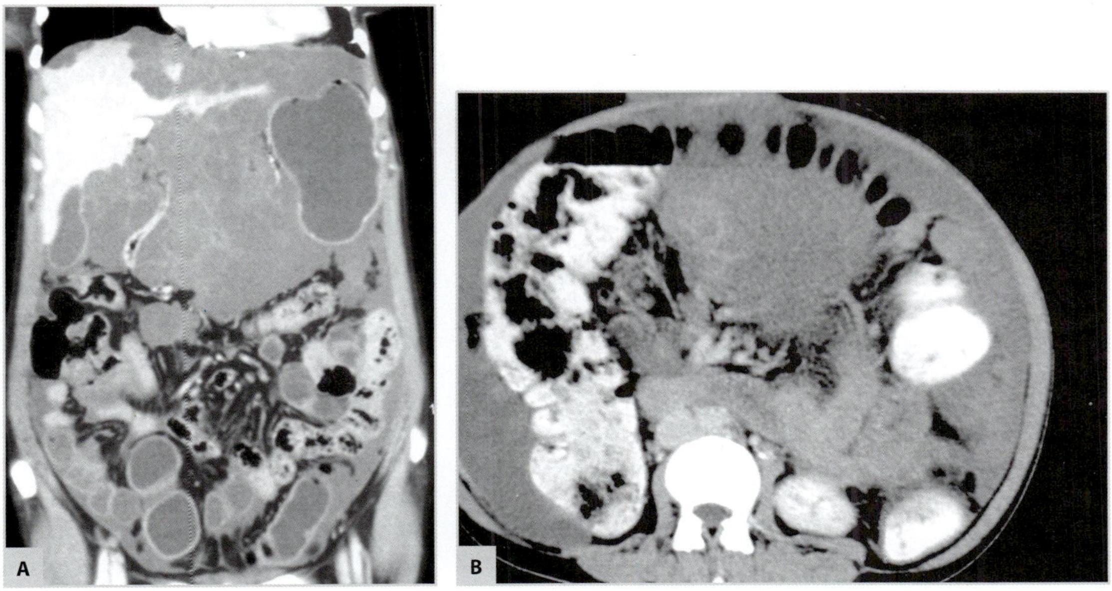

Figs 3A and B: (A) Computed tomography (CT) scan of a patient with pseudomyxoma peritonei showing tumor around the transverse colon; (B) Pseudomyxoma peritonei showing tumor infiltration in the transverse mesocolon

(stomach, small or large bowel, spleen, segments of liver, uterus and ovaries). Optimal treatment for mucinous cystadenocarcinoma involving the appendix is a right hemicolectomy with aggressive tumor debulking. Even after complete cytoreduction has been performed with no macroscopically visible tumor, microscopic tumor will always remain. Hence, hyperthermic intraperitoneal chemotherapy (HIPEC), which was described by Sugarbaker,[10-14] is effective in eradicating cancer with emboli with maximal diameter less than 2–3 mm. This is used in locally advanced cancers as an adjuvant treatment after cytoreductive surgery. The rationale for intraperitoneal chemotherapy is that after cytoreductive surgery the site of tumor (peritoneal cavity) receives sustained exposure to high concentrations of antitumor agents while the normal tissues (bone marrow) are spared. After cytoreduction, before the closure of the abdomen, intraperitoneal chemotherapy at high temperature (41–43°C) is instilled for 90 minutes. Supposedly, this destroys the residual tumor cells in the peritoneum. This entire procedure is time consuming (7–8 hours) with significant morbidities, with variable results and not routinely practised. It should be used only in tertiary centers with experience in the ambit of clinical research trials. At times debulking surgery is necessary to alleviate the patient's symptoms and make them more comfortable. Chances of recurrence are usually high and repeated surgeries may be needed.

Conservative Approach

A small lesion can be kept under observation as they are slow growing. Risks versus benefits of major debulking surgery should be carefully weighed. Close follow-up is necessary as recurrence is almost a rule.

CHEMOTHERAPY

Mitomycin C is used intraperitoneally during HIPEC. Sometimes, ports are inserted to instill perioperative intraperitoneal chemotherapy drugs (Mitomycin C or 5-fluorouracil), which are administered in multiple cycles.[15] Systemic chemotherapy can also be administered as an adjuvant therapy. Radiotherapy is ineffective as the lesion is radioresistant and widespread.

REFERENCES

1. Wikipedia Free Encyclopaedia—Pseudomyxoma peritonei
2. Sleisenger and Fordtran's Gastrointestinal and Liver Disease, ninth edition. Chapter 37—Surgical Peritonitis and other Diseases of the Peritoneum, Mesentery, Omentum and Diaphragm—Pg. 619.
3. Long RT, Spratt JS, Dowling E. Pseudomyxoma peritonei: new concepts in management with a report of 17 patients. Am J Surg. 1969;117(2):162-9.
4. Little JM, Halliday JP, Glenn DC. Pseudomyxoma peritonei. Lancet. 1969;2:659-63.
5. Young RH, Gilks CB, Scully RE. Mucinous tumors of the appendix associated with mucinous tumors of the ovary and pseudomyxoma peritonei: a clinicopathological analysis of 22 cases supporting an origin in the appendix. Am J Surg Pathol. 1991;15(5):415-29.
6. Pai RK, Longacre TA. Appendiceal mucinous tumors and pseudomyxoma peritonei: histologic features, diagnostic problems, and proposed classification. Adv Anat Pathol. 2005;12(6):291-311.
7. Ronnett BM, Zahn CM, Kurman RJ, et al. Disseminated peritoneal adenomucinosis and peritoneal mucinous carcinomatosis: a clinicopathologic analysis of 109 cases with emphasis on distinguishing pathologic features, site of origin, prognosis, and relationship to "pseudomyxoma peritonei." Am J Surg Pathol. 1995;19(12):1390-408.
8. Qu ZB, Liu LX. Management of pseudomyxoma peritonei. World J Gastroenterol. 2006;12(38):6124-7.
9. Sugarbaker Oncology Associates. Sugarbaker Oncology Associates Speciality Section for the Treatment of Pseudomyxoma Peritonei Syndrome. [online] Available from www.surgicaloncology.com [Accessed January, 2014].
10. Young RH. Pseudomyxoma peritonei and selected other aspects of the spread of appendiceal neoplasms. Semin Diagn Pathol. 2004;21(2):134-50.
11. Sugarbaker PH. New standard of care for appendiceal epithelial neoplasms and pseudomyxoma peritonei syndrome. Lancet Oncol. 2006;7(1):69-76.
12. Bryant J, Clegg AJ, Sidhu MK, et al. Systematic review of the Sugarbaker procedure for pseudomyxoma peritonei. Br J Surg. 2005;92(2):153-8.
13. Miner TJ, Shia J, Jaques DP, et al. Long-term survival following treatment of pseudomyxoma peritonei: an analysis of surgical therapy. Ann Surg. 2005;241(2):300-8.
14. Complete cytoreduction for pseudomyxoma peritonei (Sugarbaker technique): April 2004. National Institute for Health and Clinical Excellence (NICE).
15. Culliford AT, Brooks AD, Sharma S, et al. Surgical debulking and intraperitoneal chemotherapy for established peritoneal metastases from colon and appendix cancer. Ann Surg Oncol. 2001;8(10):787-95.

31 Gastrointestinal Stromal Tumors

Praful Desai, Keyuri Patel

INTRODUCTION

Gastrointestinal stromal tumors (GISTs) are very rare tumors arising in the gastrointestinal (GI) tract forming only 1–3%[1] of alimentary tract cancers, with a worldwide incidence of 10–15 million cases. They are unique in the sense that it provides a classic example of a highly effective translational research directly leading to effective targeted therapy. The gastrointestinal stromal tumor (GIST) histopathology and its biologic understanding has indeed added to the biological therapy armamentarium; possibly a portent of future targeted cancer therapies in our quest for control and cure of cancer. In the United States of America, around 4,000–5,000 cases are reported annually.[1] The stomach is the most common site forming nearly 65%, followed by small bowel (25%), colon and rectum (10%). Very rarely esophageal GIST has been reported.

PATHOLOGY

Though uncommon, GIST remains a classic example of translational research based on understanding of molecular pathogenesis of cancer therapy which targets main pathways of proliferation. In GIST, the nuances of molecular biology and histopathologic understanding have led to the first molecular based therapy by tyrosine kinase inhibitor Gleevac (imatinib mesylate). Gastrointestinal stromal tumor is a subset of leiomyosarcomas with unique histologic features and is a well-defined distinct clinical entity, arising in the mesenchymal tissues first so christened by Mazur and Clark in 1983. Modern immunohistochemical (IHC) techniques have greatly helped in our understanding of GIST.

Gastrointestinal stromal tumor is the most common mesenchymal tumor of GI tract. It occurs anywhere along GI tract (stomach: 60%, small intestine: 30%, rectum: 3%, colon: 1–2%, esophagus: < 1%, omentum/mesentery: Rare). Eighty-five percent of stromal tumors (GISTs), contain oncogenic mutations in one of the two receptor tyrosine kinases—KIT or platelet-derived growth factor receptor alpha (PDGFRA). Activation of either of these plays a central role in pathogenesis of GIST. Most tumors (85–90%) express c-kit. Five percent tumors do not express c-kit, but exhibit mutations in PDGFRA and are more likely to have epithelioid morphology. Five to ten percent of tumors are negative for both mutations. Correct identification of GIST is very important because of availability of specific molecular targeted therapy with KIT/PDGFRA tyrosine kinase inhibitors such as imatinib mesylate. Generally tumors that are c-kit (CD 117) positive by immunohistochemistry will respond to imatinib.

Gross

Circumscribed nodular tumors ranging in size from less than 1 cm to more than 40 cm, forming subserosal, intramural or polypoid intraluminal masses. Cut surface is solid and pinkish white. It may show areas of hemorrhage, necrosis or cystic change. Biologic behavior cannot be predicted based on gross examination findings.

Microscopy

Varied morphology is seen. Spindle cell type (70%) (Fig. 1), epithelioid type (20%) (Fig. 2) and mixed (10%). Epithelioid type is more common in stomach and omentum.

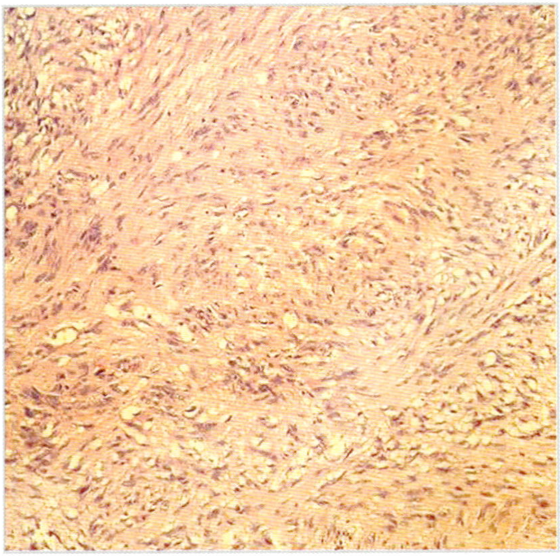

Fig. 1: Spindle cell type

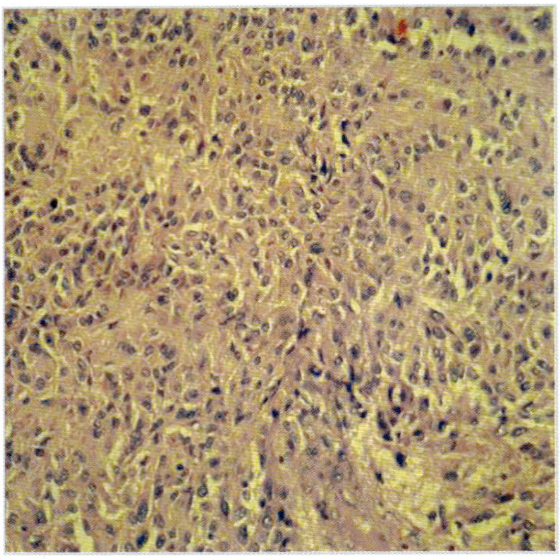

Fig. 2: Epithelioid type

TABLE 1: Guidelines for relative risk of malignant behavior

Tumor Parameters		*Risk of Progressive Disease (Percent)*			
Mitotic Index	*Size (cm)*	*Stomach*	*Duodenum*	*Jejunum/Ileum*	*Rectum*
≤ 5/50 hpf	≤ 2	None (0)	None (0)	None (0)	None (0)
	> 2 but ≤ 5	Very low (1.9)	Low (8.3)	Low (4.3)	Low (8.5)
	> 5 but ≤ 10	Low (3.6)	Insufficient data	Moderate (24)	Insufficient data
	> 10	Moderate (10)	High (34)	High (52)	High (57)
> 5/50 hpf	≤ 2	None	Insufficient data	High	High (54)
	> 2 but ≤ 5	Moderate (16)	High (50)	High (73)	High (52)
	> 5 but ≤ 10	High (55)	Insufficient data	High (85)	Insufficient data
	> 10	High (86)	High (86)	High (90)	High (71)

Source: Adapted from Reference 3

Immunohistochemistry

Ninety-five percent of tumors express CD117, Bcl2: 80%, CD34: 60%, SMA: 30%, S-100 protein: 10% and desmin: 5%. After treatment with imatinib, GISTs undergo regressive changes with areas of necrosis, old hemorrhage and dense hyalinization.

Biologic Behavior

The neoplasms exhibit a broad spectrum of biologic behavior with a potential for aggressive biologic behavior. Risk stratification is based on size, mitotic rate and location. Asymptomatic incidentally detected GISTs almost always behave in a benign fashion.[2] The following guidelines provide relative risk of malignant behavior (Table 1).[3]

Long-term follow-up of malignant GISTs is necessary as recurrences and metastasis can develop over a long period of time, sometimes years later.[2]

CLINICAL

Majority of lesions are asymptomatic to begin with resulting in late presentation with either an abdominal mass, symptoms resulting therefrom like abdominal pain, vomiting (if obstructive) and very rarely bleeding (hematemesis or melena). Incidental findings on imaging the abdomen for other causes may also define a GIST. Very rarely a large tumor may perforate and may bleed intraperitoneally with an acute abdomen. Majority of these mesenchymal tumors grow in an exophytic manner and

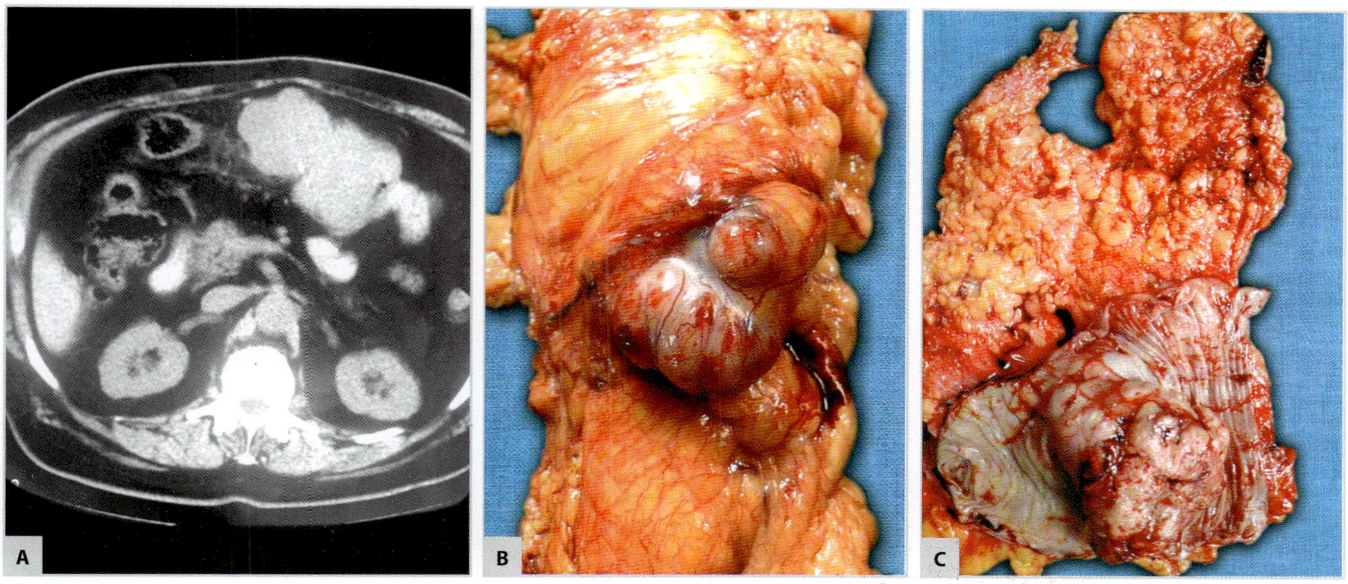

Figs 3A to C: (A) Computed tomography (CT) scan of a patient with extreme emaciation showing lesion in the transverse colon. Fine-needle aspiration cytology (FNAC) revealed a gastrointestinal stromal tumor (GIST); (B) Operative specimen; (C) Specimen opened to see the mucosal extent of the lesion

may involve adjacent organs (stomach to colon or to liver). Involvement of the omentum is uncommon and peritoneal deposits are disseminated or multicentric nodules rather than lymphatic nodal spread. Retroperitoneal sarcoma and leiomyosarcomas are the main differential diagnosis.

INVESTIGATIONS

Imaging by a computed tomography (CT) scan is the major diagnostic tool and relevant endoscopic evaluations will be helpful. Endoscopic biopsy may be negative because of its exophytic nature. Endoscopic ultrasound, fine-needle aspiration cytology (FNAC), may be helpful for a cytologic diagnosis. Routine investigations will include routine liver and kidney profiles, routine urine and stool examination and other relevant studies as indicated in a given patient. C-kit estimations are important—either pretherapy or after surgical excision (Figs 3A to C).

MANAGEMENT

The therapy of choice is a surgical excision of the lesion which may necessitate resection of infiltrated surrounding organs like colon, stomach, small bowel, omentum and rarely pancreas (body or tail) as needed depending on a given clinical setting. Very large lesions, which may appear nonresectable, neoadjuvant[4] therapy after c-kit studies with Gleevac (Imatinib) is indicated in the doses of 400–600 mg daily for 4–6 months and assessing the response by imaging. Tumors do shrink and resection is thereafter feasible. This is particularly significant when organs like pancreas are infiltrated to be able to salvage them after size reduction due to neoadjuvant therapy. Adjuvant Gleevac[5] is standard therapy which should last for a long time (1–2 years). Overall complete responses with Gleevac reported are about 5% and partial responses in about 60% of cases. The alternative therapy in nonresponsive resistant cases is Sutent,[6] another tyrosine kinase inhibitor which may show marginal to moderate response, a little less than Gleevac (Figs 4A to E).

The larger the lesions (it can assume a large size filling more than half of the abdominal cavity) the greater are the chances of recurrence. Most series in long follow-ups report recurrence up to 65–70%.[7] A 2–3 cm margin should be aimed at surgical excision and adjuvant chemotherapy (Gleevac) after c-kit positivity. The dose of Gleevac is usually (400–600 mg) administered for at least 2 years or more.

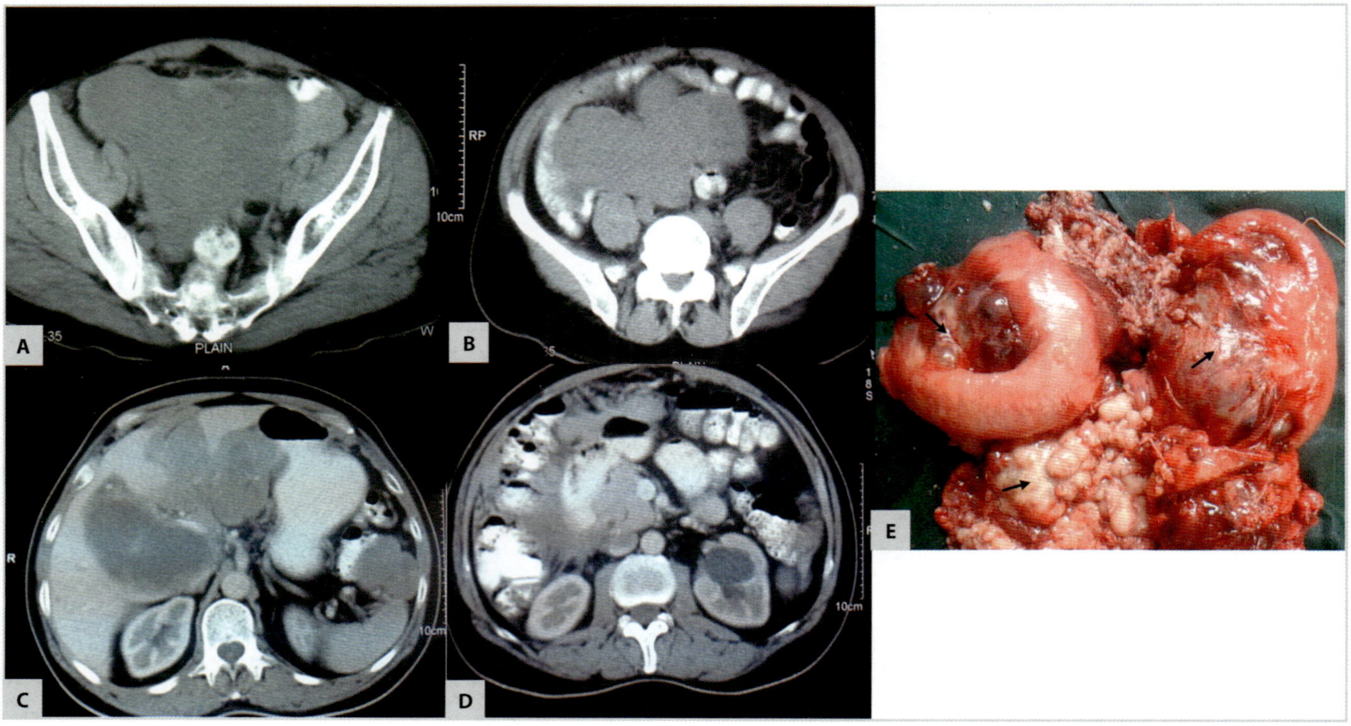

Figs 4A to E: A large pelvic and abdominal GIST in a male (51 years) widely excised (2009) (A, B). Good control on Gleevac for 4½ years. Large recurrence in abdomen 4½ years later with bowel entrapment and large masses straddling but not infiltrating the liver surface (C, D). Extensive surgical debulking which required resection of two segments of the small bowel (2014). The operative specimen shows recurrent GIST infiltrating the bowel mesentery (E). The nodules are individual small GIST lesions and not lymph nodes or omentum. Uneventful recovery and patient now on adjuvant Sorafenib, further reasonable remission can be expected

REFERENCES

1. Cassier PA, Ducimetière F, Lurkin A, et al. A prospective epidemiological study of new incident GISTs during two consecutive years in Rhône Alpes region: incidence and molecular distribution of GIST in a European region. Br J Cancer. 2010:103(2)165-70.
2. Miettinen M, El-Rifai W, Sobin LH, et al. Evaluation of malignancy and prognosis of gastrointestinal stromal tumors: a review. Hum Pathol. 2002;33(5):478-83.
3. Rubin BP, Blanke CD, Demetri GD, et al. Protocol for the examination of specimens from patients with gastrointestinal stromal tumor. Arch Pathol Lab Med. 2010;134 (2):165-70.
4. Dematteo RP, Ballman KV, et al. Adjuvant and Neo-adjuvant imatinib after resection of localised primary GIST. Lancet. 2720(9688):1058-60.
5. Demetri GD, von Mehren M, Blanke CD, et al. Efficacy and safety of imatinib mesylate in advanced gastrointestinal stromal tumors. N Engl J Med. 2002;347(7):472-80.
6. Demetri GD, van Oosterom AT, Garrett CR, et al. Efficacy and safety of sunitinib in patients with advanced gastrointestinal stromal tumour after failure of imatinib: a randomised controlled trial. Lancet. 2006;368(9544):1329-38.
7. Eisenberg BL, Harris J, Blanke CD, et al. Phase II trial of neoadjuvant/adjuvant imatinib mesylate (IM) for advanced primary and metastatic/recurrent operable gastrointestinal stromal tumor (GIST): early results of RTOG 0132/ACRIN 6665. J Surg Oncol. 2009;99(1):42-7.

32 Hepatic Malignancies

Deepak Chhabra, Palepu Jagannath

INTRODUCTION

Liver cancer in men is the fifth most frequently diagnosed cancer worldwide; however, it is the second most frequent cause of cancer death. In women, it is the seventh most commonly diagnosed cancer and the sixth leading cause of cancer death.[1] A variety of primary malignant tumors arise in the liver. These may be of the epithelial or nonepithelial type (Table 1).

The most frequent and important hepatic neoplasm is the primary hepatocellular carcinoma (HCC). HCC, a primary malignancy of the hepatocyte, represents the major histological subtype, accounting for 70–85% of the total liver cancer burden worldwide. Cholangiocarcinomas arise primarily from the epithelial lining of the bile ducts (intra- and extrahepatic) and occur with much less frequency than HCC. Angiosarcoma, lymphoma and primary neuroendocrine tumors are rare primary liver tumors. Hepatoblastomas are found exclusively in children below the age of 5 years and these rare tumors are not discussed in this chapter.

HEPATOCELLULAR CARCINOMA

Introduction

High incidence rates of HCC (120 cases per 100,000)[2] in parts of Asia and sub-Saharan Africa largely reflect the increased prevalence of chronic hepatitis B virus (HBV) infection, with over 8% of the populations in these regions chronically infected with the virus.[3] HBV infection accounts for about 60% and 23% of HCCs in developing and developed countries respectively, while corresponding percentages for hepatitis C virus (HCV) infection are 33% and 20% respectively.[4] Interaction of aflatoxin B1 (AFB1) exposure with chronic HBV infection has been noted to increase liver cancers. However, the contribution of AFB1 exposure to the liver cancer burden in parts of Africa and Asia, where the exposure is prevalent, is unknown. In the United States and several other low-risk Western countries, alcohol-related cirrhosis and possibly nonalcoholic fatty liver disease (NAFLD), associated with obesity, are thought to account for the majority of HCC. With respect to Asian population, the Asian Pacific Association for the Study of

TABLE 1: Classification of malignant liver tumors

Epithelial tumors	*Nonepithelial tumors*
Hepatocellular carcinoma (liver cell carcinoma)	Epithelioid hemangioendothelioma
Intrahepatic cholangiocarcinoma (peripheral bile duct carcinoma)	Angiosarcoma
Bile duct cystadenocarcinoma	Embryonal sarcoma (undifferentiated sarcoma)
Combined hepatocellular and cholangiocarcinoma	Rhabdomyosarcoma
Hepatoblastoma	
Undifferentiated carcinoma	

the Liver (APASL) guidelines[5] outlined the following risk factors:

- Patients with cirrhosis due to HBV or HCV are at the highest risk for HCC
- The incidence of HCC is significantly higher in those who were hepatitis B e-antigen (HBeAg) positive or have HBV DNA with high loads (> 10 copies/mL) and older than 40 years
- Male sex, aging and familial history are independent risk factors for HCC
- Chronic and heavy alcohol intake, high body mass index (BMI > 25) and diabetes mellitus leading to liver disease increases the risk for HCC.

Natural History of Hepatocellular Carcinoma

Hepatocellular carcinoma generally leads to death within 6–20 months. These tumors frequently arise in the setting of cirrhosis, appearing 20–30 years following the initial insult to the liver.[6] Infection with HBV can clearly lead to HCC without the intermediate step of cirrhosis, although majority of patients with HBV-related HCC have cirrhotic disease. Conversely, HCV-related HCC almost always arises in the setting of advanced fibrosis or cirrhosis, though a direct hepatocarcinogenic role of HCV has not been clearly proven. However, 25% of patients have no history or risk factors for the development of cirrhosis. The extent of hepatic dysfunction limits treatment options, as many patients die of liver failure as from tumor progression.

Carcinogenesis in patients with cirrhosis is a stepwise process that begins with the development of dysplastic nodules (DNs). These nodules are evident on gross examination of the liver as distinct lesions more than 1 mm in size that differ from the surrounding hepatic parenchyma in terms of size, color, texture or degree of bulging at the cut surface. DNs are classified as low-grade or high-grade on the basis of cytological and architectural atypia on microscopic examination. Over a 2-year follow-up period, about one-third of high-grade DN will progress to HCC and at 5 years the risk of HCC increases to 81%.[7] The distinction between high-grade DN and very early HCC can be difficult, and different pathologists might classify the same lesion differently. Identification of stromal invasion is the key to identify this transition.[8] Early HCC (i.e. 2 cm in diameter or smaller) is typically nodular and well-differentiated. As disease progression occurs, microscopic vascular invasion begins, leading to intrahepatic invasion and ultimately to systemic dissemination, typically as the tumor reaches a diameter of around 3 cm.[9] With further progression, the tumor can extend into larger hepatic vessels, most commonly portal, but also hepatic veins. Once this occurs, curative treatment is rarely possible.

Pretherapy Work-up and Investigation

Biochemistry

Simple tests such as a complete blood count and liver function tests are robust baseline tests for an overall evaluation of the liver status. A low platelet count can be an indicator of underlying cirrhosis. Aspartate aminotransferase (AST), formerly serum glutamic-oxaloacetic transaminase (SGOT) and alanine aminotransferase (ALT), formerly serum glutamate-pyruvate transaminase (SGPT) levels tend to be higher in cirrhotic patients with continuing inflammation or necrosis than in those without continuing liver injury. Serum albumin level is an index of liver synthetic capacity and a reversal of albumin to globulin ratio (A:G) is a strong indicator of compromised synthetic capacity of the liver. The liver synthesizes blood clotting factors II, V, VII, IX and X. The prothrombin time (PT) does not become abnormal until more than 80% of liver synthetic capacity is lost. Thus an abnormal PT prolongation may be a sign of serious liver dysfunction. The liver function tests form an integral component of the Child-Pugh classification (Table 2) for grading the severity of liver dysfunction.

TABLE 2: Modified Child-Pugh classification

Parameter	*Points assigned*		
	1	*2*	*3*
Ascites	Absent	Slight	Moderate
Bilirubin (mg/dL)	< 2	2–3	> 3
Albumin (g/dL)	> 3.5	2.8–3.5	< 2.8
Prothrombin time			
Seconds over control	1–3	4–6	> 6
INR	< 1.7	1.8–2.3	> 2.3
Encephalopathy	None	Grade 1–2	Grade 3–4

Abbreviation: INR, international normalized ratio

Modified Child-Pugh classification of the severity of liver disease according to the degree of ascites, plasma concentrations of bilirubin and albumin, PT and the degree of encephalopathy. A total score of 5–6 is considered grade A (well-compensated disease); 7–9 is grade B (significant functional compromise); and 10–15 is grade C (decompensated disease). These grades correlate with 1 and 2-year survival; grade A: 100% and 65%; grade B: 80% and 60%; and grade C: 45% and 35%.

Tumor Markers

Serum alpha-fetoprotein (AFP) is the most commonly used serum biomarker in conjunction with ultrasound in screening programs. AFP is elevated in 60–70% of patients with HCC, but has low sensitivity (45%).[10] Normally, levels of AFP are below 10 ng/mL, but marginal elevations are common in patients with chronic hepatitis or cirrhosis. However, all patients with elevated AFP should be screened for HCC with imaging, especially if there has been an increasing trend from baseline level. AFP has to be significantly elevated (400 ng/mL) to be of any value as a screening tool. It is also usually not elevated in patients with small HCCs. Analysis of recent studies shows that AFP determination lacks adequate sensitivity and specificity for effective surveillance and diagnosis.[11]

Des-gamma-carboxy prothrombin (DCP) has been used widely in Japan for HCC diagnosis and surveillance. DCP is an abnormal prothrombin molecule that is generated as a result of an acquired defect in the posttranslational carboxylation of the prothrombin precursor in malignant cells; this prothrombin defect in malignant cells is similar to the deficit in vitamin K deficiency and has been called prothrombin induced by vitamin K absence (PIVKA). Experience with DCP in western countries, and in India particularly, is limited.

Radiological Imaging

Ultrasound (US) is usually the first-line investigation within a surveillance plan or within the standard evaluation of patients with suspected or known liver disease. Upon US detection of a hepatic nodule, the next step is to characterize the nodule and establish its diagnosis. Dynamic imaging [contrast-enhanced computed tomography (CECT) and magnetic resonance imaging (MRI)] with gadolinium injection, with follow-up computed tomography (CT) usually allows a confident diagnosis to be made. High resolution triple-phase CT scan (CT in non-contrast, hepatic-arterial, portal-venous and delayed phases) is a mandatory investigation. Similarly, if MRI is used, pre-contrast, arterial, venous and delayed phases are essential.

Consensus guidelines have been drafted by several large international working groups on different occasions in an attempt to standardize the diagnosis and management of HCC. The major working groups included the European Association for the Study of the Liver (EASL), the American Association for Study of Liver Diseases (AASLD) and the APASL.

The "classical imaging features" generally considered to be highly specific for the diagnosis of HCC are the presence of arterial hypervascularity and washout (Fig. 1).[12] In particular, this enables differentiation from intrahepatic cholangiocarcinoma, which shows delayed enhancement. Despite the abundant use of multidetector row technology, CT may underestimate the extent of disease in around 50%

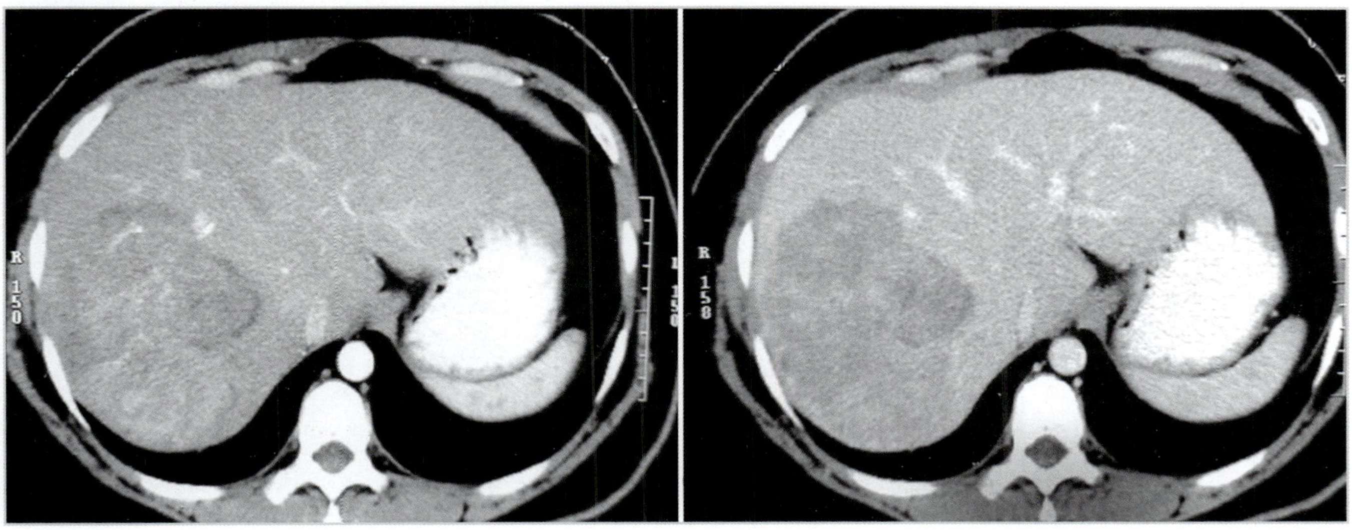

Fig. 1: A classical feature of hepatocellular carcinoma (HCC) with arterial enhancement and washout

of cases.[13] Although it has been established that MRI is superior in the detection of HCCs, particularly the lesions smaller than 2 cm in size,[14,15] neither the APASL nor the AASLD recommends the use of MRI over CT for staging of disease. In the study by Pitton et al., direct comparison between MRI and 64-row CT, MRI was significantly more sensitive in detecting tumor nodules.[16] In the presence of atypical findings from a single imaging test (CT or MRI), the AASLD recommends a different imaging modality (CT or MRI) for further assessment. However, if atypical findings are again demonstrated, biopsy is recommended. Biopsy restores the specificity of imaging to 100% where any of the findings are atypical.[17] A contrast-enhanced ultrasound (CEUS) is not considered to be specific enough (besides the fact that the CEUS agents are not commercially available) and is excluded from the revised AASLD guidelines.

Diffusion Weighted MRI studies the random motion of water molecules and shows promise for detection and characterization as well as post (local and ablative) treatment assessment of tumors.[18] It improves MR detection of HCCs, particularly in lesions smaller than 2 cm,[19] with sensitivities of 84–98% compared to 76–85% for multiphasic MRI alone.[20] Its role in the diagnostic algorithm is not certain at this point, although, given the promising results and its ease of implementation in routine clinical practice incorporation into future guidelines is anticipated. F-18 fluorodeoxyglucose (FDG) PET has low sensitivity (50–68%) for intrahepatic HCC[21] and is, therefore, not considered to be useful for diagnosis of HCC.

To Biopsy or Not to Biopsy

The role of hepatic fine-needle aspiration (FNA) biopsy has been debated. Advances in imaging modalities have obviated the need for tissue confirmation in most HCCs. Moreover, there is risk of needle-tract seeding. Diagnostic challenges associated with cirrhosis include distinction of benign hepatocellular nodules (regenerative nodules and dysplastic nodules) from reactive hepatocytes; and distinction of well-differentiated HCCs from benign hepatocellular nodules.

Nodules larger than 2 cm occurring in cirrhotic livers are diagnosed as HCC if they show characteristic intense arterial profile with contrast washout in delayed venous phase on one dynamic imaging modality. Nodules measuring between 1 and 2 cm in cirrhotic livers require concurrence of two coincidental imaging modalities; otherwise, biopsy is recommended. The dilemma is whether to biopsy nodules less than 1 cm. The EASL guidelines recommend the "wait and see" policy with 3-monthly ultrasound surveillance. However, this view is not easily accepted. According to Caturelli et al., the prognostic implications of early diagnosis and treatment of HCC cannot justify this policy of "masterly inactivity".[22] Firstly, it is incongruous to work on increasing detection of small nodules in high-risk patients and then recommend "masterly inactivity". Secondly, more than half of the nodules less than 1 cm in cirrhotic livers prove to be HCCs (68%). Thirdly, US-guided FNA biopsies of hepatic nodules less than 1 cm in experienced hands with the use of novel biomarkers and interpreted by an expert reader yield correct diagnoses in about 90% of cases.[23]

Whilst some studies have shown that preoperative FNA has no statistically adverse effect on the operability, possibility of tumor spread, or long-term survival of HCC patients,[24] there are others who strongly maintain that pretransplant FNA diagnosis of HCC is not necessary.[25] There is, however, no clear evidence that independent of tumor stage, patients who undergo FNA biopsy are at higher risk of tumor recurrence and post-transplantation recurrence due to biopsy-induced hematogenous dissemination of tumor cells.[26,27]

Details of cytological features of HCV vary with tumor differentiation and are beyond the scope of this chapter. The commonly found moderately differentiated HCC typically shows broad tongues of cohesive malignant hepatocytes wrapped by peripheral endothelium (Fig. 2).

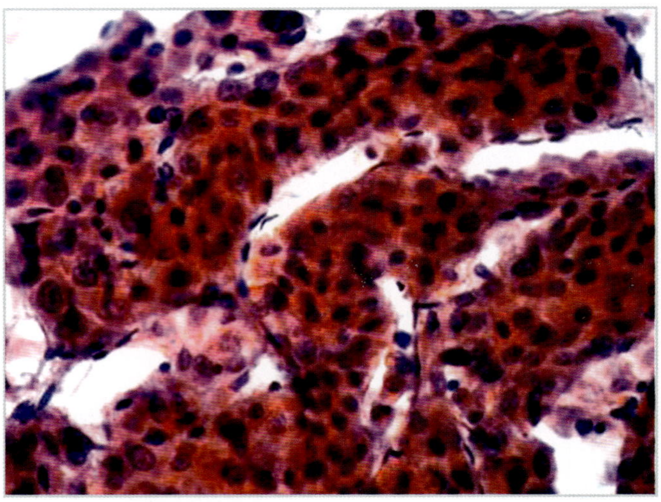

Fig. 2: Fine-needle aspiration (FNA) of moderately differentiated hepatocellular carcinoma. Broad tongues of cohesive malignant hepatocytes wrapped by peripheral endothelium (Papanicolaou, ×400)

Staging

A staging system for HCC poses problems because the presence of liver disease and tumor varies due to the different epidemiological backgrounds and risk factors. An ideal staging system needs to include prognostic information regarding both the cancer and liver functional status and take account of clinical factors that influence response to treatment. The tumor-node-metastasis (TNM) classification does not take into account the liver functional status. The Okuda staging system uses four criteria of: (1) ascites; (2) albumin; (3) bilirubin; and (4) tumor size to assess liver functional status and tumor stage. It is a good system for stratifying advanced or symptomatic disease, but less useful in early stage to guide treatment choices. Other available systems are the French classification, the Cancer of the Liver Italian Program (CLIP) classification, the Barcelona-Clinic Liver Cancer (BCLC) staging system, the Chinese University Prognostic Index (CUPI score) and the Japan Integrated Staging (JIS) or biomarker combined JIS (bm-JIS) if biomarkers are included.[28] The BCLC is emerging as the standard staging system for HCC in the West and has been externally validated. The BCLC classification incorporates not only the prognostic variables related to tumor (size, number, vascular invasion, N1 and M1), liver function (Child-Pugh) and health status [Eastern Cooperative Oncology Group Performance Status (ECOG)], but also incorporates variables that influence therapy such as bilirubin, portal hypertension and presence of symptoms to assist in treatment decision-making (Flow chart 1).

The BCLC classification has been endorsed by an EASL panel of experts and the AASLD guidelines.[29,30] Practises in Asia, particularly in Japan, are somewhat different, and the recently published APASL recommendations[5] on HCC mirror current clinical practice in Asian countries (Flow chart 2).

SURGICAL TREATMENT OF HEPATOCELLULAR CARCINOMA

Hepatocellular carcinoma has proven to be a difficult target for systemic therapies. The mainstays of treatment are, thus, physical treatments that in one way or another directly attack the tumor or its blood supply. The additional challenge posed by the fact that most cases of HCC develop in the setting of cirrhosis with impaired liver function, makes the selection of treatment a challenge in itself. In the absence of treatment, the overall 5-year survival is less than 10%.

Surgical resection and liver transplantation are the only chances of cure but have limited applicability.

Flow chart 1: The Barcelona-Clinic Liver Cancer staging and treatment schedule

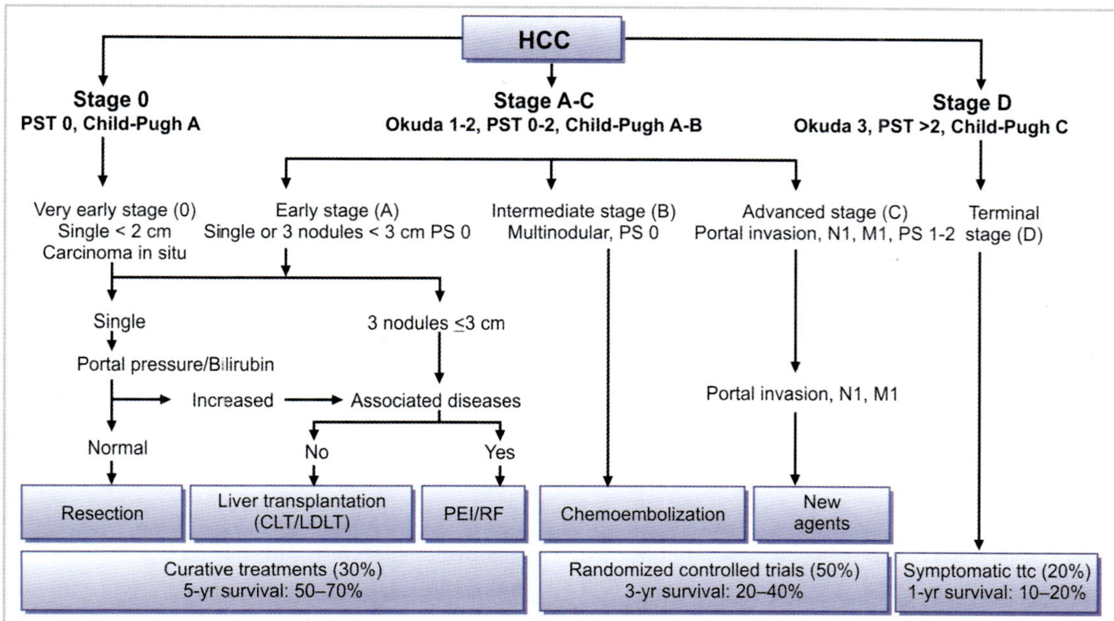

Abbreviations: HCC, hepatocellular carcinoma; PST, performance status test; CLT, cadaveric liver transplant; LDLT, live donor liver transplant; PEI, percutaneous ethanol injection; RF, radiofrequency ablation

Flow chart 2: The Asia-Pacific Association for the Study of the Liver (APASL) treatment algorithm of hepatocellular carcinoma (HCC)

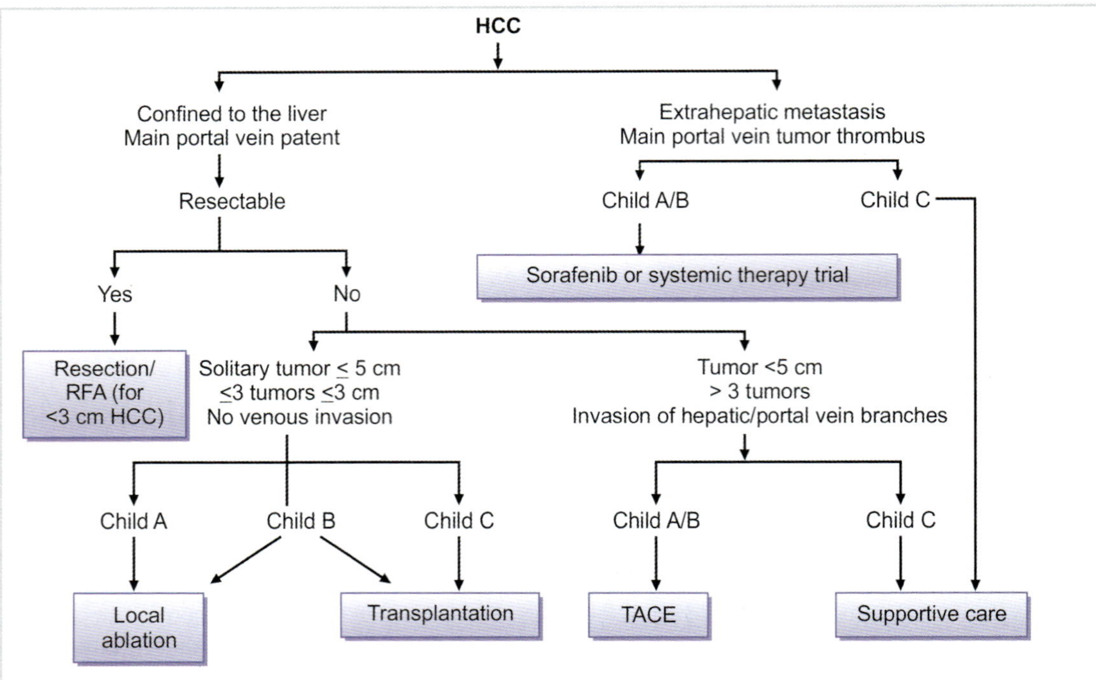

Abbreviation: TACE, transarterial chemoembolization

Liver Resection

In the minority of patients with HCC, who do not have cirrhosis, resection is the treatment of choice. Major hepatic resections involving removal of at least one hemiliver (Figs 3 and 4) are now reported to carry an operative mortality of less than 10% in cirrhotic patients. While some cirrhotic patients with HCC are also best treated with resection, the decision in these cases is not straightforward. A preoperative assessment of liver function and prediction of postoperative residual functional liver remnant are of paramount importance to minimize the surgical risk. Preoperative laparoscopic inspection aids in diagnosing both the tumor and extent of cirrhosis. Cirrhosis limits resectability and especially in the setting of HCV cirrhosis, 75–80% of patients experience tumor recurrence within 5 years of resection.[31] Many tests of liver function (e.g. indocyanine green clearance) have been used to judge resectability, but none has proved more useful than the Child-Pugh classification. Portal hypertension seems to be an independent factor in determining postresection outcome; patients with Child-Pugh class A cirrhosis and minimal portal hypertension (e.g. platelet count > 100,000/ mm^3 and/or hepatic venous pressure gradient < 10 mm Hg)[32] are optimum resection candidates.

Model for End-Stage Liver Disease (MELD) is a prospectively developed and validated chronic liver disease severity scoring system that uses a patient's laboratory values for serum bilirubin, serum creatinine and the international normalized ratio (INR) for PT to predict survival. In patients with chronic liver disease, an increasing MELD score is associated with increasing severity of hepatic dysfunction and 3-month mortality risk. It has been evaluated principally for selecting patients for liver transplantation. Use of this model for predicting surgical risk in the nontransplant setting has been promising and, thus, it may possibly replace the Child's classification as the principal method for determining surgical risk in future.

Surgical Principles for Hepatic Resection

- In general, even for patients with well-compensated Child's grade A cirrhosis, one should try to limit resections to less than two segments of functional liver
- Major hepatic resections should be restricted to those who have large tumors replacing most of one hemiliver with an acceptable liver function, and no atrophy of the uninvolved hemiliver

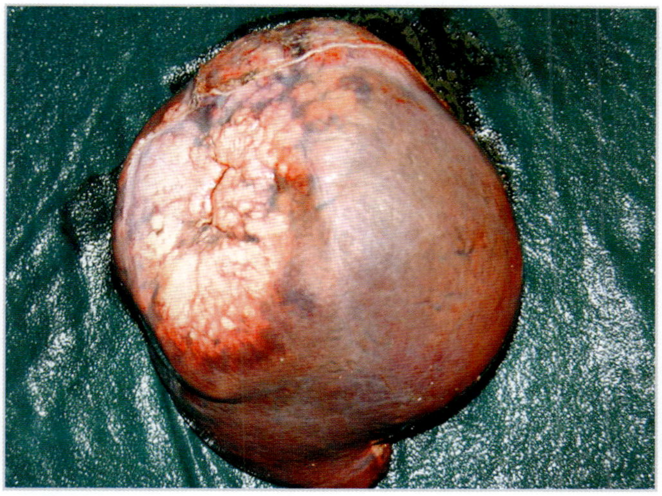

Fig. 3: Specimen of a right hepatic resection for hepatocellular carcinoma (HCC)

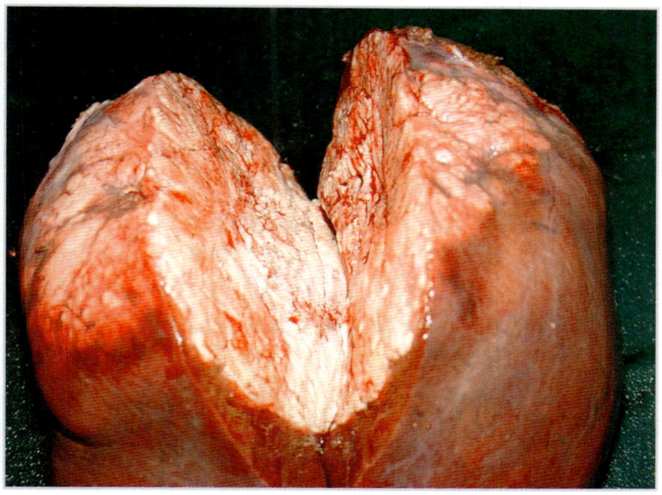

Fig. 4: Nodular pattern of hepatocellular carcinoma on gross examination

- Small tumors are often more difficult to manage. For patients with small, deeply placed tumors, whose resection would necessitate removal of a large amount of functional parenchyma, an ablative alternative might be more suitable
- Involvement of adjacent organs by HCC is no longer considered a contraindication to resectional surgery with curative intent and en bloc resection of the tumor with the adjacent organ should be attempted
- Tumor size is not relevant to resectability, but an unfavorable location may deem a tumor unresectable. By and large, patients, who have circumscribed single tumors, are potentially resectable, regardless of tumor size
- Preoperative portal vein embolization can be employed to increase future remnant liver volume to allow more extensive resections to be undertaken, but the complication rate in cirrhosis is 10–20% and its effectiveness in this patient group is not fully established
- A laparoscopic approach to resection in cirrhosis has been proposed by some to reduce the operative insult and the risk of decompensation.

Operative Technique Modifications for Hepatic Resection in Cirrhotic Patients

The guiding principle for hepatectomy in cirrhotic patients is that limited resections should be favored with as much functional parenchyma spared as possible. Certain modifications in the operative technique and the postoperative care can result in favorable outcomes.

Exposure and mobilization

Trifurcated incisions and thoracoabdominal incisions should be avoided in cirrhotic patients because of the potential for ascitic leakage externally or into the chest. The increased firmness of the cirrhotic liver and the consequent difficulty of retraction can lead to significant blood loss from retroperitoneal or phrenic collateral vessels during mobilization. To prevent such bleeding, it may be preferable to use an anterior approach in which the liver parenchyma is split within the principal scissura down to the anterior surface of the vena cava before the right hemiliver is mobilized off the retroperitoneum. The right hemiliver is then mobilized in a medial-to-lateral direction, and the right hepatic vein is secured during mobilization of the right hemiliver off the vena cava.

Inflow control

At one time, it was widely doubted whether the Pringle's maneuver was safe in cirrhotic patients. Subsequently, however, many studies verified that this maneuver can be performed for extended periods in cirrhotic patients without increasing either morbidity or mortality. Nevertheless, it is advisable to employ the Pringle's maneuver sparingly in this population so as to minimize ischemic stress.

Parenchymal transection

There are at least 10 different techniques, but there are no convincing data to demonstrate the superiority of any single technique. Various devices are available for liver transection and comparative data on transection techniques are limited by the diversity of operative procedures. "Selective techniques" such as clamp crushing (Kelly-clysis) with a Cavitron ultrasonic surgical aspirator (CUSA, Integra Radionics) is widely used for splitting the liver parenchyma. Hemostasis is achieved by bipolar coagulation, ligatures or hemoclips. Clamp-crushing technique is still favored by most experienced hepatic surgeons to transect the liver tissue during resection. In patients with cirrhosis, however, the firmness of the parenchyma makes the clamp-crushing technique less than ideal because the parenchyma is often harder than the underlying vasculature and biliary radicle. Blunt dissection is likely to tear these vessels. Accordingly, ultrasonic dissectors that coagulate and seal vessels during dissection may be more suitable for parenchymal transection in this population. In nonselective techniques, mass coagulating devices such as radiofrequency ablation (RFA) aided Habib® 4X, TissueLink® and LigaSure® have been used for liver split by a "pre-coagulation strategy". The inherent disadvantage of these methods is necrosis of liver parenchyma that can result from lack of precision and biliary leaks as major complications. The authors have recently published a simple and efficient "fusion technique" of Focus-clysis utilizing a single instrument.[33] In fusion technique, the Harmonic FOCUS* is used and all the steps in the liver split, i.e. clamp-crush, post coagulation and transection are done utilizing the same technology in a single instrument. Whatever be the choice of transection technique, it should be carefully selected in cirrhotic livers and be based on the institutional protocols and the surgeon's preference.

Closure and drainage

Because of the likelihood of postoperative ascites, the abdominal wall is closed with a heavy continuous absorbable monofilament suture to create a watertight closure. To prevent major fluid and protein losses and ascending infections, abdominal drains generally are not used.

Postoperative Care in Cirrhotic Patients

- Transient hepatic insufficiency develops postoperatively in most cirrhotic patients, who undergo hepatic resection, and is reflected with hyperbilirubinemia, ascites formation, hypoalbuminemia, edema and worsening of the baseline coagulopathy
- In the first 24 hours after the procedure, crystalloid must be administered at a level sufficient to maintain adequate portal perfusion
- If patients are stable after the first 24 hours, they are subjected to water and sodium restriction and should receive liberal amounts of salt-poor albumin for volume expansion, if needed
- Spironolactone is started in all patients as soon as oral diet is resumed, and furosemide is added as needed
- The PT is checked twice daily during the immediate postoperative period; a PT longer than 17 seconds should be corrected by administering fresh frozen plasma.

The General Criteria of Unresectability of HCC Commonly Employed by Surgeons

- Large size of tumor with insufficient hepatic remnant after liver resection
- Extensive and multifocal bilobar tumors
- Extrahepatic metastases of the disease
- Tumor with main portal vein tumor thrombus or hepatic vein or inferior vena cava involvement.

Patients with multiple tumors, however, are not ideal resection candidates, as, in most cases, the presence of multiple tumors implies intrahepatic metastasis.[34] Macroscopic vascular invasion is a strong risk factor for recurrence, but in selected cases with normal liver function, without portal hypertension, and with a unilateral intraportal tumor thrombus that does not completely occlude the portal bifurcation, resection and portal tumor extraction can yield long-term survival in 25–30% of patients.[35]

Downstaging locoregional therapy can be employed to facilitate resection in disease which is initially regarded as unresectable and can achieve reasonable outcome, with 5-year survivals of 25–67%, with the possibility of cure.[36] In general, postresection survival rates are in the range 80–92% at 1 year, 61–86% at 3 years and 41–74% at 5 years. Five-year survival for tumors less than or equal to 2 cm, 2–5 cm and greater than 5 cm are 66%, 52% and 37% respectively.[37,38]

Recurrence after Resection: Metastases or New Primary?

Tumor recurrence occurs in approximately 20%, 50% and 75% of patients at 1 year, 3 years and 5 years respectively.[39] Predictors of recurrence include tumor grade, microscopic and macroscopic vascular invasion, tumor size, number of tumors, presence of satellites, AFP levels and positive surgical margins. The most common site of post-resection recurrence is the remaining liver. Intrahepatic recurrences could be either unrecognized metastases from the resected HCC or a de novo development of a new primary HCC. In the past, the distinction was based on clinical grounds: multiple small nodules that develop early after resection in the same anatomic region as a large resected tumor, for example, are likely to be metastases, while a solitary nodule that presents late after resection in the opposite lobe is more likely to be a new primary HCC. With the advent of molecular techniques such as the analysis of patterns of integration of HBV into the host genome and analysis of microsatellite allelic imbalance, it is now possible to accurately identify recurrent HCC as either metastatic or de novo. On the basis of such analyses, it has become clear that, even among recurrences clinically judged as being de novo, the majority are, in fact, metastatic lesions.[40,41] At present, there is no evidence that neoadjuvant or adjuvant therapy has any efficacy in reducing recurrence after resection.[42]

LIVER TRANSPLANTATION

Liver transplantation (LT) seems an attractive treatment option as it treats both the cancer and underlying liver disease. In the 1980s, patients presenting with large HCC were considered good candidates for LT as they were in better condition than patients with chronic liver disease and were more likely to survive the perioperative period as they had large or multifocal tumors. This resulted in a high recurrence rate of upto 65%, a 5-year survival of 10–35%, and a median survival of 6 months in those with recurrence.[43] This coupled with increasing demand for donor livers led to a more restrictive selection process for LT. Recognition that small tumors appeared to fare better after LT led Mazzaferro to introduce the Milan criteria to select patients leading to improved survival with low rates of tumor recurrence.[44] By adhering to the Milan criteria of undertaking LT for HCC with a solitary tumor less than 5 cm or 3 tumors less than 3 cm each, a 5-year survival greater than 70% and recurrence rates of less than 10% were achieved. The major limitation to LT as treatment for HCC is the scarcity of cadaveric donors and the associated waiting time that results in a 20% dropout rate and potentially increases the risk of recurrence from extension or vascular invasion.

A number of groups have tried to expand indications beyond the Milan criteria and claim to achieve similar survival rates. The University of California San Francisco (UCSF) criteria include one tumor less than 6.5 cm or multiple tumors, of which the largest is 4.5 cm and the sum of all diameters is less than or equal to 8 cm. More recently, the "up-to-seven criteria," where the HCC scores 7 based on the sum of the largest tumor (diameter in cm) and the total number of tumors, have been introduced by Mazaferro et al.[45] Once again, majority of the studies supporting extension of the Milan criteria is based on retrospective histological analysis of the tumor burden in the explant liver and has not been validated prospectively.

In many countries, especially in Asia, where HCC is prevalent and cadaveric livers are scarce, liver resection remains the preferred curative treatment of choice for HCC.

LOCOREGIONAL THERAPY

Nonsurgical modalities include percutaneous ethanol injection (PEI), RFA, transarterial chemoembolization (TACE) and transarterial radioembolization (TARE). All these modalities have well-documented antitumor effects.

Percutaneous Ethanol Injection

Percutaneous ethanol injection was the first chemical ablative technique utilized. Performed under percutaneous ultrasound guidance, a needle is placed into the tumor and absolute alcohol is injected. The physical characteristics of a soft HCC within a firm cirrhotic liver facilitate diffusion of the alcohol within the tumor, while limiting extranodular diffusion. When applied to small tumors less than 2 cm, PEI produces 90% necrosis and a 5-year survival of 47–53% but is limited by high recurrence rates of approximately 40%. Chemical ablation has now been superseded by thermal techniques such as RFA.

Radiofrequency Ablation

Over recent years, RFA has largely replaced PEI at most centers as it produces better local tumor control with a 2-year recurrence of 2–18% and a 5-year survival of 40–70% or better when the treatment groups have been selected.[46] Meta-analyses of randomized control trials have confirmed that RFA is a more effective way to obtain local tumor control and survival benefit compared to PEI, establishing it as a standard locoregional treatment.[47,48]

Radiofrequency ablation can be performed percutaneously, laparoscopically or at open surgery, depending on tumor location. Overall 10–25% of tumors will not be suitable for RFA because of location such as subcapsular, adjacent to the gall bladder or major vessels which increases the risk of complication and inadequate ablation because of heat sink. RFA is effective for early small HCC less than 3 cm whereas larger tumors may be inadequately treated. The recurrence rate after RFA for selected early small HCC can be comparable to that of surgery.[49] However, randomized control trials of RFA against resection for small HCC less than 3 cm have failed to show that RFA is as effective as resection, but the majority of studies was underpowered or had incomplete follow-up. Increasingly, RFA is being considered as an alternative initial "curative" treatment option for small centrally placed HCC as it offers the advantages of preserving parenchyma, potentially removes competition from the transplant waiting list and, based on location, effective tumor necrosis can be obtained.[50]

Radiofrequency ablation is less effective for solitary HCC greater than 3 cm but less than 5 cm. But when TACE followed by RFA for this size tumor is applied, the therapeutic effect of RFA is significantly increased and reduces tumor progression rate to 6% compared to 39% for RFA alone. However, no advantage has been demonstrated by combining therapies in larger HCC greater than 5 cm that are outside LT criteria or not suitable for resection.[51,52]

Transarterial Chemoembolization

As the name suggests, TACE is a treatment procedure using the transarterial route of the hepatic artery to inject chemotherapeutic and embolizing agents in the treatment of liver cancer. There is no standardized protocol in the choice of the chemotherapeutic agents, the dosage, the dilution, the rate of injection and the time interval between the treatments. Similarly, there is no agreement on the choice of the embolizing agent, the degree of embolization and whether the chemotherapeutic agent should be given before, or together with the embolizing agent. Commonly performed TACE involves hydrophilic chemotherapeutic agents mixed in an emulsion with ethiodized oil (Lipiodol®) subsequent to which an embolization of the hepatic artery is performed. For optimal results, TACE needs to be as selective as possible, producing sustained and high localized concentrations within the tumor minimizing systemic exposure. Alternatively, chemotherapy can be delivered through drug-eluting bead. A randomized control trial, comparing drug-eluting beads with doxorubicin to conventional TACE with doxorubicin found it was better tolerated, with reduced liver toxicity and improved treatment response.[53] HCC have been shown to shrink with TACE and unresectable HCC has become resectable in many instances. A partial response of 15–55% has been observed producing a survival benefit, increasing median survival time from 16 months to 20 months with 49% survival at 2 years.[54] Though TACE has demonstrated improved survival compared to best supportive care, the results have not been consistent. It needs to be understood that good results with TACE are achieved when it is used on a selective basis. Perhaps the beneficial effects of TACE in a certain subgroup of patients are offset by the toxic side-effects of the treatment on another subgroup so that the impact on the overall survival of the whole patient group is dismal. TACE is not suitable in the setting of a portal vein thrombosis or decompensated liver disease where there is ascites or jaundice.

Transarterial Radioembolization

Conventional external radiotherapy has a limited role in the treatment of HCC because of the adverse effects of irradiation to the surrounding nontumorous liver tissue, leading to radiation hepatitis. The aim of TARE is to deliver radioisotopes to the tumor, where it must reside for a sufficient period to deliver the scheduled dose of radiation. The amount of radiation delivered to the nontumorous liver parenchyma and other organs should be as low as possible. Based on the rationale of regional therapy and taking advantage of the better arterial blood supply of HCC, most radioactive substances injected through the hepatic artery can be delivered to the tumor, thus giving a favorable uptake ratio of tumor to normal tissue. This is called selective internal irradiation. Patients can be considered for TARE if they have an unresectable HCC, but without extrahepatic disease and satisfactory liver function. Two isotopes which have been studied extensively are iodine-131 which can be used with Lipiodol®, and yttrium-90 (90Y) which can be incorporated into resin-based or glass microspheres. 90Y is a pure β-emitter and decays to stable zirconium-90 with a physical half-life of 64.2 hours. The average energy of beta emission is 0.935 MeV (maximum energy, 2.27 MeV), with a mean tissue penetration of 2.5 mm and a maximum penetration of 11 mm. The mean energy and mean penetration of 90Y is great, so it can be used to treat larger tumors. 90Y microspheres can be delivered either through an angiographic catheter during hepatic angiography or an implantable arterial port. There are two absolute contraindications to 90Y microspheres treatment: exaggerated hepatopulmonary shunting, and reflux into the arteries that supply the gastroduodenal region. The toxicity profile of 90Y microspheres therapy remains low and the treatment is generally well-tolerated. The most common side-effects associated with 90Y microspheres are transient elevations in liver enzymes.

Other side-effects include gastrointestinal symptoms (including abdominal pain, nausea, vomiting, anorexia and gastritis) and, occasionally, gastric and duodenal ulcers. There is a minimal embolic effect. So when there is main portal vein involvement and TACE is contraindicated, radioembolization with 90Y may be a good option.

TARGETED THERAPY

Hepatocellular carcinoma is a unique chemoresistant tumor. In the early 1990s, a number of randomized controlled studies assessed the role of adjuvant chemotherapy. A systematic review and meta-analysis of published randomized studies have failed to show any survival benefit of systemic chemotherapy for HCC patients. Systemic chemotherapy is not recommended as standard therapy outside a clinical trial protocol. Since 2007, sorafenib tosylate, an oral tyrosine kinase inhibitor was approved for use in patients with unresectable HCC. Sorafenib blocks tumor cell proliferation by targeting the Raf/mitogen-activated protein kinase/extracellular signal regulated kinase (Raf/MEK/ERK) signaling pathway and exerts an antiangiogenic effect by targeting the tyrosine kinases (TKs), vascular endothelial growth factor receptor 2 (VEGFR-2), VEGFR-3 and platelet-derived growth factor receptor beta (PDGFR-beta). The approval of this drug was based on the results of an international, multicenter, randomized, double-blind, placebo-controlled trial referred to as the Sorafenib Hepatocellular Carcinoma Assessment Randomized Protocol (SHARP) trial in patients with unresectable, biopsy-proven HCC.[55] The study demonstrated that Sorafenib improved median survival from 7.9 months to 10.7 months and slowed time to progression from 2.8 months to 5.5 months. Sorafenib can be considered standard of care for patients with advanced and metastatic HCC, who are not candidates for curative or locoregional therapies, but, at present, only patients with good liver function have been rigorously studied.

PREVENTION AND SURVEILLANCE

Although HCC is currently one of the most common worldwide causes of cancer death, a major impact on the incidence of HCC should be achieved through current vaccination strategies for HBV infection, screening and treatment for HCV infections, and from the reduction of alcoholic liver disease. There are about 350 million carriers of HBV worldwide. Hepatitis B vaccine has been proven to be safe and effective. The vaccine is 95% effective in preventing children and adults from developing chronic infection if they have not been infected. Since 1991, the World Health Organization (WHO) has called for all countries to add hepatitis B vaccine to their national immunization programs.[56] By March 2000, 116 countries had included hepatitis B vaccine in their national program, including most countries in Asia. In Taiwan area, the national vaccination of infants between 1984 and 1986 reduced the prevalence of HBV carriers in childhood from 15% to 1% and that of HCC by 60% when compared with nonimmunized children.[57] Globally, an estimated 170 million persons are chronically infected with hepatitis C and 3–4 million persons are newly infected each year, but no vaccine is currently available. In the absence of an effective vaccine, all precautions to prevent infection must be taken including screening of blood and organ donors, virus inactivation of plasma-derived products, implementation and maintenance of infection control practice in the healthcare setting, promotion of healthy behavior change in the general public, such as prevention of sharing of needles for injection and safe sexual practice. However, because the latency period from hepatic damage to HCC development is very long, it may be many years until the incidence of HCC decreases as a result of these interventions.

A surveillance program in cirrhotic patients has the potential advantage of detection of HCC at early stages, when the tumors are amenable to curative treatments. However, its cost-effectiveness is still debated. Although there is still no strong evidence that screening in HCC improves survival, many physicians advocate screening patients in high-risk groups with either serum AFP or ultrasound of the liver, or both. If surveillance is offered, it should be performed at 6-month intervals. Some investigators have suggested that, because of the unpredictable tumor growth rate, screening should be done more frequently (3-month intervals) in a high-risk population.

OTHER PRIMARY MALIGNANT LIVER TUMORS

Intrahepatic Cholangiocarcinoma

Intrahepatic cholangiocarcinoma (ICC) is a rare, malignant tumor, which arises from the epithelial cells of intrahepatic bile ducts (beyond the second order bile ducts). The incidence of ICC is reported to be only about 10% of primary liver cancers. A recent study reported that, in addition to the established risk factors such as choledochal cysts, chronic cholangitis, inflammatory bowel disease, primary sclerosing cholangitis (PSC) parasitic infections, drug or toxin exposure, and genetic risks, other conditions such as biliary cirrhosis, cholelithiasis, alcoholic liver disease, nonspecific cirrhosis are significantly associated with ICC.[58] ICC has the worst prognosis of any tumor arising in the liver; its 5-year survival is poor, and accompanied by a high recurrence rate. The overall 5-year survival rate ranges from 13 to 42%.[59,60]

Intrahepatic cholangiocarcinoma arises from cholangiocytes and is usually a moderate to well-differentiated tubular adenocarcinoma. The most outstanding histological feature is the presence of abundant desmoplastic stroma in ICC compared with HCC, leading to a low diagnostic yield of random biopsies. Desmoplasia may also cause capsular retraction. This capsular retraction may be seen on radiological imaging and is a diagnostic feature of ICC. CT scans may demonstrate irregular mass often with segmental biliary ductal dilatation because of obstruction. With the intravenous administration of iodinated contrast material, the mass may demonstrate a variable enhancement pattern. Delayed enhancement with increasing attenuation may be seen on images in as many as 74% of patients. This pattern of enhancement may be useful in differentiating HCC from cholangiocarcinomas. Often serum carcinoembryonic antigen (CEA) and serum carbohydrate antigen 19-9 (CA 19-9) are elevated while AFP levels are normal in cases of ICC.

Three types of ICC have been established using the TNM staging system and the classification system established by the Liver Cancer Study Group of Japan: mass-forming (MF) type, periductal infiltrating (PI) type and intraductal growth (IG) type. MF type forms a definite round-shaped mass with an expansive growth pattern, but without fibrous capsule, and locates in the liver parenchyma. The border between cancerous and noncancerous portions is distinct, and this type of ICC does not invade the major branch of the portal triad. PI type is defined as a mass extending longitudinally along the bile duct, occasionally involves the surrounding blood vessels and/or hepatic parenchyma, often resulting in dilatation of the peripheral bile duct. IG type proliferates toward the lumen of bile duct papillary or like a tumor thrombus, occasionally involving superficial extension. This type of ICC is usually detected in a thick bile duct.[61]

Unlike HCC, ICC is associated with early lymphatic spread. Hepatoduodenal ligament is the most common site of nodal metastasis in ICC patients irrespective of the tumor location. ICC has no characteristic symptoms at its early stage and is often at its advanced stage when it is diagnosed. Anatomic and extended hepatectomy is the rational procedure for mass-forming ICC, while hepatectomy with extrahepatic duct excision and hilar lymph nodal resection is the rational procedure for infiltrating ICC. Consequently, the resectability rate is usually low, extended hepatectomy possibly in combination with resection of other structures (e.g. extrahepatic bile duct, portal vein and inferior vena cava) is generally required.

No consensus has been reached concerning the indications and value of lymph node dissection for ICC. Hepatectomy with extensive lymph node dissection is the standard operation for intrahepatic cholangiocarcinoma in Japan. However, lymph node dissection may not always be effective in reducing tumor recurrence. However, there are reported cases of long-term survival after extended surgical resection of intrahepatic cholangiocarcinoma with extensive lymph node metastasis.[62,63]

Liver transplant in the setting of ICC has not shown favorable results, neither has adjuvant nor neoadjuvant therapy been able to show an improved survival.

RARE PRIMARY LIVER TUMORS

Primary hepatic neuroendocrine tumors (PHNETs) are extremely rare and very little is known about the clinical features and treatment outcomes of these tumors. As liver is the most frequent metastatic site of neuroendocrine carcinomas, differential diagnosis between primary hepatic neuroendocrine carcinomas (PHNECs) and metastatic hepatic neuroendocrine carcinomas is very important for the diagnosis of PHNECs. Therefore, only with careful analysis and after excluding extrahepatic origin of neuroendocrine carcinomas with liver metastasis, can PHNETs be diagnosed.

Rare primary liver tumors include "angiosarcoma" and "lymphoma". "Hepatoblastomas" are found exclusively in children below the age of 5 years. They are beyond the scope of this chapter.

REFERENCES

1. Jemal A, Bray F, Center MM, et al. Global cancer statistics. CA Cancer J Clin. 2011;61(2):69-90.
2. Bosch FX, Ribes J, Diaz M, et al. Primary liver cancer: worldwide incidence and trends. Gastroenterology. 2004;127(5):S5-16.
3. Ferlay J, Shin HR, Bray F, et al. Estimates of worldwide burden of cancer in 2008: GLOBOCAN 2008. Int J Cancer. 2010;127: 2893-917.
4. Parkin DM. The global health burden of infection-associated cancers in the year 2002. Int J Cancer. 2006;118(12):3030-44.
5. Omata M, Lesmana LA, Tateishi R, et al. Asian Pacific association for the study of the liver consensus recommendations on hepatocellular carcinoma. Hepatol Int. 2010;4(2):439-74.
6. Tong MJ, el-Farra NS, Reikes AR, et al. Clinical outcomes after transfusion-associated hepatitis C. N Engl J Med. 1995;332(22):1463-6.
7. Kobayashi M, Ikeda K, Hosaka T, et al. Dysplastic nodules frequently develop into hepatocellular carcinoma in patients with chronic viral hepatitis and cirrhosis. Cancer. 2006;106(3): 636-47.
8. Sugihara S, Nakashima O, Kojiro M, et al. The morphologic transition in hepatocellular carcinoma: a comparison of the individual histologic features disclosed by ultrasound-guided fine-needle biopsy with those of autopsy. Cancer. 1992;70(6):1488-92.
9. Kenmochi K, Sugihara S, Kojiro M. Relationship of histologic grade of hepatocellular carcinoma (HCC) to tumor size, and demonstration of tumor cells of multiple different grades in single small HCC. Liver. 1987;7(1):18-26.
10. Forner A, Reig M, Bruix J. Alpha-fetoprotein for hepatocellular carcinoma diagnosis: the demise of a brilliant star. Gastroenterology. 2009;137(1):26-9.
11. Bruix J, Sherman M, American Association for the Study of Liver Diseases. Management of hepatocellular carcinoma: an update. Hepatology. 2011;53(3):1020-2.
12. Marrero JA, Hussain HK, Nghiem HV, et al. Improving the prediction of hepatocellular carcinoma in cirrhotic patients with an arterially-enhancing liver mass. Liver Transpl. 2005;11(3):281-9.
13. Luca A, Caruso S, Milazzo M, et al. Multidetector-row computed tomography (MDCT) for the diagnosis of hepatocellular carcinoma in cirrhotic candidates for liver transplantation: prevalence of radiological vascular patterns and histological correlation with liver explants. Eur Radiol. 2010;20(4):898–907.
14. Yu NC, Chaudhari V, Raman SS, et al. CT and MRI improve detection of hepatocellular carcinoma, compared with ultrasound alone, in patients with cirrhosis. Clin Gastroenterol Hepatol. 2011;9(2):161-7.
15. Kim YK, Kim CS, Han YM, et al. Detection of hepatocellular carcinoma: gadoxetic acid-enhanced 3-dimensional magnetic resonance imaging versus multi-detector row computed tomography. J Comput Assist Tomogr. 2009;33(6):844-50.
16. Pitton MB, Kloeckner R, Herber S, et al. MRI versus 64-row MDCT for diagnosis of hepatocellular carcinoma. World J Gastroenterol. 2009;15(48):6044-51.
17. Leoni S, Piscaglia F, Golfieri R, et al. The impact of vascular and nonvascular findings on the noninvasive diagnosis of small hepatocellular carcinoma based on the EASL and AASLD criteria. A J Gastroenterol. 2010;105(3):599-609.
18. Yu JS, Kim JH, Chung JJ, et al. Added value of diffusion-weighted imaging in the MRI assessment of perilesional tumor recurrence after chemoembolization of hepatocellular carcinomas. J Magn Reson Imaging. 2009;30(1):153-60.
19. Vandecaveye V, De Keyzer F, Verslype C, et al. Diffusion-weighted MRI provides additional value to conventional dynamic contrast-enhanced MRI for detection of hepatocellular carcinoma. Eur Radiol. 2009;19(10):2456-66.
20. Xu PJ, Yan FH, Wang JH, et al. Added value of breathhold diffusion-weighted MRI in detection of small hepatocellular carcinoma lesions compared with dynamic contrast-enhanced MRI alone using receiver operating characteristic curve analysis. J Magn Reson Imaging. 2009;29(2):341-9.
21. Park JW, Kim JH, Kim SK, et al. A prospective evaluation of 18F-FDG and 11C-acetate PET/CT for detection of primary and metastatic hepatocellular carcinoma. J Nucl Med. 2008;49(12):1912-21.
22. Caturelli E, Solmi L, Anti M, et al. Ultrasound guided fine needle biopsy of early hepatocellular carcinoma complicating liver cirrhosis: a multicentre study. Gut. 2004;53(9):1356-62.
23. Durand F, Regimbeau JM, Belghiti J, et al. Assessment of the benefits and risks of percutaneous biopsy before surgical resection of hepatocellular carcinoma. J Hepatol. 2001;35(2): 254-8.
24. Ng KK, Poon RT, Lo CM, et al. Impact of preoperative fine-needle aspiration cytologic examination on clinical outcome in patients with hepatocellular carcinoma in a tertiary referral center. Arch Surg. 2004;139(2):193-200.
25. Stigliano R, Burroughs AK. Should we biopsy each liver mass suspicious for HCC before liver transplantation?—no, please don't. J Hepatol. 2005;43(4):563-8.
26. Stigliano R, Marelli L, Yu D, et al. Seeding following percutaneous diagnostic and therapeutic approaches for hepatocellular carcinoma. What is the risk and the outcome? Seeding risk for percutaneous approach of HCC. Cancer Treat Rev. 2007;33(5):437-47.
27. Saborido BP, Díaz JC, de Los Galanes SJ, et al. Does preoperative fine needle aspiration-biopsy produce tumor recurrence in patients following liver transplantation for hepatocellular carcinoma? Transplant Proc. 2005;37(9):3874-7.
28. Olthoff KM, Forner A, Hübscher S, et al. What is the best staging system for hepatocellular carcinoma in the setting of liver transplantation? Liver Transpl. 2011;17(2):S26-33.
29. Bruix J, Sherman M, Llovet JM, et al. Clinical management of hepatocellular carcinoma. Conclusions of the Barcelona-2000 EASL conference. European Association for the Study of the Liver. J Hepatol. 2001;35(3):421-30.
30. Bruix J, Sherman M. Practice Guidelines Committee, American Association for the Study of Liver Diseases. Management of hepatocellular carcinoma. Hepatology. 2005;42(5):1208-36.
31. Llovet JM, Fuster J, Bruix J. Intention-to-treat analysis of surgical treatment for early hepatocellular carcinoma: resection versus transplantation. Hepatology. 1999;30(6):1434-40.

32. Bruix J, Castells A, Bosch J, et al. Surgical resection of hepatocellular carcinoma in cirrhotic patients: prognostic value of preoperative portal pressure. Gastroenterology. 2004;111(4):1018-22.
33. Jagannath P, Chhabra DG, Sutariya KR, et al. Fusion technique for liver transection with Kelly-clysis and harmonic technology. World J Surg. 2010;34(1):101-5.
34. Ng IO, Guan XY, Poon RT, et al. Determination of the molecular relationship between multiple tumour nodules in hepatocellular carcinoma differentiates multicentric origin from intrahepatic metastasis. J Pathol. 2003;199(3):345-53.
35. Koike Y, Nakagawa K, Shiratori Y, et al. Factors affecting the prognosis of patients with hepatocellular carcinoma invading the portal vein—a retrospective analysis using 952 consecutive HCC patients. Hepatogastroenterology. 2003;50(54):2035-9.
36. Lau WY, Lai EC. Salvage surgery following downstaging of unresectable hepatocellular carcinoma—a strategy to increase resectability. Ann Surg Oncol. 2007;14(12):3301-9.
37. Fong Y, Sun RL, Jarnagin W, et al. An analysis of 412 cases of hepatocellular carcinoma at a Western center. Ann Surg. 1999;229(6):790-9.
38. Poon RT, Fan ST, Lo CM, et al. Extended hepatic resection for hepatocellular carcinoma in patients with cirrhosis: is it justified? Ann Surg. 2002;236(5):602-11.
39. Chen WT, Chau GY, Lui WY, et al. Recurrent hepatocellular carcinoma after hepatic resection: prognostic factors and long-term outcome. Eur J Surg Oncol. 2004;30(4):414-20.
40. Chen YJ, Yeh SH, Chen JT, et al. Chromosomal changes and clonality relationship between primary and recurrent hepatocellular carcinoma. Gastroenterology. 2000;119(2): 431-40.
41. Finkelstein SD, Marsh W, Demetris AJ, et al. Microdissection-based allelotyping discriminates de novo tumor from intrahepatic spread in hepatocellular carcinoma. Hepatology. 2003;37(4):871-9.
42. Samuel M, Chow PK, E. Chan Shih-Yen E, et al. Neoadjuvant and adjuvant therapy for surgical resection of hepatocellular carcinoma. Cochrane Database Syst Rev. 2009;(1):CD001199.
43. Moreno P, Jaurrieta E, Figueras J, et al. Orthotopic liver transplantation: treatment of choice in cirrhotic patients with hepatocellular carcinoma? Transplant Proc. 1995;27(4):2296-8.
44. Mazzaferro V, Regalia E, Doci R, et al. Liver transplantation for the treatment of small hepatocellular carcinomas in patients with cirrhosis. N Engl J Med. 1996;334(11):693-9.
45. Mazzaferro V, Llovet J.M, Miceli R, et al. Predicting survival after liver transplantation in patients with hepatocellular carcinoma beyond the Milan criteria: a retrospective, exploratory analysis. Lancet Oncol. 2009;10(1):35-43.
46. Livraghi T, Meloni F, Di Stasi M, et al. Sustained complete response and complications rates after radiofrequency ablation of very early hepatocellular carcinoma in cirrhosis: is resection still the treatment of choice? Hepatology. 2008;47(1):82-9.
47. Lencioni R. Loco-regional treatment of hepatocellular carcinoma. Hepatology. 2010;52(2):762-73.
48. Tanaka S, Shimada M, Shirabe K, et al. Surgical radiofrequency ablation for treatment of hepatocellular carcinoma: an endoscopic or open approach. Hepatogastroenterology. 2009,56(93):1169-73.
49. Tateishi R, Shiina S, Teratani T, et al. Percutaneous radiofrequency ablation for hepatocellular carcinoma: an analysis of 1000 cases. Cancer. 2005;103(6):1201-9.
50. Cho YK, Kim JK, Kim WT, et al. Hepatic resection versus radiofrequency ablation for very early stage hepatocellular carcinoma: a Markov model analysis. Hepatology. 2010;51(4):1284-90.
51. Morimoto M, Numata K, Kondou M, et al. Midterm outcomes in patients with intermediate-sized hepatocellular carcinoma: a randomized controlled trial for determining the efficacy of radiofrequency ablation combined with transcatheter arterial chemoembolization. Cancer. 2010;116(23):5452-60.
52. Veltri A, Moretto P, Doriguzzi A, et al. Radiofrequency thermal ablation (RFA) after transarterial chemoembolization (TACE) as a combined therapy for unresectable non-early hepatocellular carcinoma (HCC). Eur Radiol. 2006;16(3):661-9.
53. Lammer J, Malagari K, Vogl T, et al. Prospective randomized study of doxorubicin-eluting-bead embolization in the treatment of hepatocellular carcinoma: results of the PRECISION V study. Cardiovasc Intervent Radiol. 2010;33(1):41-52.
54. Llovet JM, Bruix J. Systematic review of randomized trials for unresectable hepatocellular carcinoma: chemoembolization improves survival. Hepatology. 2003;37(2):429-42.
55. Llovet J, Ricci S, Mazzaferro V, et al. Sorafenib improves survival in advanced hepatocellular carcinoma (HCC): results of a Phase III randomized placebo-controlled trial (SHARP trial). Proceedings from the American Society of Clinical Oncology Conference; Chicago; 2007.
56. Lai EC, Lau WY. The continuing challenge of hepatic cancer in Asia. Surgeon. 2005;3(3):210-5.
57. Ni YH, Chen DS. Hepatitis B vaccination in children: the Taiwan experience. Pathol Biol (Paris). 2010;58(4):296-300.
58. Sorensen HT, Friis S, Olsen JH, et al. Risk of liver and other types of cancer in patients with cirrhosis: a nationwide cohort study in Denmark. Hepatology. 1998;28(4):921-5.
59. Lieser MJ, Barry MK, Rowland C, et al. Surgical management of intrahepatic cholangiocarcinoma: a 31-year experience. J Hepatobiliary Pancreat Surg. 1998;5(1):41-7.
60. Valverde A, Bonhomme N, Farges O, et al. Resection of intrahepatic cholangiocarcinoma: a Western experience. J Hepatobiliary Pancreat Surg. 1999;6(2):122-7.
61. Liver Cancer Study Group of Japan. Intrahepatic cholangiocarcinoma, macroscopic typing. In: Okamoto E (Ed). Classification of Primary Liver Cancer. Tokyo: Kanehara; 1997;6-7.
62. Shirabe K, Shimada M, Harimoto N, et al. Intrahepatic cholangiocarcinoma: its mode of spreading and therapeutic modalities. Surgery. 2002;131(1): S159-64.
63. Asakura H, Ohtsuka M, Ito H, et al. Long-term survival after extended surgical resection of intrahepatic cholangiocarcinoma with extensive lymph node metastasis. Hepatogastroenterology. 2005;52(63):722-4.

33 Biliary Malignancies

Deepak Chhabra, Palepu Jagannath

INTRODUCTION

Malignancies of the biliary tract have been recognized for centuries. Carcinoma of the biliary tree was first described by Durand-Fardel in 1840. Klatskin, in a classic article in 1965, first described its clinical and pathologic features that led to the eponym "Klatskin tumor". The first description of gallbladder cancer was by DeStoll in 1777 and the first resection for cancer was performed by Keen in 1891. The association between gallstones (GST) and cancer was first reported by Mayo in 1903.[1]

Despite this long-standing appreciation of these tumors, carcinomas of the gallbladder and extrahepatic bile ducts are associated with late manifestation and poor prognosis. The diagnosis is often late when the disease is at an advanced stage due to the lack of effective screening strategies, lack of symptoms, and nonspecific symptoms of early tumors. Once diagnosed, the surgical treatment of these cancers is challenged by a complex anatomy of the porta hepatis, high morbidity and mortality of extended hepatic resections, and lack of effective neoadjuvant or adjuvant therapy. Survival outcomes of these tumors show a regional variability as experience in the management of these tumors is limited to predominantly high-volume surgical centers.

An enhanced understanding of portal and biliary anatomy coupled with improved imaging modalities and interventional radiology techniques have increased the safety of hepatic resection. Thus, an increasingly aggressive surgical approach to achieve a complete tumor clearance with negative margins and an improved lymphatic clearance, along with early developments in adjuvant therapy, have improved the outlook for patients with cancer of the gallbladder and extrahepatic bile ducts.

GALLBLADDER CARCINOMA

EPIDEMIOLOGY AND RISK FACTORS FOR GALLBLADDER CARCINOMA

The incidence of gallbladder carcinoma (GBC) has a specific geographic and ethnic variation. Northern India has one of the highest reported incidences of GBC in the World. The highest incidence rates of GBC in the world are 21.5/100,000 in females in Delhi, 13.8/100,000 in Karachi, and 12.9/100,000 in Quito.[2] GST were said to play a major role. Other risk factors are obesity, multiparity, and chronic infections.

In India, GBC is most prevalent in northern and northeastern states of Uttar Pradesh, Bihar, Orissa, West Bengal, and Assam.[3] GBC is two times higher in women than men and is the leading digestive cancer in women in northern Indian cities.[4] Six cancer registries of the Indian Council of Medical Research (1990–96) show a 10 times lower incidence of GBC per 100,000 in South India compared with the North, the age-adjusted incidence rate for females being 0.8 in Chennai in the south and 8.9 in Delhi in the north.[5]

In a review of worldwide incidence, the female-to-male ratio (F:M) was reported between 2 and 3. In northern India and South America the gender discrepancy is especially pronounced with an F:M ratio of 5:1 to 6:1. The gender difference is less pronounced in Eastern Asia (Korea, Japan, China), where the F:M ratio is between 1.0 and 1.4:1.[2] There are subtle indications, including the 1:1 M:F ratio, that the epidemiology of GBC seen in East Asia (e.g. China, Japan and Korea) may differ from that seen in other high-risk areas and in other ethnic populations. One hypothesis is that this difference can be attributed to the higher frequency of anomalous pancreaticobiliary duct junction (APBDJ) seen in this population. This congenital malformation results in premature junction of the common bile duct (CBD) and the pancreatic duct (PD), which permits the regurgitation of pancreatic secretions into the gallbladder and biliary tree. The resulting bile stasis and inflammation may predispose to cancer in a manner similar to that seen for choledochal cysts in cholangiocarcinoma (CCA) of the CBD.[6]

Gallstones associated with GBC have been reported in 75–90% of patients; however, the relationship between causation and association is unclear. The incidence of GBC in a population with GST varies from 0.3 to 3% only, and it has been suggested that larger stones (greater than or equal to 3 cm) have a greater impact on the risk of developing GBC.[7] The author has been a part of multi-institutional field survey by the Gallbladder Abnormalities in Northern Gangetic Area (GANGA) study group to estimate the prevalence of gallbladder diseases (GBD) and other risk factors that may be associated with the high prevalence of GBC in Northern Indian community. The study reported a high prevalence of GBD in females and a high prevalence of GBC (but with small absolute numbers). In comparison there was a lower prevalence of GST suggesting that factors other than GST were associated with high prevalence of GBC in the north Indian regions.[8]

Other risk factors associated with GBC include race, obesity, multiparity, smoking, certain diet pattern, chronic infections like *Salmonella typhi* and *S. paratyphi*, porcelain gallbladder and anomalous pancreaticobiliary ductal junction. Solitary polyps with a size greater than 1 cm are recognized as a predisposing factor for GBC.[9]

CLINICAL PRESENTATION

The symptoms associated with GBC are usually nonspecific, and as a result, most patients present at an advanced, inoperable stage. Abdominal pain and biliary colic may predominate and may be misinterpreted as cholecystitis. An asymmetric mass may be detected on a routine ultrasound (US) in the work-up of biliary symptoms. A palpable mass is present in a minority of patients at presentation. In advanced cases of invasion or compression of the porta hepatis, jaundice may ensue and the patients may have systemic signs, such as malaise and weight loss. Jaundice is an ominous finding. In a series from the Memorial Sloan-Kettering Cancer Center (MSKCC) from 1995 through 2005, one-third of patients presented with jaundice and only 7% had resectable disease.[10]

PATHOLOGY AND PATTERNS OF SPREAD

Approximately 60% of cancers arise in the fundus of the gland, with 30% developing in the body, and 10% in the neck.[11] Based on macroscopic features, cancers can be categorized into infiltrative, nodular, papillary, or mixed forms. The infiltrative form is the most common and often exhibits early and extensive infiltration of the subserosal layer leading to involvement of the entire gallbladder wall. The margins of these tumors are often poorly defined, making the surgical management of these cases more challenging. Nodular tumors are characterized by early invasion through the gallbladder wall into adjacent organs and liver. The growth of papillary tumors is predominantly intraluminal, resulting in a polypoid or cauliflower-like lesion. These tumors are less prone to local invasion and lymph node metastases and are therefore associated with a better prognosis.[12]

Gallbladder carcinoma spreads in four modes: (i) local invasion to liver or adjacent organs; (ii) lymphatic spread, (iii) peritoneal dissemination, (iv) hematogenous spread, and (v) Intraductal spread in papillary type of tumors. Understanding these modes of spread is important in considering an approach to surgical resection of these tumors. The gallbladder lymphatics drain first into the cystic duct node and the nodal chain along the CBD. Subsequent drainage is to the pancreaticoduodenal lymph nodes as well as the nodes posterior to the portal vein and along the common hepatic artery. From there, lymphatic drainage proceeds to the celiac, superior mesenteric and para-aortic lymph nodes. Involvement of para-aortic nodes indicates incurable metastatic disease with no better survival than patients without resection or distant metastases.[13] Adjacent liver involvement occurs via direct invasion or by invasion of veins that drain from the gallbladder into the adjacent liver segment. Helical CT observations during superselective injection of contrast medium into cholecystic artery has shown 96% of gallbladder veins end in the intrahepatic portal branches of segment V, 93% of gallbladder veins end in the intrahepatic portal branches of segment IV.[14] Direct invasion of the cancers can also occur along the hilar plate and Glisson's capsule toward the liver hilum; this mode of spread is particularly challenging when considering surgical resection and can often render tumors unresectable based on early hepatic vascular invasion. Other organs that can become involved by direct invasion include the anterior abdominal wall, duodenum, colon, diaphragm,

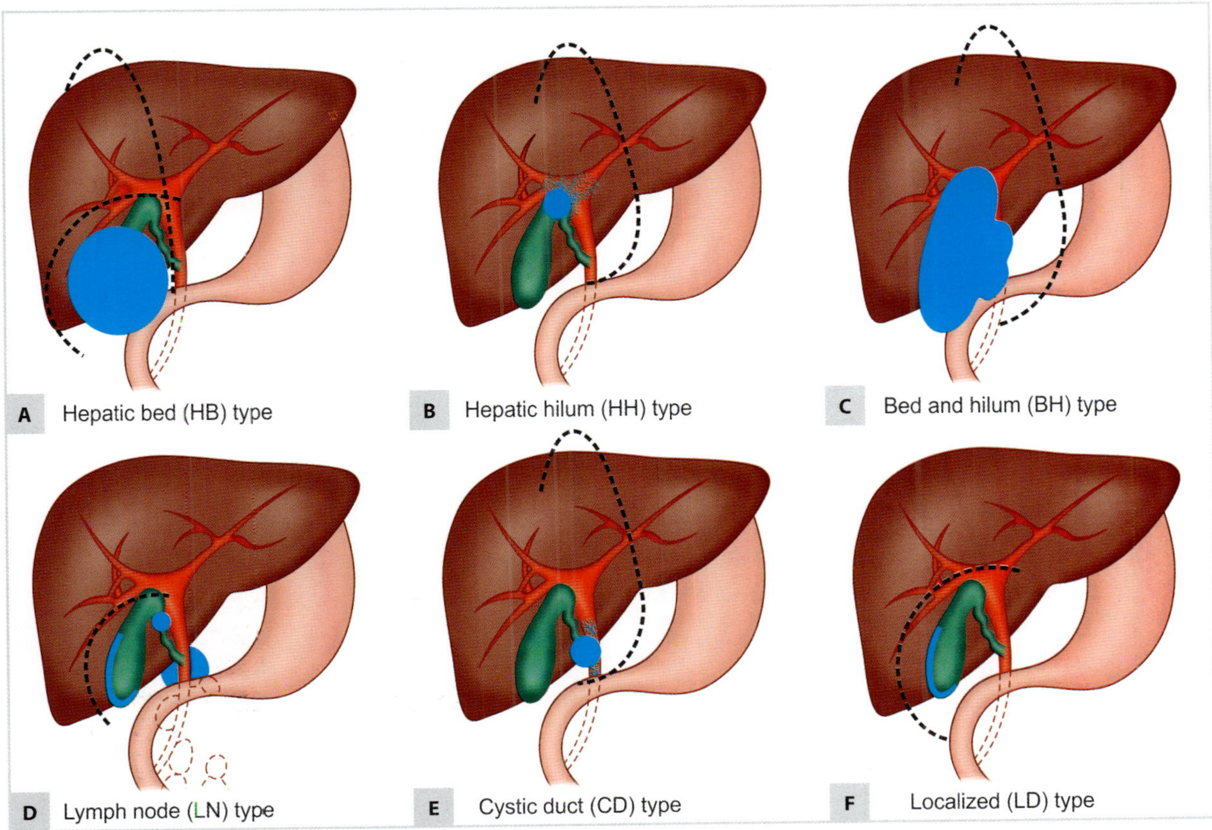

Figs 1A to F: Schematic illustrations showing the six types of the mode and degree of tumor spread in gallbladder cancer. Interrupted lines represent the type of hepatic resection that should be performed. In addition a portal/hepato-duodenal nodal clearance is a must

[*Source:* Kondo S, Nimura Y, Kamiya J, et al. Mode of tumor spread and surgical strategy in gallbladder carcinoma. Langenbecks Arch Surg. 2002;387(5-6):222-8.]

and hepatic ducts. Intraductal spread is commonly seen in papillary cancers, and perineural spread often follows the course of the arterial anatomy of the region.

Kondo et al. have identified six types of presentation of GBC on basis of patterns of dissemination.[15] The study classified the mode and degree of tumor spread macroscopically using surgical specimens from patients who underwent radical resection. This information should assist the surgeon in the choice of operation and predict outcome. The patterns identified were hepatic bed (HB) type, hepatic hilum (HH) type, bed and hilum (BH) type, lymph node (LN) type, cystic duct (CD) type and the localized (LC) type. These are summarized in Figures 1A to F. HB, HH, BH, and LN are grouped as (locally) advanced tumors.

STAGING

Multiple tumor staging systems [Nevin staging, Japanese Biliary Surgical Society staging system, TNM staging system of the American Joint Committee on Cancer (AJCC)/Union for International Cancer Control (UICC)] have been described for GBC. According to the most recent revised AJCC staging algorithm (Table 1), GBCAs are staged according to tumor depth of invasion (T), presence of lymph node metastasis (N) and presence of distant metastasis (M).[16] T stage describes how deeply the primary tumor invades through the layers of the gallbladder wall and into adjacent structures. In general, tumors confined to the gallbladder wall are classified as T1 or T2 whereas T3 and T4 tumors have extended beyond the gallbladder.

In the 7th edition of TNM staging, N differentiation is probably the most notable point; the lymph nodes of GBC are divided into the hilar/hepatoduodenal lymph nodes and other regional lymph nodes. In the absence of lymph node evaluation, radical resection might not provide benefits over simple cholecystectomy.[17] A study from the MSKCC demonstrated that distant and nodal metastases increased progressively from 16 to 79% and from 33 to 69%, respectively, in going from T2 to T4 tumors.[18]

INVESTIGATIONS

Ultrasonography and CT scan are commonly used to demonstrate the primary lesion and local spread of GBC. In addition, magnetic resonance imaging (MRI)

TABLE 1: UICC/AJCC staging system for gallbladder cancer, 7th edition, 2010

T stage			
T0	No evidence of primary tumor		
Tis	Carcinoma in situ		
T1	Tumor invades lamina propria or muscle layer		
	T1a Tumor invades lamina propria		
	T1b Tumor invades muscle layer		
T2	Tumor invades perimuscular connective tissue with no extension beyond serosa or into liver		
T3	Tumor perforates serosa (visceral peritoneum) and/or directly invades liver and/or invades adjacent or structure, such as duodenum, stomach, colon, pancreas, omentum or bile ducts		
T4	Tumor invades main portal vein or hepatic artery or multiple extrahepatic organs or structures		
N stage			
Nx	Regional lymph nodes cannot be assessed		
N0	No regional lymph node metastasis		
N1	Metastases to nodes along the cystic duct, common bile duct, hepatic artery, and/or portal vein		
N2	Metastases to periaortic, pericaval, superior mesenteric artery, and/or celiac artery lymph nodes		
M stage			
Mx	Distant metastases cannot be assessed		
M0	No distant metastases		
M1	Distant metastases		
UICC/AJCC stage grouping for gallbladder cancer, 7th edition, 2010			
Stage 0	Tis	N0	M0
Stage 1	T1	N0	M0
Stage 2	T2	N0	M0
Stage 3A	T3	N0	M0
Stage 3B	T1–3	N1	M0
Stage 4A	T4	N0–1	M0
Stage 4B	Any T	N2	M0
	Any T	N0	M1

with magnetic resonance cholangiography (MRC) or endoscopic retrograde cholangiopancreatography (ERCP) provide additional information for tumor staging and resectability: (i) distant metastases; (ii) hepatic invasion, (iii) bile duct invasion; (iv) lymph node metastasis, and (v) vascular invasion.[19-25] The overall accuracy of CT scan for staging GBC has been reported in the range of as 71–93%.[26] However, they are limited for detecting biliary invasion. Recent MR techniques, such as MRC and MR angiography (MRA), have improved the evaluation of bile ducts and vascular structures. Several recent studies describe the usefulness of MRI in the evaluation of GBC (Fig. 2). The sensitivity and specificity of MRI with MRC/MRA have been reported as 80–100% and 89–100% for bile duct invasion, 87% and 100% for vascular invasion, 67–100% and 86–89% for hepatic invasion, and 56–92% and 89–90% for lymph node metastasis, respectively.[27]

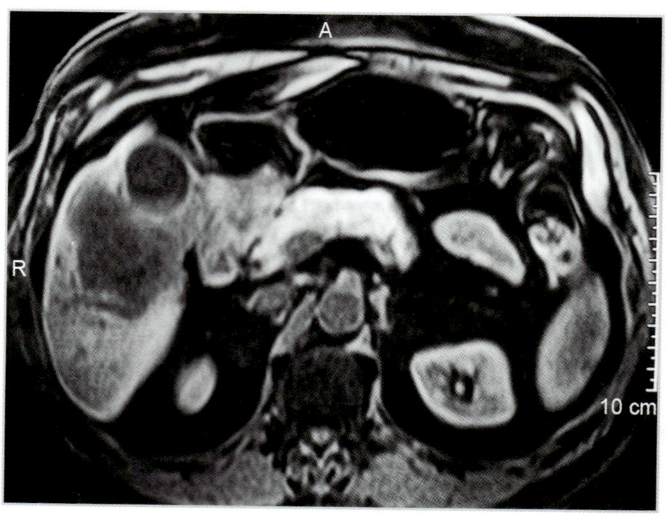

Fig. 2: Magnetic resonance imaging showing a locally advanced gallbladder carcinoma (GBC) with duodenal infiltration

Though 18-fluorodeoxyglucose positron emission tomography (FDG-PET) scans are increasingly being used in primary and metastatic disease, overall evidence supporting the use of PET in GBC is still limited and larger studies are necessary to determine the potential of these techniques to influence patient outcomes. In cases where there is suspicion of metastatic disease that is not completely appreciated on conventional cross-sectional studies, it may be helpful in delineating suspicious masses as malignant or benign. According to one study additional information from PET alters management in 23% of selected patients with GBC who were preoperatively staged using US/CT/MRI.[28]

Ca 19-9 has been increasingly used as a surrogate marker for the diagnosis and follow up of patients with GBC. However, there are no studies in literature to support the use of Ca 19-9 as a sole marker for diagnosis of GBC. CA19-9 is unfortunately increased not only in patients with pancreatic or biliary cancers but also in benign biliary diseases, which often present with jaundice and is therefore often misleading, reducing significantly the diagnostic accuracy of this marker.[29]

A staging laparoscopy is recommended prior to an exploration for GBC. A recent prospective study from an Indian center evaluating the role of staging laparoscopy in 409 patients with GBC reported an overall yield of 23.2% (95/409) for metastatic disease and obviated the need for a laparotomy.[30]

MANAGEMENT

Patients generally present in one of the three different ways: (i) GBC suspected preoperatively, (ii) GBC found intraoperatively at the time of cholecystectomy for presumed benign disease, and finally, (iii) a common situation wherein GBC is diagnosed incidentally on pathologic examination after cholecystectomy.[31]

Known or Suspected Gallbladder Cancer before Operation

Laparoscopic cholecystectomy is absolutely contraindicated when GBC is known or suspected preoperatively. Bile spillage and injuries to the biliary system occur more often during the laparoscopic procedure than during the conventional open method, and can convert potentially curable GBC to an incurable disease.[12] Thus, patients with preoperative findings suspicious for GBC should undergo open exploration with an intent to perform a radical cancer operation as a primary procedure if the diagnosis is confirmed intraoperatively.[32] In addition, the biological properties of the tumor, tumor stage, operative maneuvers and impact of pneumoperitoneum pressure may be involved in the onset of peritoneal and port site recurrence.[33]

Complete surgical resection is the only potential curative treatment of GBC. If GBC is suspected preoperatively, an open cholecystectomy should be performed to enable a complete evaluation and radical resection.[34]

Incidental Carcinoma of Gallbladder

Gallbladder carcinoma is diagnosed during or after cholecystectomy for presumed benign disease in 0.3–2% of cases.[35] A thickened gallbladder and obscured tissue planes should be looked with suspicion. This scenario presents an oncologic dilemma since dissection in a routine cholecystectomy usually occurs in a subserosal plane. This subserosal dissection would violate the tumor plane for lesions that penetrate the muscularis (T2 or greater) of the gallbladder. Therefore, if an incidental cancer is encountered intraoperatively, it is recommended that a radical resection is performed. In the event of a lack of experience, the procedure should be terminated and the patient referred to a tertiary surgical center with hepatobiliary specialization for appropriate staging and curative resection. Alternatively, if the surgeon has adequate experience and training, and the patient and surgical team are prepared for extensive surgery, a curative en bloc resection can be undertaken along with excision of the port sites. In most cases, GBC is diagnosed at histological examination following simple cholecystectomy, i.e. incidental GBC.

For those patients with Tis or T1a disease with clear resection margins, no further surgical intervention is needed. Perineural invasion, vascular invasion and lymph node metastases are extremely rare with T1a lesions, but their presence along with bile spillage during cholecystectomy are negative prognostic features and increase the rate of local recurrence. The addition of radical resection following cholecystectomy for T1a lesions has not improved the long-term survival of these patients.[36] There is controversy regarding the optimum management of incidentally detected T1b disease. Many authors reported long-term survival (95–100% 10-year survival) after simple cholecystectomy alone and did not recommend radical resection for T1b disease patients.[37] Many others reported treatment failure with locoregional recurrence after simple cholecystectomy for T1b disease and with 5-year survival of 37.5–68%[38] indicating that some patients with T1b disease were undertreated. As a consequence, some authors advocate aggressive surgery (extended cholecystectomy, wedge resection of gallbladder bed or segment IVb and V resection, N1 lymph node dissection) for pT1b disease.

For incidentally detected T2 or advanced GBC, a completion second radical operation is the only chance for long-term survival. There has also been a debate about the timing of revision surgery depending on the referral patterns. Completion second radical operation should be undertaken at the earliest following diagnosis of GBC, although there is no comparative study on the impact of the different intervals between initial cholecystectomy and second radical operation and the long-term survival.

EXTENT OF LIVER RESECTION FOR GALLBLADDER CANCERS

The extent of resection required in varies from a cholecystectomy with a wedge resection of the liver to extended right hepatectomy. A thorough understanding of the location of the tumor, the extent of local invasion, involvement of adjacent liver, lymph nodes, bile duct and vascular structures, patterns of disease spread, and tumor biology are critical to the surgical management of GBC. Liver involvement is most common in the adjacent segments IVB and V although involvement of the hilum can lead to extension beyond this area, even to the caudate lobe. It is necessary to achieve negative surgical margins of 2 cm around the tumor. The distance from the gallbladder neck to the right hepatic duct can be as little as 2 mm and the distance to the right sectoral ducts can be as little as 6 mm.[39] This proximity and the associated proximity of the gallbladder neck to the right portal pedicle poses limitation on the surgical margins in this area without compromising the integrity of the right liver. Thus some form of liver resection is necessary to achieve a R0 resection for tumors beyond stage T1a.

A variety of operations are performed for GBC.

Extended cholecystectomy: An extended cholecystectomy involves en bloc resection of the gallbladder in combination with a wedge resection of approximately 2 cm of adjacent liver tissue. Since this technique employs a nonanatomic resection of segments IVB and V, it has the potential limitations of increased blood loss, increased morbidity, and higher rates of positive surgical margins. In addition, the proximity of the gallbladder neck to the right hepatic duct and the bifurcation of the right portal vein limit the margin that can be achieved by this technique in this location. Therefore, the extended cholecystectomy should be reserved for T1b lesions and selected cases of nodular type T2 lesions where there is little or no hepatic invasion.

S4b + S5 resection: A formal anatomic resection of segments IVB and V has been advocated for early GBC and has the advantage of assuring a wider clearance of the tumor as well as proceeding along an anatomic plane of dissection, limiting the potential for blood loss and bile leak.

This resection may be appropriate for T2 lesions of the fundus and should be combined with a portal lymphadenectomy to resect local lymph nodes. Bile duct resection and reconstruction may be required to achieve R0 status. In cases where direct extension of tumor into adjacent organs (duodenum, stomach, or colon) is suspected, en bloc resection should be performed as it can be difficult to distinguish inflammation from invasion, especially in cases where there has been a prior cholecystectomy.

Surgical Steps of S4b + S5 Resection

After a laparotomy and assessment of resectability, the hepatoduodenal area is skeletonized and a complete nodal dissection is performed. The bile duct is identified and encircled with a yellow vessel loop. The hilum is dissected to skeletonize the portal vein and hepatic artery. The hepatic artery should preferably be isolated up to the right second-order branch.

The left portal vein is dissected and isolated from the horizontal portion to the umbilical fissure. The branches of the portal vein into the hepatic S4b originate from the right wall of the umbilical portion of the portal vein. The dissection and clamp/ligation of the S4b branch vein reveals a clear demarcation on the liver surface (Fig. 3).

The border of the S4b should be marked on the liver surface by electrocautery (Fig. 4).

The portal vein and hepatic artery branches into the right posterior segment of the liver are clamped with a vascular clip, which might reveal the demarcation line between the right anterior and the right posterior segments. This border is also marked by electrocautery (Fig. 5).

The hepatic S5 area can be identified by extending the upper border of S4b to the right until reaching the border between the right anterior and posterior segments (Figs 6 and 7).

Hepatic parenchymal transection is then started from the right or the left side. A vascular control is achieved

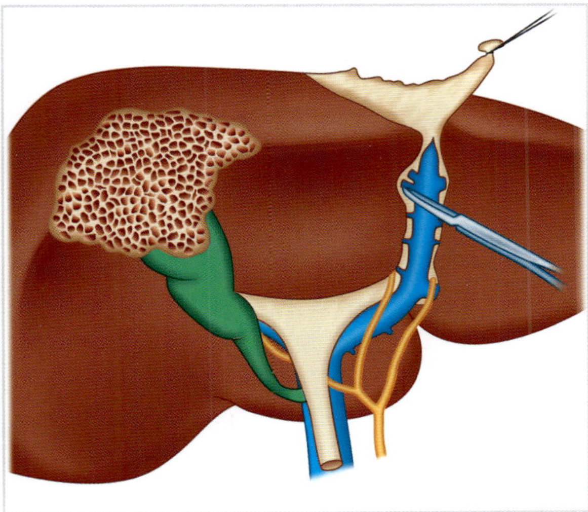

Fig. 3: S4b branch vein at the umbilical fissure

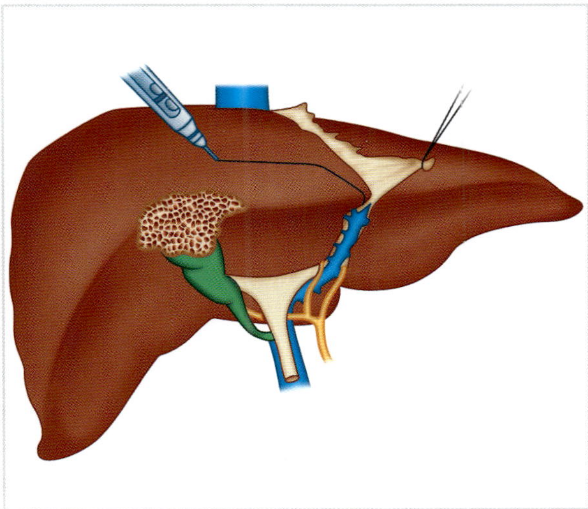

Fig. 4: S4b surface marking with electrocautery

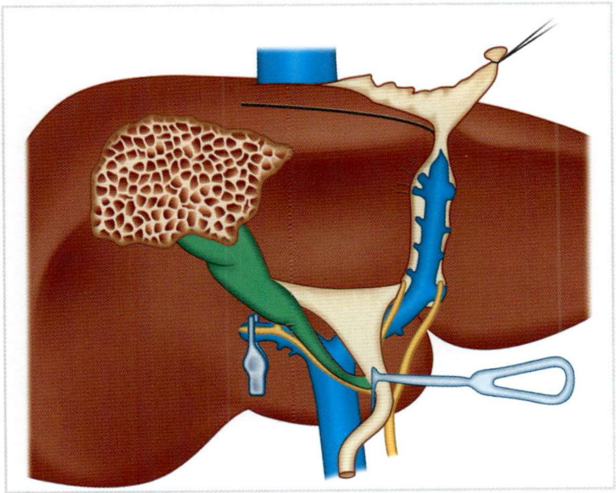

Fig. 5: Right posterior portal vein clamp

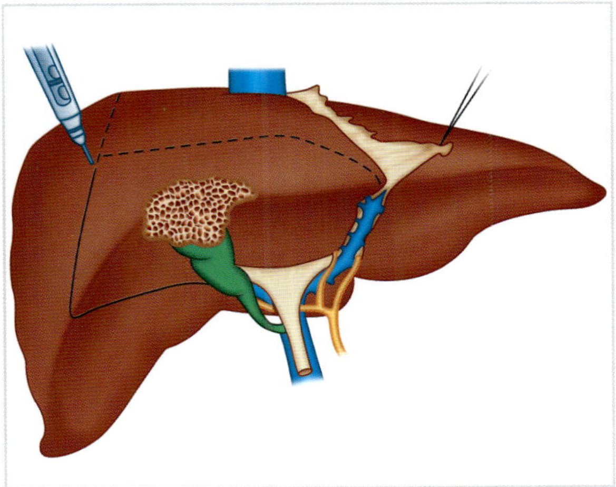

Fig. 6: Surface marking of S5 and joining 4b

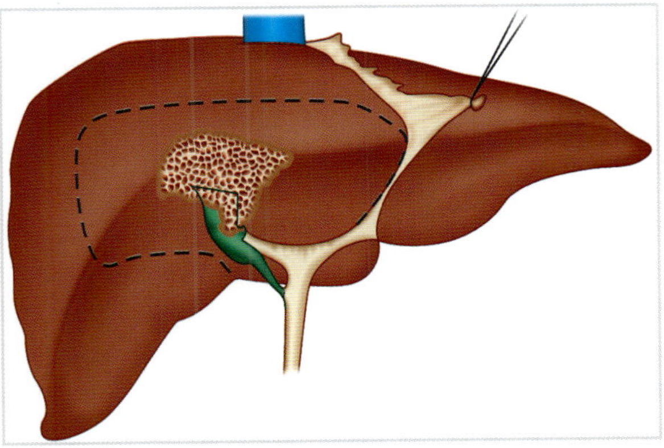

Fig. 7: Final transection area

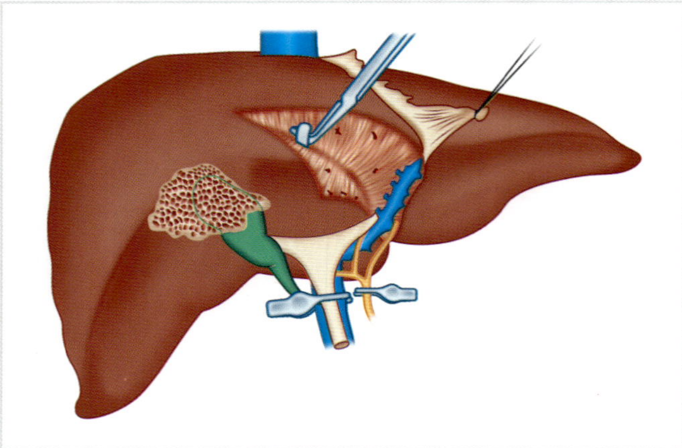

Fig. 8: Middle hepatic vein at the apex of transection

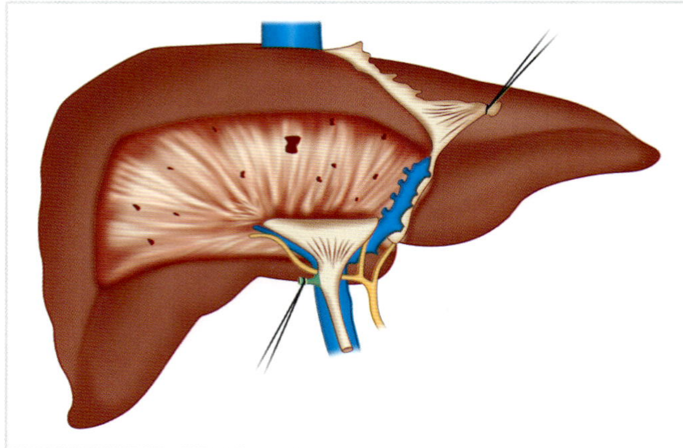

Fig. 9: S4b + 5 resection completed

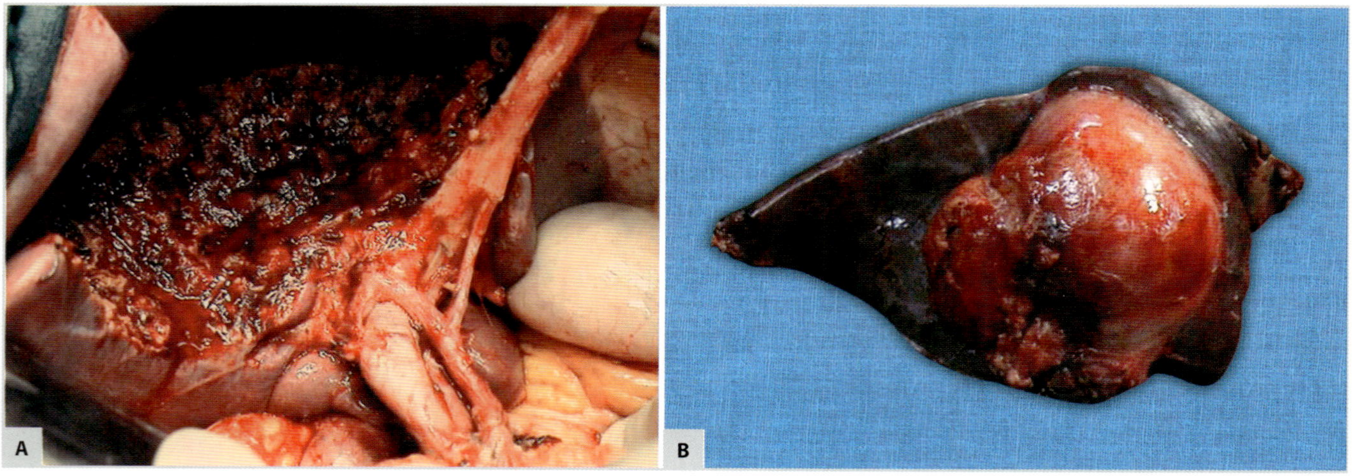

Figs 10A and B: S4b + 5 resection in situ

by clamping the main portal vein and the proper hepatic artery. Care should be taken to avoid any injury to the left hepatic duct.

The middle hepatic vein (MHV) usually comes into view at the apex of the resection and this should be carefully encircled and ligated (Fig. 8). Division of the MHV usually eases the exposure of the Glisson sheath of S5 where it branches from the right anterior Glisson sheath. This is the divided.

On releasing the vascular clamp on the portal vein and the hepatic artery, the demarcated area of S4b + 5 can be seen more clearly on the liver parenchymal surface (Figs 9 and 10).

Extended hepatic resection: T2 tumors of the body and neck as well as T3 tumors are likely to require resection of the right portal triad to achieve adequate tumor clearance and therefore an extended right hepatectomy with lymphadenectomy is necessary. Inclusion of the caudate lobe in the resection specimen may be required if there is suspicion of tumor invasion posterior to the porta hepatis and into segment I.

Combined hepatic resection with pancreatoduodenectomy: Japanese groups have been aggressive with resections for GBC and have often combined hepatectomy with pancreatoduodenectomy to achieve R0 resection in GBC with direct invasion of the duodenum or pancreas and the presence of peripancreatic lymph node involvement.[40] They report an acceptable morbidity and mortality; however, these results have not been reproduced at Western centers. Based on the available evidence, hepato-pancreatoduodenectomy cannot be recommended as a routine practice.

EXTENT OF LYMPHADENECTOMY

Lymph node involvement is an important prognostic factor in patients with GBC. Significant differences in survival have been observed in patients with or nodal metastases (5-year survival, 0–45% vs 58–77%).[41,42] The extent of lymph node dissection remains controversial and there is no randomized controlled trial (RCT) comparing the extent of lymph node dissection with survival. Based on the lymphatic spread pathways and the frequency of regional lymph node involvement in T2 and T3/T4 GBC, N1 and N2 regional lymph node dissection is indicated for T2–T4 disease. The role of para-aortic lymph node dissection in advanced GBC is not known. A retrospective analysis by Kondo, et al. showed that the routine para-aortic lymph node dissection provided no survival benefit for patients with para-aortic disease and the postoperative survival for patients with positive para-aortic lymph nodes without distant metastases was as poor as those patients with distant metastases.[43]

BILE DUCT RESECTION

It is important to know the status of cystic duct margin for patients with incidental detection of GBC. If it was negative for malignant cells, a bile duct resection cans safely be avoided. However, if the cystic duct margin was positive, the common duct is usually resected with the portal nodes and liver bed to optimize surgical margins, and a roux-en-y hepaticojejunostomy is fashioned. Removing the bile duct may also improve node clearance, and some surgeons prefer to do this routinely. A recent study did not show any survival benefit associated with elective bile duct resection.[44]

NEOADJUVANT AND ADJUVANT TREATMENTS FOR GBC

There is still no effective adjuvant therapy for GBC. The use of radiotherapy with or without chemotherapy in the adjuvant setting remains controversial. The roles of radiation, chemoradiation, and chemotherapy in the neoadjuvant settings remain to be better defined in prospective studies. Over the last decade, gemcitabine has been used in various combinations with cisplatin, oxaliplatin, 5-FU and capecitabine. A recent phase III study, conducted in 410 patients, including 149 patients with GBC, demonstrated that the addition of cisplatin to gemcitabine afforded significant progression-free survival (PFS) (median, 8.4 months versus 6.5 months.[45] Neoadjuvant chemotherapy has thus been used in locally advanced GBC with good responses documented in single centers. Preoperative chemotherapy enables the downsizing of initially unresectable locally advanced BTC, with radical resection made possible in a certain proportion of patients. Downsizing chemotherapy should be proactively carried out as a multidisciplinary treatment strategy for patients with initially unresectable GBC with the aim of expanding the surgical indication.[46] Molecularly targeted agents that inhibit angiogenesis and epidermal growth factor receptor (EGFR) pathways are entering clinical trials. Further understanding of the molecular mechanism of carcinogenesis coupled with more extensive genetic profiling of GBC patients will help to assess the therapeutic relevance of targeting a specific pathway.

PALLIATIVE CARE

Most patients with GBC present with advanced, incurable disease and are not candidates for surgical resection. Omental spread and distant disease can be readily seen on CT scans in many cases. The median survival of patients with advanced GBC who are deemed inoperable is only 2–4 months.[47] Thus, palliation of symptoms should be the primary goal. These patients typically suffer from jaundice, pain and gastrointestinal obstruction. Jaundice is best managed by percutaneous transhepatic cholangiography (PTC) decompression, with internalization if possible. Once jaundice resolves, palliative gemcitabine/capecitabine may be offered occasionally in conjunction with radiotherapy. The prognosis, however, remains dismal and a symptomatic care may possibly be a better option in such patients.

HILAR CHOLANGIOCARCINOMA

INTRODUCTION

Cholangiocarcinoma (CCA) arises from the malignant transformation of the bile duct epithelium and represents approximately 10% of all primary hepatobiliary cancers. These tumors occur most commonly in the proximal bile duct, at the hepatic duct confluence [hilar cholangiocarcinoma (HCCA) or Klatskin tumor], or in the distal CBD near the papilla (distal CCA) and pose a major challenge in the management due to close proximity to the vascular structures at the hilum and hepatodudodenal area. This chapter focuses on management issues specific to HCCA.

In earlier decades, surgical management of HCCA was primarily palliative with generally poor outcomes. Early reports of resection of HCCA typically involved resection of the biliary tree with hepaticojejunostomy. In the last two decades, surgical management of HCCA has been refined due to improvements in preoperative imaging and an enhanced appreciation of tumor growth characteristics. It is now recognized that liver resection is necessary to manage both direct hepatic invasion and the longitudinal intraductal extension that typically characterize HCCA.

EPIDEMIOLOGY AND RISK FACTORS FOR CHOLANGIOCARCIOMA

The incidence of CCA shows a large geographic variation. Moreover many registries have combined CCAs with primitive liver tumors and often peri-HCCA and the intrahepatic CCA have been considered as one and the same. Very high incidence rates (85/100,000) have been reported in northeast Thailand (where CCA represents approximately 85% of total primitive liver cancers) and other Asian countries such as China and Korea.[48,49] The Taiwan and Japanese population have relatively higher rates of CCA incidence (Hiroshima 3.05, Osaka 3.4, Taiwan 4.7/100,000) than others Asian populations such as Singapore, Philippines and Vietnam (1.45/100,000, 1.2/100,000 and 0.15/100,000 respectively). In comparison with the eastern countries, lower incidence rates occur in all Western countries.[49,50]

While the exact etiology of CCAs is unknown there are several conditions that are associated with an increased risk.

Primary sclerosing cholangitis (PSC): An autoimmune disease characterized by inflammation of the periductal tissues, ultimately resulting in multifocal strictures of the intrahepatic and extrahepatic bile ducts. The diagnosis of cancer in these patients can be extremely challenging since differentiating between benign and malignant strictures can be very difficult. The lifetime risk of CCA in patients with PSC is 10–40% and patients with PSC and bile duct cancer tend to be younger (30–50 years of age) than sporadic cases.[51]

Parasitic infections: Epidemiologic studies of high-incidence areas in Asia have demonstrated an association between liver fluke infection and CCA. These liver flukes (Opisthorcis viverrini infection in Thailand and Clonorchis sinensis in Japan, China and Korea) inhabit the biliary tree and gallbladder; eggs are secreted in bile and feces where they infect snails (first intermediate host) followed by fish (second intermediate host). Human infection occurs through ingestion of raw or undercooked fish.[52]

Congenital biliary cystic diseases: Choledochal cysts and Caroli's disease are associated with increased risk of CCA. Malignant degeneration is uncommon in choledochal cysts that have been completely excised early. The cancer risk is related to the duration of disease, with a 15% incidence after 20 years and an overall incidence in untreated cysts of 28%.[53,54] High incidence of cancer in patients with cystic diseases appears to be related to an abnormal choledochopancreatic duct junction that predisposes to reflux of pancreatic secretions into the biliary tree, bacterial contamination and chronic inflammation.[55]

Hepatolithiasis: Also known as recurrent pyogenic cholangiohepatitis or oriental cholangiohepatitis, is prevalent in Japan and parts of Southeast Asia. Obstruction of intrahepatic ducts leads to chronic recurrent episodes of cholangitis and stricture formation. Approximately 10% of patients will develop CCA.[56]

PATHOLOGY AND PATTERNS OF SPREAD

Adenocarcinoma is the most common histologic subtype. Three morphologic subtypes of CCA have been described: (i) sclerosing (infiltrating type: 70%), (ii) nodular (mass-forming type: 20%), and (iii) papillary (intraductal type: 5%) (Fig. 11).[19,20] Characteristics of the growth pattern of HCCA include (i) transmural invasion of bile ducts with radial extension into periductal tissue and adjacent structures and (ii) longitudinal extension along the bile ducts in the submucosa.[21] Mucosal extension is predominantly seen with papillary (intraductal) and nodular (mass-forming) tumors, while submucosal extension is mainly seen with sclerosing (infiltrating) tumors.[22]

The length of longitudinal extension is determined by the type of invasion, with a mean length of 6–10 mm for the submucosal spread and 10–20 mm for the mucosal spread.[23] Therefore, a gross surgical margin of more than 1 cm in the infiltrating type and more than 2 cm in the papillary and nodular types is recommended to achieve negative microscopic resection margins. Perineural invasion is a poor prognostic factor for survival and is seen in about 75% of cases of HCCA.[24,25] A gross similarity

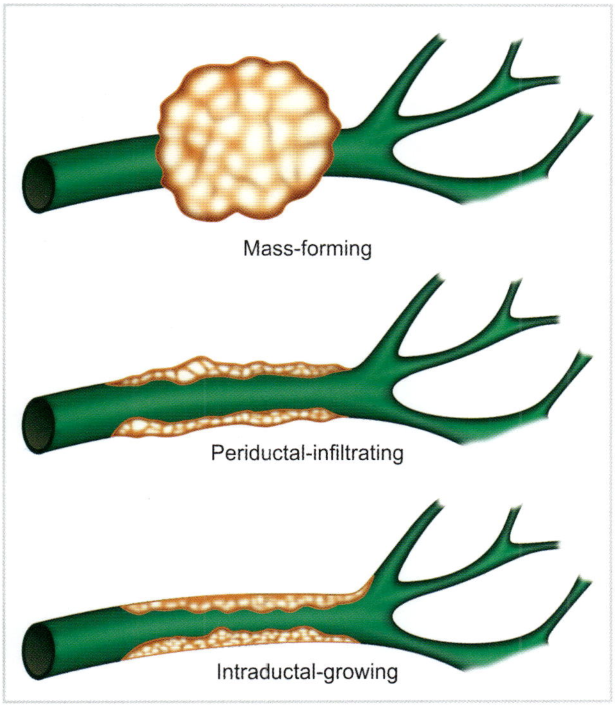

Fig. 11: Depiction of the morphology of the three classes of cholangiocarcinoma that have been proposed by the Liver Cancer Study Group of Japan

[*Source:* Hammill CW, Wong LL. Intrahepatic cholangiocarcinoma: A malignancy of increasing importance. J Am Coll Surg. 2008;207(4):594-603.]

between tumor and peritumoral inflammatory changes can make preoperative and intraoperative biopsies diagnostically challenging.

Radial extension of HCCA is very common and often results in invasion of the portal vein, hepatic arteries and the hepatic parenchyma adjacent to the hilar plate. Anatomically the caudate lobe (Segment I) lies in close proximity to the ductal confluence and is involved by either direct invasion or ductal extension. Some series have identified microscopic tumor infiltration into the caudate lobe in nearly all patients in with HCCA.[57]

Tumors at the biliary confluence involve the portal vein in 30% of cases and often result in hepatic lobar atrophy.[58,59] Though portal vein involvement may indicate an infiltrative tumor and have some negative impact, it translates into a therapeutic advantage as patients may tolerate more extensive surgical resections due to a hypertrophied contralateral lobe thereby decreasing the risk of perioperative mortality and enhancing the chances of negative resection margins.

Lymphatic metastases are found in 30–50% of patients undergoing resection. Hilar and pericholedochal lymph nodes are most commonly involved, followed by periportal, common hepatic, posterior pancreaticoduodenal, celiac and preaortic nodes.[60]

STAGING

So far there have been three classification systems that are used to evaluate HCCA. They are (a) modified Bismuth-Corlette system, (b) the AJCC/UICC TNM classification and (c) the MSKCC classification.

The Bismuth-Corlette classification system is most commonly used worldwide.[61,62] This classification, proposed by Bismuth and Corlette focuses exclusively on the level and extension of the tumor invasion along the biliary tree (Fig. 12).

The classification however fails to provide key information such as vascular encasement, lymph node involvement, distant metastases and atrophy of a part of the liver. In addition, variations in the anatomy of the branches often change the applicability of the Bismuth-Corlette system. Thus, it does not correlate with patient survival. This classification may serve only as a rough guide for surgical strategy (e.g. types I and II indicate local resection, type III indicates associated liver resection, and type IV indicates unresectability).

The AJCC staging is based largely on pathologic criteria (Table 2) and has little clinical applicability. In the current AJCC/UICC edition,[16] vessel invasion does affect the tumor category (T3 or T4), but it fails to indicate local resectability of the tumor. Moreover, patients with involvement of N1- and N2-lymph nodes are staged similarly. This is inappropriate since patients with metastatic disease to N2-level lymph nodes (celiac, periduodenal, or retroperitoneal) are not candidates for resection and should be considered to have M1 disease.

Although this classification fits within the standard TNM system for all cancers and appears simple, it is mostly used postoperatively and therefore fails to distinguish between the various surgical options. Its usefulness in the preoperative setting is thus limited.

The MSKCC classification made a specific attempt to predict resectability (Table 3).[58]

This staging system classifies HCCA according to three factors related to the local extension of the tumor, the location of bile duct involvement, and the presence of portal vein invasion and hepatic lobar atrophy. This staging system seems complicated. It does not evaluate the presence of nodal or distant metastases or the involvement of the artery. The MSKCC staging system was designed

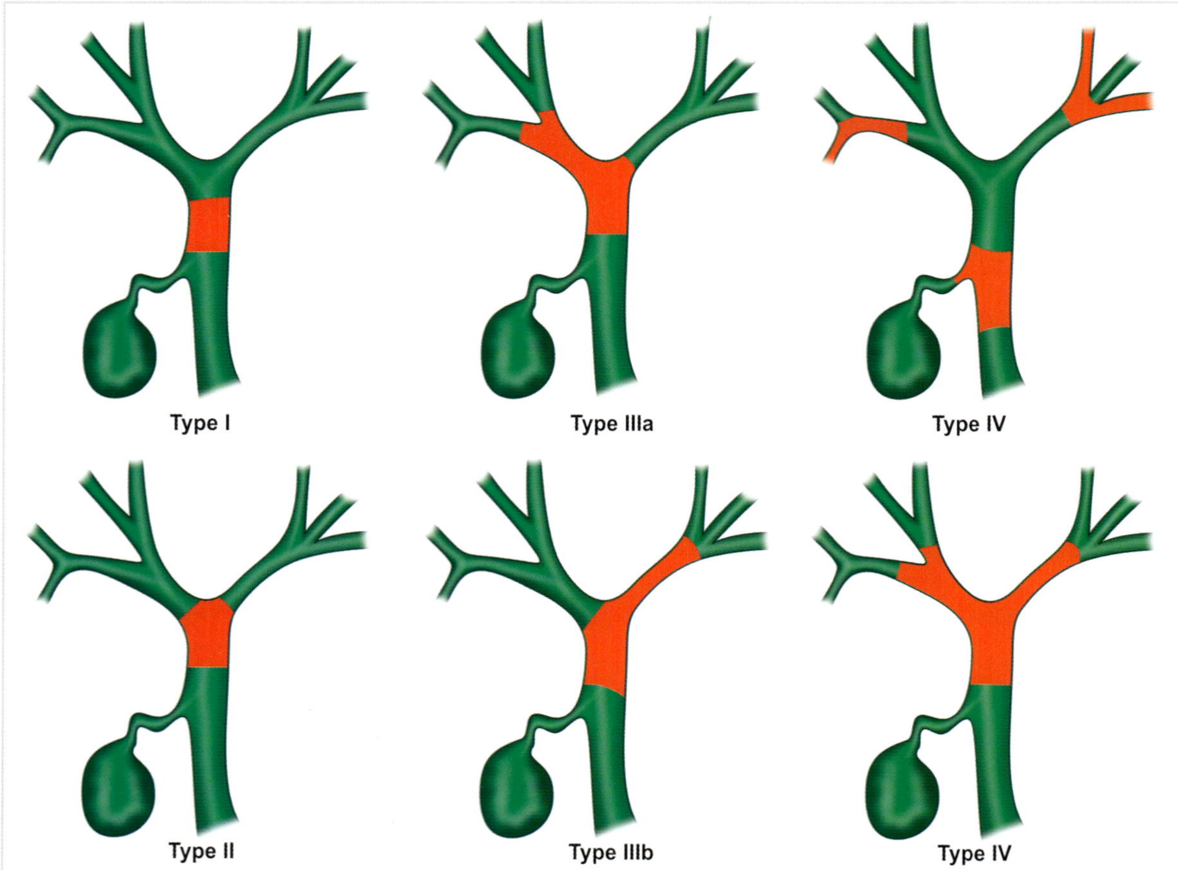

Fig. 12: Bismuth-Corlette classification for hilar cholangiocarcinoma. Type I: The tumor involves only the common hepatic duct below the confluence of the left and right hepatic duct; Type II: The tumor involves the hepatic bile duct confluence, but there is no invasion above the confluence; Type III: The tumor affects the right or left hepatic duct in addition to the biliary confluence; Type IIIa refers to the right hepatic duct, and Type IIIb refers to the left one; Type IV: The tumor involves both the right and left hepatic ducts and the confluence and reaches the secondary intrahepatic biliary system or involves multiple discontinuous sites in the right and left ducts

TABLE 2: TNM classification of extrahepatic bile duct tumors according to the AJCC/UICC, 7th edition

Stage	Tumor	Node	Metastases
Stage 0	Tis	N0	M0
Stage I	T1	N0	M0
Stage II	T2a/b	N0	M0
Stage IIIA	T3	N0	M0
Stage IIIB	T1–T3	N1	M0
Stage IVA	T4	Any N	M0
Stage IVB	Any T	N2	M0
	Any T	Any N	M1

Abbreviations: T0 = no evidence of a primary tumor; Tis = Carcinoma in situ; T1 = tumor is confined to the bile duct histologically; T2a = tumor invades the adipose tissue beyond the wall of the bile duct; T2b = tumor invades the adjacent hepatic parenchyma; T3 = tumor invades unilateral branches of the portal vein or hepatic artery; T4 = tumor invades the main portal vein or its branches bilaterally, the common hepatic artery, the second-order biliary radicals bilaterally, or the unilateral second-order biliary radicals with contralateral portal vein or hepatic vein involvement.

N0 = no regional lymph node metastasis; N1 = regional lymph node metastasis (cystic duct, CBD, hepatic artery, and portal vein); N2 metastasis to periaortic, pericaval, superior mesentery artery, and/or celiac artery nodes

M0 = no distant metastasis; M1 = distant metastasis

TABLE 3: Memorial Sloan-Kettering Cancer Center (MSKCC) classification for hilar cholangiocarcinoma

T Stage	Description
T1	The tumor involves the biliary confluence with unilateral involvement up to secondary biliary radicles. There is no portal vein involvement or liver atrophy
T2	The tumor involves the biliary confluence with unilateral involvement up to secondary biliary radicles. There is ipsilateral portal vein involvement or ipsilateral hepatic lobar atrophy
T3	The tumor involves the biliary confluence with bilateral involvement up to secondary biliary radicles, unilateral extension to secondary biliary radicles with contralateral portal vein involvement, unilateral involvement up to secondary biliary radicles with contralateral hepatic lobar atrophy, or main/bilateral portal vein involvement

exclusively on the basis of the criteria of resectability from a single institution, which may not correspond to the current concept of resectability for HCCA at many other centers.

A new staging system has been proposed by the International CCA group.[63] The proposed staging system provides information about the anatomical location of the tumor along the bile duct, the involvement of the portal vein, the involvement of the hepatic artery, the volume of the future remnant liver, the lymph node, and metastases status. Additionally, the tumor size, the tumor form, and the underlying disease are important pieces of information that are included to stage the HCCA better. The Bismuth-Corlette classification, the AJCC TNM classification as well as the Japanese Society of Biliary Surgery classification[64] is incorporated in this proposed staging. Though this staging system looks impressive and incorporates all parameters for data acquisition, it has not yet been validated.

PREOPERATIVE EVALUATION

As resectability is the prime motive behind evaluating patients with HCCA, the preoperative evaluation must address four critical determinants of resectability: (1) tumor extent within the biliary tree, (2) vascular invasion, (3) hepatic lobar atrophy, and (4) metastatic disease.[65]

Patients with HCCA often present with jaundice of varying degrees and most of the patients need some form of biliary drainage. It is imperative that an imaging should be performed prior to any intervention as placement of endobiliary stents and catheters may obscure critical information obtained on scans. Numerous reports in literature debate the superiority of MRI and MRCP over a triphasic CT scan and CT cholangiography, however both these modalities are complimentary from the clinical practice point of view. MRI with concurrent MRCP and three dimensional reconstruction of the biliary tree has been reported to have diagnostic accuracy comparable to invasive cholangiographic techniques such as ERCP or PTC.[66] Triple-phase CT scan provides valuable information regarding local spread, vascular invasion, lymph node involvement, lobar atrophy and presence of distant metastases.[67]

Cholangiography can provide detailed and accurate information on the anatomy of the biliary tree and can be performed via percutaneous transhepatic rout or retrograde endoscopic approaches ERCP and PTC provide dynamic images but require invasive access to the biliary system. Both techniques can detect biliary abnormalities and determine the location and extent of disease within the biliary tree. The choice between PTC and ERCP is generally dictated by the availability of local expertise and the anatomical characteristics of the tumor.[68] Selective cholangiography via endoscopic nasobiliary drainage (ENBD) and/or percutaneous transhepatic biliary drainage (PTBD) catheters provides precise information about the complicated segmental anatomy of the intrahepatic bile ducts and extent of cancer along the separated segmental bile ducts, which contributes toward designing a type of resection.[69] Both techniques have the capability of obtaining a cytologic diagnosis by bile duct brushings and can relieve jaundice by the placement of biliary stents. The sensitivity of biopsy and brush cytology for diagnosing CC has been low due to the desmoplastic reaction associated with the tumor which is characterized by the presence of few malignant cholangiocytes within an extensive fibrous stroma.[70] In a large prospective study, the sensitivity of routine cytology varied from 9% to 24% and the specificity varied from 61% to 100% with a high rate of inter-pathologist variation.[71]

Use of per-oral cholangioscopy, choledochoscopy and intraductal ultrasound (IDUS) have been limited to a very few centers in patients presenting with biliary strictures with no mass being detected on a CT scan. These modalities are more helpful in the setting of PSC that is relatively uncommon in a country like India. Experience with 18-FDG-PET is limited in HCCAs.

Serum tumor markers [CA 19-9 and S. carcinoembryonic antigen (CEA)] may support the diagnosis of a CCA. These tumors are not sensitive enough and are not very specific as well. In patients without PSC, serum Ca 19-9 values above 100 U/mL have a sensitivity of 53% and specificity of 75–90% for the diagnosis of a CCA.[72] In patients with PSC, serum Ca 19-9 levels above 100 U/mL have sensitivity of 75–89% and specificity of 80–86% for the diagnosis of CCA.[73]

The following clinical and radiological criteria define unresectability in patients with HCCA.[74-76]

Patient Factors

- Medically unfit for operation
- Cirrhosis/portal hypertension.

Local Tumor Invasion

- Bilateral hepatic duct involvement up to secondary biliary radicles
- Encasement or occlusion of the main portal vein

- Unilateral tumor extension to secondary biliary radicles with contralateral portal vein or hepatic artery encasement or occlusion
- Hepatic lobar atrophy with contralateral portal vein or hepatic artery encasement or occlusion
- Hepatic lobar atrophy with contralateral tumor extension to secondary biliary radicles.

Metastatic Disease

- Lymph node metastases beyond the hepatoduodenal ligament (N2 lymph nodes)
- Distant metastasis (e.g. lung, liver, peritoneal).

MANAGEMENT

Preoperative Biliary Drainage

The role of preoperative biliary drainage (PBD) in jaundiced patients remains controversial. Three RCTs have revealed that preoperative PTBD does not improve perioperative results.[77-79] A meta-analysis on PBD has failed to demonstrate any benefit and on the contrary reported that it may increase the risk of perioperative infections and a lengthen the postoperative hospital stay.[80] Nevertheless, PBD has been shown to be beneficial in the presence of cholangitis, severe malnutrition and coagulation abnormalities.[81] PTBD catheter is usually placed in the side that will remain after the resection, this drain is usually internalized, and the operation performed 4–6 weeks later once jaundice has resolved and the patient is fit for resection.

Portal Vein Embolization

Quite often, resection of a HCCA involves extended hepatic resections. Portal vein embolization (PVE) is a valuable preoperative measure when anticipating extensive liver resections with subsequent small hepatic residual volume.[82] Selective PVE can induce a compensatory hypertrophy of the remnant hepatic parenchyma and increase the volume of the anticipated future liver remnant (FLR) by 12–20%.[83] Currently, there is no evidence to support routine use of PVE for HCCA, but PVE should be considered for potentially resectable patients with normal liver function when anticipated FLR less than 20% of the total liver volume, or patients with compromised liver function when anticipated FLR less than 40% of the total liver volume. Most patients with HCCA present with jaundice and are considered to have cholestasis-induced compromised liver function.

Staging Laparoscopy

In a recent study of 195 patients treated from 2000 to 2010, the yield and accuracy of staging laparoscopy were considerably lower than those reported in previous studies. Laparoscopy avoided unnecessary laparotomy in only 14% of patients, with an accuracy of only 32%. A major limitation of laparoscopy is the inability to detect vascular or nodal involvement that is an important determinant of resectability. The use of staging laparoscopy for HCCA is thus not widely accepted.[84]

PRINCIPLES OF SURGICAL RESECTION IN HILAR CHOLANGIOCARCINOMA

The only chance of a cure for this type of cancer is complete surgical resection of the tumor (and perhaps liver transplantation in highly select cases). Most of these cancers have a dismal prognosis, and the current 5-year survival rate after surgery, even in select cases, rarely exceeds 30%.[85,86] Currently, no effective neoadjuvant or adjuvant therapy is available for enhancing the results of complete resection.[87]

Surgical management of HCCA has evolved in the last 20 years. Earlier reports of surgery for HCCA typically involved resection of the biliary tree with hepaticojejunostomy. The management was primarily palliative with generally poor outcomes. An improvement in preoperative imaging and an enhanced appreciation of tumor growth characteristics has resulted in the recognition that liver resection is necessary to manage both direct hepatic invasion and the longitudinal intraductal extension. Incorporation of major hepatic resection as a fundamental surgical strategy for this disease has increased the proportion of R0 resection with improved recurrence-free survival outcomes.[88]

A resection of the caudate lobe and part of segment IV, combined with a right or left hepatectomy, bile duct resection, lymphadenectomy of the hepatic hilum and sometimes vascular resection, is the standard surgical procedure for HCCA.

Intraoperative Frozen Section

Intraoperative frozen section should be performed whenever possible to confirm histologically negative margins. In a study from MSKCC intraoperative frozen section was shown to be 71.4% sensitive, 100% specific, and with a positive predictive value of 100% and negative predictive value of 80.2%.[89]

Should Caudate Lobe be Routinely Resected?

Most institutions perform caudate lobe resection selectively, depending on tumor location and a routine caudate lobe resection remains controversial. Japanese centers have been advocating a routine resection of the caudate lobe to improve margin clearance and overall survival. The caudate lobe ducts join the left and right hepatic ducts near their confluence, although the primary drainage is to the left hepatic duct.[20,21] This anatomic relationship explains the observation that the caudate lobe is involved by HCCA in 40–98% of patients.[90]

Portal Vein Resections

The philosophy that portal vein invasion is a contraindication to surgery has become outdated. Combined portal vein resection (PVR) and reconstruction may be necessary to obtain a negative surgical margin. PVR should be performed only when the vessel adheres to and cannot be freed from the tumor during the skeletonization of the hepatoduodenal ligament. Recently published results from an international, multicenter database of seven major hepatobiliary centers found that 30-d postoperative mortality was higher in the cohort of patients who underwent concomitant PVR (17.6% vs 10.6%, P = 0.03). However, no differences in long-term outcome were observed compared to patients who underwent hepatectomy without vein resection. The authors concluded that PVR should be undertaken when necessary to extirpate all disease.[91] PVR is more commonly performed in right-sided hepatectomy due to its technical feasibility. However, a vascular resection is often required in cases of left-sided hepatectomy for advanced tumors with left-sided predominance.[92]

No Touch Technique

Usually, resection of the portal vein is carried out when the vein is adherent to the tumor and cannot be freed. However, Neuhaus et al.[93] recommend routine resection of the portal vein to achieve more radical surgery. The concept is based on the fact that majority of hilar malignancies have microscopic perineural infiltration and the distance between the tumor and the outer layer of the adventitia of the portal vein is less than 1 mm even in cases without portal infiltration.[94] Thus, an attempt at portal dissection may result in exposure of the tumor even in a case without microscopic infiltration. In the "no-touch technique", an en bloc resection is achieved by placing vascular clamps on the left portal vein branch within the umbilical fissure as well as on the portal vein trunk, directly above the pancreatic head. The two vessels are the divided without dissecting the portal vein bifurcation. After this, an end-to-end venous anastomosis is performed. This reconstruction straightens the portal vein, avoiding the kinking frequently observed after right hepatic resections. According to Nagino,[95] this technique lacks scientific validation as mortality in patients who underwent hepatectomy with PVR was as high as 17% and that the cancer invasion of the resected portal vein was histologically observed in only 22% of patients who underwent combined resection. Under the concept of "no-touch technique", these findings strongly indicated that unnecessary PVR was performed in many patients.

Arterial resections: Recent advances in surgical techniques and experiences gained with liver transplantation have encouraged some aggressive hepatobiliary surgeons for the performance of hepatic artery resection with reconstruction. In a recently reported series of 53 patients undergoing concomitant hepatic artery resection with or without PVR, only one patient died in the postoperative period and two survived more than 5 years after surgery.[96]

Lymphadenectomy: Lymphadenectomy associated with resection of HCCA must include lymph nodes, lymphatic channels and nerves surrounding the portal vein and hepatic artery. Nodal invasion beyond the hepatoduodenal ligament, including para-aortic nodal metastases, has a dismal prognosis with a 5-year survival of 0–12%. In one study, the 5-year survival was 30% for node-negative patients, 15% for the patients with regional nodal metastases and 12% for those with para-aortic nodal metastases.[97] Therefore, routine lymph node dissection beyond the hepatoduodenal ligament is not generally recommended.[98]

Parenchyma preserving surgery: Minor liver resection (three segments or fewer, according to the Couinaud's nomenclature) may be one way to resolve the problem of the high morbidity and mortality after major liver resections. With the understanding that the hilar bifurcation of the bile ducts is near to liver segments IV, V and I; adequate liver resection of these segments (a central liver resection) together with the bile ducts has been performed for early stage tumors. Such a resection can preserve up to 35% more functional liver parenchyma than an extended hepatectomy. However, it has not been widely accepted as an alternative to extended hepatectomy because of its uncertain oncological equivalence and greater technical complexity.[99]

Hepatopancreatoduodenectomy (HPD): The concept of HPD was first introduced by Takasaki et al. for treatment of locally advanced gallbladder in 1980. HPD for biliary cancer remains controversial and is the most challenging operation employed by hepatobiliary surgeons. High mortality rates have precluded HPB surgeons from performing this procedure. However, data from a single Japanese center demonstrates that HPD can be performed with a low-mortality rate and offers an improved chance of long-term survival in selected patients.[95]

Liver Transplantation

Many cases of HCCA are often considered unresectable due to bilateral liver involvement and/or vascular encasement and since some cases of CCA arise on a background of PSC, liver transplantation has been suggested as a viable treatment option. If CCA is truly confined to the liver, transplantation offers the theoretical ability to achieve complete tumor clearance. The results of liver transplant for HCCA have been disappointing. The Cincinnati Transplant Tumor Registry reported 28% 5-year survival with a 51% tumor recurrence rate.[100] A protocol was developed at the Mayo Clinic (Mayo protocol) to treat selected patients with unresectable HCCA or HCCA arising in a setting of PSC. This protocol followed a strict regimen of preoperative staging and neoadjuvant treatment followed by orthotopic liver transplantation (OLT).[101] In 38 patients who underwent this protocol, the 5-year survival reported was 82%[102] and is purely due to a rigorous selection bias in favor of patients with biologically favorable disease. At present, OLT cannot be considered a standard form of therapy for HCCA for patients with resectable disease, but it does offer a potential option for patients with underlying PSC.

PALLIATION

For patients with HCCA who are not candidates for resection, the primary goal of therapy is to palliate the effects of biliary obstruction, such as intractable pruritus and cholangitis. Patients who may be offered nonoperative therapies such as chemotherapy and radiation therapy also require optimal hepatic function prior to beginning treatment, and thus often require biliary drainage as well. Palliation of jaundice can be accomplished by operative biliary-enteric bypass or endoscopic/percutaneous stenting of the biliary tree. Endoscopic intervention for proximal bile duct tumors is challenging as there may be an involvement of multiple bile ducts requiring two or more stents. PTBD is generally preferred. In the absence of cholangitis, unilateral biliary stenting is usually sufficient for relieving jaundice which can be subsequently internalized. Biliary drainage through an atrophic lobe usually does not relieve jaundice and should be avoided unless performed for cholangitis.[75] For patients with unresectable disease, metallic stents are preferred because of their superior long-term patency and relative cost-effectiveness compared with plastic stents.

SYSTEMIC AND OTHER TREATMENTS

There is no robust data supporting the use of neoadjuvant therapy, adjuvant therapy, photodynamic therapy or intraluminal brachytherapy in patients with HCCA. External radiation therapy alone has been disappointing in prolonging survival of patients with CCA. Both gemcitabine and cisplatin have been shown to have some activity against HCCA but more studies need to be done to define the role of systemic chemotherapy in the palliative treatment of HCCAs.

REFERENCES

1. Cleary SP, Dawson LA, Knox JJ, et al. Cancer of the gallbladder and extrahepatic bile ducts. Curr Probl Surg. 2007;44(7):396-482.
2. Randi G, Franceschi S, La Vecchia C. Gallbladder cancer worldwide: geographical distribution and risk factors. Int J Cancer. 2006;118:1591-602.
3. Nandakumar A, Gupta PC, Gangadharan P, et al. Geographic pathology revisited: development of an atlas of cancer in India. Int J Cancer. 2005;116:740-54.
4. Dhir V, Mohandas KM. Epidemiology of digestive tract cancers in India IV. Gallbladder and pancreas. Indian J Gastroenterol. 1999;18:24-8.
5. National Cancer Registry Programme. Consolidated Report of the Population Based Cancer Registries 1990–96. New Delhi: Indian Council of Medical Research; 2001.
6. Wistuba II, Gazdar AF. Gallbladder cancer: lessons from a rare tumour. Nat Rev Cancer. 2004;4:695-706.
7. Lowenfels AB, Walker AM, Althaus DP, et al. Gallstone growth, size, and risk of gallbladder cancer: an interracial study. Int J Epidemiol. 1989;18:50-4.
8. Unisa S, Jagannath P, Dhir V, et al. Population-based study to estimate prevalence and determine risk factors of gallbladder diseases in the rural Gangetic basin of North India. HPB. 2011; 13:117-25.

9. Mainprize KS, Gould SW, Gilbert JM. Surgical management of polypoid lesions of the gallbladder. Br J Surg. 2000;87:414-7.
10. Hawkins WG, DeMatteo RP, Jarnagin WR, et al. Jaundice predicts advanced disease and early mortality in patients with gallbladder cancer. Ann Surg Oncol. 2004;11(3):310-5.
11. Levy AD, Murakata LA, Rohrmann CA,. Gallbladder carcinoma: radiologicpathologic correlation. Radiographics. 2001;21:295-314.
12. Sumiyoshi K, Nagai E, Chij iwa K, et al. Pathology of carcinoma of the gallbladder. World J Surg. 1991;15:315-21.
13. Wakabayashi H, Ishimura K, Hashimoto N, et al. Analysis of prognostic factors after surgery for stage III and IV gallbladder cancer. Eur J Surg Oncol. 2004;30(8):842-6.
14. Yoshimitsu K, Honda H, Kaneko K, et al. Anatomy and clinical importance of cholecystic venous drainage: helical CT observations during injection of contrast medium into the cholecystic artery. AJR Am J Roentgenol. 1997;169(2):505-10.
15. Kondo S, Nimura Y, Kamiya J, et al. Mode of tumor spread and surgical strategy in gallbladder carcinoma. Langenbecks Arch Surg. 2002;387(5-6):222-8.
16. Edge SB, Byrd DR, Compton CC, et al. Perihilar Bile Ducts. In: AJCC Cancer Staging Handbook, 7th edition. Chicago, IL: Springer; 2010. p. 718.
17. Cziupka K, Partecke LI, Mirow L, et al. Outcomes and prognostic factors in gallbladder cancer: a single-centre experience. Langenbecks Arch Surg. 2012;397(6):899-907.
18. Fong Y, Jarnagin W, Blumgart LH. Gallbladder cancer: comparison of patients presenting initially for definitive operation with those presenting after prior noncurative intervention. Ann Surg. 2000;232(4):557-69.
19. Weinbren K, Mutum SS. Pathological aspects of cholangiocarcinoma. J Pathol. 1983;139:217-38.
20. Hammill CW, Wong LL. Intrahepatic Cholangiocarcinoma: A Malignancy of Increasing Importance. J Am Coll Surg. 2008;207(4):594-603.
21. Hayashi S, Miyazaki M, Kondo Y, et al. Invasive growth patterns of hepatic hilar ductal carcinoma. A histologic analysis of 18 surgical cases. Cancer. 1994;73:2922-9.
22. Sakamoto E, Nimura Y, Hayakawa N, et al. The pattern of infiltration at the proximal border of hilar bile duct carcinoma: a histologic analysis of 62 resected cases. Ann Surg. 1998;227: 405-11.
23. Ebata T, Watanabe H, Ajioka Y, et al. Pathological appraisal of lines of resection for bile duct carcinoma. Br J Surg. 2002;89:1260-7.
24. Yamaguchi K, Chijiiwa K, Saiki S, et al. Carcinoma of the extrahepatic bile duct: mode of spread and its prognostic implications. Hepatogastroenterology. 1997;44:1256-61.
25. He P, Shi JS, Chen WK, et al. Multivariate statistical analysis of clinicopathologic factors influencing survival of patients with bile duct carcinoma. World J Gastroenterol. 2002;8:943-6.
26. Kalra N, Suri S, Gupta R, et al. MDCT in the staging of gallbladder carcinoma. AJR Am J Roentgenol. 2006;186:758-62.
27. Kaza RK, Gulati M, Wig JD, et al. Evaluation of gallbladder carcinoma with dynamic magnetic resonance imaging and magnetic resonance cholangiopancreatography. Australas Radiol. 2006;50:212-7.
28. Corvera CU, Blumgart LH, Akhurst T, et al. 18F-fluorodeoxyglucose positron emission tomography influences management decisions in patients with biliary cancer. J Am Coll Surg. 2008;206(1):57-65.
29. Marrelli D, Caruso S, Pedrazzani C, et al. CA19-9 serum levels in obstructive jaundice: clinical value in benign and malignant conditions. Am J Surg. 2009;198:333-9.
30. Agarwal AK, Kalayarasan R, Javed A, et al. The role of staging laparoscopy in primary gallbladder cancer—an analysis of 409 patients: a prospective study to evaluate the role of staging laparoscopy in the management of gallbladder cancer. Ann Surg. 2013;258(2):318-23.
31. de Aretxabala X, Roa I, Burgos L, et al. Gallbladder cancer: an analysis of a series of 139 patients with invasion restricted to the subserosal layer. J Gastrointest Surg. 2006;10(2):186-92.
32. Weiland ST, Mahvi DM, Niederhuber JE, et al. Should suspected early gallbladder cancer be treated laparoscopically? J Gastrointest Surg. 2002;6:50-6.
33. Kondo S, Takada T, Miyazaki M, et al. Guidelines for the management of biliary tract and ampullary carcinomas: surgical treatment. J Hepatobiliary Pancreat Surg. 2008;15:41-54.
34. Sikora SS, Singh RK. Surgical strategies in patients with gallbladder cancer: nihilism to optimism. J Surg Oncol. 2006;93:670-81.
35. Misra S, Chaturvedi A, Misra NC, et al. Carcinoma of the gallbladder [comment]. Lancet Oncol. 2003;4:167-76.
36. Taner CB, Nagorney DM, Donohue JH. Surgical treatment of gallbladder cancer. J Gastrointest Surg. 2004;8:83-9.
37. Wakai T, Shirai Y, Yokoyama N, et al. Early gallbladder carcinoma does not warrant radical resection. Br J Surg. 2001;88:675-8.
38. Rodriguez Otero JC, Proske A, Vallilengua C, et al. Gallbladder cancer: surgical results after cholecystectomy in 25 patients with lamina propria invasion and 26 patients with muscular layer invasion. J Hepatobiliary Pancreat Surg. 2006;13:562-6.
39. Yamaguchi K, Chijiiwa K, Shimizu S, et al. Anatomical limit of extended cholecystectomy for gallbladder carcinoma involving the neck of the gallbladder. Int Surg. 1998;83:21-3.
40. Sasaki R, Itabashi H, Fujita T, et al. Significance of extensive surgery including resection of the pancreas head for the treatment of gallbladder cancer--from the perspective of mode of lymph node involvement and surgical outcome. World J Surg. 2006;30:36-42.
41. Shimada H, Endo I, Fujii Y, et al. Appraisal of surgical resection of gallbladder cancer with special reference to lymph node dissection. Langenbecks Arch Surg. 2000;385:509-14.
42. Chijiiwa K, Noshiro H, Nakano K, et al. Role of surgery for gallbladder carcinoma with special reference to lymph node metastasis and stage using Western and Japanese classification systems. World J Surg. 2000;24:1271-6.
43. Kondo S, Nimura Y, Hayakawa N, et al. Regional and para-aortic lymphadenectomy in radical surgery for advanced gallbladder carcinoma. Br J Surg. 2000;87:418-22.
44. Yokomizo H, Yamane T, Hirata T, et al. Surgical treatment of pT2 gallbladder carcinoma: A reevaluation of the therapeutic effect

of hepatectomy and extrahepatic bile duct resection based on the long-term outcome. Ann Surg Oncol. 2007;14:1366-73.

45. Valle JW, Wasan HS, Palmer DD, et al. Gemcitabine with or without cisplatin in patients (pts) with advanced or metastatic biliary tract cancer (ABC): Results of a multicenter, randomized phase III trial (the UK ABC-02 trial). J Clin Oncol. 2009;27(15 suppl):4503.
46. Kato A, Shimizu H, Ohtsuka M, et al. Surgical resection after downsizing chemotherapy for initially unresectable locally advanced biliary tract cancer: a retrospective single-center study. Ann Surg Oncol. 2013;20(1):318-24.
47. Ito H, Matros E, Brooks DC, et al. Treatment outcomes associated with surgery for gallbladder cancer: a 20-year experience. J Gastrointest Surg. 2004;8(2):183-90.
48. Poomphakwaen K, Promthet S, Kamsa-Ard S, et al. Risk factors for cholangiocarcinoma in Khon Kaen, Thailand: a nested case-control study. Asian Pac J Cancer Prev. 2009;10:251-8.
49. Shin HR, Oh JK, Masuyer E, et al. Comparison of incidence of intrahepatic and extrahepatic cholangiocarcinoma--focus on East and South-Eastern Asia. Asian Pac J Cancer Prev. 2010;11:1159-66.
50. Ferlay J, Shin HR, Bray F, et al. GLOBOCAN 2008 v2.0, Cancer Incidence and Mortality Worldwide: IARC Cancer Base No. 10 [Internet]. Lyon, France: International Agency for Research on Cancer; 2010.
51. Broome U, Olsson R, Loof L, et al. Natural history and prognostic factors in 305 Swedish patients with primary sclerosing cholangitis. Gut. 1996;38:610-5.
52. Watanapa P, Watanapa WB. Liver fluke-associated cholangiocarcinoma. Br J Surg. 2002;89:962-70.
53. Lipsett PA, Pitt HA, Colombani PM, et al. Choledochal cyst disease. A changing pattern of presentation. Ann Surg. 1994;220:644-52.
54. Chijiiwa K, Koga A. Surgical management and long-term follow-up of patients with choledochal cysts. Am J Surg. 1993;165: 238-42.
55. Tanaka K, Ikoma A, Hamada N, et al. Biliary tract cancer accompanied by anomalous junction of pancreaticobiliary ductal system in adults. Am J Surg. 1998;175:218-20.
56. Chu KM, Lo CM, Liu CL et al. Malignancy associated with hepatolithiasis. Hepatogastroenterology. 1997;44:352-7.
57. Nimura Y, Hayakawa N, Kamiya J, et al. Hepatic segmentectomy with caudate lobe resection for bile duct carcinoma of the hepatic hilus. World J Surg. 1990;14:535-43.
58. Jarnagin WR, Fong Y, DeMatteo RP, et al. Staging, resectability, and outcome in 225 patients with hilar cholangiocarcinoma. Ann Surg. 2001;234:507-17.
59. Nagorney DM, Kendrick ML. Hepatic resection in the treatment of hilar cholangiocarcinoma. Adv Surg. 2006;40:159-71.
60. Kitagawa Y, Nagino M, Kamiya J, et al. Lymph node metastasis from hilarcholangiocarcinoma: audit of 110 patients who underwent regional and para-aortic node dissection. Ann Surg. 2001;233:385-92.
61. Bismuth H, Corlette MB. Intrahepatic cholangioenteric anastomosis in carcinoma of the hilus of the liver. Surg Gynecol Obstet. 1975;140:170-8.
62. Bismuth H, Nakache R, Diamond T. Management strategies in resection for hilar cholangiocarcinoma. Ann Surg. 1992;21 5:31-8.
63. DeOliveira ML, Schulick RD, Nimura Y, et al. New staging system and a registry for perihilar cholangiocarcinoma. Hepatology. 2011;53:1363-71.
64. Japanese Society of Biliary Surgery. General Rules for Surgical and Pathological Studies on Cancer of Biliary Tract, 5th edition. Tokyo, Japan: Kanehara Publishers; 2003.
65. Burke EC, Jarnagin WR, Hochwald SN, et al. Hilar cholangiocarcinoma: patterns of spread, the importance of hepatic resection for curative operation, and a presurgical clinical staging system. Ann Surg. 1998;228:385-94.
66. Rösch T, Meining A, Frühmorgen S, et al. A prospective comparison of the diagnostic accuracy of ERCP, MRCP, CT, and EUS in biliary strictures. Gastrointest Endosc. 2002;55:870-6.
67. Tillich M, Mischinger HJ, Preisegger KH, et al. Multiphasic helical CT in diagnosis and staging of hilar cholangiocarcinoma. AJR Am J Roentgenol. 1998;171:651-8.
68. Khan SA, Davidson BR, Goldin R, et al. Guidelines for the diagnosis and treatment of cholangiocarcinoma: consensus document. Gut. 2002;51(Suppl 6):VI1-9.
69. Nimura Y. Preoperative biliary drainage before resection for cholangiocarcinoma (Pro). HPB (Oxford). 2008;10:130-3.
70. Lazaridis KN, Gores GJ. Cholangiocarcinoma. Gastroenterology. 2005;128:1655-67.
71. Harewood GC, Baron TH, Stadheim LM, et al. Prospective, blinded assessment of factors influencing the accuracy of biliary cytology interpretation. Am J Gastroenterol. 2004;99:1464-9.
72. Lamerz R. Role of tumour markers, cytogenetics. Ann Oncol. 1999;10(Suppl 4):145-9.
73. Chalasani N, Baluyut A, Ismail A, et al. Cholangiocarcinoma in patients with primary sclerosing cholangitis: a multicenter case-control study. Hepatology. 2000;31:7-11.
74. Nathan H, Aloia TA, Vauthey JN, et al. A proposed staging system for intrahepatic cholangiocarcinoma. Ann Surg Oncol. 2009;16:14-22.
75. Jarnagin WR, Shoup M. Surgical management of cholangiocarcinoma. Semin Liver Dis. 2004;24:189-99.
76. Burke EC, Jarnagin WR, Hochwald SN, et al. Hilar Cholangiocarcinoma: patterns of spread, the importance of hepatic resection for curative operation, and a presurgical clinical staging system. Ann Surg. 1998;228:385-94.
77. Hatfield AR, Tobias R, Terblanche J, et al. Preoperative external biliary drainage in obstructive jaundice. A prospective controlled clinical trial. Lancet. 1982;2:896-9.
78. McPherson GA, Benjamin IS, Hodgson HJ. Pre-operative percutaneous transhepatic biliary drainage: the results of a controlled trial. Br J Surg. 1984;71:371-5.
79. Pitt HA, Gomes AS, Lois JF, et al. Does preoperative percutaneous biliary drainage reduce operative risk or increase hospital cost? Ann Surg. 1985;201:545-53.
80. Sewnath ME, Karsten TM, Prins MH, et al. A meta-analysis on the efficacy of preoperative biliary drainage for tumors causing obstructive jaundice. Ann Surg. 2002;236:17-27.

81. Aly EA, Johnson CD. Preoperative biliary drainage before resection in obstructive jaundice. Dig Surg. 2001;18:84-9.

82. Nagino M, Kamiya J, Nishio H, et al. Two hundred forty consecutive portal vein embolizations before extended hepatectomy for biliary cancer: surgical outcome and long-term follow-up. Ann Surg. 2006;243:364-72.

83. Abdalla EK, Barnett CC, Doherty D, et al. Extended hepatectomy in patients with hepatobiliary malignancies with and without preoperative portal vein embolization. Arch Surg. 2002;137: 675-80.

84. Ruys AT, Busch OR, Gouma DJ, et al. Staging laparoscopy for hilar cholangiocarcinoma: is it still worthwhile? Ann Surg Oncol. 2011;18:2647-53.

85. DeOliveira ML, Cunningham SC, Cameron JL, et al. Cholangiocarcinoma: thirty-one-year experience with 564 patients at a single institution. Ann Surg. 2007;245:755-62.

86. Aljiffry M, Abdulelah A, Walsh M, et al. Evidence-based approach to cholangiocarcinoma: a systematic review of the current literature. J Am Coll Surg. 2009;208:134-47.

87. Lazaridis KN, Gores GJ. Cholangiocarcinoma. Gastroenterology. 2005;128:1655-67.

88. Ito F, Agni R, Rettammel RJ, et al. Resection of hilar cholangiocarcinoma: concomitant liver resection decreases hepatic recurrence. Ann Surg. 2008;248:273-9.

89. Endo I, House MG, Klimstra DS, et al. Clinical significance of intraoperative bile duct margin assessment for hilar cholangiocarcinoma. Ann Surg Oncol. 2008;15:2104-12.

90. Nimura Y, Hayakawa N, Kamiya J, et al. Hepatic segmentectomy with caudate lobe resection for bile duct carcinoma of the hepatic hilus. World J Surg. 1990;14:535-43.

91. de Jong MC, Marques H, Clary BM, et al. The impact of portal vein resection on outcomes for hilar cholangiocarcinoma: a multi-institutional analysis of 305 cases. Cancer. 2012;118:4737-47.

92. Nagino M, Nimura Y, Nishio H, et al. Hepatectomy with simultaneous resection of the portal vein and hepatic artery for advanced perihilar cholangiocarcinoma: an audit of 50 consecutive cases. Ann Surg. 2010;252:115-23.

93. Neuhaus P, Thelen A, Jonas S, et al. Oncological superiority of hilar en bloc resection for the treatment of hilar cholangiocarcinoma. Ann Surg Oncol. 2012;19:1602-8.

94. Ebata T, Nagino M, Kamiya J, et al. Hepatectomy with portal vein resection for hilar cholangiocarcinoma: audit of 52 consecutive cases. Ann Surg. 2003;238:720-7.

95. Nagino M. Cutting edge of an aggressive surgical approach for perihilar cholangiocarcinoma. Updates Surg. 2013;65:81-3.

96. Igami T, Nishio H, Ebata T, et al. Surgical treatment of hilar cholangiocarcinoma in the "new era": the Nagoya University experience. J Hepatobiliary Pancreat Sci. 2010;17:449-54.

97. Kitagawa Y, Nagino M, Kamiya J, et al. Lymph node metastasis from hilar cholangiocarcinoma: audit of 110 patients who underwent regional and paraaortic node dissection. Ann Surg. 2001;233:385-92.

98. Schiffman SC, Reuter NP, McMasters KM, et al. Overall survival peri-hilar cholangiocarcinoma: R1 resection with curative intent compared to primary endoscopic therapy. J Surg Oncol. 2012;105:91-6.

99. Sotiropoulos GC, Lang H, Molmenti EP, et al. Partial or complete mesohepatectomy combined with resection of the hilar bifurcation in cases of Klatskin tumors: a reasonable strategy? Am J Surg. 2009;198:297-8.

100. Meyer CG, Penn I, James L. Liver transplantation for cholangiocarcinoma: results in 207 patients. Transplantation. 2000;69:1633-7.

101. Shimoda M, Farmer DG, Colquhoun SD. et al. Liver transplantation for cholangiocellular carcinoma: analysis of a single-center experience and review of the literature. Liver Transpl. 2001;7:1023-33.

102. Rea DJ, Heimbach JK, Rosen CB, et al. Liver transplantation with neoadjuvant chemoradiation is more effective than resection for hilar cholangiocarcinoma. Ann Surg. 2005;242:451-8.

34 Pancreatic Malignancies

Shailesh V Shrikhande, Palepu Jagannath

INTRODUCTION

Pancreatic cancer (PC) is a malignancy with a dismal prognosis in which the mortality rate nearly equals its incidence. Incidence of PC in South-Central and South-West Asia versus Western countries is 0.2–6/100,000 versus 1.5–12.6/100,000 persons per year, respectively.[1–3] The approximate annual burden of PC in India is 14,230 and the incidence of 2.4/100,000 persons per year is low compared with Europe, America and Japan.[4] The 5 year relative survival rate was 4.1% for PC in a population-based study from Mumbai.[5]

While the management of PC is increasingly multimodal, radical surgery remains the only treatment option with a chance of cure.

Ductal adenocarcinoma is the most frequent tumor of the pancreas with predominant localization within the pancreatic head. This chapter mainly deals with periampullary tumors (i.e. tumors that arise within 2 cm of the major papilla in the duodenum) including classical pancreatic ductal adenocarcinoma of the head.[6] However, it also completes the spectrum of pancreatic malignancies by covering PC of body and tail and other uncommon pancreatic tumors.

RISK FACTORS AND MOLECULAR BIOLOGY

The precise cause of PC remains unknown. Though environmental factors have been implicated, evidence exists of a causative role only for tobacco use. Smokers have a 2.5–3.6% increased risk as compared to nonsmokers; the greater and longer exposure to smoke, the greater the risk.[7] Other possible risk factors are alcohol, coffee, and use of aspirin. Some studies have shown an increased incidence in those with a history of diabetes or chronic pancreatitis (CP), and some evidence exists that cirrhosis, a high-fat, high-cholesterol diet, and previous history of cholecystectomy are associated with an increased incidence.[8-11] Approximately, 5–10% of patients with PC have a family history of PC.[12] An increased risk has been observed with blood group A, B, or AB as compared with blood group O.[13]

The cell type of origin of pancreatic ductal adenocarcinoma has been controversial. Molecular analysis has demonstrated a step by step accumulation of certain genetic and epigenetic alterations from pancreatic intraepithelial neoplasms to invasive ductal adenocarcinoma.[14,15]

CLINICAL FEATURES

Tumor location dictates the symptomatology and timing of presentation of patients with PC. Ampullary carcinomas tend to present the earliest owing to the relatively early obstruction of the bile duct and the resultant painless obstructive jaundice—often the first point of contact between the patient and the surgeon. In this location, "waxing and waning" of obstructive jaundice may be noted in approximately 30% of patients.[16] Pancreatic head cancer may also present as painless, progressive, obstructive jaundice. In contrast, tumors of the body and tail tend to present rather late with recent onset upper abdominal pain with or without a palpable abdominal mass.[17] A majority of body and tail PCs are locally advanced or metastatic at the time of presentation. Other common presenting symptoms of carcinomas of the pancreatic head, neck, body and tail are asthenia (> 80%), anorexia (> 80%), weight loss (> 80%) and upper abdominal pain (70–80%).[18] Features suggestive of gastric outlet obstruction may be encountered in advanced carcinomas of the pancreas.

Upper abdominal pain radiating to the back, though not always, is often a sign of an advanced tumor. New symptoms developing over an established case of CP should arouse suspicion of PC.[18]

Clinical signs vary from jaundice in ampullary and pancreatic head cancer with a palpable gallbladder (Courvoisier's law) to a hard, fixed palpable lump in the left hypochondrium in tumors of the body and tail. Patients may have enlarged supraclavicular lymph nodes or even peritoneal deposits on per rectal examination (Blumer's shelf) in advanced cases. Ascites is a sign of advanced disease.

PRETHERAPY INVESTIGATIONS

Apart from routine laboratory blood tests, an obstructive pattern of liver function tests is encountered in pancreatic head and ampullary lesions obstructing the lower common bile duct. Assessment of coagulation profile (bleeding time, clotting time, international normalized ratio) in obstructive jaundice is crucial prior to referral for biopsy (if indicated) and even prior to definitive resectional surgery. A deranged coagulation profile warrants correction with injection of vitamin K for three consecutive days. Specific attention needs to be given to the renal function as well as blood sugar levels. The tumor marker, serum CA 19-9, is routinely measured in pancreatic carcinomas. Its overall sensitivity is approximately 80% with a specificity of 90%.[19] In terms of predicting unresectability, levels greater than 1,000 U/mL have been found to be linked to unresectable disease.[19] However, elevated CA 19-9 levels are also encountered in nonmalignant obstructive jaundice, liver cirrhosis, pancreatitis, gastric cancer and even cholecystitis.[18] Thus, raised CA 19-9 levels can be more specific for advanced or metastatic disease in a nonjaundiced patient. In such situations, it can be a good complementary test to guide treatment pathways. To cite an example, a staging laparoscopy would be indicated in a PC that appears to be localized and resectable on imaging but the patient has high serum CA 19-9 levels in the absence of obstructive jaundice. Serum CA 19-9 levels are also useful (in combination with objective radiologic criteria) to monitor response to chemotherapy and radiotherapy.

Anemia (sometimes associated with waxing and waning jaundice) may be encountered in patients with periampullary carcinoma where repeated sloughing off of the tumor can cause gastrointestinal bleeding and melena.[20]

Imaging and Staging of Pancreatic Cancer

Accurate preoperative imaging and staging of PC helps avoid unnecessary and unsuccessful surgical explorations. The modalities commonly employed are multidetector computed tomography (MDCT) scans as well as magnetic resonance imaging (MRI) and magnetic resonance cholangiopancreatography (MRCP) scans. In a small subset of patients, endosonography (EUS) and positron emission tomography (PET) scans may also be used to guide treatment. The aim of imaging should be to objectively classify PC into one of the four categories mentioned below:

- Resectable PC
- Borderline resectable PC[21](see section later)
- Locally advanced and unresectable PC
- Metastatic PC

In a recent systematic review by the first author evaluating 66 studies from 1990–2011,[22] MDCT and MRI/MRCP were shown to have comparable sensitivity and specificity rates for diagnosis and staging of PC. EUS offered the best sensitivity (approaching 100%) and specificity rates (approaching 95%) for lesions less than 2 cm, lesions that were not clearly detected/delineated but yet strongly suspected, and to assess response of borderline resectable PC following neoadjuvant chemoradiation with regards to vascular involvement. Improved staging was noted when PET-CT scans were added to pretreatment evaluation of borderline resectable and locally advanced PC.

Furthermore, high quality imaging forewarns pancreatic surgeons regarding aberrant anatomy which is a fairly common feature in the hepatic-pancreatic-biliary (HPB) region.

In India, ultrasonography is amongst the most widely available and often the first investigative imaging modality used to assess patients with jaundice or even nonspecific abdominal pain. The presence of obvious hepatic metastases, para-aortic lymph nodes or ascites on ultrasonography can obviate the need for further imaging. However, the retroperitoneal location of the pancreas obscured often by bowel gas, as well as the operator-dependent nature of the investigation preclude the use of ultrasonography as an accurate staging modality in this era of modern imaging.

CONFIRMATION OF DIAGNOSIS

A confirmation of diagnosis by biopsy in a resectable pancreatic mass suspected to be PC is not indicated. Percutaneous fine needle aspiration cytology/biopsy has been shown to be associated with needle tract seeding. However, a tissue diagnosis is a necessity in borderline resectable (EUS guided) and locally advanced unresectable (percutaneous) PC following which appropriate chemoradiotherapy can be administered. A negative biopsy in a lesion with a high suspicion of malignancy, should always be questioned and should not preclude resection.[6]

OBSTRUCTIVE JAUNDICE IN RESECTABLE PANCREATIC HEAD AND PERIAMPULLARY CANCER: MANAGEMENT APPROACH

Drainage of obstructive jaundice in a resectable case of PC should be considered in the following situations:

- Signs and symptoms of cholangitis (viz. fever with chills coupled raised white blood cell counts)
- Deranged synthetic function and coagulation profile (viz. raised prothrombin activity)
- Serum bilirubin above 15 mg% even in an symptomatic patient with otherwise well maintained laboratory parameters
- Major associated comorbidities/frail patient/poor nutritional status
- When time taken for specialist referral and for investigations is likely to result in delay in surgery.

The above mentioned situations are not absolute indications but can serve as best available guiding principles based on data that has been accumulated over the years and the need to be selective while considering drainage of obstructive jaundice prior to surgery cannot be over emphasized. The benefits of routine preoperative stenting over nonstenting had been unclear for many years.[23] A recent randomized trial from Netherlands confirmed that routine preoperative biliary drainage by endoscopic retrograde cholangiopancreatography with stenting in pancreas head cancer is not indicated and was associated with increased rate of complications.[24]

Endoscopic retrograde cholangiopancreatography with plastic stenting (higher chances of stent block) is commonly performed in cases that are likely to be resected within a few weeks of stenting; in borderline resectable PC requiring neoadjuvant treatment prior to surgery and in those where the delay in surgery is anticipated to be over 6 weeks,[25,26] a self-expanding metal stent (SEMS) is increasingly preferred (lower chances of stent block).

Effect of Biliary Stenting on Outcomes of Pancreaticoduodenectomy

There is evidence to suggest that biliary stenting may be harmful since their placement inevitably contaminates the bile.[27] The senior author examined the effects of preoperative biliary stenting on early outcome after pancreaticoduodenectomy (PD).[28] In a series of 144 PDs, it was observed that positive intraoperative bile culture was associated with higher morbidity and mortality rates following PD. A positive culture in the stented group was related only to complicated stenting and if duration of stenting was less than 6 weeks. Uncomplicated stenting was not associated with increased morbidity or mortality.[28] In view of these findings and considering the inflammation associated with stenting, it seems prudent to wait for 4–6 weeks following biliary stenting prior to proceeding with PD.

TREATMENT

Surgery for Pancreatic Cancer

Radical surgical resection is the only treatment option with a chance of cure in resectable and borderline resectable PC.

Pancreatic Head and Periampullary Cancer

Codivilla was the first surgeon to perform an en-bloc excision of the head of the pancreas and a major portion of the duodenum for a patient suffering from pancreatic carcinoma in.[29,30] However, it was Walther Kausch from Germany who was credited with the first successful PD in the world in 1909. To this day, the PD or the Whipple's operation (named after Allen Oldfather Whipple's successful report of a series of PDs in 1934) [31] continues to be the operation of choice for carcinomas involving the head, neck and/or uncinate process of the pancreas. This operation, widely regarded as the most complex and challenging of abdominal surgeries, involves the following principles:

- An initial intraoperative assessment prior to proceeding with resection. This assessment involves a wide Kocher maneuver after complete mobilization of the hepatic flexure of the colon. Only when a wide Kocher maneuver is performed and the gastrocolic omentum divided, is a complete assessment for ensuring an R0 resection possible viz. involvement of the superior mesenteric vessels, the extent of the pancreatic head lesion (whether the neck is free or otherwise) and involvement of the common hepatic artery and gastroduodenal artery (GDA). Furthermore an assessment of porta hepatis structures should also be done by finger palpation through the foramen of Winslow.

- En-bloc removal of the pancreatic head along with the duodenum (with or without the antrum of stomach), the distal common bile duct and the gallbladder.
- A standard lymphadenectomy that involves removal of lymph nodes around the common hepatic artery, portal vein (PV), the distal common bile duct, the duodenum (superior and inferior pancreaticoduodenal lymph nodes) and the lymph nodes on the head of the pancreas in the region of the right gastroepiploic artery and the superior mesenteric vein (SMV) as it courses under the pancreatic neck (Fig. 1).
- A complex reconstruction to ensure a pancreatic, biliary and digestive continuity (viz. pancreaticojejunostomy (PJ) or pancreaticogastrostomy (PG)/hepaticojejunostomy/duodenojejunostomy or gastrojejunostomy).

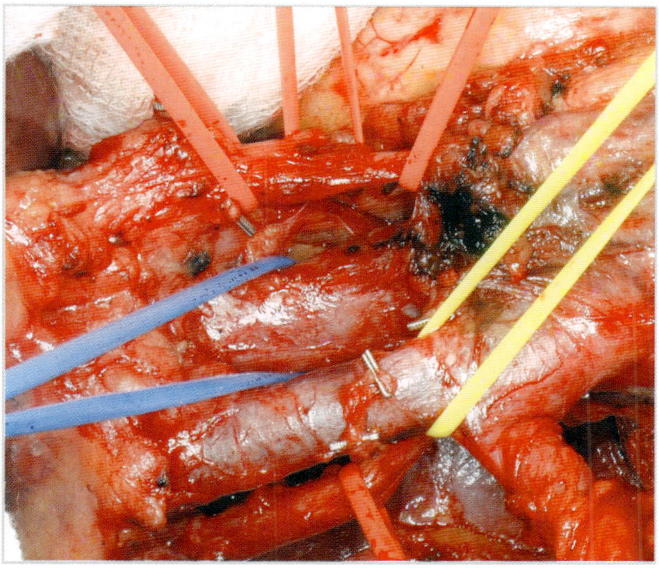

Fig. 1: Intraoperative photograph of the extent of portal lymphadenectomy during Whipple's resection. The yellow loop shows the cystic and bile duct clearance, the blue loop shows the portal vein clearance and the red loops show the clearance along the right hepatic, hepatic artery proper, the common hepatic and gastroduodenal arteries

Technical Modifications of Pancreaticoduodenectomy: Evidence-based Concepts

Pylorus preserving pancreaticoduodenectomy versus classic whipple (with Antrectomy)

A number of trials have failed to show superiority of one technique over the other. A Cochrane review has shown no oncologic benefit separating the two procedures.[32] From a practical standpoint, a classic Whipple procedure is more often considered in large pancreatic head or duodenal tumors while a pylorus preserving pancreaticoduodenectomy is reserved for smaller head lesions and periampullary tumors.

Standard versus extended lymphadenectomy

Extended lymphadenectomy entails, in addition to a standard lymphadenectomy described above, removal of lymph nodes all around the superior mesenteric artery (SMA) and around the coeliac axis and in the interaortocaval groove. However, a landmark meta-analysis based on a number of trials observed no difference in 3 year survival when standard and extended lymphadenectomy were compared.[33] Furthermore, the morbidity was higher in those who underwent extended lymphadenectomy. Currently, extended lymphadenectomy cannot be recommended outside of clinical trials.

Pancreatic Anastomosis

Pancreaticojejunostomy versus pancreaticogastrostomy: The pancreatic anastomosis is widely considered as the Achilles heel of PD. A well done and meticulous anastomosis has a direct bearing on perioperative outcomes of PD. A number of techniques have been described in the literature and are beyond the scope of this chapter. The most commonly performed anastomoses are PJ and PG. A number of randomized clinical trials (RCTs) have evaluated the two techniques and no apparent superiority of one technique over the other was established.[34-36] Soon after these RCTs, two meta-analyses conclusively confirmed that both procedures can be performed with comparable outcomes.[37,38] From a practical standpoint, it must be appreciated that multiple factors have to be considered while performing a good leak proof pancreatic anastomosis—amongst others, tumor location and the associated presence or absence of pancreatic ductal dilation, the texture of the gland, pancreatic juice output and surgeon experience are perhaps most crucial.

The following principles of pancreatic anastomosis are most likely to yield excellent outcomes:[39]

- Good blood supply
- Perfect duct to mucosa approximation
- Use of fine sutures (4-0/5-0 PDS sutures)
- Absence of tension
- Absence of distal obstruction
- Gentle handling by an experienced pancreatic surgeon in a high volume center.

Digestive Anastomosis

Antecolic versus retrocolic gastrojejunostomy/duodenojejunostomy: Delayed gastric emptying (DGE) after PD has been a vexing issue since long. Well known causes of DGE is the development of intra-abdominal complications after surgery such as infected collections or postoperative pancreatic fistula (POPF). However, other causes that can contribute to DGE remain unclear. Performance of an antecolic gastrojejunostomy/duodenojejunostomy has been shown to be associated with a significantly reduced rate of DGE.[40-42] Possible explanations could be the avoidance of torsion or angulation that may occur with a retrocolic anastomosis.

Vascular Resections

The vast majority of pancreatic head cancers are not resectable by conventional PD. The proximity of pancreatic head cancer to the SMV-PV complex has been increasingly recognized as a cause of unresectability in the last few decades. This observation prompted surgeons to further push the limits of an already challenging operation by addition of vascular resections[43-45] with an aim to remove the tumor completely and thus give the patient a chance of cure. While venous resection and reconstruction has been performed in many series, the resistance to arterial resections (hepatic artery or celiac trunk) is almost universal.[46,47] The premise and the perceived benefit of performing a venous resection over an arterial resection in cancer is that the portal venous system, unlike the arterial system, is not surrounded by perivascular neural plexus and lymphatic tissue. Hence, PV involvement potentially remains the only barrier to radical tumor removal.[47] However, the argument against venous resection and reconstruction is that by the time the tumor infiltrates the SMV/PV, the incidence of lymph nodal involvement is very high thus reducing the possibility of cure despite a supramajor resection. On the other hand, this argument has been challenged by a number of surgeons, especially from high volume centers, who have observed that vein involvement is mainly due to tumor location and it is not the venous resection per se that is a determinant of poor long-term outcomes but disease biology that dictates long term survival.

Siriwardena et al. in 2006[48] reviewed 1,646 patients with vein resections and reconstruction and noted that while the procedure could be performed with acceptable morbidity (42%) and mortality (6%), the benefit in terms of overall survival was lacking. Lymph node involvement was also high leading credence to the argument that the disease is usually beyond cure by the time venous involvement takes place in PC. However, the same study documented that in 40% of patients the resection margin was positive, thus precluding an accurate analysis of the benefit of the venous resection in terms of overall survival. This has been shown by other studies[49,50] that followed soon after the systematic review by Siriwardena.[48] As long as an R0 resection could be achieved, they demonstrated no difference in outcomes when venous involvement was documented on histology as compared to absence of venous involvement.[49,50] From a practical standpoint, vein resections and reconstruction should be performed only when an R0 resection can be achieved. The current evidence does not support arterial resections in PC outside of clinical trials.

Complications of Pancreaticoduodenectomy and their Management

Even in the era of modern pancreatic surgery, PD remains a demanding operation. While the mortality has progressively declined over the last decade and a half, the morbidity still remains high between 25% and 52% even in high volume centers.[51-53] The common complications after PD are hemorrhage, fistula and DGE.

Post-pancreatectomy Hemorrhage

There have been numerous studies and publications on this subject. However in 2013, postpancreatectomy hemorrhage is defined by three parameters: onset, location, and severity. The onset is considered early if it is within 24 hours of surgery and it is considered late if it is after 24 hours of surgery. The location is defined as intraluminal or extraluminal and the severity can be categorized as mild or severe. Based on these parameters, three grades of hemorrhage A, B and C are defined wherein the clinical impact worsens from Grade A to Grade C.[54]

Early hemorrhage: Early hemorrhage is almost always due to technical failure and the bleeding can be intraluminal (pancreatic anastomosis or digestive anastomosis) or extraluminal (GDA stump, inferior pancreaticoduodenal artery stump, unnamed vessels along the superior mesenteric vessels, gallbladder fossa, etc.). Irrespective of the site, the cause is lack of attention to finer details of surgery—slipped ligatures, inadequate or incomplete transfixation sutures, wider distance between successive sutures and smaller vessels that can spontaneously open up postoperatively once the vasospasm gets relieved which prevents their intraoperative detection in the first place during surgery. Early hemorrhage is best detected by close monitoring of the patient in the immediate postoperative period and the best way to control early hemorrhage is to return to the operating theater without delay for a re-laparotomy for source control. It is important to realize that once a diagnosis of early hemorrhage is reached, it is better to act without delay rather than convert a semi-emergent situation with a stable patient into an emergent one with an unstable patient. Intraluminal early postoperative hemorrhage from the pancreatic anastomosis can pose a challenge. An elegant approach[55] is to open the jejunal limb on the side opposite to the pancreatic anastomosis (or the stomach from the anterior wall in case of a PG), identify the bleeding point and control it with fine polypropylene sutures without disturbing the pancreatic anastomosis.

Late hemorrhage: Late hemorrhage is invariably a consequence of postoperative pancreatic fistula (POPF) in a setting of local or even systemic sepsis and the consequences can be devastating with high morbidity and even mortality. The most common sites of late hemorrhage are pseudoaneurysms of GDA, pancreaticoduodenal vessels or the initial branches of the splenic artery. In contrast to early hemorrhage, late hemorrhage is an event that is to be anticipated in a patient who develops a POPF grade B or C (see below). Sentinel bleed as an entity deserves specific mention. It is seen in up to 30% patients sometime during the 2nd or 3rd postoperative week in an otherwise hemodynamically stable patient who has an apparently controlled POPF. The sentinel bleed is an indication for CT angiography and localization of possible sources of hemorrhage. It is an ominous sign and often precedes major and life-threatening hemorrhage. The ideal treatment option of late hemorrhage is by angiographic stenting or embolization and surgery is usually reserved as a last option.[56] During surgery, the aims should be two fold, control of hemorrhage by suture ligation of extremely friable tissues and also control of local sepsis by thorough abdominal lavage, drainage of collections and addressing the pancreatic anastomosis (resuture and drainage/disconnection with controlled external pancreatic fistula/completion pancreatectomy). It is obvious that surgery in these conditions is a demanding and high-risk undertaking. The best treatment of late hemorrhage is to prevent its occurrence by active and dedicated management of a POPF and preventing/minimizing/controlling the local sepsis associated with it right from the time of its onset and detection.

Postoperative Pancreatic Fistula

The single most significant cause of morbidity and mortality after PD is the development of POPF and rates even up to 20% are reported from experienced centers of pancreatic surgery.[57-59] While the best way to prevent a POPF is by constructing a safe and standardized pancreatic anastomosis (refer above to the section on pancreatic anastomosis), it is crucial that early recognition of a POPF and prompt institution of appropriate treatment is the key to preventing its potentially devastating consequences—namely sepsis and life threatening late hemorrhage. The most widely accepted definition of a POPF is the International Study Group on Pancreatic Fistula (ISGPF) definition (Table 1).[60] The definition focuses on the presence of a high drain amylase (> 3 times the upper normal serum value) of any volume (at any time after the 3rd postoperative day) as an essential component in deciding

TABLE 1: International study group on pancreatic fistula definition of postoperative pancreatic fistula

Grade		*Degree of impact*	*Imaging/change in manegement*	*Treatment outcome*
Grade A	"Transient fistula"	No clinical impact	No peripancreatic collections on CT scan; little/no change in management	Clinically well; no sepsis; no prolongation of hospital stay; slow removal of operatively placed drains
Grade B		Clinical impact	Peripancreatic drains in place or repositioned to drain collections; change in management is required	Clinically fairly well; degree of infection requiring specific treatment; prolongation of hospital stay; patients often discharged with drains in situ and observed in outpatient setting
Grade C		Severe clinical impact	Worrisome peripancreatic collections that require percutaneous drains; Major change in management usually in ICU setting; possible re-surgery to salvage a difficult situation (completion pancreatectomy, etc.)	Clinical unwell; associated sepsis requiring aggressive antibiotic, octreotide and other intensive care support; major prolongation of hospital stay; associated complications and possibility of mortality

the presence or absence of a pancreatic anastomotic leak. The ISGPF definition also grades POPF into grade A, B and C depending on the clinical impact on the patient's hospital course and eventual outcome with grade A being the best and grade C being the worst of POPFs. Based on this validated definition, the treatment approach to different grades of POPF can be tailored appropriately in most situations.[61] A conservative approach is successful in over 90% cases.[62,63] These include maintenance of enteral nutrition (via peroperatively placed nasojejunal tube or a feeding jejunostomy), prolonged nasogastric suction (only if associated DGE), and appropriate antibiotic cover based on culture sensitivity reports of drain effluent/aspirated collections. In situations where the oral intake is poor or the patient is not tolerating the nasojejunal/jejunostomy feeding, total parenteral nutrition may have to be considered. All along careful clinical evaluation at frequent short intervals is the need of the hour. If there is no fever, tachycardia or leukocytosis, no major wound infection, and the abdomen is soft (with bowels functioning) without signs of spreading peritonitis, it is safe and ideal to continue these conservative measures.[61] A contrast-enhanced CT scan at an interval of a week is an invaluable aid in guiding the above mentioned approach. Furthermore, it detects undrained collections and also gives a clear idea of the regional vascular anatomy with regards to development of pseudoaneurysms. Failure of conservative management (viz. spreading peritonitis, severe wound infection, silent abdomen, burst abdomen, worsening clinical signs and laboratory parameters) should prompt the surgeon to consider re-exploration with an aim to achieve source control that could include a range of procedures such as abdominal lavage with re-positioning of drains, addition of a feeding jejunostomy (if not done at the apex operation), disconnection of pancreatic anastomosis or even a completion pancreatectomy. Late hemorrhage is perhaps the worst manifestation of a POPF (usually grade C) and occurs in a setting of severe sepsis and inflammation. Its management has been described in the preceding section.

To reduce complications of pancreatic resections, namely, POPF, somatostatin analogs are used and advocated by many surgeons. While a number of European trial reported benefits, American trials did not and the issue remains a matter of debate. More recently, a Cochrane review evaluated 19 randomized trials involving 2,245 patients and concluded that somatostatin analogs may reduce perioperative complications but do not reduce perioperative mortality and while based on current evidence it does appear that somatostatin and it analogs should be used in pancreatic surgery, adequately powered trials with low risk of bias are still necessary to settle this controversial issue.[64]

Delayed Gastric Emptying

A number of preoperative (PC, pancreatic fibrosis, portal hypertension), intraoperative (neural and vascular ischemia, extent of lymph node dissection, removal of duodenum with loss of motilin, type of digestive reconstruction), and postoperative factors (intra-abdominal sepsis, enteral nutrition, somatostatin analogs) can contribute to the development of DGE.[65] In modern times, the most common cause of DGE is intra-abdominal sepsis such as infected collections or POPF. Management revolves around conservative measures such as nasogastric aspiration, maintaining electrolyte balance, patient reassurance, ensuring local control of sepsis if any, and perhaps use of erythromycin lactobionate. With antecolic form of digestive anastomosis (discussed above), the incidence of DGE has decreased markedly. Similar to the hemorrhage and POPF definitions, a unifying definition was published by the ISGPS in 2007 grading DGE into grades A, B and C.[66]

Indications for Re-exploration Following Complications of Pancreaticoduodenectomy

It is clear from the preceding sections that surgical re-explorations have gone down in this era of safe pancreatic surgery coupled with improvements in perioperative and critical care and interventional radiology guided drainage of infected collections and management of POPFs.[67,68] Nevertheless, there still remain situations in a small subgroup of patients where re-explorations are indicated. The first author, evaluating a series of 157 consecutive PDs identified that early hemorrhage (from the pancreatic stump or anastomotic line), clinically significant pancreatic anastomotic leak with discharge from the main wound (not controlled by conservative measures, i.e. POPF grade B going to grade C), and an early postoperative biliary anastomotic leak are the prime indications for re-exploration in patients with complications following PD.[68]

Pancreatic Body and Tail Cancer

Approximately two-thirds of all ductal adenocarinomas arise in the pancreatic head, neck or uncinate process. The remaining one-third arise within the body or tail or diffusely throughout the gland. A study of 3,476 patients with PC from Memorial Sloan-Kettering Cancer Center, USA, noted that 23% patients had disease in either the body or tail.[69] Laparoscopy has become increasingly common especially for the preoperative evaluation and staging of PC of the body and tail. Laparoscopy, in combination with CT scans, improves staging and assessment of resectability in a safe, accurate and cost-effective manner. This approach is particularly useful in PC of the body and tail because of their late presentation and the high rate of metastasis observed in these tumors. In these instances, staging laparoscopy reveals unsuspected metastases and avoids a laparotomy.[70]

The procedure of choice for body and tail PC is distal pancreaticosplenectomy with standard lymphadenectomy. Even if spleen preservation is possible, it is not recommended given the malignant nature of the disease. While this procedure may carry medium morbidity ("bland" POPFs and undrained collections), the mortality rates are very low. The POPF after distal pancreaticosplenectomy is "bland" in the sense that compared to the activated enzymes that leak after a pancreatic anastomosis following head resection, the leaking enzymes following distal pancreaticosplenectomy are not activated with less severe consequences. Re-exploration is hardly ever required for this complication which is best managed by interventional radiology guided aspirations/pig-tail drainage. Postoperative and long term management of diabetes and pancreatic enzyme insufficiency is more often necessary compared to pancreatic head resection.

Technical Modifications of Distal Pancreaticosplenectomy[71]

Spleen preserving distal pancreatectomy: Spleen preservation should be attempted for low grade pancreatic malignancies such as cystic pancreatic tumors (Fig. 2A) or small neuroendocrine tumors but is not recommended for pancreatic ductal adenocarcinoma due to inferior oncologic clearance. However, in low grade malignancies, spleen preservation is associated with lesser rate of infectious complications and reduced length of postoperative stay.[72]

Radical antegrade pancreatosplenectomy: This technique provides improved visibility during dissection, removes N1 nodes, has advantage of early vascular control and allows better assessment of posterior extent of dissection. The exposure is similar to conventional distal pancreatectomy but transection at the pancreatic neck occurs early followed by retropancreatic node dissection (Fig. 2B) and then the dissection proceeds to the left in either of the two planes—in front of or behind the adrenal gland.[73]

Management of pancreatic remnant after distal pancreatectomy: Postoperative pancreatic fistula is the single major cause of morbidity after distal pancreatectomy. Appropriate method of closure of pancreatic remnant is still debated. A variety of procedures are used[71] to manage the pancreatic remnant—hand sewn closure with fine sutures, stapled closure, fibrin glue application, serosal patch, PJ and even patch of ligamentum teres. The variety

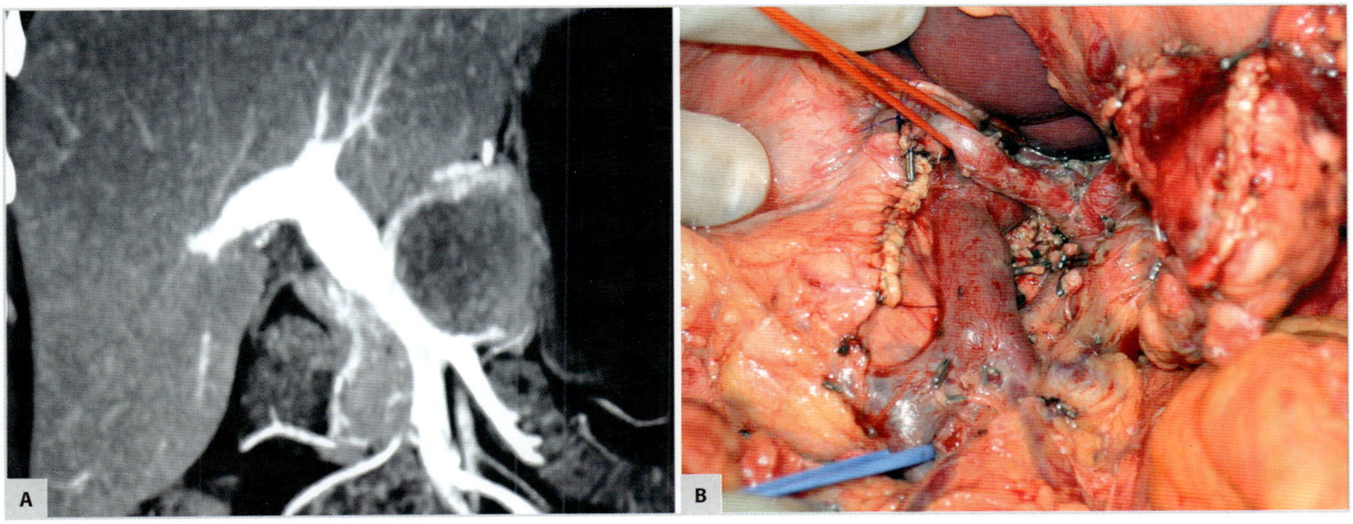

Figs 2A and B: (A) CT scan image of a solid and cystic pancreatic tumor abutting the main portal vein close to the neck-body of the pancreas; (B) Pancreatic transection at the neck with all major vessels (superior mesenteric vein/portal vein, common hepatic artery, splenic artery and coeliac trunk) exposed after regional lymph nodes have been cleared in the initial part of a distal pancreatectomy in the same patient of techniques used clearly suggests that no superiority of any one technique has been established. A meta-analysis of six studies comparing stapler versus hand sewn closure of remnant seemed to suggest stapler closure as a superior method.[74] However, a recent multicenter RCT concluded that stapler closure did not reduce the rate of pancreatic fistula compared with hand-sewn closure for distal pancreatectomy and novel strategies is the need of the hour to reduce this adverse outcome.[75]

Newer Concepts in Pancreatic Cancer

Borderline Resectable Pancreatic Cancer

This distinct subset has evolved in the past years thanks to the superior imaging and dedicated attempts to improve the pool of patients with PC who can be offered aggressive treatment with a chance to improve survival.[21,76-79] Borderline resectable PC is defined when any of the following criteria are met:

- Less than or equal to 180° tumor abutment with SMA
- Short segment encasement or occlusion of PV/SMV
- Encasement of short segment of hepatic artery, but not up to celiac axis
- Encasement of GDA up to hepatic arterial origin
- Less than or equal to 180 tumor abutment with PV, SMV.

While upfront surgery is recommended for resectable PC, multimodality treatment with chemotherapy and radiotherapy is being extensively investigated in this group for two reasons:

- To improve chances of R0 resection in this complex group of tumors
- Neoadjuvant protocols may perhaps help identify those patients with better tumor biology who are more likely to benefit from major radical surgery.

The assessment of resectability in this group revolves around high quality MDCT images that evaluate circumferential contact (CC), length of contact (LC) and extent of venous deformity (VD) when major vessels, i.e. SMV/PV and SMA are evaluated. The first author, in a small series from Tata Memorial Centre, Mumbai, observed that greater the CC and VD, higher were the chances of vein resection but LC did not influence the chances of vein resection and reconstruction.[80] The ability to resect (with or without vein resection) this complex group of tumors has been greatly enhanced by recent advances in technical concepts in the performance of PD. The uncinate first approach, long practiced by the senior author, and the SMA first approach can both greatly facilitate these resections (Fig. 3).[81,82]

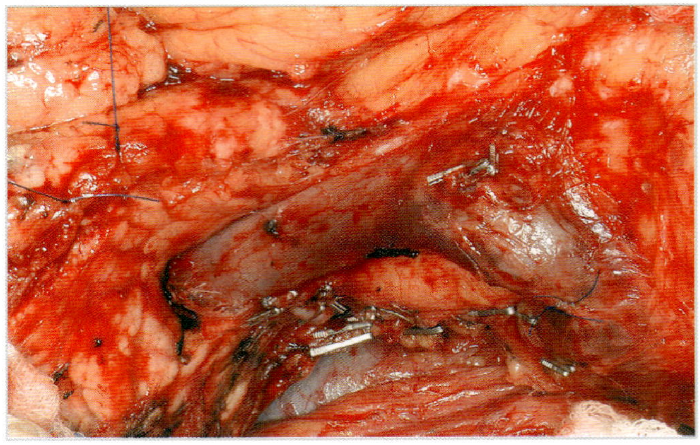

Fig. 3: The right lateral approach of superior mesenteric artery first technique and the uncinate first approach often go hand in hand and is a useful technical modification in large uncinate process tumors and in portal vein resections

Centralization of Pancreatic Resections

The benefits of high volume have been well documented over a decade ago by the inverse relationships between hospital volume and mortality and even long term survival. Furthermore, surgeon volume and operative mortality is also relevant. These observations have been recognized best in various high-risk surgical procedures including PD.[83,84] The first author, evaluating 917 patients from 17 studies from India,[85] highlighted the fact that there exist islands of excellence in India but surgical audits and databases are not really forthcoming in a large country like India and are the need of the hour.[85] The Tata Memorial Centre recently published their series of 500 PDs demonstrating the impact of increasing volume and service reconfiguration on decreasing morbidity and a mortality rate approaching 3% despite increasingly complex resections.[86] This study also documented a 2-year disease-free survival of 75%. Centralization of pancreatic resections has already been established in the UK and other countries are also following suit. In this era of specialization, especially in a country of low incidence of pancreatic and periampullary cancer coupled with varied infrastructure, centralization of complex pancreatic resections is perhaps the way forward to improve standards of care.

Laparoscopic and Robotic Pancreatic Resections

Minimal access surgery has made inroads in all abdominal surgery and pancreatic surgery is no exception. A number of studies have been published demonstrating the feasibility of laparoscopic PD and distal pancreatectomy.[87,88] It is obvious that this procedure is feasible in skilled hands with acceptable results. However, feasibility should not be confused with benefit is the current thinking with regards to laparoscopic PD. This is based on the understanding that the complexity of the procedure is immense and no real advantage in terms of shorter hospital stay or earlier recovery has been convincingly documented. Furthermore, this procedure has a learning curve of 60 open procedures and it is difficult to ensure widespread acceptance of this procedure in the immediate future in this era of evidence-based surgery. Laparoscopic distal pancreatectomy, on the other hand, is an ideal approach for small tumors of the left pancreas and is expected to receive widespread acceptance in the coming years.[89]

ADJUVANT THERAPY IN PANCREATIC CANCER

Three large RCTs have firmly established the role of adjuvant treatment in patients with resected PC.[90-92] The results of the European Study Group for Pancreatic Cancer Trial 1 (ESPAC 1) and the Charite Onkologie 1 trial showed that adjuvant chemotherapy with either fluorouracil and leucovorin or gemcitabine, improves progression-free and overall survival. Through a practice standpoint, all patients staged above T2 and node positive resections should be offered adjuvant chemotherapy. Chemoradiation therapy in the adjuvant setting has not been established with a high level of evidence as yet. The evidence to support use of adjuvant chemoradiation, even in margin positive resections, has not been convincing and cannot be routinely recommended.

NEOADJUVANT APPROACHES IN PANCREATIC CANCER

With the recognition of borderline resectable PC as a distinct entity, neoadjuvant approaches have gained in prominence and gradual acceptance in recent years. Studies suggest that the neoadjuvant approach is as effective as adjuvant treatment and may decrease the rate of local failures and positive resection margins after surgery.[78,93] Thus, these findings are particularly relevant for borderline resectable tumors where preoperative treatment may result in increased R0 resection rates.[78]

PALLIATION IN PANCREATIC CANCER

Majority of PC patients unfortunately present late in the course of the disease when the disease is unresectable. At initial presentation only 50% are free of distant metastases and only 20% have disease amenable to curative resection.[94,95] The median survival of patients with advanced PC is anywhere between 3 months and 18 months and every effort should be made to palliate patient symptoms and improve their quality of life. Amongst others, the major areas that need the attention of a multidisciplinary team are palliation of obstructive jaundice, palliation of gastroduodenal obstruction and management of intractable abdominal pain.[96,97] Obstructive jaundice in isolation is best treated by endoscopic placement of SEMS. While these stents have the advantage of not getting blocked in majority of cases, they are expensive compared to the inexpensive plastic stents that are widely available but run the risk of getting blocked early and frequently. If life expectancy is good and patient has biliodigestive obstruction in a locally advanced disease, a gastrojejunostomy with hepaticojejunostomy and jejunojejunostomy is the best option. On the other hand if the life expectancy is expected to be short in those with biliodigestive obstruction, patients can be offered endotherapy in the form of common bile duct and duodenal stenting.

Intractable abdominal pain of PC can be debilitating, unrelenting and can rapidly erode the quality of life of a patient. This pain is usually in the upper abdomen and in the back and is mainly due to infiltration of the retroperitoneal nerves by tumor. Non opiod analgesics and narcotic analgesics form the backbone for management of this pain where the goal should be to keep the patient pain free round the clock during rest and activity on one hand and yet avoid the side effects of these medications on the other. When pain is not relieved even by 50% despite medications, celiac plexus blocks should be considered[98] since they can often provide satisfactory long-term pain relief.

UNCOMMON PANCREATIC TUMORS

Other uncommon pancreatic malignancies are cystic tumors of the pancreas[99] and neuroendocrine tumors of the pancreas.[100] Their prognosis is much superior compared to the dismal pancreatic adenocarcinoma. While they are separate topics by themselves, broad information is provided below.

Cystic tumors are increasingly detected due to increasing awareness and improved imaging technology. In majority of cases, the diagnosis is reached by a combination of MDCT or MRI/MRCP coupled with EUS and EUS-guided aspiration of cyst fluid for assessment of

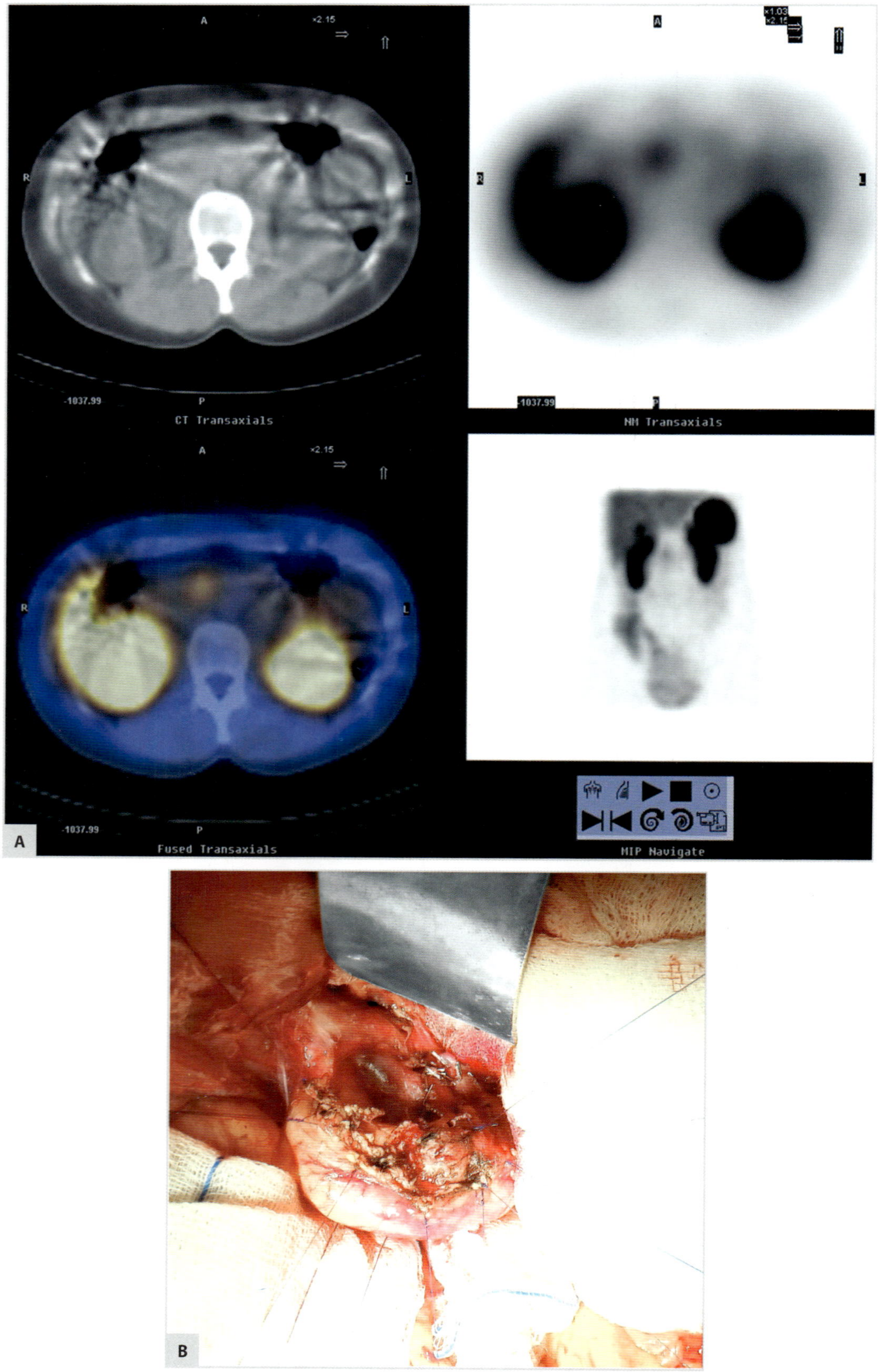

Figs 4A and B: (A) DOTATOC scan localizing neuroendocrine tumor in the region of the body and neck of the pancreas; (B) Enucleation of a G1, localized pancreatic neuroendocrine neoplasm on the posterosuperior aspect of the junction of the neck and body of pancreas in the same patient. The pancreas neck has been dissected away from the common hepatic and gastroduodenal arteries and from the portal vein posteriorly mucin and cyst fluid carcinoembryonic antigen (CEA). It is also crucial to avoid labeling a cystic neoplasm as a "pseudocyst of the pancreas" in the absence of positive and documented history of abdominal pain and attacks of pancreatitis. While serous cystadenoma is a benign condition that should be observed unless the patient is symptomatic from it, mucinous tumors and intraductal papillary mucinous neoplasms (IPMNs) and solid papillary epithelial neoplasms (SPEN) should be offered pancreatic resection. Appropriate resections ensure excellent long term survival.

Neuroendocrine tumors of the pancreas (pNETs) account for less than 5% of pancreatic malignancies and are thought to arise from pancreatic islets. They can be functioning (uncommon) or nonfunctioning (more common). Diagnosis and staging revolves around histopathology involving immunohistochemistry based on which tumors are graded as G1, G2 (neuroendocrine neoplasms) or G3 (neuroendocrine carcinoma). Imaging and localization is dependent on MDCT scans and nuclear medicine scans—somatostatin receptor scintigraphy and 68Ga-DOTA(0)-Phe(1)-Tyr(3)-octreotide (68Ga-DOTATOC) PET-CT scans (Fig. 4A). Treatment is multidisciplinary involving surgery, medical oncology and nuclear medicine. Surgery for localized, resectable disease offers the best chance of cure especially when an R0 resection can be achieved. While larger tumors should be resected by conventional PD for head lesions and by distal pancreatectomy (with or without spleen preservation) for body and tail lesions, lesions less than 2 cm in size, especially those away from the main pancreatic duct can be offered parenchyma preserving pancreatic resections such as enucleation (Fig. 4B) or a median pancreatectomy. Liver limited metastases also warrants an aggressive approach for G1 and G2 neoplasms by a combination of surgery and liver directed therapies (transarterial chemoembolization, transarterial radioembolization, etc.) liver resections and even transplantation in highly selected cases. The treatment of advanced or unresectable disease involves cytotoxic chemotherapy (streptozotocin, doxorubicin, temozolamide, etc.), long acting octreotide and peptide receptor radionuclide therapy (PRRT).

REFERENCES

1. Salim EI, Moore MA, Bener A, et al. Cancer epidemiology in south-west asia—past, present and future. Asian Pac J Cancer Prev. 2010;11 (Suppl 2):33-48.
2. Anderson K, Mack T, Silverman D. Cancer of the pancreas. In: Schottenfeld D, Fraumeni Jr JF (Eds). Cancer Epidemiology and Prevention. New York: Oxford University Press. 2006.
3. Curado M, Edwards B, Shin H, et al. Cancer incidence in five continents. Volume IX. IARC Sci Publ. 2008;(160):1-837.
4. Dhir V, Mohandas KM. Epidemiology of digestive tract cancers in India iv. Gall bladder and pancreas. Indian J Gastroenterol. 1999;18:24-8.
5. Yeole B, Kumar A. Population-based survival from cancers having a poor prognosis in Mumbai (Bombay), India. Asian Pac J Cancer Prev. 2004;5(2):175-82.
6. Shrikhande SV, Jagannath P. Current Options in diagnosis and management of Ampullary Carcinoma. Indian Journal of Surgery. 2003;65:347-53.
7. Hassan MM, Bondy ML, Wolff RA, et al. Risk factors for pancreatic cancer: casecontrol study. Am J Gastroenterol. 2007;102:2696-707.
8. Batty GD, Kivimaki M, Morrison D, et al. Risk factors for pancreatic cancer mortality: extended follow-up of the original Whitehall Study. Cancer Epidemiol Biomarkers Prev. 2009;18:673-5.
9. Landi S. Genetic predisposition and environmental risk factors to pancreatic cancer: A review of the literature. Mutat Res. 2009;681:299-307.
10. Lowenfels AB, Maisonneuve P. Epidemiology and risk factors for pancreatic cancer. Best Pract Res Clin Gastroenterol. 2006;20:197-209.
11. Genkinger JM, Spiegelman D, Anderson KE, et al. Alcohol intake and pancreatic cancer risk: a pooled analysis of fourteen cohort studies. Cancer Epidemiol Biomarkers Prev. 2009;18:765-76.
12. Shi C, Hruban RH, Klein AP. Familial pancreatic cancer. Arch Pathol Lab Med. 2009;133:365-74.
13. Wolpin BM, Chan AT, Hartge P, et al. ABO blood group and the risk of pancreatic cancer. J Natl Cancer Inst. 2009;101:424-31.
14. Hruban RH, Maitra A, Goggins M. Update on pancreatic intraepithelial neoplasia. Int J Clin Exp Patho . 2008;1:306-16.
15. Hidalgo M. Pancreatic cancer. N Engl J Med. 2010;362:1605-17.
16. Barreto SG, Shukla PJ, Shrikhande SV. Periampullary carcinoma. In: Shrikhande SV, Friess H, Buechler MW (Eds). Surgery of Pancreatic Tumors. New Delhi: BI Publications; 2007. pp. 206-15.
17. Barreto SG, Shukla PJ, Shrikhande SV. Tumors of the pancreatic body and tail. World J Oncol. 2010;1:52-65.
18. Shrikhande SV, Shrikhande VN. Pancreatic cancer. In: Haribhakti S (Ed). Clinical GI Surgery. Ahmedabad: Haribhakti Education Foundation; 2008. pp. 627-41.
19. Steinberg W. The clinical utility of the CA 19-9 tumor-associated antigen. Am J Gastroenterol. 1990;85:350-5.
20. Shrikhande SV, Barreto SG. Surgery for pancreatic carcinoma: state of the art. Indian J Surg. 2012;74:79-86.

21. Varadhachary GR, Tamm EP, Abbruzzese JL, et al. Borderline resectable pancreatic cancer: definitions, management, and role of preoperative therapy. Ann Surg Oncol. 2006;13:1035-46.
22. Shrikhande SV, Barreto SG, Goel M, et al. Multimodality imaging of pancreatic ductal adenocarcinoma: a review of the literature. HPB. 2012;14:658-68.
23. Sewnath ME, Birjmohun RS, Rauws EA, et al. The effect of preoperative biliary drainage on postoperative complications after pancreaticoduodenectomy. J Am Coll Surg. 2001; 192:726-34.
24. Van Der Gaag NA, Rauws EA, Van Eijck CH, et al. Preoperative biliary drainage for cancer of the head of the pancreas. N Eng J Med. 2010;362:129-37.
25. Mullen JT, Lee JH, Gomez HF, et al. Pancreaticoduodenectomy after placement of endobiliary metal stents. J Gastrointest Surg. 2005;9:1094-104.
26. Wasan SM, Ross WA, Staerkel GA, et al. Use of expandable metallic biliary stents in resectable pancreatic cancer. Am J Gastroenterol. 2005;100:2056-61.
27. Blenkharn JI, McPhearson GA, Blumgart LH. Septic complications of percutaneous transhepatic drainage. Evaluation of a new closed drainage system. Am J Surg. 1984;147:318-21.
28. Jagannath P, Dhir V, Shrikhande S, et al. Effect of preoperative biliary stenting on immediate outcome after pancreaticoduodenectomy. Br J Surg. 2005;92:356-61.
29. Modlin IM, Kidd M, Champaneria MC, et al. Historical Perspectives of surgery for pancreatic tumors. In: Shrikhande SV, Friess H, Buechler MW (Eds). Surgery of Pancreatic Tumors. New Delhi: BI Publications; 2007. pp. 1-13
30. Shukla PJ, Barreto SG, Shrikhande SV. The evolution of pancreatoduodenectomy. Hepatogastroenterology. 2011;58: 1409-12.
31. Whipple AO, Parsons WB, Mullins CR. Treatment of carcinoma of the ampulla of vater. Ann Surg. 1935;102:763-79.
32. Diener MK, Fitzmaurice C, Schwarzer G, et al. Pylorus-preserving pancreaticoduodenectomy (pp Whipple) versus pancreaticoduodenectomy (classic Whipple) for surgical treatment of periampullary and pancreatic carcinoma. Cochrane Database Syst Rev. 2011;5:CD006053.
33. Michalski CW, Kleeff J, Wente MN, et al. Systematic review and meta-analysis of standard and extended lymphadenectomy in pancreaticoduodenectomy for pancreatic cancer. Br J Surg. 2007;94:265-73.
34. Yeo CJ, Cameron JL, Maher MM, et al. A prospective randomized trial of pancreaticogastrostomy versus pancreaticojejunostomy after pancreaticoduodenectomy. Ann Surg. 1995;222:580-8.
35. Duffas JP, Suc B, Msika S, et al. A controlled randomized multicenter trial of pancreatogastrostomy or pancreatojejunostomy after pancreatoduodenectomy. Am J Surg. 2005;189:720-9.
36. Bassi C, Falconi M, Molinari E, et al. Reconstruction by pancreaticojejunostomy versus pancreaticogastrostomy following pancreatectomy: results of a comparative study. Ann Surg. 2005;242:767-71.
37. McKay A, Mackenzie S, Sutherland FR, et al. Meta-analysis of pancreaticojejunostomy versus pancreaticogastrostomy reconstruction after pancreaticoduodenectomy. Br J Surg. 2006;93:929-36.
38. Wente MN, Shrikhande SV, Muller MW, et al. Pancreaticojejunostomy versus pancreaticogastrostomy: systematic review and meta-analysis. Am J Surg. 2007;193:171-83.
39. Shrikhande SV, Qureshi SS, Rajneesh N, et al. Pancreatic anastomoses after pancreaticoduodenectomy: do we need further studies? World J Surg. 2005;29:1642-9.
40. Hartel M, Wente MN, Hinz U, et al. Effect of antecolic reconstruction on delayed gastric emptying after the pylorus-preserving Whipple procedure. Arch Surg. 2005;140:1094-9.
41. Tani M, Terasawa H, Kawai M, et al. Improvement of delayed gastric emptying in pylorus-preserving pancreaticoduodenectomy: results of a prospective, randomized, controlled trial. Ann Surg. 2006;243:316-20.
42. Chijiiwa K, Imamura N, Ohuchida J, et al. Prospective randomized controlled study of gastric emptying assessed by (13)C-acetate breath test after pylorus-preserving pancreaticoduodenectomy: comparison between antecolic and vertical retrocolic duodenojejunostomy. J Hepatobiliary Pancreat Surg. 2009;16:49-55.
43. Fortner JG, Kim DK, Cubilla A, et al. Regional pancreatectomy: en bloc pancreatic, portal vein and lymph node resection. Ann Surg. 1977;186:42-50.
44. Martin RC, Scoggins CR, Egnatashvili V, et al. Arterial and venous resection for pancreatic adenocarcinoma: operative and long-term outcomes. Arch Surg. 2009;144:154-9.
45. Abramson MA, Swanson EW, Whang EE. Surgical resection versus palliative chemoradiotherapy for the management of pancreatic cancer with local venous invasion: a decision analysis. J Gastrointest Surg. 2009;13:26-34.
46. Shrikhande SV, Barreto SG. Extended pancreatic resections and lymphadenectomy: an appraisal of the current evidence. World J Gastrointest Surg. 2010;2:39-46.
47. Amano H, Miura F, Toyota N, et al. Is pancreatectomy with arterial reconstruction a safe and useful procedure for locally advanced pancreatic cancer? J Hepatobiliary Pancreat Surg. 2009. [Epub ahead of print].
48. Siriwardena HP, Siriwardena AK. Systematic review of outcome of synchronous portal-superior mesenteric vein resection during pancreatectomy for cancer. Br J Surg. 2006;93:662-73.
49. Toomey P, Hernandez J, Morton C, et al. Resection of portovenous structures to obtain microscopically negative margins during pancreaticoduodenectomy for pancreatic adenocarcinoma is worthwhile. Am Surg. 2009;75:804-9.
50. Kaneoka Y, Yamaguchi A, Isogai M. Portal or superior mesenteric vein resection for pancreatic head adenocarcinoma: prognostic value of the length of venous resection. Surgery. 2009;145:417-25.
51. Yeo CJ, Cameron JL, Sohn TA, et al. Six hundred fifty consecutive pancreaticoduodenectomies in the 1990's: pathology, complications, and outcomes. Ann Surg. 1997;226:248-57.
52. Yeo CJ. Management of complications following pancreaticoduodenectomy. Surg Clin N Am. 1995;75:913-24.
53. Buchler MW, Friess H, Wagner M, et al. Pancreatic fistula after pancreatic head resection. Br J Surg. 2000;87:883-9.

54. Wente MN, Veit JA, Bassi C, et al. Postpancreatectomy haemorrhage (PPH): an International Study Group of Pancreatic Surgery (ISGPS) definition. Surgery. 2007;142:20-5.
55. Wente MN, Shrikhande SV, Kleeff J, et al. Management of early haemorrhage from pancreatic anastomosis after pancreaticoduodenectomy. Dig Surg. 2006;23:203-8.
56. Singh RK, Baijal SS, Kapoor VK. Management of delayed haemorrhage following pancreaticoduodenectomy. In: Shrikhande SV, Friess H, Buechler MW (Eds). Surgery of Pancreatic Tumors. New Delhi: BI Publications; 2007. pp. 174-89
57. Schmidt CM, Powell ES, Yiannoutsos CT, et al. Pancreaticoduodenectomy: a 20-year experience in 516 patients. Arch Surg. 2C04;139:718-25.
58. Bassi C, Falconi M, Salvia R, et al. Management of complications after pancreaticoduodenectomy in a high volume centre: results on 150 consecutive patients. Dig Surg. 2001;18:453-57
59. Balcom JH, Rattner DW, Warshaw AL, et al. Ten-year experience with 733 pancreatic resections: changing indications, older patients, and decreasing length of hospitalization. Arch Surg. 2001;136:391-8.
60. Bassi C, Dervenis C, Butturini G, et al. Postoperative pancreatic fistula: an internationa study group (ISGPF) definition. Surgery. 2005;138:8-13.
61. Shrikhande SV, D'Souza MA. Pancreatic fistula after pancreatectomy: Evolving definitions, preventive strategies and modern management. World J Gastroenterol. 2008;14:5789-96.
62. Kazanjian KK, Hines OJ, Eibl G, et al. Management of pancreatic fistulas after pancreaticoduodenectomy: results in 437 consecutive patients. Arch Surg. 2005;140:849-54.
63. Munoz-Bongrand N, Sauvanet A, Denys A, et al. Conservative management of pancreatic fistula after pancreatico-duodenectomy with pancreaticogastrostomy. J Am Coll Surg. 2004;199:198-203.
64. Gurusamy KS, Koti R, Fusai G, et al. Somatostatin analogues for pancreatic surgery. Cochrane Database Syst Rev. 2012;6:CD008370.
65. Vij V, Chaudhary A. Delayed gastric emptying after pancreaticoduodenectomy. In: Shrikhande SV, Friess H, Buechler MW (Eds). Surgery of Pancreatic Tumors. New Delhi: BI Publications; 2007. pp. 190-6.
66. Wente MN, Bassi C, Dervenis C, et al. Delayed gastric emptying (DGE) after pancreatic surgery: a suggested definition by the International Study Group of Pancreatic Surgery (ISGPS). Surgery. 2007;142:761-8.
67. Myatra S, Divatia JV, Jibhkate B, et al. Preoperative assessment and optimization in periampullary and pancreatic cancer. Indian J Cancer. 2011;1:86-93.
68. Shukla PJ, Barreto SG, Mohandas KM, et al. Defining the role of surgery for complications after pancreaticoduodenectomy. ANZ J Surg. 2009;79:33-7.
69. Conlon KC, Brennan MF. Management of adenocarcinoma of the body and tail of the pancreas. In: Cameron JL (Ed). Pancreatic Cancer. London: BC Decker; 2001. pp. 255-63.
70. Jimenez RE, Warshaw AL, Rattner DW, et al. Impact of laparoscopic staging in the treatment of pancreatic cancer. Arch Surg. 2000;135:409-15.
71. Navadgi S, Jagannath P. Distal pancreatectomy: technical considerations. In: Shrikhande SV, Friess H, Buechler MW (Eds). Surgery of Pancreatic Tumors. New Delhi: BI Publications; 2007. pp. 234-9.
72. Shoup M, Brennan MF, McWhite K, et al. The value of splenic preservation with distal pancreatectomy. Arch Surg. 2002;137:164-8
73. Strasberg SM, Drebin JA, Linehan D. Radical antegrade modular pancreatosplenectomy. Surgery. 2003;133:521-7.
74. Knaebel HP, Diener MK, Wente MN, et al. Sytematic review and meta-analysis of technique for closure of the pancreatic remnant after distal pancreatectomy. Br J Surg. 2005;92:539-46.
75. Diener MK, Seiler CM, Rossion I, et al. Efficacy of stapler versus hand-sewn closure after distal pancreatectomy (DISPACT): a randomized, controlled multicenter trial. Lancet. 2011;377:1514-22.
76. Kuvshinoff BW, Bryer MP. Treatment of resectable and locally advanced pancreatic cancer. Cancer Control. 2000;7:428-36.
77. National Comprehensive Cancer Network (NCCN) Guidelines Version 1. 2013. Pancreatic Adenocarcinoma.
78. Katz MH, Pisters PW, Evans DB, et al. Borderline resectable pancreatic cancer: the importance of this emerging stage of disease. J Am Coll Surg. 2008;206:833-46.
79. Springett GM, Hoffe SE. Borderline resectable pancreatic cancer: on the edge of survival. Cancer Control. 2008;15:295-307.
80. Shrikhande SV, Arya S, Barreto SG, et al. Borderline resectable pancreatic tumors: Is there a need for further refinement of this stage? Hepatobiliary Pancreat Dis Int. 2011;10:319-24.
81. Shrikhande SV, Barreto SG, Bodhankar YD, et al. Superior mesenteric artery first combined with uncinate process approach versus uncinate process first approach in pancreatoduodenectomy: a comparative study evaluating perioperative outcomes. Langenbecks Arch Surg. 2011;396:1205-12.
82. Sanjay P, Takaori K, Govil S, et al. 'Artery-first' approaches to pancreatoduodenectomy. Br J Surg. 2012;99:1027-35.
83. Birkmeyer JD, Siewers AE, Finlayson EV, et al. Hospital volume and surgical mortality in the United States. N Engl J Med. 2002;346:1128-37.
84. Birkmeyer JD, Stukel TA, Siewers AE, et al. Surgeon volume and operative mortality in the United States. N Engl J Med. 2003;349:2117-27.
85. Shrikhande SV, D'Souza MA, Wente MN. Pancreaticoduodenectomy in India: how far are we from centralization? Pancreas. 2009;38:473-5.
86. Shrikhande SV, Barreto SG, Somashekar BA. et al. Evolution of pancreatoduodenectomy in a tertiary cancer center in India: improved results from service reconfiguration. Pancreatology. 2013;13:63-71.
87. Palanivelu C, Jani K, Senthinathan P, et al. Laparoscopic pancreaticoduodenectomy: techniques and outcomes. J Am Coll Surg. 2007;205:222-30.
88. Kendrick ML, Cusati D. Total laparoscopic pancreaticoduodenectomy: feasibility and outcome in an early experience. Arch Surg. 2010;145:19-23.

89. Michalski CW, Kong B, Erkan M, et al. Laparoscopic pancreatic resection for pancreatic cancer—How good is the evidence? In: Shrikhande SV, Buchler MW (Eds). Pancreatic Cancer. New Delhi: Elsevier; 2011. pp. 245-56.

90. Neoptolemos JP, Stocken DD, Friess H, et al. A randomized trial of chemoradiotherapy and chemotherapy after resection of pancreatic cancer. N Engl J Med. 2004;350:1200-10.

91. Oettle H, Post S, Neuhaus P, et al. Adjuvant chemotherapy with gemcitabine vs observation in patients undergoing curative-intent resection of pancreatic cancer: a randomized controlled trial. JAMA. 2007;297:267-77.

92. Regine WF, Winter KA, Abrams RA, et al. Fluorouracil vs gemcitabine chemotherapy before and after fluorouracil based chemoradiation following resection of pancreatic adenocarcinoma: a randomized controlled trial. JAMA. 2008;299:1019-26.

93. Evans DB, Varadhachary GR, Crane CH, et al. Preoperative gemcitabine-based chemoradiation for patients with resectable adenocarcinoma of the pancreatic head. J Clin Oncol. 2008;26:3496-502.

94. Kalser MH, Barkin J, MacIntyre JM. Pancreatic cancer: assessment of prognosis by clinical presentation. Cancer. 1985;56:397-402.

95. Ahrendt SA, Pitt HA. Surgical management of pancreatic cancer. Oncology (Huntingt). 2002;16:725-34.

96. Mehta S. Endoscopic palliation in pancreatic tumors. In: Shrikhande SV, Friess H, Buechler MW (Eds). Surgery of Pancreatic Tumors. New Delhi: BI Publications; (2007). pp. 386-98.

97. Jain PN. Management of pain and palliative care in advanced pancreatic cancer. In: Shrikhande SV, Friess H, Buechler MW (Eds). Surgery of Pancreatic Tumors. New Delhi: BI Publications; (2007). pp. 399-408.

98. Jain PN, Shrikhande S, Myatra SN, et al. Neurolytic celiac plexus block: A better alternative to opioid treatment in upper abdominal malignancies: An Indian experience. J Pain Palliat Care Pharmacother. 2005;19:15-20.

99. Barreto SG, Shukla PJ, Ramadwar M, et al. Cystic tumours of the pancreas. HPB. 2007;9:259-66.

100. Shrikhande SV, Sirohi B, Goel M, et al. Pancreatic neuroendocrine tumors. Indian J Gastroenterol. 2013;32:3-17.

35 Breast Cancer

Ratna Parikh, Praful Desai, Anita Borges, Sarabjeet Kaur Arneja, Nagraj G Huilgol, Bhavin Jankharia, Bhavna Parikh, Ganesh Balasubramaniam

EPIDEMIOLOGY

Breast cancer is the most common female cancer worldwide with an estimated 1.38 million new cancer cases diagnosed in 2008 representing 23% of all cancers in women.[1] Data from National Cancer Registry Program shows that in all urban areas of India, breast cancer has now surpassed cervical cancer as the most frequently diagnosed cancer in women and accounts for 25–32% of all female cancers.[2] The age-standardized incidence rate (ASR) 22.9 per 100,000 (Fig. 1).[1] The most recent data available from the National Cancer Registry Program shows a wide variation in ASR observed between rural and urban populations ranging from 36.1 per 100,000 in Bengaluru to 7.2 per 100,000 in the state of Sikkim.[2]

Age at Diagnosis

It is important to note that the incidence rates in urban cities have risen remarkably over the last three decades, while in rural areas it has not changed significantly. The incidence rates have increased from 20.7 per 100,000 in 1983 to 32.3 per 100,000 in 2008 in Mumbai, while it has increased from 18.2 per 100,000 in 1983 to 31.5 per 100,000 in 2008 in Chennai; however, the rates in Barshi (rural) have increased from 6.9 per 100,000 in 1983 to 8.8 per 100,000 in 2008.[2]

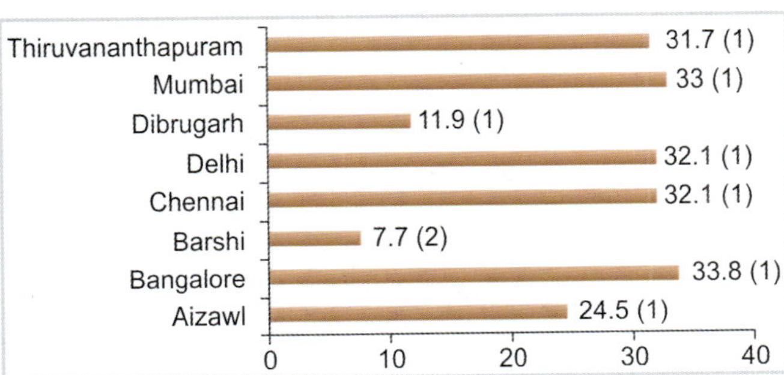

Fig. 1: Age-standardized incidence rate (ASR) (per 100,000) of breast cancer in Indian registries

As per the National Cancer Registry Reports breast cancer occurs a decade earlier in Indian patients compared to their Western counterparts, with premenopausal patients constituting about 50% of all patients [Sanjay Gandhi Postgraduate Institute of Medical Sciences (SGPGIMS), Lucknow data)].[3] The average age of patients in six hospital-based registries ranges from 44 years to 53 years.[4] Population-based registry data shows 50–53 years as the average age. A significant proportion of Indian breast cancer patients are younger than 35 years of age and the incidence rate varies between 11% (Tata Memorial Hospital, Mumbai)[5] to 26% (SGPGIMS, Lucknow). Younger age has been associated with larger tumor size, higher number of metastatic lymph nodes, higher tumor grade, low rates of hormone receptor-positive status, earlier and more frequent locoregional recurrences and poorer overall survival (OS).[6,7]

From the Tata Hospital Registry data, it is observed that the proportion of patients diagnosed before the age of 50 years has decreased from 57.5% in 1985 to 40.4% in 2007, while proportion of those diagnosed at and above the age of 50 years has increased from 42.5% in 1985 to 59.6% in 2007, clearly indicating that there is definite shift in the age at diagnosis and more patients are diagnosed in the postmenopausal stage which is a characteristic observation in the Western countries.

Stage of Disease at Presentation

Agarwal and Ramakant[8] reported a summary of tumor, node and metastasis (TNM) stage at presentation at four major cancer centers in India. Maximum proportion of stage II cancer patients were reported from Mumbai, while Chennai reported maximum proportion of stage III patients. Almost 50% of patients present with locally advanced disease. Majority of patients from SGPGIMS, Lucknow presented in stages IIIb (35%) and IIIa (27%).[9] In another study, 6–25% of Indian breast cancer patients had distant metastatic disease at presentation, with a higher incidence of skeletal metastases.[3,8,10]

Associated Factors

One of the foremost studies on breast cancer in India, a case control study in Mumbai, indicated that compared to married women, single women had a four to five-fold higher risk for developing breast cancer in the age group of 40–54 years and above.[11] Another study from Mumbai, reported risk factors like marital status and age at first pregnancy. Nulliparous women had a 2.2-fold higher risk than parous women.[12] Reproductive history, age at menarche or at marriage, first pregnancy, parity, use of contraceptives and other exogenous hormones, as well as differences in weight, exercise, diet and alcohol consumption, are associated known factors for breast cancer. The role of diet in the etiology of breast cancer remains controversial; alcohol intake and obesity are also associated with a higher incidence of breast cancer. It is believed that women with dense breast have higher risk of developing breast cancer, four to six-fold increase risk of breast cancer.[13]

Genetic Predisposition in Breast Cancer (BRCA1 and BRCA2)

Hereditary (familial) breast cancer syndromes account for about 5–10% of all breast cancers. The rest 90–95% are "sporadic". About 80% hereditary cancers are due to mutations of either BRCA1 (40–45%) or BRCA2 (35–40%).[14] This helps identify high-risk women for breast and ovarian cancers, who should be counseled regarding risk-reducing options. The strongest risk factor for developing breast cancer is a positive family history. If there is a first-degree relative with early onset of breast cancer, a woman's risk of breast cancer doubles with BRCA1 gene. There is increased risk for breast and ovarian cancer syndrome in women with a positive family history. The lifetime risk of breast cancer development in mutation carriers ranges from 37 to 87% by age of 70 years for breast cancer and risk of ovarian cancer from 16 to 63% and from 10 to 27%, especially for carriers of BRCA1 and BRCA2. Appropriate genetic studies are therefore worthwhile in selected cases though not generally available yet in India; Positive mutation findings can lead to primary prevention by prophylactic bilateral mastectomy/reconstruction or secondary prevention (early diagnosis) by appropriate screening. Our knowledge is still evolving and a positive or negative mutation has limitations which need to be understood. In vitro and in vivo, mechanisms are not yet clearly understood. A positive mutation (BRCA1-2) may not produce cancer and the reverse may be true. Tamoxifen and bilateral oophorectomy are options in BRCA1 and BRCA2 positive women for prevention of breast cancer.

PATHOLOGY

In the last two decades, the practice of surgical pathology in oncology has changed considerably. This has been driven by technology, trends in cancer management and the increasing emphasis on genomics and personalized medicine. Breast cancer is no exception. Whereas, the basic classification of breast cancer has not changed much from what it was 20 years ago, a greater understanding of the biology of the disease and its impact on diagnosis, management and prognosis has significantly changed the way a pathologist looks at breast cancer.

Classification of Carcinoma of the Breast

Carcinomas of the breast are classified into two main categories: invasive and noninvasive. The latter are often referred to as in situ carcinomas. Invasive carcinomas are further subdivided into two groups: invasive carcinoma of no special type, often referred to as infiltrating duct carcinoma, and special subtypes (Figs 2A and B). Of the latter, invasive lobular carcinoma is the most often encountered variant. Other less common variants are tubular carcinoma, medullary carcinoma, papillary carcinoma and mucinous carcinoma.

Invasive Breast Carcinoma

Invasive breast carcinoma of no special type [infiltrating duct carcinoma, not otherwise specified (NOS)] accounts for more than two-thirds of all breast carcinomas. It is difficult to describe the histological appearances of this group of tumors because it is a heterogeneous entity defined by exclusion of tumors of recognized special types. The tumors may be of high or low grade. They may also coexist with tumors of special type. The heterogeneous

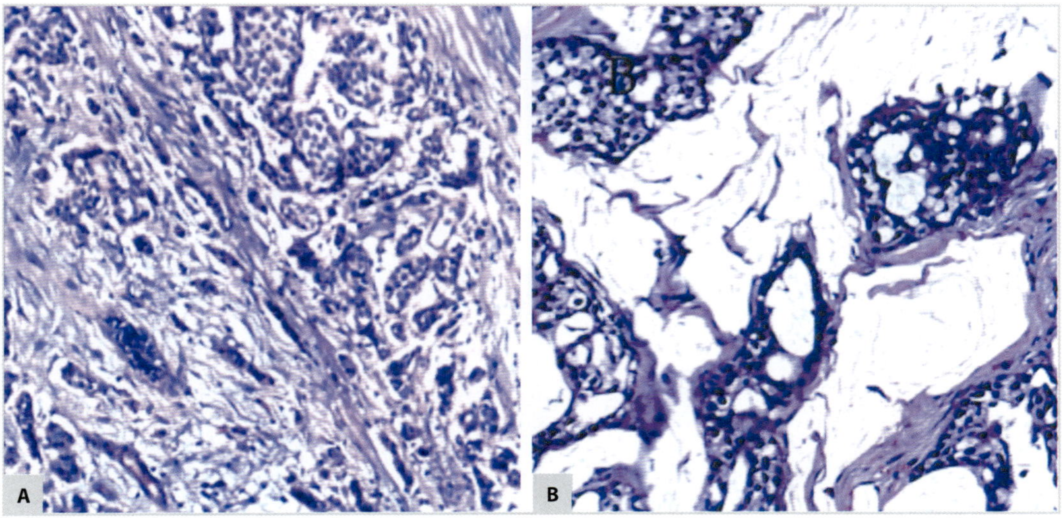

Figs 2A and B: (A) Invasive ductal carcinoma (IDC), not otherwise specified (NOS); (B) IDC, mucinous type

nature of this entity is also reflected in its molecular make-up. Attempts to correlate morphology with particular molecular profiles have only been partially successful. For instance, low-grade tumors more often express estrogen receptors (ER), and high-grade tumors with solid growth patterns are more likely to be negative for ER, progesterone receptor (PR) and human epidermal growth factor receptor 2 HER2 neu, the so-called "triple negative phenotype".

Invasive Lobular Carcinoma

Invasive lobular carcinoma is composed of noncohesive cells, often arranged in a linear-single file pattern, fancifully called the Indian-file pattern of infiltration, after the native American-Indian style of advancing on an enemy. Approximately 5–15% of all breast carcinomas are of this type. The noncohesive pattern of growth is a reflection of the loss of the adhesion molecule E-cadherin in 80–90% of these tumors. Immunohistochemistry (IHC) can be used to demonstrate the lack of expression of this molecule if this is diagnostically important. The frequency of contralateral tumors is higher than with invasive carcinoma of no special type, the reported frequency being of the order of 5–19%.

Duct Carcinoma In Situ

Duct carcinoma in situ (DCIS) is also referred to as intraductal carcinoma. The cancer is limited to and grows within the ductal system. Invasion cannot be demonstrated on careful evaluation of multiple sections of the tumor. This may require the use of immunostains to demonstrate that the outer layer of myoepithelial cells which is present in normal duct is still intact, i.e. microscopic foci of invasion are not present. On occasion, this is difficult to establish and a pathologist may have to issue equivocal report with regard to the presence or absence of invasion.

Duct carcinoma in situ may be of low, intermediate or high grade. The latter is often of the comedo type. Many palpable lesions reported as DCIS are of this variety and may be associated with microinvasion. This form of DCIS, more than any other, is associated with the rare phenomenon of lymph node metastasis in what is believed to be a noninvasive carcinoma. It is often assumed that microscopic foci of invasion were missed by the pathologist. However, some authors believe that the palpable form of DCIS of the high-grade type may actually represent an extremely differentiated form of invasive duct carcinoma that has a marked tendency to recapitulate a ductal pattern of growth. Microscopic foci of invasion may not impact adversely on prognosis. However, the presence of such foci must be noted and their size measured. Microinvasive carcinoma is defined as one or more foci of invasive carcinoma, each less than 1 mm in size, in a setting of DCIS. The latter is often of high-grade type. The low-grade variants of DCIS are difficult to distinguish from atypical ductal hyperplasia. Criteria for the distinction are not uniformly applied or accepted. The majority are detected by screening mammography or incidentally found in breast tissue excised for other reasons. DCIS is a potential but not an obligate precursor of invasive carcinoma. When an invasive carcinoma occurs on follow up, it is almost always in the area or quadrant that was previously affected. The interval and incidence of subsequent recurrent DCIS and/or invasive carcinoma is often said to be related to the grade of the preceding DCIS. However, it is possible that relapse is more size-

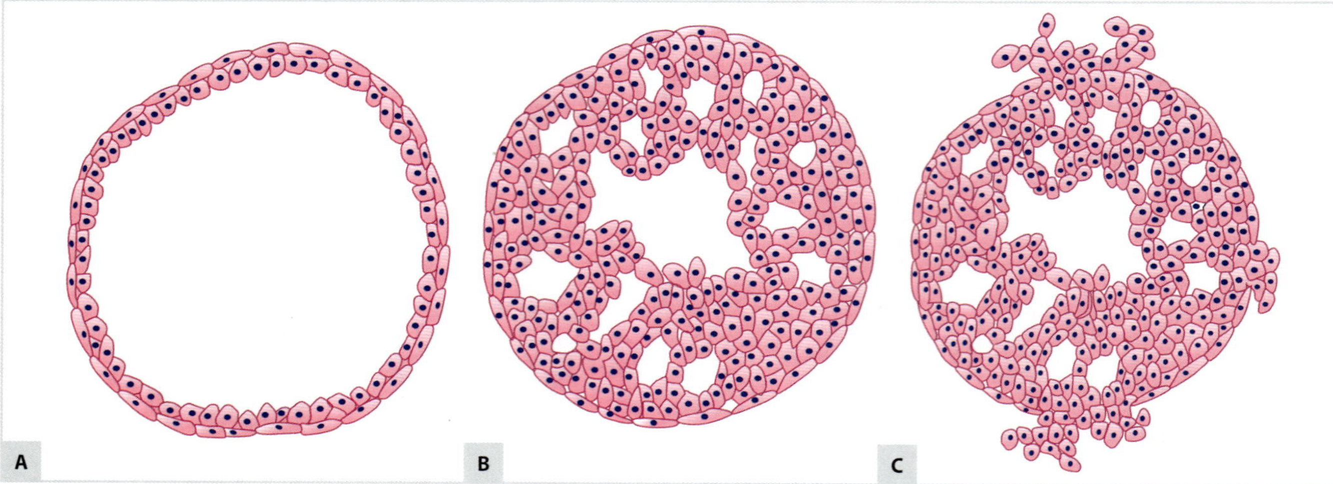

Figs 3A to C: Progression from (A) normal duct cells to (B) a ductal carcinoma in situ (DCIS) and (C) invasive ductal carcinoma (IDC)

Box 1: Consensus Committee recommendation for nuclear grading of intraductal carcinoma[14]

- *Low nuclear grade (nuclear grade 1):*
  - Monomorphic appearance
  - Size of ductal epithelial nuclei or 1.5–2.0 times that of RBC
  - Chromatin finely dispersed, occasional nucleoli
  - Occasional mitosis
- *High nuclear grade (nuclear grade 3):*
  - Markedly pleomorphic
  - Size more than 2.5 times that of ductal epithelial nuclei
  - Chromatin vesicular with prominent nucleoli
  - Mitoses may be conspicuous
- *Intermediate nuclear grade (nuclear grade 2):*
  - Nuclei that are neither grade 1 or grade 3

Abbreviation: RBC, red blood cells

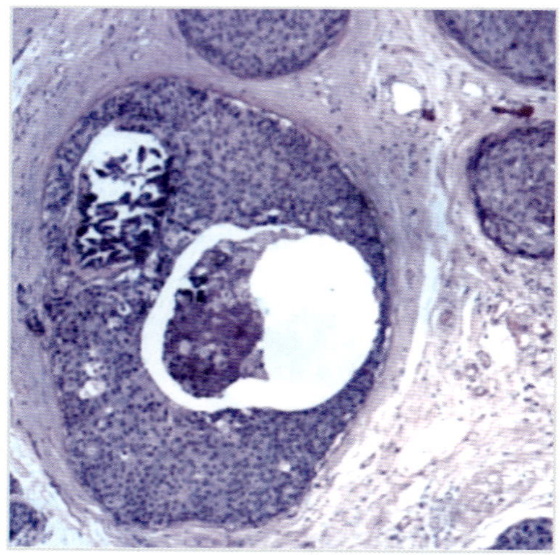

Fig. 4: High-grade ductal carcinoma in situ (DCIS) with comedonecrosis and intraluminal microcalcification

dependent than grade-dependent. Numerous morphologic variants of DCIS exist such as solid, cribriform, papillary, micropapillary, clinging and cystic hypersecretory. Based on the cytologic criteria, a three-tier grading system (Box 1) has been defined.[15]

Duct carcinoma in situ presenting as a large palpable mass has a significantly higher possibility of occult invasion, axillary nodal metastasis, multicentricity, chances of local recurrence. This group has an overall worse prognosis than nonpalpable, mammographically discovered small, microscopic lesions (Figs 3 and 4).

Lobular Neoplasia

This term encompasses all atypical epithelial lesions arising in the terminal duct lobular unit composed of small discohesive cells. Lobular carcinoma in situ (LCIS) is the most extreme end of the spectrum. Whereas DCIS is considered as a precursor of invasive carcinoma, lobular neoplasia (LN) is believed to be a marker of risk for invasive carcinoma in both breasts. The distinction lies in the fact that the invasive carcinoma which follows LN may affect any quadrant of the ipsilateral breast.

GRADING OF BREAST CARCINOMA

All invasive carcinomas are graded on the basis of tubule/gland formation, nuclear pleomorphism and mitotic count. The Elston and Ellis modification of the Bloom and Richardson grading system is currently accepted grading system (Box 2). It is best applied to invasive carcinoma of no special type. However, its application to

Box 2: **Modified Scarff-Bloom-Richardson grading system**

- *Tubule/gland formation:*
  - Score 1: Tubule formation > 75%
  - Score 2: Tubule formation 10–75%
  - Score 3: Tubule formation < 10%
- Nuclear size:
  - Score 1: Tumor nuclei same as normal duct cell nuclei
  - Score 2: Intermediate-size nuclei
  - Score 3: Large vesicular nuclei with prominent nucleoli
- *Mitotic count [per 10 hpf at the edge of tumor (40 × objective)]:*
  - Score 1: 0–7 mitoses/10 hpf
  - Score 2: 8–14 mitoses/10 hpf
  - Score 3: > 15 mitoses/10 hpf

Abbreviation: hpf, high power fields

invasive lobular carcinoma is more controversial. Grade has a definite bearing on prognosis and is used in various prognostic indices along with T size and lymph node status.

HORMONE RECEPTOR

The presence of hormone (estrogen and progesterone) receptors in the tumor tissue determined on IHC correlates with response to hormone therapy. The two parameters evaluated in immunohistochemical preparations of hormone receptors are the percentage of tumor cell nuclei stained and the intensity of the reaction. The two parameters are combined into a scoring system.[16]

HER2 neu

With the availability of trastuzumab (Herceptin) as a therapeutic agent,[17] the need to find HER2 neu expression in breast tumors has great significance. According to the recent American Society of Clinical Oncology and College of American Pathologist Guideline Recommendations for HER2 neu testing in breast cancer:[18]

- A positive HER2 neu result is:
  - An immunohistochemical staining scored as 3+
  - Dual-probe HER2 neu/CEP17 ratio with an average HER2 neu copy number ≥ 4.0 signals/cell
  - Dual-probe HER2 neu/CEP17 ratio ≥ 2.0 with an average HER2 neu copy number < 4.0 signals/cell
  - Dual-probe HER2 neu/CEP17 ratio < 2.0; c, e with an average HER2 neu copy number ≥ 6.0 signals/cell.
- A negative HER2 neu result is:
  - An immunohistochemical staining scored as 0 or 1+
  - Dual-probe HER2 neu/CEP17 ratio < 2.0 with an average HER2 neu copy number < 4.0 signals/cell (Table 1).

Tumors that are negative for all the three markers, i.e. ER, PR and HER2 neu are termed "triple negative tumors". They are usually high-grade invasive ductal carcinoma (IDC), NOS type with a higher propensity to metastasize.[19]

MOLECULAR CLASSIFICATION

The breast cancers have been segregated into molecular subgroups based on similarities in the gene expression profiles.[20] The subtypes of breast cancers recognized by their gene signature are: luminal A, luminal B, HER2 neu type, basal-like and normal breast-like. The salient features of the molecular subtypes are summarized in Table 2. Among the various subtypes, the basal-like subtype is associated with the worst prognosis.[21]

TABLE 1: **Grading of human epidermal growth factor receptor 2 [HER2 (neu)] overexpression by immunohistochemical staining**

Staining pattern	*Score*	*HER2 neu protein overexpression assessment*
No staining or membrane staining in < 10% of the tumor cells	0	Negative
A faint to barely perceptible membrane staining in > 10% of the tumor cells	1^+	Negative
A weak to moderate complete membrane staining in > 10% of the tumor cells	2^+	Weakly positive
A strong complete membrane staining in > 10% of the tumor cells	3^+	Strongly positive

Abbreviation: HER2 neu, human epidermal growth factor receptor 2

TABLE 2: **Major molecular subtypes of breast cancer determined by gene expression profiling**

Luminal A	*Luminal B*	*HER2 neu*	*Basal-like*
• ER/PR positive • HER2 neu negative • Low Ki-67 (< 14%)	• ER/PR positive • HER2 neu expression may be positive or negative • Ki-67 ≥ 14%	• ER/PR negative • HER2 neu positive	• Most ER/PR and HER2 neu negative (triple negative) • CK 5/6 and/or $EGFR^+$

Abbreviations: ER, estrogen receptor; PR, progesterone receptor; HER2 neu, human epidermal growth factor receptor 2; CK 5/6, cytokeratin 5/6; $EGFR^+$, epidermal growth factor receptor-positive

Biologic Subtyping in Early-Stage Disease

- High grade/proliferation: Low ER level
- Low grade/proliferation: High ER level.

Ki-67

It is a predictive and a prognostic marker. It is an antibody marker to a tumor antigen found in breast cancer cells. High scores, greater than 20% mean that the cancer cells are growing and dividing at a rapid pace. High-grade tumors have a higher Ki-67 score.

SCREENING

Breast imaging plays an integral role in screening patients for early diagnosis of breast cancer. It helps detect a clinically occult lesion in an asymptomatic woman. Mammogram detects approximately 40% of lesions, half of these are invasive cancers less than 1 cm. Meta-analysis reveals a statistically significant decrease in mortality from breast cancer mainly due to mammogram studies. Hendrick et al.[22] analyzed eight randomized-controlled trials of mammogram screening and found an 18% reduction in mortality in women in their 40s. Combined data from five Swedish trials yielded a statistically significant mortality decrease of 29%.

Guidelines for Screening Mammography

- Baseline mammography at 40–45 years, thereafter every 1–2 years
- Annual mammography for women, 50 years and above
- If genetic testing is positive (BRCA1 or BRCA2) annual screening mammography is advisable at age 25–35 years
- In a first-degree relative (mother/sister) with premenopausal breast cancer, annual screening mammogram should be done at an age 10 years younger than the age at which relative developed breast cancer (generally, around 30 years)
- Women who have had breast cancer or a biopsy diagnosis of LCIS, annual screening mammography is recommended
- Previous radiation to chest or surrounding areas, screening mammogram begins 8–10 years after completion of radiation
- Screening mammogram after 70 years is debatable, but can be done in individuals in good health or if any abnormality is detected
- Magnetic resonance imaging (MRI) may be considered in mutation carriers and women with dense glandular tissue on mammogram.

PREVENTION

- *Primary prevention* of breast cancer remains an important goal for which prophylactic bilateral mastectomy and chemoprevention are major considerations. Prophylactic bilateral mastectomies may be considered in women with the diagnosis of LCIS, in women with a significant family history of breast cancer and who are known carriers of genetic mutation of BRCA1 and BRCA2. Though prophylactic bilateral total mastectomy will reduce the development of breast cancer in high-risk women, it is a heavy price to pay as all are not likely to develop the disease. A more frequent surveillance may be a cautious option. The high incidence of mastectomies in the West is the result of easily available reconstructive surgeries (transverse rectus abdominis myocutaneous flap and latissimus dorsi flap) and frequent use of tissue expanders/implants with excellent cosmetic results. In India, few women may opt for reconstruction but majority avoid it due to socioeconomic reasons. Bilateral oophorectomy reduces incidence of breast cancer by 50%. Reduction in obesity in postmenopausal women offers protection against breast cancer. Chemoprevention should therefore be considered for all high-risk women (Table 3). The National Surgical Adjuvant Breast and Bowel Project (NSABP) trial proved the role of tamoxifen with a 50% reduction in development of invasive and noninvasive breast cancer. Tamoxifen has an anti-estrogen effect and significantly reduces the number of contralateral breast cancers. Tamoxifen still remains the gold standard against which other anti-estrogens are evaluated. It is cheaper, a fact of relevance in developing countries. Raloxifene is a selective estrogen receptor modulator and is being investigated to define its role in breast cancer chemoprevention
- *Secondary prevention* is aimed at early diagnosis of breast cancer which decreases mortality. Breast examination (Table 4) and screening mammography fall into this category.

DIAGNOSIS

- Complete history and physical examination
- Routine blood, hepatorenal profile
- Chest radiograph

TABLE 3: Risk factors

No.	Risk factor	Category at risk
1.	Early menarche	• Younger than 12 years
2.	Late menopause	• Older than 55 years
3.	Age at first childbirth	• Older than 30 years
4.	Family history	• First-degree relative with breast cancer • Breast-ovarian cancer syndrome
5.	Germ-line mutation	• $BRCA_1$ and $BRCA_2$
6.	• Personal history of breast cancer • Ionizing radiation exposure	• Invasive breast cancer • Hodgkin's disease
7.	Proliferative breast cancer lesions	• Lobular carcinoma in situ (LCIS) • Ductal carcinoma in situ (DCIS)
8.	Hormone replacement therapy (HRT) with estrogen and progesterone	• Unopposed use for at least 5 years

TABLE 4: American Cancer Society (ACS) recommendation for the early detection of breast cancer in average risk, asymptomatic individuals

Examination pattern	Outcomes
Breast self-examination (BSE)	• Beginning in early 20s, women should be advised about the benefits and limitations of BSE, every 3–4 months • The importance of prompt reporting of any new breast symptoms to a health professional should be emphasized
Clinical breast examination (CBE)	• For women in their 20s and 30s, it is recommended that CBE be a part of periodic health examination at least every 3 years • Asymptomatic women aged ≥ 40 years, should continue to receive a CBE as part of a periodic health examination annually

- Ultrasound of the abdomen and pelvis
- Mammography and sonomammogram
- Bone scan (optional)—only if recent skeletal symptoms
- Computed tomography (CT) of chest/abdomen or positron emission tomography with CT (PET-CT) (optional or as indicated)—worthwhile in stage III lesions.

Mammography

The advent of modern imaging techniques for early diagnosis and multimodality therapy has made a significant difference in the overall survival (OS). According to the Surveillance Epidemiology and End Result (SEER) data screening mammography has reduced mortality by 29%, which is highly significant. Conventional film-screen mammography has been the mainstay in the initial diagnosis of breast cancer and is widely used for screening as well. About 15–20% of breast cancer is not visible on mammography. Recently, full-field digital mammography (FFDM) and computed radiography (CR) systems are frequently used. Standard views in mammography include mediolateral oblique (MLO) and craniocaudal (CC) views (Figs 5A and B). Breast tomosynthesis, an advanced application of digital mammography, could develop into a promising solution to resolve the problem of tissue overlap with its three-dimensional capabilities.[23] In radiologically-dense breast digital, breast, tomosynthesis is the future of mammography (Box 3); this will replace two-dimensional (2-D) mammography in 5 years. However, digital tomosynthesis does not replace MRI.

Mammographic findings that raise a suspicion of malignancy include new or asymmetric masses or densities. Spiculated margins of a mass and fine, linear branching microcalcifications are considered to be the two most important signs of malignancy (Fig. 6). Ill-defined masses, increased number of microlobulations, architectural distortion, nipple retraction and enlarged axillary nodes are other ancillary findings (Figs 7 to 9).[24] Along with the branching pattern, amorphous and pleomorphic pattern of calcification should also be viewed with concern and may warrant a biopsy.[25] Five or more microcalcifications within a 1 cm^3 volume (defined as cluster) on the mammogram, should be regarded with suspicion for malignancy, with more compact clusters being ominous (Figs 10 and 11).[26]

Breast Ultrasound

Breast ultrasound may be preferred to mammography in younger females needing breast imaging, to avoid radiation. By and large, it is used to complement mammography than as a stand alone investigation.[27] About 28% more cancers were detected when ultrasound was added to

Box 3: Oslo tomosynthesis screening trial

- 40% increase in the detection of invasive breast cancers
- 27% increase in the detection of all cancers (invasive and in situ cancers combined)
- 15% decrease in false-positive rates
- No increase in detection of duct carcinoma in situ (DCIS)

Source: Radiology; January 2013.

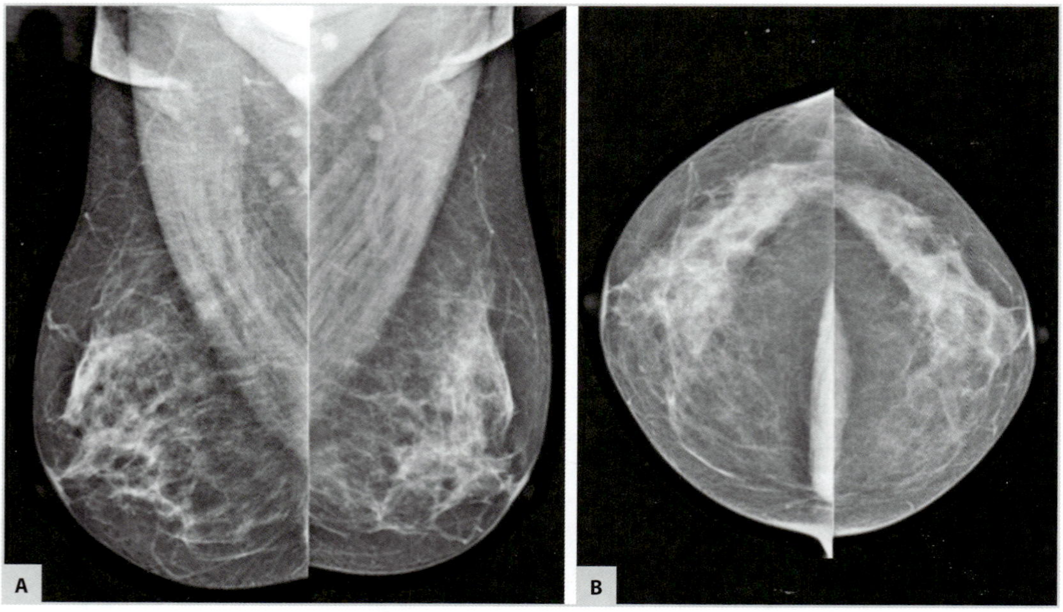

Figs 5A and B: (A) Standard mediolateral oblique (MLO); (B) Craniocaudal (CC) views in a normal mammogram

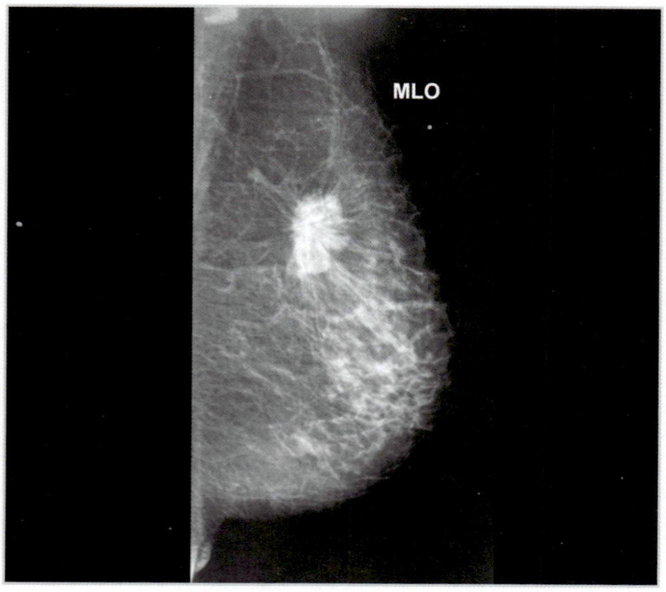

Fig. 6: A spiculated mass lesion with linear branching. Not an ideal candidate for breast conservation surgery (BCS) due to linear branching

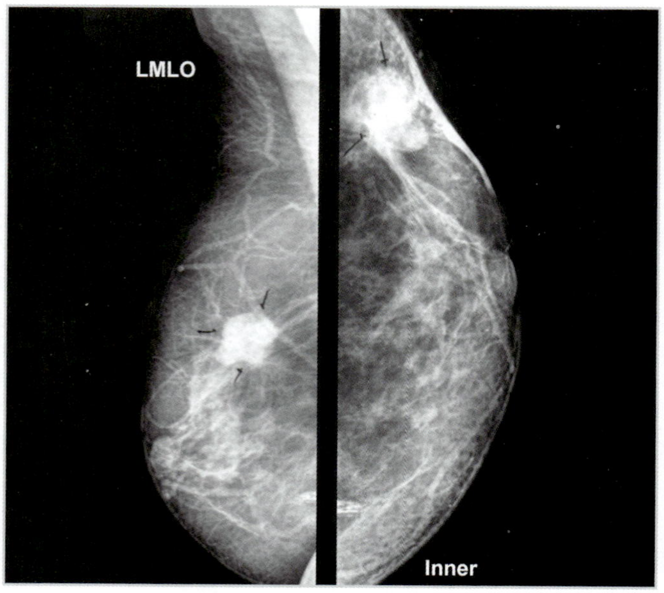

Fig. 7: Mediolateral oblique (MLO) view of breast showing an ill-defined mass

mammography. It will find three to four additional cancers per 1,000 women. In 91% breast cancer was detected when ultrasound and mammography were combined, while 78% were detected when only mammography was used [American College of Radiology Imaging Network (ACRIN) 6666 Trial]. There is a high false-positive in young women. Primarily, ultrasound helps to distinguish between solid and cystic lesions (Figs 12A and B). The solid lesions can be further characterized to decide if a short-interval follow-up can be opted for instead of immediate biopsy.[28] Also, ultrasound may give an advantage over mammography in imaging of dense breasts. Features of malignant solid mass include marked hypoechogenicity, ill-defined or spiculated margins, mass depth greater than width, microcalcifications and posterior acoustic shadowing.[28,29] Finally, ultrasound is useful for image-guided procedures such as aspiration of cysts, drainage of abscesses, breast biopsies and preoperative needle

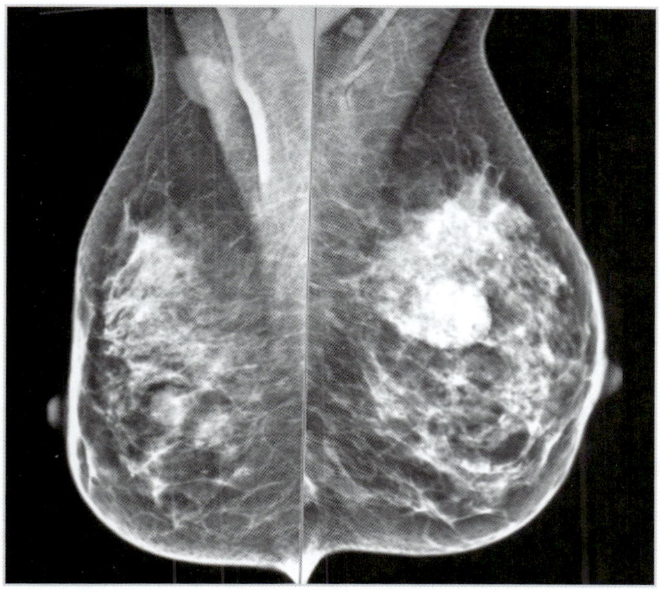

Fig. 8: Mediolateral oblique (MLO) view of breast showing a mass lesion in the left breast, which was histologically benign. Most dense breast lesions are usually suspect for a mitotic lesion

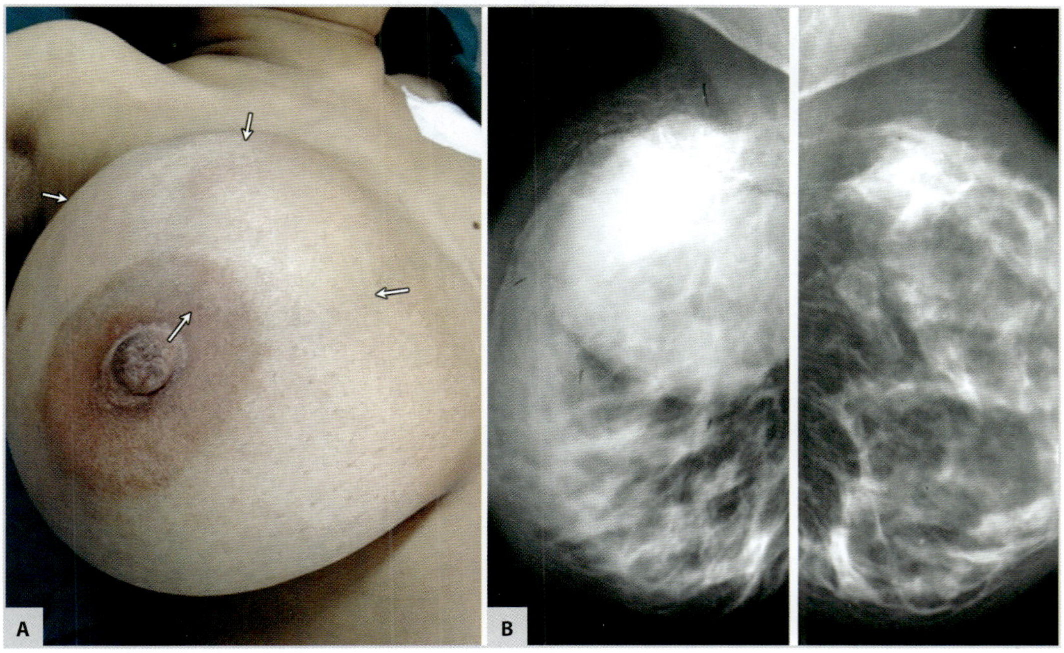

Figs 9A and B: (A) A 34-year-old woman with a large breast lump occupying almost half of the breast. Typical clinical setting for a neoadjuvant chemotherapy; (B) Mammography of the same patient. Biopsy showed a metaplastic carcinoma with sarcomatoid element

localization. Ultrasonography (USG) elastography can be useful for breast mass characterization, as breast cancers are stiffer than benign lesions.[30] This must be supported by a good clinical examination to rule out a suspicious mitotic lesion despite Breast Imaging Reporting and Data System [BI-RADS (I-III)] (Table 5). Based on imaging data, a long-term or a short-term surveillance is recommended. Lesions which are BI-RADS III, a short-term follow-up at 6–12 months is worthwhile.

Breast MRI

The value of contrast-enhanced MRI in breast imaging lies in the cross-sectional detailing, T_1 and T_2 characterizing and mapping of enhancement kinetics that it enables.[31,32]

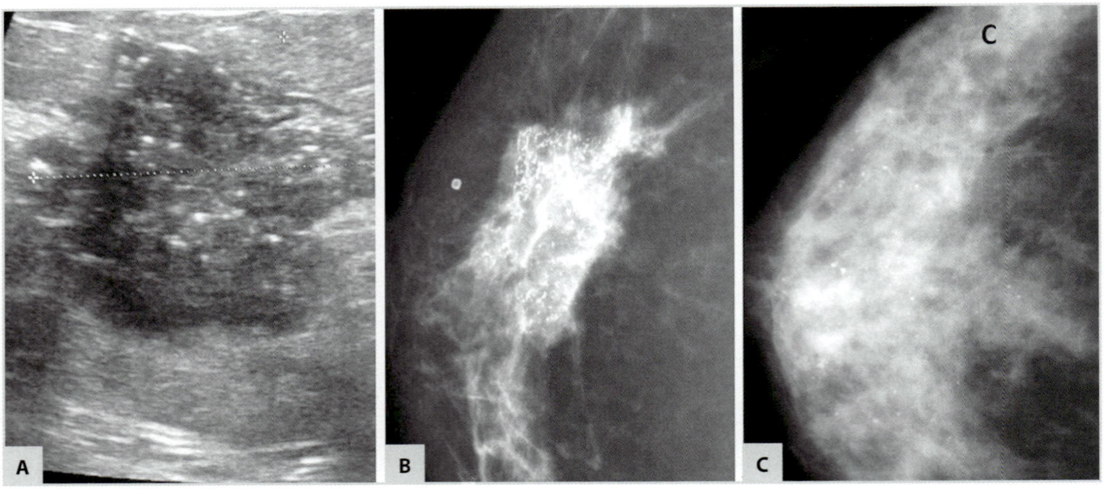

Figs 10A to C: (A) Ultrasonography (USG) of breast showing a malignant mass with microcalcification; (B) Mammography showing a mass with microcalcification of the same patient; (C) Mammography showing benign calcification

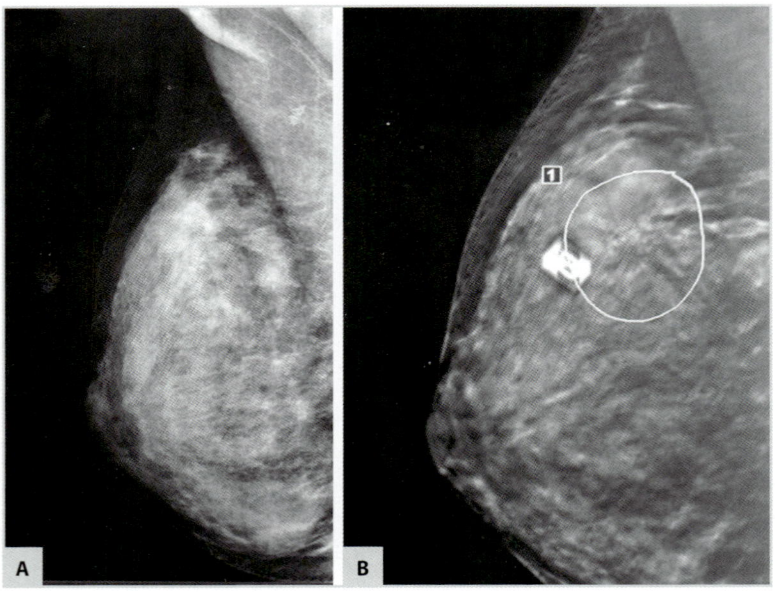

Figs 11A and B: (A) Female (28 years) with a firm 3 cm lump in upper quadrant of the right breast. Dense glandular tissue prevented precise interpretation on mammography. Fine-needle aspirate cytology (FNAC) revealed atypical ductal hyperplasia; (B) Breast tomosynthesis shows tiny suspect spiculations—Breast Imaging Reporting and Data System (BIRADS) IV. Excision biopsy showed an infiltrating duct carcinoma. Previous history of fibrocystic disease, histologically proven 4 years ago on the opposite side

TABLE 5: Breast Imaging Reporting and Data System (BI-RADS)—The American College of Radiology

BI-RADS	*Findings*
I	Negative (no findings)
II	Benign appearance
III	Probably benign appearance (< 2% chance of malignancy)
IV	Suspicious for breast cancer
V	Highly suspicious for breast cancer

Abbreviation: BI-RADS, Breast Imaging Reporting and Data System

MRI is indicated when mammography findings are indeterminate (Fig. 13). It is also useful for local staging of breast cancer; diagnosing a postoperative recurrence, evaluating postchemotherapy patients or as a problem-solving tool for mammography findings in which malignancy could be a differential diagnosis. Spiculated borders, peripheral enhancement, irregular shape of mass lesions and enhancement with ductal or segmental pattern in non-mass lesions are highly suspicious for malignancy.[33] Other ominous findings include

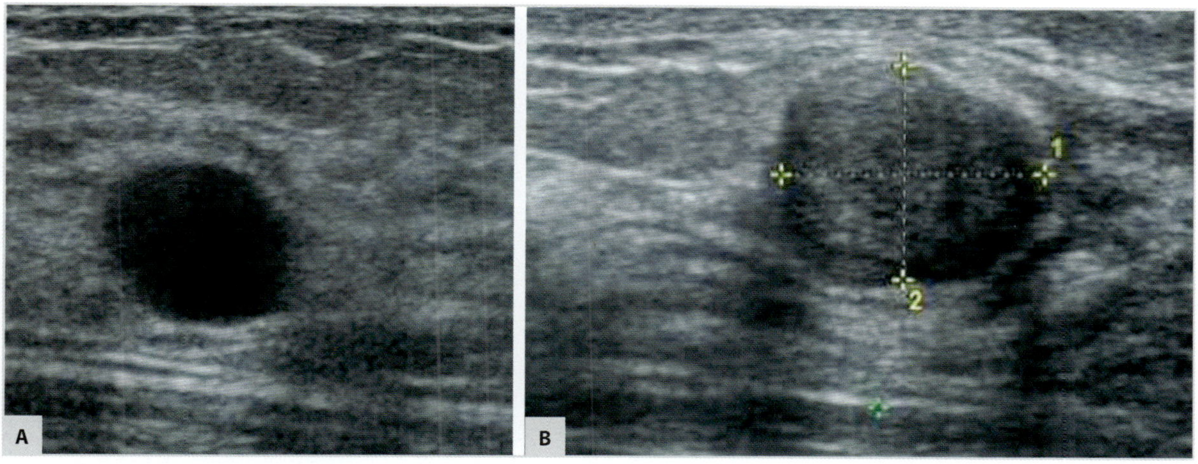

Figs 12A and B: Cystic (A) versus solid (B) mass seen on ultrasonography (USG) of breast

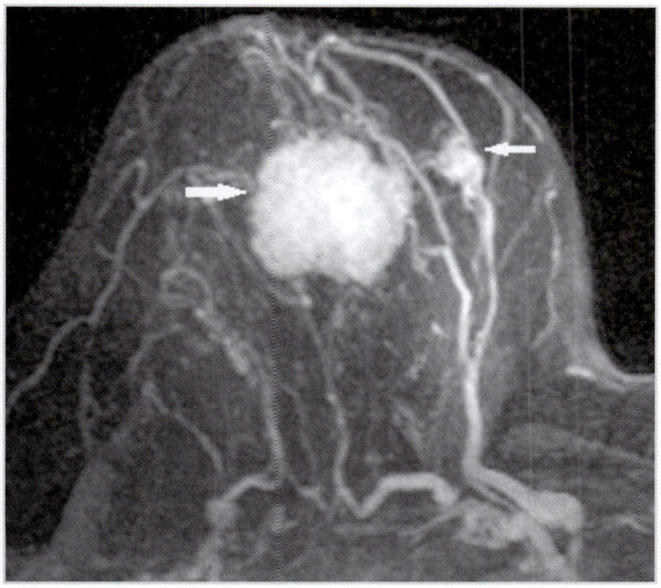

Fig. 13: Multifocal malignancy in magnetic resonance imaging (MRI) of breast

heterogenous enhancement and enhancing septae.[34] In general, on T_2-weighted, non-fat suppressed sequences, high T_2-signal intensity has been associated with benign disease and low T_2-signal intensity with carcinoma.

PET-CT Scan

Positron emission tomography with CT scan is used for staging, restaging and monitoring therapy response in patients treated by chemo/radiotherapy (Figs 14A to D).[35] Fluorodeoxyglucose (FDG)-PET has limited diagnostic utility in detection of small primary tumors, in staging the axilla and in detecting osteoblastic metastatic lesions. It helps in detecting distant metastasis, recurrent disease and in monitoring therapy response. In T_3N_1 disease PET/CT is worthwhile though mediastinal and paratracheal adenopathy may yield a false-negative result. In early cases $T_{1,2}N_0$, the use of PET/CT is optional, though chest and abdomen CT studies may be indicated.[36]

Tissue Diagnosis

- Fine-needle aspirate cytology (FNAC)
- Core-needle biopsy (CNB)
- Surgical biopsy (incisional biopsy/excisional biopsy)
- Wire localization (for nonpalpable lesions or calcification).

Fine-needle aspirate cytology for palpable lesions is an office procedure; however, for smaller lesions ultrasound-guided FNAC is preferred. This can only indicate presence of cancer cells without any details of architecture or invasive component. Hence, mammography or ultrasound-guided CNB will help in evaluating precise histopathology and biologic factors of the lesion based on which therapy can be planned. Due to heterogenous distribution of antigens in breast cancer tumors, HER2 neu activity does not appear to be adequately detected on CNB. There is good concordance between CNB and surgical specimens in regard to tumor type, ER and PR for most patients. Data suggest that IHC testing on the CNB alone may not be adequate to tailor targeted therapy in all patients. It was hence recommended retesting HER2 neu in the surgical specimen.[37]

Ultrasound-guided wire localization with hook wires is simple and precisely locates calcifications or an

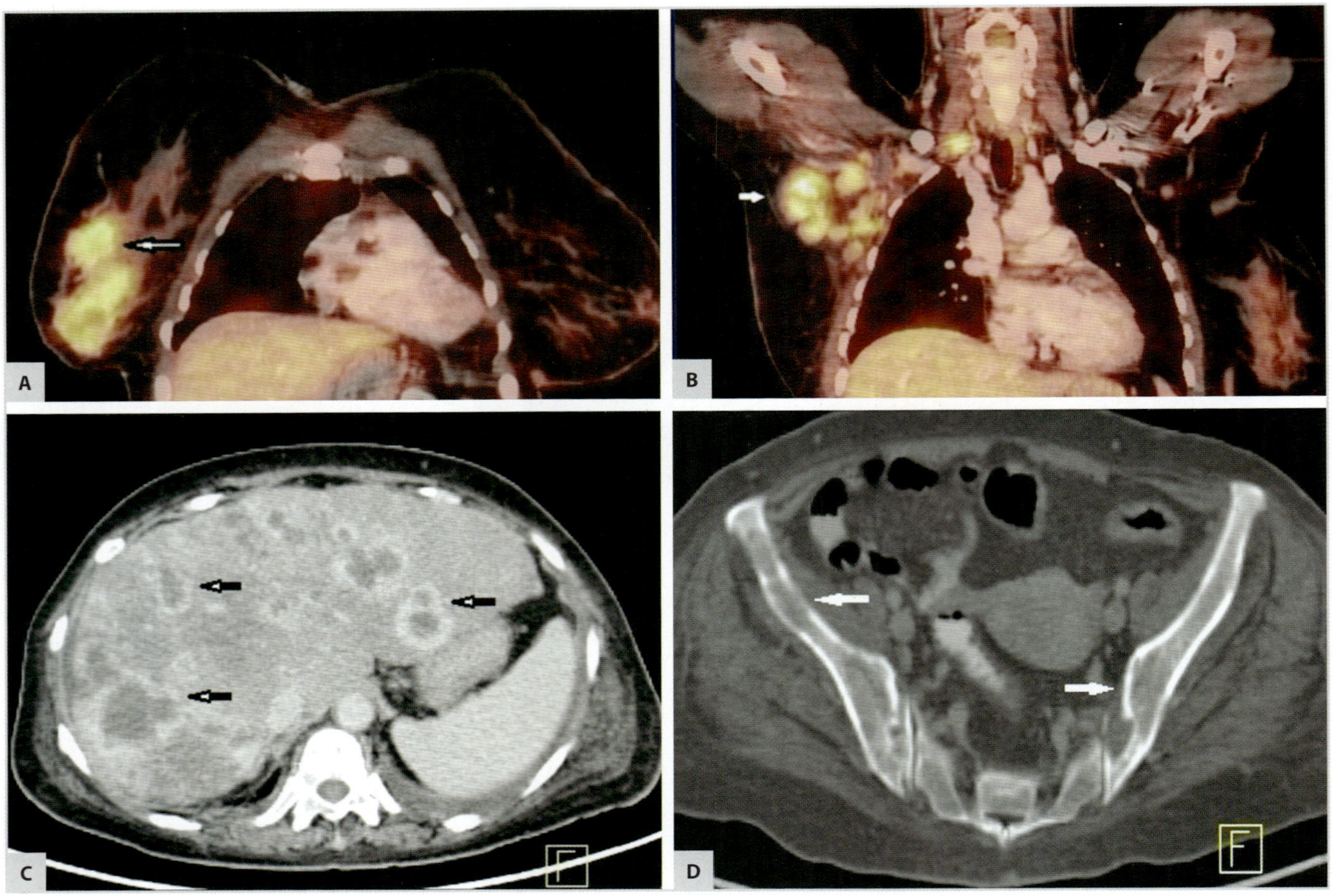

Figs 14A to D: Positron emission tomography (PET)/computed tomography (CT) studies showing (A) Metabolically active breast mass (arrow); (B) Metastatic axillary nodes (arrow); (C) Metastases in liver (arrow); and (D) Bones (arrow) of the same patient

impalpable mass enabling the surgeon to widely excise the area (Figs 15 to 17). Gross-free margins should then be confirmed by an X-ray of the specimen. This is then sent for histopathology (Table 6).

NONINVASIVE BREAST CANCER

Ductal Carcinoma In Situ

This is a "mammographic disease" entity in asymptomatic individuals. It is a heterogeneous group of lesions rather than a simple entity.[38] DCIS mostly manifests on a routine mammographic study by localized or diffuse tiny calcifications. Not all microscopic DCIS will progress to clinical cancer; however untreated DCIS has the propensity to progress to invasive breast cancer. The widespread use of screening mammography has resulted in a significant increase in the detection of DCIS. In the United States (US), the incidence is 25–35 per 100,000 woman years. DCIS accounts for 25% of all new screen-detected neoplasms in the US with 1.7 cases of DCIS-detected per 1000 screening mammograms.[39] As in the west, the incidence of DCIS in India is definitely on the rise due to increased use of screening mammographies. The proportion of women with mammographically-detected DCIS in whom invasive carcinoma will develop is uncertain. The peak incidence of DCIS, 96.7 per 100,000 women, occurs around 65–69 years. Studies reveal that 25–30% untreated patients with non-comedo DCIS will develop invasive cancer within 10 years.[40-42]

Detection and Diagnosis

More than 90% of DCIS is detected on routine-screening mammogram; however, 5–15% will have a lump.[43] Before the advent of routine-screening mammography, patients with DCIS presented with a palpable mass, nipple thickening or Paget's disease. In patients with palpable lesions, about 25% demonstrated foci of invasive carcinoma. DCIS can present as microcalcification (8–90%), a soft-tissue density

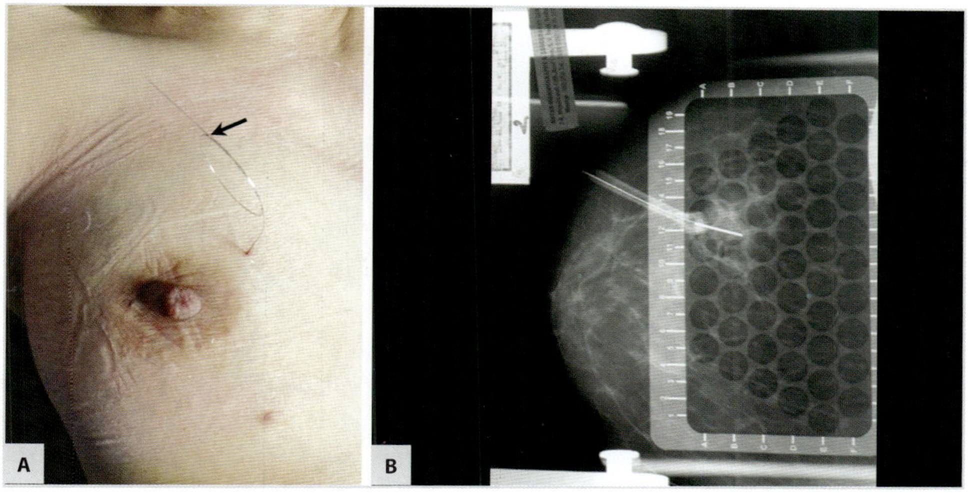

Figs 15A and B: (A) Wire localization in another patient with mammographically detected microcalcification; (B) Mammography-guided wire localization in a patient with almost complete regression of the tumor, after neoadjuvant chemotherapy

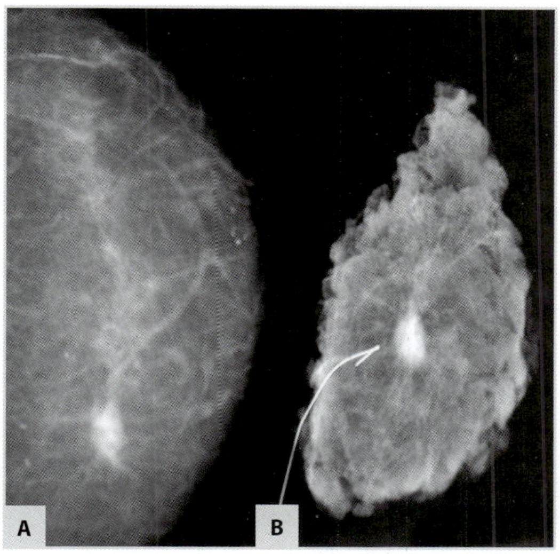

Figs 16A and B: (A) Nonpalpable lesion detected on mammography; (B) Hook-wire localization for nonpalpable lesion. It is necessary to radiograph the excised lesion to confirm wide-margins before studying histopathology

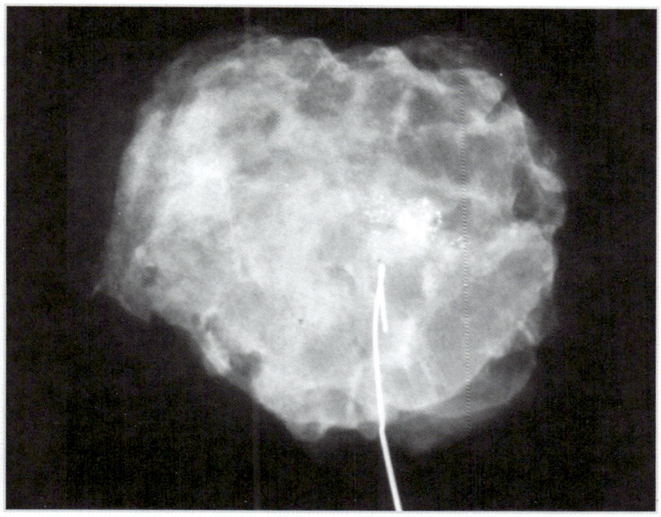

Fig. 17: Radiography of a surgical specimen with the hook-wire within microcalcifications indicating a safe margin of excision (3–4 cm)

TABLE 6: Tumor, node and metastasis (TNM) staging

Stage	*TNM staging*
Stage 0	Carcinoma in situ
Stage I	T_1 (< 2 cm) N_0
Stage IIA	T_1 (< 2 cm) N_1 T_2 (2–5 cm) N_0
Stage IIB	T_2 N_1 T_3 (> 5 cm) N_0
Stage IIIA	(T_0–T_3) fixed axillary lymph nodes (ALNs)
Stage IIIB	LABC or inflammatory cancer or tumors with metastasis to the internal mammary lymph nodes
Stage IV	Distant or supraclavicular metastasis

Abbreviations: TNM, tumor, node and metastasis; LABC, locally advanced breast cancer or both. For evaluation of DCIS mammography remains the gold standard; however, MRI is beneficial in patients at high risk and those with very dense breasts. DCIS can mimic fibrocystic changes and often benign findings on MRI and can also lead to unnecessary biopsies. MRI is also useful to identify multicentric lesions.[44,45]

Treatment Options

Mastectomy in DCIS

- Extensive microcalcifications
- Multicentricity (Multiquadrant disease) 20–30%
- Unicentric DCIS lesions too large to achieve free margins, which is nearly impossible in diffuse lesions
- Unacceptable cosmetic results with breast conservation
- Patients with DCIS with local recurrence after breast conservation.

Breast conservation surgery in DCIS

Patients with localized DCIS are treated with wire localization, breast conservation and radiation therapy (XRT) with excellent local control with negative margins.[46-50] The crucial factor in breast conservation surgery (BCS) is an optimally free margin of the excised specimen to prevent local recurrence. Excessively wide margins should be avoided to ensure good cosmesis. An appropriately done BCS with free margins consistently ensures very low recurrence rates of around 3–5% at 10 years. Randomized Clinical Trials have demonstrated that adding radiation treatment after surgical excision reduces risk of developing local recurrence and invasive local recurrence by approximately 50%. Use of radiation in DCIS should be judicious, since DCIS is not a killer disease and 20 years survival is 98% (Tables 7 and 8).

Management of the axilla in DCIS

In 1987, NSABP studies made axillary node dissection for patients with DCIS optional, at the discretion of the surgeons. Since, then literature evidence indicates that axillary lymph node dissection (ALND) can be dispensed

TABLE 7: The University of South California/Van Nuys Prognostic Index (USC/VNPI) Scoring System

Score	1	2	3
Size (mm)	≤ 15	16–40	≥ 41
Margins (mm)	≥ 10	1–9	< 1
Pathological classification	Non-high grade without necrosis	Non-high grade with necrosis	High grade with or without necrosis
Age (years)	≥ 61	40–60	≤ 39

TABLE 8: Treatment guidelines for DCIS based on University of South California (USC)/Van Nuys Prognostic Index (VNPI)[57]

USC/VNPI Score	Recommended treatment
4–6	Excision only
7–9	Excision + radiation
10–12	Mastectomy

in patients with DCIS. DCIS and DCIS with microinvasion (DCIS-M) have become frequent with screen-detected breast cancers. Sentinel lymph node biopsy (SLNB), which is now the gold standard, remains controversial for this clinicopathological entity. Positive SLNs are however reported in 8–16% with pure DCIS or DCIS-M.[51-56]

Indications for sentinel lymph node biopsy (SLNB) in DCIS

- Patients undergoing mastectomy for DCIS with or without reconstruction
- Easy accessibility if DCIS in upper-outer quadrant
- Palpable DCIS more than 4 cm as there is a chance of microinvasion

Patients with DCIS are prescribed hormonal therapy with tamoxifen for 5 years, if the tumor is hormone receptor positive. No other systemic therapy is necessary.

Lobular Carcinoma In Situ (LCIS)

Lobular carcinoma in situ is a rare but a distinct form of clinicopathological entity. Atypical lobular hyperplasia (ALH) and LCIS are proliferative lesions of the breast.[58] ALH and LCIS are risk factors for development of malignancy. The risk of development of an ipsilateral or contralateral breast cancer is reported to be four to five-fold more in patients with ALH and nine to twelve-fold more with LCIS.[59] LCIS occurs around 40–50 years and is generally not accompanied with any mammographic changes, calcification or a mass. LCIS is often diagnosed incidentally with other breast lesion biopsies. The incidence is 0.5–3.8% and is often bilateral, multicentric and multifocal. 50% of LCIS have multiple foci in the ipsilateral breast and 30% have LCIS in the contralateral breast.[60] This should be evaluated at diagnosis and excluded.

Management[61,62]

- Surveillance is probably the most appropriate option and rational approach
- Chemoprevention can be offered for risk reduction

- Prophylactic bilateral mastectomy reduces risk by 90% (usually for high-risk patients with family history or other factors)
- If LCIS is found in an excised tissue, it is not necessary to obtain negative margins of resection
- There is no role of radiation after local excision of LCIS
- It is recommended to excise a LCIS identified on CNB to rule out an associated malignancy.[63]

INVASIVE BREAST CANCER

Changing Paradigms—Management of Breast Cancer

It took almost a little less than a millennium before the Halsted management of breast cancer was modified and yet it would be unfair to say that the Halsted principle should be confined to the dustbin of history. It was probably the finest operation ever devised, based on the lymphatic drainage and removal of metastatic nodes in the drainage basin. The Halsted principle has remained steadfast, despite modifications in our approach to the lymphatic system. Our increasing knowledge about cell biology, genetics, chemo/radiotherapy and the seminal contributions of Randomized Clinical Trials (Fisher) has revolutionized our current approach to breast cancer management, which is based on robust evidence, and is rapidly accepted as a "standard of care" globally.

Tables 9 and 10 sum up the events that have lead us to the current standard of care in breast cancer management.

Modified Radical Mastectomy

Modified radical mastectomy (MRM) remained a gold standard for surgical treatment for decades; however, with an early diagnosis there has been a shift toward breast conversation surgery (BCS). Our approach to axillary lymph node dissection (ALND) is rapidly changing to conservation normal axillary nodes by frequent use of SLNB techniques. In the current milieu, mastectomy can be questioned; however, MRM will still remain in our armamentarium in the following conditions:

- Multicentric lesions with high nodal burden (local)
- When chemo/radiotherapy facilities are not at hand
- Socioeconomic reasons
- Patient refusal for radio/chemotherapy
- Poor response to chemo/radiotherapy with residual tumor
- In the Indian context, mastectomy will survive (Fig. 18).

TABLE 9: Therapeutic evolution

Landmarks	*Year*
Beatson-hormonal manipulation	1895
Radical mastectomy (Halsted)	1896
Conservation breast surgery	1938
The McWhirter regime	1952
Supervoltage therapy (Co^{60})	1958
Bonadonna and Veronesi (CMF)	1970–80
The Fisher hypothesis: NSABP trials	1975
Hormonal therapy revolution	1980
Improved chemo/radiation therapy (XRT)	1985
Cons surgery consolidation	1985
The sentinel node story	1995
Neoadjuvant chemotherapy/XRT-Impact (LABC/early carcinoma)	1998
The tamoxifen era—recent revisitation	2000
Newer chemotherapy molecules (paclitaxel, gemcitabine, vinorelbine)	2000
Molecular biology revolution (targeted therapies)	2000
Genomics (*$BRCA_{1-2}$* genes)	2000
Aromatase inhibitors (AI)	2002
Partial breast irradiation	2005
Intraoperative XRT	2005
Oncotype Dx® genomic score	2010
Mammaprint Tomosynthesis	2011

Abbreviations: CMF, cyclophosphamide, methotrexate, and fluorouracil; NSABP, National Surgical Adjuvant Breast and Bowel Project; LABC, locally advanced breast cancer

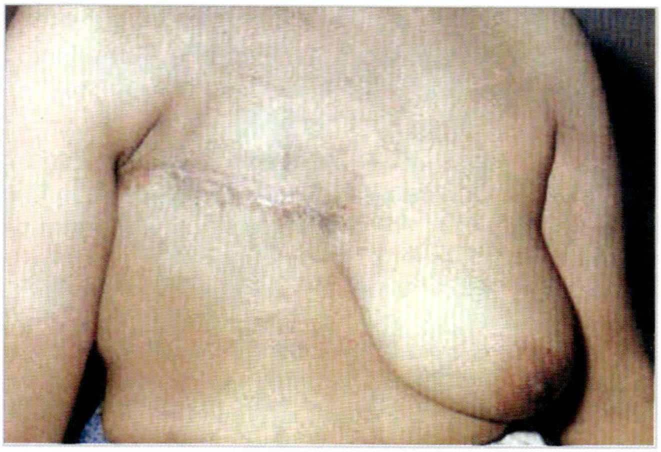

Fig. 18: Mastectomy—relics of the past?

TABLE 10: Selected National Surgical Adjuvant Breast and Bowel Project (NSABP) Trials impacting on management

Trial	Treatment	Outcome
NSABP B-32	SLN biopsy followed by axillary dissection vs SLN biopsy alone for clinically node-negative patients	SLN identification rate was similar in both groups, accuracy was high for both, negative predictive values were high for both
NSABP B-21	Lumpectomy plus tamoxifen vs lumpectomy plus tamoxifen plus XRT vs lumpectomy plus XRT for node-negative tumors < 1 cm	Combination of XRT and tamoxifen was more effective than either alone in reducing ipsilateral breast tumor recurrence
NSABP B-14	Surgery alone vs Surgery plus adjuvant tamoxifen in node-negative patients with estrogen receptor-positive tumors	Improved DFS rate for adjuvant tamoxifen group
NSABP B-13	Surgery alone vs surgery plus adjuvant chemotherapy in node-negative patients with estrogen receptor-negative tumors	Improved DFS rate for adjuvant chemotherapy group
NSABP B-06	Total mastectomy vs lumpectomy vs lumpectomy with XRT	No significant difference in DFS or OS rates; addition of XRT to lumpectomy reduced local recurrence rate from 39 to 10%
NSABP B-04	Total mastectomy vs total mastectomy with XRT vs radical mastectomy	Disease-free survival (DFS) or overall survival (OS) rates, no difference

Abbreviations: NSABP, National Surgical Adjuvant Breast and Bowel Project; XRT, radiation therapy; AC, doxorubicin (adriamycin), cyclophosphamide; SLN, sentinel lymph node

Breast Conservation Surgery (BCS)

This entails removing the tumor with an adequate (2 cm) surrounding margin free of tumor. This is followed by XRT which could be conventional whole breast radiation, intraoperative at the end of surgery or accelerated partial breast irradiation. Axillary radiation is avoided in $N_{0,1}$ cases as determined by SLNB to prevent arm edema. Since axillary recurrence is rare after a good ALND, radiotherapy to the axilla is best avoided unless the nodal (metastatic) burden is high, greater than 5–6 nodes. Since local recurrence after BCS mainly (90%) occurs in the index area, even whole breast irradiation could be avoided to reduce the morbidity unless the primary tumor was a locally advanced breast cancer (LABC) which was downstaged with chemotherapy. In early-stage breast cancer, multiple large prospective, randomized trials have shown BCS to be equivalent to mastectomy for OS. Local recurrence in the ipsilateral breast has been reported to occur at a rate of 3–9% at 5 years and 14–20% at 20 years following BCS with breast radiotherapy. Neoadjuvant chemotherapy is often considered in large tumors to downstage the disease, to enable a BCS (Figs 19A and B).

Contraindications for BCS

Absolute contraindications include:

- Multicentric disease
- Positive margins after multiple attempts to obtain negative margins
- A large tumor with sparse breast parenchyma as the cosmetic outcome is suboptimal
- Diffuse suspicious malignant microcalcifications
- Prior radiotherapy to the chest wall
- When XRT facilities are not available or patient's refusal to XRT
- Therapy resolved LABC when mammography does not show a localized lesion.

Relative contraindications include:

- Multifocal disease (in the same quadrant)
- Active connective tissue disease (scleroderma, systemic lupus erythematosus)
- Tumor size greater than 5 cm. The size of the lesion is relative to the size of the breast, an important consideration for BCS. Larger lesions could be considered for BCS in a large breast parenchyma if adequate margins are ensured.

Axillary Staging

Despite molecular profiling of the primary lesion, axillary lymph node (ALN) status still remains the single most important prognostic factor in patients with invasive breast cancer. The biological behavior of the tumor determines nodal involvement. A large lesion may not involve the nodes and a small primary lesion can disseminate rapidly to the nodes and elsewhere. In surgical oncology, the technique is the prince, selection is the queen but biology is the king.[64] ALND was once considered to be the gold standard for assessing the nodal basin for lymph node metastasis.[65] However, currently SLNB is the standard of care for assessing axillary node involvement as sentinel lymph nodes (SLNs) are the initial recipients of metastasis. A negative SLN is a very reliable indication of a

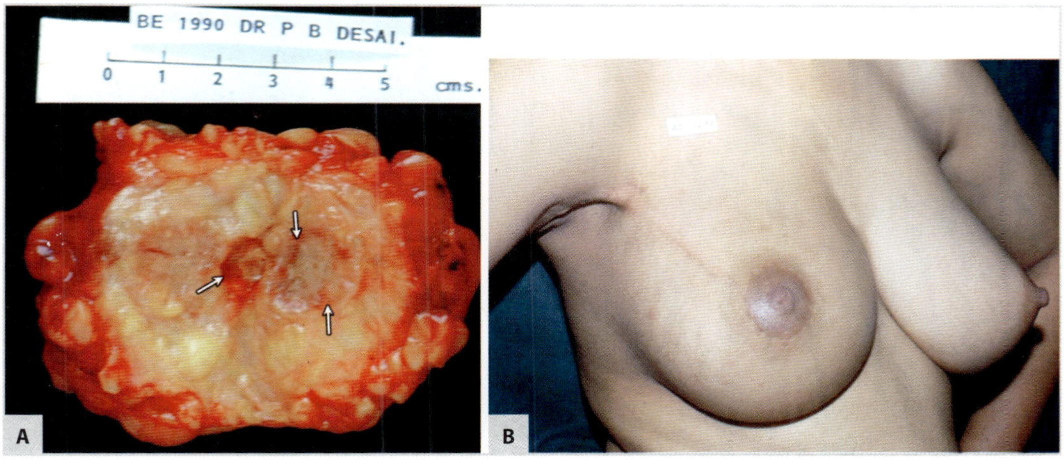

Figs 19A and B: (A) Surgical specimen after breast conservation surgery (BCS) showing the tumor with wide and adequate margins; (B) Same patient disease-free survival (DFS) after 23 years

negative axilla as proven by large multicenter studies.[66,67] Removal of large number of normal axillary nodes is a disservice to the patients and is a strong predisposing factor for arm edema producing significant morbidity.[68-71] Nearly 50–60% of patients with a positive SLN have no axillary disease. If the SLN is positive on frozen section one generally proceeds to complete ALND; patients with a negative SLN are spared the morbidity of this procedure; however, grossly palpable axillary nodes during surgery are best removed (Table 11).

Large clinical trials the (NSABP) B32 and the American College of Surgeons Oncology Group (ACOSOG) Z0010 studies have firmly established SLNB as an accurate method for axillary staging.[72] ACOSOG Z0010 trial was a prospective evaluation of occult metastases in SLNs and bone marrow of patients with T_{1-2} clinically node negative breast cancer planned for BCS and whole breast irradiation. Patients with Hematoxylin and Eosin (H&E) negative SLNs, did not receive any axilla-specific treatment. The overall and disease-free survival (DFS) were found to be similar in patients with H&E negative SLNs and those with H&E negative nodes found to have occult metastases on immunohistochemistry (IHC) evaluations. A recent study reported that local regional recurrences are rare in early breast cancer with H&E negative SLNs. Younger age and hormone receptor negative disease are associated with higher recurrence rates and a local recurrence is associated with reduced OS.

Axillary lymph node dissection is yet justified in:

- Clinically positive axilla
- Primary tumor greater than 5 cm

TABLE 11: Imaging sensitivity and specificity in axillary metastatic nodal disease

Imaging modality	*Sensitivity (%)*	*Specificity (%)*
Ultrasound	25–92	49–100
Color Doppler	71–96	53–75
MRI	65–100	54–100
CT scan	60–94	60–90
PET scan	40–94	96–100

Abbreviations: MRI, magnetic resonance imaging; CT, computed tomography; PET, positron emission tomography

Source: Summarized data derived from single and multicenter studies. Presented at Breast Cancer Symposium, 2013, San Francisco.

- Chemotherapy resistant axillary nodes
- Clinically negative axilla with positive SLNs
- SLNs cannot be identified.

The ACOSOG Z0011 trial was designed to determine whether ALND would impact survival in SLN positive patients. The trial enrolled patients with clinical $T_{1-2}N_0M_0$ breast cancer undergoing BCS, adjuvant whole breast radiotherapy and chemotherapy who were found to have one or two positive SLNs on standard H&E staining. At median follow-up of 6.3 years, there were no differences in locoregional recurrence or OS between the two groups.[73-77] There have been some concerns regarding ACOSOG Z0011 that the radiation oncologists treated the axilla and it was highly favorable in selected population and results are not generally acceptable.

The other logical area for discussion is whether patients who undergo mastectomy for invasive breast cancer require ALND if SLN shows metastasis. Results

TABLE 12: Stage-wise incidence of axillary lymph node (ALN) metastasis in breast cancer and its impact on ALN dissection (ALND)

Stage	Incidence of lymph node metastases	ALND avoided
I	15%	85%
II	33%	66%
III	60%	40%

Abbreviation: ALND, axillary lymph node dissection

from a recent large clinical trial to address this question are anticipated in the near future, based on the ACOSOG Z0011 trials. It is reasonable to presume that chemotherapy can control low volume nodal disease in the axilla, in patients who do not undergo adjuvant radiation.[78-80] There is a possibility that ALND, in the future may be performed less frequently and may become an archive in the history of breast cancer treatment in appropriately selected cases (Table 12).

Beyond Z-11 new trials

Sound trial: Sentinel node versus observation after axillary ultrasound.[81]

Can ultrasound identify clinically relevant nodal burden?

- Multicenter, randomized-controlled trial
- Less than 2 cm breast cancer
- Single lymph node on axillary ultrasound: Fine-needle aspiration (FNA) negative: SLNB ± ALND arm 1 or no axillary surgery.

Observation

- Endpoint: DFS
- Secondary: Axillary recurrence, OS.

Techniques for Identification of SLNs

The SLNs can be localized by injecting radioactive colloid and/or the blue dye. The simplicity of injection of blue dye for the identification of SLN in breast cancer is an accepted method of identification because it eliminates preoperative injection of radioisotope, is less uncomfortable for patients, takes less operative time and reduces hospital costs. The accuracy of breast lymphatic mapping and SLN identification (Fig. 20) using isosulfan blue dye has ranged from 65 to 94%. With the dye only technique there is a limitation as non-axillary nodes, particularly internal mammary nodes (IMNs) cannot be identified. This is of little significance as only 0.3–4% patients have isolated IMNs drainage. Identification rate of SLNs significantly improves when both the techniques are used together.

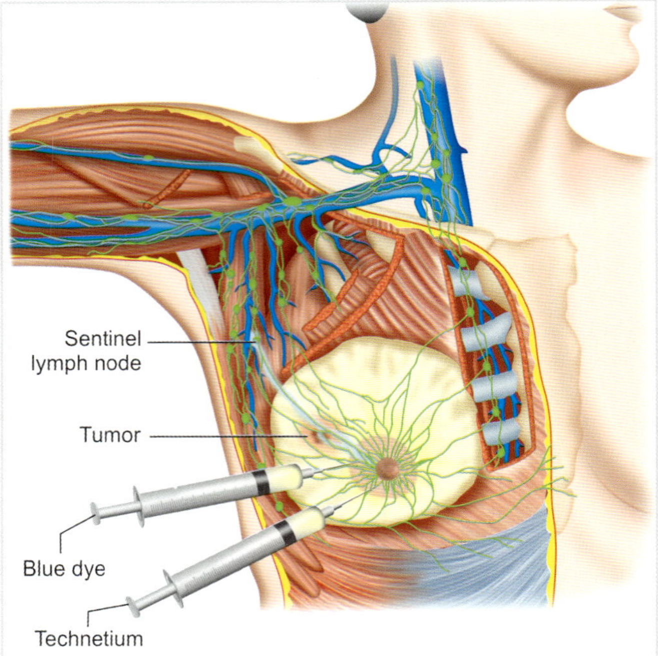

Fig. 20: Techniques of identification of sentinel lymph nodes (SLNs)

Radioactive Colloid

Just prior to surgery, an injection of 0.5 cc of filtered $^{99m}T_c$ sulfur colloid in a volume of 0.5 mL is used. This is injected into the skin, subdermal, subareolar or peritumoral into the breast parenchyma. A lymphoscintigraphy is then performed to identify the nodal basin, i.e. axillary or IMNs. The gamma probe is used intraoperatively to locate the SLNs which are identified as hot spots or those with the greatest signal.

Blue Dye

Three to five milliliter of isosulfan blue dye (lymphazurin 1%) is injected intraoperatively, subdermal, subareolar or peritumoral. The breast is massaged for 5 minutes; the blue dye migrates to the SLNs. If the lesion has been excised, the blue dye is injected subareolar or in the breast parenchyma around the cavity. If the lesion is not palpable then blue dye is injected in the surrounding parenchyma at the site of wire localization. The SLNs is located by visual identification of a blue lymphatic or a blue-stained node, on an average 2–3 SLNs are identified (Figs 21A and B).

A study by Ashraf Nour[82] from Egypt used methylene blue for the identification of SLNs as an alternative to lymphazurin or isosulfan blue dye (Fig. 22). Methylene blue is easily available and is cost effective. This is very important in developing countries. However, few authors believe that methylene blue dye is not optimal in SLN localization due to its small particle size; hence sometimes even the non-sentinel axillary nodes get stained blue.

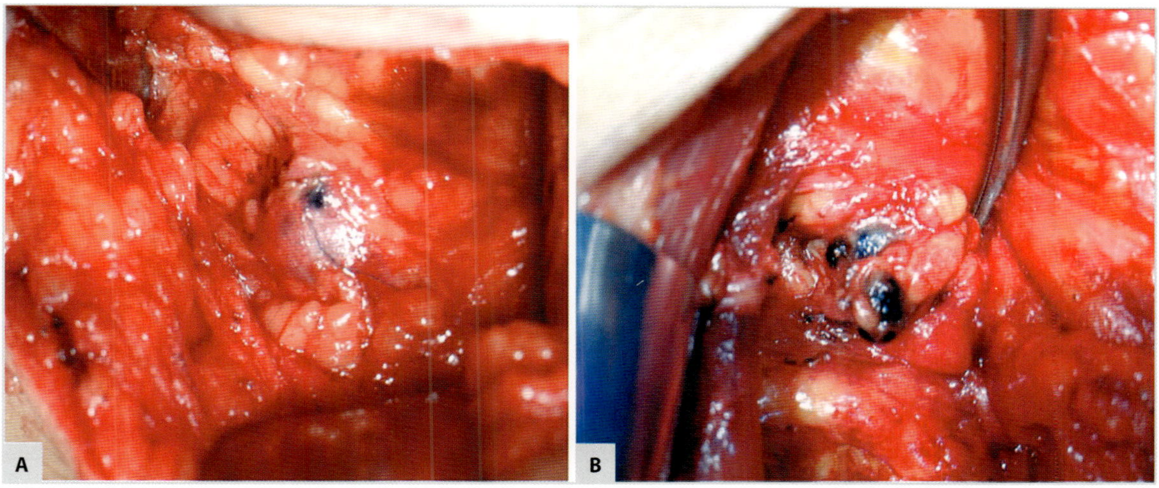

Figs 21A and B: The sentinel lymph node (SLN) which appears blue with blue lymphatics

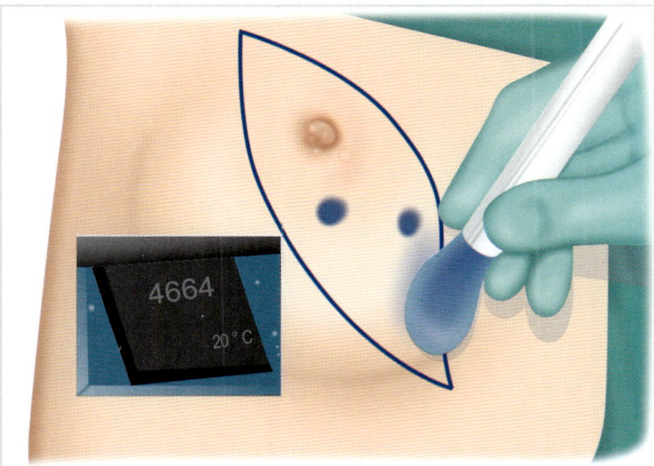

Fig. 22: Technique for identification of sentinel lymph node (SLN) using blue dye and radioactive colloid with gamma probe

SENTINEL LYMPH NODE RETRIEVAL IN BREAST CANCER (SANS TECHNOLOGY)

(*R Parikh, P Desai, et al. Personal series*)

A major therapeutic paradigm shift in surgical oncology is organ and function preservation. The cause of morbidity in standard surgical therapy of breast cancer is due to mastectomy and ALND. With the advent of high quality screening mammography many breast cancers are now detected at an early stage, thus offering an option of breast-conserving therapy (BCT) and the need for less invasive methods for evaluating regional nodal status. SLN retrieval will undoubtedly replace standard ALND in selected patients. Recent studies[83,84] have conclusively shown that when the sentinel node is negative for metastasis the axillary nodes are non-metastatic. In these cases, ALND can be safely avoided. This will prevent the morbidities of lymphedema, neuralgias sensory deficit, restricted mobility and seroma formation.[85,86] Studies[87-90] have shown that with the use of radioactive colloid injection and/or the blue dye, it is possible to locate the SLNs for biopsy, at the time of surgery in 66–100% of cases. This is widely practiced in many centers globally.[91] However, this technique is expensive, time consuming and has a learning curve, the blue dye can rarely cause anaphylaxis (0.6–2.5%)[92,93] and has cosmetic issues. SLNs are the first to receive lymphatic drainage from a specific area of the breast, so if a tumor has metastasized the SLN is most likely to contain metastasis. Proper localization and retrieval of these nodes is therefore important. We devised a simple technique to retrieve the SLNs based on an anatomical approach without the use of any technology. This technique can be easily performed by all surgeons practicing in either urban or rural setting.

A total of 400 women with breast cancer ($T_{1-2}N_0$) were enrolled at two hospitals in Mumbai. BCS was performed in 160 patients and mastectomy in 240 patients. SLNs were identified during surgery using only anatomical approach, without the use of any technology.

Technique

A curvilinear incision between the lower hair margin and the upper outer quadrant margin of the breast is taken. The excess fat is denuded (for access) if necessary. Delineate the margins of the pectoralis major and minor. Slowly tease the tissue around the upper and middle one-third of the pectoral muscle margin. Incise the clavipectoral fascia. The SLN appears as a brownish spot amongst the pad of fat. The intercostobrachial nerves are inferior to the sentinel group. 1–3 SLNs are generally retrieved for frozen section. It is good to resist dissection of fatty tissue which contains low axillary nodes. However, any firm or large lymph nodes should be removed and sent for examination (frozen) (Figs 23A to C).

Follow up over 11 years

4/384 (1.04%) patients with a negative SLN retrieval developed, ALNs between 1 year and 4 years (Tables 13A and B).

Evidence-based medicine has proven that retrieval and histopathologic evaluation of sentinel nodes is the "standard of care" in the surgical management of breast cancer. A histologic negative sentinel node precludes the necessity of an axillary dissection to prevent arm morbidity, a major cause of dysfunction in patients undergoing mastectomy or BCS.

TABLE 13A: Results

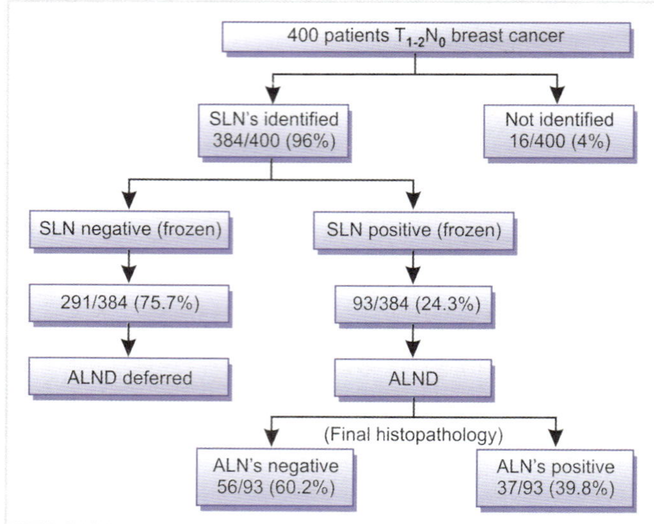

Abbreviations: SLN, Sentinel lymph node; ALND, axillary lymph node dissection; ALN, axillary lymph node

TABLE 13B: Functional results

Sl. No.		*SLNB (291)*	*ALND (109)*
1.	Lymphedema	None	24 (22%)
2.	Seroma	1 (0.26%)	82 (75.2%)
3.	Restricted movement at the shoulder joint	None	22 (20.1%)
4.	Neuralgias and paresthesias	1 (0.26%)	106 (97.2%)

Abbreviations: SLNB, sentinel lymph node biopsy; ALND, axillary lymph node dissection

LOCALLY ADVANCED BREAST CANCER

This is an important and a challenging problem, especially in India. Patients from rural area with poor socioeconomic and low education levels are more often affected. Occasionally, educated population with self-denial also present with LABC. LABC is a large primary tumor [> 5 cm T_3, American Joint Committee on Cancer (AJCC) staging] with edema, occasional chest wall involvement, with or without lymph nodal involvement of the axilla or supraclavicular region or peau d'orange changes in the breast parenchyma which often involves the whole breast. Even a moderate sized tumor (3–5 cm) located in a small breast behave like a LABC and needs to be treated accordingly. Surgery plays a less important role in stage III breast cancer. Majority of patients at diagnosis will have ALN involvement or distant metastasis at diagnosis (PET-CT). Multiple reports have, however, documented the effectiveness of primary systemic therapy in patients

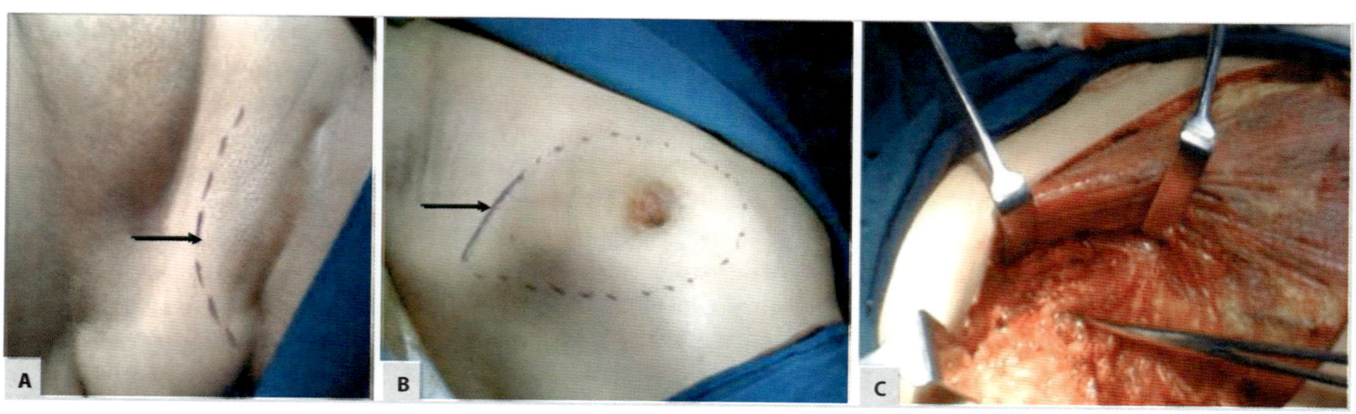

Figs 23A to C: (A) Curvilinear incision between the lower hair margin and the upper outer quadrant margin of the breast for sentinel lymph node (SLN) retrieval; (B) During mastectomy, SLN can be retrieved first through the same transverse incision near the axilla; (C) Location of SLN at the junction of upper and middle one-third of the pectoral muscle margin (retracted cephaled and medially). SLNs are often seen or felt within the pad of fat with LABC (Figs 24A and B). Appropriate management may result in a 5-year survival rate of greater than 30% (Flow chart 1).[94-96]

INFLAMMATORY BREAST CANCER

Inflammatory breast cancer (IBC) is a rare and an aggressive form of invasive breast cancer accounting for 2.5% of all breast cancers. It is characterized by rapid progression, local and distant metastasis, younger age at onset and a lower OS compared with other breast cancers. IBC is a lethal disease with a dismal less than 5% survival rate at 5 years when treated with surgery/chemotherapy and XRT. It is often misdiagnosed as mastitis or generalized dermatitis. There is diffuse edema and brawny erythema of the skin with or without an underlying breast mass. It is usually an infiltrative ductal cancer. The pathognomic feature of this disease is "dermal lymphatic invasion" in a skin biopsy (Table 14).

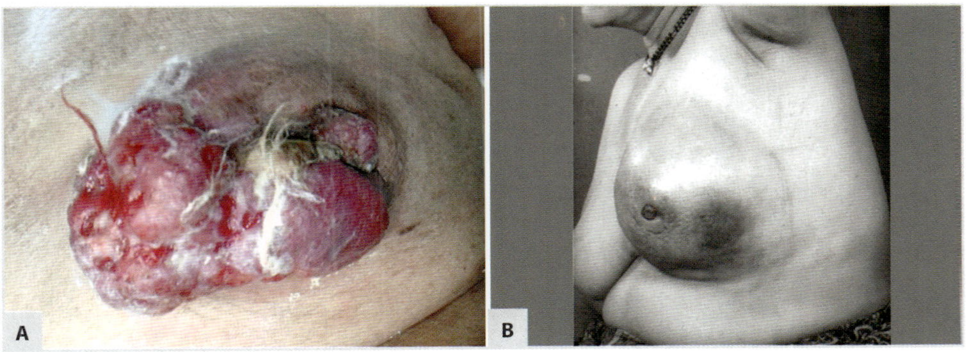

Figs 24A and B: (A) Locally advanced fungating breast cancer; (B) Typical locally advanced breast cancer (LABC)

Flow chart 1: Management of locally advanced breast cancer (LABC)

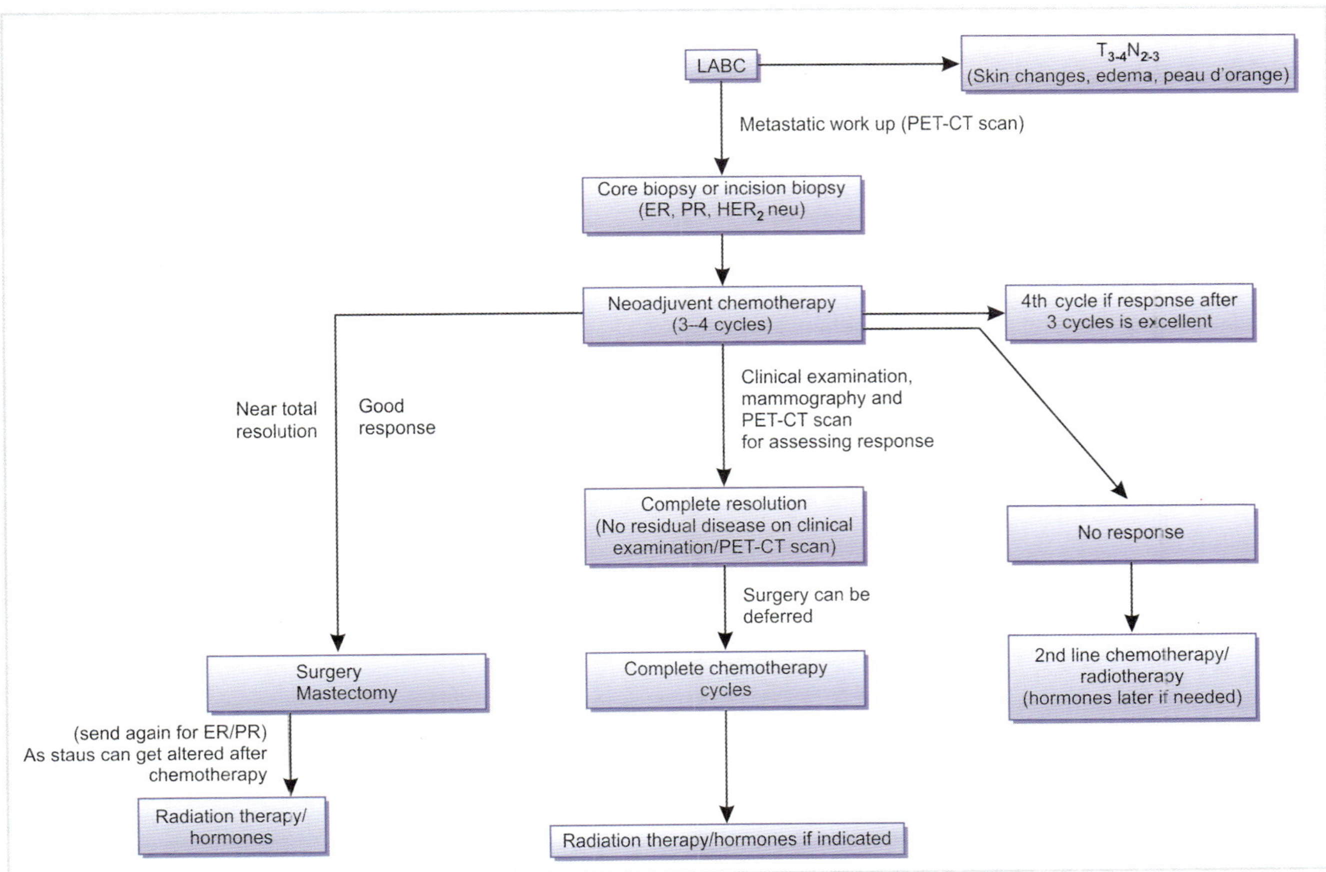

Abbreviations: LABC, locally advanced breast cancer; PET-CT, positron emission tomography with computed tomography; ER, estrogen receptor; PR, progesterone receptor; HER2 neu, human epidermal growth factor receptor 2; BCS, breast conservation surgery

TABLE 14: Comparison of primary and secondary inflammatory breast cancers (IBCs)

Primary inflammatory breast cancer (IBC)	*Secondary IBC*
• De novo development of IBC in a previously normal breast	• Skin changes that mimic primary IBC either in a breast that already had cancer or on the chest wall after mastectomy for non-IBC

BILATERAL BREAST CANCER

In patients with a unilateral breast cancer, there is a 2.6–5 times increased risk of developing a second primary tumor in the normal breast. Bilateral breast cancer represents 2–5% of all breast cancer cases. A second primary in the contralateral breast may be synchronous or metachronous. Most studies consider a tumor to be synchronous, if it is diagnosed within 6 months. A contralateral breast tumor may be a second primary or metastatic. Metastasis to the other breast can occur through lymphatic channels across the midline or by lymphatic dissemination. Generally, in the absence of widespread metastases, contralateral breast tumor should be considered as on independent primary tumors.

Treatment

Synchronous bilateral breast cancer

Therapy options include mastectomy or BCS depending upon the clinical setting. Bilateral breast radiation is safe when indicated.

Metachronous bilateral breast cancer

Therapy of second breast cancer is based on the same principle as treating an independent breast cancer. Women who develop metachronous contralateral breast cancer on tamoxifen will receive no benefit on continuing the drug. Aromatase inhibitors (AIs) are useful. A metachronous second breast cancer after completion of 5 years on tamoxifen should be treated as an independent primary tumor. Chemotherapy should be used when indicated.

MUCINOUS BREAST CANCER (COLLOID OR GRANULOMATOUS CARCINOMA)

Pure mucinous cancer is a low-grade mammary cancer and represents 2% of all breast tumors. Pure and mixed patterns of mucinous tumors show important clinical and pathological differences. These tumors are most common in the elderly and are of average size. Pure mucinous cancer is described as a circumscribed mass lesion which is devoid of microcalcification on mammography. The differential diagnosis includes benign lesions like fibroadenomas; higher the content of mucin, the more benign is the mammographic appearance. To distinguish a benign from a malignant lesion is difficult on FNAC and these can be diagnosed accurately only on a CNB. Upto 75% of mucinous carcinomas have intraductal cancer at the periphery.[97-99] They are usually estrogen-receptor positive and HER2 neu negative. Despite pure mucinous tumors having a lower incidence of nodal metastases, there is always a small risk even in tumors less than 1 cm. Breast conservation in eligible patients provides adequate local treatment. In patients with pure mucinous lesions 10-year survival is 90%. Patients with mixed mucinous tumor, or nodal metastases have survival similar to infiltrating duct carcinoma (IDC). For mucinous carcinoma, chemotherapy is not very effective. It may be beneficial to some extent in mixed mucinous histology or in node positive patients.

TUBULAR CARCINOMA

These are also rare variants and the incidence ranges from 0.7 to 10%. These are characterized as having a low metastatic potential. It is known to occur in the elderly, have a higher incidence of multicentricity and bilaterality, and are usually smaller in size. The majority of tubular carcinomas express positive hormone receptors. Treatment with local excision followed by XRT provides excellent local control. Nodal metastases may occur; however it does not adversely impact on survival. Role of adjuvant therapy for this malignancy is debatable.[100]

PAPILLARY CARCINOMA

They represent 1–2% of all breast cancers. They may be either intracystic or non-cystic and may be associated with nipple discharge in about one-third of patients. The incidence of lymph node metastases ranges in the literature from 20 to 35% depending on the size of tumor. Generally, they have a favorable prognosis.

MEDULLARY CARCINOMA

The incidence is about 3–10% and occurs at a younger age. Recent reports have identified a strong predisposition toward medullary carcinoma in patients with BRCA1 mutation. On mammography, they are circumscribed or present as a distinct mass which can be confused with a fibroadenoma. Hormone receptors are usually negative and the lesion is nonresponsive to endocrine therapy. MRM or BCS will depend on the clinical setting. Staging of the axilla is important because a significant number of patients may develop metastases in the axilla.

MALE BREAST CANCER

The pathology of male breast cancer is predominantly ductal and 85% of cases are invasive type; the remainders are DCIS. Paget's disease can also occur in males. The staging and treatment is on similar lines as female breast cancer. Hormone therapy is recommended for hormone receptor positive lesions. Tamoxifen is the only drug approved for hormonal therapy.

PHYLLODES TUMOR (CYSTOSARCOMA PHYLLODES)

This is an uncommon fibroepithelial breast neoplasm and accounts for 0.5–1%[101] of all breast cancers and is common between 35 years and 55 years. Phyllodes are usually large and have a mean diameter of 4–5 cm; mammographically they are difficult to distinguish from fibroadenomas. When indicated a wide excision with surrounding normal breast tissue rather than enucleation is the preferred primary therapy. Local recurrences are common and ranges from 5 to 15% for benign tumors and from 20 to 30% for malignant tumors (Table 15). Local recurrences are salvageable with a total mastectomy and do not affect the OS rate. The low incidence of axillary nodal metastasis (< 1%) obviates lymphadenectomy, though metastasis can occur in the malignant variant (< 7%). The reported rate of distant metastases with a rare malignant phyllodes tumor ranges from 25 to 40%, particularly in large tumors. XRT, chemotherapy or hormonal therapies are of no proven value in a phyllodes tumor (Figs 25A and B).

TABLE 15: Phyllodes tumor—survival[101]

Survival	*Benign phyllodes*	*Malignant phyllodes*
5 years	91%	82%
10 years	79%	42%

PAGET'S DISEASE

Paget's disease of the nipple was first described by Sir James Paget in 1874. It is an uncommon form of breast cancer; incidence varies from 1 to 4% of all breast tumors.[102-104] Microscopically, large cells with clear cytoplasm and atypical nuclei are seen within the epidermis, more so along the basal layer. Nonhealing recurrent eczematous ulceration of the nipple and areola is the most common presentation with or without a retroareolar mass. Patients present without a clinical mass in 66–86% and a mammogram will have DCIS alone. Some patients will present with a palpable or mammographic mass and will have an underlying invasive carcinoma. Prognosis is determined by the presence or absence of an invasive component. Clinically Paget's disease is characterized by a superficial tumor infiltration of the nipple and surrounding skin. Disease presentation is usually unilateral; bilateral symptoms are more consistent with benign etiologies like dermatitis or eczema. Initial signs include an erythematous exudate or nipple scaling

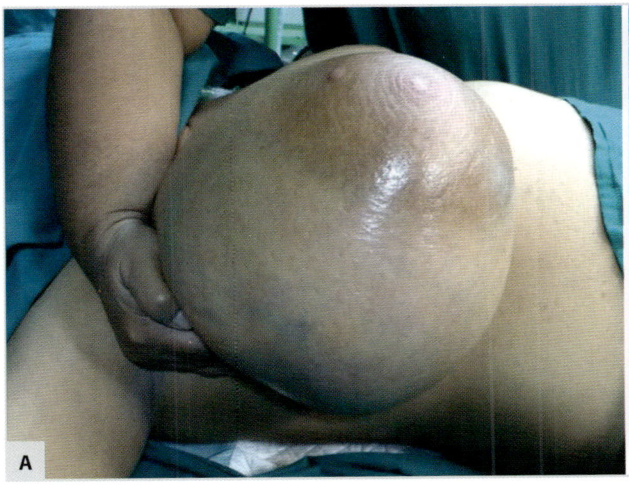

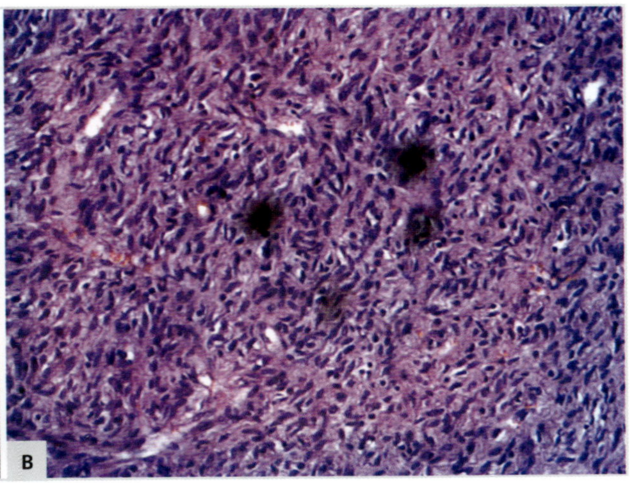

Figs 25A and B: (A) Massive neglected cystosarcoma phyllodes (*Courtesy:* Dr Tehemton Udwadia and Dr Rushad Udwadia); (B) Phyllodes tumor, a characteristic biphasic tumor. In this case, it showed malignant features including marked stromal cellularity, invasive borders and nuclear atypia

Box 4: An interesting case report

- Eczematous pagetoid lesion right breast since 13 years (2000).
- Surgery twice including mastectomy with skin grafting (2007). Histology—high-grade intraductal carcinoma, no invasive component. 6 cycles of chemotherapy.
- Recurrence in the chest wall (2010), defaulted follow-up.
- Extensive recurrent skin lesion involving the whole right chest wall area (2013)—Figures 26A to C. Postexcision defect (R) chest wall (L) breast seen superiorly.
- Wide excision of the chest wall lesion with reconstruction by a transverse thoracoabdominal, fasciocutaneous flap, skin grafting and left breast mobilization as shown in the Figure 26D.
- Final histopathology showed recurrent carcinoma grade III, involving skin of the chest wall infiltrating deep dermis and shows Pagetoid involvement of the overlying squamous epithelium as shown in the Figure 26E.

and symptoms of itching and burning; discharge may or may not be present. Nonhealing chronic ulceration is a typical clinical presentation. Nipple retraction, thickening and bleeding are less common signs and are present only with a retroareolar mass. A punch biopsy, scrape cytology, wedge incisional biopsy or a complete nipple excision will establish the diagnosis. Mastectomy has been the standard therapy for Paget's disease. However, current trials indicate that breast conservative surgery (removal of nipple areola complex) and postoperative radiotherapy to be an acceptable and preferable option for an early-stage invasive lesion.[105] Axillary staging should be offered to those with invasive carcinoma and SLNB may be indicated on the histology and the status of ALNs (Box 4).

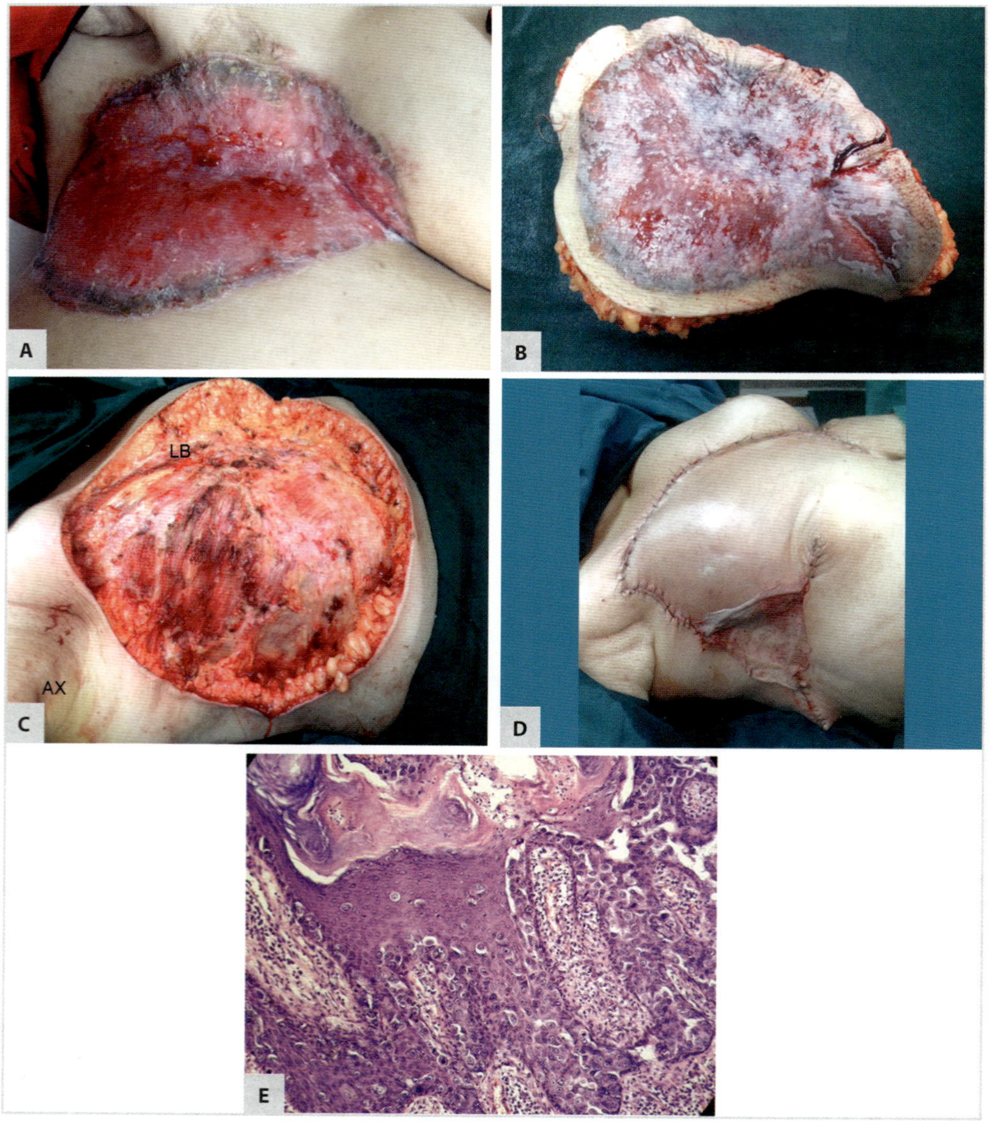

Figs 26A to E: (A to D) A recurrent extensive chest wall skin involvement after a right modified radical mastectomy (4 years ago) for a slow growing Pagetoid high-grade infiltrating duct carcinoma. The initial skin Pagetoid lesion started 23 years ago. Result after a very wide excision of the recurrent lesion, and primary reconstruction by mobilization of the left breast, left abdominal lower flap, axillary and lateral flaps with a very small split thickness skin graft. The final histopathology was (E) (*Courtesy*: Dr Keyuri Patel) Pagetoid involvement of epidermis by duct carcinoma (chest wall recurrence)

BREAST CANCER AND PREGNANCY

Breast cancer diagnosed during pregnancy, lactation or during the 1st postpartum year is defined as pregnancy associated breast cancer. The incidence is low (1.8%). Diagnosis is difficult, due to a low level of suspicion in the young; pregnancy-associated nodular changes and increased density during pregnancy often confuse the clinician. The treatment goal should be curative with preservation of pregnancy without fetal injury. All first trimester pregnancies should be terminated as organogenesis has not yet commenced. MRM or BCS with ALND when indicated as primary therapy can be undertaken during pregnancy without any risk to the mother or fetus. It is better to defer therapy until the 12th gestational week to avoid the risk of spontaneous abortion. For lesions detected in the third trimester, it is preferable to delay primary treatment for upto 4 weeks to allow delivery before surgery is planned. During pregnancy radiation is generally contraindicated, hence BCS is inadvisable. However, in the third trimester, BCS lumpectomy with SLNB can be performed and radiation can be considered postpartum.

- Administration of chemotherapy can occasionally lead to congenital malformations as believed earlier
- Current studies, however have demonstrated a safety profile and there is generally no risk of fetal malformation. For patients in the second and third trimester cyclophosphamide, adriamycin and fluorouracil (CAF) combination is approved
- Patients with pregnancy-associated breast cancer have similar survivals to the nonpregnant group.

Nipple Discharge

It is a common symptom, may be unilateral or occasionally bilateral. Most non-bloody discharges are due to benign duct ectasia and may be uni- or bilateral. Serum like, greenish, brownish yellow, blackish in color are generally benign. Any bloody discharge in the presence of duct carcinoma in the periareolar region may show presence of malignant cells in the smear. Bloody discharge often indicates a benign papilloma or occasionally a papillary type of duct carcinoma. BCS is always worthwhile in a duct papillary carcinoma. Sonomammography will indicate duct ectasia—diffuse or localized. No mammographic changes will help to diagnose a carcinoma. Clinically accurate localization (if localized to a sector or segment) of the bleeding is generally possible and will require a microdochectomy or a segment excision of the involved area.

Occult Carcinoma Breast Clinically Presenting Only with Axillary Node Metastasis

Occult breast cancer with a metastatic ALN with no identifiable breast lesion is known but rare. It accounts for 0.3–0.8% of breast cancers.[106] The other causes of a solitary malignant ALN include lymphoma, melanoma and rarely carcinoma lung, thyroid, ovary, gastrointestinal tract, liver, pancreas or kidney. Standard breast imaging (mammography and sonography) may be normal. In 25% of patients, mammography may indicate a breast tumor not clinically discernible. FNAC, core biopsy or an excisional biopsy of the ALN is necessary. Histologic studies, including hormone receptors and HER2 neu status and IHC are generally indicated. These patients are considered to have AJCC stage II (T_0N_1 or T_0N_2). If no suspicious lesion is seen on imaging, treatment options are ALND with whole breast irradiation, MRM or careful observation and follow up. Adjuvant chemotherapy/hormone therapy and radiotherapy is advised, if indicated. A suspicious lesion, on imaging should have an image-guided biopsy if positive, it should be treated as stage II breast cancer. In 50–60% of mastectomy specimens, a previously occult lesion is generally identified.[107]

Tumor Markers

Cancer Antigen 15-3

Cancer antigen (CA) 15-3 is an important prognostic marker in breast cancer. It is a large transmembrane glycoprotein frequently overexpressed and frequently glycosylated in cancer.[108] CA 15-3 is produced by normal breast cells. In many patients there is increased production of CA 15-3, which is shed by the tumor cells and enters the blood stream. It is elevated in about 10% with early localized lesions and in about 70% with metastatic disease. CA 15-3 may be elevated in healthy people and also in individuals with other cancers like colorectal and lung cancers, cirrhosis, hepatitis and benign breast diseases. It helps estimate the tumor burden. Very high levels indicate skeletal and liver metastases. Even in 25–30% with advanced disease CA 15-3 may be normal. Increasing concentration of CA 15-3 despite therapy indicates a poor prognosis with spread or recurrence of the disease. Normal range is less than 30 μ/mL.

Carcinoembryonic Antigen

The importance of this antigen was recognized first for colorectal carcinomas and then for solid tumors in general.

The carcinoembryonic antigen (CEA) value is directly proportional to the tumor burden. It is a useful monitor during follow-up period after therapy. It is elevated in 30% with demonstrable metastases. Rising CA 15-3 and CEA values may precede the onset of metastatic disease. Rising levels in the follow-up period indicates onset of metastasis. The need for a specific early serologic diagnosis of breast cancer continues.

Neither of the tumor markers is useful in recurrent disease and is not advised as part of any evidence-based guidelines.

RECURRENT DISEASE

Local Recurrence

After BCS a physical examination and/or mammography can detect a recurrence (Flow chart 2). This is usually subtle and difficult to distinguish due to the effects of surgery and radiation. Finding of a small firm lump or a nodule around the scar within 5 cm and occurring within or more than 2 years after completion of radiation are considered suspicious. Recurrences after BCS are reported to be around 5–10% and 90% are generally around the original lesion. Recurrence after BCT carries a 5-year survival of about 50%. Properly managed, local scar recurrence (after mastectomy) (Flow chart 3) and local recurrence after BCS do not impact on long-term survival rates. A repeat wide excision often suffices to control the local recurrence. Rarely a mastectomy may be necessary depending on the clinical setting or attitude of the patient.

METASTATIC BREAST CANCER

The development of metastasis in a given case of breast cancer will generally depend on the stage at presentation; most importantly, it will be the biologic behavior of a given lesion which will dictate metastatic disease. It is known, though rare, that a large primary lesion, even fungating, may not metastasize and a small T_1N_0 lesion could present with distant spread. Presence of metastasis is generally directly proportional to the invasive component, the T and N stage, the grade and the histological type of the lesion. Needless to state that the clinician is often called upon to treat metastasis, often years later after the primary disease has remained controlled for many years, even sometimes longer than 15–20 years.

The role of surgery

Solitary metastasis developing in bone, liver, lung, brain, ovaries or uterus/cervix or any other anatomic site, which lends itself to a safe surgical excision should remain the therapy of choice and probably a standard of care; particularly so, if the primary disease is controlled and the metastatic event comes after 3–4 years or more.[109] Rapid onset of metastasis within a year conveys aggressive disease and chemotherapy should precede any surgical intervention. Palliative effective surgical treatment often results in 25–30% 5-year survival. More often metastatic disease is multicentric and chemotherapy will remain the therapy of choice and hormonal therapy as indicated with positive hormone receptors.

Brain metastasis often presents with a solitary lesion which if amenable to surgical excision should be

Flow chart 2: Local recurrence after breast conservation surgery (BCS)

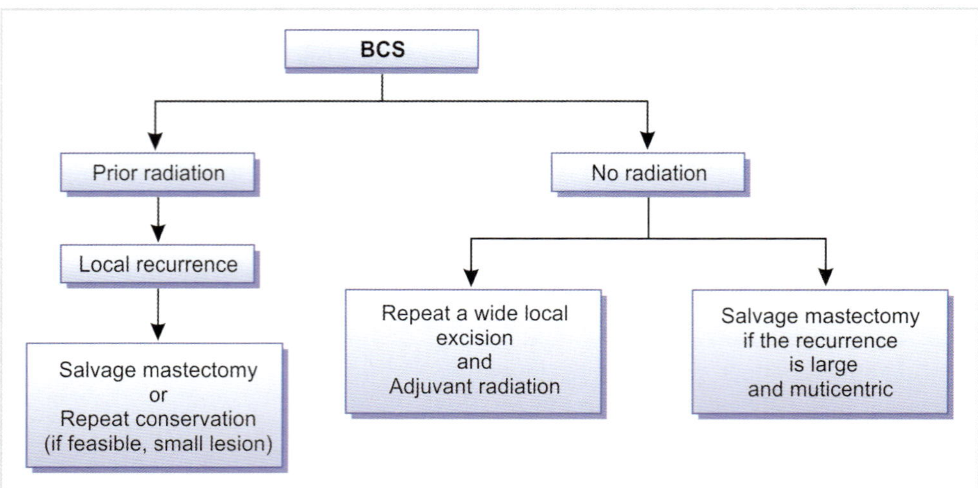

Flow chart 3: Local scar recurrence (after mastectomy)

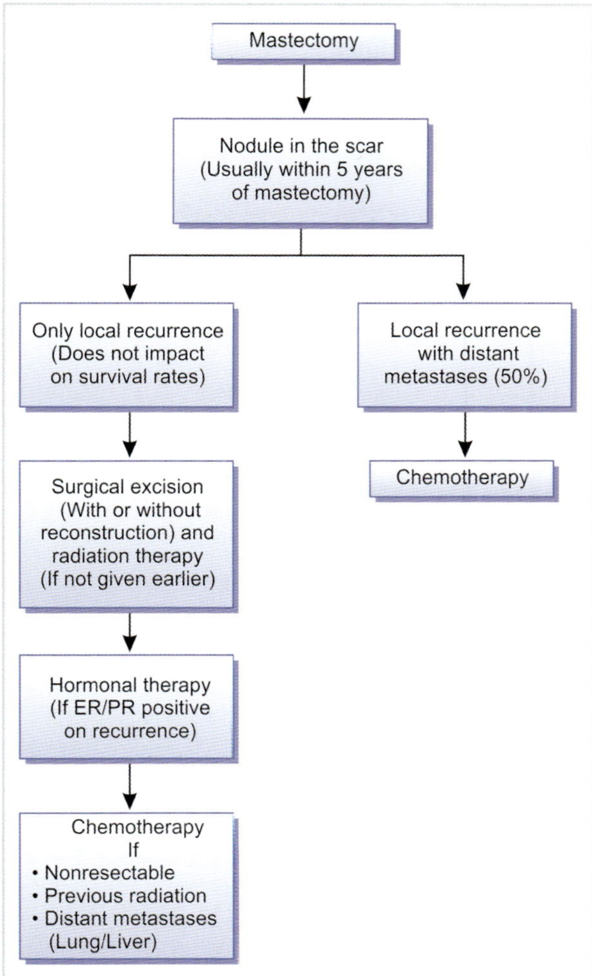

Abbreviations: ER, estrogen receptor; PR, progesterone receptor

excised followed by whole brain irradiation as chances of multicentric foci are high. The issue of blood-brain barrier is still debatable; recent studies with "lapatinib" with HER2 neu positivity are reported to have better results. The overall outlook is grim with a reported survival of only 3–6 months. Though blood-brain barrier conveys ineffectiveness of chemotherapy, it is often used as an adjunct as more lesions are likely to develop in the brain or elsewhere in the following period.

Localized spinal or dural metastasis, when feasible, should be surgically excised to prevent impending paraplegia. Postoperative radiotherapy is often considered after surgical excision. Overall data suggest better outcomes with surgery; often decompression surgery followed by radiotherapy and steroids are indicated. Generally, in vast majority of cases systemic therapy is indicated. Krukenberg's (ovarian) tumors are best managed by a panhysterectomy and follow-up chemotherapy. Localized radiotherapy can be considered if the disease is localized to two or three vertebrae for pain relief and followed by systemic therapy and bisphosphonates (zoledronic acid) which should be given on monthly basis for 12 months. Newer drug, injection denosumab can be given in the dose of 120 mg subcutaneously every month. These agents prevent skeletal-related events like hypercalcemia, fractures and bone pain. Palliative radiotherapy must be considered for painful bone metastasis and for lesions in weight-bearing areas to prevent fractures.

Lymphedema

Arm lymphedema is a feared complication after axillary surgery and radiotherapy for breast cancer (Fig. 27). The reported incidence is 6–70%. The true incidence is difficult to determine as it may take years to develop. However, 90% of women will develop lymphedema within 3 years of breast cancer surgery. It is a chronic, dysfunctional, disfiguring and a potentially disabling condition due to accumulation of protein-rich fluid, resulting in varying degree of edema, hypertrophy and eventually fibrosis of the extremity, which can very rarely lead to lymphangiosarcoma of the extremity. There can be physical impairment, alteration in lifestyle, musculoskeletal pain and restriction of shoulder mobility depending on the severity of lymphedema (Table 16).[110-116] Determinants of lymphedema are axillary radiation, obesity, recurrent lymphangitis after ALND.

Prevention

- Healing by first intention without infection or wound breakdown is the most important goal and can be achieved by appropriate planning of flaps, and proper surgical technique
- SLNB in early breast cancer is preferred as rate of lymphedema is only 0–3% and there is hardly any seroma formation. Avoidance of ALND based on SLNB findings. Complete axillary dissection (level III) and stripping the adventitia of the axillary vein is best avoided
- Radiation to a dissected axilla significantly increases the rate of lymphedema to almost 45%.[117] XRT to axilla should be considered only if the nodal burden is large, (> 4 nodes). A properly dissected axilla, is very rarely (< 5%) the site of a local recurrence
- Control of diabetes: Pre- and postoperative phase.

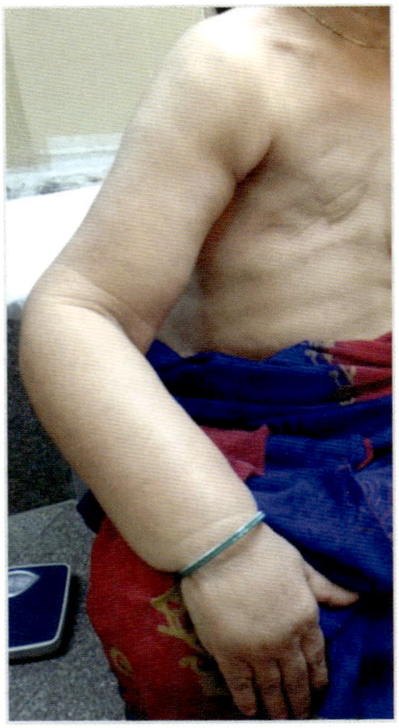

Fig. 27: A frequent consequence of complete axillary lymph node dissection (ALND), along with failure of primary healing and radiotherapy are other causes

TABLE 16: Classification of lymphedema

Grade	Presentation
I	Swelling, pits on pressure
II	Firm, non-pitting, skin changes, alteration of nails
III	Thickened skin with huge skin folds

Precautions

Aggressive skin care to avoid trauma or injury [avoidance of needle puncture, blood withdrawal or intravenous (IV) lines], avoidance of limb constriction [blood pressure (BP) cuff inflation, tight clothing], avoidance of extreme temperatures and frequent use of compression garments (especially for air-travel).[118]

Treatment

Elevation, specific exercises for the arm, compression garments, stroking and retrograde massage performed by a trained therapist, and a sequential compression chambers pneumatic pump may be beneficial to reduce lymphedema. Moderate physiotherapy, reduction of excess weight, arm elevation on pillows at night helps significantly.

Follow-up after Primary Treatment of Invasive Breast Cancer

Studies report that recurrences usually occur even within 5 years after primary therapy, yet it can also recur after 20 years after primary treatment. There is still debate about the frequency of follow ups. Individualization is recommended depending upon the stage of the disease. Too frequent follow ups and investigations can be a source of unnecessary anxiety in patients and relatives. There is still debate about the frequency of follow ups. Investigation is recommended depending upon the stage of the disease. Randomized evidence supports that investigation on follow up in asymptomatic patients does not save lives (Tables 17 and 18).

TABLE 17: Published guidelines from the American Society of Clinical Oncology (ASCO) for follow-up recommended scheduled visits

Frequency of visits	Duration from primary treatment
Between 3 months and 6 months	1–3 years
Between 6 months and 12 months	For 4th and 5th year
Once in every 12 months	Thereafter

TABLE 18: Examination/investigation of invasive breast cancer

Examination/investigation	
Breast self-examination (BSE)	Monthly:
Mammogram	• 6 months after BCT, then yearly • Yearly mammogram in patients who have undergone mastectomy—less frequently in later years
Routine blood investigations, USG of abdomen, pelvis and chest skiagram	Yearly then: • Once in 18 months (after 5 years) • Once in 2 years (after 10 years)

Abbreviations: USG, ultrasonography; BCT, breast-conserving therapy

SYSTEMIC THERAPY OF BREAST CANCER

Breast cancer can often be a systemic disease. This was realized by pioneers like Bonadonna and Fisher as radical and supraradical surgeries did not prevent metastatic disease. In the last three to four decades, many newer and effective chemotherapeutic drugs have been discovered for breast cancer. Anthracyclines were introduced in late 1960s, cisplatin in 1980s while taxanes were introduced in 1990s. These drugs have significantly improved survival for breast cancer patients.

Role of Gene Profiling in Risk Assessment for Future Recurrence

Gene profiling is the latest tool in the risk assessment for breast cancer. These are now commercially available. These

TABLE 19: Oncotype Dx® recurrence score

Recurrence score	Risk	Outcome
< 18	Minimal	Chemotherapy avoided
> 30	High risk	Chemotherapy recommended
18–30	Inconclusive	May or may not give chemotherapy

tools help a subgroup of patients to avoid chemotherapy. Acute and long-term toxicities can be avoided. These tools are used for early-stage breast cancer, which are hormone receptor positive and lymph node negative tumors. It is not 100% specific or sensitive but acts as a reasonable guide. Oncotype Dx®[119] consists of 21 gene assay and results are given as recurrence score (Table 19).

In a recent study by Cuzick et al.[120] suggested that the amount of prognostic information contained in four widely performed IHC assays: (1) ER, (2) PR, (3) HER2 neu and (4) Ki-67 (IHC 4) is similar to oncotype Dx®.

The systemic therapy of breast cancer consists of three groups of drugs:

1. Chemotherapy
2. Hormonal therapy
3. Targeted therapy.

Chemotherapy

It involves administration of various cytotoxic drugs in different combinations. The choices of drugs depend on many factors, viz.: tumor size, nodal burden, high-grade tumor, high-risk pathological features, like lymphovascular emboli, perinodal infiltration, hormonal receptor positivity, HER2 nue status, comorbid conditions and performance status of the patients. In a patient who has undergone ALND, the operated arm side should not be used for IV access. Patients should be counseled for long-term venous access for a subcutaneous venous port on the chest wall. This is a sophisticated venous access tool, which will avoid extravasation, venous pigmentation and ulceration. It is easy and comforting to the patient who has poor venous access in the extremity. It is moderately expensive.

Adjuvant chemotherapy

Indications:

- All patients with positive ALNs
- Node negative but tumor size greater than 2 cm and/or a high-grade tumor
- *PR negative, HER2 neu positive*, triple receptor ER, negative, tumors with high-risk features (lymphovascular invasion, perineural infiltration).

Usually 4–8 cycles of chemotherapy is generally planned, based on the various factors as described earlier.[121]

The protocols:

- CAF: Cyclophosphamide, adriamycin and 5-fluorouracil (5-FU)
- FEC: 5-FU, epirubicine, cyclophosphamide
- AC/EC: Adriamycin/epirubicine with cyclophosphamide
- TC: Taxotere (docetaxel), cyclophosphamide
- CMF: Cyclophosphamide, methotrexate and 5-FU
- TAC: Taxotere (docetaxel), adriamycin, cyclophosphamide
- Paclitaxel-based regimen.

Chemotherapy for locally advanced breast cancer

In India, majority of patients report in this stage to the oncologist, especially in rural population. In urban population, this stage is seen less frequently due to increased awareness. LABC patients present with large primary tumors and/or large lymph node burden. This is mainly due to delay in diagnosis. These patients will undergo thorough staging as chances of metastasis are high at this stage of the disease. It is recommended to start chemotherapy first so as to shrink the tumor to achieve better surgical outcome and to prevent metastasis. This is called as neoadjuvant chemotherapy.

It is strongly recommended to do breast mass biopsy before starting chemotherapy. As many patients will achieve good response to chemotherapy, lot of necrosis takes place. It is not possible for a pathologist to perform IHC for hormone status and HER2 neu status. Hence, breast tissue must be obtained before starting the chemotherapy.

For this clinical setting, taxane-anthracycline combination is the preferred combination. Single-agent chemotherapy can be given if the patient is unfit for aggressive chemotherapy. These patients are advised to undergo 3–6 cycles of chemotherapy depending on the response. The chemotherapy is continued till maximum response is achieved. After achieving maximum response to chemotherapy, surgery is planned. After studying the pathology report closely, further treatment is planned with chemo/radio/hormonal/targeted therapy.

Chemotherapy for metastatic breast cancer

Though this is an incurable stage of the disease, good control of the disease can be achieved by giving palliative chemotherapy (salvage chemotherapy). This will help to control the symptoms and prolong the survival. For a patient with minimum symptoms, either hormonal therapy or single agent can be planned. For a patient with rapidly progressing disease, combination chemotherapy will be required. Apart from the various drugs mentioned in the previous section, many additional drugs can be used as a salvage therapy, viz: gemcitabine, cisplatin, carboplatin, ixabepilone, capecitabine, vinorelbine, etc. If a patient is able to maintain good performance status, multiple lines of chemotherapy can be given as long as the disease remains chemosensitive.

Hormonal Therapy

Ever since Beatson (1896) suggested oophorectomy for estrogen suppression in breast cancer therapy, this procedure has remained a sheet anchor as an important adjunctive therapy. Improvement in XRT brought forth ovarian-ablation by radiation after the middle of the last century. Tamoxifen burst upon the therapeutic scene in mid 1980s and has now continued to be a gold standard against which other estrogen suppressors are measured for their efficacy (Aromatase inhibitiors-AI). The patients are broadly classified into premenopausal and postmenopausal tumors. For premenopausal patients, tamoxifen is the drug of choice. It is a partial agonist and antagonist of estrogen. In adjuvant setting, tamoxifen is given in the dose of 20 mg/day for 5 years. This drug can lead to abnormal vaginal bleeding. It also has a real risk of causing endometrial cancer, cardiovascular and thrombotic issues and other side effects like cataract development. For postmenopausal patients, AIs are the drug of choice as they have more efficacy with decreased toxicity compared to tamoxifen in this clinical setting.[122] AIs are classified into nonsteroidal (anastrozole and letrozole) and steroidal (exemestane). All the three agents are approved for adjuvant use. The duration of adjuvant therapy is 5 years.

Toxicities of aromatase inhibitors

These drugs may increase osteoporosis and cardiac risks. Hence, patients are advised to undergo bone densitometry and osteoporosis must be treated if found on bone densitometry. All the patients on AI are advised to take calcium supplements. For metastatic disease, any of these drugs can be used sequentially till progression of the disease. Exemestane has a very strong data as a second-line hormonal therapy.

Concept of switch therapy

Many perimenopausal women are started on tamoxifen in adjuvant setting. If their menopausal status converts into postmenopausal during this adjuvant therapy, they are shifted to AIs for remaining period of time. This is called as switch therapy. This helps the patient get benefits of the both groups of drugs.

Concept of extended adjuvant therapy

The landmark trial of MA 17 demonstrated benefit of extending adjuvant therapy beyond 5 years upto 10 years. Women who are started on tamoxifen for 5 years can be considered for letrozole if they have turned postmenopausal at that time. Letrozole can be given for another 5 years, thus protecting these women against delayed recurrences.

Role of fulvestrant

This is an injectable hormonal preparation which is used as a salvage therapy after failure of other lines of therapy. It is a monthly intramuscular injection in the dose of 250 mg or 500 mg per month till progression.

Role of oophorectomy

Oophorectomy was considered as an important tool against metastatic breast cancer. With the availability of various hormonal preparations, role of oophorectomy has drastically reduced. It is not indicated for adjuvant therapy as chemotherapy-induced amenorrhea is highly beneficial. A revisitation of oophorectomy is still considered effective where cost-constraint is significant.

Use of single injection progesterone before surgery

The appropriate use of progesterone is a new entrant in the hormone therapy armamentarium against breast cancer, based on a large study recently reported from India. A single injection of hydroxy-progesterone before a surgery in women who were node positive showed a significant improvement. However, it did not improve outcomes in all women with operable breast cancer. This is a simple and inexpensive intervention, especially in developing countries where the incidence of lymph node metastasis is high.[123]

Targeted Therapy

Anti-estrogen therapy was the first targeted therapy for breast cancer.

HER2 neu as a target

This is one of the important antigens found on breast cancer cells. About one-third of the breast cancer tissues will express this antigen. It belongs to the family of epidermal growth factor receptor (EGFR) family. The expression can be of various degrees. The IHC would report it as +1, +2 or +3. The patient with +3 is eligible for antibody therapy while those with +1 report are not eligible for the same. Those patients with +2 expressions will be advised to carry out confirmation with FISH technique. If FISH confirms the expression, the patient will be eligible for antibody therapy.

The antibody to HER2 neu is called trastuzumab.[124] This is an IV preparation and given as a loading dose of 8 mg/kg followed by 6 mg/kg every 3 weeks. The toxicities include allergic reactions during first infusion and importantly, cardiac dysfunction as a cumulative toxicity.[125] This drug can lead to cardiomyopathy, hence cardiac function needs to be monitored every 3 months. Most important clinical implication is that anthracyclines, i.e. doxorubicin or epirubicine cannot be combined with trastuzumab.[126]

Another agent approved for HER2 neu positive patients is lapatinib. This is an oral drug and can be given to the patient who fails on trastuzumab. The dose of lapatinib is 1,250 mg/day daily. This drug can cross blood-brain barrier; hence, it is useful for patients with brain metastasis. It has peculiar side effects like diarrhea and hand-foot syndrome (painful erythematous rash over tips of fingers and toes, peeling of skin and dryness of skin). These side effects require close monitoring and dose adjustments. Lapatinib is combined with capecitabine for metastatic breast cancer.[127] This drug is also being tried with hormonal therapy in neoadjuvant setting.

RADIATION THERAPY

Radiation Therapy is an integral treatment modality in the comprehensive management of breast cancer. XRT has been used since decades to reduce locoregional failure and palliation. It is rarely employed singly as a comprehensive treatment. Patients have been treated with photon of different energy, cobalt-60 (CO^{60}) beam, electrons and interstitial radiation. Introduction of Co^{60} machines made a significant improvement in treating bulky women. Photon of 4, 6 and higher energies have been utilized with no difference in outcome. High-energy photons may be required to treat very large pendulous breast. Three-dimensional conformal radiation (Figs 28A and B) has the advantage of reducing the volume of normal tissue involved in the treatment.

This generally translates into reduction in immediate and delayed side-effects. Electrons of varying energy or temporary Ir^{92} implants have been used to boost tumor bed. Radiation with intensity modulated radiation therapy (IMRT) (Figs 29A and B) may be considered investigational. IMRT can deliver more homogenous radiation following lumpectomy or mastectomy. This comes at a cost of increased integral dose to lungs and heart.

Radiation therapy is indicated following BCS and in selected patients after mastectomy. BCS became a standard of care in stages I and II following the publication of recommendation by a consensus development conference in 1992.[128] It involves surgical excision with adequate margins, attention to axillary nodes. Whole breast radiation, to a dose of 45–50 Gy, followed by a boost of 10–20 Gy to the tumor bed is administered. Axilla is spared, if the numbers of nodes are less than 4. There is no consensus or irradiating supraclavicular fossa (SCF) and internal mammary nodes (IMN) routinely. Clinical recurrence in IMN rarely exceeds 3% in most series. Inclusion of IMN may increase cardiac and lung toxicity but without proportionate increase in survival benefit. There is no consensus on the routine inclusion of SCF as well. However, it is prudent to include SCF in patient with more than 4 axillary nodes, a large primary poorly differentiated tumor and the presence of lymphovascular invasion. Axilla is not radiated if there is no nodal metastasis, or the numbers of metastatic nodes are less than 4 and without perinodal extension. Whole breast radiation following BCS has been practiced on the premise that most patient harbor multicentric sites of cancer in the breast. However for most patients detectable cancer rarely goes few centimeters of the epicenter. Hulland and colleagues have conclusively demonstrated following serial section that cancer cells are rarely found 2 cm beyond the tumor. Besides 70–90% of recurrences are seen within the tumor bed even when surgery is followed by radiation.[129] This has prompted the practice of partial breast radiation (PBI) with accelerated or hypofractionated radiation. PBI is a relatively new innovation with a limited data.[130] Hence, PBI should be recommended with care and circumspection. External beam partial breast irradiation, interstitial brachytherapy, intracavitary mammosite, interstitial seed implant, intraoperative soft X-rays of 50 Kev (intrabeam) are some of the technique for PBI to avoid morbidity.

Brachytherapy

Brachytherapy (Fig. 30) interstitial implantation; this technique involves placing hollow plastic tubes in single or multiple layers within the tumor bed during or after surgery. A margin of 3–4 cm is recommended for inclusion for radiation. A dose of 45 Gy in 3–6 days administered in low-dose rate mode (LDR), while 32 Gy in 8 fractions or 34 Gy in 8 fractions over 4 day is administered in high-dose rate mode (HDR). Local control and cosmetic results are comparable with conventional whole breast radiation. In one of the studies done at William Beaumont hospital

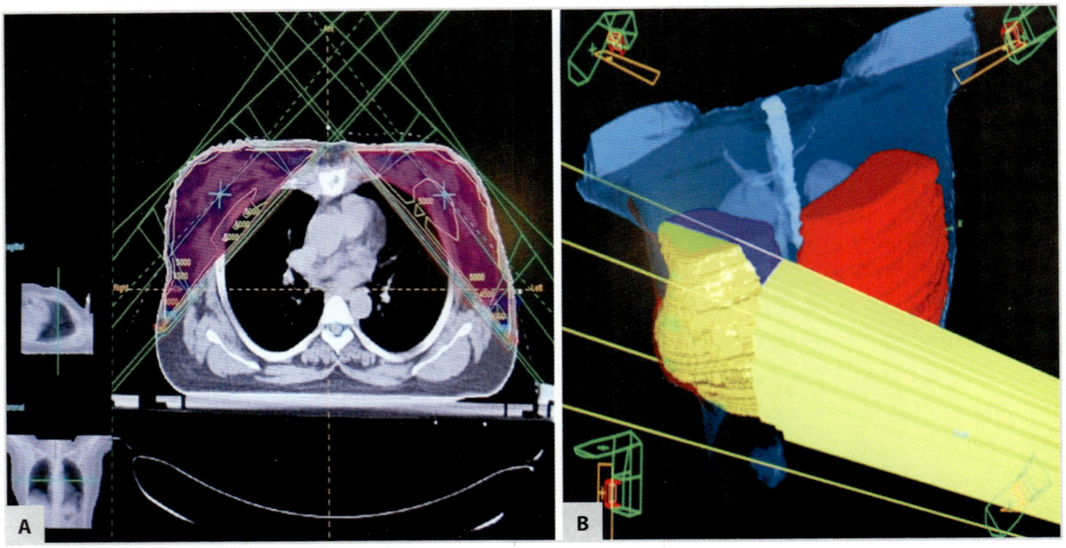

Figs 28A and B: Three-dimensional (3D) conformal radiation

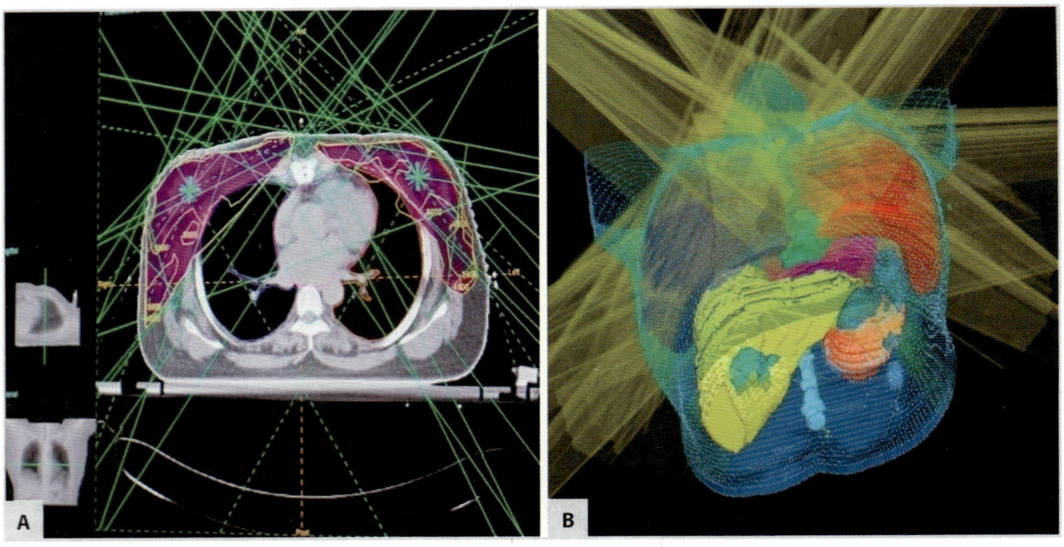

Figs 29A and B: Intensity modulated radiation therapy (IMRT)

in Detroit documented an incidence of 4% fat necrosis and fibrosis while 6% of patient developed grade I or II breast edema.[131] Interstitial radiation requires substantial skill and complex quality assurance studies. The other techniques like seed implants and intracavitary, i.e. tumor bed radiation with mammosite are not widely available, hence not routinely used.

External beam radiation therapy

External beam radiation therapy (EBRT) with or without IMRT is another technique and an option for PBI. The technique of IMRT is less operator-dependent but both complex and expensive. It involves a dose of 34 Gy in 25 fractions, or 38.5 Gy in 10 fractions twice daily, over 1 week. Treatment is well tolerated with no major dose limiting toxicities. Intraoperative radiation has been resurrected for PBI. European Institute of Oncology in Milan treated 237 patients to a dose of 17–21 Gy in single session with 3–9 MeV electrons. A mobile linear accelerator was used widely and others from United Kingdom (UK) have developed intraoperative radiation with "intrabeam". It is a 50 Kev X-ray with a limited depth of penetration. A surface dose of 20 Gy was delivered in a study which included 185 patients. It is purported to be a cost effective treatment in a community hospital set-up.

Locoregional radiation is offered to most patients with BCT. However, all patients following mastectomy do not require postoperative radiation. Postmastectomy

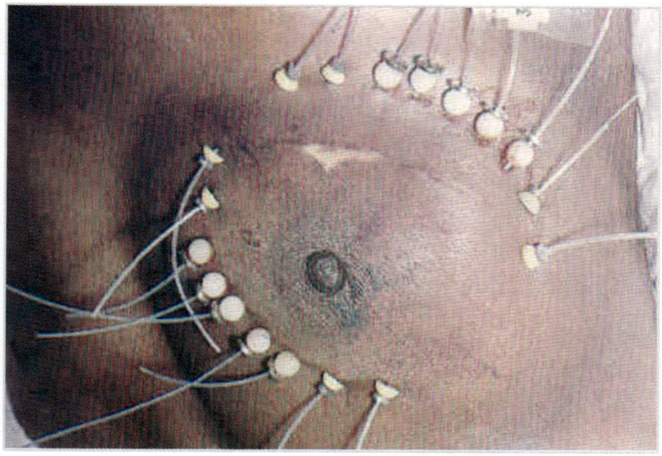

Fig. 30: Brachytherapy

TABLE 20: Indications and contraindications of postmastectomy radiation therapy (PMRT)

Indications	*Contraindications*
Breast conservation surgery (BCS): All patients	• Previous radiation to the involved side
Post-MRM: T > 5 cm • Skin/chest wall involvement • Axillary node metastasis > 4	• Pregnancy
Inoperable (Haagensen and Stout criteria) • Skin ulceration • Edema • Fixation to the chest wall	• Collagen vascular disease: Increase the severity of radiation reaction
	• Persistent pathological positive margin

Abbreviation: MRM, modified radical mastectomy

radiation therapy (PMRT) in high-risk patient is based on the premise that islands of occult foci may survive surgery and systemic therapy. The occult foci on regrowth can cause distressing local recurrence and can be a reservoir from which, cells can metastasize to other organs. In 2005, Oxford Early Breast Cancer Trialists Collaborative Group published a data of 8,505 women, with lymph node metastasis who underwent mastectomy and PMRT demonstrated a reduction of local recurrence from 22.8 to 5.8% at 5 years and a survival benefit of 4.4% at 15 years. PMRT is indicated in patients with tumor size greater than 5 cm, more than 4 lymph nodes and with metastatic foci, perinodal extension, skin and pectoral fascia involvement. Local recurrence in chest wall, axilla or supraclavicular nodes is another indication for locoregional radiation. Patients need to be radiated with Co^{60}, or higher energy of photons. A total dose of 50 Gy in 5 weeks or its equivalent is delivered. Table 20 shows indications for PMRT. Indications for PMRT following neoadjuvant chemotherapy are governed by prechemotherapy parameters.

The immediate toxicities due to radiation include dry or wet desquamation of skin, particularly under axilla and analgesic pigmentation. These are managed easily with appropriate local emollients or antibacterial ointments. Late radiation sequels include arm lymphedema, brachial plexopathy, cardiac toxicity, pneumonitis, and rib fracture. Radiation-induced neoplasm though rare, is relevant, in younger patients with early disease with a potential for long survival. Second primaries are known to occur in esophagus, lung and contralateral breast. Local radiation of metastatic deposits in brain and bone can effectively ameliorate symptoms and improve quality of life. Whole brain radiation therapy (WBRT), 30 Gy in 10 fractions is the standard of care. Solitary metastasis in brain can be effectively radiated with stereotactic hypofractionated radiation. Metastasis in appendicular skeleton should be radiated promptly to manage alleviate pain and prevent pathological fracture.

Survival Rates

A report by American Society of Clinical Oncology (ASCO) in 2009 shows the improvements in the overall 5-year survival for various cancers in the US[132] and reports that the overall 5-year survival for breast cancer had increased from 75% in 1970s to almost 89% presently, which meant that out of every 100 women with breast cancer in the US, 89 women are likely to survive for at least 5 years. A study conducted in Tata Memorial Hospital, Mumbai reported an overall 5-year survival rate of 77%;[133] they reported a 5-year survival rate of 81% for those "less than or equal to 50 years" of age and 67% for those "greater than 50 years" of age; the study showed an inverse relationship of stage-of disease with survival which has been shown in earlier studies (Tables 21 to 23).[10,134-137]

TABLE 21: Five-year survival rate of various stages of cancer

Stage	*5-year survival rate*
T_1	85%
T_2	63%
T_3	32%
T_4	21%

Source: Adapted from reference 10.

TABLE 22: Survival rates[10,139]

Stage	10-year survival (Western data) (%)	5-year survival (Indian data) (%)
Stage 0	99	
Stage I	80–90	90
Stage II A-B	60	65
Stage III A	50	33
Stage III B	30	33
Stage IV	10	6

TABLE 23: Future scenario in breast cancer

Pattern	1995	2020
Prophylaxis	Tamoxifen	Genetic engineering
Early diagnosis	Screening mammography	DNA testing/online digital mammography
Histology	FNAC or surgical biopsy	Robotics—virtual reality
Therapy	Lumpectomy—MRM Axillary dissection	Laser destruction Precision beam radiotherapy/IORT
Adjuvant therapy	Chemotherapy	Targeted chemotherapy—biological agent

Abbreviations: FNAC, fine-needle aspirate cytology; MRM, modified radical mastectomy; DNA, deoxyribonucleic acid; IORT, intraoperative radiotherapy

REFERENCES

1. Ferlay J, Shin HR, Bray F, et al. (2012). GLOBOCAN 2008 v2.0, Cancer Incidence and Mortality Worldwide: IARC Cancer Base No 10. Lyon, France: International Agency for Research on Cancer; 2010. [online] Available from globocan.iarc.fr/Default.aspx. [Accessed January, 2014].
2. NCRP(a). Two-year Report of the Population Based Cancer Registries (2006-2008). National Cancer Registry Programme, Indian Council of Medical Research, 2009, Bangalore, India.
3. Agarwal G, Pradeep PV, Aggarwal V, et al. Spectrum of breast cancer in Asian women. World J Surg. 2007;31:1031-40.
4. NCRP(b). National Cancer Registry Programme Consolidated report of the population based cancer registries (1990–1996). 2001. Indian Council of Medical Research, India.
5. Dinshaw KA, Sarin R, Budrukkar AN, et al. Safety and feasibility of breast conserving therapy in Indian women: two decades of experience at Tata Memorial Hospital. J Surg Oncol. 2006;94:105-13.
6. Mathew A, Pandey M, Rajan B. Do younger women with non-metastatic and non-inflammatory breast carcinoma have poor prognosis? World J Surg Oncol. 2004;2:2.
7. Shavers VL, Harlan LC, Stevens JL. Racial/ethnic variation in clinical presentation, treatment, and survival among breast cancer patients less than age 35 years. Cancer. 2003;97:134-47.
8. Agarwal G, Ramakant P. Breast cancer care in India: The current scenario and the challenges for the future. Breast Care (Basel). 2008;3(1):21-7.
9. Saxena S, Rekhi B, Bansal A, et al. Clinico-morphological patterns of breast cancer including family history in a New Delhi hospital, India – a cross-sectional study. World J Surg Oncol. 2005;3:67.
10. Nair MK, Sankaranarayanan R, Nair KS, et al. Overall survival from breast cancer in Kerala, India, in relation to menstrual, reproductive, and clinical factors. Cancer. 1993;71:1791-6.
11. Paymaster JC, Gangadharan P. Some observations on the epidemiology of cancer of breast in women in western India. Int J Cancer. 1972;10:443-50.
12. Rao DN, Ganesh B, Desai PB. Role of reproductive factors in breast cancer in a low-risk area: a case-control study. Br J Cancer. 1994;70:129-32.
13. Boyd NF, Guo H, Martin LJ, et al. Mammographic density and the risk and detection of breast cancer. N Engl J Med. 2007;356(3):227-36.
14. Miki Y, Swensen J, Shattuck-Eidens D, et al. A strong candidate for the breast and ovarian cancer susceptibility gene BRCA1. Science. 1994;266:66-71.
15. Consensus Conference on the classification of ductal carcinoma in situ. The Consensus Conference Committee. Cancer. 1997;80(9):1798-802.
16. Harvey JM, Clark GM, Osborne CK, et al. Estrogen receptor status by immunohistochemistry is superior to the ligand-binding assay for predicting response to adjuvant endocrine therapy in breast cancer. J Clin Oncol. 1999;17:1474-81.

17. Barron JJ, Cziraky MJ, Weisman T, et al. HER2 testing and subsequent trastuzumab treatment for breast cancer in a managed care environment. Oncologist. 2009;14:760-8.
18. Wolff AC, Hammond ME, Schwartz JN, et al. American Society of Clinical Oncology/College of American Pathologists guideline recommendations for human epidermal growth factor receptor 2 testing in breast cancer. J Clin Oncol. 2007;25:118-45.
19. Foulkes WD, Smith IE, Reis-Filho JS. Triple-negative breast cancer. N Engl J Med. 2010;363:1938-48.
20. Perou CM, Sorlie T, Eisen MB, et al. Molecular portraits of human breast tumours. Nature. 2000;406:747-52.
21. Sorlie T, Perou CM, Tibshirani R, et al. Gene expression patterns of breast carcinomas distinguish tumor subclasses with clinical implications. Proc Natl Acad Sci U S A. 2001;98:10869-74.
22. Hendrick RE, Smith RA, Rutledge JH, et al. Benefits of screening mammography in women aged 40-49: a new meta-analysis of randomized controlled trials. Monog Nat Cancer Institute. 1997;22:87-92.
23. Park JM, Franken EA, Garg M, et al. Breast tomosynthesis: present considerations and future applications. Radiographics. 2007;27:S231-40.
24. Popli MB. Pictorial essay: mammographic features of breast cancer. Indian J Radiol Imaging. 2001;11:175-9.
25. Nalawade YV. Evaluation of breast calcifications. Indian J Radiol Imaging. 2009;19:282-6.
26. Park JM, Choi HK, Bae SJ, et al. Clustering of breast microcalcifications: revisited. Clin Radiol. 2000;55:114-8.
27. Shah G, Jankharia B. Pictorial essay: Breast USG. Indian J Radiol Imaging. 2010;20:98-104.
28. Gokhale S. Ultrasound characterization of breast masses. Indian J Radiol Imaging. 2009;19(3):242-7.
29. Stavros AT. Benign solid nodules: Specific pathologic diagnosis. In: Breast Ultrasound. Philadelphia, USA: Lippincott Williams and Wilkins; 2004. pp. 528-96.
30. Zhi H, Ou B, Luo BM, et al. Comparison of ultrasound elastography, mammography, and sonography in the diagnosis of solid breast lesions. J Ultrasound Med. 2007;26(6):807-15.
31. Kuhl C. The current status of breast MR imaging. Part I. Choice of technique, image interpretation, diagnostic accuracy, and transfer to clinical practice. Radiology. 2007;244(2):356-78.
32. Kuhl CK, Klaschik S, Mielcareck P, et al. Do T2-weighted pulse sequences help with the differential diagnosis of enhancing lesions in dynamic breast MRI? J Magn Reson Imaging. 1999;9:187-96.
33. Liberman L, Morris EA, Lee MJ, et al. Breast lesions detected on MR imaging: Features and positive predictive value. AJR Am J Roentgenol. 2002;179(1):171-8.
34. Macura KJ, Ouwerkerk R, Jacobs MA, et al. Patterns of enhancement on breast MR images: Interpretation and imaging pitfalls. Radiographics. 2006;26:1719-34.
35. Rosen EL, Eubank WB, Mankoff DA. FDG PET, PET/CT, and Breast cancer imaging. Radiographics. 2007;27:S215-29.
36. Groves AM, Shastry M, Ben-Haim S, et al. Defining the role of PET-CT in staging early breast cancer. Oncologist. 2012;17(5):613-9.
37. Greer LT, Rosman M, Mylander WC, et al. Does breast tumor heterogeneity necessitate further immunohistochemical staining on surgical specimens? J Am Surg. 2013;216(2):239-51.
38. Patchefsky AS, Schwartz GF, Finkelstein SD, et al. Heterogeneity of intraductal carcinoma of the breast. Cancer. 1989;63(4): 731-41.
39. Feig BW, Ching DC. Invasive breast cancer. In: The MD Anderson Surgical Oncology Handbook, 5th edition. Philadelphia, PA: Lippincott Williams and Wilkins; 2011.
40. Page D, Rogers L, Schuyler P, et al. The natural history of ductal carcinoma in situ of the breast. In: Silverstein MJ, Recht A, Lagios M (Eds). Ductal carcinoma in situ of the breast. Philadelphia, USA: Lippincott Williams and Wilkins; 2002. pp. 17-21.
41. Sanders M, Schuyler P, Dupont W, et al. The natural history of low grade ductal carcinoma in situ of the breast in women treated by biopsy only revealed over 30 years of long-term follow-up cancer. 2005:2481-4.
42. Moran MS, Bai HX, Harris EE, et al. ACR appropriateness criteria® ductal carcinoma in situ. Breast J. 2012;18(1):8-15.
43. Silverstein M, Lagios M, Recht A, et al. Image detected breast cancer: state of art diagnosis and treatment. J Am Coll Surg. 2005;201:586-97.
44. Silverstein MJ. Ductal carcinoma in situ of the breast. Ann Rev Med. 2000;51:17-32.
45. Swain SM. Noninvasive breast cancer: Part 1. Ductal carcinoma in situ--incidence, presentation, and guidelines to treatment. Oncology (Williston Park). 1989;3(3):25-31.
46. Fisher B, Land S, Mamounas E, et al. Prevention of invasive breast cancer in women with ductal carcinoma in situ: An update of the National Surgical Adjuvant Breast and Bowel Project experience. Semin Oncol. 2001;28(4):400-18.
47. UK Coordinating committee on Cancer Research (UKCCCR). Ductal carcinoma in situ (DCIS) working party, radiotherapy and tamoxifens in women with completely excised ductal carcinoma in situ of breast in the UK, Australia, and New Zealand: randomized controlled trial. Lancet. 2003;362:95-102.
48. Fisher B, Constantino J, Redmond C, et al. Lumpectomy compared with Lumpectomy and Radiation therapy for treatment of intraductal Breast Cancer. N Engl J Med. 1993;328: 1581-6.
49. Fisher B, Dignam J, Wolmark N, et al. Lumpectomy and Radiation therapy for the treatment of intraductal breast cancer : findings from National Surgical Adjuvant Breast and Bowel project B-17 Clin Oncol. 1998;16(2):441-452.
50. Julein J, Bijker N, Fentiman I, et al. Radiotherapy in breast conserving treatment for ductal carcinoma in situ: first results of EORTC randomised phase III trials 10853. Lancet. 2000;355: 528-33.
51. Meretoja TJ, Heikkilä PS, Salmenkivi K, et al. Outcome of patients with ductal carcinoma in situ and sentinel node biopsy. Ann Surg Oncol. 2012;19(7):2345-51.
52. Klauber-Demore N, Tan LK, Liberman L, et al. Sentinel lymph node biopsy: is it indicated in patients with high risk ductal carcinoma in situ, a ductal carcinoma in situ with microinvasion. Ann Surg Oncol. 2000;7:636-42.

53. Mittendorf EA, Arciero CA, Gutchell V, et al. Core biopsy diagnosis of ductal carcinoma in situ: an indication for sentinel lymph node biopsy. Curr Surgery. 2005;62:253-7.
54. Yen TW, Hunt KK, Ross MI, et al. Predictions of invasive breasts cancer in patients with an initial diagnosis of ductal carcinoma in situ: a guide to selective use of sentinel lymph node biopsy in management of ductal carcinoma in situ. J Am Coll Surg. 2005;200:516-26.
55. Zavagno G, Carcoforo P, Marconato R, et al. Role of axillary sentinel lymph node biopsy in patients with pure ductal carcinoma in situ of the breast. BMC Cancer. 2005;5:28.
56. Giuliano AE, Hawes D, Ballma KV, et al. Association of occult metastases in sentinel lymph nodes and bone marrow with survival among women with early-stage invasive breast cancer. JAMA. 2011;306:385-93.
57. Gilleard O, Goodman A, Cooper M, et al. The significance of the Van Nuys prognostic index in the management of ductal carcinoma in situ. World J Surg Oncol. 2008 6:61.
58. Haagensen CD, Lane N, Lattes R, et al. Lobular neoplasia (so-called lobular carcinoma in situ) of the breast. Cancer. 1978;42(2):737-69.
59. Page DL, Kidd TE, Dupont WD, et al. Lobular neoplasia of the breast: higher risk for subsequent invasive cancer predicted by more extensive disease. Hum Pathol. 1991;22:1232-9.
60. Harris JR, Lippman ME, Osborne CK, Marow M (Eds). Lobular cancer in situ biology and pathology. In: Disease of the Breast, 4th edition. Philadelphia, USA: Lippincott Williams and Wilkins; 2009.
61. Oppong BA, King TA. Recommendations for women with lobular carcinoma in situ (LCIS). Oncology (Williston Park). 2011;25(11):1051-6, 1058.
62. Hussain M, Cunnick GH. Management of lobular carcinoma in-situ and atypical hyperplasia of the breast--a review. Eur J Surg Oncol. 2011;37(4):279-89.
63. Polat AK, Kanbour-Shakir A, Andacoglu O, et al. Atypical hyperplasia on core biopsy: is further surgery needed? Am J Med Sci. 2012;344(1):28-31.
64. Aphorisms and quotations – Blake and Cady.
65. Imoto S, Isaka H, Sakemura N, et al. Paradigm shift in axilla surgery for breast cancer patients treated with sentinel node biopsy. Breast Cancer. 2012;19(2):104-9.
66. Yi M, Giordano S, meric-Bernstam F, et al. Trends in and outcomes from sentinel lymph node biopsy (SLNB) alone v/s SLNB with axillary lymph node dissection for node positive breast cancer patients: experince from the SEER database. Ann Surg Oncol. 2010;17.
67. Viviana G, Camelia C, et al. Positive axillary sentinel lymph node: is axillary dissection always necessary? Breast. 2011;20(Suppl 3):S96-8.
68. Ivens D, Hoe AL, Podd TJ, et al. Assessment of morbidity from complete axillary dissection. Br J Cancer. 1992;66:136-8.
69. Golshan M, Martin W, Dowlastshahi K. Sentinel lymph node biopsy lowers the rate of lymphedema when compared with standard axillary lymph node dissection. Am Surg. 2003;69:209-12.
70. Langer I, Guller U, Besclaz G, et al. Morbidity of sentinel lymph node biopsy (SLN) alone versus SLN and completion of axillary lymph node dissection after breast cancer surgery. A prospective Swiss multicenter study on 659 patients. Ann Surg. 2007;245:452-61.
71. Aitken RJ, Gaze MN, Rodger A et al. Arm morbidity within a trial of mastectomy and either nodal sample with selective radiotherapy or axillary clearance. Br J Surg. 1989;76:568-71.
72. Giuliano A, Hunt K, Ballman K, et al. Axillary dissection v/s no axillary dissection in women with invasive breast cancer and sentinel node metastases. JAMA. 2011;305(6):569-75.
73. Morrow M, Giuliano A. To cut is to cure can be really apply All in practice? Ann Surg Oncol. 2011;18(9):2413-5.
74. Caudle A, Hunt K, Keuren H, et al. Multidisciplinary considerations in the implementation of the findings from the American college of surgeons oncology group (ACOSOG) Z0011 study: a practice changing trial. Ann Surg Oncol. 2011;19(8):2407-12.
75. Hunt KK, Ballman KV. Factors associated with loco-regional recurrence after a negative sentinel node dissection. Ann Surg. 2012;256:428-36.
76. Caudle A, Hunt K. American College of Surgeons Oncology Group (ACOSOG) Z0011: Impact on Surgeon practice patterns. Ann Surg Oncol. 2012;19(10):3144-51.
77. Gainer S, Hunt K, et al. Changing behaviour in clinical practice in response to the ACOSOG Z0011 Trial: A survey of the American Society of Breast Surgeons. Ann Surg Oncol. 2012;19(10):3152-8.
78. Weber WP, Barry M, et al. A 10-year trend analysis of sentinel lymph node frozen section and completion axillary dissection for breast cancer: are these procedures becoming obsolate? Ann Surg Oncol. 2012;19:225-32.
79. Viviana G, Camelia C, et al. Positive axillary sentinel lymph node: Is axillary dissection always necessary? Breast. 2011;20.
80. Jeremy S, Hiram C, et al. Radiation field design and regional control in sentinel lymph node-positive breast cancer patients with omission of axillary dissection. Cancer. 2012:1994-2003.
81. Gentilini O, Veronesi U. Abandoning Sentinel lymph node biopsy in early breast cancer? A new trial in progress in the European Institute of Oncology of Milan (SOUND: Sentinel Node Vs Observation after Axillary Ultrasound). Breast. 2012;21:678-81.
82. Nour A. Efficacy of methylene blue dye in localization of sentinel lymph node in breast cancer patients. Breast J. 2004;10(5): 388-91.
83. Nwariaku FE, Euhus DM, Beitsch PD, et al. Sentinel lymph node biopsy, an alternative to elective axillary dissection for breast cancer. Am J Surg. 1998;176:529-31.
84. Barnwell JM, Arredondo MA, Kollmorgen D, et al. Sentinel node biopsy in breast cancer. Ann Surg Oncol. 1998;5:126-30.
85. Haid A, Kuehn T, Konstantinivk P, et al. Shoulder--arm morbidity following axillary dissection and sentinel node biopsy for breast cancer. Eur J Surg Oncol. 2002;28:705-10.
86. Ivens D, Hoe AL, Podd TJ, et al. Assessment of morbidity from complete axillary dissection. Br J Cancer. 1992;66:136-8.
87. Krag DN, Weaver DL, Alex JC, et al. Surgical resection and radio localization of the sentinel lymph node in breast cancer using a gamma probe. Surg Oncol. 1993;2:335-40.
88. Giuliano AE, Kirgan DM, Guenther DM, et al. Lymphatic mapping and sentinel lymphadenectomy for breast cancer. Ann Surg. 1994;220:391-401.

89. Albertini JJ, Lyman GH, Cox C, et al. lymphatic mapping and sentinel node biopsy in the patient with breast cancer. JAMA. 1996;276:1818-22.

90. Veronesi U, Paganelli G, et al. Sentinel lymph node biopsy and axillary dissection in breast cancer: results in a large series. J Natl Cancer Inst. 1999:91:368-73.

91. Tafra L, Lannin DR, Swanson MS, et al. Multicenter trial of sentinel node biopsy for breast for breast cancer using technetium sulfur colloid and isosulfan blue dye. Ann Surg. 2001;233:51-9.

92. Albo D, Wayne JD, Hunt KK, et al. Anaphylactic reactions to isosulfan blue dye during sentinel lymph node biopsy for breast cancer. Am J Surg. 2001;182:393-8.

93. Leong SP, Donegan E, Heffernon, et al. Adverse reactions to isosulfan blue during selective sentinel lymph node dissection in melanoma. Ann S Surg Oncol. 2000;7:361-6.

94. Hortobagyi GN, Buzdar AU. Locally advanced cancer: a review including the MD Anderson experience. In: Ragaz J, Anel IM (Eds). High-risk Breast Cancer. Berlin, Germany: Springer Verlag; 1991. pp. 382-415.

95. Valagussa P, Zambetti M, Bignami PD et al. T3b – T4 breast cancer: factors affecting rsults in combined modality treatment. Clin Exp Metastasis. 1983;1:191-202.

96. Kuerer H, Newman L, et al. Role of Axillary Lymph Node Dissection After Tumor Downstaging With Induction Chemotherapy for Locally Breast Cancer. Ann. Surg. Oncol. 1998;5(8):673-80.

97. Isabelle Bedrosian, et al. Tubular, mucinous and medullary carcinoma. In: Singletary, Robb, Hortobagyi (Eds). Advanced Therapy of Breast Disease, 2nd edition. pp. 705-12.

98. Rasmussen BB, Rose C, Christensen IB. Prognostic factors in primary mucinous breast carcinoma. Am J Clin Pathol. 1987;87:155-60.

99. Fentiman IS, Millis RR, Smith P, et al. Mucoid breast carcinomas: histology and prognosis. Br J cancer. 1997;75:1061-5.

100. Diab SG, Clark GM, Osborne CK, et al. Tumor characteristics and clinical outcome of tubular and mucinous breast carcinomas. J Clin Oncol. 1999;17-14.

101. Chaney A, Pollack A et al. Primary Treatment of Cystosarcoma Phyllodes of the Breast. Cancer. 2000;89(7):1502-11.

102. Dixon AR, Galea MH, Ellis IO, et al. Paget's disease of the nipple. Br J Surg. 1991;78:722-3.

103. Pierce LJ, Haffty BG, Solin LJ, et al. The conservative management of Paget's disease of the breast with radiotherapy. Cancer. 1997;80:1065-72.

104. Sheen-Chen S, Chen H, et al. Paget's Disease of the Breast – an Easily Overlooked Disease? J Surg Oncol. 2001;76:261-5.

105. Marshall J, Griffith K, et al. Conservative Management of Paget Disease of the Breast with Radiotherapy. Cancer. 2003;97(9): 2142-9.

106. Foroudi F, Tiver KW. Occult breast carcinoma presenting as axillary metastases. Int J Radiat Oncol Biol Phys. 2000;47:143-7.

107. Baron PL, Moore MP, Kinne DW et al. Occult breast cancer presenting with axillary metastasis: updated management. Arch Surg. 1990;125:210-4.

108. Duffy M, Shering S, et al. CA 15-3: a prognostic marker in breast cancer. Int J Biol Majors. 2000;15(4):330-3.

109. Singletary, et al. A Role for curative surgery in the treatment of selected patients with metastatic breast cancer – Oncologist. 2003;8:241-51.

110. Lymphoedema – May Quan et al. In: Singletary, Robb, Hortobagyi (Eds). Advanced Therapy of Breast Disease, 2nd edition. pp. 772-80.

111. Casley-Smith JR, Foldi M, Ryan TJ, et al. Summary of the 10th International Congress of Lymphology working group discussions and recommendations, Adelaide, Australia, August 10-17, 1985. Lymphology. 1985;18:175-80.

112. Mortiner PS. The pathophysiology of lymphedema. Cancer. 1998;83:2798-802.

113. Aitken RJ, Gaze MN, Rodger A, et al. Arm morbidity within a trial of mastectomy and either nodal sample with selective radiotherapy or axillary clearance. Br J Surg. 1989;76:568-71.

114. Ivens D, Hoe AL, Podd TJ, et al. Assessment of morbidity from complete axillary dissection. Br J Cancer. 1992;66:136-8.

115. Golshan M, Martin W, Dowlastshahi K. Sentinel lymph node biopsy lowers the rate of lymphedema when compared with standard axillary lymph node dissection. Am Surg. 2003;69: 209-12.

116. Langer I, Guller U, Besclaz G, et al. Morbidity of sentinel lymph node biopsy (SLN) alone versus SLN and completion of axillary lymph node dissection after breast cancer surgery. A prospective Swiss multicenter study on 659 patients. Ann Surg. 2007;245:452-61.

117. Goffman T, Laronga C, et al. Lymphedema of the Arm and Breast in Irradiated Breast Cancer Patients: Risks in an Era of Dramatically Changing Axillary Surgery. Breast J. 2004;10(5): 405-11.

118. Trends in risk reduction practices for the prevention of lymphedema in the first 12 months after breast cancer surgery. J Am Coll Surg. 2013;216:380-9.

119. Markopoulos C, Xepapadakis G, et al. Clinical experience of using oncotype Dx as an additional treatment decision tool in early breast cancer – A retrospective analysis from 4 Greek institutions. EJSO J Cancer Surg. 2012;38(2012):413-9.

120. Jack Cuzick, et al. Prognostic Value of a combined estrogen receptor, progesterone receptor, Ki-67 and Human Epidermal Growth Factor Receptor 2. Immunohistochemical score and comparison with the Genomic Health Recurrence Score in early breast cancer. J Clin Oncol. 2011.

121. De Laurentiis M, Cancello G, D'Agostino D, et al. Taxane-based combinations as adjuvant chemotherapy of early breast cancer: a meta-analysis of randomized trials. J Clin Oncol. 2008;26(1): 44-53.

122. Winer EP, Hudis C, Burstein HJ, et al. ASCO technology assessment on the use of aromatase inhibitors as adjuvant therapy for post-menopausal women with hormone receptor-positive breast cancer: status report 2004. J Clin Oncol. 2005;23(3):619-29.

123. Badwe, et al. Single injection depot progesterone before surgery and survival in women with operable breast cancer: A randomized control trial. J Clin Oncol. 2011.

124. Hudis CA. Trastuzumab-mechanism of action and use in clinical practice. N Eng J Med. 2007;357(1):39-51.

125. Piccart-Gebhart M, Procter M, Leyland-Jones B, et al. Trastuzumab after adjuvant chemotherapy in HER-positive breast cancer. N Eng J Med. 2005;353(16):659-72.

126. Romond EH, Perez EA, Bryant J, et al. Trastuzumab plus adjuvant chemotherapy for operable HER2-positive breast cancer. N Engl J Med. 2005;353(16):1673-84.

127. Geyer CE, Foster J, Lindquist D, et al. Lapatinib plus capecitabine for HER2-positive advanced breast cancer. N Engl J Med. 2006;355(26):2733-43.

128. Ribeiro GG, Mayee B, Swindell R, et al. The Ehristic Hospital breast conservation trail: an update at 8 yearsfrom inception.

129. Host H. Brennhovd 10, Loeb M. Postoperative radiotherapy in breast cancer long term results from the Oslo study. Inj J Radiat Oncol Biol Phy. 1986;12:727-32.

130. Bagakan KL, sharpe MB, Jaffny D. et al. Accelerated partial breast irradiation using 3D conformal radiation therapy (3D-CRT). Int J Radiat Oncol Phy. 2003;55:302-11.

131. Wazer DE, Lowther D, Bayle T, et al. clinically evident fat necrosis in women treated with high dose rate brachytherapy alone for early breast cancer. Inj J Radiat Oncol Biol Phys. 2001;50:107-11.

132. Petrelli NJ, Winer EP, Brahmer J, et al. Clinical Cancer Advances 2009: Major Research Advances in Cancer Treatment, Prevention, and Screening—A Report From the American Society of Clinical Oncology: JCO. 2009;27(35).

133. Ganesh B, Talole SD, Dikshit R, et al. Dinshaw Estimation of Survival Rates of Breast Cancer Patients - an Hospital-Based Study from Mumbai. Asian Pac J Cancer Prev. 2008;9(1):53-57.

134. Nandakumar A, Anantha N, Venugopal TC, et al. Survival in breast cancer: population-based study in Bangalore, India. Int J Cancer. 1995;60:593-96.

135. Gajalakshmi CK, Shanta V, Swaminathan R, et al. A population-based survival study on female breast cancer in Madras, India. Br J Cancer. 1997;75:771-75.

136. Shanta V, Gajalakshmi CK, Swaminathan R. Cancer survival in developing countries. In Cancer Survival in Chennai (Madras), India. Chapter 12. Ed: R Sankarnarayanan, RJ Black and DM Parkin. IARC Scientific Publication No 145. 1999.

137. Yeole BB, Jussawalla DJ, Sabnis SD, et al. Cancer survival in developing countries. Survival from breast and cervical cancer in Mumbai (Bombay), India (2001). Chapter11. Ed: R Sankarnarayanan, RJ Black and DM Parkin. IARC Scientific Publication No 145. 1999.

138. Hoque LW. Pathology, progression and staging in breast cancer. In: Borgen PI, Hill AD (Eds). Breast Diseases. Georgetown, Texas, USA: Landes Bioscience; 2000. pp. 88-99.

36 Ovarian Cancer

Ratna Parikh, Praful Desai, Ganesh Balasubramaniam, Bhavna Parikh, Sarabjeet Kaur Arneja

INTRODUCTION

Ovarian cancer is the second most common gynecologic cancer globally. It is generally diagnosed late which results in poor overall outcomes. In India, it is also the second most common cancer of the genital tract and the third most common cancer in women, next to breast and cervix. Early symptoms are vague with inconstant and variable abdominal pain, anorexia and sense of fullness in the abdomen. Vague symptoms are the main reasons for a late diagnosis in most patients ovarian cancer therefore is a distressing and challenging problem and forms about 23% of all gynecological malignancies. It accounts for 47% of deaths due to female genital tract cancers. In the United States of America (USA), one out of 70 women will develop the disease.[1] Epithelial ovarian cancers form 90% of all ovarian cancers, the median age being 61 years.[2]

EPIDEMIOLOGY

As per the Global Burden of Cancer (GLOBOCAN) study estimates, there were nearly 12.7 million new cancer cases and 7.6 million deaths in 2008 worldwide.[3] It is estimated that globally 0.2 million (224,747) new ovarian cancer cases were diagnosed with an age-standardized rate (ASR) of 6.3 per 10^5. It is the 7th leading malignancy among women's cancers. Ovarian cancers are on the rise as breast cancer and both are hormone dependent. There are differences in incidence rates between more developed and less developed regions; a total of 99,521 new cases in more developed (ASR = 9.3 per 10^5) and 28,080 new cases (ASR = 4.6 per 10^5) in the less developed regions have been recorded.

In India, there are 0.88 million cancer cases with an incidence rate (ASR) of 105.5 per 100,000 in women; Annually 28,000 new ovarian cancer cases are diagnosed in India with ASR of 5.7 per 10^5. It is the third leading malignancy after cervix and breast cancer in India. As per the reports of the Indian registries age-adjusted rates of ovarian cancer does not vary much and is 7.8, 7.4 and 7.1 in Mangalore, Chennai and Mumbai, respectively;[4] it is the third most common in all these registries among women.

ASSOCIATED FACTORS

Age

The risk of developing ovarian cancer rises with age. It is rare in women younger than 40 and most develop after menopause. Half of all ovarian cancers occur around 63 years of age or beyond.

Obesity

Various studies show the relationship of obesity and ovarian cancer. Overall, obese women [those with a body mass index (BMI) of at least 30] have a higher risk of developing ovarian cancer. In a pooled analysis of recent studies of the Ovarian Cancer Consortium, an evaluation of the association between BMI and ovarian cancer risk in young adults using original data from 15 case-control studies, reported a high BMI (all time-points) associated with an increased risk. This was most pronounced for borderline serous [pooled odds ratio (OR) = 1.24], invasive endometrioid (OR = 1.17) and invasive mucinous (OR = 1.19) cancers.[5]

Reproductive History

Pregnancy carried to term has a lower risk of ovarian cancer than women who have not. The risk reduces with each full-term pregnancy. Breastfeeding may lower the risk even further. In the self-reported history of endometriosis from 4 population-based case-controlled studies indicated a higher risk of incident epithelial ovarian cancer, women with endometriosis were at an increased risk of ovarian cancer (OR = 1.32).[6] The use of oral contraceptives, child-bearing tubal ligation or hysterectomy were associated with a reduced risk, irrespective of endometriosis.

Gynecologic Surgery

Tubal ligation may reduce the chance of developing ovarian cancer by two-thirds. A hysterectomy may reduce the risk of ovarian cancer by about one-third. Case-control and cohort studies indicate that gynecologic surgeries reduce the risk of ovarian cancer but it is unclear whether it will reduce the risk in BRCA1 and BRCA2 mutation carriers. A study on Jewish women with incident ovarian cancer and tested for an Ashkenazi founder mutation (185delAG and 5382insC in BRCA1 and/or 6174delT in BRCA2) reported a reduced risk by 45% compared to women without a gynecologic surgery (OR = 0.55);[7] the risk estimate for BRCA1 and BRCA2 mutation carriers with gynecologic surgery compared to the controls was also protective (OR = 0.51).

Fertility Drugs

Controversy surrounds the relations among infertility, fertility drug use, and the risk of ovarian cancer. The authors pooled interview data on infertility and fertility drug use from eight case-control studies conducted in the USA, Denmark, Canada and Australia.[8] Among nulligravid women, attempts at pregnancy for more than 5 years compared to less than 1 year increased the risk of ovarian cancer 2.67-fold. In another Hormones and Ovarian Cancer Prediction (HOPE) study, the results provided further evidence that fertility drug use does not significantly contribute to ovarian cancer risk among the majority;[9] however, women who still remain nulligravid, may have an elevated risk for ovarian cancer and similar findings were reported in another study.[10]

Hormone Therapy

Some recent studies suggest women using unopposed estrogens after menopause have an increased risk. It seems to be higher in women taking estrogen for a prolonged time (at least 5 or 10 years). The increased risk is less for women taking both estrogen and progesterone.[11]

Family History of Ovarian Cancer, Breast Cancer, or Colorectal Cancer

Up to 10% of ovarian cancers are due to an inherited tendency. A family history of other types of cancer caused by an inherited mutation (change) in certain genes can increase the risk.[12] Mutations of BRCA1 and BRCA2 genes increase the risk of breast or ovarian cancer; family history of breast cancer increases the risk. The risk of developing ovarian cancer for BRCA1 mutation carriers by age 70 is 39–54% in contrast to 22–27% among BRCA2 mutation carriers.[13,14] Association with hereditary nonpoylposis colorectal carcinoma (HNPCC-mutations) or Lynch II syndrome accounts for a 2% risk of ovarian cancer and 60% of endometrial cancer. Breast cancer in a first- or second-degree relative was associated with increased risk of ovarian cancer.[15]

Talcum Powder

In a review article, it has been reported that talcum powder applied directly to the genital area or on sanitary napkins may be carcinogenic (cancer-causing) to the ovaries.[16] Some studies suggest a very slight increase in risk of ovarian cancer in women who used talc on the genital area. In the past, talcum powder was sometimes contaminated with asbestos, a known cancer-causing mineral.

Diet

The precise etiology of epithelial ovarian cancer remains unknown. Reports suggest high dietary fat intake has an increased risk, although this is speculative. A meta-analysis examining the association of high versus low dietary fat indicates a relative risk (RR) of 1.24 for a high fat intake.[17] In a population-based case-control study in Canada, the association and risk of ovarian cancer was associated with higher consumption of dietary cholesterol and eggs and inversely associated with higher intake of total cruciferous vegetables and supplementation of vitamin E, β-carotene, and B-complex vitamins.[18]

Analgesics

The role of analgesic drug use in development of ovarian cancer is not fully understood. Use of any analgesics (OR = 0.72) or aspirin (OR = 0.60) resulted in a statistically significant decreased risk of serous ovarian cancer but not mucinous or other ovarian tumors.[19] There was a statistically significant inverse association between paracetamol use and ovarian cancer risk;[20] there was a modest nonsignificant inverse association with aspirin use and ovarian cancer and no association with ibuprofen use.

Smoking and Alcohol Use

Smoking, caffeine, and alcohol intake are all potentially modifiable factors that have an unclear association with ovarian cancer risk. The results of a study suggested that intake was not associated with risk;[21] however, an inverse association was observed between caffeine intake and ovarian cancer risk, particularly in women not using hormones and similar findings were also reported in another study.[22]

SURVEILLANCE

Considering the overall poor survival rates, attempts at prevention and early diagnosis needs to be emphasized in presence of a family history of ovarian, uterine or breast cancer. Personal history of breast cancer is a strong predisposing factor for per se ovarian cancer or metastatic spread (Breast-ovarian cancer syndrome). A study of BRCA 1-2 genetic mutations need to be studied in appropriate groups of women with a positive family history.

In the presence of predisposing factors aforementioned, appropriate clinical examination should begin between 30 years and 35 years or earlier if indicated by any symptoms. Imaging ultrasound of abdomen and pelvis and tumor markers [carcinoma antigen 125 (CA-125), carcinoembryonic antigen (CEA)] cannot really screen ovarian cancers for early diagnosis; however, markers and ultrasound studies should begin earlier in the offsprings and careful surveillance should, therefore begin after 30 years every year or 18 months.

CHEMOPREVENTION

Oral contraceptives have been used for chemoprevention for hereditary BRCA mutation carriers. The risks and benefits, however, should be carefully weighed as there is an increased risk of breast cancer. Fenretinide, a synthetic vitamin A analog (200 mg daily) has an antitumor effect and high potency progestins is known to reduce the incidence of ovarian cancer during the course of treatment.[23]

PROPHYLACTIC SURGERY

Bilateral salpingo-oophorectomy reduces the risk of ovarian cancer by 85–90% in women with BRCA mutations.[24] Protection is maximal in premenopausal women. The timing of salpingo-oophorectomy will depend on the desire for fertility. At prophylactic surgery, approximately 5% of women with BRCA mutations are reported to have an occult carcinoma.[25] Panhysterectomy is optional.

PATHOLOGY

The classification of ovarian tumors is based on the embryogenesis of ovary, and they are classified into three main categories based on the postulated cell of origin:

1. Surface or celomic epithelium
2. Germ cells
3. Sex cords and stromal tumors

Surface Epithelial Tumors

They are postulated to derive from the epithelium on the surface of the ovary.[26] They are the most common form of ovarian cancer account for nearly 80% of all tumors and are referred to as surface epithelial tumors. Surface epithelial tumors are subcategorized into benign, borderline (low-malignant potential) and malignant (Table 1). The behavior of benign and malignant tumors is fairly well-understood, but there is a considerable controversy pertaining to the diagnosis, prognosis and treatment of borderline tumors. Surface epithelial tumors are also subclassified based on their line of cellular differentiation that is serous, endometrioid, mucinous, clear cell and transitional cell type.

Classification of surface epithelial tumors based on behavior has been given in the following Table 1.

Serous: An increasing spectrum of proliferation exists in these tumors, represented at one end by benign serous cystadenoma or cystadenofibroma, in which the cyst and the papillae, if present are lined by a single layer of cells, devoid of atypia or architectural complexity. At the

TABLE 1: Classification of surface epithelial tumors based on behavior

Degree of benignancy/ malignancy	*Pathologic features*
Benign	Simple, non-stratified epithelium, no cytologic atypia
Borderline (low malignant potential)	Epithelial proliferation with stratification and cellular tufting, variable degree of mitotic activity and nuclear atypia, no stromal invasion
Malignant	Cytologic atypia and stromal invasion

other end are the serous adenocarcinoma, characterized by nuclear atypia, mitotic activity, cellular stratification, glandular complexity, branching papillary structures and stromal invasion (Fig. 1A). In between are tumors that show some or all of the features of carcinoma but lack stromal invasion.[27] These tumors are known as borderline or of low malignant potential.[28]

Immunohistochemically, the keratin profile of serous tumors is cytokeratin (CK)7+/CK20-. Wilm's tumor suppressor gene 1 (WT1) is diffusely positive in most ovarian serous carcinomas. It less frequently stains ovarian endometrioid carcinoma and is usually negative in ovarian mucinous carcinoma.

Mucinous: Mucinous neoplasms have been divided into benign (mucinous cystadenoma), malignant (mucinous adenocarcinoma) and borderline mucinous tumors. Microscopically, single layer of tall columnar mucinous cells with small regular basally situated nuclei lines the benign tumors. Malignant tumors are characterized by nuclear atypia, epithelial stratification, greater complexity of the glands and areas of stromal invasion.[29] Because of a continuum from benign to malignant, it is common to see an admixture of graded morphological patterns (benign, borderline, borderline with intraepithelial carcinoma, microinvasive, malignant) within the same tumor. Borderline tumors with severe nuclear atypia are designated as intraepithelial carcinoma.[30] Microinvasive carcinoma is characterized by the presence of small foci of invasive carcinoma (<5 mm). Invasion in primary ovarian mucinous carcinomas can be either expansile (nondestructive or confluent glandular) or infiltrative (destructive). The former is more common and is associated with a relatively good prognosis. Most primary ovarian mucinous tumors are typically diffusely positive

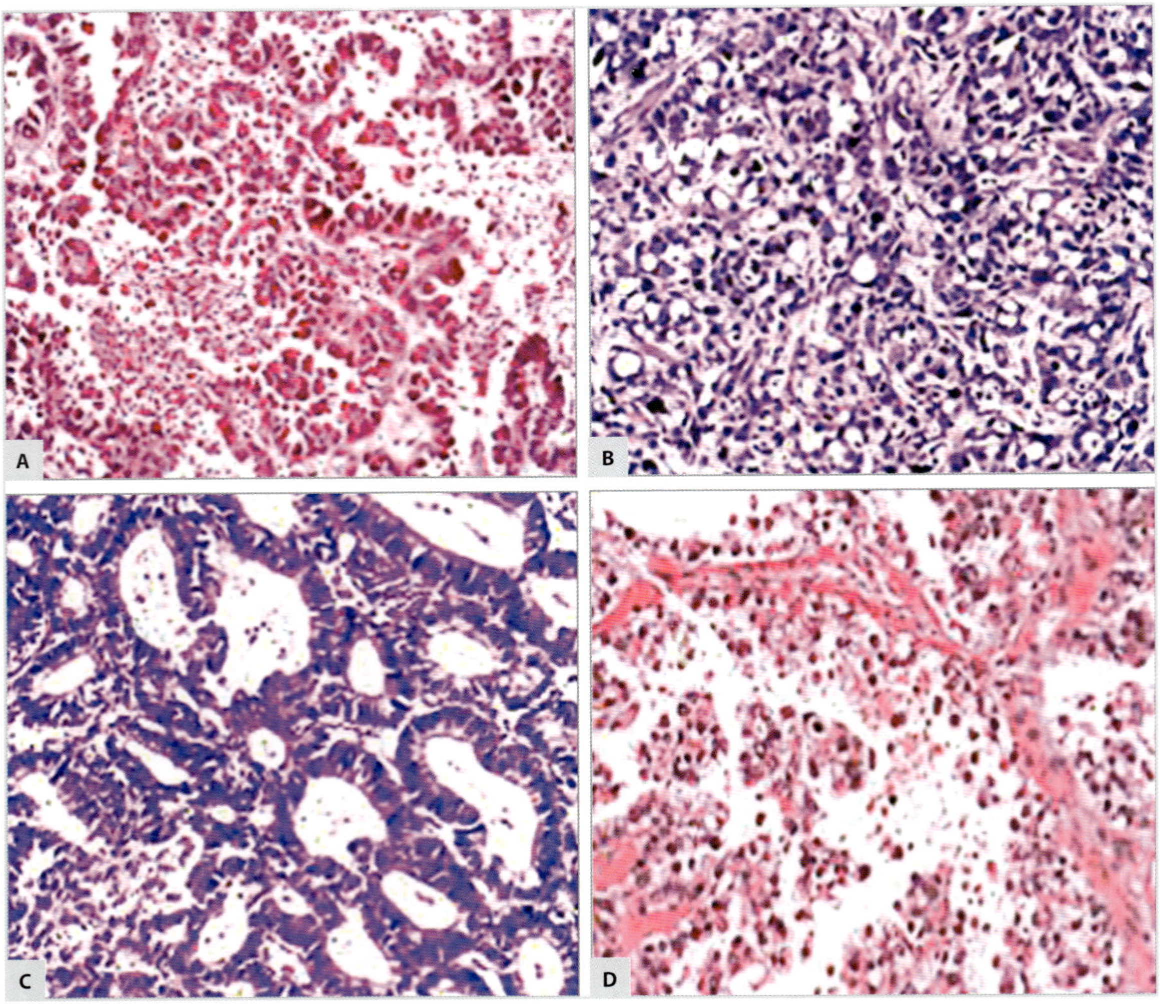

Figs 1A to D: (A) Serous carcinoma, papillary pattern with cellular tufting and marked nuclear atypia; (B) Mucinous carcinoma with destructive stromal invasion. Intraepithelial mucin vacuoles are evident; (C) Endometrioid carcinoma; (D) Clear cell carcinoma, tubulopapillary pattern. Cells have enlarged nuclei, cytoplasm is abundant, nuclear hobnailing is seen with CK7 but may also express, focally or diffusely, enteric markers such as CK20 and caudal type homeobox (CDX) 2. This is helpful in differentiating metastatic mucinous carcinoma from large bowel cancers which are usually negative for CK7 and positive for CK20. The tumors are negative for estrogen receptor (ER), progesterone receptor (PR) and WT1.

Endometrioid: Benign, borderline and malignant types of endometrioid ovarian tumors exist. The benign variants are included with the cystadenofibromas. In the atypical category, the epithelial changes are equivalent to those of atypical endometrial hyperplasia without stromal invasion. Endometrioid carcinoma may present as a cystic or solid mass. The contents of tumor when cystic are more often hemorrhagic, than serous or mucinous. Microscopically, the tumors resemble endometrial adenocarcinoma (Fig. 1C) of uterine origin.[31]

Clear cell: This is a distinctive type of ovarian tumor with a grossly spongy to cystic appearance. Microscopically, it can grow in tubulocystic, papillary, and solid-sheet pattern (Fig. 1D).[32] Microscopically, tumor cells are large with clear cytoplasm, the nuclei often protrude into the lumina, resulting in a "hobnail" configuration.

Transitional cell (Brenner): Microscopically, the benign tumors consist of solid and cystic nests of epithelial cells resembling transitional epithelium surrounded by abundant dense fibroblastic stroma. When this pattern is associated with a greater degree of atypia, equivalent to high-grade transitional cell carcinoma, but stromal invasion is not seen, the term borderline or low malignant potential is proposed.[33]

Malignant mixed Müllerian tumor (MMMT): These tumors resembles its more common uterine counterpart. A homologous variety, with nonspecific malignant stroma and a heterologous variety, with malignant heterologous stromal elements are known.[34] The latter may have the morphologic appearance of a known sarcoma, i.e. chondrosarcoma, osteosarcoma, rhabdomyosarcoma or angiosarcoma. The carcinomatous component may be of serous, endometrioid or clear cell type.

Germ Cell Tumors

They are believed to be derived from germ cells of the gonad and constitute the second largest group of ovarian tumors. They may occur in women at any age, but peak incidence is in the early 20s.

Classification of germ cell neoplasms:

- Mature cystic teratoma (dermoid cyst)
- Immature teratoma
- Monodermal teratoma (e.g. struma ovarii)
- Dysgerminoma
- Yolk sac tumor
- Embryonal carcinoma
- Choriocarcinoma.

The vast majority of benign germ cell tumors are constituted by mature cystic teratomas (dermoid cyst). Dysgerminoma is the most common malignant germ cell tumor, accounting for 50% of all germ cell tumor cases. Yolk sac tumors, also known as endodermal sinus tumors, are the second most common and account for 20% of all cases. Less common germ cell tumors are embryonal carcinoma, immature teratoma, choriocarcinoma, polyembryomas, and mixed germ cell tumors.

Sex Cord—Stromal Tumors

They account for approximately 10% of all ovarian tumors. They are composed of different cell types derived from gonadal stroma and sex cords. They account for most of the hormonally active ovarian tumors.

Sex cord-stromal tumors could be classified as:

- Fibroma
- Thecoma
- Granulosa cell tumor
- Sertoli cell tumor
- Leydig cell tumor
- Sertoli-Leydig cell tumor
- Sclerosing stromal tumor.

Granulosa cell tumors preponderantly occur in postmenopausal women. Microscopically, they display a variety of patterns, microfollicular, macrofollicular, insular, trabecular and diffuse. Characteristic features include Call-Exner bodies and nuclei with "coffee bean" (longitudinal grooves) appearance. Sertoli-Leydig cell tumors are relatively rare, the average age of patients diagnosed with these tumors is 25, and only 10% of patients are over 50. Approximately, one-third of these tumors produce signs of virilism, hoarse voice, appearance of facial hair, infrequent menstrual periods or cessation of menstrual periods before menopause. Microscopically, they can range from well-differentiated to poorly differentiated. Well-differentiated forms are constituted by tubular structures resembling seminiferous tubules lined by Sertoli cells. The behavior of tumor correlates with degree of differentiation.

CLINICAL FEATURES

Diverse ovarian tumors clinically manifest in a like manner. Diagnosis of early ovarian cancer is difficult and often incidental. Majority present in an advanced stage. Symptoms like vague abdominal discomfort, dyspepsia and flatulence should not be ignored, and especially in women above 40 years, it should raise an index of suspicion. Very occasionally pain, torsion (due to large size), rupture or infection may be the presenting symptom. Diagnosis is generally delayed in 65% of patients when dissemination has occurred. A moderate to severe ascites, urinary or bowel complaints, pleural effusion with cough or dyspnea are often initial symptoms. Per vaginal/per rectal examination may reveal a mass in the pelvis. Rectal infiltration is rare but known and more often there is evidence of external pressure with a normal rectal mucosa (Figs 2A and B).

INVESTIGATIONS

Routine blood chemistry, liver and renal profile, marker studies with CA-125 and CEA may be significantly elevated, α-fetoproteins, beta-human chorionic gonadotropin (β-hCG) and lactate dehydrogenase (LDH) can effectively screen women for ovarian germ cell tumors (Figs 3A and B). Pap smear may be obtained as a routine. Imaging with computed tomography (CT)/magnetic resonance imaging (MRI)/positron emission tomography (PET) scan as needed to delineate the extent of the disease and to help

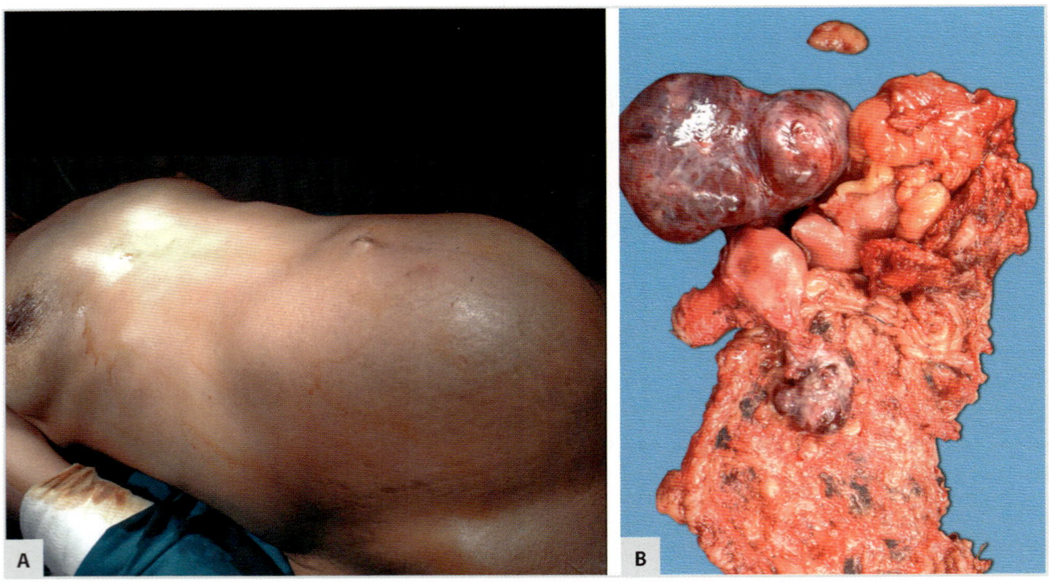

Figs 2A and B: (A) A middle-aged lady with a large ovarian mass; (B) Resected specimen ovarian carcinoma with omentectomy

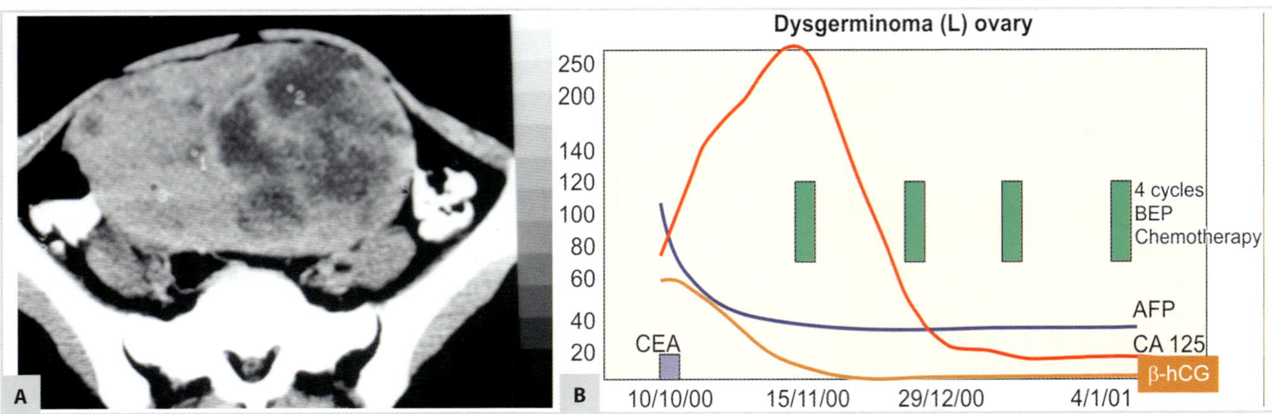

Figs 3A and B: (A) Computed tomography (CT) scan of a 19-year-old young female showing a large ovarian mass for which a left oophorectomy and omentectomy was performed. The final histopathology was a dysgerminoma; (B) Rising tumor markers in the same patient despite being asymptomatic. Appropriate chemotherapy resulted in markers reaching normal values. Survival free of disease 13 years

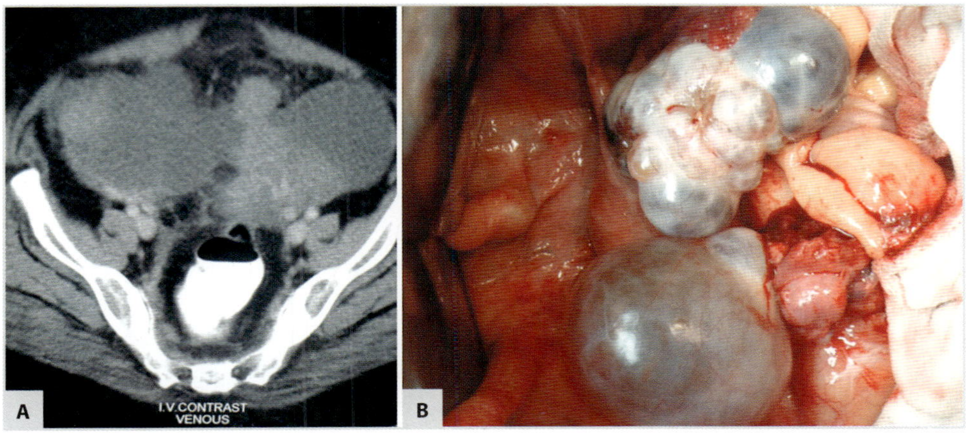

Figs 4A and B: (A) Bilateral ovarian tumors: computed tomography (CT) scan; (B) Same patient surgical exposure

plan therapy (Figs 4A and B). Ascitic fluid cytology and a fine needle aspiration cytology (FNAC) from the omental mass will clinch cytologic or histologic diagnosis before neoadjuvant chemotherapy (NACT) can be initiated in most patients.

In a very few cases, laparoscopy may be needed to confirm the diagnosis. Most patients with stage III-IV will clinically present with moderate or massive ascites and/or pleural effusion. Imaging may demonstrate the extent of celomic involvement from the pelvis to diaphragmatic surfaces. Miliary carcinomatosis may not be detected on imaging but ascites generally conveys peritoneal surface involvement.

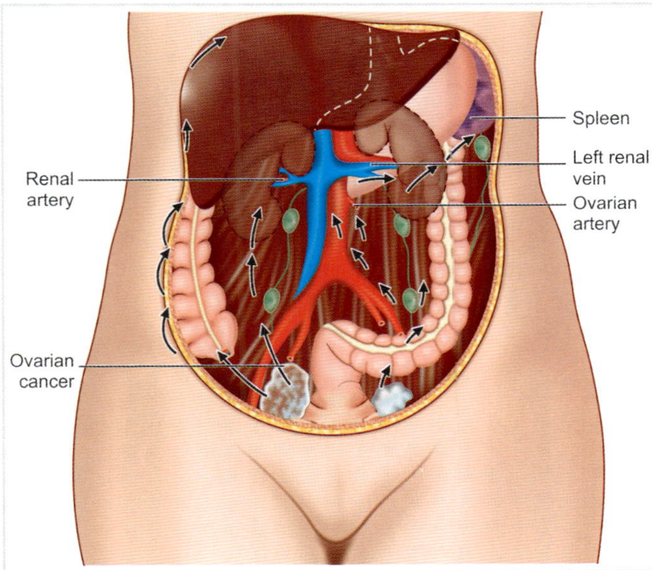

Fig. 5: Spread of ovarian cancer. As the primary tumor develops, cells shed from the tumor, circulate within the peritoneal cavity and implant on peritoneal surfaces within the abdomen and/or pelvis. This can happen even when the primary tumor is small in volume

Carcinoma Antigen 125 (CA 125)

This is an antigen produced by serous carcinoma of the ovary (which forms 40% of ovarian cancers). Its normal range is less than 35 IU/mL. CA-125 is an important tumor marker which can be elevated even in other non-malignant gynecologic conditions, such as uterine fibroids and endometriosis.[35] CA-125 values begin to rise months before cancer is found clinically. It is an important marker to assess the response to treatment or a recurrence of the disease. Values are often higher in tubercular and inflammatory lesions.

MODE OF SPREAD

Ovarian cancer spreads either by direct extension, peritoneal dissemination, retroperitoneal lymphatics and hematogenous dissemination. The right paracolic gutter is the most frequent site of peritoneal deposits and tumor nodules, as malignant cells in the ascitic fluid get deposited along the path of its circulation (Fig. 5). Two main lymphatic routes drain the ovaries, those in the broad ligament which go to the pelvic nodes and the other through the infundibulopelvic ligaments to the aortocaval area (Fig. 6).[36] Lymph node metastases can obstruct lymph flow and can lead to retrograde metastases which appear to skip regional chains. Thus, some patients with ovarian cancer can have an isolated para-aortic lymph node

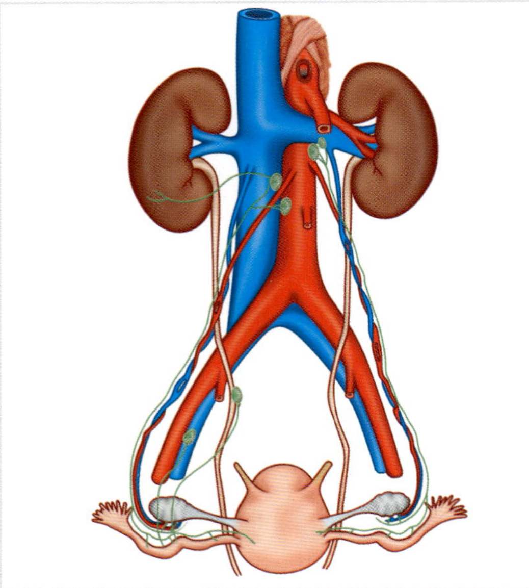

Fig. 6: Lymphatic drainage in ovarian cancer

spread through the lymph vessels of the infundibulopelvic ligament and show a retrograde lymphatic spread. Burghardt and colleagues[37] reported a 25–30% risk of nodal metastases even in early ovarian cancer which is on the higher side, though in retrospective series, the rates of lymph nodes vary between 11% and 20%.[38-42]

Staging (Table 2)

Ten percent of patients with ovarian carcinoma extend beyond the pelvis with exclusive retroperitoneal lymph node involvement and have a better prognosis than tumors with peritoneal involvement. Overall survival (OS) of patients with stage IIIC (retroperitoneal lymph node metastases without peritoneal carcinomatosis) is 58–84% compared with 18–36% for those with macroscopic peritoneal carcinomatosis.[43]

Onda et al.[44] showed that patients upstaged from stage I/II to stage IIIC based on lymph node metastases had survival of 84% at 5 years, compared to women diagnosed as stage IIIC due to presence of peritoneal carcinomatosis (26%). Women with stage I/II who were upstaged due to positive lymph nodes had a similar survival to those with stage I/II with negative nodes.

SURGERY

Panhysterectomy with omentectomy is the standard therapeutic procedure of choice. Peritoneal washings and/or ascitic fluid is sent for cytology. In patients with mucinous neoplasm an appendicectomy is worthwhile. Decision about nodal dissections should be individualized. Careful palpation of the pelvis, the lower reaches of the aortocaval and paracaval region will indicate the need for biopsy or dissection. Suspect nodes are generally firm to feel; softish and oblong nodes are usually normal; however, they can rarely harbor microscopic metastasis. Any suspect node should have a frozen section and if positive a nodal dissection should be proceeded with. The dissection should extend up to the renal vein on the left side and the site of drainage of the ovarian vein in the vena cava

TABLE 2: Stages of ovarian carcinoma

Stage	*Extent of disease*
I	Tumors limited to the ovaries (one or both)
IA	Tumor limited to one ovary
IB	Tumor limited to both ovaries
IC	Surface seedling and malignant cells in abdominal fluid or peritoneal washings
II	Involves one or both ovaries with pelvic extension
IIA	Implants on uterus and/or adnexa
IIB	Tumors extends to other pelvic tissues
IIC	Stage IIA and/or IIB with malignant cells in the abdominal fluid or peritoneal washing
III	Growth involving one or both ovaries, with peritoneal implants outside the pelvis and/or positive retroperitoneal or inguinal lymph nodes
IIIA	Evidence of microscopic peritoneal metastases beyond the pelvis
IIIB	Evidence of macroscopic peritoneal metastases beyond the pelvis
IIIC	Peritoneal metastases beyond the pelvis greater than 2 cm and/or lymph node metastases
IV	Distant metastases, positive cytology from pleural effusion or liver metastases

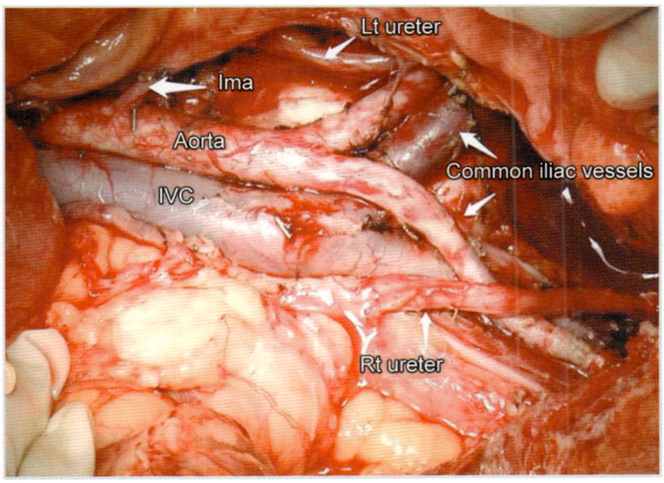

Fig. 7: Retroperitoneal lymph node dissection

Source: Dr Sanket Mehta

on the right side, particularly if lower nodes are suspect. The femoral ring constitutes the caudal limit of pelvic node dissection. Removal of negative normal nodes is a disservice to patients and is compatible with complications and morbidities like edema of the extremities or recurrent thrombophlebitis, repeated seromas and infection. In stage III and IV disease, nodal dissections are mandatory as the nodal involvement is high (Fig. 7).

Young and nulliparous women with a stage IA may undergo a unilateral salpingo-oophorectomy if the opposite ovary is normal. Even in patients with a tumor of low malignant potential a conservative therapy is usually possible. Data show improved survivals after complete resections.[45,46] A close follow-up is advisable and excision of the second ovary can be considered after completion of the family.

Cytoreductive Surgery (CRS)

This is an important component in the surgical treatment of epithelial, advanced or recurrent ovarian cancers. Patients with metastatic disease hardly ever achieve a cure; however, current therapies (chemotherapy + cytoreductive surgery) can significantly help in palliation and extended remissions which can convert advanced "solid" cancers into a chronic condition. The indication for aggressive surgery should be individualized. In an advanced ovarian cancer, neoadjuvant chemotherapy (NACT) with subsequent CRS is recommended. Only 20% of women exhibit localized disease in the pelvis at the time of diagnosis. CRS ($\leq$ 1 cm residual disease) is a difficult and prolonged procedure, if it becomes necessary. Griffith's study[47] showed that there was an inverse correlation between patient outcome and left over residual tumor diameter. Chi et al.[48] reviewed 282 patients with advanced stage ovarian cancer at Memorial Sloan-Kettering Cancer Center (MSKCC) in a retrospective analysis. The prognostic factors for survival were age, ascites and residual disease less than or equal to 1 cm. Survival results were 55 months versus 28 months for residual disease less than 1 cm or more than 1 cm, respectively.

In advanced ovarian cancers, the most significant factors affecting long-term survival are high volume surgeons and high volume hospitals, where data shows better outcomes. There is definitely a high negative correlation of survival with high volume of residual disease.[49] There are arguments against CRS as the morbidity is high, and the quality of life is worse after such radical surgery. Initiation of chemotherapy is delayed, increased blood loss and longer hospitalization occur. Complications like bowel obstruction, ileus, infections and thromboembolism are not infrequent. Moderate increase in disease free survival and overall survival (OS) are reported proportional to the extent of debulking. In the presence of miliary mesentric and bowel implants, the wisdom of extensive debulking procedures is debatable and can be questioned as it may not substantially add to survival benefit. Involved and obstructive bowel lesions have to be resected.

SYSTEMIC THERAPY OF EPITHELIAL OVARIAN CANCER

Neoadjuvant Chemotherapy

Most patients presenting with an advanced ovarian cancer are candidates for NACT as effective debulking primarily is ineffective and difficult because of large disease volume. Reduction of tumor volume facilitates proper excision of the residual tumor mass and CRS at the same time. Effective tumor burden reduction occurs in nearly 80% of patients after NACT. Surgery after NACT is usually carried out 3–4 weeks after 3 or 4 cycles after assessing all the blood and other preoperative parameters. Surgery after NACT is more effective, complete and cleaner.[50-52] The tissue removed show severe necrosis (chemotherapy induced) and little mitotic activity. CA-125 is an excellent marker of the effects of chemotherapy.

The drug of choice will be a combination of paclitaxel and carboplatin. The patients are usually advised about three cycle's paclitaxel and carboplatin followed by CRS. Adjunctive three cycles of chemotherapy are given postoperatively.

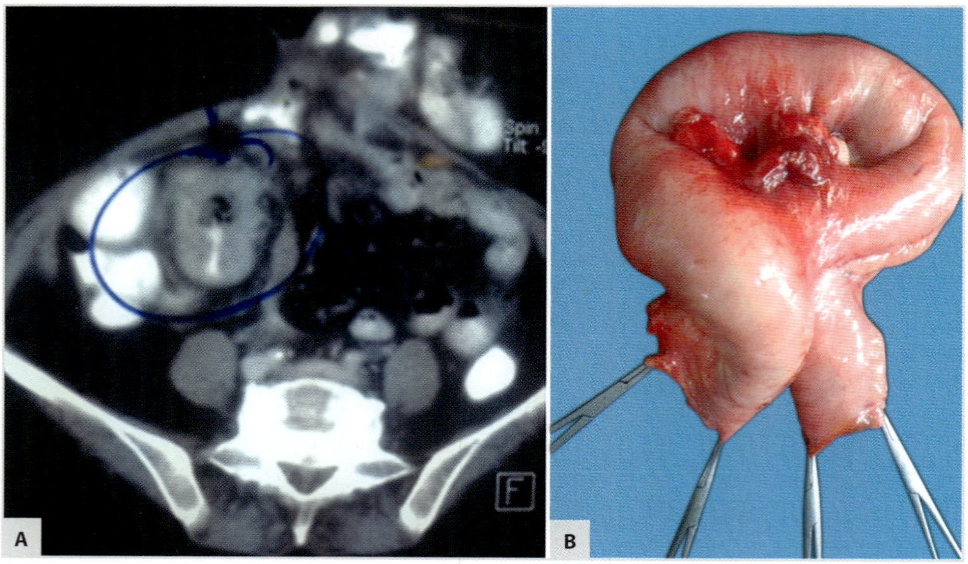

Figs 8A and B: (A) Recurrent carcinoma of the ovary with metastasis in the mid-ileum; (B) Resected specimen

Adjuvant Chemotherapy

Primary CRS is preferred as far as possible. Postoperatively patients with stage I grade III, stage IC or stage II disease (or higher stage) are advised adjuvant chemotherapy. The results of two randomized trials published in 2003 confirmed the benefit of adjuvant treatment. These trials involved 925 patients.[53] The data confirmed superior OS in patients who received platinum-based chemotherapy. The combination of injection paclitaxel + injection carboplatin is the Standard of Care for adjuvant treatment. Gynecologic Oncologic Group (GOG) performed a study to compare three cycles versus six cycles of chemotherapy.[54] There was a 35% reduction in the risk of recurrence in the group of patients who received six cycles of chemotherapy. Hence, six cycles of adjuvant chemotherapy is the Standard of care for Ovarian Cancer.

Advanced Ovarian Cancer

Surgical intervention and systemic therapy are both important in advanced stages of disease. Primary CRS or interval CRS can be planned depending on condition of the patient, comorbid conditions, extent of involvement of vital organs (lung, liver). Ovarian cancer is a chemosensitive disease and responds well to treatment even in an advanced stage of disease. It offers reasonably good prolongation of survival, improved quality of life and relief of symptoms (e.g. malignant ascites).

Among all the chemotherapy drugs, platinum group of drugs are the most effective. Injection cisplatin was the standard of care since 1970s. Injection carboplatin was equally efficacious with less toxicities especially neuropathy, nephropathy and emesis. A combination of injection paclitaxel and injection carboplatin is the standard of care. In 1996, McGuire WP et al. published a trial comparing injection cyclophosphamide + injection cisplatin versus injection paclitaxel + injection cisplatin in patients with advanced ovarian cancer.[55] Taxane based arm produced complete clinical response (CCR) to the tune of 51% versus 31% in the comparative arm. The median OS was 38 months versus 24 months.

Ozols RF et al.[56] conducted a phase III trial involving about 792 patients comparing paclitaxel and carboplatin versus paclitaxel and cisplatin. The median progression-free survival (PFS) was 20.7 months versus 19.4 months. Median OS was 57.4 months versus 48.7 months, respectively. Paclitaxel + carboplatin are currently established as a Standard of Care for ovarian cancer.

MANAGEMENT OF RECURRENT DISEASE

The concept of second look surgery which was prevalent in the 70s and 80s receded into background because of more efficient chemotherapy generally used for recurrent disease. Despite this, localized or organal local recurrence after a reasonably long latent period of disease free period can be considered for a surgical excision if feasible. Classic examples may be localized involvement of rectum, colon or the small bowel due to obstructive pathology or hemorrhage (Figs 8A and B). It will result in effective palliation and a good quality of life with improvement in disease free survival.

Advanced stage ovarian cancer has a significant risk of recurrence in spite of an initial good response to chemotherapy. The disease can have "Biochemical recurrence" or "Clinical recurrence". Some of the patients may present with isolated CA-125 elevations. These patients are asymptomatic, healthy and show no evidence of disease recurrence clinically or by imaging. This is described a "Biochemical recurrence". It has been shown in various clinical studies that early treatment of biochemical recurrence does not prolong survival hence no treatment is offered to these patients; however, close follow-up and regular monitoring is necessary as these patients would eventually develop obvious recurrence. These patients can benefit from hormonal therapy with tamoxifen or aromatase inhibitor for a short period of time[57] or megace 160 mg/day in a slowly escalating dose.

Patients with clinical recurrence are defined as patients with symptoms, objective evidence on CT scan or failure of hormonal therapy. Platinum-free interval (PFI) is the most important factor in deciding treatment. Patients with PFI less than 6 months are "Platinum-Refractory" patients. They show poor response to second line drugs with platinum-based chemotherapy. Treatment with non-platinum compounds like liposomal doxorubicin, paclitaxel, docetaxel, topotecan, gemcitabine, oral etoposide, and nanoparticle albumin based paclitaxel (nab-paclitaxel: abraxane) and trabectidine. Liposomal doxorubicin is given in the dose of 40 mg/m^2 every 4 weeks. The toxicity profile includes palmer-planar erythrodysesthesia (Hand-foot syndrome) and mucositis which may require dose reduction.

Topotecan can lead to myelosuppression, fatigue, nausea and vomiting. The advantage of topotecan is that it is available both in intravenous (IV) preparation and oral form. The bioavailability of both the forms is equivalent. IV preparation is better tolerated in a weekly schedule.[58] It has been observed that the response rates to any of these agents is not more that 20% and median PFS is in the range of 4–6 months.

Patients with PFI more than 6 months are considered as platinum sensitive patients. For patients with PFI between 6 months to 24 months, the response rates are about 30% while patients with PFI more than 24 months, have response rates of 60–70%. These platinum sensitive patients are either treated with a single platinum compound or a combination with paclitaxel or gemcitabine or liposomal doxorubicin.

International Collaborative Ovarian Neoplasm (ICON) 4 clinical trial[59] compared platinum sensitive patients either receiving paclitaxel with platinum or only platinum agent. There was a statistically significant difference in OS at 2 years favoring the combination arm. This study has been criticized as significant percentage of patients on single agent arm never received paclitaxel. Another trial by German group[60] randomized patients with platinum sensitive relapse into two arms, one offering gemcitabine + carboplatin versus one offering only carboplatin. This study demonstrated improved PFS in combination arm but there was no change in OS. The decision to use combination chemotherapy will depend on patient's age, general condition, extent of disease, kinetics of relapse and patient preference. Single agent therapy can be used for elderly asymptomatic patients and those with small volume disease. Single agent liposomal doxorubicin is also a good option for these patients.

COMMON PROTOCOLS

- Standard of care
  - Injection paclitaxel 175 mg/m^2
  - Injection carboplatin AUC 6 or injection cisplatin 75 mg/m^2 q3w for 6 cycles
- For recurrent disease
  - Injection liposomal doxorubicin 40 mg/m^2 every 4 weeks
  - Injection gemcitabine 1–1.2 g/m^2 per week* 2/3 weeks depending on protocol
  - Oral topotecal 2.3 mg/m^2 per day D1 to D5 every 21 days
  - Injection nab-paclitaxel 100–130 mg/m^2/week (depending on tolerability)

Intraperitoneal Chemotherapy

A combination of CRS and chemotherapy [intravenous (IV) and intraperitoneal (IP)] is the treatment of choice for stage III ovarian cancer. The advantage of IP chemotherapy; however, is that a more concentrated dose of chemotherapy is delivered to the peritoneum thus ensuring better tissue penetration and limited systemic toxicity. IP ports are preferred over percutaneous catheters, as it decreases the risk of colonization and infection. Three large, randomized multicenter trials comparing cisplatin-combination IP chemotherapy to standard IV therapy for patients who underwent optimal cytoreduction. The study revealed an 8–16 months survival benefit in the group with IP and IV chemotherapy. There was a 21% reduction in mortality.[61-63]

Due to the natural history of the disease, recurrence is generally confined to peritoneal cavity. IP chemotherapy has been studied after optimal cytoreduction of residual

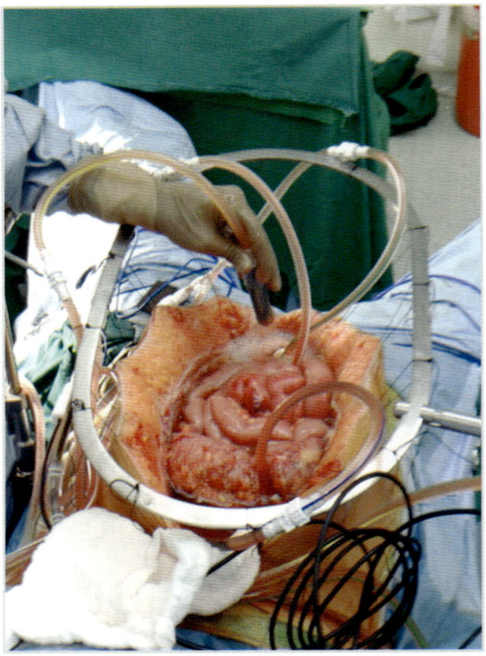

Fig. 9: Hyperthermic intraperitoneal chemotherapy (HIPEC)
Source: Dr Sanket Mehta

disease (< 1 cm). Most trials combine IP cisplatin and IP/IV paclitaxel. Results have been contradictory. A meta-analysis showed that IP chemotherapy was associated with a 21.6% reduction in risk of death with a significant morbidity.[64] It is possible that using better tolerated protocols, IP chemotherapy can be used safely.

Hyperthermic Intraperitoneal Chemotherapy (HIPEC)

Despite the high chemosensitivity of ovarian cancers, with often a near complete response of 80%, majority of patients will develop recurrence and long term survivals are poor. Microscopic tumor always remains and recurs on the peritoneal surface, even after complete cytoreduction. IP chemotherapy is effective in eradicating cancer emboli with a maximal diameter less than 2–3 mm. Hyperthermic intraperitoneal chemotherapy (HIPEC) has been used intraoperatively in advanced epithelial ovarian cancers after CRS with promising results.[65-67] HIPEC can be performed using the Coliseum technique (open abdomen technique)[68,69] for 90 minutes, when cisplatin (50 mg/m^2) and doxorubicin (15 mg/m^2) were instilled; for 60 minutes for gemcitabine (1,000 mg/m^2) and 30 minutes for oxaliplatin (460 mg/m^2) at 42–43°C. The Coliseum technique (Fig. 9) ensures uniform distribution of heat and cytostatic drugs in the abdominal cavity. It appears to improve long-term survival in patients with advanced ovarian cancer. HIPEC is associated with a high rate of complications and therefore should be offered in the ambit of clinical research trials. CRS with HIPEC demonstrates significant survival benefit, 60% at 2 years and 40% at 5 years.[70] These figures are not reproducible at all centers.

Gonzales Bayon L et al.[71] conducted a prospective study involving 42 patients. Fifteen patients were treated upfront, 19 at first recurrence and second or subsequent recurrence. After a median follow-up of 24 months, median OS was 77.8 months for patients treated upfront, 62.8 months for those treated at the first recurrence and 35.7 months for patients treated at second or subsequent recurrence. Disease free survival was 21.1 months, 18 months, 5.7 months, respectively. OS was statistically lower for the third group. The authors concluded that the therapy should be considered upfront and at first recurrence. The percentage of mortality and morbidity was 26% and 7%, respectively. These results warrant further randomized trials. There are many other ongoing studies. It seems that patient selection and cytoreductive score are the two most important factors deciding the outcome after HIPEC.

Role of Antiangiogenic Agents

Bevacizumab is a humanized antibody to vascular endothelial growth factor (VEGF), secreted by ovarian cancer cells. As a single agent, it has shown to produce recurrence rate of 18% with PFS of 39% at 6 months.[72] It may be used even in platinum refractory patients but the risk of bowel perforation is high. Heavily pretreated patients and those with bowel involvement or obstruction have greater chances of bowel perforation with bevacizumab. It can be used in combination with other drugs.

Radiotherapy

Role of radiotherapy is limited in ovarian cancers. Localized residual mass or distant (skeletal, chest, brain) metastasis nonresponsive to chemotherapy should be considered for radiotherapy. Dysgerminoma is a highly radiosensitive and often radiocurable tumor (response to chemotherapy is equally satisfactory).

Recommended Follow-up

Initially patients are followed up every 3–4 months for the first 2 years, then every 6 months for the next 3 years, then annually after 5 years. Monitoring should be with marker studies of CA-125, α-fetoproteins, β-hCG and LDH in case with high initial levels (pretherapy). Ultrasound of abdomen/pelvis is usually recommended and if needed a CT scan with/without PET scan should be advised in appropriate cases (Table 3).

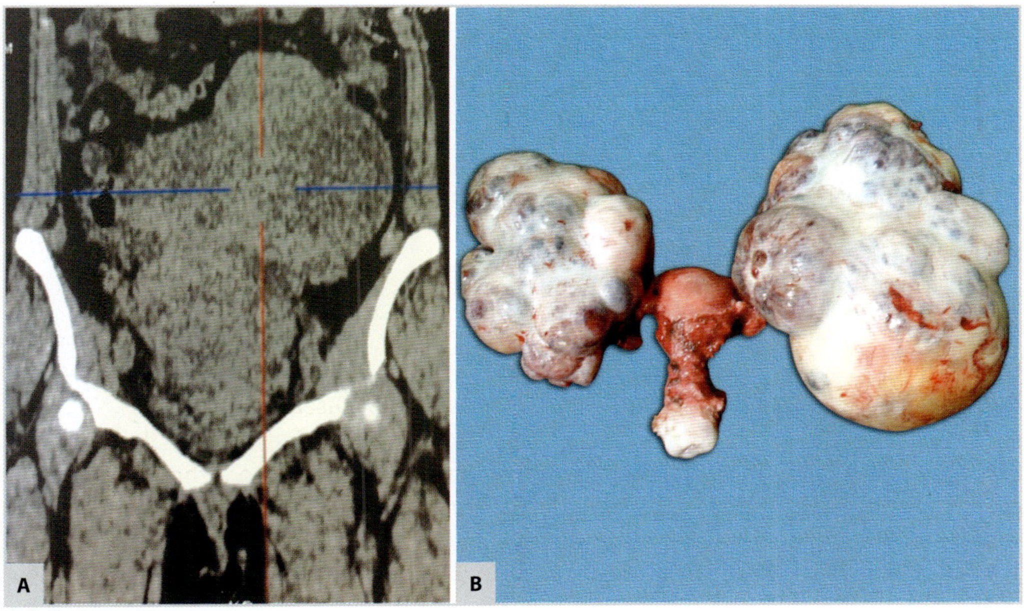

Figs 10A and B: (A) Magnetic resonance imaging (MRI) of a 40 years female showing bilateral ovarian tumors; (B) Surgical specimen of the same patient showing bilateral ovarian tumors. Final histopathology was metastatic neuroendocrine tumor of the ovary. Lung was the primary site of disease

TABLE 3: International Federation of Gynecology and Obstetrics (FIGO) staging system for epithelial ovarian cancer

Stage	*Five years survival*
Stage I	50–90%
Stage II	20–80%
Stage III	20–58%
Stage IV	6–14%

Source: Adapted from NCCN Clinical Practice Guidelines – Coukos G, Rubin SG – Early Ovarian Cancer[73,74]

Krukenberg's Tumor

The classically used term Krukenberg tumor is used to designate a bilateral metastatic ovarian tumor. This is a rare clinical entity and accounts for 1–2% of ovarian cancers (Figs 10A and B).[75] Metastases to the ovaries commonly occur from stomach, breast, colon, rectum, small bowel, gallbladder, pancreas, biliary tract and the appendix.[76] The spread usually occurs by duct seedling or via the lymphatics. The tumor is grossly characterized by solid multinodular enlargement of the ovaries. Microscopically, it is seen as diffuse infiltration by signet ring cells containing intracytoplasmic mucins, in a dense stromal proliferation. Immunohistochemistry helps in diagnosing Krukenberg's tumor from a primary ovarian neoplasm. If the primary cancer is controlled it is worthwhile doing a panhysterectomy, followed by chemotherapy.

Borderline Ovarian Tumors

Borderline ovarian tumors (BOT) comprise 15–20% of all epithelial ovarian malignancies.[77,78] These form a separate entity within the epithelial ovarian tumors (BOT) first described by Taylor in 1929 as a separate group. They form a heterogenous group of noninvasive tumors of uncertain malignant potential, have a characteristic histology and are usually seen in the younger age group around 40 years. They usually represent borderline tumors, tumors of low malignant potential and atypical proliferative tumor.[79] They can be histologically distinguished from ovarian carcinomas by the absence of stromal invasion. In spite of that cells can be shed into the peritoneal cavity and can eventually form serosal implants in advanced cancer. Ten to fifteen percent may develop aggressive and invasive carcinoma. They have the potential to spread beyond the ovary and have the ability to recur as carcinoma, with a poor prognosis.[80]

Women usually have nonspecific gastrointestinal complaints, pelvic pain or a mass in the abdomen. Borderline tumors are difficult to diagnose preoperatively using imaging methods. Conservative treatment can be planned, in view of the younger age and desire for childbearing. Borderline tumors which spread to lymph nodes or are invasive require chemotherapy; evidence is insufficient to determine exactly which therapy is indicated for BOT. Platinum based agents are used but with varying results. BOT with noninvasive implants do not require any further therapy and should be observed.

REFERENCES

1. DiSaia PJ, Creasman WT (Eds). Advanced epithelial ovarian cancers. Clinical Gynecologic Oncology, 3rd edition. p. 325.
2. Feig BW, Ching D. The MD Anderson surgical oncology handbook. Gynecologic Cancers, 5th edition. Philadelphia, PA: Lippincott-Williams and Wilkins; 2002. p. 636.
3. Ferlay J, Shin HR, Bray F, et al. GLOBOCAN 2008 v2.0, Cancer Incidence and Mortality Worldwide: IARC Cancer Base No. 10. Lyon, France: International Agency for Research on Cancer; 2010.
4. NCRP. Two-year Report of the Population Based Cancer Registries-2006-2008. National Cancer Registry Program, Indian Council of Medical Research, Bangalore, India. 2009.
5. Olsen CM, Nagle CM, Whiteman DC, et al. Ovarian Cancer Association Consortium. Obesity and risk of ovarian cancer subtypes: evidence from the Ovarian Cancer Association Consortium. Endocr Relat Cancer. 2013;20(2):251-62.
6. Modugno F, Ness RB, Allen GO, et al. Oral contraceptive use, reproductive history, and risk of epithelial ovarian cancer in women with and without endometriosis. Am J Obstet Gynecol. 2004;191(3):733-40.
7. Rutter JL, Wacholder S, Chetrit A, et al. Gynecologic surgeries and risk of ovarian cancer in carriers and non-carriers of the BRCA1 and BRCA2 ashkenazi founder mutations: an Israeli population-based case-control study. J Natl Cancer Inst. 2003;95(14):1072-8.
8. Ness RB, Cramer DW, Goodman MT, et al. Infertility, fertility drugs, and ovarian cancer: a pooled analysis of case-control studies. Am J Epidemiol. 2002;155(3):217-24.
9. Kurta ML, Moysich KB, Weissfeld JL, et al. Use of fertility drugs and risk of ovarian cancer: results from a US-based case-control study. Cancer Epidemiol Biomarkers Prev. 2012;21(8):1282-92.
10. Jensen A, Sharif H, v K, et al. Use of fertility drugs and risk of ovarian cancer: Danish population based cohort study. BMJ. 2009;338:249.
11. Simpkins F, Garcia-Soto A, Slingerland J. New insights on the role of hormonal therapy in ovarian cancer. Steroids. 2013;78(6): 530-7.
12. Srivastava A, McKinnon W, Wood ME. Risk of breast and ovarian cancer in women with strong family histories. Oncology. 2001;15(7):889-902.
13. King MC, Marks JH, Mandell JB, et al. Breast and ovarian cancer risks due to inherited mutations in BRCA1 and BRCA2. Science. 2003;302(5645):643-6.
14. Chen S, Iversen ES, Friebel T, et al. Characterization of BRCA1 and BRCA2 mutations in a large United States sample. J Clin Oncol. 2006;24(6):863-71.
15. Kazerouni N, Greene MH, Lacey JV, et al. Family history of breast cancer as a risk factor for ovarian cancer in a prospective study. Cancer. 2006;107(5):1075-83.
16. Muscat JE, Huncharek MS. Perineal talc use and ovarian cancer: a critical review. Eur J Cancer Prev. 2008;17(2):139-46.
17. Huncharek M, Kupelnick B. Dietary fat intake and risk of epithelial ovarian cancer: a meta-analysis of 6,689 subjects from 8 observational studies. Nutr Cancer. 2001;40(2):87-91.
18. Pan SY, Ugnat AM, Mao Y. A case-control study of diet and the risk of ovarian cancer. Cancer Epidemiol Biomarkers Prev. 2004;13(9):1521-7.
19. Ammundsen HB, Faber MT, Jensen A, et al. Use of analgesic drugs and risk of ovarian cancer: results from a Danish case-control study. Acta Obstet Gynecol Scand. 2012;91(9):1094-102.
20. Cramer DW, Harlow BL, Titus-Ernstoff L, et al. Over-the-counter analgesics and risk of ovarian cancer. Lancet. 1998;351(9096): 104-7.
21. Tworoger SS, Gertig DM, Gates MA, et al. Caffeine, alcohol, smoking, and the risk of incident epithelial ovarian cancer. Cancer. 2008;112(5):1169-77.
22. Kelemen LE, Bandera EV, Terry KL, et al. Recent alcohol consumption and risk of incident ovarian carcinoma: a pooled analysis of 5,342 cases and 10,358 controls from the Ovarian Cancer Association Consortium. BMC Cancer. 2013;13:28.
23. De Palo G, Mariani L, Camerini T, et al. Effect of fenretinide on ovarian carcinoma occurrence. Gynecol Oncol. 2002;86(1):24-7.
24. Rebbeck TR, Lynch HT, Neuhausen SL, et al. Prophylactic oophorectomy in carriers of BRCA 1 or BRCA 2 mutations. N Eng J Med. 2002;346(21):1616-22.
25. Leeper K, Garcia R, Swisher E, et al. Pathologic findings in prophylactic oophorectomy specimens in high risk women. Gynecol Oncol. 2002;87(1):52-6.
26. Godwin AK, Testa JR, Hamilton TC. The biology of ovarian cancer development. Cancer. 1993;71(Suppl 2):530-6.
27. Colgan TJ, Norris HJ. Ovarian epithelial tumors of low malignant potential: a review. Int J Gynecol Pathol. 1983;1:367-82.
28. Silva EG, Kurman RJ, Russell P, et al. Symposium: ovarian tumors of borderline malignancy. Int J Gynecol Pathol. 1996;15:281-307.
29. Hoerl HD, Hart WR. Primary ovarian mucinous cystadenocarcinomas: a clinicopathologic study of 49 cases with long-term follow-up. Am J Surg Pathol. 1998;22:1449-62.
30. Ronnett BM, Kajdacsy-Balla A, Gilks CB, et al. Mucinous borderline ovarian tumors: points of general agreement and persistent controversies regarding nomenclature, diagnostic criteria, and behavior. Hum Pathol. 2004;35:959-60.
31. Czernobilsky B, Silverman BB, Mikuta JJ. Endometrioid carcinoma of the ovary: a clinicopathologic study of 75 cases. Cancer. 1970;26:1141-52.
32. Matias-Guiu X, Lerma E, Prat J. Clear cell tumors of the female genital tract. Semin Diagn Pathol. 1998;14:233-9.
33. Roth LM, Dallenbach-Hellweg G, Czernobilsky B. Ovarian Brenner tumors. I. Metaplastic, proliferating, and of low malignant potential. Cancer. 1985;56:582-91.
34. Dictor M. Malignant mixed mesodermal tumor of the ovary: a report of 22 cases. Obstet Gynecol. 1985;65:720-4.
35. Karlan BY, Markman MA, et al. Ovarian cancer, peritoneal carcinoma and fallopian tube carcinoma. In: DeVita VT, Hellman S, Rosenberg SA (Eds). Cancer: Principles and Practice of Oncology, 7th edition. Philadelphia, PA: Lippincott-Williams and Wilkins; 2006. pp. 1364-97.

36. Plentl AA, Friedman EA. Lymphatic system of the female genitalia. Philadelphia, PA: WB Saunders; 1971.

37. Burghardt E, Pickel H, Lahousen M, et al. Pelvic lymphadenectomy in operative treatment of ovarian cancer. Am J Obstet Gynecol. 1986;155:315-9.

38. Ayhan A, Gultekin M, Taskiran C, et al. Lymphatic metastasis in epithelial ovarian carcinoma with respect to clinicopathological variable. Gynecol Oncol. 2005;97(2);400-4.

39. Crouet H, De Ranieri J, Heron JF, et al. Para-aortic lymphadenectomy in the surgical evaluation of ovarian cancer. Press Med. 1986;15(2):61-4.

40. Petru E, Lahousen M, Tamussino K, et al. In stage I ovarian cancer. Am J Obstet Gynecol. 1994;170(2):656-62.

41. Zinzindohoue C, Lujan R, Boulet S, et al. Pelvic and para-aortic lymphadenectomy in epithelial ovarian cancer. Report of a series of 86 cases. Ann Chir. 2000;125(2):163-70.

42. Harter P, Gnauert K, H ls R, et al. Pattern and clinical predictors of lymph nodes metastases in epithelial ovarian cancer. Int J Gynecol Cancer. 2007;17:1238-44.

43. Berek JS. Lymph node positive stage III C ovarian cancer: a separate entity? Int J Gynecol Cancer. 2009;19:518-20.

44. Onda T, Yoshikawa H, Yasugi T, et al. Patients with ovarian carcinoma upstaged to stage III after systematic lymphadenctomy have similar survival to stage I/II patients and superior survival to other stage III patients. Cancer. 1998;83(8):1555-60.

45. Munnell EW. The changing prognosis and treatment in cancer of the ovary: a report of 235 patients with primary ovarian carcinoma 1952-1961. Am J Obstet Gynecol. 1968;100(6):790-805.

46. Zanetta G, Chiari S, Rota S, et al. Conservative surgery for stage I ovarian carcinoma in women of childbearing age. Br J Obstet Gynecol. 1997;104(9):1030-45.

47. Griffiths CR. Surgical resection of tumor bulk in the primary treatment of ovarian carcinoma. Nat Cancer Inst Monogram. 1975;42:101-4.

48. Chi DS, Liao JB, Leon LF, et al. Identifications of prognostic factors in advanced epithelial ovarian carcinoma. Gynecol Oncol. 2001;82(3):532-7.

49. Eisenkop SM, Spirtos NM, Montag TW, et al. The impact of subspecialty training on the management of advanced ovarian cancer. Gynecol Oncol. 1992:47:203-9.

50. Schwartz PE, Rutherford TJ, Chambers JT, et al. Neoadjuvant chemotherapy for advanced ovarian cancer: long-term survival. Gynecol Oncol. 1999;72(1):93-9.

51. Vergote I, De Wever. Neoadjuvant chemotherapy or primary debulking surgery in advanced ovarian carcinoma: a retrospective analysis of 285 patients. Gynecol Oncol. 1998;71(3):431-6.

52. Schwartz PE. Cytoreductive surgery for the management of stage IV ovarian cancer. Gynecol Oncol. 1997;64(1):1-3.

53. Trimbos JB, Parmar M, Vergote I, et al. International collaborative ovarian neoplasm trial I and adjuvant chemotherapy in ovarian neoplasm trial: two parallel randomized phase III trials of adjuvant chemotherapy in patients with early stage ovarian carcinoma. J Nalt Cancer Institute. 2003;95:105.

54. Bell J, Brady M, Large JM, et al. A randomized phase III trial of three versus six cycles of carboplatin and paclitaxel as adjuvant treatment in early stage ovarian epithelial carcinoma. Gynecol Oncol. 2003;88:156.

55. McGuire WP, Hoskins WJ, Brady MF, et al. Cyclophosphamide and cisplatin compared with paclitaxel and cisplatin in patients with stage III and stage IV ovarian cancer. N Engl J Med. 1996;334(1): 1-6.

56. Ozols RF, Bundy BN, Greer BE, et al. Phase III trial of carboplatin and paclitaxel compared with cisplatin and paclitaxel in patients with optimally resected stage III ovarian cancer. J Clin Oncol. 2003;21:3194.

57. Ahlgren JD, Ellison NM, Gottlieb RJ, et al. Hormonal palliation of chemoresistant ovarian cancer: three consecutive phase II trials of the Mid-Atlantic Oncology Program. J Clin Oncol. 1993;11(10):1957-68.

58. Homesley HD, Hall DJ, Martin DA, et al. A cose escalating study of weekly bolus topotecan in previously treated ovarian cancer patients. Gynecol Oncol. 2001;83:394-9.

59. Parmar MK, Lederman JA, Columbo N, et al. Paclitaxel plus platinum based chemotherapy versus conventional platinum based chemotherapy in women with relapsed ovarian cancer: the ICON4/AGO-OVAR-2.2 trial. Lancet. 2003;361:2099-106.

60. Pfisterer J, Plante M, Vergote I, et al. Gemcitabine plus carboplatin compared with carboplatin in patients with platinum-sensitive recurrent ovarian cancer: an intergroup trial of the AGO-OVAR, the NCI CTG and the EORTC GCG. J Clin Oncol. 2006;24: 4699-707.

61. Alberts DS, Liu PY, Hannigan EV, et al. Intraperitoneal cisplatin plus intravenous cyclophosphamide vs intravenous cisplatin plus intravenous cyclophosphamide for stage III ovarian cancer. N Eng J Med. 1996;335(26):1950-5.

62. Markman M, Bundy BN, Alberts DS, et al. Phase III trial of standard-dose intravenous cisplatin plus paclitaxel versus moderately high-dose carboplatin toll by intravenous paclitaxel and intraperitoneal cisplatin in small-volume stage III ovarian carcinoma. J. Clin Oncology. 2001;19:1001-7.

63. Armstrong DK, Bundy B, Wenzel L, et al. Intraperitoneal cisplatin and paclitaxel in ovarian cancer. N Eng J Med. 2006;354(1):34-43.

64. Jaaback K, Johnson N, Lawrie TA. Intraperitoneal chemotherapy for the initial management of primary epithelial ovarian cancer. Cochrane Database Syst Rev. 2006;25(1):CD005340.

65. Piso P, McQuellon R, Gavazzi C, et al. Cytoreductive surgery and hyperthermic intraperitoneal chemotherapy in peritoneal carcinomatosis from ovarian cancer. World J Surg Oncol. 2004;2(21).

66. Look M, Chang D, Sugarbaker PH, et al. Long-term results of cytoreductive surgery for advanced and recurrent epithelial ovarian cancers and papillary serous carcinoma of the peritoneum. Int J Gynecol Cancer. 2004;14(1) 35-41.

67. Li Giorgio A, Naticchioni, et al. Cytoreductive surgery (peritonectomy procedures) combined with HIPEC in the treatment of diffuse peritoneal carcinomatosis from ovarian cancer. Cancer. 2008;113(2):315-25.

68. Sugarbaker PH. Management of peritoneal surface malignancy using intraperitoneal chemotherapy and cytoreductive surgery. A Manual for Physicians and Nurses, 3rd edition. USA: Ludann Company; 1998.

69. Sugarbaker PH. Management of peritoneal surface malignancy: the surgeon's role. Langenbecks Arch Surg. 1999;384(6):576-87.

70. Surgical Oncology Clinics of North America. Patient selection for cytoreductive surgery and hyperthermic intraperitoneal chemotherapy. 2012;21(14):515-31.

71. Gonzalez Bayon L, Steiner MA, Vasquez Jimenez W, et al. Cytoreductive surgery and hyperthermic intraperitoneal chemotherapy for the treatment of advanced epithelial ovarian carcinoma: upfront therapy, at first recurrence or later? Eur J Surg Oncol. 2013;39(10):1109-15.

72. Burger RA, Sill M, Monk BJ, et al. Phase II trial of bevacizumab in persistent or recurrent epithelial ovarian cancer (EOC) or primary peritoneal cancer. Proc Am Soc Clin Oncol. 2005;23:457s.

73. Coukos G, Rubin SC. Early ovarian cancer. Curr Treat Options Oncol. 2000;1:129-37.

74. National Comprehensive Cancer Network (2009). NCCN Clinical Practice Guidelines. Ovarian Cancer. V2. [online]. Available from www.nccn.org/professionals/physician_gls/PDF/Ovarian.pdf-Accessed September 17 [Accessed January, 2014].

75. Al-Agha OM, Nicastri AD. An in depth look at Kreukenberg tumor: an overview. Arch Pathol Lab Med. 2006;130(1):1725-30.

76. Woodruff JD, Novak ER. The Krukenberg tumor. Study of 48 cases from the Ovarian Tumor Registry. Obstet Gynecol. 1960;15:351-60.

77. Katusbe Y, Berg JW, Silverberg SG. Epidemiologic pathology of ovarian tumors: a histopathologic review of primary ovarian neoplasms diagnosed in the Denver Standard Metropolitan Statistical Area, 1 July-31 December 1969 and 1 July-31 December 1979. Int J Gynecol Pathol. 1982;1(1):3-16.

78. Skirnisdottir I, Garmo H, Wilander E, et al. Borderline ovarian tumors in Sweden 1960-2005: trends in incidence and age at diagnosis compared to ovarian cancer. Int J Cancer. 2008;123:1897-901.

79. Sutton GP. Ovarian tumors of low malignant potential. In: Rubin SC, Sutton GP (Eds). Ovarian Cancer, 2nd edition. Philadelphia, PA: Lippincott Williams and Wilkins, 2001. PP. 399-417.

80. Fischerova D, Zikan M, Dundr P, et al. Diagnosis, treatment and follow-up of borderline ovarian tumors. Oncologist. 2012;17(12):1515-33.

37 Carcinoma of the Cervix

Praful Desai, Keyuri Patel, Bhavna Parikh,
Nagraj G Huilgol, Ganesh Balasubramaniam

INTRODUCTION

Cancer cervix is the commonest cancer affecting Indian women except in the metropolitan areas like Mumbai and Delhi, where incidence of breast cancer is higher.[1] With easy access to "Pap" smear facilities, greater awareness and education, diagnosis is in earlier stages in now the urban population. Globally, there is now a significant decrease in the death rates due to cervix cancer because of routine cervical screening in most Western countries leading to early diagnosis.[2] In India, cervical cancer is still a late diagnosis due to paucity of medical facilities (availability of Pap smear) in the rural and semi-urban population, ignorance and low awareness. It mostly occurs in women of low socioeconomic strata, with early marriages and multiple pregnancies with poor genital hygiene and also multiple sex partners. Infection with human papillomavirus (HPV) is common in this group in developing countries.

Most lesions are squamous cell cancers. The use of diethylstilbesterol (DES) in early stages of pregnancy is known to produce adenocarcinoma of the vagina and cervix.[3] Rarer verities are small cell cancer and a carcinosarcoma. The section on pathology discusses this in greater details including HPV infection.

EPIDEMIOLOGY

Cervical cancer is the second most common cancer in women, and the seventh overall, with an estimated 530, 232 new cases in 2008 in the world; more than 85% of the global burden occurs in developing countries (n=453,531), where it accounts for 13% of all female cancers.[4] The age-standardized incidence rates in the world is 8.8 per 10^5, while it is 17.7 in less-developed regions. High-risk regions are Eastern and Western Africa (ASR > 30 per 10^5), Southern Africa (26.8 per 10^5), South-Central Asia (24.6 per 10^5), South America (23.9 per 10^5) and Middle Africa (23.0 per 10^5). Rates are lowest in Western Asia, Northern America and Australia/New Zealand (ASRs less than 6 per 10^5). Cervical cancer remains the most common cancer in women only in Eastern Africa, South-Central Asia and Melanesia. Overall, the mortality: incidence ratio is 52%, and cervical cancer was responsible for 275,000 deaths in 2008, about 88% of which occured in developing countries: 53,000 in Africa, 31,700 in Latin America and the Caribbean, and 159,800 in Asia.

In India, the incidence rates (per 10^5) are 21.4 in Bangalore, 16.5 in Barshi, 20.6 in Chennai and 14.5 in Mumbai; overall the rates are higher in rural areas.[5] It is estimated that there were 134,420 new cervix cancer cases in India in the year 2008 with an age-standardized incidence rate of 27.0 per 10^5, which is threefold compared to world rates (Fig. 1).

HUMAN PAPILLOMA VIRUS INFECTION

The most important risk factor for cervical cancer is infection by the HPV. HPV is a group of more than 100 related viruses, some of which cause a type of growth called a papilloma, which are more commonly known as warts. HPV can infect cells on the surface of the skin and those lining the genitals, anus, mouth and throat. HPV is generally sexually transmitted.

Human papilloma virus is responsible for nearly 70% of cervical cancer worldwide.[6] The large majority of patients belong to developing world due to multifactorial reasons. Globally, the incidence of HPV infection is rising

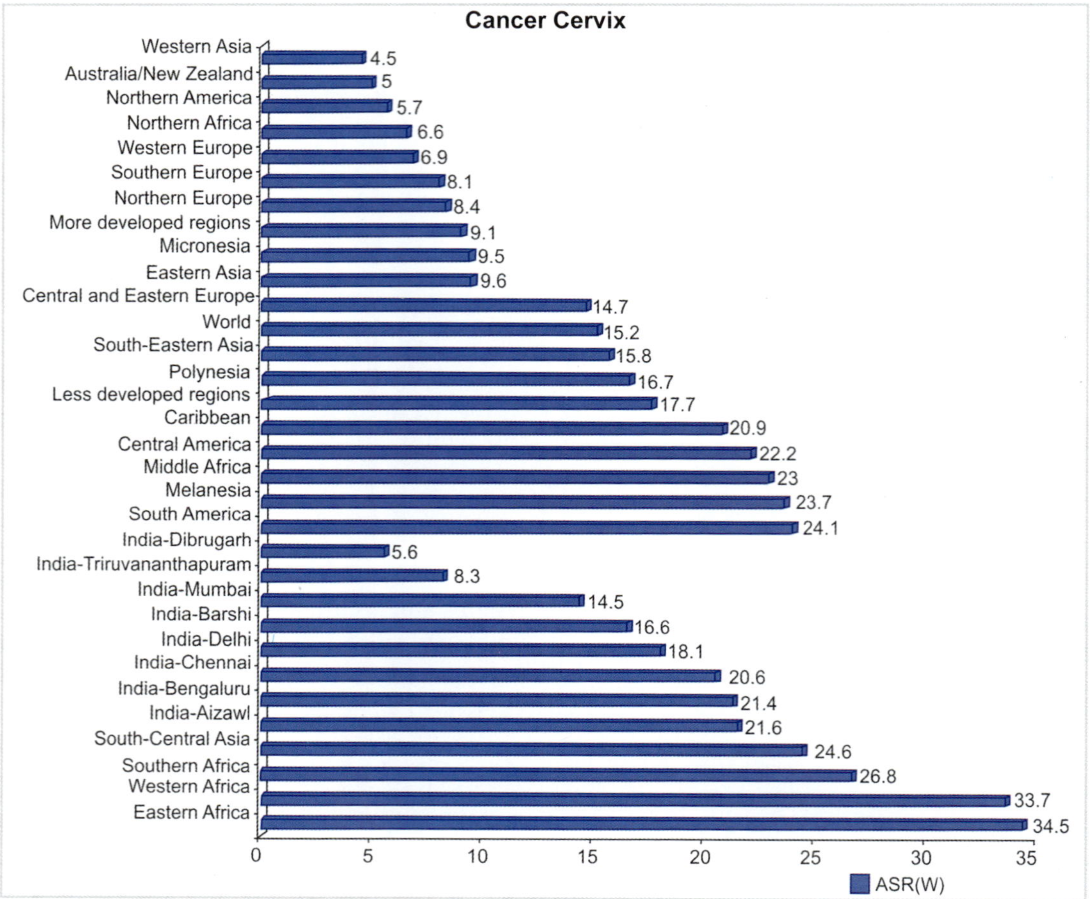

Fig. 1: Age standardized incidence rates in the different regions of the world

with almost 6.2 million cases annually.[7] This may result in an increase of low or high grade squamous epithelial lesions (CIN II and III), anorectal or genital warts which are all precursors of cancer of the cervix in women and anal cancer in men. Recent studies have evaluated two vaccines (bivalent and quadrivalent) approved by the US food and drug administration.[8]

It will be a long way off before the vaccines can positively impact on the incidence of cervical cancer, may be 20–25 years; however, prevention of precancerous or dysplastic lesions of the cervix (CIN II and III) may be the first step towards the final goal of cancer prevention. It cannot substitute routine cervical screening in the near future. Recommendation for HPV vaccination in India should be selective and should be advised in a population prone to cervix cancer by virtue of their habits and lifestyle. Since cervix cancer can be a sexually transmitted disease, male vaccination is also advisable in appropriate groups.

Smoking

Moutinho[9] published an article in 2011, which reviewed smoking and cervix cancer. In 2004, International Agency for Research on Cancer (IARC) listed cervical cancer among those causally related to smoking. Smoking interferes with incidence and prevalence of HPV infection and is associated with cervical intraepithelial neoplasia (CIN) and invasive cervical cancer. Multiple factors seem to intervene in cervical carcinogenesis related with tobacco, especially by direct local carcinogenic effect and local immunosuppression. Women who smoke are about twice more likely than non-smokers to get cervical cancer.

Immunosuppression

Human immunodeficiency virus (HIV), the virus that causes AIDS, damages the immune system and puts women at higher risk for HPV infections. This might explain why women with AIDS have an increased risk for cervical cancer. The immune system is important in destroying cancer cells and slowing their growth and spread. In women with HIV, a cervical pre-cancer might develop into an invasive cancer faster than it normally would. Another group of women at risk of cervical cancer are women receiving drugs to suppress their immune response, such as those being treated for an autoimmune disease.

Diet

Women whose diet does not include enough fruits and vegetables may be at increased risk for cervical cancer. Overweight women are more likely to develop adenocarcinoma of the cervix. Though the HPV has been demonstrated to be a causative agent for this cancer, a variety of other risk factors are in play, such as sexual and reproductive patterns, socioeconomic, hygienic practices, and diet. The dietary intake of antioxidants and vitamins like vitamin A, carotenoids, vitamin C, folacin and tocopherol is found to have protective effects against cancer of the cervix; however dietary data regarding cervical cancer are still scanty.

In an Indian study enrolled from a referral hospital including the food frequency pattern and 24-hour dietary recall on the food consumption pattern along with other important factors showed that the mean intake of energy, protein, vitamins, etc., between the cases and controls was not significantly different except for the vitamin C level but serum vitamin E was found to have lower average in patients as compared to controls.[10] The nutrient intake of cervical cancer patients and controls was grossly deficient in the low socioeconomic group studied and with regard to the macronutrient intake; calorie and protein intakes showed a deficit of around 50%. The food consumption profile was not found to be significantly different between cervical cancer patients and normal controls in this study. Other major factors include poor socioeconomic conditions, multiple pregnancies, due to early marriage and poor hygiene particularly in rural areas.

Oral Contraceptives

There is evidence that prolonged oral contraceptives (OC), intake increases the risk of cancer of the cervix; however the risk reduces after the OC are withdrawn.

Intrauterine Device Use

A recent study found that women who had never used an intrauterine device (IUD) had a lower risk of cervical cancer. Risk was seen even in women who had an IUD for less than a year; however, protective effect persists after the use of IUD was withdrawn.

Multiple Full-term Pregnancies

High parity has long been suspected of being associated with an increased risk of cervical cancer. Women who have had three or more full-term pregnancies have an increased risk of developing cervical cancer. Studies have pointed to hormonal changes during pregnancy making women more susceptible to HPV infection and cancer. A general decline in parity might therefore partly explain the reduction in cervical cancer recently seen in most countries. Poverty is also a risk factor for cervical cancer. Many low-income women do not have ready access to adequate health care services, including Pap tests. Screening programs in rural areas need to be strengthened.

Diethylstilbestrol (DES)

Diethylstilbestrol is a hormone administered to women to prevent miscarriage. Intake of DES during pregnancy predisposes daughters to a clear-cell adenocarcinoma of the vagina or cervix more often than would normally be expected. This type of cancer is extremely rare in women who have not been exposed to DES. A follow-up to evaluate long-term cancer risks for women prescribed DES while pregnant found no increased risk for any other cancers, including endometrial, cervix or ovarian cancer.[11]

Family History of Cervical Cancer

Cervical cancer may run in some families and chances of developing the disease are two to three times higher. Some researchers suspect that some instances of this familial tendency are caused by an inherited condition that makes some women less able to fight off HPV infection than others. In other instances, women with family history are more likely to have one or more of other non-genetic risk factors. A study from Gwalior, India to understand the factors influencing acceptance of Cervical Cancer Screening among Women in India reported that limited knowledge of cervical cancer, the necessity of cervical cancer screening, inadequate public health education, lack of patient-friendly health services, sociocultural health beliefs and personal difficulties were the few salient barriers to screening.[12]

To reduce the incidence of cervical cancer a concerted and organized control measures are necessary. Primary prevention through a prophylactic vaccine is still far away in the future, though a beginning has been made. Control of cervical cancer through secondary preventive measures is the only viable solution now.

PATHOLOGY

Human papilloma virus is an important factor in cervical oncogenesis. HPV DNA is detected in 95% of cervix cancer. HPV is divided into two major categories depending on the level of association with carcinoma in-situ (CIS) and invasive squamous carcinoma.

- High-risk types (associated with carcinoma), are primarily 16 and 18;[13] however, many other types are associated.
- Low-risk types (associated with condyloma and low grade [squamous intraepithelial lesion (SIL)] are 6, 11 and many other types.

Association between HPV and cervical neoplasia is strong for squamous cell carcinoma, CIS, invasive adenocarcinoma and adenosquamous carcinoma.

Precancerous Squamous Lesions

Nearly all invasive squamous carcinomas are preceded by a stage in which abnormal cells are confined to the epithelium (intraepithelial stage) (Fig. 2). Carcinomatous change generally occurs at the transformation zone. It may exist in non-invasive stage for as long as 20 years. It will not invariably progress to cancer and may spontaneously regress. Association with HPV types 16 and 18 is strongly associated with higher grade lesions and has greatest risk of progression.

Microinvasive Squamous Carcinoma

Depth of stromal invasion is 5 mm or less and maximum width is 7 mm [International Federation of Gynecology and Obstetrics (FIGO) Stage Ia].[14] It is subdivided into FIGO Stage Ia1 (< 3 mm stromal invasion)-lymph node metastasis in 0.9% and FIGO Stage Ia2 (3–5 mm depth of stromal invasion)—lymph node metastasis occurs in 13%. Natural history is different from ordinary invasive squamous carcinoma and almost resembles CIN III/CIS; it is thus amenable to conservative treatment. Diagnosis can be made only on specimen containing entire lesion (excision biopsy).

Squamous Carcinoma

It is the commonest type of cervical cancer. It constitutes 70–78% of cervical malignancies. Most evolve from precancerous lesions and persistent HPV infection.[15] It is classified according to the degree of squamous differentiation (well, moderate and poorly differentiated) or according to cell type [large cell keratinizing type with intercellular bridges and keratin pearls, large cell non-keratinizing type (Fig. 3) and small cell squamous carcinoma]. However, treatment is not significantly influenced by histologic patterns.

Variants of Squamous Carcinoma

- *Verrucous carcinoma*: Very rare in cervix.[16] Large sessile condylomatous lesion, which is locally invasive but does not metastasize. Cytologically very well differentiated.
- *Spindle cell (sarcomatoid) carcinoma*: Aggressive tumor, which often recurs; spindle cell morphology.
- *Papillary/transitional cell carcinoma*: Resembles urothelial carcinoma of bladder; aggressive tumor with local recurrence and late metastasis.
- *Lymphoepithelioma like carcinoma*: Morphologically resembles nasopharyngeal counterpart; EBV association in Asians; low stage at presentation and hence better outcome than conventional squamous carcinoma.
- *Condylomatous (warty) carcinoma*: Very rare tumor with condylomatous appearance and koilocytotic atypia. Less aggressive than well differentiated squamous carcinoma.
- *Basaloid squamous carcinoma*: Aggressive behavior.

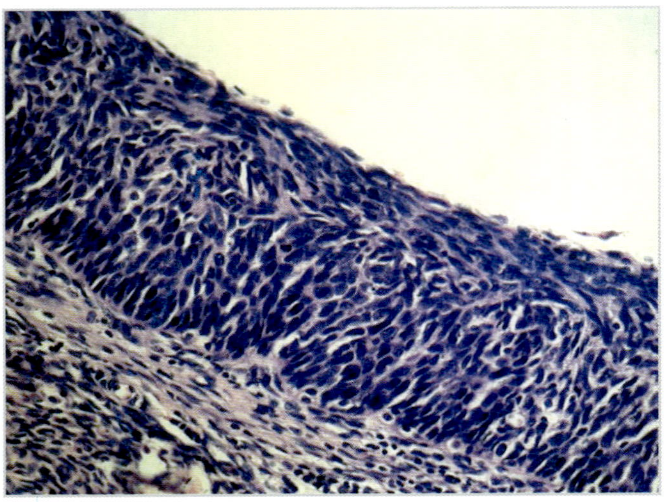

Fig. 2: Intraepithelial stage

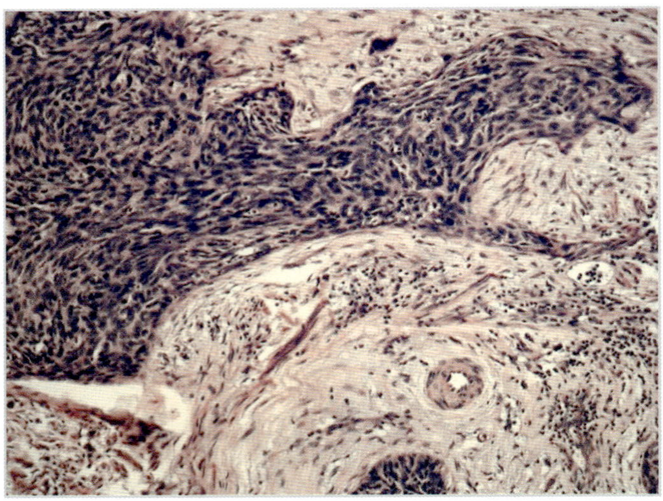

Fig. 3: Large cell non-keratinizing type

Adenocarcinoma

It constitutes 15% of invasive carcinomas of cervix. Endocervical (mucin secreting type) constitutes 70% of adenocarcinoma of cervix.[17] Most express HPV 16 and 18. Rare variants include colloid carcinoma,[18] intestinal carcinoma and signet-ring type carcinoma.[19]

- *Endometrioid adenocarcinoma* (Fig. 4). It is second in frequency to endocervical adenocarcinoma. Resembles its endometrial counterpart. Immunohistochemistry is useful in differentiating between endometrial and cervical adenocarcinoma (Endocervical adenocarcinoma expresses p16 and CEA and is negative for Vimentin and Estrogen receptor).
- *Minimal deviation adenocarcinoma* (adenoma malignum) constitute 1–2% of all cervical adenocarcinomas.[20] It may be associated with Peutz Jeghers syndrome or may be sporadic. Diagnosis on small biopsies can be challenging since cytologic and architectural features are subtle and mimic benign lesions. Histologic features consist of haphazard infiltration of irregular or "claw shaped", often cystically dilated, very well differentiated glands, deep in the cervical stroma. It has a worse prognosis than other cervical adenocarcinomas due to difficulty in detection and diagnosis at a late stage.
- *Villoglandular papillary adenocarcinoma*: It is well differentiated and has a good prognosis.[21,22]
- *Clear cell carcinoma* of Müllerian origin. Rare in cervix and occurs in young females, associated with in utero DES exposure. Good survival.[23]
- *Serous papillary adenocarcinoma*:[24] Rare primary adenocarcinoma of cervix. It is a high grade, aggressive tumor, resembles counterpart in ovary/endometrium. In young females it is HPV associated and usually constitutes a focal component of conventional adenocarcinoma. In postmenopausal females, it may represent a "drop metastasis" from endometrial or upper genital tract tumor.
- *Adenosquamous carcinoma*: Biphasic pattern of well defined malignant glands and squamous component. Most are high grade and carry a worse prognosis than other cervical carcinomas. "Glassy cell" variant, shows a solid growth of large tumor cells with abundant eosinophilic cytoplasm and intratumoral eosinophilic infiltrate.
- *Adenoid basal carcinoma*: It is an uncommon indolent tumor in the elderly. No visible mass is detected. It has a favorable prognosis.
- *Adenoid cystic carcinoma*: Rare. Poor prognosis due to high frequency of local recurrence and distant metastasis.

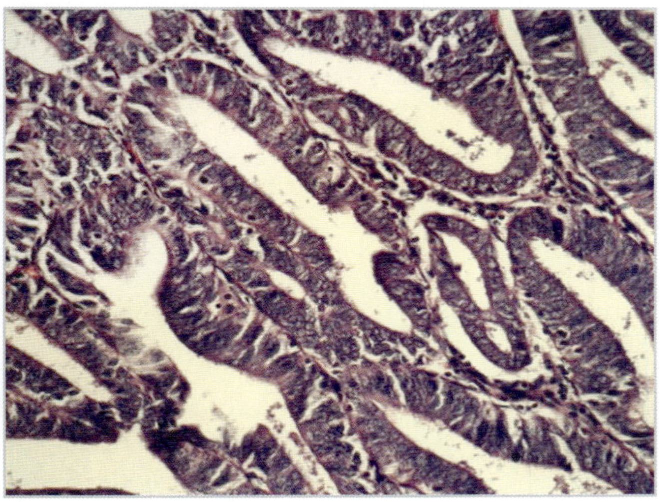

Fig. 4: Endometrioid adenocarcinoma

Neuroendocrine Carcinoma

Spectrum of tumors ranging from well differentiated neuroendocrine tumors (carcinoid) to small cell neuroendocrine carcinoma (oat cell type) are known. The latter reveals sheets of medium sized tumor cells, with hyperchromatic mitotically active nuclei, frequently showing broad zones of necrosis. Rosette formation may be seen. It is positive for neuroendocrine markers on immunohistochemistry and has a strong association with HPV 18.[25] It is an aggressive tumor with poor prognosis.

SCREENING FOR CERVICAL CANCER

The low incidence of cervical cancer and reduction in death rates in the developed Western world is the direct consequence of well planned screening programs. Developing countries like India, should create this infrastructure, at least for the "Prone" groups as mentioned above in semi-urban and rural population around the age of 20 or above in married women at least once in 2 years. Routine Pap smear in urban population is probably not indicated in asymptomatic population until the age of 25–30 years. Pap smears are strongly indicated in symptomatic population at any age and once in 2 years after the age of 40 years even in an asymptomatic population.

PAPANICOLAOU SMEARS

George Papanicolaou in 1928[26] first reported on the cytologic studies of exfoliated cervical cells (PAP smears) which can also be observed in human endocervical and vaginal smears and even endometrial cells could be identified in the exfoliated cells.[26] Even earlier, Ameli Babes[27] reported similar findings 2 years before Papnicolaou. Since then the Pap smear study has remained the gold standard for early diagnosis of cervical cancer.

PROBLEMS AND CHALLENGES

Though an invaluable aid in controlling and curing cervical cancer the availability of Pap smear facility in developing countries remains a serious challenge particularly in the underprivileged rural areas. The appropriate method of collecting and processing and even more importantly an appropriate interpretation of the smears still remain major issues in developing countries, though a steady improvement is now a feature even in Afro-Asian countries.[28] Training of cytotechnicians and cytopathologists are vital issues in creating a major impact on early detection of cervical cancers and subsequent reduction in deaths due to this highly preventable and curable disease.

Cervical Intraepithelial Neoplasia

It is a common term now used to encompass all epithelial abnormalities of the cervix. It is classified into grades I to III based on the abnormal epithelial changes. In fact, it is a continuum from initial mild abnormalities of mild dysplasia to full blown cancer of the cervix (Class V-Cervical smears). The Pap smears are generally classified from class I to V. Different nomenclature for the same pathology often creates confusion in interpretation. Table 1 summarizes the progression and genesis from a normal epithelium to early dysplasia and the final culmination towards a full-blown squamous cell cancer of the cervix. Various nomenclatures are best simplified as follows (Table 1):[29]

Classification: Pap Smear/WHO/CIN

Interpretation and Management of CIN/ Abnormal Smears (Preinvasive Lesions)

Effective and appropriate management of pre-cancer CIN (III to V) or class III to V Pap smears in a symptomatic patient is easier where the cervix shows a lesion in the form of severe inflammation or an ulceration from where a tissue biopsy or cytology could be obtained for histopathologic studies.

TABLE 1: Classification of Pap smear

Class	*WHO*	*CIN*	*Bethesda*
I	Normal	Normal	Infection/ Reparative
II	Atypical	Inflammation	Marked inflammation
III	Mild dysplasia Moderate dysplasia Severe dysplasia	CIN–I CIN–II CIN–III	LGSIL* HGSIL** HGSIL
IV	CIS	CIS	HGSIL
V	Cancer	Cancer	Squamous cell CA

Abbreviations: *LGSIL, low grade squamous epithelial lesion; **HGSIL, high grade squamous epithelial lesion; CIN, cervical intraepithelial neoplasia; CIS, carcinoma-in-situ.

Colposcopy

For abnormal smears from a normal appearing cervix without any lesion when the woman is asymptomatic in a routine screening program, a colposcopic assessment and appropriate biopsy needs to be obtained. Hinselmann (1925) devised the colposcope, an optical device which magnifies more than 10–15 fold to define changes in the morphology of the cervix, details of hyper-vascular changes (Fig. 5) and nodularity in the surface epithelium—The "WHITE" epithelium particularly in the transformation zone[29] (Fig. 5). This area is a highly suspect region and colposcope directed biopsies needs to be performed to identify an early invasive cancer. The colposcope, however,

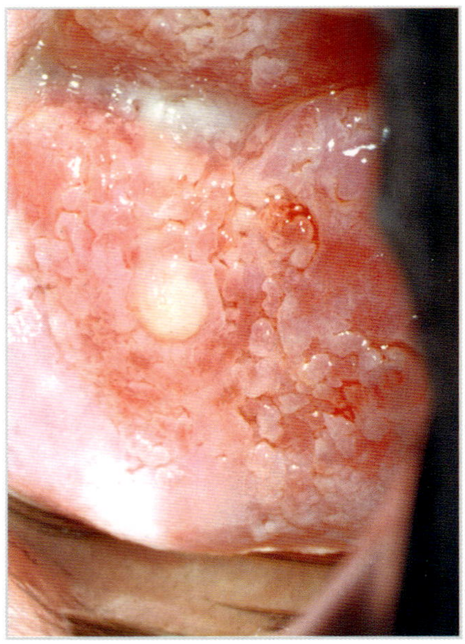

Fig. 5: Cervix showing hypertrophied papillae with dense acetowhitening suggestive of high-grade lesion

is not frequently used as most cases manifest clinically. It is important to have a well trained colposcopist to monitor a well organized screening program for cervical cancer.

Management of Patients with Abnormal Pap Smear (Class III to V)/ HGSIL (Preinvasive Disease)

The procedure loop electro excision (LEEP) can be considered as an office/out patient procedure for patients with high grade squamous epithelial lesion (HGSIL). It helps in fertility preservation. Therapeutic conization is another procedure to preserve fertility for microinvasive disease. Hemorrhage, sepsis and stenosis of the cervix-endocervix are known complications and a clear scalpel conization is preferred to thermal cautery conization. These group of patients will require careful follow up surveillance after treatment.

Preinvasive disease of the cervix should therefore be treated carefully to prevent its progress to invasive carcinoma and recurrence. Multiple outpatient procedures are considered adequate management as noted above like electrocautery, cryosurgery and even laserization. Conization will require in patient therapy and can be performed without blood loss by laser. It is a technically demanding procedure and hemorrhage, infection and stenosis are known. The cone size and type can be defined by the abnormal epithelial extent as determined by Colposcopy. Besides the procedures mentioned above a simple vaginal hysterectomy is often preferred and widely accepted by patients for preinvasive lesions, particularly if the family has been completed.

CLINICAL FEATURES AND PRE-THERAPY WORK-UP

Most patients present with bleeding per vaginum, foul discharges (leukorrhic) or with complaints of post-coital frictional bleeding or spotting. In patients with early marriages, multiple pregnancies and poor genital hygiene the onset is often earlier and careful clinical examination and essential investigations as indicated (Pap smear, biopsy) should be expedited. In the more frequent scenarios of an advanced lesion additional symptoms of pain in the lower abdomen, back or along the extremities may be a feature due to entrapment of ureters or infiltration of the obturator nerves on the pelvic wall. Infiltration of bladder and rectum (Stage IV) will result in hematuria or melena.

Clinical Examination

Apart from the usual general examination, a careful per vaginum and per rectal examination gives a mine of information regarding the type of cervical lesion (ulcerative or proliferative), its extent into the cervix and fornices, involvement of parametrium and fixity or otherwise to the pelvic wall. This also gives an idea of staging with fair accuracy. A speculum examination will indicate involvement of the vaginal walls and helps to stage the disease. A tissue diagnosis by a punch biopsy is sufficient for interpretation.

Cystocopy

This is optional and may be carried out if clinical symptoms so dictate. Ureteric catheterization can be considered in case of ureteric encasement before therapy.

Imaging

A routine chest skiagram, ultrasound of the abdomen and pelvis and an abdominal computed tomography (CT) study should be done as a routine. Magnetic resonance imaging (MRI) is optional for better delineation of soft-tissue masses.

Staging

Armed with these investigations, cervical cancer could be staged and appropriate therapeutic procedure could be planned.

The FIGO (2009) classification could be simplified as under:

Stage I: Lesion localized to cervix (extension to corpus-still stage I).

Stage II A.B: Lesions beyond cervix–Parametria, fornices, upper 1/3 vagina (II B).

Stage III A.B: Invasion of the pelvic wall, hydronephrosis, lower 1/3 vagina.

Stage IV: Invasion of organs (bladder, rectum and beyond pelvis).

INVASIVE CARCINOMA OF THE CERVIX: SURGICAL MANAGEMENT

Traditionally surgery was the mainstay for localized (Stage I/II) cancers of the cervix ever since Ernest Wertheim (1903) described radical hysterectomy and popularized

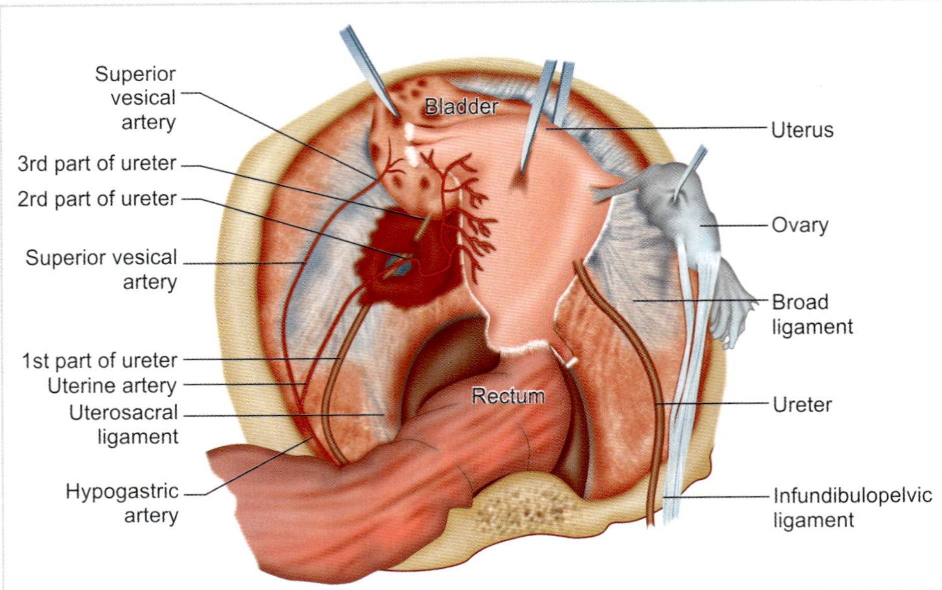

Fig. 6: Diagrammatic representation of surgical anatomy of the pelvis for Wertheim-Meigs radical hysterectomy

by Meigs in 1944 (Fig. 6). This involved removal of the uterus and adnexa, with a good 2 to 3 cm margin of the upper vagina to avoid vault recurrence. The lymph nodes draining the cervical and upper vaginal area includes paracervical, parametrial and pelvic external and internal iliac group of nodes which are removed en-mass with the main specimen—Wertheim's operation (radical hysterectomy).

Surgical Treatment

The surgical approach was frequently and widely accepted because of the dissatisfaction and limitation of radiotherapy in the earlier era. Some lesions were radio resistant and metastatic lesions in the nodes were reported to be radiation resistant. With the advent of more effective radiotherapy techniques in the latter half of the last century besides effective chemotherapy, the surgical approach for stage I and II cancer needs to be selective. Every operable lesion does not require very radical surgery. Sentinel node evaluation in cervical cancer surgery is in a clinical research state; however, in the next 5–10 years with a large database, it may become a practice changing paradigm.[30] In a recent study by Chereau of 66 patients, a false negative sentinel node biopsy was detected in 20% and positive pelvic nodes were found in 40%. Para-aortic skip metastases were noted in 6%. The main determinant of disease free survival (DFS) and overall survival (OS) was para-aortic node involvement ($P < 0.001$).[31]

A selective surgical approach was first described by Piver and Rutledge[32] classifying radical hysterectomy (Wertheim's operation) in types I, II and III with increasing radicality depending upon the extent of disease (Figs 6 to 9).

The current dispensation of avoiding removal of non-involved normal pelvic nodes to avoid morbidities like lymphorrhea, extremity edema and bladder dysfunction has revised our approach to radical lymph node dissection as has happened in breast cancer and melanoma. Sentinel node biopsy in cancer cervix is therefore currently an important surgical clinical research area to avoid removal of normal uninvolved lymph nodes in surgery for cancer cervix.

Class I Hysterectomy is indicated for in-situ and microinvasive carcinomas and is often referred to as extra fascial hysterectomy. Pelvic node dissection is avoided and the ureters are not extensively mobilized; the procedure generally involves removal of all cervical tissue with a good free margin of the upper vagina. The para-cervical tissue is clamped away from the uterine and cervical margin to ensure removal of adjacent para-cervical tissues. Preservation of ovarian function at younger age is feasible as direct metastasis to ovary is very infrequent.

Class II hysterectomy is also classified as moderately extended hysterectomy by removing a greater amount of paracervical tissues with medial half of cardinal and uterosacral ligaments and upper 1/3rd of vagina.

Class III hysterectomy consists of removal of entire cardinal and uterosacral ligaments with upper 1/3rd of

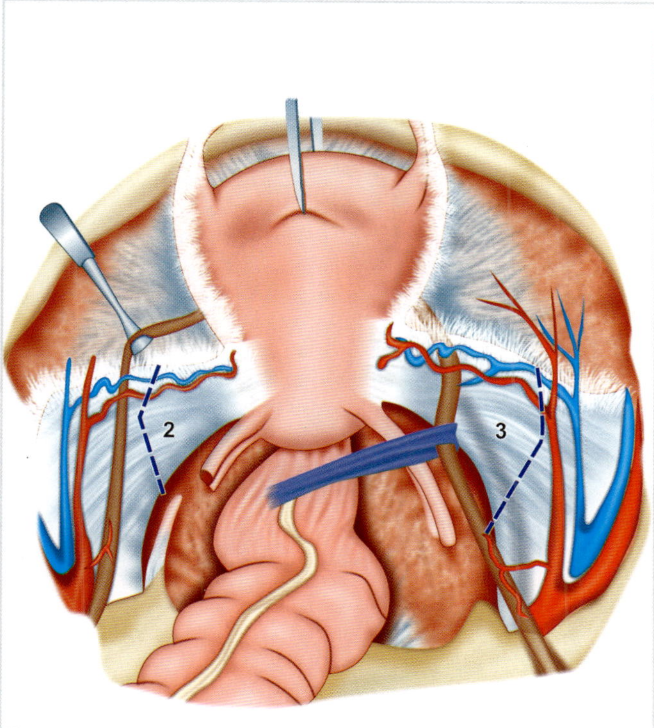

Fig. 7: Broken lines identify the point of transaction for the cardinal ligaments in class II and class III radical hysterectomy

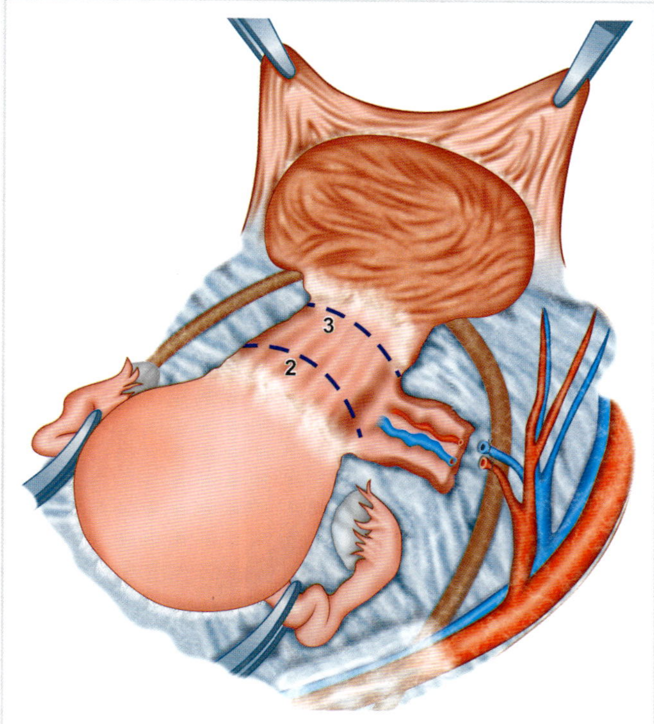

Fig. 9: Broken lines illustrate level of vaginal removal in class II and class III radical hysterectomy

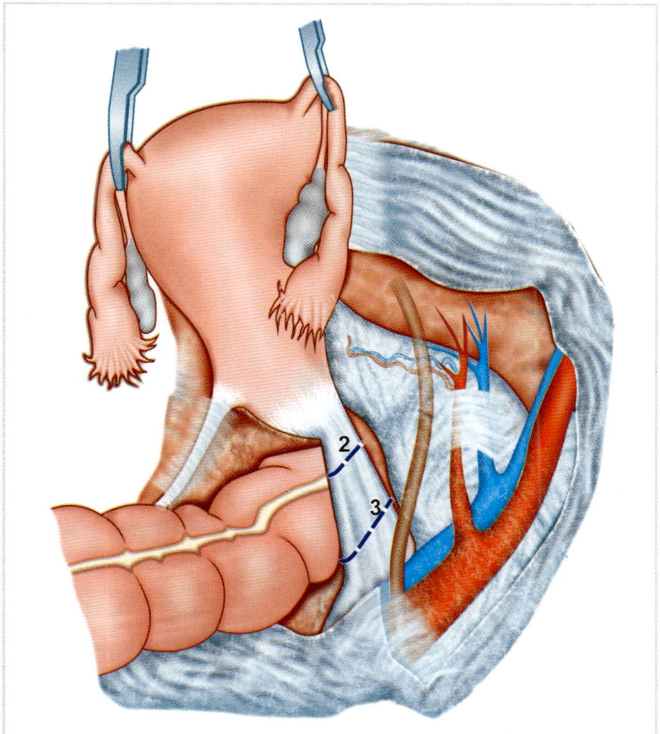

Fig. 8: Broken lines identify the point of transection of the uterosacral ligaments in class II and class III radical hysterectomy

vagina and complete pelvic node dissection (iliac group, obturator and node of Cloquet) from the inguinal ligament area on the pelvic brim. Assessment of bifurcation node, sacral and periaortic node region should be assessed and dissected if suspect. Stage IV disease may require an anterior or posterior pelvic exenteration with removal of the bladder or rectum respectively. A total pelvic exenteration will mean removal of all organs with a permanent colostomy and ileal urinary diversion.

Radiation Therapy

For all patients with stage IIb, III the therapy of choice is radiation therapy (RT). Even patients in early stage (I and II), who are obese with comorbidities, can be effectively treated with radiotherapy—external and interstitial (brachytherapy). The results stage-wise are favorably comparable and radiotherapy remains the treatment of choice in appropriate clinical settings. As early as 1972 Fletcher[33] reported 91% five year cure rate for stage I disease.

Chemoradiotherapy[35]

A study by E Saibish kumar and Patel from India[34,35] in a phase II trial of concurrent chemoradiation therapy (CRT) in treatment of locally advanced cancer of the uterine cervix, the authors found that CRT was not superior to RT alone. The study was based on small numbers, suboptimal chemotherapy doses and limitations of a non-randomized trial, the authors maintained that these restraints may have impacted on the findings.

Cisplatin based chemotherapy along with concurrent or sequential radiotherapy is another standard of care in patients with locally advanced stage IIb and III cervix cancer. Rapid down-staging occurs and occasionally stage IIa and b could be considered for subsequent surgery or continued with radical radiotherapy.[34] This neoadjuvant chemoradiotherapy and subsequent surgery if planned should be discussed by the surgeon, chemotherapist and radiotherapist. Treatment decisions should be based on a number of factors like stage of the disease, patient's medical status, obesity and other co-morbidities. Patients with significant obesity and comorbidities at any stage are better managed by chemoradiotherapy.

Total Pelvic Exenteration

Pelvic organs including involved bladder and the rectum along with the uterus, cervix and upper 3/4th of the vagina, a permanent end colostomy and urinary diversion becomes mandatory. Reported 5 years survival rates for such extensive procedures range from 15% to 30%. Morbidities and complications are significant and prolonged hospitalization is not unusual. These procedures are now uncommon because of early diagnosis and effective chemoradiotherapy.

Extent of Lymph Node Dissection

Metastasis to the lymph nodes follows a predictable spread in cervix, uterine and ovarian cancers based on the lymphovascular drainage. In cervical cancer, the nodal spread starts from the parametrial nodes to the pelvic (external and internal iliac, obturator nodes) space to the bifurcation node (bifurcation of the common iliac to external and internal iliac artery) sacral node and proximally towards the aortocaval, periaortic and retroperitoneal nodes (Fig. 10). The incidence at various nodal site is directly proportional to the increasing stage of the disease. Table 2 shows reported incidence of periaortic nodes in literature. If indicated, nodal dissection and clearance should be extended to the para-aortic regions. In an advanced or untreated case, the nodal metastasis can disseminate into the mediastinum, neck and inguinal region. Organal spread into the liver, lungs, spleen, adrenal,

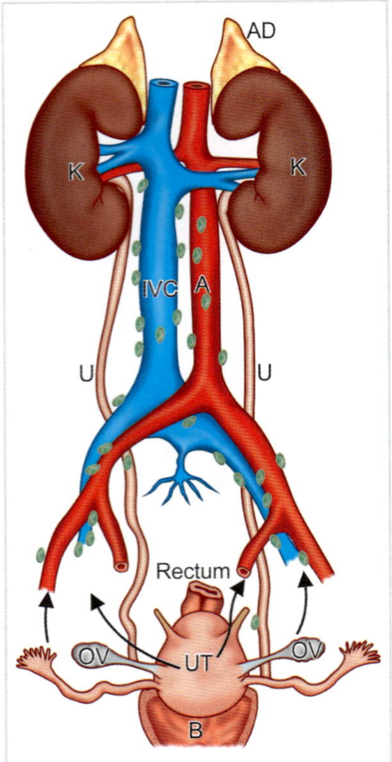

Fig. 10: The common lymphatic drainage pathways from cancer of the ovary, endometrium and cervix

TABLE 2: Incidence of periaortic nodes by clinical stage

Stage	*Positive nodes percentage*
I b	5.6
II a	18.2
II b	31.7
III a	33.3
III b	31.1
IV a	33.3

Source: Henriksen E. The lymphatic spread of carcinoma of the cervix and of the body of the uterus; a study of 420 necropsies. Am J Obstet Gynecol. 1949;58:924-42.

kidney and even thyroid are known. The importance of sentinel node biopsy evaluation has been referred to and will help to avoid unnecessary dissections and help to obviate morbidities. It is still an investigative research.

Recurrent Carcinoma of Cervix

Recurrence after definitive surgical or RT are not uncommon. The patient usually presents with bleeding per vaginum (vault recurrence) due to recurrence on the cervix and surrounding fornices and vagina after surgery or radiotherapy. Pain in the lower abdomen and lower extremities can result after pelvic recurrences which involve the pelvic space and the pelvic wall. Encasement of the ureters leads to pain in the loins, lower abdomen and back. Infiltration of the bladder or rectum will produce related symptoms. Appropriate clinical examination, investigations and tissue biopsies are mandatory before a precise diagnosis is reached relating to the site and extent of the disease.

Recurrence after Previous Surgery

Large pelvic recurrences are generally treated by combined radiochemotherapy,[37] which can lead to good palliation of symptoms apart from excellent results obtained as in primary definitive therapy for cervical cancer. Intracavitary radiation is effective for cervical and vaginal recurrences. Isolated distant skeletal metastasis with pain can also be effectively controlled with radiotherapy. Encasement of ureters and proximal obstructive uropathy can be palliated, if possible, with ureteric stenting before chemoradiotherapy. Repeat surgery is generally contraindicated and neither worthwhile or possible.

Recurrence after Previous Chemoradiotherapy: Salvage Surgery

Appropriate investigations will determine whether any salvage surgery is feasible. Appropriate surgical assessment should be done whether the surgical approach will allow a near complete clearance of the recurrent disease. Anteroposterior, (involvement of bladder, rectum) or central recurrences which are localized and devoid of extra pelvic spread beyond pelvic brim can be managed by anterior, posterior or total pelvic exenterations with urinary and fecal diversions as needed. Three and five years survivals are reported between 20% and 60% at 5 years and 3 years in appropriately selected patients for anterior or total pelvic exenteration.[38] Postoperative complications are not uncommon and hospital stay is often prolonged from 4 weeks to 6 weeks.

Localized isolated recurrences at a resectable site and amenable to surgical excision should be considered for a surgical approach. This is particularly so if the recurrence occurs after a latent period of 3–4 years or more after control of the primary cervical lesion by chemoradiotherapy. Pelvic and inguinal node metastases are known to occur after a lapse of time and are generally amenable to surgical removal.

CHEMOTHERAPY

Management of cervical cancer requires a multimodality approach. The role of systemic therapy is threefold.

1. Neoadjuvant chemotherapy (NACT)
2. Adjuvant
3. For recurrent and metastatic disease

NEOADJUVANT CHEMOTHERAPY

The concept of NACT was introduced for patients with locally advanced disease, i.e. stage III and IV/A before considering them for local treatment (surgery or radiotherapy). It was postulated that NACT may help in better progression-free survival (PFS) and overall survival (OS) for these patients, though robust evidence is lacking.

Neoadjuvant Chemotherapy Followed by Radiotherapy

The result of randomized trials of NACT followed by RT versus RT alone have been disappointing.[39] A meta-analysis of 18 randomized clinical trials included 2,074 patients. There was no advantage of NACT with regards to PFS, or locoregional DFS, metastasis-free survival or OS. Concurrent chemoradiotherapy is being used in patients with good health and advanced disease.

Neoadjuvant Chemotherapy Followed by Surgery

In 1990s, there were many non-randomized studies suggesting benefit of NACT followed by surgery. Some of the randomized trials showed a trend favoring NACT. A meta-analysis of five randomized clinical trials involving 872 patients who received NACT followed by surgery plus RT was compared to RT alone. There was a significant improvement in disease-free survival (DFS), locoregional DFS, metastasis free-survival and OS for those who became resectable following NACT; however, the role of NACT is not yet *confirmed* based on available data.

Katsumata et al. conducted a Phase III trial[40] of NACT consisting of bleomycin, vincristine, mitomycin and cisplatin (BOMO) regimen every 3 weeks for 2–4 cycles followed by radical surgery. It did not improve 5 year OS in the NACT arm (NACT+Surgery–70.0% vs. surgery 70.4%). Another retrospective study of 65 patients[41] involved NACT followed by surgery. Patients also received adjuvant treatment if histopathology report revealed pelvic lymph node involvement, parametrial infiltration or a positive surgical margin. About 70% of stage IB2-IIB could be cured by NACT followed by surgery. Those with pelvic lymph node involvement had a worse outcome. In an Indian study, Singh et al.[42] conducted a pilot study to find out the benefit of weekly paclitaxel plus carboplatin followed by definitive CT+RT. Twenty-eight patients with locally advanced cervical cancer received paclitaxel 60 mg/m^2 and carboplatin area under control (AUC) 2 weeks for 6 doses. After a period of 2 weeks, weekly cisplatin 40 mg/m^2 (six times) with RT. Following NACT, response rate of -67.8% with 7.1% of complete response was observed. This increased to 90% complete response at the end of CT+RT. NACT is a feasible approach which can result in high response rates; however, neoadjuvant chemotherapy remains an investigational treatment modality.

ADJUVANT CHEMOTHERAPY

Adjuvant chemotherapy for cervical cancer is generally administered as concurrent chemoradiation. Injection cisplatin in the dose of 35–40 mg/m^2/weeks for 6 weeks is administered along with radiation. There are many large randomized control trials, which have confirmed the beneficial effect of concurrent chemoradiation. One of the landmark trials is radiation therapy oncology group (RTOG) 90-01[5] which involved comparing RT alone vs. RT with concurrent cisplatin + 5FU. This is the only study where chemotherapy was given during both brachytherapy and external beam components of RT. The first report of this trial was published in 1991 as the authors found highly significant differences in the rate of local control, distant metastasis, DFS and OS favoring Chemotherapy arm.[43] In 2004, the update of the same study confirmed significant improvement in all stages (stage I B to IV) with concurrent CT+RT. The role of cisplatin based CT+RT has proved beneficial. The only question is whether a combination of more than one drug adds to any benefit. Various drugs used are cisplatin, 5FU, epirubicine, mitomycin-C and hydroxyurea.

Recently, newer agents like paclitaxel, carboplatin have been studied. Till today, cisplatin remains the gold standard of care along with radiotherapy. The practical problem is safety of cisplatin in patients with poor performance status, comorbid conditions (cardiac dysfunction, renal dysfunction). The role of full dose adjuvant systemic therapy is investigational.

SALVAGE CHEMOTHERAPY FOR METASTATIC AND RECURRENT DISEASE

In incurable stages of the disease, palliative care (e.g. pain control) is an important issue. Single agent studies have utilized cisplatin, ifosfomide, carboplatin, irinotecan and paclitaxel. The response to non-cisplatin based treatment was 10–20%. It is observed that non-irradiated tissues, like lungs respond better than irradiated areas like pelvis.

Combination chemotherapy: Moore et al.[44] compared cisplatin and paclitaxel vs. cisplatin in a randomized phase III trial, demonstrating improved PFS. Another trial compared cisplatin with or without topotecan, which also showed and improved PFS and OS. The combination of paclitaxel + platinum is a standard of care for this group of patients.

STANDARD PROTOCOLS

Concurrent Chemotherapy: Radiation

- Injection Cisplatin (six doses) 35–40 mg/m^2/week, till completion of radiation.

Advanced Stage Disease

- Injection cisplatin 60–80 mg/m^2/injection carboplatin AUC 4–6
- With injection paclitaxel 175 mg/m^2
- (The cycle to be repeated once every 21 days. The disease status should be reassessed after three cycles and to continue for further three cycles, if a good response is documented).

Role of systemic therapy in the management of cervical cancer:

- Concurrent chemotherapy and radiation. Every patient receiving radiation must receive platinum concurrently to improve local as well as distant disease control
- Palliative chemotherapy with platinum with paclitaxel is the standard of care
- Neoadjuvant chemotherapy before surgery or radiation is investigational.

RADIOTHERAPY

Radiation therapy for cervical cancer is a complementary treatment modality with surgery in all stages of cancer. Historically, brachytherapy with radioactive radium capsules ushered in a new technique of treating cervical cancer. Development in technology of external radiation and brachytherapy have ensured safe and effective delivery of radiation to a radical dose. RT alone was a standard of care till the concept of chemoradiation treatment strategies evolved. Neoadjuvant therapy, chemoradiation and adjunctive RT have been standard of care as a combined modality. Indications for RT are stage specific as discussed hereafter.

STAGE IA–C FIGO

The standard treatment for this stage of disease is surgery; however, those with comorbid conditions, which preclude surgery can be treated effectively with radiation. Treatment usually consists of administering 6,500 cGy to 7,500 cGy to point A in two or three brachytherapy sessions of low dose radiation or its equivalent with high-dose brachytherapy. Nearly all patients survive at 10 years after treatment.[45]

STAGE IA 2

Patients who are poor surgical candidates or those who refuse surgery can be effectively treated with a combination of external pelvic RT and brachytherapy. A dose of 4,500 cGy to 5,000 cGy in 4–5 weeks to pelvic cavity followed by a boost to point A to a dose of 7,500 cGy to 8,000 cGy, with brachytherapy ensures a 95% 5 year survival.[46]

FIGO–STAGE IBI, AND IIA A

Radical RT is an effective modality of treatment. RT consists of combination of external RT to entire pelvis to include primary site, parametrium and pelvic nodes and brachytherapy to boost the point. A dose to 8,000 cGy. Brachytherapy can be administered with low dose rate application or fractionated high dose rate technique. External radiation is restricted to 4,500–5,000 cGy. Patients with clinically evident metastatic lymph node benefit from chemoradiation or by the addition of weekly hyperthermia. The 5-year survival rate following RT or chemoradiation verges on 95 percent.

ADJUVANT POSTOPERATIVE RADIATION THERAPY

Patients with poor prognostic indicators seen following radical hysterectomy for stage 2 BI and II A benefit from postoperative radiation. Involvement of regional nodes, parametrium and positive margins definitely benefit from postoperative RT. Gynecology oncology group (GOG) has clearly demonstrated a significant decrease in local recurrence and improvement at 2 years. Patients with negative lymph nodes but tumor larger than 4 cm, capillary lymphatic space involvement and stromal invasion of more than 1/3rd thickness also require postoperative RT.

Radiation therapy involves 4,500–5,000 cGy to pelvis followed by intra vaginal radiation to boost local radiation by 1,500 cGy. External beam RT is delivered on megavoltage teleradiation equipments. Intensity modulated radiation therapy (IMRT) is a preferred technique as there a strong evidence of reduction in acute gastrointestinal toxicities as compared to three dimensional conformal radiation or conventional RT. Fractionated high dose rate and continuous low dose rate brachytherapy are biologically equivalent. High dose rate (HDR) endocavitary radiation is quick with a more reliable dosimetry.[47]

Locally, advanced disease (FIGO/B2-IV A) are effectively treated with chemoradiation with variable, stage dependent outcome. External beam radiation therapy (EBRT) generally precedes intracavitory radiation to reduce the bulk and improve geometry. This facilitates the optimum application of brachytherapy. Boost with brachytherapy has been a standard of care for decades. However, Low et al. have demonstrated superiority of IMRT over brachytherapy at point A. Coverage was as good as brachytherapy insertion with a less bladder and rectal dose. Extended field radiation of parametrial nodes is not practiced routinely.

Chemoradiation was announced as a standard of care in 1999 by National Cancer Institute. This announcement was based on randomized trials conducted by GOG, RTOG and National Cancer Institute of Canada (NCIC). The randomized trial by NCIC however did not show any benefit with chemo radiation arm. All five positive trials included cisplatin and 5FU or hydroxyurea. Patients who received chemoradiation are at a higher risk of neutropenia and gastrointestinal toxicities. Most of these toxicities are reversible.

The biological rationale for chemoradiation are hypoxic cell sensitization, additive effects, inhibition of cellular repair following damage due to radiation and recruitment of quiescent cells into the proliferating pool. Proliferating cells are more sensitive to radiation.

Drugs other than 5FU and cisplatin have been used but without a strong positive outcome. Mitomycin-C is one of the other drugs.[48] Addition of hypoxic cell sensitizers like senazole and nimorazole also have shown improved outcomes. Zee has similarly demonstrated an improved survival following external locoregional hyperthermia.

Neoadjuvant chemotherapy also has been attempted in stages from IB2, IIA and II B. Randomized trials have not shown any benefit in progression free survival or OS.[49] Neoadjuvant chemotherapy generally enhances the toxicity of RT. Similarly, radiation prior to surgery also has not shown any significant benefit.[50] Patient with stage IV B cervical cancer benefit from brief hypo fractionated radiation with systemic chemotherapy; vesicovaginal or rectovaginal fistula preclude any meaningful local radiation. Local pelvic RT plays a significant role in recurrent cervical cancer following surgery.[51] RT is planned and scheduled according to the extent of recurrence. Chemoradiation must be considered if there are no comorbid conditions.

ACUTE SIDE-EFFECTS

Nausea, vomiting, colicky pain and diarrhea are the most frequent acute side effects seen during external beam radiation. Most of the above side effects can be managed easily with antispasmodics and antiemetics. Clinicians should periodically monitor the nutritional status and intervene at the earliest sign of nutrient depletion. One should guard against the patient slipping into dehydration or electrolyte imbalance. Hypoglycemic attacks are common in diabetics if ant-diabetic agents are not administered and monitored carefully. Erythema and patchy desquamation is seen in some patients. Perivulval reaction in patients with low vaginal disease on occasions can be distressing. Local therapeutic interventions may be required for adequate healing.

LATE SIDE-EFFECTS

Delayed side effects due to radiation are seen in 3–8 % of patients. Technique of comorbid conditions like diabetes mellitus, scleroderma, smoking, prior pelvic infection and surgery enhance the incidence of late side effects like severe proctitis, cystitis and bowel obstruction. Vesicovaginal and rectovaginal fistula is seen in less than 2% of patients. Unsatisfactory application of brachytherapy is a risk factor for development of a fistula.

REFERENCES

1. Population based cancer registry (2008) – ICMR
2. Disaia P, William T. Clinical Gynec Oncology. CV. Mosby and Co; 1969. p. 2
3. Disaia P, William T. Management of the female exposed to Diethylstilbesterol. Clinical Gynec Oncology. CV Mosby and Co; 1969. p. 49
4. Ferlay J, Shin HR, Bray F, et al. GLOBOCAN 2008 v2.0, Cancer Incidence and Mortality Worldwide: IARC CancerBase No. 10 [Internet]. Lyon, France: International Agency for Research on Cancer; 2010.
5. NCRP. Two-year Report of the Population Based Cancer Registries. 2006-2008. National Cancer Registry Programme, Indian Council of Medical Research, 2009, Bangalore, India.
6. Weinstock H, Berman S, Cates W. Sexually transmitted diseases among American youth – Perspects Sex reproduction health - 2004Weinstock H, Bernuan S – Sexually transmitted diseases among American youth. Perspect Sex Reprod Health. 2004;36:6-10.
7. Medeiros LR, Rosa DD, da Rosa MI, et al. Efficacy of human papillomavirus vaccines: a systematic quantitative review. Int J Gynecol Cancer. 2009;19:1166-76.
8. Zimmerman RK. HPV vaccination and its recommendation. J Fam Practice 2007:56(Suppl 1-5).
9. José Alberto Fonseca-Moutinho. Smoking and Cervical Cancer. Obstet Gynecol. 2011;84(7):684.
10. Labani L, Andallu B, Satyanarayana L. Food consumption pattern in cervical carcinoma patients and controls. Indian J Med Paediatr Oncol. 2009;30(2):71-5.
11. Titus-Ernstoff L, Hatch EE, Hoover RN, et al. Long-term cancer risk in women given diethylstilbestrol (DES) during pregnancy. Br J Cancer. 2001;84:126-33.
12. Singh S, Badaya S. Factors Influencing uptake of cervical cancer screening among women in India: A hospital based pilot study. J Community Med Health Educ.2012;2:157.
13. Munger K, Howley PM. Human papillomavirus immortalization and transformation function. Virus Res. 2002;89:213-28.
14. Benedet JL, Bender H, Jones H, et al. FIGO staging, classification and clinical practice guidelines in the management of gynaecologic cancers: FIGO committee on Gynaecologic Oncology. Int J Gynaecol Obstet. 2000;70:209-62.
15. Ylitalo N, Josefsson A, Melbye M, et al. A prospective study showing long term infection with human papillomavirus 16 before the development of cervical carcinoma in situ. Cancer Res. 2000;60:6027-32.
16. Spratt DW, Lee SC. Verrucous carcinoma of the cervix. Am J Obstet Gynaecol. 1977;129:699-700.
17. Young RH, Clement PB, Scully RE. Premalignant and malignant glandular lesions of the uterine cervix. In: Clement PB, Young RH, (eds). Corpus and Cervix. New York: Churchill Livingstone; 1993.

18. Lewis TLT. Colloid (mucus secreting) carcinoma of the cervix. Br J Obstet Gynaecol. 1971;78:1128-32.
19. Moll UM, Chumas JC. Mann WJ, et al. Primary signet-ring cell carcinoma of uterine cervix. N Y State J Med. 1990;90:559-60.
20. Gilks CB, Young RH, Aguirre P, et al. Adenoma malignum (minimal deviation adenocarcinoma) of the uterine cervix : a clinicopathologic and immunohistochemical analysis of 26 cases. Am J Surg Pathol. 1989;13:717-29.
21. Jones MW, Silverberg SG, Kurman J. Well differentiated villoglandular adenocarcinoma of uterine cervix: a clinicopathologic study of 24 cases. Int J of Gynaecol Pathol. 1993;12:1-7.
22. Young RH, Scully RE. Villoglandular adenocarcinoma of uterine cervix: a clinicopathologic analysis of 13 cases. Cancer. 1989;63:1773-9.
23. Kaminski PF, Maier RC. Clear cell adenocarcinoma of cervix unrelated to diethylstilbesterol exposure. Obstet Gynaecol. 1983;62:720-7.
24. Zhou C, Gilks CB, Hayes M, et al. Papillary serous carcinoma of uterine cervix: a clinicopathologic study of 17 cases. Am J Surg Pathol. 1998;22:113-20.
25. Stoler M, Mills SE, Gersell DJ, et al. Small cell neuroendocrine carcinoma of cervix : a human papillomavirus type 18 associated cancer. Am J Surg Pathol. 1991;15:28-32.
26. Papanicolay G. New cancer diagnosis. In: Proceedings of Third race betterment conference. Battle Creek, MI: Race Betterment Foundation. 1928. pp. 528-34.
27. Babes A. Diagnostione du cancer uterion Par les. Prese Med. 1928;36:451-4.
28. Shankarnarayanan A, Neue BM, Shastri SS, et al. HPV screening for cervical cancer in rural India. New Eng J Med. 2009;360:1385.
29. Philips S, Disai A, William T, et al. Preinvasive disease of the cervix, vagina and vulva. Clinical Gynec Oncology. CV Mosby and Co. 1989. p. 19.
30. Eiriksson R, Corens A. Sentinel lymph node biopsy in cervical cancer–The future? Int J Obst Gyne. 2011:129-133
31. Chereau E, Feron JG, Ballestor M, et al. Contribution of Pelvic and Para-aortic lymphadenopathy with Sentinel node biopsy in patients with IB2-IIb cervical cancer. BJ Cancer. 2012:106:39-44.
32. Piver MS, Rutledge FN, Smith PJ. Five classes of extended hysterectomy for women with cervical cancer. Obstet Gynecol. 1974;44:265.
Courtesy: American College of Obstetrician and Gynecologist
33. Fletcher GH, Rutledge FN. Extended field technique in the Management of cancers of the uterine cervix. Am Journ of Roertgeology. 1972;114:116.
34. Rose PG. Chemoradiotherapy for cervical cancer. Eur J Cancer. 2002;38:270-8.
35. Rose PG. Combination therapy: New treatment paradigm for locally advanced cancer? Nat Rev Clin Onc. 2011;388-90.
36. Saibishkumar E, Patel F, Sharma C. Results of a phase II trial of concurrent chemo-radiation in treatment of locally advanced cancer of uterine cervix: an experience from India. Bull Cancer. 2005 92(1) E 7-12
37. Chemo-Radiotherapy for Cervical Cancer Meta analysis Collaboration. Reducing uncertainties about the effects of chemoradiotherapy for cervical cancer: a systematic review and meta-analysis of individual patient data from 18 randomized trials. J Clin Oncol. 2008;26(35):5802-12.
38. Berek JS, Howe C, Lagasse LD, et al. Pelvic exenteration for recurrent gynecologic malignancy: survival and morbidity analysis of the 45-year experience at UCLA. 2005:99:153-9.
39. The neoadjuvant Chemotherapy for Cervical Cancer. Meta-analysis Collaboration. Neoadjuvant Chemotherapy for locally advanced Cervical Cancer: A systematic review and Meta-analysis of individual patient data from 21 randomized trials; Eur J Cancer. 2003;39:2470-86.
40. Katsumata N, Yoshikawa H, Kobayashi H, et al. Phase III Randomized control trial of Neoadjuvant chemotherapy plus radical surgery versus radical surgery alone for stage IB2, IIA2,IIB cervical cancer :a Japan Clinical Oncology Group Trial.(JCOG 0102). Br J Cancer. 2013;108:1957-63.
41. Uegaki K, Shimada M, Sato S, et al. Outcome of stage IB2-II B patients with bulky Uterine cervical cancer who underwent Neoadjuvant Chemotherapy followed by radical hysterectomy. Int J Clin Oncol. 2013 Apr 17 (Epub ahead of print).
42. Singh RB, Chander S, Mohanti BK, et al. Neoadjuvant Chemotherapy with weekly Paclitaxel + Carboplatin followed by Chemo radiation in locally advanced cervical carcinoma: a pilot study. Gynaecol Oncol. 2013; 129(1):124-8.
43. Eifel PJ, Winter K, Morris M, et al. Pelvic irradiation with concurrent chemotherapy versus pelvic to para-aortic irradiation for high-risk cervical cancer: an update of Radiation Therapy Oncology Group trial (RTOG) 90-01. J Clin Oncol. 2004 22(5): 872-80.
44. Moore DH, Blessing JA, McQuellon RP, et al. Phase III study of Cisplatin with or without Paclitaxel in stage IV B, recurrent or persistent Squamous cell Carcinoma of the Cervix; A GOG study. J Clin Oncol. 2004;22:3113-9.
45. Rotman M, Sedlis A, Piedmonte MR, et al. A phase III randomized trial of postoperative pelvic irradiation in Stage IB cervical carcinoma with poor prognostic features: follow-up of a gynecologic oncology group study.Int J Radiat Oncol Biol Phys. 2006;65:169-76.
46. Peters WA 3rd, Liu PY, Barrett RJ 2nd, et al. Concurrent chemotherapy and pelvic radiation therapy compared with pelvic radiation therapy alone as adjuvant therapy after radical surgery in high-risk early-stage cancer of the cervix. J Clin Oncol. 2000;18:1606-13.
47. Eifel PJ. Uterine Cervix, in Radiation Oncology, Rationals, Technique, Result, 8th Edition. JD Cox, Ang KK (Eds). 2002. St.Louis, Mo Mastry.
48. Peter WA. III. Liu PY, Baret RJ, et al. Cisplatinum plus 5 flurouracil plus radiation therapy are superior to radiation therapy as adjuvant in high risk early stage carcinoma of the cervix after radical hysterectomy and pelvic lymphadenectomy : Report of a phase III intergroup study. J Clin Onu. 2000;18:781-6.
49. Green JA, Kirshna JM, Trerney JF, et al, survival and recurrence after concomitant chemotherapy and radiotherapy for cancer of uterine cervix: A systematic review and meta analysis. Lancet. 2001;358:781-6.
50. Tobia J Buxton EJ Blackledger G, et al. Neoadjuvant bleomycin, ifosfamide and cisplatinum in cervical cancer. Cancer Chemother Pharmacol. 1990;26 (suppl.):S59-62.
51. Landoni F, Maneo A, Colombo A, et al. Randomised study of radical surgery versus radiotherapy for stage Ib-IIa cervical cancer. Lancet. 19997:350:535-40.

38 Endometrial Cancer

Praful Desai, Keyuri Patel, Bhavna Parikh, Nagraj G Huilgol, Ganesh Balasubramaniam

INTRODUCTION

Malignancy of the uterine body is the second commonest genital cancer in Indian women after cervical cancer; it is the commonest genital cancer in Western women. Essentially a postmenopausal event, around 10% of premenopausal women are also afflicted by endometrial cancer (EC). Major predisposing factors are obesity, diabetes and hypertension, though genetic predisposition and familial incidence is known. In rare cases of Lynch syndrome (HNPCC; hereditary nonpolyposis colorectal cancer), it is known to be associated with colonic cancers. Exogenous factors of intake of tamoxifen in patients with breast cancer can cause endometrial hyperplasia and thickening and rarely can lead to EC. Unopposed and continual use of estrogen can also predispose toEC. Perimenopausal endometrial hyperplasia, particularly adenomatous and complex hyperplasia is an important premalignant state which needs to be carefully observed and treated.

EPIDEMIOLOGY

Worldwide in 2008, 288,000 women were diagnosed with uterine cancer, the most common gynecologic malignancy in developed countries, with an incidence of 12.9 per 100,000 women and a mortality rate of 2.4 per 100,000.[1] In developing countries, it is the second most common gynecologic malignancy next only to cervical cancer, with an incidence of 5.9 per 100,000 and a mortality rate of 1.7 per 100,000. In India, there are 0.88 million cancer cases with an incidence rate (age-adjusted standardized rate-ASR) of 105.5 per 100,000 in women. It is estimated that there are about 8,800 new ECs annually with an age-adjusted incidence rate of 1.9 per 10^5; thus the incidence of EC is very low in India. The Network of Indian cancer registries reported variation in rates between the registries;[2] the highest rates were observed in Bangalore (4.2 per 10^5) and in Delhi (4.3 per 10^5), while in Mumbai it was 2.8 per 10^5 indicating that this not a major cancer concern.

Associated Factors

There are several risk factors which contribute to the development of EC.

Age: Old age is a known risk factor for all cancers and EC is no exception

Hormones and Contraceptives

It is known that a shift in the balance of estrogen and progesterone with increased estrogen raises a woman's risk for developing EC. In a nationwide population-based case-control study among postmenopausal women aged 50–74 years in a Swedish study on hormonal contraceptives with oral contraceptives [combined oral contraceptives (COCs)] and EC risk, it was found that the use of any oral contraceptive decreased the risk of EC by 30%, while oral progestin reduced the risk significantly and concluded that COC use confers a long-lasting protection against EC. This is particularly so for long-term users[3] and similar findings were reported in a systematic review of EC consisting of more than 15 case-control studies and four large cohort studies.[4] Similarly, in a case-control study conducted to study the association of tamoxifen with EC, it was reported that the risk of EC (Odd's Ratio: OR = 2.4) for tamoxifen users increased with longer usage, extending beyond 5 years (OR = 3.6).[5]

Obesity

Obesity increases EC risk independent of other factors but was not associated with stage or grade of disease.[6] Obese women (BMI > or = 30 kg/m^2) had an increased risk of both [Hazard Rate Ratio (HRR) = 1.6, 95% CI 1.0–2.5] EC (HRR = 2.0) and mortality, compared with nonoverweight women (BMI < 25 kg/m^2).[7]

Early Menarche and Late Menopause

A reduction in EC risk was observed in women with late menarche, early menopause, past oral contraceptive use, high parity and a shorter time since last full-term pregnancy but no association was observed for duration of breast feeding.[8] One of the large cohort study of postmenopausal women from Iowa. USA, reported a positive association with early age at menarche, late age at natural menopause, total length of ovulation span and induced abortion (OR = 2.5).[9]

Family History

It is known that those with a family history of cancer are at a higher risk even for other cancers. In women with no family history, the ORs were 2.1 for those with family history and 1.8 for those without[10] a family history of intestinal cancer was directly associated with EC risk (OR = 1.6) concluding that a family history of endometrial or intestinal cancer in first-degree relatives is associated with an increased risk of EC.

Diabetes and Hypertension

Endometrial cancer with diabetes had an increased risk of all-cause mortality compared with nondiabetic women (HRR = 1.7), although there was no association with EC mortality. History of obesity and diabetes may increase the risk of mortality after EC diagnosis.[11] The relative risk for the association of EC with diabetes was 4.1 and with hypertension 1.6. Diabetics and hypertensives are identifiable risk groups for EC in Finland. Diabetics form a suitable target population for a trial of the efficacy of screening for EC. In another study, history of diabetes was associated with a twofold increased risk of EC among hypertensive women, but no association was observed among nonhypertensive women.[12]

Nulliparity and Infertility

In a large postmenopausal, Caucasian, nulliparous women (360 EC) and Caucasian, parous women (1,378 ECs) from four US prospective studies, EC was higher among nulliparous women;[13] stratified association between EC and hormone-related risk factors did not differ between nulliparous versus parous women. For both groups, oral contraceptives and earlier menopause were associated with a reduced risk. The highest hazard ratio (HR) were for obesity; a BMI of 30 kg/m^2 (versus less than 25 kg/m^2), which increased the risk of EC threefold among nulliparous women (HR = 3.04) and parous women (HR = 2.88).

Dietary red meat and animal fat have been linked to EC risk. In a large, population-based, case-control study in Shanghai, animal-derived iron intake was positively associated with EC risk (OR = 1.9) predominantly after menopause (OR = 2.2) and also in obese women with BMI more than or equal to 25 kg/m^2(OR = 3.2) with EC risk (OR = 1.7).[14] In another Greek study, consumption of pulses, nuts, and seeds was significantly and inversely related to the risk for EC; no other significant association with food groups was detected, although a protective effect of added lipids, which in the Greek diet are primarily represented by olive oil, was highly suggestive and retinol, nicotinic acid, vitamin B-6, and riboflavin were inversely associated with the disease.[15] In evaluating the role of tea and coffee and added substances (sugar/honey, creamers, and milk) on EC risk in a population-based case-control study in six counties in New Jersey reported a moderate inverse association with coffee consumption (OR = 0.65) for women who reported more than two cups/day of coffee compared to none.[16] Tea consumption was not statistically significant (OR = 1.77) and similar finding was reported in another study.[17]

Physical Activity

It is known that physical activity is related to obesity index; among many studies; findings from a study suggested that total physical activity had a weak inverse association with EC risk and that leisure time inactivity was statistically significantly associated with increased risk for EC.[18]

There are many other factors like Lynch syndrome, BRCA, other genetic syndromes, endometrial hyperplasia, etc. which have a higher risk of developing EC.

Survival Rates

There are several studies in India as well from Western countries on survival rate for EC. In a recent study conducted at Tata Memorial Hospital on EC, the 5-year overall survival rate was 92%;[19] the five-year rates indicated better prognosis for those less than 50 years (97%), non-tobacco-chewers (94%), with no family history of cancer (93%), localized disease (93%) and those treated with surgery either alone or as a combination treatment (95%) had improved overall and disease-specific survival for endometrial carcinoma.

PATHOLOGY

Endometrial Hyperplasia

It is a spectrum of estrogen-dependent proliferation ranging from benign changes to premalignant disease. WHO classification[20] is based on degree of architectural complexity and cytologic features.

- Hyperplasia without atypia (simple and complex)
- Hyperplasia with atypia (simple and complex)

In a study by Kurman et al.[21] risk of progression to carcinoma was 23% for atypical hyperplasia and only 2% for nonatypical hyperplasia.

Tamoxifen-related endometrial lesions[22] are seen in patients undergoing long-term treatment with tamoxifen. Endometrial polyps are common, usually large sessile polyps frequently exhibiting metaplastic changes in glands and stroma. Malignant transformation occurs in 3% of cases and the carcinoma is most frequently of endometrioid type.

Endometrial Carcinoma

The most common malignant tumor of the uterine corpus is an Endometrioid adenocarcinoma, which constitutes more than 80% of endometrial carcinoma and shows presence of at least some glandular and villoglandular structures lined by columnar cells with elongated nuclei (Fig. 1). Higher grade lesions show less glandular differentiation and solid nests and sheets of cells. Squamous differentiation is common (Table 1).

Variants: Villoglandular, secretory and ciliated cell types are of low nuclear grade. Grading [International Federation of Gynecology and Obstetrics (FIGO)][23] of endometrioid adenocarcinoma is based on degree of architectural differentiation.

Modified FIGO Grading System

Grade 1: Five percent or less of a nonsquamous or nonmorular solid growth pattern.

Grade 2: Six to fifty percent of a nonsquamous or nonmorular solid growth pattern.

Grade 3: More than 50% of a nonsquamous or nonmorular solid growth pattern.

Cytologic features to be used in formulating final grade:

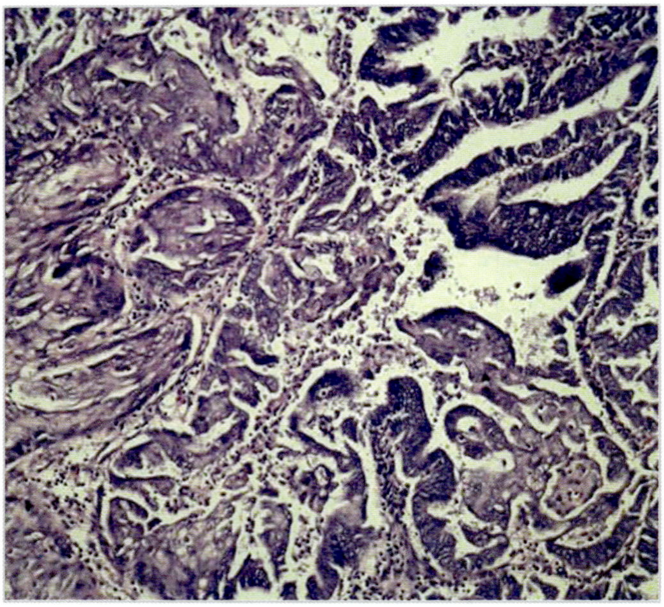

Fig. 1: Endometrioid adenocarcinoma showing the presence of glandular and villoglandular structures are lined by columnar cells with elongated nuclei

- Notable nuclear atypia inappropriate for the architectural grade raises the grade of a Grade 1 or Grade 2 tumor by one level.
- In serous adenocarcinomas, clear cell adenocarcinomas and areas of squamous differentiation, nuclear grade takes precedence over architecture.

Serous papillary carcinoma (Fig. 2) constitutes 5–10% of all endometrial carcinomas. It is characterized by complex papillary architecture, high grade nuclear features, psammomatous calcifications, lack of association with hyperestrogenism and endometrial hyperplasia and aggressive behavior. These tumors show a tendency to develop deep myometrial invasion, extensive lymphatic invasion and presentation with extrauterine spread.[24]

Clear cell adenocarcinoma constitutes 1–5% of all endometrial carcinomas. It is composed of clear or "hobnail" cells arranged in solid, tubulocystic or papillary patterns. It is frequently diagnosed in advanced clinical stage and has poor prognosis.[25] However, if limited to the uterine corpus it has a better prognosis than serous adenocarcinoma of same stage.

Mixed adenocarcinoma is a tumor composed of admixture of endometrioid carcinoma or mucinous carcinoma and serous or clear cell carcinoma in which the minor type must comprise at least 10% of the total volume of the tumor.

Squamous cell carcinoma is often associated with cervical stenosis and pyometra. Primary pure squamous

TABLE 1: Clinicopathologic types of endometrial carcinoma[26]

Type I	*Type II*
40–60 years of age	Elderly
H/o chronic anovulation or estrogen replacement therapy	No H/o hyperestrogenism
Endometrial hyperplasia common	Atrophic non-neoplastic endometrium
Endometrioid histology	Special variant carcinomas or high grade endometrioid carcinoma
Well-differentiated, Stage I, nonmyoinvasive	High stage with deep myoinvasion
ER/PR positive, p53 negative, low Ki-67	ER/PR negative, p53 strongly expressed, high Ki-67 index
Very favorable prognosis after hysterectomy	Molecular genetic abnormalities
	Often not cured by hysterectomy

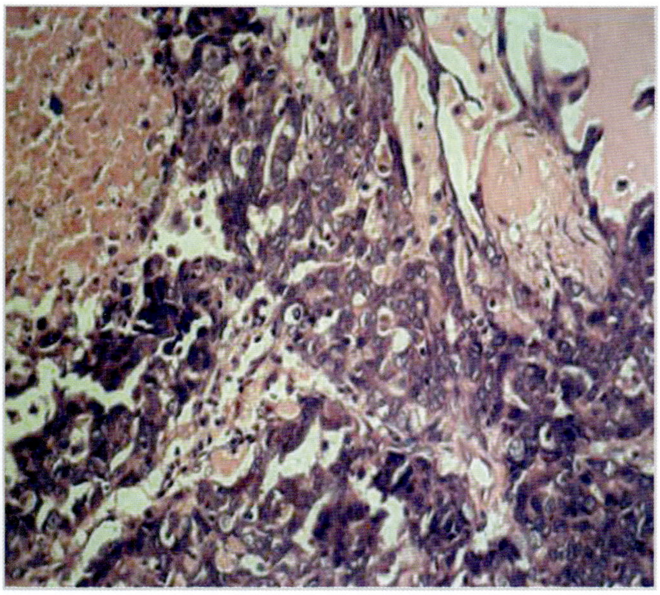

Fig. 2: Serous papillary carcinoma showing complex papillary architecture, high grade nuclear features with psammomatous calcifications

cell carcinoma of endometrium is rare and it is necessary to exclude predominantly squamous differentiation of an endometrioid adenocarcinoma and cervical squamous cell carcinoma extending into endometrium. Prognosis is poor. *Other variants* are rare and include transitional cell carcinoma, small cell carcinoma and undifferentiated carcinoma.

Very rarely secondary metastatic tumors may invade the uterus, either by hematogenous spread or by direct extension from other pelvic malignancies (sigmoid, bladder).

Malignant Mullerian Mixed Tumor (Carcinosarcoma)[27]

There is increasing evidence that these "mixed" tumors are subsets of endometrial carcinoma. Commonly seen in elderly postmenopausal females, these tumors are polypoid, bulky, necrotic and hemorrhagic, filling the endometrial cavity, exhibiting deep myoinvasion and often extending beyond the uterus. Intra-abdominal and retroperitoneal lymph node metastasis are frequent. Histologically, these high grade malignant neoplasms are composed of an admixture of malignant epithelial and mesenchymal components. Epithelial element is usually glandular (endometrioid, serous or clear cell types), rarely squamous or undifferentiated carcinoma. Sarcomatous elements are homologous (undifferentiated sarcoma, leiomyosarcoma (Figs 3A and B), endometrial stromal sarcoma), or heterologous (chondrosarcoma, rhabdomyosarcoma, osteogenic sarcoma, liposarcoma). In some cases, one or the other elements predominate and the biphasic pattern is inconspicuous especially in endometrial curettings.

Clinical Features

Typical symptomatology is postmenopausal bleeding and continuous intermenstrual bleeding in the premenopausal women. Leukorrhic discharges should be adequately investigated with pap-smears (ECs shed cells). Appropriate investigations with a good clinical speculum examination of the cervix and as needed a biopsy of the endometrium (with curettage) with or without hysteroscopy are mandatory. CA-125 estimation is worthwhile after histologic diagnosis. Rarely (10–15%) patients with advanced disease may present with abdominal pain, swelling (rare) or symptoms due to metastasis in the chest or elsewhere. Metastatic lesions may be asymptomatic and may be detected on investigations. Abdominal ultrasonography and a CT/MRI of the abdomen and pelvis are indicated in higher stages of disease, though its use in early stages is debatable (Table 2).

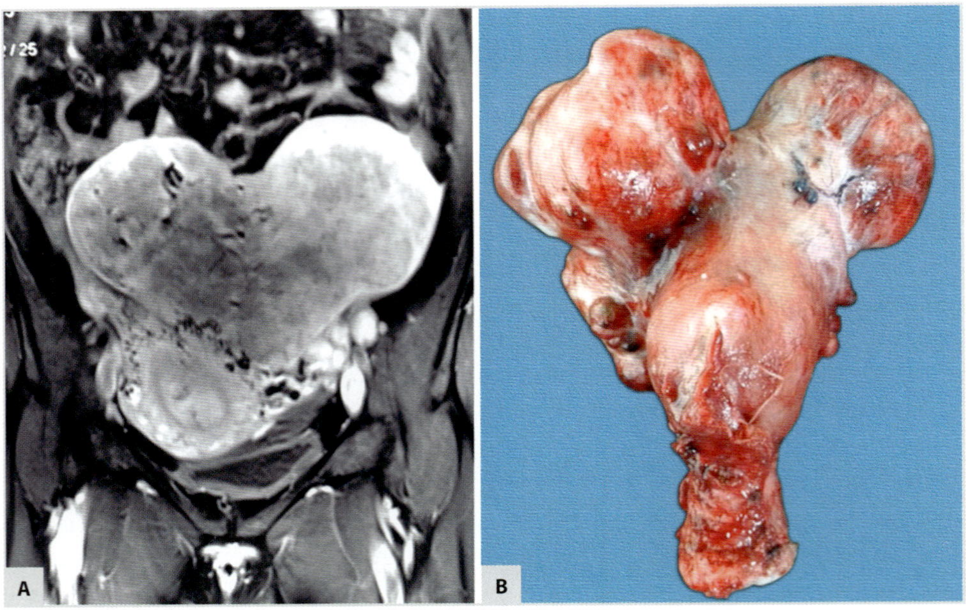

Figs 3A and B: (A) MRI scan of a large lobulated leiomyosarcoma arising from the uterus; (B) Operative specimen of multiple leiomyosarcoma of the uterus shown in the MRI scan

TABLE 2: Practical approach to staging

Staging	*Extension*
I	Lesions localized to the endometrium
I	a. Limited to the endometrial mucosa b. Infiltration into the myometrium < 50% c. Infiltration into the myometrium > 50%
II	Extension to the endocervix
III	a. Extension to parametria and the involvement of serosa of the body of uterus b. Extension to the vagina, adnexa, pelvis c. Extension beyond pelvis, nodal involvement (pelvic and para-aortic)
IV	a. Invasion of bladder, bowel b. Distant metastasis

TREATMENT

The therapy of choice is predominantly surgery though a wide panhysterectomy is worthwhile as adnexal spread is known. In younger premenopausal women the role of oophorectomy is debatable (below 35 years). The risk of adnexal metastasis in 10–15% at a later stage in the follow-up period is significant. For this reasons panhysterectomy remains the therapy of choice. A 1 to 2 cm vaginal margin is necessary as vault recurrences are known.

Lymphadenectomy

Lymphatic spread is mainly limited to pelvic and para-aortic nodes; spread along the broad ligament and round ligament may produce inguinal node metastasis in locally advanced lesions. Lymphovascular spread is predominantly to the para-aortic and para-caval nodes from the fundus and to the pelvis from the body and lower segments of the uterus. The possibility of lymphatic spread in stage I and II disease is minimal (less than 10%); however, in a locally advanced disease (stage III), the incidence of nodal metastasis is significant to merit a pelvic and para-aortic dissection.

Routine lymphadenectomy in stage I and II disease is not of any benefit and can produce complications due to para-aortic and para-caval dissections. A good preoperative imaging study, PET/CT, may give significant information regarding the need for para-aortic dissection up to the level of the renal veins. It is indeed a good practice for palpating the pelvic and para-aortic regions at surgery and consider a dissection if significantly firm nodes are palpable. Sentinel node studies are a clinical research area and is not used routinely by most surgeons for the treatment of ECs. Soft nodes may harbor metastasis; large nodes can be inflammatory in nature. Dissections are justified in advanced cases.

Chemoradiation therapies are important additions for the therapy of EC. If pretherapy work up indicates a disseminated lesion, neoadjuvant chemotherapy is the therapy of choice and adjuvant (postsurgical) chemotherapy is best exhibited when the disease is locally advanced (though resectable) after the surgical treatment.

Postoperative pelvic radiotherapy (RT) is generally administered if the disease is stage II and III. It is not worthwhile in early stage Ia. Pelvic radiotherapy is indicated in stage Ic with >50% myometrial infiltration. Metastatic spread to the skeleton should be managed by RT for relief of pain as indicated and when feasible. Localized metastatic lesions after a long period of disease free survival after primary therapy can be considered for surgery—if feasible after adequate pretherapy assessment.

Systemic Therapy of Uterine Carcinoma

Role of Systemic Therapy in Early Stages (Adjuvant Therapy)

In patients with disease though confined to uterus (stage I), deeply invasive grade III disease, prognosis is relatively poor as many patients develop recurrences despite adjuvant radiation. Currently therefore, chemotherapy sequentially with radiation is advisable in this group of patients and the patients even with completely resected stage II disease.

Patients surgically staged IIIA, IIIB, IIIC, IV are considered for adjuvant systemic therapy. A trial GoG-122[28] was a phase III randomized trial comparing whole abdomen radiation versus combination chemotherapy with doxorubicin and cisplatin. This combination consists of seven cycles plus eighth cycle with cisplatin alone. This regimen produces significant hematologic, gastrointestinal and cardiac toxicities but improved progression free and overall survival in the chemotherapy arm. Adjuvant chemotherapy is therefore mandatory for patients with resected stage III and IV disease.

Systemic Therapy of Recurrent or Metastatic Disease

Hormonal therapy: This is useful only for endometroid histologies. Progestin, tamoxifen, aromatase inhibitors (letrozole), have been given in various schedules and doses. Patients with well-differentiated histology, long disease free interval and those with pulmonary metastasis, this treatment can be considered after conventional therapy is completed. High dose progestin is a preferred agent. Megestrol acetate (megace) 160 mg per day is the usual dose. The median duration of response in various studies has been about 10 months. There is also a concept of alternating tamoxifen with megestrol acetate. Tamoxifen helps upregulate progesterone receptors. This combination may prove more effective.

Role of chemotherapy: It has been proven that combination chemotherapy is a better option than a single agent therapy. Single agent therapy can be used in patients with borderline performance status. In a phase III randomized trial, GoG 177[29], two combination arms were compared. One with cisplatin + doxorubicin + paclitaxel and the other consisted of cisplatin + doxorubicin. The three drug regimen improved survival with significant toxicities; hence, both arms are recognized as approved chemotherapy regimens.

A combination of paclitaxel + carboplatin produces response rates of 40–62% with an overall survival of 13–29 months. This combination is very useful for patients with a papillary serous carcinoma. The biological behavior of this histological subtype is similar to ovarian cancer.

- The role of chemotherapy in surgically resected stage III and IV uterine cancer is well-established. Its role in high risk stage Ic and II is investigative
- For optimally selected patients with recurrent or metastatic disease, hormone therapy is indicated
- Combination chemotherapy is beneficial in patients with recurrent and metastatic disease
- Complex atypical hyperplasia has a very high risk of progressing to invasive carcinoma and requires an aggressive approach.

Protocols

- AP regimen:
  - Injection doxorubicin 60 mg/m^2
  - Injection cisplatin 50 mg/m^2
  - Once every 3 weeks for seven cycles + 1 cycle of only cisplatin
- "TAP" regimen:
  - Injection paclitaxel 160 mg/m^2
  - Injection doxorubicin 45 mg/m^2
  - Injection cisplatin 50 mg/m^2, (along with Filgrastim support)
  - Once every 3 weeks
- Injection paclitaxel 175 mg/m^2
  - Injection carboplatin AUC 6
  - Once every 3 weeks.

Radiotherapy (RT)

Adjunctive RT in early stage intermediate risk endometrial carcinoma decreases the risk of recurrence, but should be limited to patients whose risk factors fit a "high intermediate" risk definition.[30] In patients with higher risk disease-free survival rates are decreased by pelvic and distant relapse. The challenge is to effectively select these high-risk patients who would benefit from adjuvant RT. Excellent level of locoregional control has been achieved with brachytherapy alone. In addition, intermediate-risk patients with an increased risk of recurrence (Grade 3, outer third myometrial involvement, lymphovascular invasion) may be treated with cuff irradiation alone, after surgical staging and a negative lymphadenectomy.

Low-risk Disease (Stages IA and IB Grades 1–2)

There is no need of lymphadenectomy and no postoperative radiotherapy (PORT) is indicated. These patients should be followed after panhysterectomy, and RT can be used as a very effective salvage treatment for an occasional vaginal relapse. Patients with stage IA disease, grade 1-2, and stage IB, grade 1, without evidence of LVSI, have a low risk of nodal metastases and recurrence. Excellent results have been achieved with panhysterectomy alone.[31-33] In the presence of LVSI, grade IVB brachytherapy should be considered.[34]

Intermediate Risk Disease (Stage IA G3, IB G3, IC G1 and 2, Stage II Occult G 1–2, Age 60 or Over)

Omitting RT would increase risk of locoregional recurrence. There is evidence that vaginal brachytherapy reduces the risk of vaginal relapse, with less morbidity and better quality of life. The currently ongoing PORTEC-2 trial randomizes between pelvic RT and vaginal brachytherapy.

High-risk Disease (Stage IC G3, Stage IIA G3, Stage IIB any Grade)

Pelvic RT continues to be the most effective adjuvant treatment to ensure pelvic control.

Stage II

The therapy of choice is total abdominal hysterectomy with bilateral salpingo-oophorectomy. The incidence of lymph node involvement is 25–50 %.Postoperative pelvic RT up to a total dose of 50 Gy +/- vaginal cuff brachytherapy is indicated. Patients undergoing more extensive surgery (Werthiems hysterectomy with LN dissection) with RT show similar survival rates with increased morbidity.

Stage III

Stage IIIa lesions should be managed by extended panhysterectomy and adjuvant RT. Patients with stage IIIb should receive RT and chemotherapy. Salvage surgery is feasible after failure or recurrence after chemoradiotherapy. RT fields are defined by the extent of disease. Patients with positive peritoneal cytology may have a favorable outcome without adjuvant treatment. Treatment recommendations in these patients should be guided by other pathologic findings. In addition, patients with limited pelvic nodal disease or isolated adnexal disease have relatively favorable prognoses and have been historically managed with adjuvant pelvic or extended-field radiotherapy (EFRT). Options for surgical excision in limited recurrence in the pelvis should be considered, if feasible.

Stage IVA

The standard therapy is RT alone with or without chemotherapy. Occasionally some patients without pelvic wall fixation with good performance status may be considered for a surgical consult regarding limited exenterative procedure.

Stage IVB

Patients in this category are treated with palliative intent. RT with/without chemotherapy is given for relief of pain, bleeding, discharge to improve quality of life.

Preoperative Radiation

It is delivered with a tandem, ovoid and Heyman-Simon capsules. The usual dose ranges from 3,500 mg hr Eq to 4,000 mg hr Eq. Ra. to Uterus and 1,800 mg hr Eq. (60 Gy to vaginal mucosa). The vaginal vault is treated with cylinders.

Postoperative Radiation

Adjuvant external beam radiotherapy (EBRT) in early stage EC, (high grade) either after pan-hysterectomy alone or after extended surgical staging, has been shown to improve pelvic tumor control and disease-free survival, when compared with observation, without impact on overall survival.[35-38]

External Beam Radiotherapy

Normal pelvic lymph nodes are poorly visualized by a CT scan; they are better defined by encompassing the contrast-enhanced blood vessels with an expansion of 7 mm.[39] The whole pelvis is treated in patients with positive pelvic nodes to a dose between 45 Gy and 50.4 Gy with conventional fractionation.

Extended field RT including the pelvis and para-aortic region, should be considered for patients with positive pelvic and periaortic nodes. CT simulation is even more crucial when treating extended fields for accurate delineation of the kidneys, small bowel, and liver as well the clinical target volume (CTV). It should include, in addition to the pelvic CTV, the pericaval, interaortocaval and para-aortic areas, defined by contrast-enhanced blood vessels with a modified 7–10 mm margin; the planning target volume is created by expanding the CTV by 5–10 mm for microscopic disease or 10–15 mm for gross residual disease. Generally, the EBRT delivers 45 Gy when treating electively microscopic disease. If there are positive resected periaortic nodes, an additional boost of 500 cGy or higher, depending on the volume of disease and normal organ constraints, could be delivered to the high-risk area, generally using three-dimensional conformal RT or intensity-modulated radiation therapy (IMRT) techniques. The placement of intraoperative vascular clips in the areas of gross disease is very helpful in delineating the boost areas.

More recently, IMRT is being incorporated in the adjuvant treatment of EC, for those patients requiring EBRT, in an attempt to minimize acute and long-term gastrointestinal and genitourinary toxicity.[40,41] In addition, IMRT or intensity-modulated arc therapy allows significant reduction in dose to the bone marrow, which could potentially lead to enhanced hematologic tolerance in high-risk patients undergoing pelvic (with or without para-aortic) irradiation along with systemic chemotherapy.[42-44] However, this technique requires accurate target delineation (CT simulation with intravenous and gastrointestinal contrast required), highly reproducible patient immobilization, and a clear understanding of internal organ motion to achieve optimal advantage in the use of IMRT over conventional methods of post-hysterectomy pelvic radiation therapy.[40,44,45]

Volumes Radiation Therapy

Whole pelvis is treated with anterioposterior/posterio-anterior or four-field box technique. The superior border is placed at L4-L5 junction. Inferiorly the border is placed to include up to upper half of vagina. Laterally the field is placed so as to include 1.5–2 cm lateral to pelvic wall. The anterior border of lateral fields is placed up to pubic symphysis. The posterior border is placed at S2-S3 junction. The superior and inferior borders are the same as the AP/PA field. All the fields are treated on all days. The dose delivered is 1.8–2 Gy per #, 1# per day up to a total dose of 45–50 Gy.

CT scan simulation with oral and intravenous contrast is encouraged. A vaginal marker should be placed in the vagina in addition to seed markers at the most distal tumor extent in the vagina. The gross tumor volume (GTV) includes the entire uterus and cervix as well, and vaginal extension as well as any gross regional lymphadenopathy. The CTV includes the GTV as well as the pelvic lymph node areas which can potentially harbor microscopic disease in the obturator, external, and internal iliac and the lower common iliac region. Careful attention should be paid to include the external iliac anteriorly as well as the presacral nodes posteriorly (S2-S3 level) in the lateral fields as these nodal areas are at high risk in the presence of gross cervical involvement.[46] Generally, patients receive a dose between 45 Gy and 50 Gy (200 cGy/fraction), with a four-field technique (anteroposterior/posteroanterior and lateral fields).

REFERENCES

1. Ferlay J, Shin HR, Bray F, et al. GLOBOCAN 2008 v2.0, Cancer Incidence and Mortality Worldwide: IARC Cancer Base No. 10 [Internet]. Lyon, France: International Agency for Research on Cancer; 2010.
2. NCRP. Two-year Report of the Population Based Cancer Registries- 2006-2008. National Cancer Registry Programme, Indian Council of Medical Research, 2009, Bangalore, India.
3. Weiderpass E, Adami HO, Baron JA, et al. Use of oral contraceptives and endometrial cancer risk (Sweden). Cancer Causes Control. 1999;10(4):277-84.
4. Mueck AO, Seeger H, Rabe T. Hormonal contraception and risk of endometrial cancer: a systematic review. Endocr Relat Cancer. 2010;17(4):R263-71.
5. Swerdlow AJ, Jones ME; British Tamoxifen Second Cancer Study Group. Tamoxifen treatment for breast cancer and risk of endometrial cancer: a case-control study. J Natl Cancer Inst. 2005;97 (5):375-84.
6. Reeves KW, Carter GC, Rodabough RJ, et al. Obesity in relation to endometrial cancer risk and disease characteristics in the Women's Health Initiative. Gynecol Oncol. 2011;121(2):376-82.
7. Chia VM, Newcomb PA, Trentham-Dietz A, et al. Obesity, diabetes, and other factors in relation to survival after endometrial cancer diagnosis. Int J Gynecol Cancer. 2007;17(2):441-6.
8. Dossus L, Allen N, Kaaks R, et al. Reproductive risk factors and endometrial cancer: the European Prospective Investigation into Cancer and Nutrition. Int J Cancer. 2010;127(2):442-51.
9. McPherson CP, Sellers TA, Potter JD, et al. Reproductive factors and risk of endometrial cancer. The Iowa Women's Health Study. Am J Epidemiol. 1996;143(12):1195-202.
10. Lucenteforte E, Talamini R, Montella M, et al. Family history of cancer and the risk of endometrial cancer. Eur J Cancer Prev. 2009;18(2):95-9.
11. Maatela J, Aromaa A, Salmi T, et al. The risk of endometrial cancer in diabetic and hypertensive patients: a nationwide record-linkage study in Finland. Ann Chir Gynaecol Suppl. 1994;208:20-24.
12. Saltzman BS, Doherty JA, Hill DA, et al. Diabetes and endometrial cancer: an evaluation of the modifying effects of other known risk factors. Am J Epidemiol. 2008;167(5):607-14.
13. Schonfeld SJ, Hartge P, Pfeiffer RM, et al. An aggregated analysis of hormonal factors and endometrial cancer risk by parity. Cancer. 2013;119(7):1393-40.

14. Kallianpur AR, Lee SA, Xu WH, et al. Dietary iron intake and risk of endometrial cancer: a population-based case-control study in Shanghai, China. Nutr Cancer. 2010;62(1):40-50.
15. Petridou E, Kedikoglou S, Koukoulomatis P, et al. Diet in relation to endometrial cancer risk: a case-control study in Greece. Nutr Cancer. 2002;44(1):16-22.
16. Bandera EV, Williams-King MG, Sima C, et al. Coffee and tea consumption and endometrial cancer risk in a population-based study in New Jersey. Cancer Causes Control. 2010;21(9):1467-73.
17. Je Y, Hankinson SE, Tworoger SS, et al. A prospective cohort study of coffee consumption and risk of endometrial cancer over a 26-year follow-up. Cancer. Epidemiol Biomarkers Prev. 2011;20(12):2487-95.
18. Friberg E, Mantzoros CS, Wolk A. Physical activity and risk of endometrial cancer: a population-based prospective cohort study. Cancer Epidemiol Biomarkers Prev. 2006;15(11):2136-40.
19. Balasubramaniam G, Sushama S, Rasika B, et al. Hospital-based study of endometrial cancer survival in Mumbai, India. Asian Pacific J Cancer Prev. 2013;14(2):977-80.
20. Scully RE, Bonfiglio TA, Kurman RJ, Silverberg SG, Wilkinson EJ. Uterine corpus. In: World Health Organization: Histologic Typing of Female Genital Tract Tumors. New York: Springer Verlag; 1994. pp. 13-31.
21. Kurman RJ, Kaminski PF, Norris HJ. The behaviour of endometrial hyperplasia. A long term study of 'untreated' hyperplasia in 170 patients. Cancer. 1985;56(2):403-12.
22. Cohen I, Atlaras MM, Shapira J, et al. Time dependent effect of tamoxifen therapy on endometrial pathology in asymptomatic postmenopausal breast cancer patients. Int J Gynecol Pathol. 1996;15(2):152-7.
23. Creasman WT. New gynecologic cancer staging. Obstet Gynecol. 1990;75(2):287-8.
24. Jordan LB, Abdul Kader M, al Nafussi A. Uterine serous papillary carcinoma: histopathologic changes within the female genital tract. Int J Gynecol Cancer. 2001;11:283-9.
25. Abeler VM, Vergote IB, Kjorstad KE, et al. Clear cell carcinoma of the endometrium. Prognosis and metastatic pattern. Cancer. 1996;78(8):1740-7.
26. Bokhman JV. Two pathogenetic types of endometrial carcinoma. Gynecol Oncol. 1983;15(1):10-7.
27. Silverberg S, Major F, Blessing J, et al. Carcinosarcoma (malignant mixed mesodermal tumor) of the uterus. A Gynecologic Oncology Group pathologic study of 203 cases. Int J Gynecol Pathol. 1990;9(1):1-19.
28. Randall ME, et al. Randomized phase III trial of whole abdominal irradiation versus doxorubicin and cisplatin. Chemotherapy in advanced endometrial carcinoma: a Gynecologic oncologic group study. J Clin Oncol. 2006;24(1):36-44.
29. Fleming GF, Brunetto VL, Cella D, et al. Phase III trial of doxorubicin plus cisplatin with or without paclitaxel plus filgrastim in advanced endometrial carcinoma: a Gynecologic Oncology Group Study. J Clin Oncol. 2004;22(11):2159-66
30. Keys HM, Roberts JA, Brunetto VL, et al. A phase III trial of surgery with or without adjunctive external pelvic radiation therapy in intermediate risk endometrial adenocarcinoma: a Gynecologic Oncology Group study. Gynecologic Oncology. 2004;92(3):744-51.
31. Creasman WT, Morrow CP, Bundy BN, et al. Surgical pathologic spread patterns of endometrial cancer. A Gynecologic Oncology Group Study. Cancer. 1987;60(8 Suppl):2035-41.
32. Mariani A, Webb MJ, Keeney GL, et al. Low-risk corpus cancer: is lymphadenectomy or radiotherapy necessary? Am J Obstet Gynecol. 2000;182(6):1506-19.
33. Morrow CP, Bundy BN, Kurman RJ, et al. Relationship between surgical-pathological risk factors and outcome in clinical stage I and II carcinoma of the endometrium: a Gynecologic Oncology Group study. Gynecol Oncol. 1991;40(1):55-65.
34. Mariani A, Dowdy SC, Keeney GL, et al. Predictors of vaginal relapse in stage I endometrial cancer. Gynecol Oncol. 2005;97(3):820-27.
35. Aalders J, Abeler V, Kolstad P, et al. Postoperative external irradiation and prognostic parameters in stage I endometrial carcinoma: clinical and histopathologic study of 540 patients. Obstet Gynecology. 1980;56:419-27.
36. Creutzberg CL, van Putten WL, Koper PC, et al. Surgery and postoperative radiotherapy versus surgery alone for patients with stage-1 endometrial carcinoma: multicentre randomised trial. PORTEC Study Group. Post Operative Radiation Therapy in Endometrial Carcinoma. Lancet. 2000;355:1404-11.
37. Creutzberg CL, van Putten WL, Koper PC, et al. Survival after relapse in patients with endometrial cancer: results from a randomized trial. Gynecol Oncol. 2003;89(2):201-9.
38. Keys HM, Roberts JA, Brunetto VL, et al. A phase III trial of surgery with or without adjunctive external pelvic radiation therapy in intermediate risk endometrial adenocarcinoma: a Gynecologic Oncology Group study [erratum appears in Gynecol Oncol 2004;94:241-242]. Gynecol Oncol. 2004;92:744-51.
39. Taylor A, Rockall AG, Reznek RH, et al. Mapping pelvic lymph nodes: guidelines for delineation in intensity-modulated radiotherapy. Int J Radiat Oncol Biol Phys. 2005;63(5):1604-12.
40. Ahamad A, D'Souza W, Salehpour M, et al. Intensity-modulated radiation therapy after hysterectomy: comparison with conventional treatment and sensitivity of the normal-tissue-sparing effect to margin size. Int J Radiat Oncol Biol Phys. 2005;62:1117-24.
41. Mundt AJ, Mell LK, Roeske JC. Preliminary analysis of chronic gastrointestinal toxicity in gynecology patients treated with intensity-modulated whole pelvic radiation therapy. Int J Radiat Oncol Biol Phys. 2003;56(5):1354-60.
42. Brixey CJ, Roeske JC, Lujan AE, et al. Impact of intensity-modulated radiotherapy on acute hematologic toxicity in women with gynecologic malignancies. Int J Radiat Oncol Biol Phys. 2002;54(5):1388-96.
43. Lujan AE, Mundt AJ, Yamada SD, et al. Intensity-modulated radiotherapy as a means of reducing dose to bone marrow in gynecologic patients receiving whole pelvic radiotherapy. Int J Radiat Oncol Biol Phys. 2003;57(2):516-21.
44. Wong E, D'Souza DP, Chen JZ, et al. Intensity-modulated arc therapy for treatment of high-risk endometrial malignancies. Int J Radiat Oncol Biol Phys. 2005;61(3):830-41.
45. Mundt AJ, Lujan AE, Rotmensch J, et al. Intensity-modulated whole pelvic radiotherapy in women with gynecologic malignancies. Int J Radiat Oncol Biol Phys. 2002;52(5):1330-7.
46. Henriksen E. The lymphatic spread of carcinoma of the cervix and the body of the uterus: a study of 420 necropsies. Am J Obstet Gynecol. 1949;58(5):924-42.

39 Management of Lung Cancer

Ramakant Deshpande, Tanveer Abdul Majeed

INTRODUCTION

Lung cancer ranks among the most common and most lethal malignancies, worldwide. Only about 15.6% of all lung cancer patients live 5 years or more after diagnosis. With the advent of video-assisted thoracic surgery, there has been significant decrease in postoperative morbidity, analgesic requirement and hospital stay. Lobectomy with mediastinal lymph node dissection is considered the optimum surgical procedure, however, in patients with poor pulmonary reserve sublobar resections can be considered. Prognostic and predictive biomarkers like epidermal growth factor receptor (EGFR), excision repair cross-complementation 1 (ERCC 1), Kras oncogene, ribonucleotide reductase M 1 (RRM 1) and echinoderm microtubule-associated protein like-4 (EML 4) anaplastic lymphoma kinase (ALK) fusion oncogene has revolutionized treatment of lung cancer. Radiofrequency ablation techniques have become a useful modality for medically inoperable lung cancer in a selected group of patients.

EPIDEMIOLOGY

India

In India Lung cancer was initially thought to be extremely rare.[1] However, currently the frequency is higher. Earlier studies quoted the incidence as follows: 14.4% of 9,210 consecutive autopsies by Banker (1957)[2], Sirsat (1958) reported that lung cancer formed 1% of all cancers in Tata Cancer Hospital.[3] The National Cancer Registry Program of the Indian Council of Medical Research (ICMR) which collected data from six different parts of the country, both rural and urban areas, showed varying figures at different areas.[4] While cancer of the trachea, bronchus and lungs was the most common form of malignancy in males in 1989 from Bombay, Delhi and Bhopal, it was the second most common in Madras and third in Bangalore, and was most unusual in Barshi, a rural area. The disease was most uncommon in females and in Bombay, it was the sixth common malignancy and Bhopal it was the seventh. Recent International GLOBOCAN study (2008), has shown that in India, lung cancer is the commonest cancer in men with an incidence of 10.9%, mortality of 13% and 5 years prevalence of 3.5%, where as in women, it is fifth most common cancer with an incidence of 2.2%, mortality of 2.5% and 5 years prevalence of 0.5%. Recent study by Noronha V, Dikshit et al. (2012), from Tata Memorial Hospital, Mumbai has shown that the male:female ratio of 3.5:1.[5]

International

Lung cancer is the most common cancer globally for several decades, and by 2008, there was an estimated 1.61 million new cases, representing 12.7% of all new cancers. The majority of cases now occur in developing countries (55%). In 2012 (226,000) new cases (116,000 in men and 110,000 women) of lung and bronchial cancer will be diagnosed and 160,000 deaths are estimated to occur because of disease.[6] During 2005, approximately 500,000 lung cancers were diagnosed in China.[7] Recently, Sano and Marugame[8] determined cumulative risks of lung cancer incidence from data derived from 22 cancer registries from five continents. In all registries, cumulative lung cancer risks were higher in males than females. Globally, the incidence is highest among both African-American men and women, lowest among Swedish men, French and Korean women. The global rise in lung cancer incidence, together with the fact that the overall 5-year survival of patients with this disease is less than 15%, underscores the magnitude of the lung cancer epidemic.

ETIOLOGY

Smoking is the most important causal factor for development of non-small-cell lung carcinoma (NSCLC). The risk of lung cancer is directly dependent on number of packs and pack years of cigarette smoking. Cigarette smoke contains more than 300 chemicals, 40 of which are known to be potent carcinogens. Of particular significance, 4-(methylnitrosamino)-I-(3-pyridil)-1-butanone nicotine-derived nitrosamine ketone (NNK), polyaromatic hydrocarbons (PAH) such as benzo-A-pyrene induced pulmonary carcinomas.[9] PAHs in tobacco smoke form deoxyribonucleic acid (DNA) adducts,[10] which induce mutations within tumor suppressor genes such as the p53, Ras-association domain family 1 isoform A (RASSF1A), and fragile histidine triad (FHIT), thereby, disrupting cell cycle regulation, DNA repair and apoptosis. The carcinogenic effects of tobacco smoke are not simply related to NNK and PAH, but are also directly attributable to nicotine as well as inorganic metals such as nickel, arsenic and chromium. Bidi is more carcinogenic as shown by other studies by Jussawalla and Jain (1979)[11] and Pakhala et al. (1990).[12] Hooka smoking has been associated with lung cancer by Nafae et al. (1973).[13] Smoking of bidi and hooka as well as cigarettes had similar overall risks.[14] Most cigarettes consumed in industrialized nations contain filters, which reduce tar within inhaled smoke, resulting in deposition of carcinogens deeper in the lungs and accounts, for the emergence of adenocarcinomas as the dominant lung cancer. Peto et al.[15] reported a 16-fold increase in cumulative lung cancer risk in persistent smokers; this risk is doubled for individuals who initiate smoking before age 15, which means the risk is dependent on duration and intensity of smoking. The risk decreases following cessation of smoking.

Individuals exposed to environmental tobacco smoke (ETS) inhale tobacco carcinogens at levels significantly lower than active smokers. Nevertheless, ETS is genotoxic,[16] and case-control as well as cohort studies indicate that ETS increases lung cancer risk, and contributes to 25% of all lung cancers in nonsmokers.[17,18]

Occupational and Environmental Exposure

A variety of occupational and environmental exposures have been implicated in the pathogenesis of lung cancer.

Asbestos

In individual exposed to asbestos studies as early as 1950s have demonstrated seven to tenfold increase in lung cancer risk,[19] is dose-related and with smoking exhibit multiplicative effects. It usually follows 30–35 years after exposure.

Heavy Metals

Including nickel, cobalt, cadmium and chromium have been implicated as potential pulmonary carcinogens.[20,21] Exposure to these metals typically occurs among foundry workers and welders, with lung cancer risk appearing to be increased in individuals with high levels of exposure.

Ionizing Radiation

Exposures to high energy transfer agents such as neutrons, plutonium or radon, as well as low energy transfer sources such as X-rays and gamma rays increase lung cancer risk. An increased incidence of lung cancer has been observed among atomic bomb survivors.[22] Radon, an inert gas resulting from radioactive decay of uranium, is associated with increased rates of lung cancer and cigarette smoking exhibits synergistic effects.[23]

Genetic Predisposition

Smokers with germline mutations in Li-Fraumeni syndrome have a threefold increase in lung cancer risk.[24] Vineis et al.[25] examined the cumulative effects of cytochrome P450, family 1, member A1 (CYP1A1), Glutathione S-transferase Mu 1 (GSTM1) and glutathione S-transferase theta 1 (GSTT1), and observed that risk of lung cancer was nearly eightfold higher in patients with CYPA1*23 or CYP1A1*4 with double deletion of GSTM1 and GSTT1. Wang et al.[26] observed that a polymorphism of X-ray repair complementing defective repair in Chinese hamster cells 3 (XRCC3) producing a variant T allele genotype was significantly associated with lung cancer risk in African-Americans and Mexican-Americans (odds ratio = 5.2, 1.6–17).

Diet and Lung Cancer

β-carotene was hypothesized to have a protective role. However, none of the three large subsequent trials showed a chemoprotective effect from beta-carotene or vitamins A or E dietary supplements.[27-30] Two of the trials [Alpha-Tocopherol, Beta-Carotene Cancer Prevention (ATBC) trial and Beta Carotene and Retinol Efficacy Trial (CARET)] showed an increased risk for lung cancer in the study participants who received beta-carotene. Case control studies from China have shown that vegetable intake is a protective factor for lung cancer.[31] Plant carotenoids alpha-carotene (found in carrots and tomatoes) and lycopene (found in tomatoes) are associated with 20–25% lower risk of lung cancer.[32] Flavinoids (found in apples) and isothiocyanates (found in cruciferous vegetables) has also been found to reduce the risk for lung cancer.[33]

PATHOLOGY

Adenocarcinoma

Adenocarcinoma are the most common types of lung cancer, they arise in smaller airways are most often located in the periphery of the lung. The precursor lesion for pulmonary adenocarcinoma is considered to be atypical alveolar hyperplasia (AAH).[34]

Bronchoalveolar Carcinoma

This has two variants, multifocal fatal mucinous variant and nonmucinous composed type II pneumocytes or Clara cells. These cancers, particularly those arising in nonsmoking females of Asian descent exhibit unique EGFR mutations that confer exquisite sensitivity to EGFR-tyrosine kinase inhibitors (EGFR-TKI) such as erlotinib and gefitinib.[35] There are five subtypes, A to E of bronchoalveolar carcinoma.

Large Cell Carcinoma

Account for approximately 15% of all lung cancers. The World Health organization (WHO) classification recognizes basaloid, lymphoepithelioma like, and clear cell types, they differ little clinically.[36,37] The prognosis of large cell undifferentiated carcinoma is similar to that of adenocarcinomas.

Squamous Cell Carcinoma

Classically arises in proximal segmental bronchi via progression through stages of dysplasia. Histologically, they are composed of sheets of epithelial cells with individual cell keratinization, intercellular bridges, or pearl formation.[38] They tend to be slow-growing, and progression of in situ carcinoma to a clinically apparent tumor takes 3–4 years.

Adenosquamous Carcinomas

Adenosquamous carcinomas have histologic areas differentiated as both squamous cell carcinoma and adenocarcinoma. They are predominantly found in the periphery of the lung and behave like adenocarcinoma. Studies suggest that they are a cytogenetically distinct entity.[39]

Carcinoids

Carcinoids manifest a prominent neuroendocrine phenotype in morphology, immunohistochemistry, and ultrastructural features. Typical carcinoids are usually found in large bronchi and feature an organoid pattern. Peripheral carcinoids are often peripheral and spindle-cell tumors. Both are low-grade tumors with a low incidence of metastases. Anaplastic carcinoids are classified as large cell neuroendocrine carcinomas, and have a very poor prognosis.[40]

Small Cell Carcinoma

It is a different entity belonging to neuroendocrine group characterized by very rapid growth and advanced stage at presentation. It is classified based on Veterans' Administration Lung Study Group (VALSG) as limited stage and extensive disease. The most common presentation is extensive disease. It has a spectrum of paraneoplastic disease differing from adenocarcinoma lung. The vast majority of patients in whom the syndrome of inappropriate antidiuretic hormone (SIADH), Cushing's syndrome or neurologic paraneoplastic syndrome develops have small cell lung cancer (SCLC). Prognosis is dismal inspite of aggressive treatment regimes which include aggressive chemotherapy and radiotherapy (RT) for limited disease. Prophylactic cranial irradiation is usually given in both limited and extensive stage disease. Rarely surgery is offered for limited disease usually presenting as peripheral nodule less than 2 cm in diameter.

Other rare types are pleomorphic carcinomas and carcinomas of salivary gland type.

MODES OF DISSEMINATION

Lymphatic Dissemination (Fig. 1)[42]

In the lung tissue, lymphatic drainage parallels the bronchoarterial system, with lymph nodes situated

TABLE 1: Staging of lung cancer [American Joint Committee on Cancer (AJCC) 7th Staging System][41]

T stage	*Primary tumor*	*N Stage*	*Regional lymph nodes*	*Anatomic Stage / Prognostic Group*
Tx	Primary tumor cannot be assessed	Nx	Regional lymph nodes not assessed	Occult Carcinoma: TxN0M0
T0	No evidence of primary tumor	N0	No regional lymph node metastasis	Stage O: TisN0M0
Tis	Carcinoma in situ	N1	Metastasis in ipsilateral peribronchial and/or ipsilateral hilar lymph nodes and intrapulmonary nodes	Stage IA: T1aN0M0 T1bN0M0
T1	Tumor 3 cm or less in greatest dimension surrounded by lung or visceral pleura without bronchoscopic invasion of proximal lobar bronchus	N2	Metastasis in ipsilateral mediastinal and/or subcarinal lymph nodes	Stage IB: T2aN0M0
T1a	Tumor 2 cm or less in greatest dimension	N3	Metastasis in contralateral mediastinal, contralateral hilar, ipsilateral or contralateral scalene or supraclavicular lymph node	Stage IIA: T2bN0M0 T1aN1M0 T1bN1M0 T2aN1M0
T1b	Tumor more than 2 cm but 3 cm or less in greatest dimension	[M]	Metastasis	Stage IIB: T2bN1M0 T3N0M0
T2	Tumor more than 3–7 cm or less, involves main bronchus, 2 cm or more distal to carina; invades visceral pleura; associated with atelectasis or obstructive pneumonitis that extends to the hilar region but does not involve the entire lung	M0	No distant metastasis	Stage IIIA: T1a-1b N2M0 T2a-2b N2M0 T3 N1M0 T3 N2M0 T4 N0M0 T4 N1M0
T2a	Tumor more than 3 cm but 5 cm or less in greatest dimension	M1	Distant metastasis	Stage IIIB: T1a-1b N3M0 T2a-2b N3M0 T3 N3M0 T4 N2M0 T4 N3M0
T2b	Tumor more than 5 cm but 7 cm or less in greatest dimension	M1a	Separate tumor nodule(s) in a contralateral lobe, tumor with pleural nodules or malignant pleural/pericardial effusion	Stage IV: AnyT, AnyN, M1a AnyT, AnyN, M1b
T3	Tumor more than 7 cm or one that directly invades any of the following: parietal pleura, chest wall (Including superior sulcus tumors), diaphragm, phrenic nerve, mediastinal pleura, parietal pericardium or tumor within the main bronchus less than 2 cm distal to carina but without involvement of the carina; or associated atelectasis or obstructive pneumonitis of the entire lung or separate tumor nodule in the same lobe	M1b	Distant metastasis (in extra thoracic organs)	The uncommon superficial spreading tumor of any size with its invasive component limited to bronchial wall, which may extend proximally in to main bronchus, is also classified as T1a
T4	Tumor of any size that invades any of the following: mediastinum, heart, great vessels, trachea, recurrent laryngeal nerve, esophagus, vertebral body, carina, separate tumor nodule in a different ipsilateral lobe			In case after repeated pleural/pericardial aspiration cytological diagnosis is negative, fluid is non hemorrhagic and not an exudates, it should be classified as M0

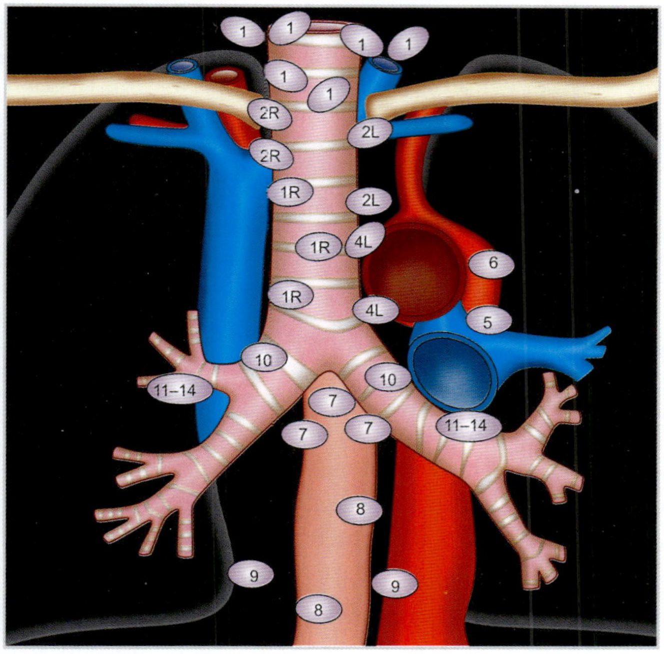

Fig. 1: Mediastinal lymph node stations

(*Courtesy:* Photographs taken from Radiology Assistant website. With kind permission for reprint from Robin Smithus, Radiology Department of the Rijnland Hospital, Leiderdorp, Netherlands)[42]

adjacent to the segmental or lobar bronchi. Lower lobe lymphatics drain to the posterior mediastinum and the subcarinal lymph nodes. Right upper lobe lymphatics drain toward the superior mediastinum. Left upper lobe lymphatics typically course lateral to the aorta and subclavian artery in the anterior mediastinum, as well as along the left main bronchus to the superior mediastinum.

Finally all of these lymphatic channels drain into the right lymphatic or left thoracic ducts, which empty into the subclavian veins. Although skip metastases can occur, antegrade lymphatic metastases most commonly exhibit sequential involvement of bronchopulmonary (N1), mediastinal (N2 and N3), and supraclavicular (N3) lymph nodes. Retrograde lymphatic spread to the pleural surface can occur, particularly with peripheral tumors.

Direct Extension

The primary tumor can invade contiguous structures, such as the bronchus, mediastinal pleura, great vessels, heart, esophagus, diaphragm or chest wall. Once vascular or lymphatic invasions occur, metastatic dissemination to distant sites is common. The most common sites of metastases are bone, liver, adrenals and brain.

Metastases within the lung result from a variety of mechanisms including endobronchial embolization, retrograde lymphatic, as well as hematogenous dissemination.

CLINICAL FEATURES

The signs and symptoms manifested by patients suffering from lung cancer depend on the location, size, number of metastases, histology and extent of locoregional invasion.

Many patients present with an asymptomatic lesion discovered incidentally on chest radiography or computed tomography (CT) scan.

- A persistent cough for a period of 8 weeks or longer. The cough may be dry or may be associated with expectoration and/or hemoptysis
- Dyspnea is a predominant symptom in presence of pleural effusion or bilateral carcinomatosis
- Involvement of recurrent laryngeal nerve may produce hoarseness
- Repeated lung infections such as bronchitis or pneumonia may be due to associated endobronchial tumor causing complete or partial blockage to drainage of lung segment
- Metastatic lesions in the brain, pathological fractures may be the first symptoms at presentation, sometimes there may be pyrexia of unknown origin.

Paraneoplastic syndrome is seen occasionally with lung cancer and consists of a group of symptoms caused by hormone-like substances secreted by tumors. It is seen most often with SCLCs, squamous cell lung cancers and large cell carcinomas. Paraneoplastic symptoms may include an elevated calcium level in the blood (hypercalcemia), a low sodium level, weakness in the upper limbs, loss of coordination and muscle cramps among other symptoms. Secretion of adrenocorticotropic hormone (ACTH) may produce Cushing's syndrome, like symptoms of raised blood pressure, obesity.

DIAGNOSIS OF LUNG CANCER

History and Physical Examination

History and physical examination remains the most important steps of assessing a patient with lung cancer. Smoking history, occupational/environmental exposures, and family history should be documented. Physical examination should determine the presence of clubbing (pulmonary osteoarthopathy), supraclavicular, cervical axillary lymphadenopathy and deep vein thrombosis. Systemic examination should focus on symptoms of advanced locoregional or metastatic disease.

Imaging

X-ray Chest [Posterioanterior (PA) and Lateral films]

X-ray chest is the most common initial investigation performed for lung cancer which usually reveals large peripheral lesions or central obstructing lesions; however, a normal chest X-ray does not exclude a primary lung cancer. In fact, conventional chest radiographs fail to detect nearly 80% of the histologically proven CT-detected lung cancers 2.0 cm or more in diameter.[43]

Contrast enhanced CT scan (Figs 2A and B) should include (chest and upper abdomen to rule out adrenal metastases), conventional CT scans have a sensitivity of 60% and specificity of approximately 80% for the detection of lung cancer. The diagnostic accuracy of CT scans can be further improved by utilization of super high-resolution scanning techniques, which have a sensitivity and specificity of approximately, 85–100%, respectively, for the detection of malignant endoluminal or obstructive lesions involving the airway.[44] CT scans are unreliable for detection of mediastinal lymph node metastases as lymph nodes more than 1 cm in transverse diameter suggests malignant lymphadenopathy, enlarged but histologically benign lymph nodes are frequently observed. Similarly, about 15% lymph nodes less than 1 cm may contain foci of malignant cells.

Fludeoxyglucose positron emission tomography (FDG-PET) scans are extremely useful for the detection of mediastinal lymph node as well as visceral and bony metastases due to the avid uptake of the FDG by most common lung cancer histologies. The overall accuracy, sensitivity and specificity of PET scans approximates 70%, 70% and 80%, respectively, compared with 70%, 50% and 70%, for CT scans in detection of histologically confirmed mediastinal lymph node metastases. Furthermore, FDG-PET scans are considerably superior to CT scans for the detection of N1 disease (42% versus 13%; P = 0.017) in patients with potentially operable lung cancers. The positive predictive value of PET scans for detection of N1 or N2 nodal metastases is only 60%, however, the negative predictive value of PET imaging approximates 90%.[45,46] False positive PET results are high in India due to associated granulomatous inflammation (tuberculosis, silicosis) and in tumors with low metabolic activity (bronchoalveolar or mucoepidermoid carcinomas). Integrated PET-CT scans are superior to either of these modalities for staging lung cancers (sensitivity, specificity and accuracy approximating 80%, 95% and 90%, respectively).[47-49]

Endoscopic ultrasound (EUS) has evolved as an important relatively noninvasive method for evaluating mediastinal lymph nodes in lung cancer patients.[50] It can detect lesions 3 mm or more, however, cannot assess pretracheal (station 3) or ascending aorta (station 6) lymph node status. Studies have confirmed that EUS detected more lymph nodes than either CT or PET, and that the sensitivities, specificities and accuracies were as follows: 57%, 74% and 67%, for CT scans, 73%, 83% and 79% for PET scans, and 94%, 71% and 92% for EUS.[50,51]

Magnetic resonance imaging (MRI) scans of the chest is useful for evaluation of tumors invading the spine, great vessels or brachial plexus. In asymptomatic patients with early-stage NSCLC, gadolinium-enhanced brain MRI scans are superior to CT scans for the detection of occult intracranial metastases with suspected stage III/IV disease.[52]

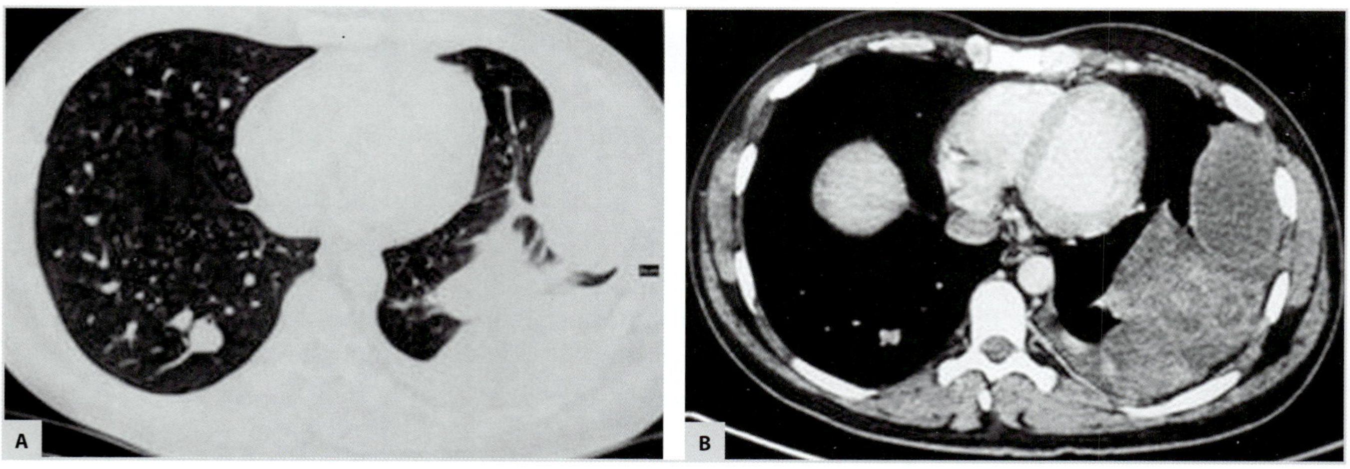

Figs 2A and B: Computed tomography (CT) scan showing lung mass in left lower lobe with left pleural effusion: (A) Lung window; and (B) Mediastinal window

Tissue Diagnosis

Sputum Cytology

Sputum cytology is based on the cytological analysis of exfoliated respiratory cells in sputum. It is rapid, inexpensive method for establishing tissue diagnosis. The sensitivity of sputum cytology is 65% (range, 22–98%) in the setting of established cancer. The diagnostic yield is enhanced in centrally located lesions, squamous cell carcinomas, and large tumors, particularly if multiple sputum samples are examined.[53] The diagnostic yield is also increased using a various molecular techniques such as nuclear image analysis, immunohistochemical evaluation of p53 and many more.

Percutaneous fine-needle aspiration (FNA) is an excellent method for establishing tissue diagnosis of pulmonary nodules. This can be performed using fluoroscopic or CT-guided techniques. The positive yield in experienced hands exceeds 95% even if lesions are less than 1 cm in diameter. However, negative and indeterminate biopsies must be interpreted with caution when there is high degree of clinical suspicion. FNA is suitable for more peripherally located lesions and metastatic disease. Core needle biopsy is preferred for diagnosis as the tissue yield can be used for study of molecular markers prior to therapy. FNA and Core-needle biopsy are contraindicated in central lesions or those lesions deeply embedded in the lung parenchyma due to proximity of great vessels; in such circumstances, a bronchoscopic biopsy is a suitable alternative.

Fiberoptic bronchoscopy (FOB) is an important investigation in patients suspected of having lung cancer. It is performed usually via transtracheal anesthesia by instilling 4% lignocaine by cricothyroid membrane puncture. FOB enables visualization of the tracheobronchial tree to the second or third segmental divisions. It is useful for obtaining cytologic or histologic specimens and planning the extent of lung resection—sleeve lobectomy (SL) and tracheal resection. The diagnostic yield of bronchoscopy is 90% if the lesion is visible and even in cases when no visible lesion is identified, the bronchus draining the area of suspicion can be lavaged, and effluent obtained for cytologic analysis. FOB is also used in transbronchoscopic needle aspiration (TBNA) using FOB can be used in evaluating mediastinal lymph nodes and is a suitable alternative to mediastinoscopy, mediastinotomy and EUS-FNA.

Mediastinoscopy is the most accurate but invasive technique to assess mediastinal lymph nodes and safe in experienced hands. It is indicated in all patients of lung cancer prior to surgical resection, locally advanced disease lung cancer extending in to mediastinum, enlarged lymph nodes on CT scan, or mediastinal uptake on PET scan. It can assess paratracheal (stations 2, 3, 4), proximal peribronchial (station 10), and subcarinal (station 7) lymph nodes in lung cancer patients. Lymph nodes within the aortopulmonary window and along the ascending aorta (stations 5 and 6) are not accessible by standard mediastinoscopy techniques but can be evaluated by extended mediastinoscopy. It is not a routine investigation for all patients.

It is mandatory to perform mediastinoscopy in those patients requiring pneumonectomy, to rule out N3 disease, and to identify individuals with multistation N2 disease in whom induction therapy should be considered prior to surgery. It can be safely excluded in PET avid lesion with N1 nodes and no uptake in N2 station nodes in the mediastinum.

Thoracentesis: Needle drainage of a pleural effusion associated with a presumed lung cancer can identify inoperable, pleural disease. Typically, a bloody pleural effusion is malignant. The diagnosis of cancer can be established in 70% of malignant effusions by thoracentesis.

Thoracoscopy: Video-assisted thoracoscopy (VATS) is frequently used for the diagnosis, staging, and resection of lung cancer. It can be used to simultaneously collect pleural fluid for cytologic examination, and obtain pleural as well as lymph node biopsies for tissue diagnosis. Peripheral nodules can be identified, resected and subjected for histologic examination. VATS is also extremely valuable for evaluation and palliation of suspected pleural disease, particularly when thoracentesis has been nondiagnostic. Thoracoscopy is ideal for assessment of mediastinal nodes not accessible by standard mediastinoscopy or EUS-FNA techniques, and for evaluation of suspected T4 lesions.

Thoracotomy: More than 95% of tumors can be accurately diagnosed and staged prior to thoracotomy. Nevertheless, in a small minority of individuals, the diagnosis of lung cancer is made only at thoracotomy. In general, these are cases in which there is a large, inflammatory component associated with a small focus of cancer that obscures diagnosis.

Treatment of Lung Cancer

The three modalities used to treat lung cancer are: (1) surgery, (2) chemotherapy and (3) radiation therapy, which are used alone or in combination depending on stage of disease.

Patient Selection

The preoperative evaluation of patients considered for surgical management of lung cancer includes the following: clinical staging of the disease to determine resectability and assessment of cardiopulmonary reserve to ascertain if the intended pulmonary resection can be performed with acceptable perioperative risk. Important studies to assess cardiopulmonary reserve include spirometry with diffusion capacity, arterial blood gases echocardiography, quantitative ventilation-perfusion scans, oxygen consumption studies, cardiac radionuclide scans, and cardiac MRI[54] of which the last three are not regularly performed. Patients are suitable candidates for pulmonary resection if the predicted postoperative forced expiratory volume in one second (FEV_1) and/or carbon monoxide diffusion capacity (DLCO) equals or exceeds 40% of the predicted, and patient does not suffer from hypercapnia or pulmonary hypertension (Fig. 3).

Surgery

Surgery remains a major treatment modality for patients whose lung cancers are limited to the hemithorax and can be totally encompassed by excision, this provides the best chance of cure for patients with resectable NSCLC. In stage I and stage II disease, when the tumor has not extended beyond the bronchopulmonary lymph nodes, complete (R0) resections are almost always feasible. Lobectomy is currently the standard of care, and results in complete resection of the tumor mass. If the tumor extends across a fissure, lobectomy with en bloc segmentectomy, bilobectomy, or pneumonectomy should be performed if the patient can tolerate a larger resection. Lung sparing anatomic resection (sleeve lobectomy) is preferred over pneumonectomy. Lobectomy or pneumonectomy is offered if anatomically appropriate, physiologically feasible and is able to achieve negative margin.

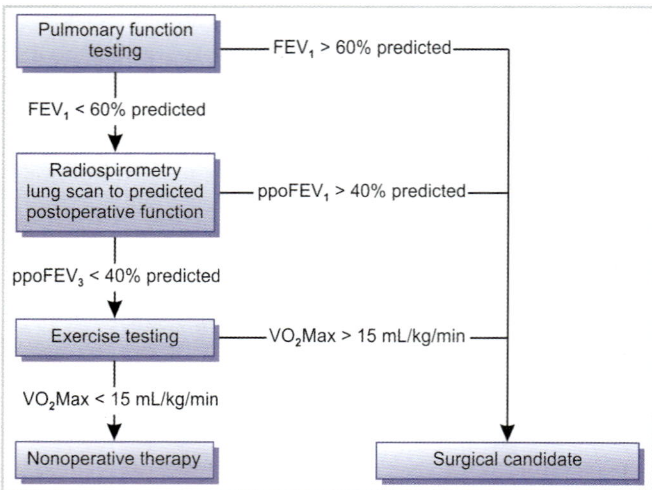

Fig. 3: Assessment of preoperative risk[55]
(*Courtesy:* Permission for reprint from Cancer News.com, Richard KJ Brown)

Video assisted thoracoscopic lobectomy is minimally invasive surgical treatment of currently being investigated management lung cancer.[56,57] Tumors larger than 5 cm in diameter, T3 lesions, and those with extensive lymph node involvement are not amenable to thoracoscopic resection. Studies have shown several advantages of thoracoscopic lobectomy over standard thoracotomy.[58-62] Thoracoscopic lobectomy is associated with minimal pain and shorter hospital stay.[63,64] Thoracoscopic lobectomy is associated with low postoperative morbidity and mortality, minimal risk of intraoperative bleeding and minimal locoregional recurrence.[65-69] Thoracoscopic lobectomy with mediastinal lymph node dissection has comparable 5-year survival rate, long-term survival and local recurrence to those achieved by routine lung resection.[70-72] Data has shown that thoracoscopic lobectomy improves the ability to complete postoperative chemotherapy regimens.[73,74]

Although lobectomy remains standard of care, sublobar resections are an option for a select group of patients. Sublobar resection includes either segmentectomy or wedge resection and is indicated in patients who are not fit for lobectomy and those with peripheral nodule less than 2 cm in diameter. Surgical procedure should achieve parenchymal resection margins of 2 cm or more. In patients of T1 category, increasing tumor size is associated with diminished survival after resection.[75] In a study by Konaka et al.[76] it was observed that lymph node metastases were noted in 18% of 171 patients (6% N1, 12% N2) peripheral clinical T1N0M0 carcinomas smaller than 2 cm in diameter; hence, it is advisable to perform lymph node dissection along with sublobar resections. There has been some conflicting data pertaining to sublobar resection where the lung cancer study group in a randomized trial[77] has shown after long-term follow-up, the locoregional recurrence rate was threefold higher with limited resection compared with lobectomy (15% vs. 5%), although morbidity and mortality rates were equal in both arms, however, retrospective studies have quoted similar survival rates for Lobectomy and sublobar resection.[78-90]

Lymph Node Dissection versus Sampling

A randomized clinical trial (ACOSOG Z0030) that compared lymph node sampling versus complete mediastinal lymphadenectomy in patients with N0 and N1 disease, demonstrated that patients with early stage disease who had negative nodes by systematic lymph node dissection, complete mediastinal lymph node dissection did not improve survival.[81-83] Thus systematic lymph node sampling is appropriate during pulmonary resection but important point is that one or more lymph nodes should be sampled from each station. Patients with N1 and N2 disease during mapping should have minimum of 3N2 node station sampled, formal ipsilateral mediastinal lymph node dissection is indicated for stage (IIIA-N2) disease.

Specific Management

Primary surgery is performed in stage I, II, peripheral T3 and N1 (IIIA). Lobectomy with mediastinal lymph node dissection is usually optimal. In patients with peripheral T3 (chest wall) or T3 (diaphragm) enbloc resection along with chest wall resection or diaphragm is feasible. It the tumor is less than 2 cm distal to carina (T3) then parenchymal preserving SL (bronchial sleeve) is optimal operation, however, in T3 (nodule in same lobe)—lobectomy is usually sufficient. If the tumor is T3 and crosses a major fissure—pneumonectomy or lobectomy combined with segmental resection of involved lung is an option. T3 parietal pericardium can be excised en bloc.

Superior Sulcus Tumors

In patients of stage III A (T3 invasion, N0–N1) neoadjuvant concurrent chemoradiation therapy followed by surgical resection has shown overall 5 year of 40%.[84] Patients with unresectable (T4 extension, N0–N1) in the superior sulcus is treated by definitive chemoradiation followed by 4 cycles of full dose chemotherapy.[85,86]

Stage III A [T4 N0-N1] [T4—metastases in ipsilateral lung in different lobe, carina, pulmonary artery (Fig. 5) and superior vena cava (SVC)] the management is as follows: [T4 ipsilateral lung—pneumonectomy], T4 carina—tracheal sleeve, T4 pulmonary artery or SVC—pulmonary artery sleeve and SVC sleeve. Fadel et al.[87] evaluated 139 patients undergoing SL with or without angioplasty for NSCLC. The overall operative mortality was 3%, and overall 5-year survival rate was 52%. Multivariate analysis revealed that nodal status (N0 or N1 vs. N2), and microscopic invasion of the bronchial stump were independent determinants of long-term survival. Deslauriers et al.,[88] De Leyn et al.[89] and Ferguson[90] confirm that SL is associated with lower perioperative mortality, affords comparable if not superior overall survival rates, and improved quality of life compared with pneumonectomy for centrally located tumors.

Stage III A-N2 disease includes microscopic and macroscopic N2 disease. Ipsilateral N2 mediastinal lymph node involvement, despite being potentially resectable, typically portends limited survival following surgery alone. N2 disease identified preoperatively has a much poorer prognosis than individuals with occult N2 disease discovered at the time of thoracotomy (less than 10% vs. 30% 5-year survival rates, respectively). Microscopic N2 is usually treated by surgery; however (macroscopic N2 node with negative mediastinum and single <3 cm node) is treated by neoadjuvant therapy either induction chemotherapy or induction chemoradiotherapy. There is no evidence that adding RT to induction regimens improves outcomes for patients with stage IIIA (N2) disease.[92] Multistation N2 lymph nodes > 3 cm are treated with definitive chemoradiotherapy followed by

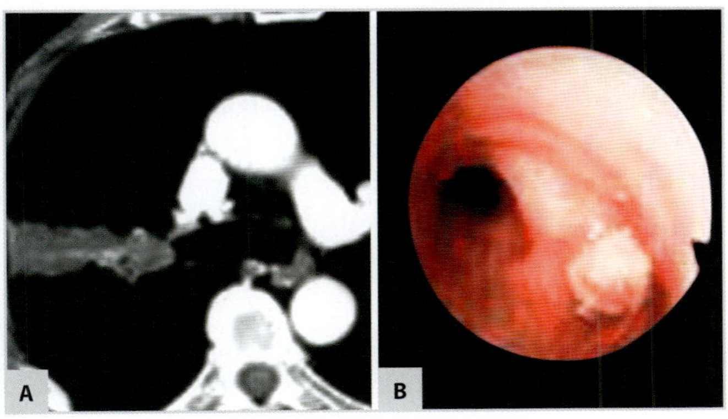

Figs 4A and B: (A) CT scan chest showing a mass lesion extending up to the hilum of right Lung;[91] (B) Bronchopscopic image showing a mass lesion in the right main bronchus[91]

(*Courtesy:* Kind permission for reprint taken from "Oxford University Press" provided by copyright clearance)

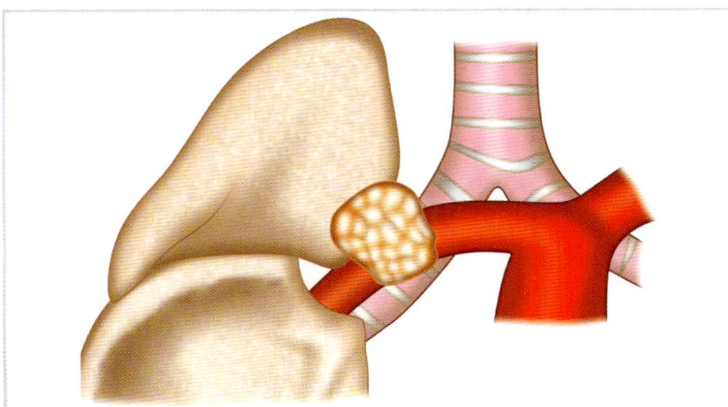

Fig. 5: Mass invading right pulmonary artery[91]

(*Courtesy:* Kind permission for reprint taken from "Oxford University Press" provided by copyright clearance)

four doses of adjuvant chemotherapy.[85,93-97] Surgery is appropriate in select patients with single station < 3 cm node who has responded to induction therapy, however, it is controversial whether pneumonectomy is appropriate after neoadjuvant therapy.[93,98-103]

Stage III-B lung cancers by virtue of contralateral (N3) lymph node metastases or invasion of vital structures such as carina, heart, or great vessels (T4), particularly in the presence of multistation N2 disease are inoperable. In cases associated with (T4 extension and ipsilateral lung) with single station N2 nodes less than 3 cm surgery can be offered after neoadjuvant chemotherapy or neoadjuvant chemoradiation. It can be tracheal sleeve, bronchial sleeve pulmonary artery and SVC sleeve or pneumonectomy. In stage III B by virtue of multistation N2 nodes are treated with definitive chemoradiation followed by four doses of adjuvant chemotherapy.[85,93,94,104-106]

Stage IV Lung Cancer is generally incurable by surgery; however, individuals with oligometastases involving brain or adrenal gland occasionally experience long-term survival following resection of the primary and metastatic lesions. M1a-pleural and pericardial effusion: all patients with cytology proven pleural effusion are treated with pleurocath insertion drainage of pleural cavity followed by pleurodesis after confirming full expansion of lung. Various agents have been used for the purpose of pleurodesis e.g. talc, bleomycin and tetracycline. Patients with pericardial effusion are treated with pleuropericardial window followed by systemic therapy. These patients are then treated with palliative chemotherapy.[107]

M1b (solitary brain metastases): Patients with solitary brain metastases may benefit from surgical resection which is followed by whole brain radiotherapy (WBRT), a reasonable alternative is stereotactic radiosurgery followed by WBRT[108,109] which is effective in patients who have surgically inaccessible and multiple brain lesions.[110] The 5-year survival rates of these patients is 10–20%[111] with a median survival of 40 weeks.[112] After treatment of brain metastases treatment options for the primary lung lesion includes surgical resection of lung lesion followed by adjuvant chemotherapy or stereotactic ablative radiotherapy (SABR) of lung lesion or additional chemotherapy followed by lung resection. Systemic therapy is an option after surgery for patients with higher stage NSCLC.

M1b (solitary adrenal metastases): About 33% patient of lung cancer have associated adrenal lesion at autopsy which may or may not be malignant, hence it is necessary to perform biopsy to rule out benign adrenal adenoma. Adrenalectomy (laparoscopic or open) has produced long-term survival when adrenal metastases has been associated with curable lung lesion.[113,114] Systemic therapy is another option for adrenal metastases.

Palliative surgery in Stage IV lung cancer: Metastatic lung cancer can present as pathological fracture of axial skeleton e.g. femur, humerus, vertebral fracture. Pathological fractures confined to axial skeleton (long bones) should undergo operative fixation followed by radiotherapy, however, fractures of central axial skeleton (vertebral bodies associated with multiple involvement are poor candidates for operative fixation and are better treated with palliative radiotherapy. In a super select group of patients with metastatic lung cancer may be subjected for primary lung surgery (lobectomy or pneumonectomy) for life-threatening hemoptysis.

Adjuvant Therapy

It is administered after primary surgical treatment. It can be in the form of adjuvant radiation therapy, adjuvant chemotherapy or chemoradiation (chemotherapy + radiation) therapy.

Adjuvant Radiation Therapy/Postoperative Radiotherapy (PORT)

Locoregional recurrence after resection of NSCLC is common, occurring in approximately 20% of patients with stage I disease[115,116] and in up to 50% of patients with stage III disease.[117-119] In a meta-analysis performed by the Medical Research Council of 2,128 patients enrolled in 9 trials.[120] PORT was associated with an increase in local control but a 7% absolute decrease in survival at 2 years (48% vs. 55%; $P = 0.001$) which was more pronounced for early-stage disease (N0-1) which led to the conclusion that PORT should not be used routinely to treat patients with completely resected early-stage NSCLC. The benefit of PORT was more pronounced in completely resected patients with N2 disease.[121] The Adjuvant Navelbine International Trialist Association (ANITA) Trial also found that PORT increased survival in patients who received adjuvant chemotherapy.[122]

Based on criticisms of the PORT meta-analysis,[123] PORT is not currently considered standard therapy despite the high risk of local recurrence after complete resection of lung cancer. PORT is considered in patients with microscopic disease at the bronchial resection margin, vascular margin, or chest wall, In addition, patients with high-risk features such as mediastinal lymph node involvement[122] inadequate mediastinal dissection, close margins, or extra capsular extension should also be considered for PORT. Conformal RT with systemic chemotherapy has shown promising results in phase 2 trials[124,125] but attempts to re-evaluate PORT in the context of a randomized trial have been difficult.

Adjuvant Chemotherapy

This is only recommended for high risk, margin negative, stage IB completely resected lung cancer. The International Adjuvant Lung Cancer Trial (IALT) statistically significant survival benefit with cisplatin based adjuvant therapy in completely resected stage I, II, III NSCLC.[126] IALT data suggest that cisplatin based adjuvant chemotherapy improves survival 5 years after treatment, however, after 7.5 years there were more number of deaths in the chemotherapy group suggesting the benefit of chemotherapy decreased over time.[127]

In National Cancer Institute of Canada Clinical Trials Group (NCIC CTG) JBR 10 trial and ANITA trial compared the effectiveness of adjuvant vinorelbine plus cisplatin versus observation in early stage NSCLC. Adjuvant chemotherapy significantly prolonged overall survival (94 vs. 73 months) and relapse free survival (not reached vs. 47 months) when compared with observation alone. The 5-year survival was 69% and 54%, respectively. However, data at 10 years shows adjuvant chemotherapy is beneficial for stage II but not IB.[128]

In the ANITA trial, it is shown that after a median follow up of 76 months, median survival was 66 months in the chemotherapy group and 44 months in the observation group.[129] Adjuvant chemotherapy significantly improved (8.6%) 5-year survival in patients with completely resected stage II and II A, although no benefit was observed in stage I.

Lung adjuvant cisplatin evaluation (LACE) meta-analysis found that postoperative cisplatin-based chemotherapy increased survival over 5 years (absolute benefit 5.4%) and there was no difference among chemotherapy regimens.[130] The benefit was greater in patients with stage II and III disease with good performance status. Postoperative adjuvant chemotherapy also benefitted elderly patients up to 80 years.[131]

In the Cancer and Leukemia Group B (CALGB) 9633 trial (Paclitaxel and Carboplatin) in patients with T2N0M0, stage IB lung cancer. After a median follow-up of 74 months show that overall survival at 6 years was not significantly different although 3 year survival was significant (80%).[132,133] Although underpowered for stage I analysis showed improved survival for stage I; however, updated results did not show improved survival (the benefit was only for more than 4 cm tumors) hence, carboplatin or paclitaxel is only recommended for patients who cannot tolerate cisplatin.[134] Presently, it is reasonable to restrict treatment to patients with good performance status and adequate end-organ function. There is no indication of adjuvant chemotherapy in patients with stage IA, as present data do not support the use of adjuvant chemotherapy in completely resected stage IB patients.

Adjuvant Concurrent Chemoradiotherapy

The rationale for examining the efficacy of adjuvant concurrent chemoradiotherapy after resection of lung cancer is based on studies that indicated concurrent chemoradiotherapy is superior to sequential therapy in nonsurgical treatment of stage III disease.[135-137] In a study by Keller et al.[138] who randomly assigned 488 patients with stage II and IIIA disease to receive either radiation alone (50.4 Gy) or radiation (50.4 Gy) administered concurrently with four cycles of cisplatin and etoposide. The median survival was 39 months for the radiation-alone arm versus 38 months for the chemotherapy plus radiotherapy arm (P = 0.56); there was no difference in overall survival between the two groups.

Inference: Although superior for bulky disease, it is not clear that concurrent chemotherapy and radiation is optimal for treating minimal residual disease in the adjuvant setting, as toxicity is more pronounced with concurrent chemoradiation therapy regimens.

Based on the trial data of Intergroup E 3590 trial[138] which showed no difference in survival between completely resected stage II and stage IIIA and received adjuvant RT alone (median survival—39 months) or RT given concurrent with chemotherapy (median survival—38 months) adjuvant chemoradiation is not recommended except in cases of stage IIIA disease and positive mediastinal lymph nodes (T1-3, N2) provided radiation is not used preoperatively and in cases where there is separate pulmonary nodule in same lobe (T3) or in another lobe of same lung (T4) and surgical resection margins are positive.

Neoadjuvant Therapy

Preoperative Radiation Therapy

It is not considered standard of care based on US Veterans Administration randomized trial[139] which showed no difference in the complete resection rate and overall survival (12.5% in the preoperative RT arm compared with 21% in the immediate resection arm) and National Cancer Institute data[140] which also failed to demonstrate an improvement in local control or survival. Given these negative findings, the area of focus has been the use of preoperative chemotherapy or chemotherapy combined with RT for patients with locally advanced, but potentially resectable, NSCLC.

Neoadjuvant Chemotherapy followed by Surgery

It is based on neoadjuvant/adjuvant paclitaxel-carboplatin hope (NATCH) phase III three arm trial of preoperative chemotherapy plus surgery versus surgery plus adjuvant chemotherapy versus surgery alone in early-stage non-small cell lung cancer using paclitaxel + carboplatin. It reflected in the trial that 90% of preoperative cohort group could complete 3 cycles of chemotherapy, whereas only 61% of postoperative cohort completed chemotherapy, however, survival was equivalent in all three arms.[141] Several trials suggest that neoadjuvant therapy is beneficial in patients with N2 disease.[142-144]

Evidence favoring neoadjuvant chemotherapy comes from various trials. Depierre et al. enrolled 355 patients with stage IB to IIIA NSCLC and compared preoperative chemotherapy followed by surgery with surgery alone. It confirmed that patients receiving neoadjuvant therapy had a median survival of 37 months compared to 26 months for surgery alone. The median disease free survival was significantly better for the neoadjuvant chemotherapy arm.[145] BLOT (bimodality lung oncology team) trial which evaluated neoadjuvant versus adjuvant chemotherapy using paclitaxel/carboplatin with stage IB–IIIA NSCLC[146] confirmed that most patients (96%) completed neoadjuvant chemotherapy compared to 45% completed postoperative therapy with 56% major objective response. At 5 years, improvement in overall survival was 9% and postoperative mortality was 3% for patients who underwent lobectomy.[146] An Intergroup Southwest Oncology Group (SWOG) trial (neoadjuvant paclitaxel or carboplatin) although closed prematurely, however, did show a trend towards improved progression-free survival (PFS, 33 months vs. 20 months) and overall survival (62 vs. 41 months) favoring neoadjuvant chemotherapy.[147] Scagliotti et al. published a phase III trial of preoperative Gemcitabine or Cisplatin versus surgery alone, although the trial closed early a significant survival benefit was seen in patients with stages IIB and IIIA disease who received chemotherapy [hazard ratio (HR) 0.63].[148]

A meta-analysis of 13 randomized trials published by Song et al. has shown improvement in overall survival favoring neoadjuvant chemotherapy arm when compared to surgery alone—[HR, 0.84; 95% confidence interval (CI), 0.77–0.92; P = 0.001][148] It has also been shown that the benefits of neoadjuvant chemotherapy is similar to that of adjuvant chemotherapy.[148,149]

Inference: Thus it can be seen that benefits of neoadjuvant chemotherapy is comparable to adjuvant chemotherapy and that neoadjuvant chemotherapy has greater patient compliance.

Preoperative Chemotherapy and Radiation Therapy

The risk of locoregional recurrence after cisplatin-based induction therapy followed by resection is 30% to 60%.[150-152] The addition of RT to chemotherapy helps to improve local control, facilitate a margin-negative resection, and help sterilize mediastinal disease. The principal drawback of preoperative chemoradiotherapy arises when a patient fails to undergo resection, and RT is resumed to a definitive dose often after a lengthy break.

In patients with unresectable stage III A and IIIB lung cancer combined modality therapy (chemoradiation is superior to radiation alone)[153-156] however, concurrent chemoradiation is superior to radiation alone.[157-160] Concurrent chemoradiation has higher rate of grade 3 or 4 esophagitis.

The Intergroup 0139 trial randomized technically resectable 396 patients with T1-3pN2 disease to induction chemotherapy (cisplatin and etoposide) and RT (45 Gy) followed by resection versus definitive RT (61 Gy) with concurrent chemotherapy. The surgical arm had a higher progression-free survival (22% vs. 11%; P = 0.017) and a trend toward improved 5-year overall survival (27% vs. 20%; P = 0.10). Surgical mortality was high (more than 20%) in patients undergoing pneumonectomy. It has been observed that the mortality for right pneumonectomy is higher after neoadjuvant chemotherapy for unexplained reasons.[161]

In a randomized controlled trial of 203 unresectable patients with either stage IIIA or IIIB NSCLC which assessed induction chemotherapy followed by either radiotherapy alone or chemoradiation using paclitaxel; median survival was 14.1 versus 18.7 months, respectively.[162]

Inference: It is based on data analyzed above it is evident in technically resectable locally advanced lung cancer that preoperative concurrent chemoradiation followed by surgery is superior to definitive radiotherapy with concurrent chemotherapy. In locally advanced inoperable stage IIIA and IIIB lung cancer induction chemotherapy followed by chemoradiation using paclitaxel is superior to radiotherapy alone. One important point which needs consideration is that patients likely to undergo resection post neoadjuvant chemoradiation the total radiation dose should not exceed 45 Gy as mediastinal landmarks get obscured at dose higher than 45 Gy.

Morbidity issues: The risks of general anesthesia and lung resection are unacceptably high in patients with significant cardiac and pulmonary comorbidities. Definitive RT has been used for many decades in these individuals. Hilton[163] and Smart[164] showed 5-year survival of 21% in 38 patients with early-stage lung cancer treated with RT with doses ranging from 50 Gy to 55 Gy for squamous cell carcinomas delivered to the primary site only, and dose from 40 Gy to 45 Gy for small cell carcinomas, delivered to the primary site and mediastinum. RT techniques are evolving to treat and manage surgically unsuitable NSCLC. The standard approach is a daily fraction of 1.8–2 Gy to a total dose of 60–70 Gy and elective nodal irradiation [ENI] is usually omitted.

Stereotactic ablative radiotherapy (SABR) is recommended for early stage NSCLC patients who refuse surgery or are medically inoperable[165] SABR is also an option for high surgical risk patients (> 75 years with poor lung function). Definitive chemoradiation is recommended for medically inoperable locally advanced (stage II and III) lung cancer.[166] In patients with advanced lung cancer (stage IV) with extensive metastases palliative RT can be used for primary or distant sites.[167]

Radiofrequency ablation: It is a reasonable option in node negative patients and medically inoperable patients. It is indicated in isolated peripheral noncavitating lesions less than 3 cm and can be used in irradiated tissue and for palliation.[168] A 2-year overall survival of 75% was reported in patients with stage I NSCLC[169] and procedure specific 30 day mortality rate is reported to be 2.6%.[170]

Palliative Chemotherapy

Patients with stage IV disease who have a good performance status benefit from chemotherapy.[171-173] These drug includes platinum agents (cisplatin/carboplatin), taxanes (paclitaxel, docetaxel), vinorelbine, vinblastine, etoposide, pemetrexed and gemcitabine. Combination agents produce better Ist year survival rates than single agents (30–40%).

Frequently used firstline regimens for nonsquamous NSCLC include pemetrexed with cisplatin/carboplatin or paclitaxel/carboplatin with or without bevacizumab.[174,175] Gemcitabine/cisplatin is used in patients with squamous cell carcinoma.[176,177] Pemetrexed based regimes are used in adenocarcinoma as Taxane based regimen are associated with more toxicity.[176,178,179] The Point break trial showed that Carboplatin/pemetrexed/bevacizumab is reasonable option and confirmed that taxane based regimens are more toxic[179] but has similar survival rates.

Single Agent Chemotherapy

In patients with poor performance status (PS-2) single agent chemotherapy or platinum based combinations are recommended.[180] They include vinorelbine, gemcitabine, pemetrexed or taxanes; combination chemotherapy regimens include carboplatin/paclitaxel or carboplatin/pemetrexed.[181-183] Recent trial data has shown that treatment with pemetrexed/carboplatin increased the median overall survival when compared to pemetrexed alone (9.1 months vs. 5.6 months).[181]

Combination Chemotherapy

Phase III randomized trials reveal that many of the platinum doublets combinations yield similar response rates and survival.[184-186] Other carboplatin based regimens include gemcitabine/carboplatin, docetaxel/carboplatin and pemetrexed/carboplatin. Nonplatinum based regimens such as gemcitabine/vinorelbine and gemcitabine/docetaxel are also options.[187-190] Inspite of the development of new chemotherapy regimens, the prognosis for advanced inoperable lung cancer remains poor. Albumin-bound paclitaxel is used in patients who are hypersensitive to paclitaxel/docetaxel inspite of use of premedications. A recent phase III randomized trial has reported that albumin-bound paclitaxel/carboplatin regimen is associated with less neurotoxicity and improved response rates when compared to standard paclitaxel/carboplatin in advanced NSCLC,[191] due to which US Food and Drug Administration (FDA) has approved albumin-bound paclitaxel/carboplatin for patients with locally advanced or metastatic NSCLC who are not candidates for curative surgery or radiotherapy and hence is recommended regimen as firstline therapy for patients of advanced NSCLC and good performance status (PS, 0–1).

Targeted Therapy

There are specific targeted therapies developed for the treatment of advanced lung cancer.[192,193]

Bevacizumab: It is a recombinant monoclonal antibody that blocks vascular endothelial growth factor (VEGF). It has been recommended in patients with unresectable locally advanced recurrent or metastatic nonsquamous NSCLC.

It is recommended in combination with paclitaxel and carboplatin based results of Eastern Cooperative Oncology Group (ECOG 4599—Point break trial)[179] phase III trial. The following criterion is to be met prior to use of bevacizumab: it should be used in nonsquamous cell histology, no recent history of bleeding, and no thrombocytopenia and PS (0–1).

Erlotinib: It is a small molecule tyrosine kinase inhibitor. Initially approved for the treatment of locally advanced or metastatic NSCLC after failure of one prior chemotherapy regimen it is also recommended as firstline in patients with advanced, recurrent or metastatic nonsquamous NSCLC who have known EGFR mutation or gene amplification regardless of PS. The recommendation is based on results of phase III randomized trial (IPASS) which showed that patients with EGFR mutation who received gefitinib had increased PFS (24.9% vs. 6.7%), response rates (71.2% vs. 47.3%) and fewer side effects when compared patients receiving carboplatin/paclitaxel.[194] The OPTIMAL trial (Phase III randomized, open label study of first line erlotinib versus gemcitabine/carboplatin in patients with EGFR—activating mutation —positive in advanced non-small cell cancer) confirmed that PFS was increased in patients with EGFR mutations who received erlotinib.[195,196] Crizotinib is approved for patients with locally advanced or metastatic NSCLC who are positive for ALK gene arrangement. This approval is based on ongoing phase II trial where (80%) patients receiving crizotinib showed dramatic response rates.

Cetuximab is a monoclonal antibody that targets EGFR. It is an option for patients with advanced NSCLC without EGFR, ALK mutations regardless of histology. It has been recommended based on results of (Flex Trial) which assessed cisplatin/vinorelbine with or without cetuximab for advanced NSCLC (stage IV).[197] Adding cetuximab slightly increased overall survival (11.3 months versus. 10.1 months). Since the result of cetuximab is not dependent on histological type of NSCLC it has been recommended as firstline therapy for adenocarcinomas as well as squamous cell carcinoma.

Palliation of Intrathoracic Disease—Surgery

A variety of surgical interventions be required to palliate symptoms in patients with advanced NSCLC. They are as follows:

- Bronchoscopic ablation of tumor to relieve endobronchial obstruction or hemoptysis
- Pleurodesis or placement of stents to relieve symptomatic malignant pleural effusions, or pericardial fenestration for malignant pericardial effusions
- On rare occasions, resection of primary tumors and lung parenchyma is required to control septic complications or massive hemoptysis
- Palliative fixation of unstable vertebral body
- Bronchoscopic removal of endobronchial tumor.

Various other techniques like endobronchial laser has been used. There has been increased use of photodynamic therapy for relieving endobronchial obstructions in the recent times.[198]

Palliation of Intrathoracic Disease with Radiation Therapy

Radiotherapy plays an important role in the palliation of symptomatic intrathoracic disease. Such symptoms include dyspnea, cough, hemoptysis, and/or chest pain. Numerous trials have demonstrated the palliative benefit of radiotherapy in patients with advanced NSCLC.[199-201] RT is especially effective in controlling hemoptysis with 75–85% of patients improving after treatment. Endobronchial brachytherapy is often used to palliate endobronchial tumors, especially in patients who have previously received external-beam radiation therapy.[202,203]

REFERENCES

1. Nath V, Grewal KS. Cancer in India. Ind J Med Res. 1935;23: 149 -90.
2. Zelicourt MD, Detournay B, Comte S, Stockemer V. Epidemiology and costs of lung cancer in France. Bull Cancer. 2001;88:753-8.
3. Zhonglua Liu Xing Bing Xue Za Zhi An analysis of incidence mortality and survival rates of lung cancer in Beijing. 1991;12: 205-7.
4. Wig KL, Lazaro EJ, Gadekar NG, Guleria JS. Bronchogenic carcinoma (clinical features and diagnosis). Ind J Chest Des. 1961;3:209-18.
5. Noronha V, Dikshit, Raut N, Joshi V. Epidemiology of Lung Cancer in India – focus on difference between smokers and non smokers: a single center experience: a single center experience. Indian Journal of Cancer. 2012;49(1):74-81.
6. Seigel R, Naishadham D, Jemal A. Cancer statistics C A. Cancer J Clin. 2012;62:10-29.
7. Wakelee HA, Chang ET, Gomez SL, et al. Lung cancer incidence in never smokers. J Clin Oncol. 2007;25(5):472.
8. Sano H, Marugame T. International comparisons of cumulative risk of lung cancer, from cancer incidence in five continents Vol. VIII. Jpn J Clin Oncol. 2006;36(5):334

9. Malkinson AM. Primary lung tumors in mice: An experimentally manipulable model of human adenocarcinoma. Cancer Res. 1992;52:2670s.
10. Vineis P, Alavanja M, Buffler P, et al. Tobacco and cancer: recent epidemiological evidence. J Natl Cancer Inst. 2004;96(2):99.
11. Notani P, Sanghavi LD. A retrospective study of lung cancer in Bombay. Br J Cancer. 1974;29:477-82.
12. Jussawala DJ, Jain DK. Lung cancer in greater Bombay correlation with religion an dsmokin habits. Br J Cancer. 1979;40:437-48.
13. Pakhale SS, Jayant A, Binde SV. Methods of reduction of harmful constituent in bidi smoke. Indian J Cest Dis and all Sci. 1985; 27:148-52.
14. Nafae A, Misra Sp, Dhar SN and Shah SNA. Bronchogenic carcinoma in Kashmir Valley. Ind J Chest Dis. 1973;15:285-95.
15. Peto R, Darby S, Deo H, et al. Smoking, smoking cessation and lung cancer in the UK since 1950: combination of national statistics with two case-control studies. BMJ. 2000; 321(7257):323.
16. Husgafvel-Pursiainen K. Genotoxicity of environmental tobacco smoke: a review. Mutat Res. 2004;567(2-3):427.
17. Gorlova OY, Zhang Y, Schabath MB, et al. Never smokers and lung cancer risk: a case-control study of epidemiological factors. Int J Cancer. 2006;118(7):1798.
18. Dhala A, Pinsker K, Prezant DJ. Respiratory health consequences of environmental tobacco smoke. Clin Occup Environ Med. 2006;5(1):139.
19. Selikoff IJ, Hammond EC, Seidman H. Mortality experience of insulation workers in the United States and Canada, 1943-1976. Ann N Y Acad Sci. 1979;330:91.
20. Boffetta P, Nyberg F. Contribution of environmental factors to cancer risk. Br Med Bull. 2003;68(1):71.
21. Gottschall EB. Occupational and environmental thoracic malignancies. J Thorac Imaging. 2002;17(3) :189.
22. Nakachi K, Harris CC, Tahara E. Japan-US Cooperative Cancer Research Seminar on molecular epidemiological characteristics of lung and colon cancer development among atomic-bomb survivors, Bethesda, USA, February 23-24, 2006. Cancer Sci 2006; 97(11):1279.
23. Leuraud K, Billon S, Bergot D, et al. Lung cancer risk associated to exposure to radon and smoking in a case-control study of French uranium miners. Health Phys. 2007;92(4):371.
24. Hwang SJ, Cheng LS, Lozano G, et al. Lung cancer risk in germline p53 mutation carriers: association between an inherited cancer predisposition, cigarette smoking, and cancer risk. Hum Genet. 2003;113(3):238.
25. Vineis P, Anttila S, Benhamou S, et al. Evidence of gene-gene interactions in lung carcinogenesis in a large pooled analysis. Carcinogenesis. 2007;28:1902.
26. Wang Y, Liang D, Spitz MR, et al. XRCC3 genetic polymorphism, smoking, and lung carcinoma risk in minority populations. Cancer. 2003;98(8):1701.
27. Shekelle RB, Lepper M, Liu S, et al: Dietary vitamin A and risk of cancer in the Western Electric study. Lancet. 1981;2:1185-90.
28. Heinonen: The effect of vitamin E and beta-carotene on the incidence of lung cancer and other cancers in male smokers: The Alpha-tocopherol, Beta-carotene Cancer Prevention Study Group. N Engl J Med. 1995;330:1029-35.
29. Hennekens CH, Buring JE, Manson JE, et al: Lack of effect of long-term supplementation with beta-carotene on the incidence of malignant neoplasm and cardiovascular disease. N Engl J Med. 1996;334:1145-9.
30. Omenn Gs, Goodman GE, Thornquist MD, et al: Effects of a combination of beta-carotene and vitamin A on lung cancer and cardiovascular disease. N Engl J Med. 1996;334:1150-5.
31. Doll R. The strategy for detection of lung cancer hazards to men. Nature 1977;265:589-95.
32. Behera D, Sharma A, Khanduja KL, Gogna ML. Beta carotene, vitamin-A, and vitamin-C levels in patients with lung cancer. (Abstract) Lung Cancer. 1998;21(Supp 1):S20.
33. Michaud DS, Feskanich D, Rimm EB. Intake of specific carotenoids and risk of lung cancer in two prospective US cohorts. Am J Clin Nutr. 2000;72:990-7.
34. Nakanishi K. Alveolar epithelial hyperplasia and adenocarcinoma of the lung. Arch Pathol Lab Med. 1990;114(4):363.
35. Lynch TJ, Bell DW, Sordella R, et al. Activating mutations in the epidermal growth factor receptor underlying responsiveness of non-small-cell lung cancer to gefitinib. N Engl J Med. 2004;350(21):2129.
36. Chan JK, Hui PK, Tsang WY, et al. Primary lymphoepithelioma-like carcinoma of the lung. A clinicopathologic study of 11 cases. Cancer. 1995;76(3):413.
37. Moro D, Brichon PY, Brambilla E, et al. Basaloid bronchial carcinoma. A histologic group with a poor prognosis. Cancer. 1994;73(11):2734.
38. Carter D. Squamous cell carcinoma of the lung: an update. Semin Diagn Pathol. 1985;2(4):226.
39. Takamori S, Noguchi M, Morinaga S, et al Clinical pathologic characteristics of adenosquamous carcinoma of the lung. Cancer. 1991;67:649.
40. Travis WD, Rush W, Flieder DB, et al. Survival analysis of 200 pulmonary neuroendocrine tumors with clarification of criteria for atypical carcinoid and its separation from typical carcinoid. Am J Surg Pathol. 1998;22(8):934.
41. Goldstraw P, Crowley J, Chansky K, et al. The IASLC Lung Cancer Staging Project: Proposals for the revision of the TNM stage groupings in the forthcoming (seventh) edition of the TNM classification of malignant tumours. J. Thorac Oncol. 2007;2: 706-14.
42. Radiology Assistant website: Courtesy – with Kind permission from Robin Smithus, Radiology Department of the Rijnland Hospital, Leiderdorp, the Netherlands.
43. Sone S, Li F, Yang ZG, et al. Characteristics of small lung cancers invisible on conventional chest radiography and detected by population based screening using spiral CT. Br J Radiol. 2000;73(866):137.
44. Finkelstein SE, Summers RM, Nguyen DM, et al. Virtual bronchoscopy for evaluation of malignant tumors of the thorax. J Thorac Cardiovasc Surg. 2002;123(5):967.

45. Reed CE, Harpole DH, Posther KE, et al. Results of the American College of Surgeons Oncology Group Z0050 trial: the utility of positron emission tomography in staging potentially operable non"small-cell lung cancer. J Thorac Cardiovasc Surg. 2003; 126(6):1943.
46. Gonzalez-Stawinski GV, Lemaire A, Merchant F, et al. A comparative analysis of positron emission tomography and mediastinoscopy in staging non"small-cell lung cancer. J Thorac Cardiovasc Surg. 2003;126(6):1900.
47. Gamez C, Rosell R, Fernandez A, et al. PET/CT fusion scan in lung cancer: current recommendations and innovations. J Thorac Oncol. 2006;1(1):74.
48. Mac Manus MP, Hicks RJ, Matthews JP, et al. Positron emission tomography is superior to computed tomography scanning for response-assessment after radical radiotherapy or chemoradiotherapy in patients with non "small-cell lung cancer. J Clin Oncol. 2003;21(7):1285.
49. Weber WA, Petersen V, Schmidt B, et al. Positron emission tomography in non "small-cell lung cancer: prediction of response to chemotherapy by quantitative assessment of glucose use. J Clin Oncol. 2003;21(14):2651.
50. Fritscher-Ravens A, Bohuslavizki KH, Brandt L, et al. Mediastinal lymph node involvement in potentially resectable lung cancer: comparison of CT, positron emission tomography, and endoscopic ultrasonography with and without fine-needle aspiration. Chest. 2003;123(2):442.
51. Fritscher-Ravens A, Davidson BL, Hauber HP, et al. Endoscopic ultrasound, positron emission tomography, and computerized tomography for lung cancer. Am J Respir Crit Care Med. 2003; 168(11):1293.
52. Hochstenbag MM, Twijnstra A, Hofman P, Wouters EF, ten Velde GP. MR-imaging of the brain of neurologic asymptomatic patients with large cell or adenocarcinoma of the lung. Does it influence prognosis and treatment? Lung Cancer. 2003; 42(2):189.
53. Petty TL. Sputum cytology for the detection of early lung cancer. Curr Opin Pulm Med. 2003;9(4):309.
54. Datta D, Lahiri B. Preoperative evaluation of patients undergoing lung resection surgery. Chest. 2003;123(6):2096.
55. Brown KJ. "Lung Cancer: Who is a candidate for Surgery? An emerging role for PET scanning" (Jules Lin MD & Andrew Chang Department of Surgery ,University of Michigan Medical Center 2120 Taubman Center 1500 E Medical Center Drive, Box 0344, Ann Arbor, Michigan 48109
56. Swanson SJ, Batirel HF Video-assisted thoracic surgery (VATS) resection for lung cancer. Surg Clin North Am. 2002;82(3): 541-59.
57. Mahtabifard A, Fuller CB, McKenna RJ Jr. Video-assisted thoracic surgery sleeve lobectomy: a case series. Ann Thorac Surg. 2008; 85(2):S729-32.
58. Shaw JP, Dembitzer FR, Wisnivesky JP et al. Video-assisted thoracoscopic lobectomy: state of the art and future directions. Ann Thorac Surg. 2008;85(2):S705-9.
59. Cheng D, Downey RJ, Kernstine K, et al. Video-Assisted Thoracic Surgery for Lung Cancer Resection: A meta-analysis and systematic review of controlled trails. Innovations: Technology & Techniques in Cardiothoracic & Vascular Surgery. 2007;2:261-92.
60. Alam N, Flores RM, et al. Video-assisted thoracic surgery (VATS) lobectomy: the evidence base. JSLS. 2007;11(3):368-74.
61. Whitson BA, Andrade RS, Boettcher A, et al. Video-assisted thoracoscopic surgery is more favorable than thoracotomy for resection of clinical stage I non-small cell lung cancer. Ann Thorac Surg. 2007;83(6):1965-70.
62. Whitson BA, Groth SS, Duval SJ, et al. Surgery for early-stage non-small cell lung cancer: a systematic review of the video-assisted thoracoscopic surgery versus thoracotomy approaches to lobectomy. Ann Thorac Surg. 2008;86(6):2008-16.
63. Scott WJ, Allen MS, Darling G, Meyers B, et. al. Video-assisted thoracic surgery versus open lobectomy for lung cancer: a secondary analysis of data from the American College of Surgeons Oncology Group Z0030 randomized clinical trial. J Thorac Cardiovasc Surg. 2010;139(4):976-81.
64. Atkins BZ, Harpole DH Jr, Mangum JH, et al. Pulmonary segmentectomy by thoracotomy or thoracoscopy: reduced hospital length of stay with a minimally-invasive approach. Ann Thorac Surg. 2007;84(4):1107-12.
65. Swanson SJ, Herndon JE 2nd, D'Amico TA. Video-assisted thoracic surgery lobectomy: report of CALGB 39802--a prospective, multi-institution feasibility study. J Clin Oncol. 2007;25(31): 4993-97.
66. Ohtsuka T, Nomori H, Horio H, Naruke T et al. Is major pulmonary resection by video-assisted thoracic surgery an adequate procedure in clinical stage I lung cancer? Chest. 2004; 125(5):1742-46.
67. McKenna RJ Jr. New approaches to the minimally invasive treatment of lung cancer. Cancer J. 2005;11(1):73-6.
68. Demmy TL, Nwogu C. Is video-assisted thoracic surgery lobectomy better? Quality of life considerations. Ann Thorac Surg. 2008;85(2):S719-28.
69. Cattaneo SM, Park BJ, Wilton AS. Use of video-assisted thoracic surgery for lobectomy in the elderly results in fewer complications. Ann Thorac Surg. 2008;85(1):231-5; discussion 235-6.
70. Thomas P, Doddoli C, Yena S. VATS is an adequate oncological operation for stage I non-small cell lung cancer. Eur J Cardiothorac Surg. 2002;21(6):1094-9.
71. Roviaro G, Varoli F, Vergani C. Long-term survival after videothoracoscopic lobectomy for stage I lung cancer. Chest. 2004;126(3):725-32.
72. Solaini L, Prusciano F, Bagioni P. Long-term results of video-assisted thoracic surgery lobectomy for stage I non-small cell lung cancer: a single-centre study of 104 cases. Interact Cardiovasc Thorac Surg. 2004;3(1):57-62.
73. Nicastri DG, Wisnivesky JP, Litle VR. Thoracoscopic lobectomy: report on safety, discharge independence, pain, and chemotherapy tolerance. J Thorac Cardiovasc Surg. 2008;135(3): 642-7.
74. Petersen RP, Pham D, Burfeind WR, Hanish SI. Thoracoscopic lobectomy facilitates the delivery of chemotherapy after resection for lung cancer Ann Thorac Surg. 2007;83(4):1245-9.

75. Gajra A, Newman N, Gamble GP, et al. Impact of tumor size on survival in stage IA non "small-cell lung cancer: a case for subdividing stage IA disease. Lung Cancer. 2003;42(1):51.

76. Konaka C, Ikeda N, Hiyoshi T, et al. Peripheral "non small-cell lung cancers 2.0 cm or less in diameter: proposed criteria for limited pulmonary resection based upon clinicopathological presentation. Lung Cancer. 1998;21(3):185.

77. Ginsberg RJ, Rubinstein LV. Randomized trial of lobectomy versus limited resection for T1 N0 non "small-cell lung cancer. Lung cancer study group. Ann Thorac Surg. 1995;60:615.

78. Warren WH, Faber LP. Segmentectomy versus lobectomy in patients with stage I pulmonary carcinoma: five-year survival and patterns of intrathoracic recurrence. J Thorac Cardiovasc Surg. 1994;107:1087.

79. Kodama K, Doi O, Higashiyama M, Yokouchi H. Intentional limited resection for selected patients with T1 N0 M0 "non small-cell lung cancer: a single-institution study. J Thorac Cardiovasc Surg. 1997;114(3):347.

80. Koike T, Yamato Y, Yoshiya K, Shimoyama T, Suzuki R. Intentional limited pulmonary resection for peripheral T1 N0 M0 small-sized lung cancer. J Thorac Cardiovasc Surg. 2003;125(4):924.

81. Darling GE, Allen MS, Decker PA. Randomized trial of mediastinal lymph node sampling versus complete lymphadenectomy during pulmonary resection in the patient with N0 or N1 (less than hilar) non-small cell carcinoma: results of the American College of Surgery Oncology Group Z0030 Trial. J Thorac Cardiovasc Surg. 2011;141(3):662-70.

82. Allen MS, Darling GE, Pechet TT. Morbidity and mortality of major pulmonary resections in patients with early-stage lung cancer: initial results of the randomized, prospective ACOSOG Z0030 trial. Ann Thorac Surg. 2006;81(3):1013-9.

83. Allen MS, Darling GE, Number of lymph nodes harvested from a mediastinal lymphadenectomy: Results of the randomized, prospective ACOSOG Z0030 trial. Journal of Clinical Oncology, 2007 ASCO Annual Meeting Proceedings (Post-Meeting Edition). 2007;25(18S)(20 Supplement):7555.

84. Rusch VW, Giroux DJ, Kraut MJ, Induction chemoradiation and surgical resection for superior sulcus non-small-cell lung carcinomas: long-term results of Southwest Oncology Group Trial 9416 (Intergroup Trial 0160). J Clin Oncol. 2007;25(3):313-8.

85. Belani CP, Choy H, Bonomi P, Scott C. Combined chemoradiotherapy regimens of paclitaxel and carboplatin for locally advanced non-small-cell lung cancer: a randomized phase II locally advanced multi-modality protocol. J Clin Oncol. 2005;23(25):5883-91. Epub 2005 Aug 8.

86. Gandara DR, Chansky K, Albain KS, Leigh BR. Consolidation docetaxel after concurrent chemoradiotherapy in stage IIIB non-small-cell lung cancer: phase II Southwest Oncology Group Study S9504. J Clin Oncol. 2003;21(10):2004-10.

87. Fadel E, Yildizeli B, Chapelier AR, et al. Sleeve lobectomy for bronchogenic cancers: factors affecting survival. Ann Thorac Surg. 2002;74(3):851.

88. Deslauriers J, Gregoire J, Jacques LF, et al. Sleeve lobectomy versus pneumonectomy for lung cancer: a comparative analysis of survival and sites or recurrences. Ann Thorac Surg. 2004;77(4): 1152.

89. De Leyn P, Rots W, Deneffe G, et al. Sleeve lobectomy for non "small-cell lung cancer. Acta Chir Belg. 2003;103(6):570.

90. Ferguson MK, Lehman AG. Sleeve lobectomy or pneumonectomy: optimal management strategy using decision analysis techniques. Ann Thorac Surg. 2003;76(6):1782.

91. Mohsen Ibrahim, Federico Venuta, et al, Bronchial and pulmonary arterial sleeve resection, doi:10.1510/mmcts.2004.000067

92. Shah AA, Berry MF, Tzao C et al. Induction Chemoradiation is not superior to induction chemotherapy alone in stage IIIA lung cancer. Ann Thorac Surg. 2012;93(6):1807-12.

93. Albain KS, Swann RS, Rusch VW et al. Radiotherapy plus chemotherapy with or without surgical resection for stage III non-small-cell lung cancer: a phase III randomized controlled trial. Lancet. 2009;374:379-86.

94. Curran WJ Jr, Paulus R, Langer CJ et al. Sequential vs. concurrent chemoradiation for stage III non-small cell lung cancer: randomized phase III trial RTOG 9410 J Natl Cancer Inst. 2011;103(19):1452-60.

95. Gandara DR, Chansky K, Albain KS et al. Long-term survival with concurrent chemoradiation therapy followed by consolidation docetaxel in stage IIIB non-small-cell lung cancer: a phase II Southwest Oncology Group Study (S9504). Clin Lung Cancer. 2006;8(2):116-21.

96. Mina LA, Neubauer MA, Ansari RH. Phase II trial of cisplatin (P) plus etoposide (E) plus concurrent chest radiation (XRT) with or without consolidation docetaxel (D) in patients (pts) with inoperable stage III non-small cell lung cancer (NSCLC). Journal of Clinical Oncology, 2008 ASCO Annual Meeting Proceedings (Post-Meeting Edition). 2008;26(15S)(20 Supplement):7519.

97. Hanna NH, Neubauer M, Ansari R, et al. Phase III trial of cisplatin (P) plus etoposide (E) plus concurrent chest radiation (XRT) with or without consolidation docetaxel (D) in patients (pts) with inoperable stage III non-small cell lung cancer (NSCLC Journal of Clinical Oncology, 2007 ASCO Annual Meeting Proceedings (Post-Meeting Edition). 2007;25(18S) (20 Supplement):7512.

98. Van Meerbeeck JP, Kramer GW, Van Schil PE et al. Randomized controlled trial of resection versus radiotherapy after induction chemotherapy in stage IIIA-N2 non-small-cell lung cancer. J Natl Cancer Inst. 2007;99(6):442-50.

99. Cerfolio RJ, Bryant AS, et al. Survival of patients with unsuspected N2 (stage IIIA) nonsmall-cell lung cancer. Ann Thorac Surg. 2008;86(2):362-6.

100. Higgins K, Chino JP, Marks LB, Ready N, et al. Preoperative chemotherapy versus preoperative chemoradiotherapy for stage III (N2) non-small-cell lung cancer. Int J Radiat Oncol Biol Phys. 2009;75(5):1462-7.

101. Shah AA, Berry MF, Tzao C, Gandhi M et al. Induction chemoradiation is not superior to induction chemotherapy alone in stage IIIA lung cancer. Ann Thorac Surg. 2012;93(6): 1807-12.

102. Stefani A, Alifano M, Bobbio A, Grigoroiu M Which patients should be operated on after induction chemotherapy for N2 non-small cell lung cancer? Analysis of a 7-year experience in 175 patients. J Thorac Cardiovasc Surg. 2010;140(2):356-63.

103. Kappers I, van Sandick JW, Burgers SA et al. Surgery after induction chemotherapy in stage IIIA-N2 non-small cell lung cancer: why pneumonectomy should be avoided. Lung Cancer. 2010;68(2):222-7.

104. Gandara DR, Chansky K, Albain KS, Gaspar L, et al. Long-term survival with concurrent chemoradiation therapy followed by consolidation docetaxel in stage IIIB non-small-cell lung cancer: a phase II Southwest Oncology Group Study (S9504). Clin Lung Cancer. 2006;8(2):116-21.

105. Mina LA, Neubauer MA, Ansari RH. Phase III trial of cisplatin (P) plus etoposide (E) plus concurrent chest radiation (XRT) with or without consolidation docetaxel (D) in patients (pts) with inoperable stage III non-small cell lung cancer (NSCLC): Journal of Clinical Oncology, 2008 ASCO Annual Meeting Proceedings (Post-Meeting Edition). 2008;26(15S)(20 Supplement):7519.

106. Hanna NH, Neubauer M, Ansari R, Phase III trial of cisplatin (P) plus etoposide (E) plus concurrent chest radiation (XRT) with or without consolidation docetaxel (D) in patients (pts) with inoperable stage III non-small cell lung cancer (NSCLC): Journal of Clinical Oncology, 2007 ASCO Annual Meeting Proceedings (Post-Meeting Edition). 2007;25(18S) (20 Supplement):7512.

107. Demmy TL, Gu L, Burkhalter JE, Toloza EM, D'Amico TA, Optimal management of malignant pleural effusions (results of CALGB 30102). J Natl Compr Canc Netw. 2012;10(8):975-82.

108. Linskey ME, Andrews DW, Asher AL. The role of stereotactic radiosurgery in the management of patients with newly diagnosed brain metastases: a systematic review and evidence-based clinical practice guideline. J Neurooncol. 2010;96(1): 45-68.

109. Aoyama H, Shirato H, Tago M, Nakagawa K. Stereotactic radiosurgery plus whole-brain radiation therapy vs stereotactic radiosurgery alone for treatment of brain metastases: a randomized controlled trial. JAMA. 2006;295(21):2483-91.

110. Alexander E 3rd, Moriarty TM, Davis RB et al. Stereotactic radiosurgery for the definitive, noninvasive treatment of brain metastases. J Natl Cancer Inst. 1995;87(1):34-40.

111. Burt M, Wronski M, Arbit E, Galicich JH. Resection of brain metastases from non-small-cell lung carcinoma. Results of therapy. Memorial Sloan-Kettering Cancer Center Thoracic Surgical Staff. J Thorac Cardiovasc Surg. 1992;103(3):399-410; discussion 410-1.

112. Patchell RA, Tibbs PA, Walsh JW. et al. A randomized trial of surgery in the treatment of single metastases to the brain. N Engl J Med. 1990;322(8):494-500.

113. Raviv G, Klein E, Yellin A, Schneebaum S, Ben-Ari G. Surgical treatment of solitary adrenal metastases from lung carcinoma J Surg Oncol. 1990;43(2):123-4.

114. NSCLC Meta-analyses Collaborative Group, Arriagada R, Auperin A, Burdett S, Higgins JP et al. Adjuvant chemotherapy, with or without postoperative radiotherapy, in operable non-small-cell lung cancer: two meta-analyses of individual patient data. Lancet. 2010;375(9722):1267-77.

115. Harpole DH, Jr., Herndon JE, Young WG, Jr., Wolfe WG, Sabiston DC, Jr. Stage I nonâ€"small-cell lung cancer. A multivariate analysis of treatment methods and patterns of recurrence. Cancer. 1995;76(5):787.

116. Trodella L, Granone P, Valente S, et al. Adjuvant radiotherapy in non-small-cell lung cancer with pathological stage I: definitive results of a phase III randomized trial. Radiother Oncol 2002;62(1):11.

117. Betticher DC, Hsu Schmitz SF, Totsch M, et al. Prognostic factors affecting long-term outcomes in patients with resected stage IIIA pN2 nonâ€"small-cell lung cancer: 5-year follow-up of a phase II study. Br J Cancer. 2006;94(8):1099.

118. Pass HI, Pogrebniak HW, Steinberg SM, Mulshine J, Minna J. Randomized trail of neoadjuvant therapy for lung cancer: Interim analysis. Ann Thorac Surg. 1992;53:992.

119. Stephens RJ, Girling DJ, Bleehen NM, et al. The role of post-operative radiotherapy in nonsmall-cell lung cancer: a multicentre randomised trial in patients witn pathologically staged T1-2, N1-2, M0 disease. Medical Research Council Lung Cancer Working Party. Br J Cancer. 1996;74(4):632.

120. Yamada M, Kudoh S, Hirata K, Nakajima T, Yoshikawa J. Risk factors of pneumonitis following chemoradictherapy for lung cancer. Eur J Cancer. 1998;34(1):71.

121. Lally BE, Zelterman D, Colasanto JM, Haffty BG. Postoperative radiotherapy for stage II or III non-small-cell lung cancer using the surveillance, epidemiology, and end results database J Clin Oncol. 2006;24(19):2998-3006.

122. Douillard JY, Rosell R, De LM, et al. Adjuvant vinorelbine plus cisplatin versus observation in patients with completely resected stage IB-IIIA non "small-cell lung cancer (Adjuvant Navelbine International Trialist Association [ANITA]): a randomised controlled trial. Lancet Oncol. 2006;7(9):719.

123. Bogart JA, Aronowitz JN. Localized non "small-cell lung cancer: adjuvant radiotherapy in the era of effective systemic therapy. Clin Cancer Res. 2005;11(13 Pt 2):5004s.

124. Bradley JD, Paulus R, Graham MV, et al. Phase II trial of postoperative adjuvant paclitaxel/carboplatin and thoracic radiotherapy in resected stage II and IIIA non "small-cell lung cancer: promising long-term results of the Radiation Therapy Oncology Group "RTOG 9705. J Clin Oncol. 2005;23(15):3480.

125. Feigenberg S, Hanlon A, Langer C, et al. A phase II trial of concurrent paclitaxel and carboplatin and thoracic radiotherapy in resected stage II and IIIA non "small-cell carcinoma. Proc ASTRO. 2006;66(3S);65.

126. Arriagada R, Bergman B, Dunant A, et al. Cisplatin-based adjuvant chemotherapy in patients with completely resected non-small-cell lung cancer. N Engl J Med. 2004;350(4):351-60.

127. Arriagada R, Dunant A, Pignon JP, et al. Long-term results of the international adjuvant lung cancer trial evaluating adjuvant Cisplatin-based chemotherapy in resected lung cancer. J Clin Oncol. 2010;28(1):35-42.

128. Butts CA, Ding K, Seymour L, Twumasi-Ankrah P, Graham B Randomized phase III trial of vinorelbine plus cisplatin compared with observation in completely resected stage IB and II non-small-cell lung cancer: updated survival analysis of JBR-10. J Clin Oncol. 2010;28(1):29-34.

129. Douillard JY, Rosell R, De Lena M. Adjuvant vinorelbine plus cisplatin versus observation in patients with completely resected stage IB-IIIA non-small-cell lung cancer (Adjuvant

Navelbine International Trialist Association [ANITA]): a randomised controlled trial. Lancet Oncol. 2006;7(9):719-27.

130. Pignon JP, Tribodet H, Scagliotti GV, et al. Lung adjuvant cisplatin evaluation: a pooled analysis by the LACE Collaborative Group. J Clin Oncol. 2008;26(21):3552-9. doi: 10.1200/JCO.2007.13.9030. Epub 2008 May 27.
131. Wisnivesky JP, Smith CB, Packer S, et al. Survival and risk of adverse events in older patients receiving postoperative adjuvant chemotherapy for resected stages II-IIIA lung cancer: observational cohort study. BMJ. 2011;343:d4013.
132. Shigematsu H, Takahashi T, Nomura M, et al. Somatic mutations of the HER2 kinase domain in lung adenocarcinomas. Cancer Res. 2005;65(5):1642-6.
133. Strauss GM, Herndon JE 2nd, Maddaus MA, et al. Adjuvant paclitaxel plus carboplatin compared with observation in stage IB non-small-cell lung cancer: CALGB 9633 with the Cancer and Leukemia Group B, Radiation Therapy Oncology Group, and North Central Cancer Treatment Group Study Groups. J Clin Oncol. 2008;26(31):5043-51.
134. Ohe Y, Ohashi Y, Kubota K, Tamura T, Nakagawa K, et al. Randomized phase III study of cisplatin plus irinotecan versus carboplatin plus paclitaxel, cisplatin plus gemcitabine, and cisplatin plus vinorelbine for advanced non-small-cell lung cancer: Four-Arm Cooperative Study in Japan. Ann Oncol. 2007;18(2):317-23.
135. Furuse K, Fukuoka M, Kawahara M, et al. Phase III study of concurrent versus sequential thoracic radiotherapy in combination with mitomycin, vindesine, and cisplatin in unresectable stage III nonâ€"small-cell lung cancer. J Clin Oncol. 1999;17(9):2692.
136. Furuse K, Kubota K, Kawahara M, et al. Phase II study of concurrent radiotherapy and chemotherapy for unresectable stage III non"small-cell lung cancer. Southern Osaka Lung Cancer Study Group. J Clin Oncol. 1995;13(4):869.
137. Pierre F, Maurice P, Gilles R, et al. A randomized phase III trial of sequential chemo-radiotherapy versus concurrent chemo-radiotherapy in locally advanced non "small-cell lung cancer: RTOG 9410. Proc Am Soc Clin Oncol. 2001;20:312a
138. Keller SM, Adak S, Wagner H, et al. A randomized trial of postoperative adjuvant therapy in patients with completely resected stage II or IIIA non "small-cell lung cancer. Eastern Cooperative Oncology Group. N Engl J Med. 2000;343(17):1217.
139. Shields TW. Preoperative radiation therapy in the treatment of bronchial carcinoma. Cancer. 1972;30:1388.
140. Warram J. Preoperative irradiation of cancer of the lung: final report of a therapeutic trial. A collaborative study. Cancer. 1975; 36(3):914.
141. Felip E, Rosell R, Maestre JA, Rodríguez-Paniagua JM, et al. Preoperative chemotherapy plus surgery versus surgery plus adjuvant chemotherapy versus surgery alone in early-stage non-small-cell lung cancer. J Clin Oncol. 2010;28(19):3138-45.
142. Martins RG, D'Amico TA, Loo BW Jr, Pinder-Schenck M, The management of patients with stage IIIA non-small cell lung cancer with N2 mediastinal node involvement. J Natl Compr Canc Netw. 2012;10(5):599-613.
143. Roth JA, Fossella F, Komaki R, Ryan MB, et al. A randomized trial comparing perioperative chemotherapy and surgery with surgery alone in resectable stage IIIA non-small-cell lung cancer. J Natl Cancer Inst. 1994;86(9):673-80.
144. Shah AA, Berry MF, Tzao C et al. Induction chemoradiation is not superior to induction chemotherapy alone in stage IIIA lung cancer. Ann Thorac Surg. 2012;93(6):1807-12.
145. Depierre A, Milleron B, Moro-Sibilot D, Chevret S. et al. Preoperative chemotherapy followed by surgery compared with primary surgery in resectable stage I (except T1N0), II, and IIIa non-small-cell lung cancer. J Clin Oncol. 2002;20(1):247-53.
146. Pisters KM, Ginsberg RJ, Giroux DJ, Putnam JB Jr, et al. Induction chemotherapy before surgery for early-stage lung cancer: A novel approach. Bimodality Lung Oncology Team. J Thorac Cardiovasc Surg. 2000;119(3):429-39.
147. Pisters KM, Vallières E, Crowley JJ, Franklin WA et al. Surgery with or without preoperative paclitaxel and carboplatin in early-stage non-small-cell lung cancer: Southwest Oncology Group Trial S9900, an intergroup, randomized, phase III trial. J Clin Oncol. 2010;28(11):1843-9.
148. Scagliotti GV, Pastorino U, Vansteenkiste JF et al. Randomized phase III study of surgery alone or surgery plus preoperative cisplatin and gemcitabine in stages IB to IIIA non-small-cell lung cancer. J Clin Oncol. 2012;30(2):172-8.
149. Pignon JP, Tribodet H, Scagliotti GV, Douillard JY, et al. Lung adjuvant cisplatin evaluation: a pooled analysis by the LACE Collaborative Group. J Clin Oncol. 2008;26(21):3552-9.
150. Rosell R, G Ãmez-Condina J, Camps C, et al. A randomized trial comparing preoperative chemotherapy plus surgery with surgery alone in patients with non "small-cell lung cancer. N Engl J Med. 1994;330(3):153.
151. Betticher DC, Hsu Schmitz SF, Totsch M, et al. Prognostic factors affecting long-term outcomes in patients with resected stage IIIA pN2 non"small-cell lung cancer: 5-year follow-up of a phase II study. Br J Cancer 2006;94(8):1099
152. Pass HI, Pogrebniak HW, Steinberg SM, Mulshine J, Minna J. Randomized trial of neoadjuvant therapy for lung cancer: Interim analysis. Ann Thorac Surg. 1992;53:992.
153. Dillman RO, Seagren SL, Propert KJ, et al. A randomized trial of induction chemotherapy plus high-dose radiation versus radiation alone in stage III non-small-cell lung cancer. N Engl J Med. 1990;323(14):940-5.
154. Le Chevalier T, Arriagada R, Quoix E, et al. Radiotherapy alone versus combined chemotherapy and radiotherapy in non resectable non-small-cell lung cancer: first analysis of a randomized trial in 353 patients. J Natl Cancer Inst. 1991; 83(6):417-23.
155. Dillman RO, Seagren SL, Hemdon J, et al. A randomized trial of induction chemotherapy plus high dose radiation versus radiation alone in stage III NCSLC: Five year follow up of Cancer and Leukemia groups (CALGB) 8433 trial. J Clin Oncol. 1993;12: 329.
156. Dillman RO, Herndon J, Seagren SL, et al. Improved survival in stage III non-small-cell lung cancer: seven-year follow-up of cancer and leukemia group B (CALGB) 8433 trial. J Natl Cancer Inst. 1996 ;88(17):1210-5.

157. Curran WJ Jr, Paulus R, Langer CJ et al. Sequential vs. concurrent chemoradiation for stage III non-small cell lung cancer: randomized phase III trial RTOG 9410. J Natl Cancer Inst. 2011; 103(19):1452-60.

158. Aupérin A, Le Péchoux C, Rolland E, et al. Meta-analysis of concomitant versus sequential radio chemotherapy in locally advanced non-small-cell lung cancer. J Clin Oncol. 2010; 28(13):2181-90.

159. Socinski MA, Rosenman JG, Halle J, et al. Dose-escalating conformal thoracic radiation therapy with induction and concurrent carboplatin/paclitaxel in unresectable stage IIIA/B nonsmall cell lung carcinoma: a modified phase I/II trial. Cancer. 2001;92(5):1213-23.

160. Furuse K, Fukuoka M, Kawahara M, et al. Phase III study of concurrent versus sequential thoracic radiotherapy in combination with mitomycin, vindesine, and cisplatin in unresectable stage III non-small-cell lung cancer. J Clin Oncol. 1999;17(9):2692-9.

161. Albain KS, Swann RS, Rusch VR, et al. Phase III study of concurrent chemotherapy and radiotherapy (CT/RT) vs. CT/RT followed by surgical resection for stage IIIA (pN2) Non small-cell lung cancer. Proc Am Soc Clin Oncol. 2005;23(16S):7014

162. Huber RM, Flentje M, Schmidt M, et al. Simultaneous chemoradiotherapy compared with radiotherapy alone after induction chemotherapy in inoperable stage IIIA or IIIB non-small-cell lung cancer: study CTRT99/97 by the Bronchial Carcinoma Therapy Group. J Clin Oncol. 2006;24(27):4397-404.

163. Hilton GL. Present position relating to cancer of the lung: Results with radiation therapy alone. Thorax. 1960;15:17.

164. Smart J. Can lung cancer be cured by irradiation alone? JAMA. 1966;195:134.

165. Timmerman R, Paulus R, Galvin J, et al. Stereotactic body radiation therapy for inoperable early stage lung cancer. JAMA. 2010;303(11):1070-6.

166. Gewanter RM, Rosenzweig KE, Chang JY, et al. ACR Appropriateness Criteria: nonsurgical treatment for non-small-cell lung cancer: good performance status/definitive intent. Curr Probl Cancer. 2010;34(3):228-49.

167. Rodrigues G, Macbeth F, Burmeister B, et al. Consensus statement on palliative lung radiotherapy: third international consensus workshop on palliative radiotherapy and symptom control. Clin Lung Cancer. 2012;13(1):1-5.

168. Decker RH, Tanoue LT, Colasanto JM, Detterbeck FC, Wilson LD, et al. Evaluation and definitive management of medically inoperable early stage non-small-cell lung cancer. Part 2: newer treatment modalities. Oncology (Williston Park). 2006;20(8): 899-905.discussion 905-8, 913.

169. Lencioni R, Crocetti L, Cioni R, Suh R, et al. Response to radiofrequency ablation of pulmonary tumours: a prospective, intention-to-treat, multicentre clinical trial (the RAPTURE study). Lancet Oncol. 2008l;9(7):621-

170. Simon CJ, Dupuy DE, DiPetrillo TA, et al. Pulmonary radiofrequency ablation: long-term safety and efficacy in 153 patients. Radiology. 2007;243(1):268 -75.

171. NSCLC Meta analysis collaborative group. Chemotherapy in addition to supportive care improves survival in Advanced NSCLC: A systematic review and meta analysis of individual patient data from 16 randomized controlled trials. J Clin Oncol. 2008;26:4617–25.

172. Souquet PJ, Chauvin F, Boissel JP, Cellerino R, et al. Polychemotherapy in advanced non small cell lung cancer: a meta-analysis. Lancet. 1993;342(8862):19-21.

173. Christopher G. Azzoli, Sherman Baker Jr, Sarah Temin . American Society of Clinical Oncology Clinical Practice Guideline Update on Chemotherapy for Stage IV Non–Small-Cell Lung Cancer. JCO December 20, 2009;27(36):6251-66.

174. Zornosa C, Vandergrift JL, Kalemkerian GP, et al. First-line systemic therapy practice patterns and concordance with NCCN guidelines for patients diagnosed with metastatic NSCLC treated at NCCN institutions. J Natl Compr Canc Netw. 2012;10(7):847-56.

175. Pennell NA Selection of chemotherapy for patients with advanced non-small cell lung cancer. Cleve Clin J Med. 2012;79 Electronic Suppl 1:eS46-50.

176. Scagliotti GV, Parikh P, von Pawel J, et al. Phase III study comparing cisplatin plus gemcitabine with cisplatin plus pemetrexed in chemotherapy-naive patients with advanced-stage non-small-cell lung cancer. J Clin Oncol. 2008;26(21):3543-51.

177. Sandler A, Gray R, Perry MC, et al. Paclitaxel-carboplatin alone or with bevacizumab for non-small-cell lung cancer. N Engl J Med. 2006;355(24):2542-50.

178. Edelman MJ, Le Chevalier T, et al. Maintenance therapy and advanced non-small-cell lung cancer: a skeptic's view. J Thorac Oncol. 2012;7(9):1331-6.

179. Patel J, Socinski MA, et al. A randomized open label phase 3 superiority study of pemetrexed + carboplatin + bevacizumab followed by maintenance Pem + Bev versus paclitaxel + carboplatin + Bev followed by maintenance B in patients with stage IIIB or IV Non squamous NSCLC. J Thoracic Oncol. 2012;7: Abstract LBPL1.

180. Felip E, Gridelli C, Baas P, Rosell R, et al. Metastatic non-small-cell lung cancer: consensus on pathology and molecular tests, first-line, second-line, and third-line therapy: 1st ESMO Consensus Conference in Lung Cancer; Lugano 2010. Ann Oncol. 2011; 22(7):1507-19.

181. Rogerio Lilenbaum, Mauro Zukin, et al. A randomized phase III trial of single-agent pemetrexed (P) versus carboplatin and pemetrexed (CP) in patients with advanced non-small cell lung cancer (NSCLC) and performance status (PS) of 2. Journal of Clinical Oncology, 2012 ASCO Annual Meeting Proceedings (Post-Meeting Edition). 30(15) suppl (May 20 Supplement), 2012:7506.

182. Langer CJ, O'Byrne KJ, Socinski MA, et al. Phase III trial comparing paclitaxel poliglumex (CT-2103, PPX) in combination with carboplatin versus standard paclitaxel and carboplatin in the treatment of PS 2 patients with chemotherapy-naïve advanced non-small cell lung cancer. J Thorac Oncol. 2008;3(6):623-30.

183. Lilenbaum R, Villaflor VM, Langer C, et al. Single-agent versus combination chemotherapy in patients with advanced non-small cell lung cancer and a performance status of 2: prognostic

factors and treatment selection based on two large randomized clinical trials. J Thorac Oncol. 2009;4(7):869-74.

184. Leighl NB. Treatment paradigms for patients with metastatic non-small-cell lung cancer: first-, second-, and third-line. Curr Oncol. 2012;19 (Suppl 1):S52-8.

185. Grossi F, Kubota K, Cappuzzo F, et al. Future scenarios for the treatment of advanced non-small cell lung cancer: focus on taxane-containing regimens. Oncologist. 2010;15(10):1102-12.

186. De Marinis, Rossi A, Di Maio M, et al. Treatment of advanced non-small-cell lung cancer: Italian Association of Thoracic Oncology (AIOT) clinical practice guidelines. Lung Cancer. 2011;73(1):1-10.

187. D'Addario G, Pintilie M, Leighl NB et al. Platinum-based versus non-platinum-based chemotherapy in advanced non-small-cell lung cancer: a meta-analysis of the published literature. J Clin Oncol. 2005;23(13):2926-36. Epub 2005 Feb 22.

188. Greco FA, Spigel DR, Kuzur ME, et al. Paclitaxel/Carboplatin/gemcitabine versus gemcitabine/vinorelbine in advanced non-small-cell lung cancer: a phase II/III study of the Minnie Pearl Cancer Research Network. Clin Lung Cancer. 2007;8(8):483-7.

189. Herbst RS, Khuri FR, Lu C, Liu DD, et al. The novel and effective nonplatinum, nontaxane combination of gemcitabine and vinorelbine in advanced non small cell lung carcinoma: potential for decreased toxicity and combination with biological therapy. Cancer. 2002;95(2):340-53.

190. Pujol JL, Breton JL, Gervais R, et al. Gemcitabine-docetaxel versus cisplatin-vinorelbine in advanced or metastatic non-small-cell lung cancer: a phase III study addressing the case for cisplatin. Ann Oncol. 2005;16(4):602-10.

191. Socinski MA, Bondarenko I, Karaseva NA, et al. Weekly nab-paclitaxel in combination with carboplatin versus solvent-based paclitaxel plus carboplatin as first-line therapy in patients with advanced non-small-cell lung cancer: final results of a phase III trial. J Clin Oncol. 2012;30(17):2055-62.

192. Sandler AB, Johnson DH, Herbst RS, et al. Anti-vascular endothelial growth factor monoclonals in non-small cell lung cancer. Clin Cancer Res. 2004;10 (12 Pt 2):4258s-62s.

193. Giaccone G. Epidermal growth factor receptor inhibitors in the treatment of non-small-cell lung cancer. J Clin Oncol. 2005;23(14):3235-42.

194. Mok TS, Wu YL, Thongprasert S, Yang CH, et al. Gefitinib or carboplatin-paclitaxel in pulmonary adenocarcinoma. N Engl J Med. 2009;361(10):947-57.

195. Zhou C, Wu YL, Chen G, Feng J, et al. Erlotinib versus chemotherapy as first-line treatment for patients with advanced EGFR mutation-positive non-small-cell lung cancer (OPTIMAL, CTONG-0802): a multicentre, open-label, randomised, phase 3 study. Lancet Oncol. 2011;12(8):735-42.

196. Zhou C, Wu YL, Chen G, et al. Updated efficacy and quality-of-life (QoL) analyses in OPTIMAL, a phase III, randomized, open-label study of first-line erlotinib versus gemcitabine/carboplatin in patients with EGFR-activating mutation-positive (EGFR Act Mut+) advanced non-small cell ung cancer (NSCLC). J Journal of Clinical Oncology, 2011 ASCO Annual Meeting Proceedings (Post-Meeting Edition). 2011;29(15_suppl) (May 20 Supplement): 7520.

197. Pirker R, Pereira JR, Szczesna A, et al. Cetuximab plus chemotherapy in patients with advanced non-small-cell lung cancer (FLEX): an open-label randomised phase III trial. Lancet. 2009;373(9674):1525-31.

198. Usuda J, Kato H, Okunaka T, et al. Photodynamic therapy (PDT) for lung cancers. J Thorac Oncol. 2006;1(5):489.

199. Macbeth FR, Bolger JJ, Hopwood P, et al. Randomized trial of palliative two-fraction versus more intensive 13-fraction radiotherapy for patients with inoperable non "small-cell lung cancer and good performance status. Medical Research Council Lung Cancer Working Party. Clin Oncol (R Coll Radiol). 1996; 8(3):167.

200. A Medical Research Council (MRC) randomized trial of palliative radiotherapy with two fractions or a single fraction in patients with inoperable non "small-cell lung cancer (NSCLC) and poor performance status. Medical Research Council Lung Cancer Working Party. Br J Cancer. 1992;65(6):934.

201. Inoperable non "small-cell lung cancer (NSCLC): a Medical Research Council randomized trial of palliative radiotherapy with two fractions or ten fractions. Report to the Medical Research Council by its Lung Cancer Working Party. Br J Cancer. 1991;63(2):265.

202. Kelly JF, Delclos ME, Morice RC, et al. High-dose rate endobronchial brachytherapy effectively palliates symptoms due to airway tumors: the 10-year MD Anderson cancer center experience. Int J Radiat Oncol Biol Phys. 2000;48(3):697.

203. Speiser BL, Spratling L. Remote After loading Brachytherapy for the Local Control of Endobronchial Carcinoma. Int J Radiat Oncol Biol Phys. 1993; 25:579.

40 Mediastinal Tumors

Ramakant Deshpande, Tanveer Abdul Majeed

INTRODUCTION

The mediastinum is a site of multiple types of tumors. They can be either primary mediastinal tumors or secondary (Metastatic). Commonly found are thymic, primary germ cell tumors, lymphomas and neurogenic tumors. Metastatic or secondary mediastinal tumors commonly are from carcinoma lung or infradiaphragmatic malignancies.

SURGICAL ANATOMY OF MEDIASTINUM

The mediastinum occupies the central portion of the thoracic cavity. It is bounded by the pleural cavities laterally, the thoracic inlet superiorly, the diaphragm inferiorly, the sternum anteriorly and by the chest wall posteriorly. It is further divided into three compartments, i.e. anterior, middle and posterior mediastinum (Fig. 1).

A large variety of tumors originate in the mediastinum:

- Anterior mediastinum: Thymus, primary germ cell tumors, thyroid and lymphomas
- Middle mediastinum: Benign cysts, cardiac tumors
- Posterior mediastinum: Neurogenic tumors
- Anterior, middle and posterior mediastinum: Lymph nodes, cysts (pericardial, thymic and bronchogenic) and mesenchymal tumors.

INCIDENCE AND PATHOLOGY

Mediastinal neoplasms are uncommon tumors that can occur at any age but are most common in the third through the fifth decades of life.[1,2] Thymic neoplasm predominate in the anterior mediastinum, pericardial cysts in the middle mediastinum, neurogenic tumors and esophageal tumors in the posterior mediastinum. A higher incidence of thymic tumors and lymphomas in adults and neurogenic tumors in children account for the age differences; however, primary mediastinal germ cells tumors are commonly seen in young adolescents.

DIAGNOSIS

A meticulous history, physical examination, imaging, serological tests and percutaneous biopsies usually

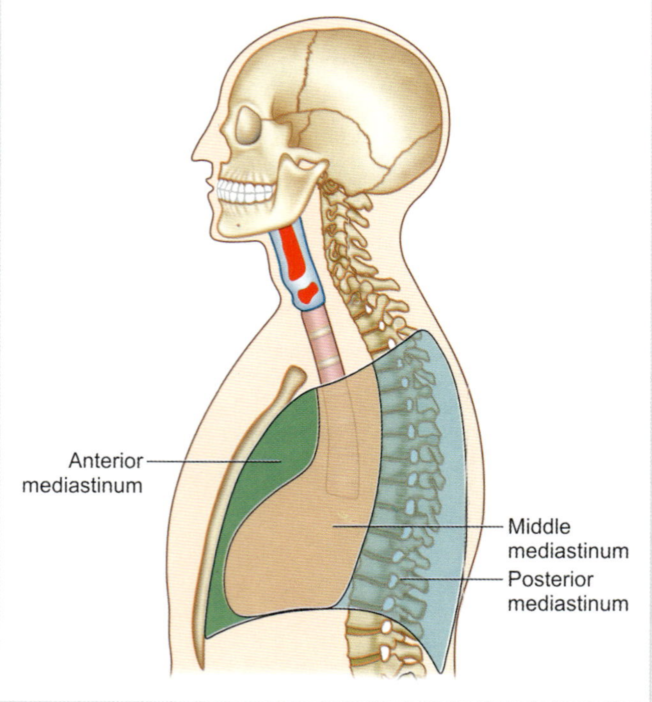

Fig. 1: Divisions of mediastinum

confirm majority of mediastinal masses, however, in certain circumstances of tuberculosis—fine-needle aspiration (FNA) and thoracoscopy are contributory especially for masses located in middle mediastinum.

SYMPTOMS AND SIGNS

Approximately, 40% of mediastinal masses are asymptomatic and discovered incidentally on routine chest imaging.[1] The remaining 60% of cases have symptoms related to either compression or direct invasion of surrounding mediastinal structures or to paraneoplastic syndromes. Asymptomatic patients are more likely to have benign lesions, whereas symptomatic patients more often harbor malignancies.[1] The most common symptoms are chest pain, cough, and dyspnea.[1] Superior vena cava syndrome, Horner's syndrome, hoarseness, and neurologic deficits are less common and often signal a malignancy.[3]

PARANEOPLASTIC SYNDROME

The common ones seen are myasthenia gravis and congenital pure cell aplasia (thymoma), multiple endocrine neoplasia (thymic carcinoid) and opsoclonus myoclonus syndrome (neuroblastoma).

Imaging and Diagnosis

Chest X-ray

It is the most common initial investigation performed and includes both posteroanterior and lateral views. It usually defines the size, density and calcification of a mass.

Contrast Enhanced CT Scan of Chest

It remains the best imaging modality to accurately assess the nature of the lesion (cystic vs solid), detect fat and calcium, determine the relationship to surrounding anatomic structures, and, in some instances, predict invasiveness of tumors (Figs 2 and 3).[4,5]

Contrast MRI of Thorax

It is superior to CT in defining vascular involvement and can detect subtle differences in tumor contour, capsule clarity and intratumoral signal (low), that correlate with the World Health Organization (WHO) classification of thymomas.[6]

Positron Emission Tomography

It is well established for the assessment of mediastinal lymphoma, and its utility in clarifying the nature of other mediastinal masses, including invasive thymoma, is gaining general acceptance.[7,8]

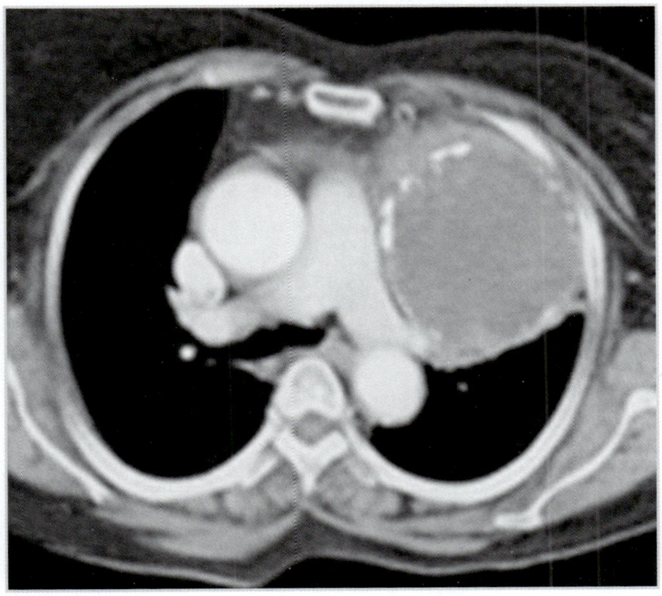

Fig. 2: Anterior mediastinal mass situated in left anterior mediastinum abutting left main pulmonary artery

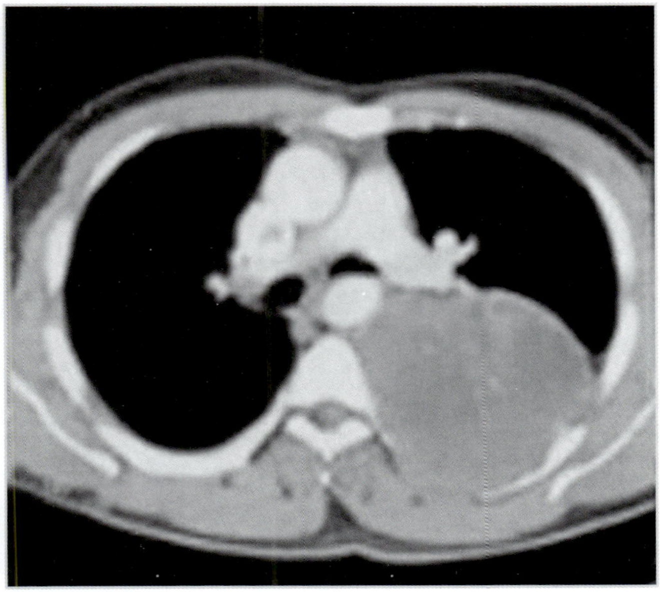

Fig. 3: Large posterior mediastinal mass located on contact with descending thoracic aorta and left main pulmonary artery

Transesophageal Ultrasonography

It can assess invasiveness of posterior mediastinal tumors.[9]

Serum Tumor Markers

Primary or secondary mediastinal germ cell tumors secrete tumor markers which have both diagnostic and prognostic utility (i.e. monitoring response to therapy and early detection of recurrence). The commonly evaluated ones are follows: α-fetoprotein (AFP), β-human chorionic gonadotropin (β-hCG), and lactate dehydrogenase (LDH).

Invasive Diagnostic Tests

It is the cornerstone for appropriate diagnosis and treatment of any mediastinal tumor. Generally, core needle biopsies are preferred over fine-needle aspiration cytology as the adequacy of tissue is better and when needed immunohistochemistry can be performed. Core needle biopsies are performed under CT scan guidance. Recent series report diagnostic yields for percutaneous needle biopsy in excess of 90%.[10] Complications include pneumothorax and hemoptysis which may occasionally require requiring chest tube placement.[10] Transesophageal ultrasonography may be used for fine-needle aspiration cytology of middle and posterior mediastinal tumors especially lymphomas and carcinomas.

THYMUS

It is an irregular, lobulated organ located in the superior aspect of anterior mediastinum. It attains its greatest relative weight at birth, but its absolute weight increases to 30–40 g by puberty. During adulthood, it slowly involutes and is replaced by adipose tissue. It is connected to the lower pole of thyroid gland by virtue of thyrothymic ligament. The thymus develops from a paired epithelial anlage in the ventral portion of the third pharyngeal pouch, and is closely associated with the developing parathyroid glands.[11] Six subtypes of epithelial cells have been identified in mature thymus.[12] Four exist primarily in the cortical region and two in the medullary region. Type 6 cells form Hassall's corpuscles that are characteristic of thymus.

THYMOMA

Thymic neoplasms (thymomas) constitute 30% and 15% of anterior mediastinal masses in adults and children, respectively.[1,2] Surveillance, epidemiology and end results (SEER) data suggest that thymomas occur in 15 of every 100,000 person-years, are more common in males and Pacific Islanders, and increase in frequency into the eighth decade of life.[13]

Pathology

Ninety percent of thymomas occur in the anterior mediastinum, and the rest arise in the neck or other areas of the mediastinum including, rarely, the heart.[14] Thymomas grossly are lobulated, firm, tan-pink to gray tumors that may contain cystic spaces, calcification or hemorrhage. They may be encapsulated, adherent to surrounding structures or frankly invasive. Microscopically, thymomas arise from thymic epithelial cells, although thymocytes/lymphocytes may predominate histologically. To unify the pathology of thymic neoplasms[15-17] the WHO adopted a new classification system for thymic neoplasm's.[17] WHO type A-B2 tumors are more likely to present with locoregional disease, compared with WHO type B3-C tumors.[18,19]

Thymomas are also classified as noninvasive and invasive thymomas. Noninvasive thymomas have an intact capsule, are movable, and are easily resected, although they can be adherent to adjacent organs. In contrast, invasive thymomas involve surrounding structures and can be difficult to remove without en bloc resection of adjacent structures, despite their benign cytologic appearance.

Clinical Features (Symptoms and Signs)

Thymomas are most commonly detected incidentally on routine chest X-ray in asymptomatic patients. Chest pain and symptoms of mediastinal compression (cough, breathlessness, hoarseness and distension of neck veins) are commonly seen in advanced stages. A significant number of patients have associated myasthenia gravis. Metastatic disease may occur and is most commonly seen as pleural implants and pulmonary nodules. Metastases to extrathoracic sites are uncommon.[20]

Associated Systemic Syndromes

The list is exhaustive, the most commonly found syndromes are myasthenia gravis, pure red cell aplasia and hypogammaglobunemia.

Myasthenia Gravis

Myasthenia gravis (MG) is the most common autoimmune disorder characterized by diplopia, ptosis, dysphagia and fatigue. It is associated with thymomas, occurring in

30–50% of patients.[21] Younger women and older men usually are affected, with a female-to-male ratio of 2:1. Myasthenia is a disorder of neuromuscular transmission. Pathologic changes in the thymus are noted in 70% of patients with MG. Lymphoid hyperplasia, characterized by the proliferation of germinal centers, is most commonly seen. Thymomas are identified in only about 15% of patients with myasthenia.[22] The treatment of MG involves the use of anticholinesterase-mimetic agents (pyridostigmine bromide). In severe cases, plasmapheresis may be required to remove high antibody titers. Thymectomy has become an increasingly accepted procedure in the treatment of MG complete remission rates vary from 7% to 63%, although the indications, timing, and surgical approach remain controversial.[23]

Red Cell Aplasia

Pure red cell aplasia is considered an autoimmune disorder and is found in approximately 5% of patients with thymomas.[24] Examination of the bone marrow reveals an absence of erythroid precursors and, in 30%, an associated decrease in platelet and leukocyte numbers. Thymectomy has produced remission in 38% of patients.

Hypogammaglobulinemia

It is seen in 5–10% of patients with thymomas, defects in both cellular and humoral immunity have been described. Thymectomy has not proven beneficial in this disorder.

Management

Surgical Resection

Complete surgical resection is the mainstay of therapy for thymomas and is the most important predictor of long-term survival.[26-29] Surgery includes total thymectomy and complete excision of tumor is recommended for patient who can tolerate surgery. The extent of surgical resection includes from ipsilateral phrenic nerve to contralateral phrenic nerve, superiorly form sternal notch to diaphragm inferiorly. There are various approaches for surgical resection namely: median sternotomy, posterolateral thoracotomy, bilateral anterolateral thoracotomies and occasionally the clam shell exposure.

Video-assisted thoracoscopy and more recently, robotic-assisted surgery have been used with acceptable outcomes, but long-term results are not available.[30] For resected stage I and II thymomas, the 10 year survival rate is excellent (approximately 90% and 70% respectively).[31,32] An important point of consideration is to avoid transpleural route for biopsy.[33,34]

Survival with aggressive resection, including lung, phrenic nerve, pericardium, pleural implants, and pulmonary metastases, is occasionally helpful.[26-28] Completely resected Stage I thymomas do not require any adjuvant radiation therapy.[35-37] The role of debulking or subtotal resection in Stage III and IV disease remains controversial.[38] Several studies have documented 5-year survival rates from 60% to 75% after subtotal resection and 24% to 40% after biopsy alone.[26,29]

Radiotherapy

Thymomas harbor variable radio sensitivity to ionizing radiation.[39] Consequently, radiation has been used to treat various tumor stages as well as recurrent disease.[26,29] A definitive total dose of 60–70 Gy is recommended for patients with unresectable disease. For adjuvant treatment, a total dose of 45–50 Gy is recommended for

TABLE 1: TNM staging of thymic tumors

World Health Organization classification of tumors of lung, pleura and heart IARC Lyon 2004[25]

T— primary tumor	N—regional lymph nodes	M—distant metastasis
TX—primary tumor cannot be assessed	NX—regional lymph nodes cannot be assessed	MX—distant metastases cannot be assessed
T0—no evidence of primary tumor	N0—no regional lymph nodes metastasis	M0—no distant metastasis
T1—completely encapsulated tumor	N1—metastasis in anterior mediastinal lymph nodes	M1—distant metastasis
T2—tumor invades pericapsular connective tissue	N2—metastasis in other intrathoracic lymph nodes (excluding anterior mediastinal lymph nodes)	
T3—tumor invades into neighboring structures (pericardium, mediastinal pleura, thoracic wall, great vessels and lung	N3—metastasis in scalene and/or supraclavicular lymph nodes	
T4—tumor with pericardial and pleural dissemination		

close margins. A total dose of 54 Gy is recommended for microscopically positive margins.[40,41] However, a total dose of 60 Gy or more (1.8–2 Gy/fraction/day) is recommended for patients with gross residual disease after surgery.[42,43] Postoperative radiation therapy can be considered in patients of thymomas and thymic carcinoma who have capsular invasion after R0 resection.[39,41,44-46] Patients with stage III thymomas or those with thymic carcinoma have a higher risk of recurrent disease and postoperative radiation is recommended to maximize local control.[47,48]

Chemotherapy

The role of chemotherapy with or without radiation therapy is defined for advanced disease.[39] Many combinations exists; however, cisplatin-/doxorubicin-based regimens seen to yield best results. Nonanthracycline regimens (e.g. cisplatin/etoposide, carboplatin/paclitaxel) may be useful for patients who cannot tolerate more aggressive regimens.[49,50] The drug of choice for thymic carcinoma is carboplatin/paclitaxel.[50,51] Induction chemotherapy followed by surgery may be useful in thymic malignancies initially considered unresectable.[52-55] Second-line systemic chemotherapy includes etoposide, ifosfamide, pemetrexed, (octreotide with or without prednisone), 5 FU, gemcitabine and paclitaxel.[49,56-61]

Molecular-Targeted Therapy

A number of molecular targets have been identified in thymic tissue. Overexpression of the EGFR has been found mostly WHO B2-B3 subtypes.[59,62,63] The overexpression of c-kit is common in thymic carcinoma, although c-kit mutations are less frequent.[62,64,65] In addition, coamplification of the HER-2/neu topoisomerase 2-α gene may correlate with response to the CAP chemotherapy regimen.[66] Somatostatin analogs have shown activity in thymic neoplasms. Response rates were seen in more than one-third (37%) of patients with tumors that were resistant to cytotoxic chemotherapy, and received octreotide plus prednisone.[67] The median and progression-free survival of 15 months and 14 months, respectively, is encouraging with somatostatin analogs. A small molecule oral, multitargeted kinase inhibitor of Bcr-Abl-Src kinases, ephrin receptor kinases, platelet-derived growth factor receptor, and c-kit (Dasatinib) has shown to have antitumor activity in thymomas.[68]

Thymic Carcinoma

Thymic carcinoma is a rare, aggressive thymic neoplasm that has a poor prognosis. It is an epithelial tumor, but cytologically it exhibits malignant features. The tumors are classified broadly as low or high grade. Low-grade tumors include squamous cell carcinoma, mucoepidermoid carcinoma, and basaloid carcinoma. High-grade neoplasms include lymphoepithelioma like carcinoma and small cell, undifferentiated, sarcomatoid and clear cell carcinomas.[69-72] They often metastasize early to regional lymph nodes and have distant metastases. Thymic carcinomas often cause pericardial and pleural effusions. Thymic carcinomas are often located in the anterior mediastinum, although like thymoma, other sites have been reported.[73] Extensive local invasion and distant metastases are common. They are commonly seen in age (10 to 76 years) and with a slight male predominance.[69] Nearly 70% of patients had symptoms of cough, chest pain or superior vena cava syndrome. Myasthenia and other thymoma-associated syndromes are rare. Low-grade tumors may have a more favorable clinical course (median survival rates of 25.4 months to more than 6.6 years) because of lower local and systemic recurrence rates, when compared with higher grade malignancies (median survival of only 11.3 to 15.0 months).[69,70] The optimal treatment of thymic carcinoma remains undefined, but currently a multimodality approach, including surgical resection, postoperative radiation and chemotherapy, is recommended. Complete surgical resection is associated with better survival than those who are incompletely resected or unresectable.[74,75] Complete resection should be attempted, but usually it is not possible.[70,76] One analysis noted a 9.5-month median survival after resection and postoperative electron-beam radiation therapy,[77] with a trend toward improved survival in other studies.[69-71] Thymic carcinomas responds poorly to chemotherapy and the highest response rates are seen with carboplatin/paclitaxel.[50] Use of neoadjuvant chemotherapy has been reported in a small number of patients.[50] The prognosis of thymic carcinoma is poor because of early metastatic involvement of pleura; lung; mediastinal, cervical and axillary lymph nodes; brain; bone; and liver.[69,78,79] The overall survival rate at 5 years is approximately 35%.[69,70] In addition, patients with stage IVa disease appear to benefit more from treatment than those with more disseminated disease (stage IVb).[65] Targeted therapy (e.g. sunitinib, sorafenib) may be useful in patients with c-Kit mutations; however these mutations are rare in thymic carcinomas.

GERM CELL TUMORS

The mediastinum is the most common site for the development of extragonadal germ cell tumors. They are most commonly seen in the anterior mediastinum and account for 10% to 15% of all primary mediastinal tumors.[1]

Etiology

Extragonadal germ cell tumors are found along the body's midline from the cranium (pineal gland) to the presacral area. This line corresponds to the embryologic urogenital ridge. It is presumed that these tumors arise from malignant transformation of germ cells that have abnormally migrated during embryonic development.[80] Mediastinal germ cell neoplasm's account for only 2–5% of all germinal tumors, but they constitute 50–70% of all extragonadal tumors.[80]

Classification (Benign or Malignant)

Benign tumors: Benign tumors (mature teratomas and mature teratomas with an immature component of less than 50%).

Malignant germ cell tumors: Seminomas (dysgerminomas) and nonseminomatous tumors. Nonseminomatous tumors include embryonal carcinomas, choriocarcinomas, yolk sac tumors, and immature teratomas.[81] Seminomas may exist in a pure form, but any elevation of AFP indicates the presence of an element of a nonseminomatous tumor.

Incidence and Clinical Presentation

It is predominantly seen in adult males; however, in pediatric population the incidence is equal in both sexes. They are commonly diagnosed in the third decade of life and affect all races equally. More than 50% of benign teratomas, are asymptomatic; however, 90–100% of patients with malignant tumors have symptoms of chest pain, dyspnea, cough, fever or other findings related to compression or invasion of surrounding mediastinal structures.[82,83]

Diagnosis

Mediastinal germ cell tumors are most often detected on standard chest radiographs, which shows a mass lesion in the anterior mediastinum, however, up to 8%, are seen in the posterior mediastinum.[83] Chest CT scans demonstrate the extent of disease, relationship to surrounding structures, and presence of cystic areas and calcification within the tumor. Recently, mediastinal sonography imaging patterns have been suggested as a means to improve the diagnostic accuracy of mediastinal teratomas.[84] Abdominal imaging should be performed to assess for possible liver metastases. Careful examination of both testes and testicular ultrasound is a must to rule out secondary mediastinal germ cell tumor (primary testis). Determination of serum tumor markers is important in the diagnosis and follow-up of mediastinal germ cell tumors. Immunoassays for β-hCG and AFP should be obtained in all patients possessing mediastinal masses suspicious for germ cell tumors. Elevations of β-hCG and AFP confirm a malignant component to the tumor which is elevated in 80–85% of nonseminomatous germ cell tumors, with AFP being detected in 60–80% of these tumors and β-hCG in 30–50%.[82] Patients with benign teratomas have normal markers and patients with pure seminoma may have low levels of β-hCG, but AFP is not detected.

Teratomas

They are the most common mediastinal germ cell tumor, accounting for 70% of the mediastinal germ cell tumors in children and 60% of those in adults. They can be seen in any age group but most commonly occur in adults from 20 years to 40 years of age. There is no gender predilection. They contain elements from all three germ cell layers, with a predominance of the ectodermal component in most tumors, including skin, hair, sweat glands, sebaceous glands, and teeth. The majority of mediastinal teratomas is composed of mature elements and exhibits a benign course. Immature teratomas phenotypically may appear as a malignancy, behave aggressively and generally are not responsive to systemic therapy. Treatment of benign mediastinal teratoma includes complete surgical resection, which results in excellent long-term cure rates. There is no role of radiotherapy and chemotherapy in the management of this tumor. Immature teratomas are potentially malignant tumors; their prognosis is influenced by the anatomic site of the tumor, patient age, and the fraction of the tumor that is immature.[81] In patients younger than 15 years, immature teratomas behave similarly to their mature counterparts. Currently, a trial of cisplatin-based combination chemotherapy (up to four cycles of cisplatin, etoposide, and bleomycin or vinblastine, ifosfamide, and cisplatin, if responding) is frequently administered before attempted surgical resection.[81]

Seminoma

Primary pure mediastinal seminoma accounts for approximately 35% of malignant mediastinal germ cell tumors; it is principally seen in men aged 20–40 years.[85] They grow slowly and metastasize later than their nonseminomatous counterparts due to which they assume a very large size by the time of diagnosis. Symptoms are usually related to compression or even invasion of surrounding mediastinal structures. Twenty to thirty percent of mediastinal seminoma is asymptomatic when discovered,[85] but metastases are present in 60–70% of patients. Pulmonary and other intrathoracic metastases are most commonly seen. Extrathoracic metastases usually involve bone.[85] Seminoma are extremely radiosensitive tumors, and for many years, high-dose mediastinal radiation has been used as initial therapy, resulting in long-term survival rates of 60–80%.[86] Thirty-five to 40 Gy are the most commonly used radiation doses.[85] Radiation portals include a shaped mediastinal field and both supraclavicular areas.[85]

Since mediastinal seminoma commonly presents as bulky, extensive, and locally invasive disease, requiring large radiotherapy portals which result in excessive irradiation of surrounding normal lung, heart and other mediastinal structures, with a resultant failure of 20–40% of patients at distant sites.[85] The use of cisplatin-based combination chemotherapy was evaluated in earlier-stage disease with encouraging results. Bokemeyer et al.[87] reported a progression-free survival and overall survival of 77% and 88% with cisplatin-based chemotherapy. Pure mediastinal seminoma, even with visceral metastases, falls into the intermediate-risk category of the new International Staging System for germ cell tumors, and these patients should be treated with curative intent. The current treatments strategies include: isolated mediastinal seminoma with minimal disease—primary radiotherapy. Locally advanced and bulky disease should be treated initially with cisplatin-based combination chemotherapy, usually four cycles of cisplatin and etoposide with or without supradiaphragmatic radiotherapy. Patients with distant metastases should undergo chemotherapy alone as initial treatment. Salvage chemotherapy (vinblastine, ifosfamide, and cisplatin) may be required for persistent or recurrent disease.[88]

The role of primary surgery followed by adjuvant treatment although with a recent report of 76.9% long-term survival has not been accepted as standard of care[89] as most authors believe that surgery does not play a role in the definitive treatment of seminoma.[86] The management of patients with postchemotherapy residual radiographic mass is controversial. Studies have shown that the residual mass is a dense scirrhous reaction in 85–90% of patients, and the presence of viable seminoma is rare whereas in others it has been shown that 25% of residual viable seminoma in these patients treated with chemotherapy followed by resection of residual masses larger than 3 cm.[89] Close observation without surgery is recommended for residual masses after chemotherapy unless the mass enlarges.[85,86] Evaluation with positron emission tomography scans has not proven to be helpful and empiric radiation therapy is not recommended.[86,88]

Nonseminomatous Germ Cell Tumors

These include choriocarcinoma, embryonal carcinoma, teratoma, and endodermal sinus (yolk sac) tumors. They may occur in pure form, but in approximately one-third of cases, multiple cell types are present. Nearly 85% of nonseminomatous germ cell tumors occur in men, with a mean age of 29 years. Karyotypic analysis have been performed on a number of these patients, and the 47XXY pattern of Klinefelter's syndrome has been found in up to 20% of patients.[83] They are most commonly found in the anterior mediastinum and appear grossly as lobulated masses with a thin capsule. They are frequently invasive at the time of diagnosis, with almost 90% of patients exhibiting symptoms. They appear on CT scans as large inhomogeneous masses containing areas of hemorrhage and necrosis. Elevated levels of β-hCG are seen in 30–50% of patients, and AFP is detected in 60–80%. These tumors fall into the poor-risk category of the new International Germ Cell Consensus Classification[90] and carry a poorer prognosis. Eighty-five percent to 95% of patients have obvious distant metastases at the time of diagnosis. Common metastatic sites include lung, pleura, lymph nodes, liver, and, less commonly, bone.[85] The diagnosis of nonseminomatous germ cell tumors can often be made without tissue biopsy.[86] The presence of an anterior mediastinal mass in a young male with elevated serum tumor markers (AFP and β-hCG) is adequate to initiate treatment. If a tissue diagnosis is deemed necessary, fine-and/or core-needle guided aspiration is used for confirmation. Treatment of nonseminomatous germ cell tumors incorporates cisplatin-based chemotherapy. Overall complete remission rates of 40–64% are obtained in most series.[81,82,85,87] Patients with relapsing mediastinal nonseminomatous germ cell tumors do extraordinarily poorly with salvage therapy, such as vinblastine, ifosfamide and cisplatin.[88] Surgical resection of residual disease despite persistently elevated tumor markers occasionally may be beneficial.[89]

Mesenchymal Tumors

These tumors originate from the connective tissue elements of the mediastinum. Mesenchymal tumors account for approximately 6% of primary mediastinal neoplasms. Approximately 55% are malignant. Treatment of malignant mesenchymal tumors involves surgical resection and radiation therapy and chemotherapy, if malignant.

Neurogenic Tumor

It occurs most commonly in the posterior mediastinum but is occasionally found in the anterior mediastinum and elsewhere. They comprise between 19% and 39% of all mediastinal tumors[91] and 75% of posterior mediastinal tumors. Lesions originate from peripheral nerves (nerves of the brachial plexus and intercostals nerves), autonomic sympathetic ganglia and, rarely, from the vagus nerve. Neurogenic tumors in the anterior mediastinum originate in chemoreceptor paragangliomas. Many of them are asymptomatic benign disease in majority of adults whereas in children they are frequently malignant and present with metastatic disease, more commonly seen in young adults equally in both sexes. They are located in paravertebral space and frequently have an occasional intraspinal extension giving rise to a dumbbell-shaped tumor, pressure symptoms are known due to their size and location. Nerve or spinal cord compression can occur in these tumors.

Neurilemoma (schwannoma)

It is the most common tumor in the paravertebral sulcus. Arising from the intercostal nerve sheath, the tumor is encapsulated, white or yellowish-pink in color, with calcifications and cystic degeneration. Histologically, it is composed of uniform slender biphasic fusiform cells with elongated, twisted nuclei that have a tendency to align in a regimented or palisaded appearance.[92]

Neurofibromas

They are most often benign and asymptomatic. They can occur as multiple lesions in von Recklinghausen's disease and inherited as an autosomal dominant trait affecting both genders equally; however, approximately half of the cases are sporadic.[93] Mediastinal neurofibromas may be multiple and appear as long plexiform masses. Histologically, they consist of large nerve fibers mixed with connective tissue stroma containing Schwann cells and fibroblasts. Surgical intervention is justified for lesions located in the spinal canal that cause spinal cord or nerve root compression. The prognosis generally is poor.[94]

Malignant Schwannoma

They are the malignant counterparts of neurilemomas and neurofibromas. Ultra structural studies, however, cannot always document Schwann cells in these tumors derived from nerve sheaths, and therefore the terms malignant nerve sheath tumor, neurogenic sarcoma, and neurofibrosarcoma are sometimes used.[94] Malignant nerve sheath tumors commonly are large. They are painful and may cause superior vena cava obstruction. Horner's syndrome, dyspnea, dysphagia, hoarseness, and invasion of the lung, bones, and aorta, depending on their location and size. The malignant nerve sheath tumors are usually large (often larger than 5 cm in diameter), partially encapsulated, soft and gray, with hemorrhage and necrosis. Histologically, they are composed of spindle cells with comma-shaped, irregular nuclei. Neural and perineural invasion, mature cartilage, bone, striated muscle, squamous differentiation, and mucin-secreting glands also may be seen.[95,96] Clinically, these tumors are aggressive, locally invasive, and highly metastatic. They often recur after resection, leading to a 75% 5-year survival rate. Patients with neurofibromatosis and a malignant nerve sheath tumor have a 15–30% 5-year survival rate. Combination chemotherapy is recommended in Stage III and IV disease.

Mediastinal Ganglioneuromas

They are found in the posterior mediastinum along the sympathetic chain in children older than 4 years and in adults in the third and fourth decades of life. They are usually asymptomatic, but sometimes present with Horner's syndrome and rarely, with diarrhea caused by production of vasoactive intestinal polypeptide. Microscopically, spindle cell proliferation is seen that appears identical to neurofibromas. They are benign tumors and require complete excision.

Neuroblastomas

Although neuroblastomas usually originate in the adrenal glands and along nerve plexuses, they can be found in any location where embryonic neuroblasts from the neural crest migrate. In the chest, they occur along the sympathetic trunk in the paravertebral sulcus. Pathology reveals lobulated gray or red tumors with hemorrhagic areas. Microscopically, small cells with scant cytoplasm and polygonal nuclei exhibit various degrees of differentiation. Intracytoplasmic neurofilaments and neurosecretory granules and extracellular material are seen on electron microscopy which differentiates it from other childhood tumors (lymphoma, Ewings and rhabdomyosarcoma). This tumor is the most common malignancy of early childhood, occurring most commonly in the first 2 years of life. Patients with mediastinal neuroblastomas usually are symptomatic and frequently have metastatic disease.[97] Symptoms are related to local compression (Horner's syndrome and heterochromia of the iris) or to systemic release of vasoactive peptides, such as catecholamines, vanillylmandelic acid, homovanillic acid and 3-methoxy-4-hydroxyphenylglycol. Encephalopathy, myasthenia, and Cushing's syndrome may be present.[98] Radiographically, a mass is seen in the posterior mediastinum with stippled calcifications, skeletal erosion, and occasional extension into the spinal canal. These tumors are highly aggressive tumors and survival depends on the age of the patient, the stage of disease, the location of the tumor, and histologic differentiation. The prognosis is better in patients younger than 1 year of age and in patients with limited, well-differentiated tumors. Treatment for Stage I and II disease is surgical resection; adjuvant postoperative radiotherapy is recommended only for Stage II tumors. For Stage III and IV, a combination of chemotherapy and radiation is advised.

Diagnosis of Posterior Mediastinal Tumors

These are predominately neurogenic, other tumors also must be considered in the differential diagnosis. Goiters, esophageal leiomyomas, solitary fibrous tumors, and bronchial/esophageal duplication cysts all have been reported. A contrast enhanced CT scan of thorax with good mediastinal window confirms the nature of these lesions, their relationship to other structures, and the presence of distant metastases. MRI scans are useful in defining vascular involvement and provide multiplanar views that are valuable in assessing tumor extension into paravertebral foramina. A iodine[131] nuclear scan may be helpful if a goiter is suspected. Histologic diagnosis is necessary, if surgery is not contemplated for further treatment planning. This can be performed by an open surgical procedure or a CT-guided core-needle biopsy.

Management

Resection is the rule in all neurogenic tumors. The standard approach uses a posterolateral thoracotomy incision, removing the tumor with normal tissue margins. More recently, thorascopic and robotic-assisted resection of small-to moderate-size tumors has been reported.[99] Complications include Horner's syndrome and chylothorax and surgery has a mortality rate of 1%. Observation is justified in a stable, asymptomatic and poor surgical candidate as neurogenic tumors grow and can cause life-threatening symptoms.

REFERENCES

1. Davis RD, Oldham HN, Sabiston DC. Primary cysts and neoplasms of the mediastinum: recent changes in clinical presentation, methods of diagnosis, management, and results. Ann Thorac Surg. 1987;44:229.-37.
2. Azarow KS, Pearl RH, Zurcher R, et al. Primary mediastinal masses: a comparison of adult and pediatric populations. J Thorac Cardiovasc Surg. 1993;106:67-72.
3. Davis RD, Oldham HN, Sabiston DC. The mediastinum. In: Sabiston DC, Spencer FC, (Eds). Surgery of the chest, 5th edition. Philadelphia: WB Saunders; 1989.
4. Bogot NR, Quint LE. Imaging of thymic disorders. Cancer Imaging. 2005;5:139-49.
5. Tomiyama H, Muller NL, Ellis SJ, et al. Invasive and noninvasive thymoma: distinctive CT features. J Comput Assist Tomogr 2001;25:388-93.
6. Inoue A, Tomiyama N, Fujimoto K, et al. MR imaging of thymic epithelial tumors: correlation with World Health Organization classification. Radiat Med. 2006;24:171-81.
7. Sung YM, Lee KS, Kim BT, et al. 18F-FDG PET/CT of thymic epithelial tumors: usefullness for distinguishing and staging tumor subgroups. J Nucl Med. 2006;47(10):1628-34.
8. El-Bawab H, Al-Sugair AA, Rafay M, et al. Role of flourine-18 fluorodeoxyglucose positron emission tomography in thymic pathology. Eur J Cardiothorac Surg. 2007;31(4):731-6.
9. Larsen SS, Krasnik M, Vilmann P, et al. Endoscopic ultrasound guided biopsy of mediastinal lesions has a major impact on patient management. Thorax. 2002;57:98-103.
10. Morrissey B, Adams H, Gibbs AR, et al. Percutaneous needle biopsy of the mediastinum: review of 94 procedures. Thorax. 1993;48:632-7.
11. Bressler EL, Kirkham JA. Mediastinal masses: alternative approaches to CT-guided needle biopsy. Radiology. 1994;191:391-6.
12. Rendina EA, Venuta F, DeGiacomo T, et al. Comparative merits of thoracoscopy, mediastinoscopy, and mediastinotomy for mediastinal biopsy. Ann Thorac Surg. 1994;57:992-5.
13. Engels EA, Pfeiffer RM. Malignant thymoma in the United States: demographic patterns in incidence and associations with subsequent malignancies. Int J Cancer. 2003;105:546.51
14. Kazemi S, Kress DC, Gal RA, et al. A rare case of intracardiac thymoma. Echocardiography. 2006;24(4):348.
15. Shimosato Y. Controversies surrounding the subclassification of thymoma. Cancer. 1994;74:542-4.
16. Suster S, Moran CA. Primary thymic epithelial neoplasms: current concepts and controversies. In: Fechner RE, Rosen PP, (Eds). Anatomic pathology. Chicago: American Society for Clinical Pathology Press. Vol 2. 1997.

17. Marx A, Müller-Hermelink HK. From basic immunobiology to the upcoming WHO-classification of tumors of the thymus. Pathol Res Pract. 1999;195:515-33.
18. Rieker RJ, Hoegel J, Morresi-Hauf A, et al. Histologic classification of thymic epithelial tumors: Comparison of established classification schemes. Int J Cancer. 2002;98:900-6.
19. Detterbeck FC. Clinical value of the WHO classification system of thymoma. Ann Thorac Surg. 2006;81:2328-34.
20. Patterson GA. Thymomas. Semin Thorac Cardiovasc Surg. 1992; 4:39-44.
21. Rinadi TP, Batocchi AP, Evoli A, et al. Thymic lesions and myasthenia gravis: diagnosis based on mediastinal imaging and pathological findings. Acta Radiol. 2002;43:380-4.
22. Berrih-Akin S, Morel E, Raimond F, et al. The role of the thymus in myasthenia gravis: immunohistological and immunological studies in 115 cases. Ann N Y Acad Sci. 1987;505:50-70.
23. Blossom GB, Ernstoff RM, Howells GA, et al. Thymectomy for myasthenia gravis. Arch Surg. 1993;128:855-62.
24. Palmieri G, Lastoria S, Cala O, et al. Successful treatment of a patient with a thymoma and pure red cell aplasia with octreotide and prednisone. N Engl J Med. 1997;336:263-5.
25. Travis WD, Brambilla E, Muller-Hermelink HK, et al. World Health Organization classification of Tumours of the Lung, Pleura, Thymus and Heart. Lyon: IARC Lyon; 2004. p.147.
26. Maggi G, Casadio C, Cavallo A, et al. Thymoma: results of 241 operated cases. Ann Thorac Surg. 1991;51:152-6.
27. Kondo K,Monden Y. Therapy for thymic epithelial tumors: a clinical study of 1,320 patients from Japan. Ann Thorac Surg. 2003;76:878-84.
28. Crucitti F, Daghetto GB, Bellantone R, et al. Effects of surgical treatment in thymoma with myasthenia gravis: our experience in 103 patients. J Surg Oncol. 1992;50:43-6.
29. Cowen D, Mornex RF, Bachelot T, et al. Thymoma: results of a multicentric retrospective series of 149 non-metastatic irradiated patients and review of the literature. Radiother Oncol. 1995; 34:9-16.
30. Rea F, Marulli G, Bortolotti L, et al. Experience with the Da Vinci robotic system for thymectomy in patients with myasthenia gravis: report of 33 cases. Ann Thorac Surg. 2006;81(2):455-9.
31. Detterbeck FC, Parsons AM. et. al. Management of stage I and II thymoma. Thorac Surg Clin. 2011;21(1):59-67.
32. Detterbeck F, Youssef S, Ruffini E. A review of prognostic factors in thymic malignancies. J Thorac Oncol. 2011;6(7 Suppl 3):S1698-704.
33. Mehran R, Ghosh R, Maziak D, et al. Surgical treatment of thymomas. Can J Surg. 2002; 45(1):25-30.
34. Murakawa T, Nakajima J, Kohno T. Results from surgical treatment for thymoma. 43 years of experience. Jpn J Thorac Cardiovasc Surg. 2000;48(2):89-95.
35. Kondo K. Optimal therapy for thymomas. J Med Invest. 2008;55(1-2):17-28.
36. Utsumi T, Shiono H, Kadota Y et al. Postoperative radiation therapy after complete resection of thymoma has little impact on survival. Cancer. 2009;115(23):5413-20.
37. Korst RJ, Kansler AL, Christos PJ, et al. Adjuvant radiotherapy for thymic epithelial tumors: a systematic review and meta-analysis. Ann Thorac Surg. 2009;87(5):1641-7.
38. Liu H-C, Chen Y-J, Tzen C-Y, et al. Debulking surgery for advanced Thymoma. Eur J Surg Oncol. 2006;32:1000-5.
39. Eng TY, Thomas CR. Radiation therapy in the management of thymic tumors. Semin Thorac Cardiovascular Surg. 2005;17(1): 32-40.
40. Gomez D, Komaki R, et al. Radiation therapy definitions and reporting guidelines for thymic malignancies. J Thorac Oncol. 2011;6(7 Suppl 3):S1743-8.
41. Gomez D, Komaki R. Technical advances of radiation therapy for thymic malignancies. J Thorac Oncol. 2010 Oct;5(10 Suppl 4):S336-43.
42. Myojin M, Choi NC, Wright CD, et al. Stage III thymoma: pattern of failure after surgery and postoperative radiotherapy and its implication for future study. Int J Radiat Oncol Biol Phys. 2000;46(4):927-33.
43. Mornex F, Resbeut M, Richaud P, et. a. Radiotherapy and chemotherapy for invasive thymomas: a multicentric retrospective review of 90 cases. The FNCLCC trialists. Fédération Nationale des Centres de Lutte Contre le Cancer. Int J Radiat Oncol Biol Phys. 1995;32(3):651-9.
44. Singhal S, Shrager JB, Rosenthal DI, et al. Comparison of stages I-II thymoma treated by complete resection with or without adjuvant radiation. Ann Thorac Surg. 2003;76(5):1635-41.
45. Rena O, Papalia E, Oliaro A, et al. Does adjuvant radiation therapy improve disease-free survival in completely resected Masaoka stage II thymoma? Eur J Cardiothorac Surg. 2007;31(1):109-13.
46. Mangi AA, Wright CD, Allan JS, et al. Adjuvant radiation therapy for stage II Thymoma. Ann Thorac Surg. 2002;74:1033-7.
47. Sugie C, Shibamoto Y, Ikeya-Hashizume C, et al. Invasive Thymoma: postoperative mediastinal irradiation, and low dose entire hemithorax irradiation in patients with pleural dissemination. J Thorac Oncolog. 2008;3:75-81.
48. Ogawa K, Uno T, Toita T, et al. Postoperative radiotherapy for patients with completely resected thymoma: a multi-institutional, retrospective review of 103 patients. Cancer. 2002;94(5):1405-13.
49. Schmitt J, Loehrer PJ. The role of chemotherapy in advanced thymoma. J Thorac Oncol. 2010;5(10 Suppl 4):S357-60.
50. Lemma GL, Lee JW, Aisner SC, et al. Phase II study of carboplatin and paclitaxel in advanced thymoma and thymic carcinoma. J Clin Oncol. 2011;29(15):2060-5.
51. Furugen M, Sekine I, Tsuta K, et al. Combination chemotherapy with carboplatin and paclitaxel for advanced thymic cancer. Jpn J Clin Oncol. 2011;41(8):1013-6.
52. Okereke IC, Kesler KA, Freeman RK, et al. Thymic carcinoma: outcomes after surgical resection. Ann Thorac Surg. 2012;93(5):1668-72.
53. Kim ES, Putnam JB, Komaki R, et. al. Phase II study of a multidisciplinary approach with induction chemotherapy, followed by surgical resection, radiation therapy, and

consolidation chemotherapy for unresectable malignant thymomas: final report. Lung Cancer. 2004;44(3):369-79.
54. Riely GJ, Huang J. Induction therapy for locally advanced thymomas. J Thorac Oncol. 2010;5(10 Suppl 4):S323-6.
55. Wright CD, Choi NC, Wain JC, et al. Induction chemoradiotherapy followed by resection for locally advanced Masaoka stage III and IVA thymic tumors. Ann Thorac Surg. 2008;85(2):385-9.
56. Girard N, Lal R, Wakelee H, et al. Chemotherapy definitions and policies for thymic malignancies. J Thorac Oncol. 2011;6(7 Suppl 3):S1749-55.
57. Girard N. Chemotherapy and targeted agents for thymic malignancies. Expert Rev Anticancer Ther. 2012;12(5):685-95.
58. Longo F, De Filippis L, Zivi A, et al. NCEfficacy and tolerability of long-acting Octreotide in the treatment of thymic tumors: results of a pilot trial. Am J Clin Oncol. 201235(2):105-9.
59. Loehrer PJ, Wang W, et al. Octreotide alone or with prednisone in patients with advanced thymoma and thymic carcinoma: an Eastern Cooperative Oncology Group Phase II Trial. J Clin Oncol. 2004;22(2):293-9.
60. Palmieri G, Merola G, Federico P, et al. Preliminary results of phase II study of capecitabine and gemcitabine (CAP-GEM) in patients with metastatic pretreated thymic epithelial tumors (TETs). Ann Oncol. 2010;21(6):1168-72.
61. Highley MS, Underhill CR, Parnis FX, et al. Treatment of invasive thymoma with single-agent ifosfamide. J Clin Oncol. 1999;17(9):2737-44.
62. Lonescu DN, Sasatomi E, Ciepley K, et al. Protein expression and gene amplification of epidermal growth factor receptor in thymomas. Cancer. 2005;103(3):630-6.
63. Strobel P, Hartmann M, Jakob A, et al. Thymic carcinoma with overexpression of mutated KIT and the response to imatinib. N Engl J Med. 2004;350(25):2625-6.
64. Pan CC, Chen PC, Chiang H. KIT (CD117) is frequently overepxressed in thymic carcinomas but is absent in thymomas. J Pathol. 2004;202:375-81.
65. Lin J-T, Wei-Shu W, Yen C-C, et al. Stage IV thymic carcinoma: a study of 2-patients. Am J Med Sci. 2005;330(4):172-5.
66. Chuah C, Lim TH, Lim AS, et al. Dasatinib induces a response in malignant thymoma. J Clin Oncol. 2006;24(34):e56-8.
67. Henley JD, Koukoulis GK, Loehrer PJ. Epidermal growth factor receptor expression in invasive thymoma. J Cancer Res Clin Oncol. 2002;128(3):167-70.
68. Nieto IP, Robledo JP, Pajuelo MC, et al. Prognostic factors for myasthenia gravis treated by thymectomy: review of 61 cases. Ann Thorac Surg. 1999;67:1568-71.
69. Suster S, Rosai J. Thymic carcinoma: a clinicopathologic study of 60 cases. Cancer. 1991;67:1025-32.
70 Hsu CP, Chan CY, Chen CL, et al. Thymic carcinoma: ten years' experience in twenty patients. J Thorac Cardiovasc Surg. 1994;107:615-20.
71. Weide LG, Ulbright TM, Loehrer PJ, et al. Thymic carcinoma: a distinct clinical entity responsive to chemotherapy. Cancer. 1993;71:1219-23.
72. Suster S, Moran CA. Spindle cell thymic carcinoma: clinicopathologic and immunohistochemical study of a distinctive variant of primary thymic epithelial neoplasm. Am J Surg Pathol. 1999;23:691-700.
73. Kadowaki T, Hamada H, Yokoyama A, et al. Thymic carcinoma originating from the mid-posterior mediastinum. Respirology. 2005;10:689-91.
74. Yano M, Sasaki H, Yokoyama T, et al. Thymic carcinoma: 30 cases at a single institution. J Thorac Oncol. 2008;3(3):265-9.
75. Okereke IC, Kesler KA, Freeman RK, et al. Thymic carcinoma: outcomes after surgical resection. Ann Thorac Surg. 2012;95(5): 1668-72.
76. Liu H, Hsu W, Chen Y, et al. Primary thymic carcinoma. Ann Thorac Surg. 2002;73:1076-81.
77. Loehrer PJ, Jiroutek M, Aisner S, et al. Phase II trial of etoposide (V), ifosfamide (I), plus cisplatin (P) in patients with advanced thymoma (T) or thymic carcinoma (TC): preliminary results from a ECOG coordinated intergroup trial. Proc Am Soc Clin Oncol. 1998;17:30 (abst 118).
78. Yano T, Hara N, Ichinose Y, et al. Treatment and prognosis of primary thymic carcinoma. Surg Oncol 1993;52:255-8.
79. Kong D-S, Lee J-I, Nam DH, et al. Cerebral involvement of metastatic thymic carcinoma. J Neuro-Oncol 2005;75:143-7.
80. Nichols CR, Fox EP. Extra-gonadal and pediatric germ cell tumors. Hematol Oncol Clin North Am. 1991;5:1189-209.
81. Dulmet EM, Macchiarini P, Suc B, et al. Germ cell tumors of the mediastinum: a 30 year experience. Cancer. 1993;72:1894-901.
82. Lemarie E, Assouline PS, Diot P, et al. Primary mediastinal germ cell tumors: results of a French retrospective study. Chest. 1992;102:1477-83.
83. Luna M, Valenzuela-Tamaritz J. Germ cell tumors of the mediastinum: postmortem findings. Am J Clin Pathol. 1976;65:450-4.
84. Wu T, Wang H, Chang Y, et al. Mature mediastinal teratoma: Sonographic imaging patterns and pathologic correlation. J Ultrasound Med. 2002;21:759-65.
85. Hainsworth JD, Greco FA. Extragonadal germ cell tumors and unrecognized germ cell tumors. Semin Oncol. 1992;19:119-27.
86. Ginsberg RJ. Mediastinal germ cell tumors: the role of surgery. Semin Thorac Cardiovasc Surg. 1992;4:51-4.
87. Bokemeyer C, Nichols CR, Draz J, et al. Extragonadal germ cell tumors of the mediastinum and retroperitoneum: results from an international analysis. J Clin Onocol. 2002;20:1864-73.
88. Ganjoo KN, Chan RJ, Sharma M, et al. Positron emission tomography scans in the evaluation of postchemotherapy residual masses in patients with seminoma. J Clin Oncol. 1999;17:3457-60.
89. Hartmann JT, Einhorn L, Nichols CR, et al. Second-line chemotherapy in patients with relapsed extragonadal nonseminomatous germ cell tumors: results of an international mutlicenter analysis. J Clin Oncol. 2001;19:1641-8.
90. International Germ Cell Collaborative Group. International germ cell consensus classification: a prognostic factor-based

staging system for metastatic germ cell cancers. J Clin Oncol. 1997;15:594-603.

91. Davidson KG, Walbaum PR, McCormack RJ. Intrathoracic neural tumors. Thorax 1978;33:359-67.
92. Wick MR, Sterenberg SS. Diagnostic surgical pathology. New York: Raven Press; 1994. p. 1141.
93. Brasfield RD, Das Gupta TK. Von Recklinghausen's disease: a clinical pathologic study. Ann Surg. 1972;175:1986.
94. Akwari OE, Payne WS, Onforio BM, et al. Dumbbell neurogenic tumors of the mediastinum. Mayo Clin Proc. 1978;53: 353-8.
95. Woodruff JM. Peripheral nerve tumors showing glandular differentiation. Cancer. 1976;37:2399-413.
96. MacKay B, Osborne BM. The contribution of electron microscopy to the diagnoses of tumors. Pathobiology annual, vol 8. New York: Raven Press; 1978. p. 359.
97. Robinson MG, McCorquodale MM. Trisomy 18 and neurogenic neoplasia. J Pediatr. 1981;99:428-9.
98. Evans AE, D'Angio GJ, Koop CE. Diagnosis and treatment of neuroblastoma. Pediatr Clin North Am. 1976;23:161-70.
99. Bodner J, Wykypiel H, Greiner A, et al. Early experience with robot-assisted surgery for mediastinal masses. Ann Thorac Surg. 2004;78(1):259-65.

41 Tumors of the Chest Wall

Ramakant Deshpande, Tanveer Abdul Majeed

INTRODUCTION

The musculoskeletal structure of the chest wall serves a critical role in the protection of intrathoracic organs and provides integrity for respiratory function. Intricate knowledge of the anatomy and physiology is mandatory prior to planning resection. Tumors of the chest wall are uncommon. They can be benign or malignant and can be divided into tumors of bony or soft tissue origin. They may be either primary or metastatic and may invade the chest wall from lung, pleura, mediastinum or breast. More than 50% of chest wall tumors are malignant, typically involving chest wall by direct invasion or metastases from distant organs. The challenges of complete resection and reconstruction have posed difficulty for surgeons attempting to minimize perioperative morbidity in the past, but advances in all these areas have greatly decreased morbidity, improved long-term survival and decreased recurrence rates.

HISTOLOGICAL TYPES

Benign Lesions

Osteochondroma

It is the most common benign bone neoplasm. The neoplasm usually begins in childhood and continues to grow until skeletal maturity. It is typically found in the femur, humerus, and tibia.[1] Osteochondroma of the chest wall is common in the rib or scapula and are normally found at the costochondral junction.[2] Osteochondromas make up 50% of benign rib tumors.[3] They frequently cause pain as they progress with growth of bony exostoses.[1] Surgical treatment is resection and provides complete pathologic evaluation, symptomatic relief and minimizes the risk of malignant transformation.[4]

Chondromas

They constitute 15% of benign neoplasms of the rib cage. Chondromas are typically found at the sternocostal junction arising from cartilaginous tissue.[5] They are relatively common, making up to 15–20% of benign chest wall lesions. Chondroma is usually painless, slow growing, present between 20 years and 30 years of age. The distinction between chondroma and low-grade chondrosarcoma is difficult, therefore, all chondromas should be considered malignant and a wide excision is recommended.[6]

Fibrous Dysplasia

It commonly presents as a solitary lesion, however, multiple lesions can be seen as a part of Albright syndrome (multiple bone cysts, skin pigmentation, and precocious sexual maturity in girls) and is associated with polyostotic fibrous dysplasia. Fibrous dysplasia typically appears in the lateral or posterior tract of the ribs and is the third most frequent benign chest wall lesion.[5] It forms a slow-growing mass, which cause pathologic fractures and result in pain. Diagnostic features on imaging include a lytic lesion with soap bubble appearance on chest radiograph. Treatment is a wide local excision for relief of symptoms and confirmation of diagnosis.[6]

Peripheral Nerve Tumors

They occur more frequently in the posterior mediastinum than in the chest wall.

Schwannomas

These arise from the nerve sheath and can be benign or malignant. Benign schwannomas appear as smooth, round lesions. Malignant schwannomas often have associated abnormalities including pleural effusions, pleural nodules and metastatic pulmonary nodules.[7] A rapid size increase, especially in neurofibromatosis should raise suspicion for malignancy.[8] Schwannomas have also been described as having a "bead-like" appearance.[9]

Neurofibroma

They arise from the nerves and are typically smoothly marginated, round or oval-shaped masses with displacement of adjacent structures rather than invasion. Neurofibromas have a low muscle-like attenuation on noncontrast computed tomography (CT) and show heterogeneous enhancement post-contrast. The magnetic resonance imaging (MRI) features include uniform low signal similar to muscle on T1 and a high signal rim-like pattern with a low signal center on T2 weighted images[10] and are associated with uniform avid enhancement following intravenous (IV) administration of gadolinium. Neurogenic tumors of the chest wall include neurofibromas and neurilemomas that arise from peripheral nerve sheaths and are usually associated with neurofibromatosis. Surgical excision is usually only recommended for cosmetic reasons for cutaneous lesions as there is a low likelihood of malignancy except in plexiform lesions that have high potential for malignant transformation.[11]

Histiocytosis X

It is a disease involving the reticuloendothelial system and includes eosinophilic granuloma, Letterer-Siwe disease, and Hand-Schuller-Christian disease. Benign soft tissue chest tumors include fibromas, lipomas, neurogenic tumors, hemangiomas, and desmoids tumors.

Lipoma

Fatty chest wall tumors are relatively common. They are sharply circumscribed tumors with uniform fat attenuation on CT and homogeneous fat signal characteristics on MRI. They may contain a few thin internal septations.

Malignant Lesions (Common)

Chondrosarcoma

These are most commonly found on the anterior chest wall and account for 30% of primary malignant bone tumors.[12] They are the most common malignant bony tumor of the chest wall. Chondrosarcoma are rarely found in patients younger than 20 years of age and are found more commonly in the third and fourth decades.[13] They usually arise in the costochondral junction or in the sternum and most commonly appear as a slowly growing mass that is generally painful. The etiology of chondrosarcoma is unknown but may include malignant degeneration of chondromas or may be associated with trauma. The diagnosis of chondrosarcoma is made after histologic studies. Radiographic appearance is typically a poorly defined mass associated with cortical destruction, and the CT usually delineates a lobulated mass of soft tissue attenuation with dense chondroid matrix calcification.[10] Synchronous or metachronous lung metastases are seen in 10% of patients at the time of presentation.[13] Pathologic distinction between chondroma and chondrosarcoma is challenging, therefore both tumors are resected with a wide 4 cm margin. Resection is the mainstay of therapy, chemotherapy is ineffective, and radiation is reserved for patients who are unresectable or with positive resection margins.[14] Five-year survival is 65–92%. Tumor-free margin is the largest predictor of local recurrence. Ten percent of patients with negative margins will have local recurrence; whereas 75% of those with positive margins will have local recurrence.[13]

Osteosarcoma

These tumors comprise of 10–15% of malignant chest wall tumors, and commonly occur in the rib, scapula, and clavicles.[10,13] They are more aggressive than chondrosarcoma and have poor prognosis. Osteosarcomas present as painful masses in young or elderly adults. Metastatic disease at the time of presentation is common, with common sites being lung, lymph nodes, and liver. Alkaline phosphatase levels are frequently elevated. Radiologically, they present as either lytic or sclerotic lesions with characteristics sunburst appearance (i.e. calcification at right angles to the cortex). Treatment is wide local excision in combination with chemotherapy. The presence of metastatic disease drastically reduces 5-year survival from more than 50% to 15% and 20%. Factors predictive of overall survival are response to chemotherapy, tumor burden, and presence of metastases.[13]

Malignant Fibrous Histiocytoma (MFH)

MFH is a common neoplasm that occurs in the chest wall. MFH is commonly found in elderly men, and there is usually a history of previous chest wall radiation.[15] These tumors tend to be invasive and spread into adjacent muscle groups. Involvement of underlying bone is not unusual in MFH. Storiform pleomorphic MFH is the most common histological form. MFH has a heterogeneous appearance on CT that can be enhancing or calcified. The MR characteristics include signal intensity similar to or lower than muscle on T1 weighted images, often inhomogeneous, and T2 weighted signal equal to or greater than adipose tissue.[16,17] They clinically present as large masses without associated pain.[18] Treatment is a wide local excision, though local recurrence rates are as high as 30%.[19] Metastatic lesions are seen in 30–50% of patients. The 5-year survival rates are around 38%.[18]

Ewing Sarcoma

They are group of tumors, which includes spectrum of small round-cell tumors including Ewing sarcoma, Askin tumor of the chest wall, and primitive neuroectodermal tumor. These tumors are the third most common malignant chest wall tumors overall and are common in the pediatric and young adult populations. The Ewing sarcoma group of lesions are aggressive with high recurrence rates and a high likelihood of metastases.[20] Neoadjuvant chemotherapy is followed by a wide local excision with good results. Response to chemotherapy is predictive of local recurrence. Metastases reduce 5-year survival to 30% from 100% with local disease at presentation.[13]

Rhabdomyosarcoma

It is the second most common chest wall soft tissue malignancy. Wide resection followed by radiotherapy and chemotherapy results in a 5-year survival of about 70%.

Metastases

Metastatic lesions to the chest wall are uncommon and are usually seen in patients with extensive metastases elsewhere. Metastatic lesions from breast, lung, or unknown primary tumors can be found in the chest wall, and the role for surgical resection is significant. Recent advances in the field of oncology, the birth of newer hormonal blocking medications and biologic therapy has totally shifted the paradigm in management of advanced metastatic disease. In these patients with limited identifiable disease (solitary skeletal metastasis) resection followed by reconstruction is a viable option, which significantly alters quality of life and improves survival.

Breast Carcinoma

It has reported rates of recurrence in the chest wall from 5% to 20%.[21,22] It may recur in the chest wall scars by direct infiltration. The occurrence of chest wall metastases is a poor prognostic indicator, associated with decreased survival rates.[21] There is paucity of formal studies; however, a large series from Chicago found an increase in survival with control of a chest wall lesion with either surgery or radiation.[23] Chest wall and sternal resection for metastatic breast cancers is associated with relief of pain, ulceration, bleeding and may contribute to increased survival in a small sub-group of patients.

Primary of Unknown Origin

In certain situations where presentation is with a chest wall tumor, the primary site remains unidentified despite of advances in imaging modalities. In these patients, the lesion in the chest wall is treated as a primary tumor with a wide resection.[24]

Malignant Lesions (Less Common)

Solitary Plasmacytoma

It is a rare tumor composed of monoclonal plasma cells. It usually presents as a discrete mass without diffuse spread or only pain often in elderly men. Surgical biopsy is followed by primary radiation therapy.[25] The 5-year survival rate is 40–60%, and overall survival is dependent on whether or not multiple myeloma develops, not on control of the primary lesion.[13] Chemotherapy is indicated as multiple sites are generally involved in most areas within 2–3 years.

Angiosarcomas of the Chest Wall

These are extremely rare vascular tumors that occur in adults and is associated with chronic lymph edema, irradiation, and chemical exposure.[16] The most common clinical presentation of angiosarcoma of the chest wall is after radiation therapy or breast conservation therapy after breast cancer. Patients commonly present 5–10 years after radiation therapy, and 5-year survival after diagnosis is only 16%.[25] Wide local excision is the only option as most patients cannot be treated with more radiation. Chemotherapy is usually ineffective in these lesions.

Liposarcoma

It is one of the most common malignant soft tissue tumors; however, they are relatively less common in the chest wall.[26] They are most common in men between age group 40 years and 60 years. The lesion is less common in children. They are usually large and frequently associated with trauma. Treatment is a wide local excision, and the

5-year survival is 60%.[27] Local recurrence rates are high. Chemotherapy and radiation therapy are ineffective.

Neurofibrosarcomas

These are typically associated with neurofibromatosis and grow along intercostal nerves. They usually occur in men in the third and fourth decades of life, with painful masses. Treatment is a wide local excision and postoperative radiation regardless of surgical margins. Currently, 5-year survival is 55%.[27]

Mesothelioma[6]

It is a primary tumor of the pleura but can present as a chest wall tumor. There is a strong causal relationship between asbestos exposure and mesothelioma. The two histologic types of mesothelioma are: (1) localized and (2) diffuse. Diffuse mesothelioma is nearly always malignant, while only 30% of localized mesothelioma are malignant. Patients with localized malignant lesions usually have symptoms, while those with localized benign lesions are asymptomatic. Symptoms include cough, pain, fever, and shortness of breath. Clubbing of the fingers and toes occurs with mesothelioma. Hematogenous spread to distant organs occurs in about one-half of patients. Symptoms of diffuse malignant mesothelioma include dyspnea, weight loss, cough, and severe pain. A hemorrhagic pleural effusion is present in some cases although a complete resection is sometimes possible in its presence.

Lung Cancer

Unusually, carcinoma of the lung by direct infiltration, can present as localized chest wall lesion; however, this is very uncommon as compared to metastases to the rib.

Lymphoma[7]

Chest wall lymphoma is rare; usually the tumor extends directly into the anterior chest wall from the mediastinum in patients with aggressive disease. Tumor tissue from lymphoma is usually of soft tissue attenuation at CT, occasionally with central areas of necrosis. The margins are usually well defined. Lymphoma tends to spread around bone and cartilage and yet may spare these structures. A variable degree of enhancement is seen postcontrast. MRI usually shows masses of isointense to mildly increased signal on T1 imaging, with hyperintensity on T2 imaging. The treatment of these tumors is primary chemotherapy.

Tumor-like Conditions of Chest Wall

Fibromatosis/Desmoids/ (Aggressive Fibromatosis)

These are often seen in the chest wall. They arise from musculoaponeurotic structures and are considered myofibroblastic or fibroblastic in origin. Histologically they are benign, but because of their aggressive growth rates and tendency to grow into nearby structures or cause compressive symptoms, hence can be considered locally malignant. They can develop anywhere in the body, but are most common in the extremities, with only 10–28% arising in the chest wall.[28] Desmoid tumors are common in females; males usually younger than 40 years and are associated with familial adenomatous polyposis (FAP), which has a mutation in the adenomatous polyposis coli (APC) gene. Desmoids can also occur in sites of previous trauma, scar, or radiation. The shoulder is the most frequently affected area. They are locally aggressive, produce large exuberant tumor growth patterns but rarely metastasize.[29,30] Extensive chest wall resection is usually required for adequate treatment. Resection with tumor-free margins is mandatory for a cure. When negative margins are not possible, radiation should be considered.[31] Recurrence rates up to 50% have been reported in the chest wall.[30] Abbas et al. reported 5-year probability of developing a local recurrence as 37%, with an 89% rate in patients who had positive margins at the time of resection.[31]

Elastofibroma Dorsi

These are muscular tumors of the posterior chest wall. They characteristically occur at the inferior angle of the scapula and have a reported prevalence of 2% in the elderly population. The treatment of these tumors is excision.

CLINICAL FEATURES

The most common presentation is an incidental mass lesion, more than 20% are detected incidentally on chest radiograph.[13] Pain is the most common symptom for both benign and malignant tumors. Extrathoracic lesions are more likely to present as a growing mass. Pain associated with malignant tumors is usually due to bony involvement and often a sign of invasion. There is a wide variation in age (18–75 years) at presentation with older patients tending to have larger and more aggressive tumors as compared to the younger patients, who are more likely to have smaller, benign tumors.[13]

DIAGNOSIS

Chest wall tumors have wide variation of histology thus making accurate diagnosis solely on individual clinical features and imaging difficult. Imaging characteristics are usually coupled with clinical findings for an accurate diagnosis.[2]

Chest Radiography

It includes both anteroposterior and lateral views; it can detect calcification, ossification, or bone destruction as well as location and size but is limited in detail.

Computed Tomography

It can accurately define type (calcification—chondrosarcoma), site, extent and vascularity of the tumor. Chest radiography (CT scan) provide information about the vascularity of a tumor, if a contrast is used, as well as a more detailed description of the extent, location, and composition of the mass (Fig. 1).

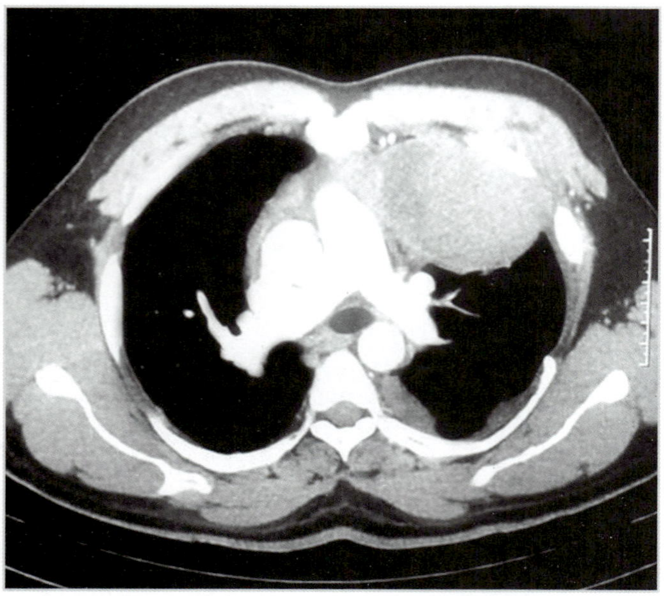

Fig. 1: Large chest wall mass extending into the anterior mediastinum flush with pulmonary artery

Magnetic Resonance Imaging

It is an important tool of assessment because of its superior tissue-resolving features and multiplanar image acquisition, which allows accurate tissue characterization.[2,32]

Positron Emission Tomography Scan

Due to the rarity of these lesions and the recent availability of positron emission tomography (PET), it has not been formally established as a diagnostic tool in the evaluation of these lesions.[33] The clinical significance of standard uptake value (SUV) may become useful in the future as more data become available.

Biopsy

In the majority of cases, radiographic features alone are insufficient to make a complete diagnosis, and therefore histologic evaluation is required. Fine-needle aspiration, incisional biopsy, or excisional biopsies are all suitable modalities to obtain a tissue diagnosis.[33] The decision of one approach over the other is usually based on the size of the lesion, extent of resection, need for reconstruction, and associated comorbidities.

Lesions less than 5 cm: Typically, lesions less than 5 cm undergo excisional biopsy *Lesions more than 5 cm* may either undergo needle aspiration, core needle biopsy or incisional biopsy. Core biopsy, incisional biopsy and excisional biopsy are usually associated with an accurate tissue diagnosis, gives accurate tissue for immunohistochemistry which in turn aids in planning preoperative treatment. This strategy is based primarily on the extent of resection and complexity of reconstruction that would be needed. A complete histopathologic diagnosis is vital prior to resection. It is important that the entire treatment plan is considered before any biopsy to ensure correct placement of skin incisions if re-excision is required.

CHEST WALL RESECTIONS AND RECONSTRUCTIONS

Preoperative Evaluation

Once the diagnosis is confirmed and decision taken for primary excision of chest wall with or without neoadjuvant therapy (radiation), preoperative evaluation is performed, which includes a detailed history and associated comorbid conditions. Availability of latissimus dorsi (LD) pedicle for reconstruction, likely surgical defects if any and the likely modality of surgical reconstruction (Fig. 2). All previous surgical scars (biopsy or incisions) should be included in the resection. The defect created after resection and modality of reconstruction is planned. Preoperative pulmonary function test (PFT), arterial blood gas analysis (ABG) and echocardiogram (Echo) is performed in patients in whom chest wall resection is contemplated. A very important aspect is a complete radiographic analysis prior to operative planning, which may delineate the need for preoperative consultation with neurosurgical or reconstructive specialists. Patients with extensive or complicated lesions are best served with a multidisciplinary approach.[34] Use of preoperative mucolytics, incentive spirometry and breathing exercises are most important factors for decreasing morbidity and hospital stay. Elective ventilation till stabilization of chest wall, epidural catheters for postoperative pain control minimize morbidity and mortality in these patients. The use of double lumen endotracheal tube for selective lung ventilation intraoperatively may be required to allow for concurrent pulmonary resection.

Surgical Management

Chest wall resection is the primary treatment modality for chest wall tumors and can be performed with low morbidity and mortality. Placing a thoracoscope in the chest, away from the lesion, may be useful to determine the extent of pulmonary involvement and exact location when the lesion is not palpable. When necessary, a needle can be inserted into the chest under thoracoscopic guidance to aid in operative planning. Adequate oncologic resection should not be compromised for concern over chest wall defect; however, the integrity of the chest wall should be maintained to avoid pulmonary complications. The treatment strategies vary based on the tumor characteristics:

- Chemosensitive tumors (osteosarcoma, rhabdomyosarcoma, Ewing sarcoma, and other small cell sarcomas) are treated with neoadjuvant chemotherapy followed by response assessment. Preoperative chemotherapy is administered to reduce the amount of tumor burden and decrease the risk of systemic failure in these patients. Resection is offered after completion of chemotherapy.
- Tumors, which are not chemosensitive (chondrosarcoma and other adult soft tissue sarcomas) are excised surgically and irradiated, if negative margins cannot be achieved. Resection can prolong survival and provide palliation for symptomatic lesions.[35] Appropriate margins are dependent on the histology of the tumor and are a key predictor of recurrence-free survival.[36]

Chondrosarcomas have a local recurrence rate of 4% after negative resection margins and 73% with positive margins.[37] For aggressive malignancies that can spread along the periosteum, the entire rib should be resected with costal articulations either posteriorly or anteriorly depending on tumor location. Sections of normal ribs above and below the tumor should be resected as well. For high-grade malignancies, 4 cm margins are adequate, and low-grade malignancies can be treated with 1–2 cm. Desmoid tumors are not technically malignant, but their behavior is so aggressive that one should use 4 cm margins for these lesions when possible. Any involved soft tissue, skin, underlying pleura, or lung tissue should be resected with the tumor, provided pulmonary function permits resection.

Reconstruction of Chest Wall (Figs 2 and 3)

Chest wall defects less than 4–5 cm or more commonly less than three rib resection and posterior defects covered with scapula do not require reconstruction.

In patients who require more than three rib resection rigid fixation using sandwich technique is often employed using marlex or prolene mesh and bone cement [polymethyl methacrylate (PMMA)]. The chest wall reconstruction is done by fixation to the rib margins (Fig. 2).

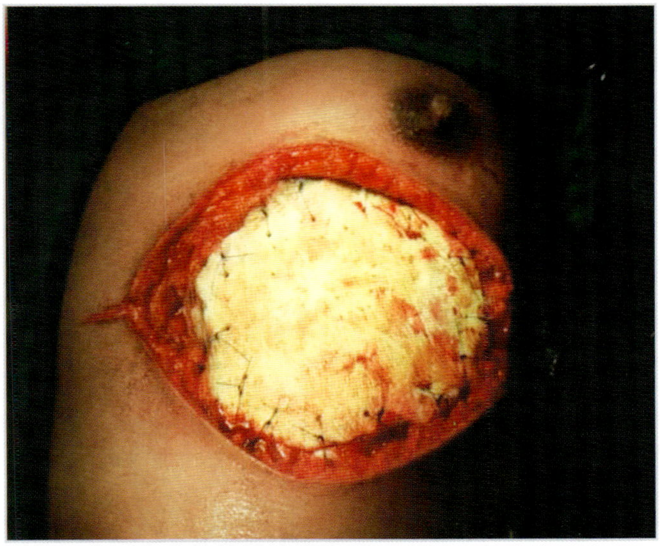

Fig. 2: Rigid chest wall reconstruction using bone cement [poly methyl methacrylate (PMMA) and prolene mesh (sandwich technique)]

Skeletal stabilization is achieved with autologous tissue (fascia lata), prolene or marlex mesh, Gore-Tex® mesh reconstruction provided adequate skin and muscle cover is available. In patients where skin and muscle is not available tissue reconstruction can be performed using pedicle or free myocutaneous flaps. The most common flap used is pedicle LD flap (Fig. 3).

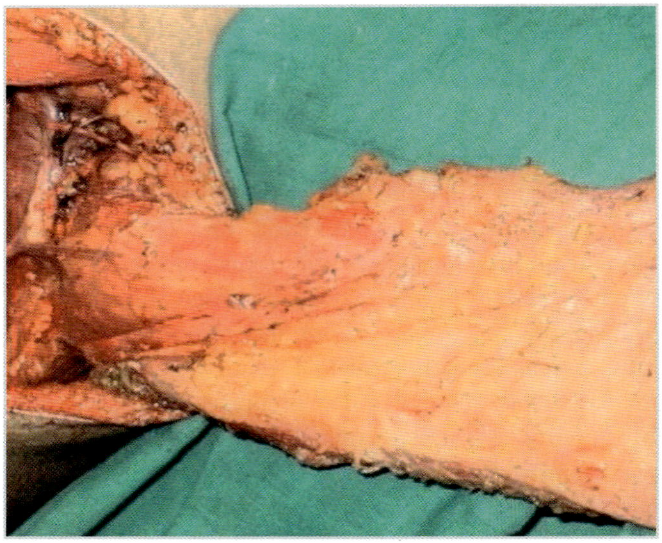

Fig. 3: Pedicle latissimus dorsi flap—used for chest wall reconstruction

Sternal resections are usually reconstructed with sandwich technique where sternum is artificially shaped using bone cement and prolene mesh and the sutured to the bony edges of ribs, Sternal end of clavicle and intervening soft tissue. Elective ventilation till stabilization of chest wall followed by aggressive postoperative pulmonary toilet is vitally important because large anterior defects can result in weak cough and inability to clear secretions. Bronchoscopy may be necessary to facilitate adequate pulmonary toilet.

REFERENCES

1. Tomo H, Ito Y, Aono M, Takaoka K. Chest wall deformity associated with osteochondroma of the scapula: a case report and review of the literature. J Shoulder Elbow Surg. 2005;14: 103-6.
2. Tateishi U, Gladish GW, Kusumoto M, et al. Chest wall tumors: radiologic findings and pathologic correlation: part 1. Benign tumors. Radiographic. 2003;23:1477-90.
3. Incarbone M, Pastorino U. Surgical treatment of chest wall tumors. World J Surg. 2001; 25:218-30.
4. Park BJ, Flores RM. Chest wall tumors. In: Shields TW, Locicero J, Reed CE, Feins RH (Eds). General Thoracic Surgery. Philadelphia, PA: Lippincott; 2009:669-78
5. P O'Sullivan, H O'Dwyer, et al. Soft tissue tumors and mass-like lesions of the chest wall: a pictorial review of CT and MR findings. B J Radiol. 2007;80:574-80.
6. Baumgartner F. Tumors of chest wall and pleura. Cardiothoracic Surgery. 375-9.
7. Moon WK, Im JG, Han MC. Malignant schwannomas of the thorax: CT findings. J Comput Assist Tomogr. 1993;17:274-6.
8. Verstraete KL, Achten E, De Schepper A, et al. Nerve sheath tumors: evaluation with CT and MR imaging. J Belge Radiol. 1992;75:311-20.
9. Tsuzuki E, Kamimura M, Kobayashi N, et al. A case of schwannoma of the chest wall showing a bead-like appearance in MRI [Article in Japanese]. Nihon Kokyuki Gakkai Zasshi. 2003;41:766-70.
10. Tateishi U, Gladish GW, Kusumoto M, et al. Chest wall tumors: radiologic findings and pathologic correlation: part 1. Benign tumors. Radiographs. 2003;23:1477-90.
11. Elizabeth A. David, M. Blair Marshall, et al. Review of Chest Wall Tumors: A Diagnostic, Therapeutic, and Reconstructive Challenge. Seminars in Plastic Surgery. 2011;25(1):16-24.
12. Stanic´ V, Vulovic´ T, Novakovic´ M, et al. Radical resection of giant chondrosarcoma of the anterior chest wall. Vojnosanit Pregl. 2008;65:64-8.
13. Shah AA, D'Amico TA. Primary chest wall tumors. J Am Coll Surg. 2010;210:360-6.
14. Somers J, Faber LP. Chondroma and chondrosarcoma. Semin Thorac Cardiovasc Surg. 1999; 11:270-7.
15. Yoshida N, Miyanari N, Yamamoto Y, et al. Successful treatment of malignant fibrous histiocytoma originating in the chest wall: report of a case. Surg Today. 2006;36:714-21.
16. Tateishi U, Gladish GW, Kusumoto M, et al. Chest wall tumors: radiologic findings and pathologic correlation: part 2.Malignant tumors. Radiographics. 2003;23:1491-508.
17. Mahajan H, Kim E, Wallace S, et al. Magnetic resonance imaging of malignant fibrous histiocytoma. Magn Reson Imaging. 1989;7:283-8.
18. Gallo AE, Coady MA. Chest wall tumors. In: Yuh DD, Vricella LA, Baumgartner WA (Eds). The Johns Hopkins Manual of Cardiothoracic Surgery. New York, NY: McGraw Hill; 2007:75-90.
19. Yoshida N, Miyanari N, Yamamoto Y, et al. Successful treatment of malignant fibrous histiocytoma originating in the chest wall: report of a case. Surg Today. 2006;36:714-21.
20. Lee WS, Kim YH, Chee HK, et al. Multimodal treatment of primary extraskeletal Ewing's sarcoma of the chest wall: report of 2 cases. Cancer Res Treat. 2009;41:108-12.
21. Haffty BG, Hauser A, Choi DH, et al. Molecular markers for prognosis after isolated post-mastectomy chest wall recurrence. Cancer. 2004;100:252-63.
22. Cuenca RE, Allison RR, Sibata C, et al. Breast cancer with chest wall progression: treatment with photodynamic therapy. Ann Surg Oncol. 2004;11:322-7.

23. Hazard HW, Gorla SR, Scholtens D, et al. Surgical resection of the primary tumor, chest wall control, and survival in women with metastatic breast cancer. Cancer. 2008;113:2011-9.

24. Haraguchi S, Hioki M, Takushima M, et al. Metastatic chest wall tumor suspected to be of lung origin by immunoreactivity for cytokeratin 7 and 20. Jpn J Thorac Cardiovasc Surg. 2006;54:132-6.

25. Styring E, Fernebro J, Jo¨nsson PE, et al. Changing clinical presentation of angiosarcomas after breast cancer: from late tumors in edematous arms to earlier tumors on the thoracic wall. Breast Cancer Res Treat. 2010;122:883-7.

26. Shoji T, Sonobe M, Okubo K, et al. Giant primary liposarcoma of the chest. Gen Thorac Cardiovasc Surg. 2009;57:159-61.

27. Gallo AE, Coady MA. Chest wall tumors. In: Yuh DD, Vricella LA, Baumgartner WA (Eds). The Johns Hopkins Manual of Cardiothoracic Surgery. New York, NY: McGraw Hill; 2007:75-90.

28. Park BJ, Flores RM. Chest wall tumors. In: Shields TW, Locicero J, Reed CE, Feins RH (Eds). General Thoracic Surgery. Philadelphia, PA: Lippincott; 2009:669-78.

29. Kabiri EH, Al Aziz S, El Maslout A, et al. Desmoid tumors of the chest wall. Eur J Cardiothoracic Surg. 2001;19:580-3.

30. Allen PJ, Schriver CD. Desmoid tumors of the chest wall. Semin Thorac Cardiovasc Surg 1999;11:264-9.

31. Abbas AE, Deschamps C, Cassivi SD, et a . Chest-wall desmoid tumors: results of surgical intervention. Ann Thorac Surg. 2004;78:1219-23; discussion 1219-23.

32. Lee TJ, Collins J. MR imaging evaluation of disorders of the chest wall. Magn Reson Imaging Clin N Am. 2008; 16:355–379.

33. Incarbone M, Pastorino U. Surgical treatment of chest wall tumors. World J Surg. 2001;25:218-30.

34. Kucharczuk JC, Kaiser LR. Chest wall resections. In: Kaiser LR, Kron IL, Spray TL (Eds). Mastery of Cardiothoracic Surgery. Philadelphia, PA: Lippincott; 2007:222-7.

35. Ryan MB, McMurtrey MJ, Roth JA. Current management of chest-wall tumors. Surg Clin North Am. 1989;69:1061-80.

36. King RM, Pairolero PC, Trastek VF, et al. Primary chest wall tumors: factors affecting survival. Ann Thorac Surg. 1986;41:597-601.

37. Widhe B, Bauer HCF; Scandinavian Sarcoma Group. Surgical treatment is decisive for outcome in chondrosarcoma of the chest wall: a population-based Scandinavian Sarcoma Group study of 106 patients. J Thorac Cardiovasc Surg. 2009;137:610-4.

42 Tumors of the Adrenal Gland

Varun Gunavanthe, Jagdeesh Kulkarni

INTRODUCTION

The adrenal or suprarenal glands are paired retroperitoneal organs, located above and medial to the kidneys in the upper abdomen (Fig. 1). They lie adjacent to the aorta, inferior vena cava (IVC) and other vital structures. The right adrenal gland is roughly triangular in shape while the left is crescent-shaped. Each gland normally weighs about 4–5 g; is 4–6 cm in length and 2–3 cm in width. Further, each gland is morphologically divided into an outer cortex and an inner medulla with an endocrine and neurocrine function which play a vital role in maintaining homeostasis.

The adrenal cortex is subdivided into three zones: (1) Zona glomerulosa, (2) zona fasciculata and (3) zona reticularis, that produce aldosterone (mineralocorticoids), cortisol (glucocorticoids) and sex steroids (androstenedione, dehydroepiandrosterone (DHEA), testosterone and estradiol], respectively (Fig. 2). The adrenal medulla is embryologically distinct and considered part of the autonomic nervous system, as it secretes epinephrine (80%) and norepinephrine (19%) (catecholamines), along with dopamine (1%). Aldosterone is a regulator of sodium and water homeostasis, regulated by the renin-angiotensin-aldosterone system and potassium levels in the body and is weakly regulated by the adrenocorticotropic hormone (ACTH). Cortisol is intricately associated to the circadian rhythm as well as metabolism, immunity, modulation of central nervous system (CNS), intravascular volume and blood pressure.

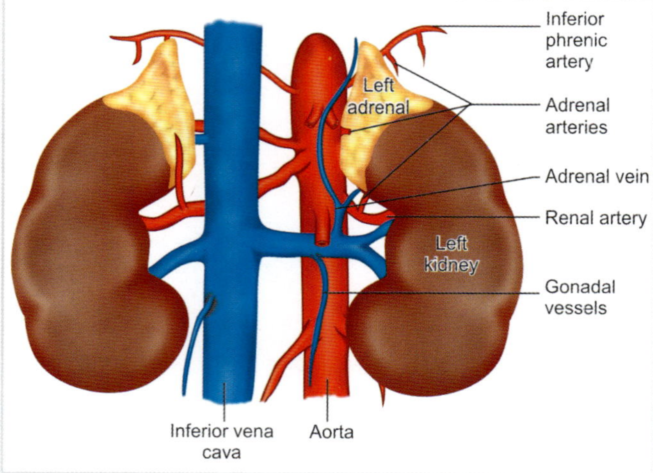

Fig. 1: Anatomy and vascularity of the adrenal glands

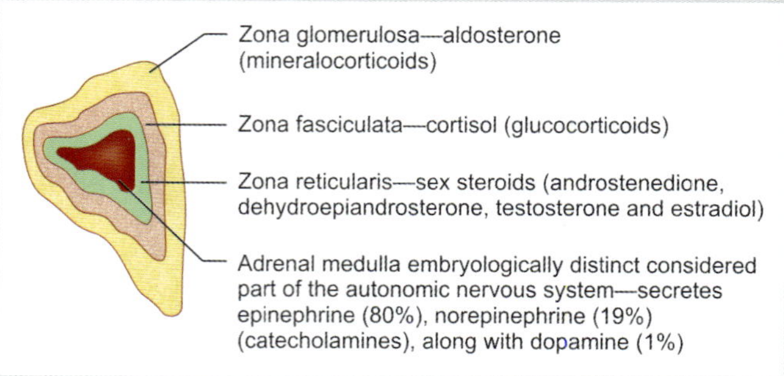

Fig. 2: Zones of the adrenal cortex, adrenal medulla and the adrenal hormones

CLINICAL PRESENTATION

Clinical symptoms due to adrenal pathology relate to either a hyperfunctioning adrenal lesion or an asymptomatic adrenal mass, incidentally detected on imaging done for some other reasons (hence called "incidentaloma") (Fig. 3). Hyperfunctioning lesions may be subclinical or may present as hypertension, electrolyte imbalance, fatigue, headaches, anxiety, palpitations, weight gain or

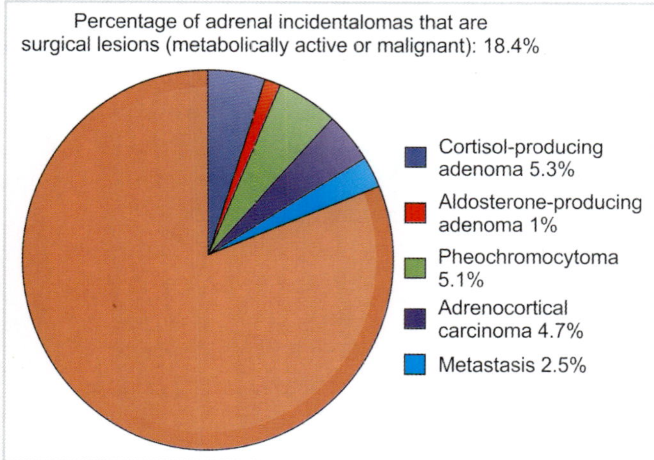

Fig. 3: Adrenal incidentalomas of surgical importance

loss depending on the nature of the lesion and excessive hormone secretion. It is important to assess the lesion by functional (Flow chart 1) and imaging studies (Flow chart 2), and plan management with a multidisciplinary approach along with an endocrinologist or internist to obtain an optimum control of the metabolic derangements in the perioperative period.

ETIOPATHOLOGY OF ADRENAL MASS

Malignant Lesions

- *Pheochromocytoma*: Incidence is about 1–2 per 100,000 population
- *Adrenal carcinoma*: 0.5–2 per 1,000,000 population

Flow chart 1: Functional evaluation of adrenal masses

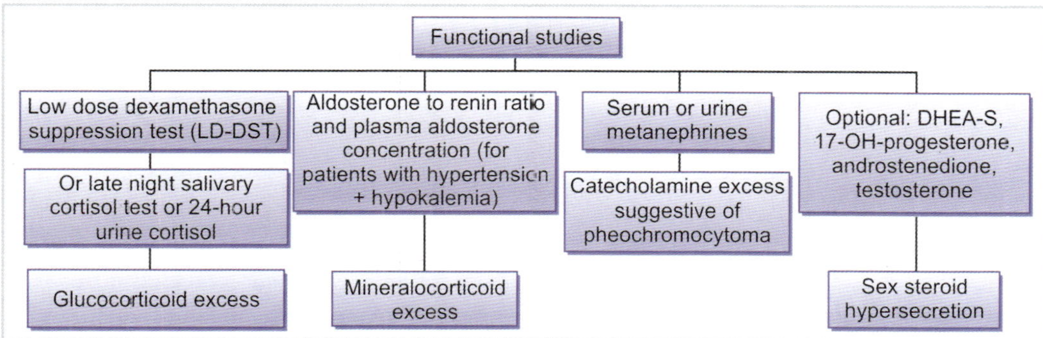

Abbreviation: DHEA-S, dehydroepiandrosterone sulfate

Flow chart 2: Radiological evaluation of adrenal tumors

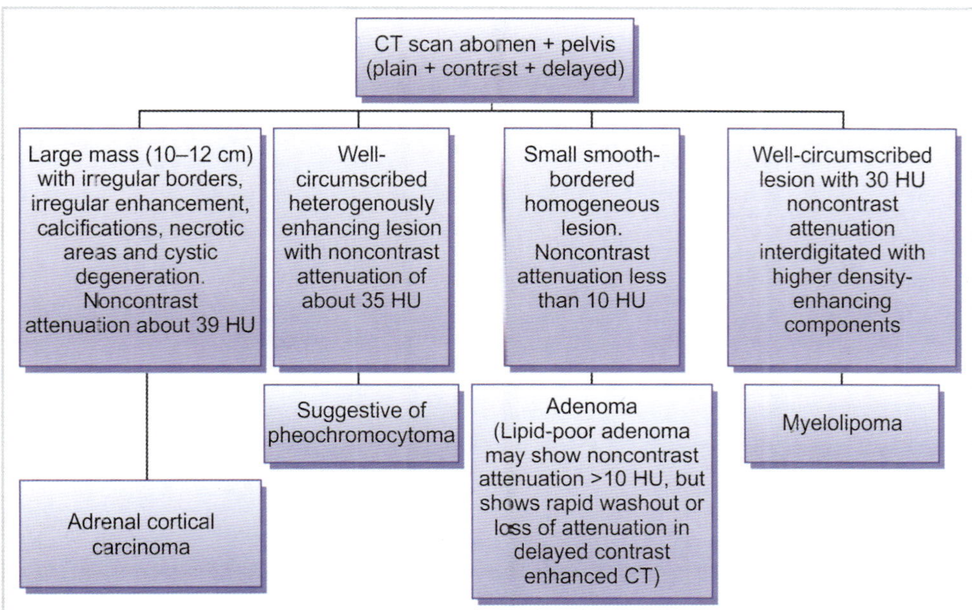

Abbreviations: CT, computed tomography; HU, Hounsfield units

- Metastasis to adrenal from melanoma, lung cancer, renal cell carcinoma (RCC), breast cancer, medullary thyroid cancer, opposite adrenal cancer, gastrointestinal, prostate, cervical and several other malignancies
- *Neuroblastoma*: In children.

Benign Lesions

- *Adenoma*: Incidence of about 6% in an autopsy series (clinically detected in about 0.5% individuals in the third decade to upto 7% in the seventh decade of life, > 85% being incidental)
- *Myelolipoma*: Less than 0.1% on autopsy series
- *Oncocytoma*: Extremely rare
- *Adrenal cysts*: 0.064–0.18%
- *Ganglioneuromas*: Extremely rare
- Nodular hyperplasia

SURGICAL INDICATIONS FOR ADRENALECTOMY[1,2] (FLOW CHART 3)

- Malignant features on imaging (lipid-poor, heterogeneous, irregular borders, infiltrates surrounding structures, etc.)
- Adrenal incidentaloma with growth greater than 1 cm on follow-up imaging
- During radical nephrectomy for RCC if: Adrenal abnormal or not visualized due to large renal tumor size on imaging/large (≥7 cm) upper pole mass/vein thrombus to level of adrenal vein
- Adrenocorticotropic hormone-independent macronodular adrenal hyperplasia (AIMAH), primary pigmented nodular adrenocortical disease (PPNAD)
- *Metastasis*: Isolated adrenal metastasis (multidisciplinary decision making required)
- *Functional adrenal mass*: Cortisol hypersecretion, pheochromocytoma, aldosterone hypersecretion
- Adrenocorticotropic hormone (ectopic ACTH) syndrome, requiring bilateral adrenalectomy
- Cushing's syndrome with failed neurosurgical treatment (requiring bilateral adrenalectomy)
- Extremely large and/or symptomatic myelolipoma (see adrenal lesions: benign: myelolipoma)
- Size greater than 4 cm (of adrenal masses) with exception of myelolipoma.

DIFFERENTIAL DIAGNOSIS OF ADRENAL TUMORS

Pheochromocytoma[1,3,4]

Pheochromocytoma is a tumor of the adrenal medulla which produces excessive catecholamines that are either self-metabolized or secreted into the circulation. It is found in 5% of all incidentally detected adrenal masses and in 0.5% patients with hypertension. Ten to twenty-five percent lesions are extra-adrenal, 10% are bilateral, 10% (upto

Flow chart 3: Algorithm for management of adrenal lesions

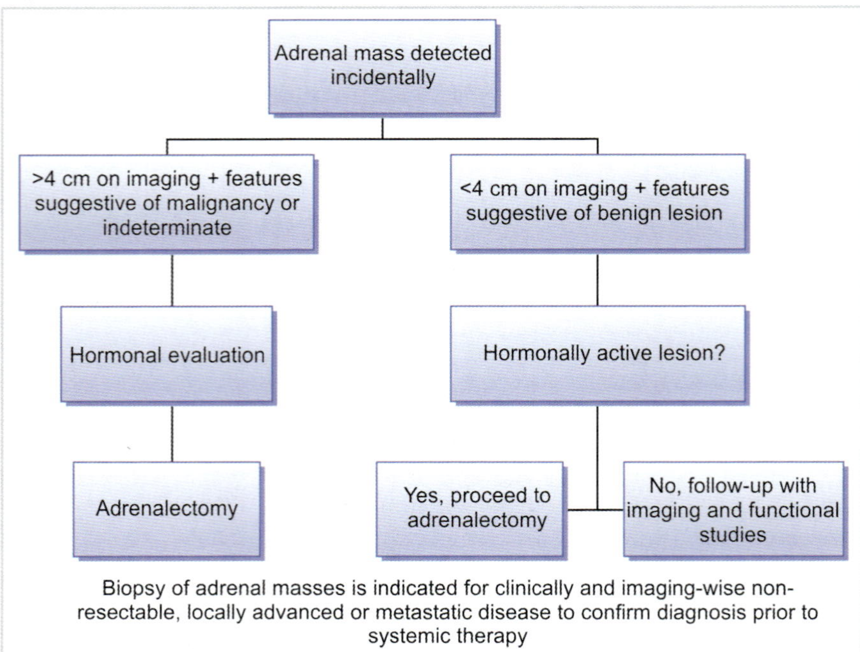

one-third) are familial, 10% occur in children and 40% are malignant. Hence it was classically described as the "10% tumor". Forty percent of pediatric pheochromocytomas are familial and more than 20% of these are bilateral. Various syndromes associated with pheochromocytoma are multiple endocrine neoplasia [multiple endocrine neoplasia (MEN) 2A and 2B] syndromes, von Hippel-Lindau syndrome (VHL type 2), neurofibromatosis type 1 and familial paraganglioma syndromes (PGL-1 and PGL-4). Hereditary pheochromocytomas occur at a younger age of about 40 years and tend to be multifocal and bilateral.

Clinical Features and Investigations

Patients usually present with headaches, palpitations and episodic sudden perspiration. They may report with nausea, hot flashes, weight loss, tiredness and anxiety. Physical examination may reveal pallor, tachycardia, sustained or paroxysmal hypertension and sometimes orthostatic hypotension. Basic laboratory tests may show hyperglycemia while specific biochemical tests indicate elevated plasma-free metanephrines (metanephrine and normetanephrine together, which are the metabolites of epinephrine and norepinephrine, respectively). Twenty four fractionated metanephrine levels are raised. Elevated plasma and urine catecholamines were used previously for diagnosis as was elevated urinary vanillylmandelic acid (VMA) levels (the end metabolite of catecholamines). Other tests like clonidine suppression test and chromogranin A are also useful. It is advisable to complete the metabolic/functional evaluation in all patients with adrenal masses planned for surgery.

Imaging

Computed tomography (CT) scan shows a well-circumscribed adrenal mass with noncontrast attenuation of about 35 Hounsfield units (HU), heterogeneously enhancing without rapid contrast washout on delayed imaging. Extra-adrenal pheochromocytomas are called PGLs.[5] Magnetic resonance imaging (MRI) shows bright signal intensity on T_2-weighted imaging on fat suppression sequences: "Light bulb" sign. Metaiodobenzylguanidine (MIBG) scan involves administration of radioactive iodine-tagged MIBG which is an analogue of norepinephrine to detect or locate extra-adrenal, metastatic or recurrent pheochromocytoma. Pheochromocytoma is called malignant only if there is evidence of metastasis to bone, lungs, liver or lymph nodes.

Surgery

Preoperatively, the patient must be referred to an Endocrinologist and the anesthetist for planning and premedication. Complete surgical resection by open, laparoscopic or robotic technique is the treatment of choice. Perioperative blood pressure control and maintenance of homeostasis is of utmost importance. Two weeks prior to the planned surgery, alpha (α)-blockers like phenoxybenzamine, terazosin or prazosin is started to maintain blood pressure in normal range. If patient develops tachycardia or arrhythmias, beta (β)-blockers like atenolol or metoprolol may be added. Alternatives are calcium-channel blockers and catecholamine synthesis blockers like metyrosine. These medications are continued until the night before surgery. Two days prior to planned surgery, patient must be admitted to the hospital and strict blood pressure control is exercised with good oral salt and fluid intake and intravenous fluid administration (to restore the intravascular volume and prevent risk of prolonged hypotension following adrenalectomy). Proper anesthetic management with arterial blood pressure monitoring, hypotensive and inotropic infusion lines is crucial for a successful surgical outcome.

Postoperatively with the withdrawal of the adrenergic stimulus following resection of pheochromocytoma, there may be rebound hypotension, hyperinsulinemia and subsequent hypoglycemia. Hence, close monitoring in the intensive care unit is necessary. Follow-up studies include repeat metabolic testing about 2 weeks postoperatively to document normalization of function. If metanephrine level remain elevated or hypertension continues, MIBG scan may help to detect previously missed or unnoticed metastases or other foci. Long-term follow-up is essential because 10-year recurrence rates are as high as 16% in some series and annual biochemical follow-up is mandatory for all patients. Subsequent imaging may be guided by results of the biochemical testing.

Patients with hereditary pheochromocytoma have a lower-risk of malignancy and tend to have bilateral disease. Hence partial cortical-sparing adrenalectomy is indicated to avoid Addison's disease and lifelong hormonal replacement and its associated morbidity. Nevertheless, counseling regarding the possible need of hormonal replacement despite a seemingly successful cortex-sparing procedure is necessary. Treatment of malignant/metastatic pheochromocytoma is largely palliative, with surgical metastasectomy whenever disease is resectable;

however, there is little evidence to demonstrate that it prolongs patient survival. An effective option is medical treatment with α/β blockade and α-methyl-paratyrosine for symptomatic relief. Local minimally invasive ablation techniques and embolization have been described.

Radioactive 131I-MIBG has been tried for the systemic treatment of metastatic patients owing to the selective uptake of MIBG by pheochromocytoma cells. About 30% of patients show tumor volume reduction, 40% exhibit a reduction in catecholamine levels and two-thirds show symptomatic response. Standard combination chemotherapy of cyclophosphamide, vincristine and dacarbazine (CVD) for malignant pheochromocytoma has a short-lived response (about 2 years). It may be used in patients who have failed MIBG therapy, or tumors that do not demonstrate MIBG uptake on initial scan.

Prognosis is good following surgical resection of pheochromocytoma with surgical mortality rates less than 3% and resolution of hypertension in most cases. However, recurrence in about 16% of patients necessitate vigilant lifelong follow-up. Studies suggest that extra-adrenal disease, hereditary pheochromocytomas, bilateral and larger tumors are more likely to recur, of which nearly 50% could be malignant. Bone metastases carry a bad prognosis. Overall 5-year survival is about 50%.

Adrenal Cortical Carcinoma[1,3,4]

Adrenocortical masses of the size (>4–6 cm) are likely to be malignant and majority of these lesions are functional at the time of presentation. Most patients with adrenal cortical carcinoma (ACC) are adults in the fourth to fifth decades of life, with a female predominance of 1.5–2.1. Children with ACC usually present in first decade of life with lower-stage functional tumors and have better survival. Most ACCs are sporadic and unilateral; however, 2–6% may be bilateral and associated with hereditary diseases. ACC is associated with various syndromes such as Li-Fraumeni syndrome (loss of TP53 function), Beckwith-Wiedemann syndrome [increased insulin-like growth factor (IGF) expression], Carney complex, MEN type 1, and McCune-Albright's syndrome. Surgical resection is the cornerstone of treatment and offers the best chance of cure for localized disease, but multimodal therapy including systemic chemotherapy and radiation therapy are often used for locally advanced and metastatic disease.

Most patients present with advanced disease and tumor-related symptoms (local or systemic) such as abdominal fullness, back pain, nausea, vomiting and other constitutional symptoms or features of hyperfunction due to hormone secretion. ACCs are now increasingly detected with the routine use of cross-sectional imaging. About 50–79% of adult and 90% of pediatric ACCs show significant metabolic activity (functional). These may be steroid precursors (patient is asymptomatic) or cortisol (most common hormone secreted presenting as ACTH-independent Cushing's syndrome with associated virilization) or 17-ketosteroids and DHEA. Androgen-secreting tumors in women can cause virilization, evident as male-pattern baldness, hirsutism and oligomenorrhea (due to elevated 17-ketosteroids). Hypersecretion of aldosterone is rare with ACC, and causes profound hypertension and hypokalemia.

Diagnostic Tests

Clinical symptoms or radiographic findings suggestive of ACC (irregular borders, irregular enhancement, calcifications, and necrotic areas with cystic degeneration with mean attenuation on noncontrast CT scan in ACC of about 39 HU compared with 8 HU as in the case of adenomas) warrant complete evaluation of the functional status of the suspicious adrenal tumor. The radiographic characteristics of ACC include larger tumors about 10–12 cm (90% being are >5 cm and 25% of tumors >6 cm are adrenal carcinomas). It is currently recommended that adrenal tumors greater than 4–6 cm should be surgically excised. Complete metastatic evaluation for lymphadenopathy and local tumor extension into the IVC and other adjacent organs should be performed as these are ominous indicators of locally advanced or distant metastatic disease. Common sites of metastases in ACC are the lung and liver. Hence cross-sectional imaging of the chest, abdomen and pelvis is a must. Bone and CNS metastases should be excluded in patients with site-specific symptoms. ACCs on MRI appear isointense relative to the liver or spleen on T_1-weighted images and demonstrate intermediate to increased intensity on T_2-weighted images. Gadolinium-enhanced images demonstrate marked contrast uptake by ACCs. In cases of suspicion for venous tumor thrombus, MRI can be an essential tool in detecting the presence of a tumor clot and delineating its extent. Experience with fluorodeoxyglucose (FDG)-positron emission tomography (PET) in diagnosing ACC is limited. Percutaneous needle biopsy is generally avoided prior to surgical excision of ACC due to a clinically unacceptable risk of needle-tract seeding and is considered only for non-resectable, locally advanced, or metastatic disease to confirm the diagnosis prior to systemic medical therapy. Surgically extirpation is justified for resectable disease, based on the information obtained from biochemical and radiographic evaluation.

Presence of distant metastasis and local invasion suggest malignancy, but in organ-confined tumors, the differentiation between benign and malignant neoplasms can be difficult. The Weiss criteria (1984) based on the higher nuclear grade (Fuhrman grade 3–4), mitotic rate [> 5 mitoses per high-power field (hpf)], presence of atypical mitoses, character of cytoplasm (low percentage of clear cells), diffuse architecture of tumor cells, presence of necrosis and the invasion of venous structures, sinusoidal structures and tumor capsule help to distinguish benign from malignant adrenal tumors (presence of three or more of the Weiss criteria).

Management

Treatment of ACC often requires a multimodal approach by the surgeons, medical oncologists, endocrinologists and radiation oncologists because most patients with ACCs present with advanced disease and those with localized disease have a high-risk of local recurrence (60–80%) and metastatic progression. Thus adjuvant therapy is often administered, but its impact on survival is not established.

Surgery: Complete surgical excision of the ACC offers the best chance of cure and control of symptoms due to hypersecretion of hormones, and other tumor-related symptoms. Regional (retroperitoneal) lymphadenectomy aids disease control and staging. Patients having venous tumor thrombus involving the IVC may require vascular bypass techniques. Open abdominal/retroperitoneal exploration is preferred due to the risk of tumor spillage, if done laparoscopically. Debulking surgery does not improve survival and is used only as a palliative measure to alleviate tumor-related side-effects or to facilitate additional therapies. Radiofrequency ablation or angioembolization may be used for locally recurrent disease and select metastatic lesions, if surgical excision cannot be performed.

Follow-up: Three-monthly CT imaging of chest, abdomen and pelvis for the first 2 years and less frequently thereafter. Measurement of elevated hormones postoperatively may help to reveal early disease recurrence despite negative radiographic studies.

Radiation: It is the treatment of choice for bone and CNS metastasis. Adjuvant radiation helps decrease local recurrence rates following complete tumor resection, with reported local recurrence rates of 14% and 79%, with and without adjuvant radiation therapy, respectively, but overall survival does not improve. Adjuvant radiation therapy may benefit those without evidence of metastatic disease and positive or indeterminant surgical margins.

Medical therapy: Mitotane is a synthetic derivative of the insecticide dichlorodiphenyltrichloroethane (DDT) and has demonstrated clinical benefit in the adjuvant setting following surgical resection and in patients with metastatic ACC. It acts by direct cytotoxicity of cells in the adrenal cortex, free-radical oxidative damage, and/or inhibition of enzymes involved with steroid synthesis. Hence, steroid replacement is typically necessary during therapy. It needs close monitoring and dosage titration according to patient tolerability and serum levels. At present, mitotane is the primary systemic therapy, as a single agent or in combination with other cytotoxic drugs (streptozotocin, etoposide, doxorubicin and cisplatin) for ACCs and for patients who are not candidates for complete tumor debulking. To control symptoms due to hypersecretion of hormones in patients with metastatic disease, adrenostatic drugs such as ketoconazole, metyrapone, aminoglutethimide and etomidate have been used in symptomatic patients to decrease cortisol levels. ACC have a poor (20–47%) overall 5-year survival, probably due to advanced stage at presentation, high rate of recurrence and the limited efficacy of current systemic therapy (Table 1).

TABLE 1: Staging of tumor, nodes and metastases (TNM) and survival

Stage	*Description*	*Incidence at diagnosis*	*5-year survival rate*
1	T1N0M0 confined to the adrenal gland <5 cm	3–4%	33–66%
2	T2N0M0 confined to the adrenal gland >5 cm	29–46%	20–58%
3	T3N0M0 extension into adjacent adipose tissue, IVC	11–19%	18–24%
	T1-2N1M0 regional lymph node involvement		
4	T3N1M0	39–49%	<5%
	T4N0-1M0 invasion of adjacent organs		
	T1-4N0-1M1 presence of distant metastasis		

Abbreviations: TNM, tumor, nodes and metastases; IVC, inferior vena cava

Metastases[1]

Owing to its vascularity, adrenal glands are a common site of metastases from lung carcinoma, RCC, breast cancer, medullary thyroid cancer, contralateral adrenocortical carcinoma, gastrointestinal, prostate, cervical cancer, basal cell, squamous cell, biliary-pancreatic, urothelial, seminoma, chronic myelogenous leukemia and several other malignancies. If patient has a history of a previous malignancy, over 50% of new adrenal lesions are metastatic. Radiographic imaging along with adrenal biopsy can diagnose metastases in the adrenal gland. RCC can have direct adrenal invasion or systemic metastases to adrenal. In melanoma and non-small cell lung carcinoma, resection of an isolated adrenal metastasis may confer survival benefit.

Adenoma[1]

Adenomas are the most common benign neoplasms arising from the adrenal gland, found in about 6% of patients at autopsy and are usually discovered incidentally on cross-sectional imaging obtained for other indications (>85%) (hence termed "incidentalomas"). Adrenal adenomas can exhibit metabolic activity (about 6% secrete cortisol, 1.1% hyperaldosteronomas) and hence require complete metabolic work-up, as they may require surgical intervention. They have yellowish color on gross pathological examination due to abundant lipid content. Histologically, they are difficult to distinguish from adenocarcinomas (Weiss criteria and modern immunohistochemical methods help in making the differentiation). Nonfunctional adrenal adenomas are thought to be associated with physiologic derangements like insulin resistance and left ventricular dysfunction. It is important to rule out the possibility of malignancy and document metabolic inactivity in all adrenal lesions greater than 1 cm in size. The growth kinetics of adrenal adenomas (>1 cm on follow-up) and likelihood of a metabolically inert adenoma to become functional on follow-up (1.7%) dictate the need for intervention.

Diagnostic Tests

Noncontrast CT scan shows most adenomas to be smooth-bordered, homogeneous tumors, less than 4 cm in diameter and due to high intracytoplasmic lipid content; they demonstrate an attenuation of less than 10 HU on unenhanced CT. About 30% of adrenal adenomas with attenuation greater than 10 HU on unenhanced CT are lipid-poor adenomas. These lesions show rapid loss of attenuation on delayed contrast-enhanced CT imaging called "washout" (>40–60% is indicative). MRI can also characterize adrenal adenomas. Pheochromocytomas may mimic adenomas on imaging, hence metanephrine testing of all adrenal lesions is recommended.

Management

Metabolically active adenomas should be completely excised in surgically fit and willing patients. Nonfunctioning adrenal masses greater than 4–6 cm have a substantial risk of malignancy (except for adrenal myelolipoma). The option of initial radiographic follow-up to ascertain growth kinetics at 6 months, 12 months and 24 months may be offered to the patient to confirm indolent growth pattern. Annual metabolic hormonal screening for 3–4 years following diagnosis is recommended, especially for masses of about 3 cm diameter. Hormone levels may return to normal within 3 months of adrenalectomy, although hypertension may continue and require medications.

Oncocytoma[1]

Oncocytomas in the adrenal glands are exceedingly rare and their evaluation is similar to an incidentaloma. The diagnosis of adrenal oncocytic tumor is usually made after surgical resection. They are histologically characterized by mitochondria-rich, large, eosinophilic cells with abundant granulations. Females are affected 2.5 times more frequently than males, and left-sided lesions predominate (3.5:1). Most lesions are metabolically inactive but about 10% may hypersecrete sex steroids, cytokines and/or cortisol. Thirty percent oncocytomas are malignant while about 23% have pathologically indeterminate behavior. On imaging, adrenal oncocytic lesions do not usually show the characteristic central stellate scar. Malignant oncocytic lesions have no recommended line of treatment but metastasectomy and radiation treatment for local recurrence have been advised. Most oncocytomas have a benign course.

Myelolipoma[1]

Myelolipomas are rare, benign, metabolically silent lesions of the adrenal gland with an incidence of less than 0.1%. Studies report that 15% of all myelolipomas are extra-adrenal. Myelolipomas are thought to result from clonal stem cell proliferation as an adrenal stress response and are composed of a mixture of mature adipose tissue and normal hematopoietic elements. These lesions do not contribute hematopoietic cells to the circulation. Etiology of these unusual tumors remains unknown. Men and women are equally affected. There is no predilection for any particular side. Tumors vary in size (average being about 5.1 cm), and may grow to sizes exceeding 10 cm. The patients are usually asymptomatic or may present with abdominal or flank pain. Spontaneous rupture of myelolipomas is rare and more likely for large lesions. Very rarely myelolipomas may demonstrate adrenal metabolic hyperactivity, commonly hypercortisolemia. CT imaging reveals a well-circumscribed adrenal lesion with varying amounts of mature adipose tissue (30 HU) interdigitated with higher-density myeloid components that enhance with contrast administration.

Over 25% of these may exhibit evidence of calcifications and areas of hemorrhage. The presence of macroscopic fat in an adrenal mass as seen by the MRI is virtually diagnostic of a myelolipoma. Standard adrenal metabolic work-up is not routinely recommended for myelolipoma. Asymptomatic myelolipomas may be treated conservatively with serial ultrasonography or CT evaluation every several years. Surgery is usually indicated for symptomatic lesions. Most lesions grow slowly or remain stable, but some may even decrease in size over time and surgical resection is considered definitive.

ILLUSTRATIVE CASE REPORTS

- A young male patient presented with a history of blurring of vision and giddiness. His blood pressure at admission was 260/180 mm Hg. With pharmacological control of hypertension, he was evaluated with imaging and functional studies. CT scan was suggestive of a right pheochromocytoma. His urine metanephrine level was 1,257 μg/day (normal range 0–350 μg/day), urine-epinephrine level was 134 μg/day (normally <20 μg/day) and plasma-free metanephrine was 787 pg/mL (normally < 90 pg/mL). With adequate preoperative adrenergic blockade, patient was explored by a transperitoneal midline approach and the irregular nodular mass was found arising from the right adrenal gland (Figs 4A and B), which was excised completely and histopathologically confirmed as a pheochromocytoma. Postoperatively patient had normal blood pressure without medications.
- A 21-year old man with complaints of intermittent headache was found to have a blood pressure of 220/100 mm Hg. CT scan of the abdomen (Figs 5A to C) revealed multiple (three) partially necrotic inhomogeneously-enhancing nodular lesions in the aortocaval and left paraaortic region at the renal hilum, abutting the adjacent vessels and compressing the duodenum and IVC. The study suggested a diagnosis of multiple PGLs. An MIBG scan confirmed the concentration of the tracer in the paraaortic region of the abdomen. His blood pressure was controlled with four antihypertensive medications. After adequate preoperative preparation, the patient had laparotomy with complete excision of the masses. After an uneventful surgery and postoperative course, the patient was able to maintain normal blood pressure without the need of antihypertensive medications.
- A 46-year old male patient reported with the complaints of dull aching pain and fullness in the left upper abdomen. CT scan revealed a huge heterogeneously enhancing mass suggestive of a left adrenal carcinoma,

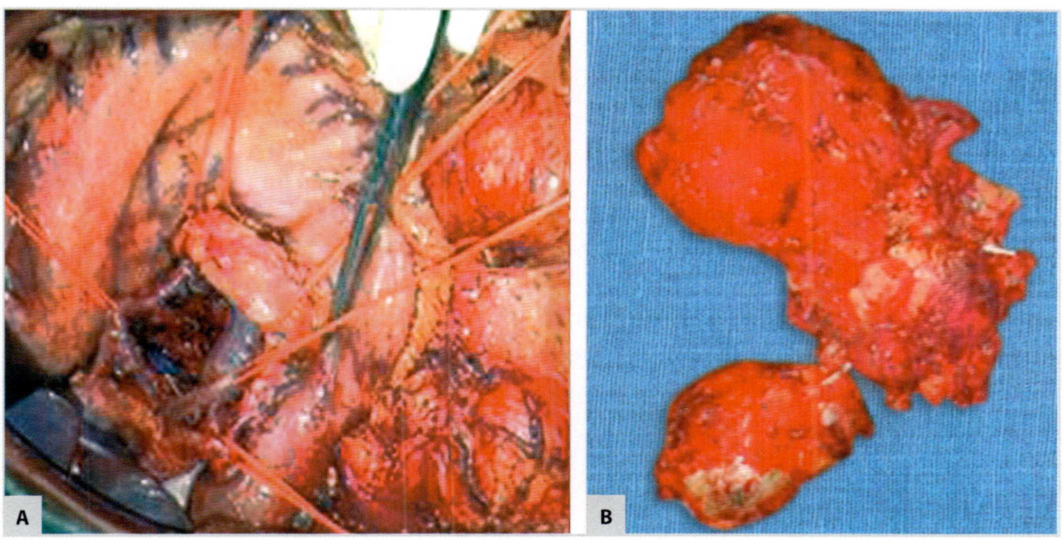

Figs 4A and B: (A) Operative picture and (B) specimen photograph of pheochromocytoma

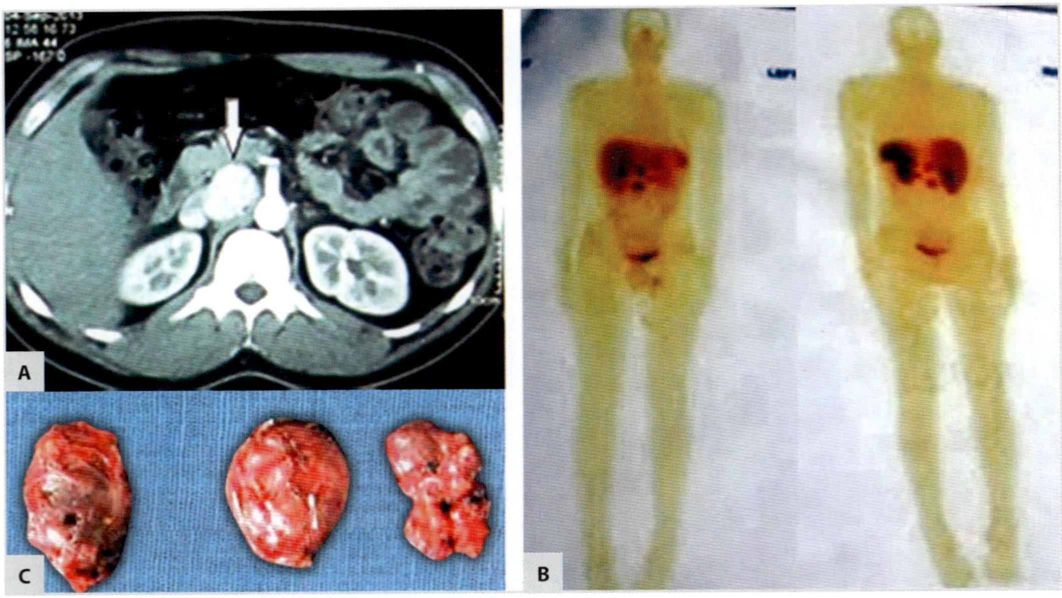

Figs 5A to C: (A) Computed tomography (CT) scan of paraganglioma (PGL) (extra-adrenal pheochromocytoma—arrow) anteromedial to inferior vena cava (IVC); (B) Metaiodobenzylguanidine (MIBG) scan; (C) Specimen photographs of paraganglioma (PGL)

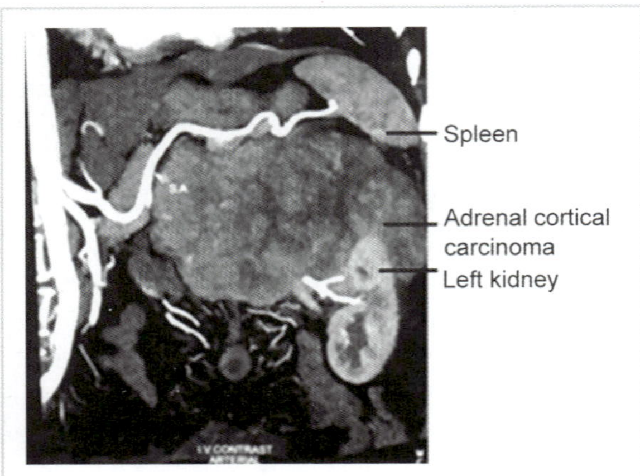

Fig. 6: Computed tomography (CT) scan image of a huge left adrenocortical carcinoma encasing the left renal vessels and an en bloc a left adrenalectomy with nephrectomy performed

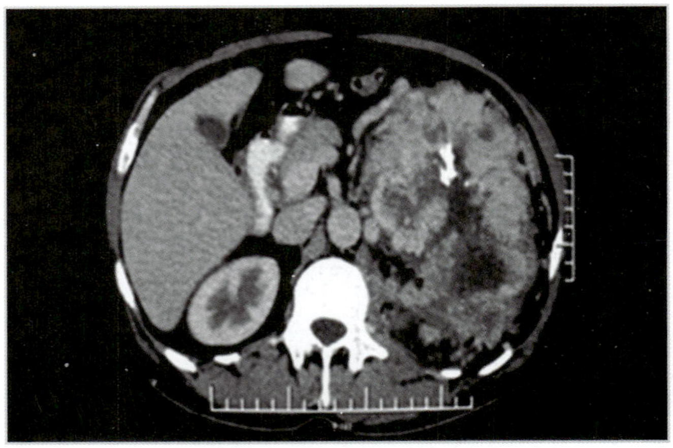

Fig. 7: Computed tomography (CT) scan showing a huge left perirenal hematoma from a myelolipoma left adrenal

pushing the left kidney downward and laterally. The left renal artery was encased by the tumor. Hence prior to surgery, consent for nephrectomy was taken. Indeed the kidney could not be salvaged due to the gross involvement of the renal vasculature with the adrenal mass and a left radical adrenalectomy with nephrectomy en bloc was done (Fig. 6). Microscopy showed high-grade adrenocortical carcinoma with involvement of upper pole of the kidney. He was counseled for adjuvant therapy with a negative response.

- A young male patient presented with acute pain in the left loin, in an emergency. CT imaging showed a huge hematoma in left suprarenal region (Figs 7 and 8). The differential diagnosis for the source of hemorrhage was thought to be either a myelolipoma of the left adrenal or angiomyolipoma from the upper pole of the left kidney. The patient was hemodynamically stabilized and explored, and the hematoma with the mass was totally excised (Figs 9A and B) and microscopy revealed a myelolipoma. Left kidney could be saved.

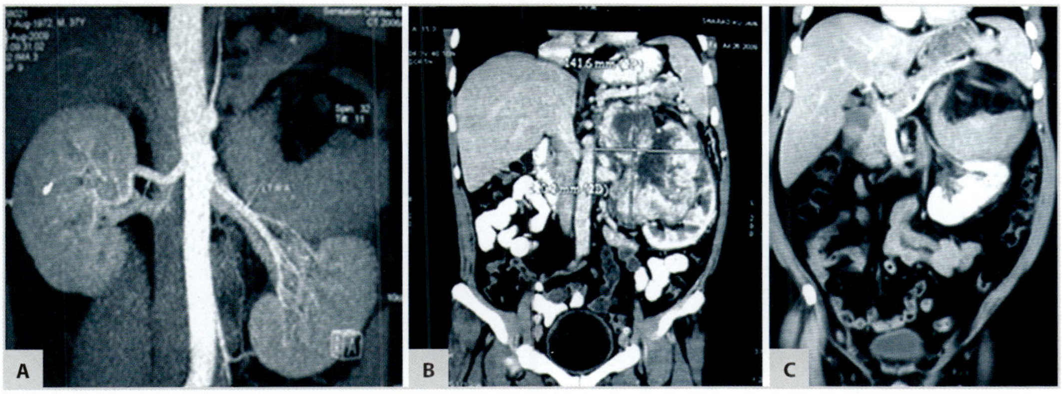

Figs 8A to C: Computed tomography (CT) scan showing a functioning left renal unit pushed downward by the hematoma

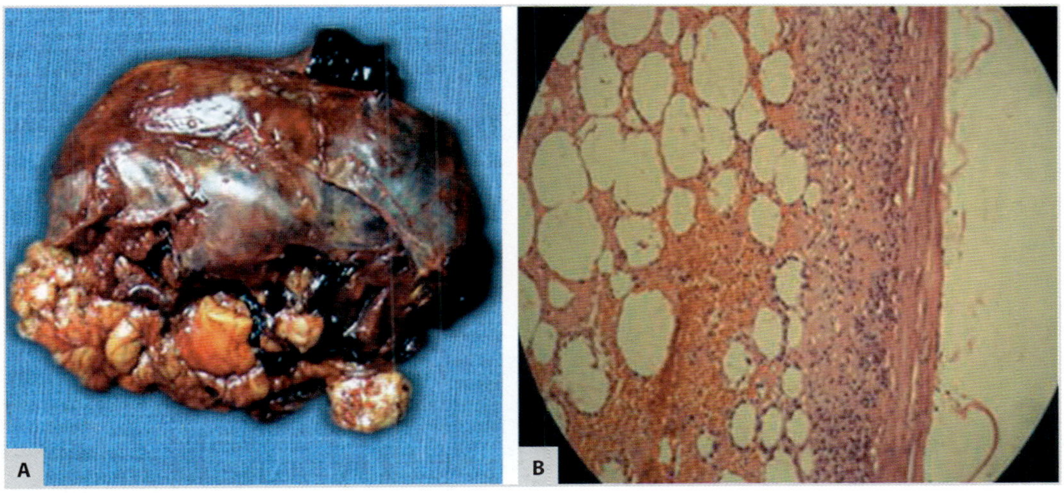

Figs 9A and B: Surgical specimen of (A) a myelolipoma with (B) hematoma. Histopathology confirms the diagnosis

REFERENCES

1. Kutikov A, Crispen PL, Jzzo RG. Pathophysiology, evaluation, and medical management of adrenal disorders. In: McDougal WS, Wein AJ, Kavoussi LR, Novick AC, Partin AW, Peters CA, Ramchandani P (Eds). Campbell-Walsh Urology, 10th edition review. Philadelphia, PA, USA: Elsevier Saunders; 2012. p. 312-9.
2. Chow GK, Blute ML. Surgery of the adrenal glands. In: McDougal WS, Wein AJ, Kavoussi LR, Novick AC, Partin AW, Peters CA, Ramchandani P (Eds). Campbell-Walsh Urology, 10th edition review. Philadelphia, PA, USA: Elsevier Saunders; 2012. pp 320-3.
3. Berruti A, Baudin E, Gelderblom H, et al. Adrenal cancer: ESMO Clinical Practice Guidelines for diagnosis, treatment and follow-up. *Ann Oncol.* 2012;23(Suppl 7):vii131-8.
4. Kane CJ. Disorders of the adrenal glands. In: Tanagho EA, McAninch JW (Eds). Smith's General Urology, 17th edition. New York, USA: McGraw-Hill Medical Publishing; 2007. p. 490-505.
5. Kulkarni JN, Tongaonkar HB, Kamat MR, et al. Extra-adrenal non-functioning paraganglioma. Tumori. 1990;76(3):258-60.

43 Renal Cell Carcinoma

Hemant B Tongaonkar, Ganesh K Bakshi, Santosh Menon, Kumar Prabhash, Amit Joshi

INTRODUCTION

The management approach to renal cell carcinoma (RCC) has undergone a paradigm shift in the last two decades. With a definite shift towards diagnosis of low stage, low-grade tumors, the treatment protocols have been redefined. This, along with better understanding of the biological behavior of RCC, refinement in diagnostic and therapeutic modalities, and the introduction of molecular targeted therapies have offered a ray of hope to patients with metastatic disease.

EPIDEMIOLOGY

Renal cell carcinoma is the third most common urological malignancy and accounts for 1.5% of all malignancies in India. It is the most lethal of all genitourinary malignancies.[1-3] It is much more common in the Western countries. Worldwide, annually there are approximately 209,000 new cases and 102,000 deaths secondary to RCC.

The incidence of RCC has been rising at a rate of 2.3–4.3% annually over the past 30 years,[4-6] partly due to a general increase in life expectancy and partly due to increased detection consequent upon the widespread use of abdominal imaging. This has been associated with an increased detection of localized incidentally detected tumors and an improved 5-year survival rates.[1,7,8] However, despite this increasing incidence, the mortality from RCC has decreased marginally.

It is more common in the elderly age group, the peak incidence being in the seventh decade,[1] with a male preponderance in the ratio of 1.5:1. RCCs are extremely uncommon in children, constituting 2.3–66.6% of all childhood renal tumors. It is equally common in children of both sexes, with a mean age of diagnosis being 8–9 years.[9,10] RCC in children is more likely to be of papillary histology, have locally advanced high-grade features and can have unfavorable histological variants. In view of this, aggressive surgery is recommended for RCC seen in children and young adults.[9,11,12]

ETIOLOGY

Although the exact etiology of RCC remains unclear, a number of environmental, hormonal, cellular, and genetic factors have been studied as possible causal factors in the development of RCC. Obesity and smoking appear to be risk factors, with relative risks of 3.6 and 2.3 respectively.[13-17] Chow et al. (2000) found a significant correlation between hypertension and RCC.[18] There have been no definitive association with occupational carcinogens. Other possible causes postulated are analgesic abuse, exposure to industrial solvents, antihypertensive medication, cadmium exposure, long-term exposure to petroleum, tar and pitch products patients of end stage renal disease (ESRD) on long-term dialysis but the evidence to the association of these factors with RCC is inconsistent and effect probably low.

Endogenous genetic risk factors include hereditary familial forms of kidney cancer such as the Von Hippel-Lindau disease (VHL), familial papillary RCC (HPRCC), hereditary leiomyoma RCC (HLRCC), the Birt-Hogg-Dube Syndrome (BHD), and tuberous sclerosis (TS).

Specific genotypic alterations have been associated with differing histological subtypes of RCC. Mutations in the VHL gene (a tumor suppressor) are responsible for most cases of conventional (clear cell) carcinoma. The VHL gene has been mapped to 3p25 and contains three axons with 852 coding nucleotides. Somatic mutations of the VHL gene are seen in approximately 50–75% of cases of sporadic clear cell renal carcinoma and are mostly point mutations, hypermethylation or rearrangement of the gene.

Other genetic alterations in clear cell RCC include frequent loss of heterozygosity (LOH) of chromosomes 8p, 14q and 9p (p16) among others suggesting other unknown tumor suppressors may be important in renal cell tumorigenesis. The most common genetic events associated with papillary RCC are trisomy of chromosomes 7 and 17 and loss of Y.

PATHOLOGY

Renal cell carcinoma originates from the renal tubular epithelium, as evidenced by electron microscopy[19] and immunohistochemical analysis.[20] They occur with equal frequency in either kidney and are randomly distributed in the upper and lower poles. RCCs originate in the cortex and tend to grow out into perinephric tissue, causing the characteristic bulge or mass effect that aids in their detection by diagnostic imaging studies. Most RCCs form a fibrous pseudocapsule when they grow and are usually not infiltrative except the collecting duct carcinomas. RCC has a number of distinct subtypes, each with a unique genetic basis and tumor biology.[21] On the basis of distinct histological and infrastructural features, RCCs are now classified into the following histological subtypes:

- Conventional clear cell
- Papillary
- Chromophobe
- Collecting duct (including medullary), and
- Unclassified.[21,22]

Histological subtyping of RCCs has become increasingly important in this era of new targeted therapies for individualization of therapy. Although traditionally thought to arise primarily from the proximal convoluted tubules, some histological subtypes like chromophobe and collecting duct RCC are derived from the more distal parts of the nephron.[23,24]

Conventional clear cell carcinoma is the most common (70%) and has characteristic gross pathological features. They are usually located at either poles of kidney and have a golden-yellow appearance owing to the abundance of lipids in the tumor cells. Cystic degeneration is seen in about 10–25% of RCCs and signifies a favorable biological behavior while calcification is seen in about 10–20% of RCCs.[25,26] Histologically, the conventional carcinoma is comprised of clear to eosinophilic granular cells in varied pattern including solid, trabecular and papillary patterns. The cellular islands are separated by delicate vascular septae. *Papillary carcinoma* (10–15%) may be multiple in up to 45% of cases[27-29] and have a variegated appearance with cystic and solid yellow and brown black areas. Microscopically, they are comprised of either cuboidal or columnar cells lining papillary fibrovascular stalks. However, solid, trabecular and glomeruloid areas may also be prominent. Presence of foam cells in the stalks is a useful diagnostic feature. *Chromophobe RCC* (3–5%) may have a characteristic central scar on cut surface and may resemble an oncocytoma. At the cellular level, it is constituted by large polygonal cells with distinct cell borders and reticulated pale eosinophilic cytoplasm, which can stain diffusely with Hale's colloidal iron.[30] Binucleate cells, nuclear border crumpling and perinuclear halo are important distinguishing microscopic features of chromophobe carcinomas. These are considered to have a favorable prognosis in most patients. *Collecting duct tumors* (<1%) are high-grade cancers with abundant desmo-inflammatory stroma rich in neutrophils and need to be delineated from the urothelial carcinomas of pelvicalyceal system. *Medullary carcinoma* occurs almost exclusively in association with the sickle cell trait and closely resembles the collecting duct variety.

Sarcomatoid change can occur in any of the aforementioned subtype of RCC and connotes a poor prognosis. It is not considered a distinct histological variety any more. Recently described renal tumors include translocation associated carcinomas, mucinous tubular and spindle-cell carcinoma, tubulocystic carcinoma, carcinoma associated with end stage renal disease and postneuroblastoma carcinoma. Of these, translocation associated carcinomas are commonly seen in children and young adults and harbor translocation involving a member of the microphthalmia transcription factor gene family most commonly involve the TFE3 gene on locus Xp11.2. The most common fusions are ASPL-TFE3 and PRCC-TFE3. A nested pattern containing cells with voluminous, clear or granular eosinophilic cytoplasm should suggest the possibility of a translocation carcinoma. Psammoma bodies and intracytoplasmic hyaline droplets are frequent findings. TFE3 translocation carcinomas seem to have a relatively indolent course, despite their often advanced stage at presentation. Mucinous tubular and spindle cell carcinoma and tubulocytic carcinomas have predilection for male (M:F ratio 7:1) and female (F:M ratio 4:1) gender respectively and have indolent behavior.[31]

In a recent description, Sukov et al. have demonstrated that translocations involving the anaplastic lymphoma kinase (ALK) locus may be even uncommonly be seen adult RCC. They found that ALK translocations may occur in about 1% of all RCC and morphologically these are more likely to have papillary architecture with clear or eosinophilic cells. Availability of targeted therapy for patients harboring this translocation further necessitates identification of these patients.[32]

Nuclear grading is done by using the Fuhrman criteria and is an independent prognostic parameter affecting survival.[1,33] However, recently experts believe that Fuhrman grade does not characterize papillary carcinomas and should not be used for chromophobe RCC. A proposal for incorporating tumor necrosis along with only the nucleolar grade has been advocated by International Society of Urological Pathology (ISUP) grading as it correlates better with survival studies.[34]

PATHOGENESIS

The majority of RCCs are sporadic and only 4% are estimated to be familial. Clear cell carcinoma of conventional type shows loss of short arm of chromosome 3 (3p-) in a vast majority of cases. This region harbors the VHL gene which acts as a tumor suppressor gene in both sporadic and familial RCC.[35,36] RCCs develop in about 50% patients with VHL disease and are characterized by early age of presentation and bilateral or multifocal involvement.[37,38] Sporadic papillary carcinomas (typically papillary type 1 and less aggressive) commonly show trisomies of chromosomes 7 and 17 and loss of Y chromosome in male patients. Familial forms (usually type 2) show trisomy 7. Chromosome 7 has a proto-oncogene MET which encodes a tyrosine kinase receptor.

Chromophobe RCCs have multiple chromosome losses and hypodiploidy, have been associated with BHD syndrome[22] and usually indicate a good prognosis.

Most sporadic RCCs are unilateral and unifocal. Bilateral involvement is uncommon (2–4%) in sporadic forms but considerably more common in the familial forms (Linehan 2003). Multicentricity seen in about 10–20% patients is again more common in familial forms and papillary histology.[39,40]

RCCs are vascular tumors that tend to spread either by direct invasion through the renal capsule into perinephric fat and adjacent visceral structures or in about 10% patients, by direct extension into the renal vein and inferior vena cava. Approximately 25–30% of patients have evidence of metastatic disease at presentation, the most common metastatic sites being the lung, liver and bone. However, other sites such as ipsilateral adjacent lymph nodes and adrenal gland, brain, the opposite kidney, and subcutaneous tissue are frequent sites of disease spread.

DIAGNOSIS AND STAGING

Many renal masses remain asymptomatic and nonpalpable until late in the natural course of the disease. Presently, more than 50% of RCCs are detected incidentally due to increased use of noninvasive imaging to evaluate a variety of nonspecific symptom complexes.[41] Incidentally detected RCCs generally tend to be smaller and of lower stage than symptomatic RCCs.

The symptom complex of RCC is due to local tumor growth, hemorrhage, metastatic disease or paraneoplastic syndrome. The most common symptoms are hematuria, flank pain or backache or palpable lump in the abdomen or flank. The classic triad of flank pain, gross hematuria and palpable abdominal mass is now rare (6–10%), but when present, signifies an advanced stage of the disease.[42-44]

Paraneoplastic syndromes are seen in about 20–30% of patients with symptomatic RCC, the most common being hypertension due to increased rennin secretion, cachexia, weight loss, pyrexia, neuromyopathy, amyloidosis, elevated erythrocyte sedimentation rate (ESR), anemia, nonmetastatic hepatic dysfunction (3–20%) hypercalcemia, polycythemia due to increased erythropoietin secretion etc.[45] These findings represent a constellation of signs and symptoms that result from the humoral release of various tumor associated proteins form the tumor cells or due to the elicited immune response. Most of these are reversible after nephrectomy but are usually not corrected by medical therapy.

20–30% of patients with RCC present with metastatic disease and some of these patients may have symptoms attributable to their metastases, such as bone pains or persistent cough.

Although physical examination has a limited role in diagnosing RCC, it is valuable in some cases and findings of importance are a palpable abdominal mass or cervical lymphadenopathy, nonreducing varicocele or bilateral lower extremity edema, both of which suggest venous involvement.

Laboratory Tests

Laboratory parameters to be studied are serum creatinine, hemoglobin, ESR, alkaline phosphatase and serum calcium. Renal function estimation is especially important in patients with tumor in solitary kidney or bilateral tumors as well as in patients having diabetes, chronic pyelonephritis, renovascular, stone or renal polycystic disease where the function of the contralateral kidney may be compromised. Abnormal preoperative laboratory values including hypercalcemia, anemia, and elevated ESR are independently associated with increased risk of cancer-specific death from clinically confined clear cell RCC.[46]

Imaging

Ultrasonography (USG) is noninvasive, accurate, and relatively inexpensive and hence is usually the first investigation carried out.[47] It helps differentiate between solid and cystic lesions and can indicate the need for further imaging studies (Fig. 1). It has a high sensitivity in diagnosing simple cysts as well as angiomyolipomas by delineating fat in the tumor. Any renal mass lesion that is not a simple cyst on USG needs further evaluation. Percutaneous aspiration and cytology of the cyst fluid as well as contrast visualization of the cyst cavity have not been proved to be very useful in diagnosing the nature of the cyst and are rarely employed at present.

A high quality contrast-enhanced spiral thin slice computed tomography (CT) scan remains the single most important radiographic test for assessment of a renal mass. A solid mass with significant heterogeneous postcontrast enhancement (due to characteristic high vascularity) less than that of the normal renal parenchyma is virtually diagnostic of a RCC[47,48] and any renal mass that enhances with contrast administration by more than 15 HU should be considered a RCC unless proved otherwise (Figs 2A and B). CT also assesses primary tumor extension with extrarenal spread, venous involvement, enlargement of locoregional lymph nodes, the adrenal and the liver (Figs 3 to 5), while also providing information about the function of the contralateral kidney. CT scan can help rule out angiomyolipomas by demonstrating areas of negative CT attenuation indicative of presence of fat in the tumor.[49] In evaluating the cystic lesions of the kidney, the CT features that need to be assessed are thickness and contour of the cyst wall, number and thickness of septae, presence of solid components or calcification and density of the cyst fluid. Based on these criteria, the cystic lesions are classified into four types by Bosniak.[50] Type I and II cysts can be observed while type III and IV require surgical intervention due to a high likelihood of malignancy in them.

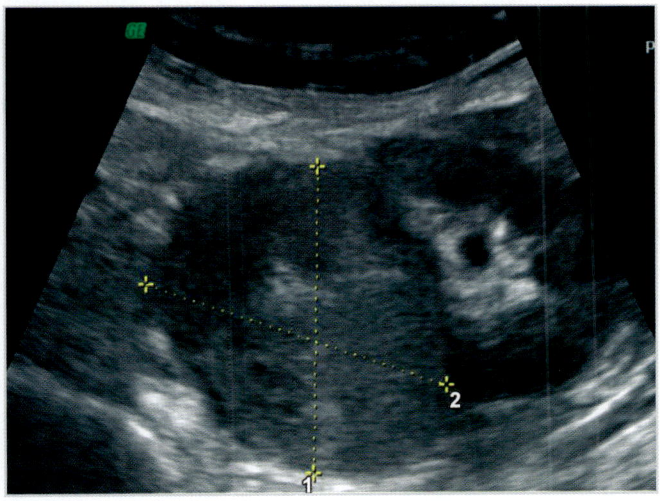

Fig. 1: Ultrasonography showing a complex heterogeneous mass in the left kidney

Magnetic resonance imaging (MRI) shows enhanced vascularity and enhancement of the mass in T1-weighted scans after administration of gadolinium contrast. This technique is most helpful in patients for whom iodinated contrast medium is contraindicated because of significant renal insufficiency or severe allergy; or to better delineate suspected or proven venous extension. MRI has better sensitivity than CT scan in evaluating the presence and extent of venous extension, differentiating a tumor thrombus from a bland one and also evaluating spread to adjacent organs (Figs 6A to C).

Venacavography is seldom performed in the present time and is only indicated in the presence of ambiguous MRI findings in cases with venous extension or in patients who cannot have MRI for some reason. Doppler-USG has limited sensitivity but a transesophageal echocardiography (echo) is a useful tool for evaluating the cephalad extent of the thrombus.

Renal arteriography has a limited role in the diagnostic evaluation of renal masses but may be useful when planning a nephron sparing surgery especially for absolute indications.

In spite of all these, it is not always possible to reliably distinguish RCC, adenoma, and oncocytoma with current diagnostic techniques and approximately 10–30% of small, solid, CT-enhancing renal masses with features suggestive of RCC prove to be benign after surgical excision.[51] Oncocytoma although being a benign tumor, associated RCC in the same or the opposite kidney has been found in as many as 30% of the patients.[52]

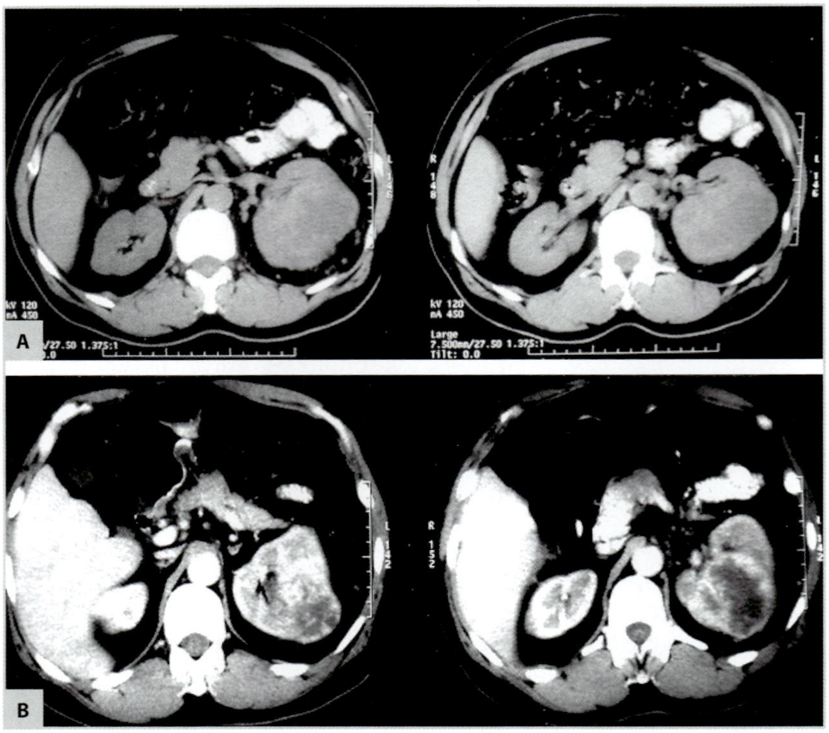

Figs 2A and B: (A) Computed tomography (CT) scan picture showing large solid heterogeneous mass in left kidney (precontrast film); and (B) Postcontrast film showing significant enhancement of the mass, suggestive of renal cell carcinoma (RCC)

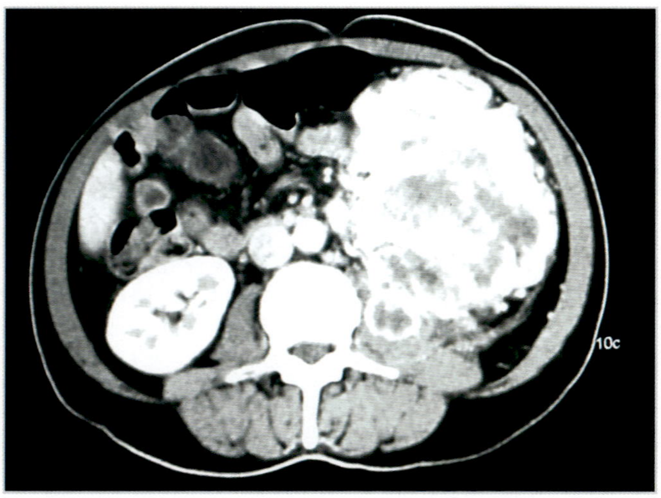

Fig. 3: Computed tomography (CT) scan film showing a left renal mass with perirenal extension in a case of renal cell carcinoma (RCC)

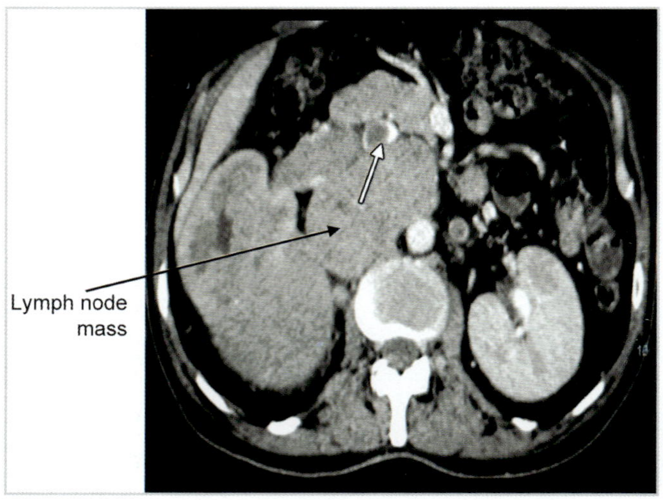

Fig. 4: Computed tomography (CT) scan film showing a left renal mass with para-aortic lymphadenopathy in a case of renal cell carcinoma (black arrow indicates the lymph node mass and the red arrow shows tumor thrombus in the inferior vena cava)

The metastatic workup includes an X-ray or CT scan of the chest (Figs 7A to C) and an isotope bone scan (in presence of skeletal-related complaints or raised serum alkaline phosphatase) and targeted skeletal radiographs or scans (Figs 8A to C), depending on the clinical circumstances. CT or MRI of brain is advised only if indicated by symptoms. The role of positron emission tomography (PET) scan for detection of metastases in

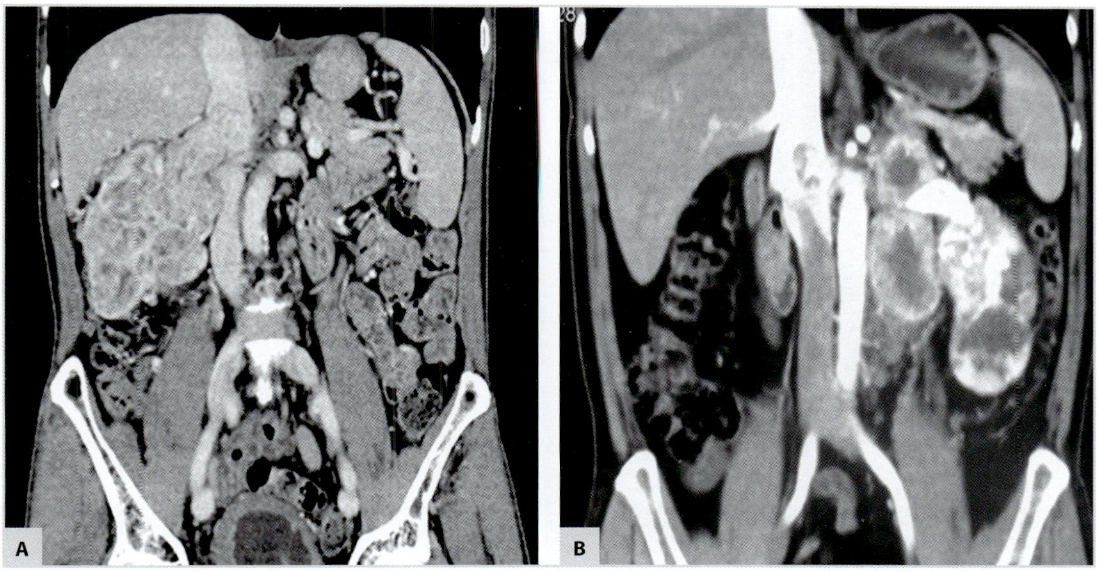

Figs 5A and B: (A) Computed tomography (CT) scan films showing a right renal mass with tumor thrombus extension to renal vein and inferior vena cava in a case of renal cell carcinoma; (B) CT scan film showing a left renal mass with extension to renal vein and inferior vena cava

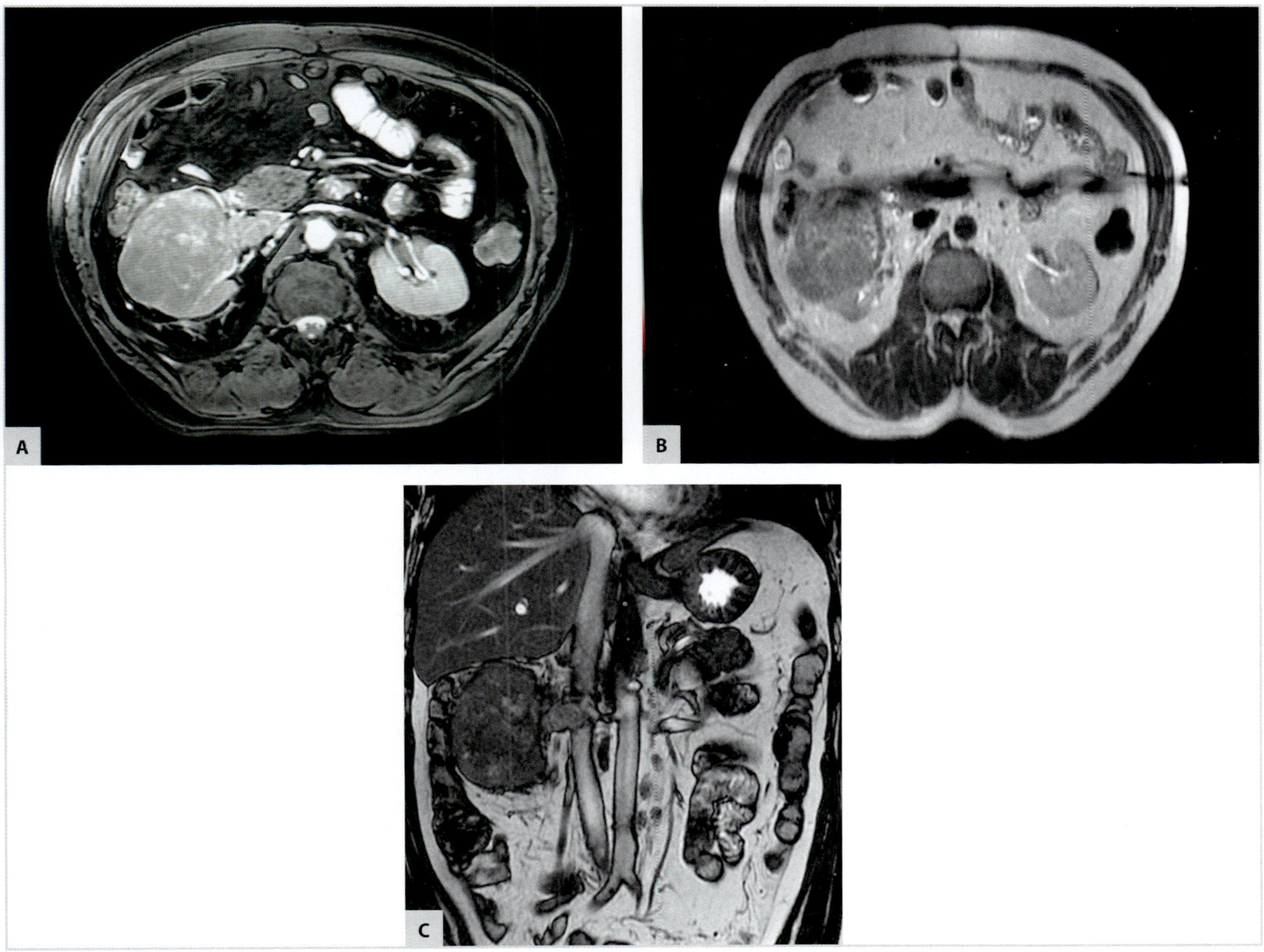

Figs 6A to C: Magnetic resonance imaging (MRI) picture showing large solid heterogeneous mass in right kidney showing significant enhancement of the mass, with evidence of tumor thrombus extension to inferior vena cava: (A) T1-weighted image; (B) T2-weighted image; (C) Coronal view

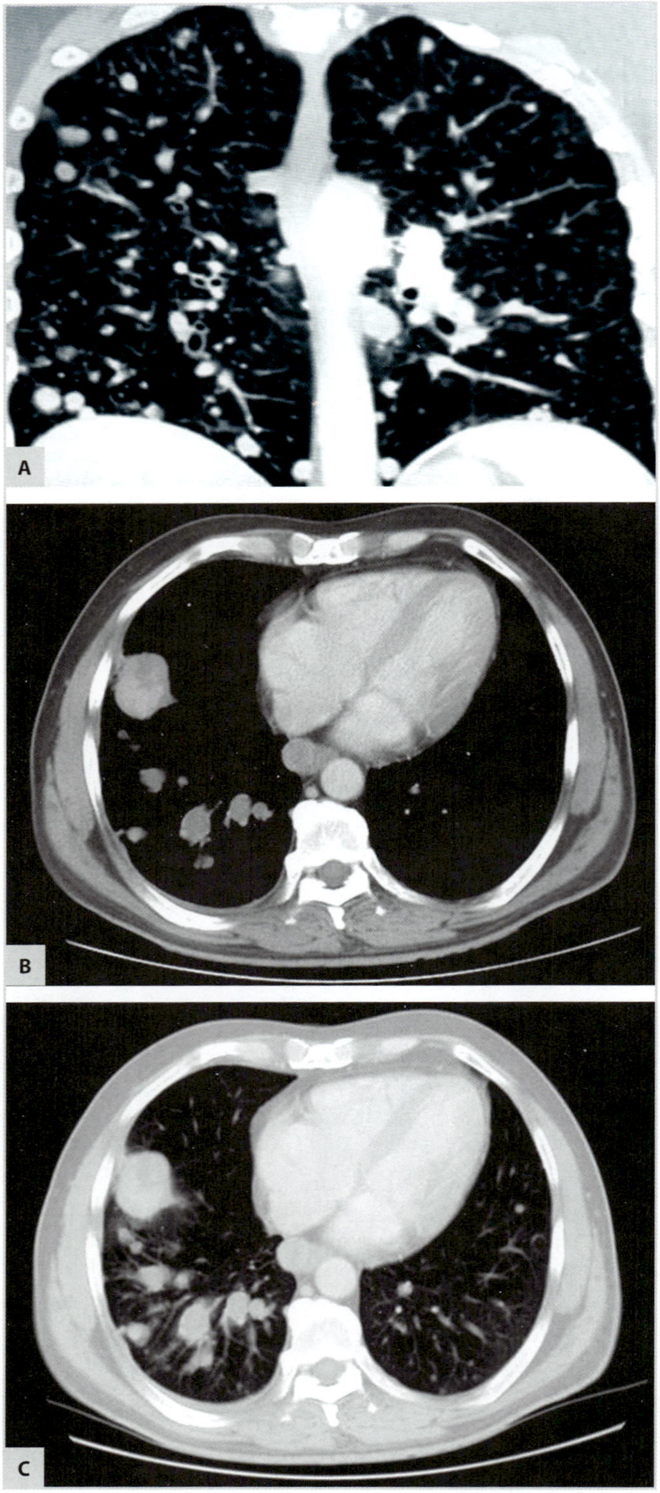

Figs 7A to C: (A) X-ray chest; and (B and C) Computed tomography (CT) scan thorax showing multiple pulmonary metastases

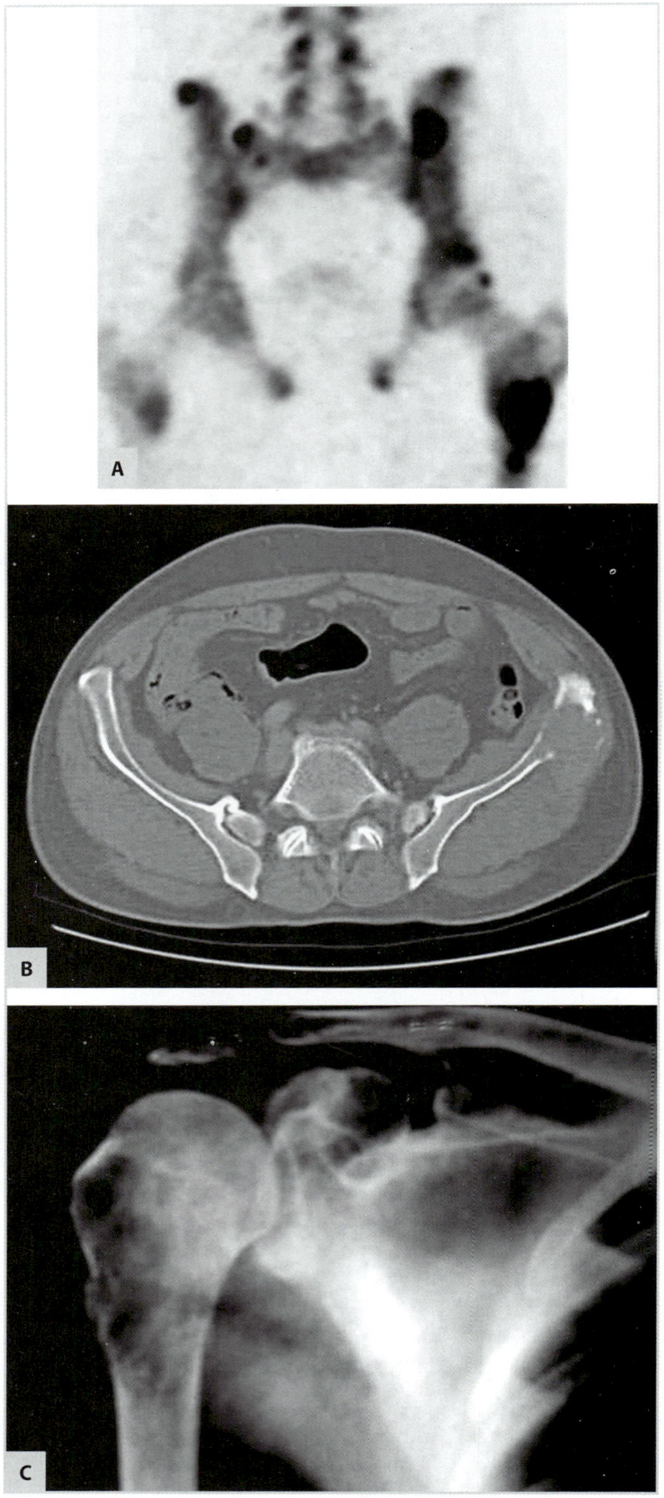

Figs 8A to C: (A) Isotope bone scan showing abnormal uptake suggestive of metastases; (B) Computed tomography (CT) scan with a bone window showing bone metastases; and (C) X-ray showing lytic area in the upper end of left humerus suggestive of metastases

RCC is investigational, with most studies showing good specificity but suboptimal sensitivity. It may have a role in patients with equivocal findings on standard imaging studies, where PET scan delineation of metastases may strongly influence further management and prognosis.[53,54]

Fine needle aspiration or biopsy of a renal mass are rarely indicated, only when a renal abscess or infected cyst is suspected and when RCC must be differentiated from metastatic malignant disease or renal lymphoma.[55,56] Needle biopsy has excellent accuracy for detecting malignant masses especially when combined with molecular analysis[57,58] but its predictive value for detecting benign masses is suboptimal.[58] Although the risk of complications like bleeding, infection, arteriovenous (AV) fistula or pneumothorax and the risk of implantation of tumor cells along the needle tract are low, its clinical impact in improving diagnostic accuracy or influencing clinical management is limited. Hence, it is seldom employed in evaluation of renal masses.

Staging

The traditional staging system of Robson has now been replaced by the American Joint Committee on Cancer (AJCC)'s tumor node metastasis (TNM) system (2010) due to better differentiation of different prognostic groups and its ability to compare data across centers more objectively (Table 1).[59]

The estimated 5-year survival rates for RCC is as follows: 96% for stage I, 82% for stage II, 64% for stage III and 23% for stage IV.[60]

TABLE 1: American Joint Committee on Cancer (AJCC) tumor-node-metastasis (TNM) staging (2010)

Primary tumor			
TX	Primary tumor cannot be assessed		
T0	No evidence of primary tumor		
T1	Tumor 7 cm or less in greatest dimension and confined to the kidney		
T1a	Tumor 4 cm or less in greatest dimension and confined to the kidney		
T1b	Tumor more than 4 cm but not more than 7 cm in greatest dimension and confined to the kidney		
T2	Tumor more than 7 cm in greatest dimension and confined to the kidney		
T2a	Tumor more than 7 cm but less than 10 cm and confined to the kidney		
T2b	Tumor more than 10 cm and confined to the kidney		
T3	Tumor extends into major veins or perinephric tissues but not into ipsilateral adrenal gland and not beyond Gerota's fascia		
T3a	Tumor grossly extends in renal vein or its segmental branches or invades perirenal and/or renal sinus fat but not beyond Gerota's fascia		
T3b	Tumor grossly extends into vena cava below the diaphragm		
T3c	Tumor grossly extends into vena cava above diaphragm or invades wall of the vena cava		
T4	Tumor invades beyond Gerota's fascia (including contiguous involvement of ipsilateral adrenal gland) (M1 if noncontiguous adrenal involvement)		
	Regional lymph nodes (N)		
NX	Regional lymph nodes cannot be assessed		
N0	No regional lymph node metastases		
N1	Metastasis in regional lymph node(s)		
	Distant metastasis (M)		
MX	Distant metastasis cannot be assessed		
M0	No distant metastasis		
M1	Distant metastasis present		
	Stage grouping		
Stage I	T1	N0	M0
Stage II	T2	N0	M0
Stage III	T1 or T2 T3	N1 Any N	M0 M0
Stage IV	T4 Any T	Any N Any N	M0 M1

Prognostic Factors

Numerous clinical, pathological and laboratory prognostic factors affecting survival in patients of RCC have been identified. Moreover, integrated prognostic systems or nomograms incorporating some of these prognostic factors have been defined and have been found to be more useful than the individual factors.[61-64]

- Clinical features such as symptomatic presentation, poor performance status and weight loss of more than 10% body weight indicate poor prognosis.[65-67] Patard et al. proposed a novel staging system for localized RCC based on tumor size and presence of symptoms and showed that this system potentially improved prognostication[68]
- Presence of paraneoplastic signs or symptoms portends a worse prognosis
- Pathological stage is probably the most important factor affecting outcome. Extragerotal spread with involvement of adjacent organs, lymph node metastases and systemic metastases all have a significant negative impact on survival; while the impact of venous involvement and its extent on survival is yet unclear.

Patients with systemic metastases are now further classified into different risk groups depending on factors such as performance status, number and site of metastases, hypercalcemia, anemia, elevated alkaline phosphatase or lactic dehydrogenase and presence of sarcomatoid histology[69-71]

- Tumor size: Various authors have shown a strong correlation between tumor size and survival but whether this is a true impact of tumor size or a reflection of higher pathologic stage and greater probability of clear cell histology and high grade features in larger tumors is debatable[72,73]
- Nuclear grade and histologic subtype: Tumor grading systems irrespective of the system used have been found to have good prognostic potential in RCC. Sarcomatoid, collecting duct and medullary histology indicate a very poor prognosis
- Several authors have combined these factors to device prognostic systems with a good predictive ability.[61,74,75] Kattan et al. proposed a prognostic system incorporating symptoms, histology, tumor size and pathologic stage to predict probability of cancer free survival after nephrectomy. They also incorporated tumor necrosis, tumor grade and vascular invasion to predict the outcome in patients with conventional RCC.[61] Parker et al. (2009) developed and evaluated a biomarker panel (BioScore™) to enhance prognostic algorithms for clear cell RCC.[76]

TREATMENT OF LOCALIZED RENAL CELL CARCINOMA

Surgery is the mainstay of treatment of RCC. Radical nephrectomy introduced by Robson (1969) still remains the gold standard of surgical treatment, with excellent cure rates of 70–92% for T1-T2 RCCs.[77] Traditionally, the principles of radical nephrectomy include early ligation of renal artery and vein, removal of kidney and ipsilateral adrenal gland surrounded by the Gerota's fascia and regional lymphadenectomy from the crus of the diaphragm to the bifurcation of aorta. Some of these tenets have now been questioned.[78] In patients without radiological abnormality of the adrenal gland, its removal may not be necessary except in patients with T3-T4 disease, locally advanced tumors and upper pole tumors.[79-82]

The need for a complete regional lymphadenectomy in all patients undergoing radical nephrectomy remains unclear and controversial. The proponents of lymphadenectomy cite the negative prognostic impact of lymph node metastases and the apparently improved survival with lymphadenectomy seen in retrospective cohorts.[83,84] The opponents of routine lymphadenectomy argue that:

- Blood-borne metastases are as common as lymph node metastases in patients with RCC and that most patients with nodal metastases would ultimately develop blood-borne metastases
- Lymphatic drainage of the kidney is variable and even an extensive lymphadenectomy template is unlikely to cover all possible sites of metastases
- The therapeutic value of lymphadenectomy has not been demonstrated in randomized clinical trials (RCTs) and is probably limited to those patients with micrometastases (<2–3%)
- Although prognostic value of lymphadenectomy is proved, there is presently no effective adjuvant therapy for patients with nodal metastases.

In view of this, there remains a lack of consensus regarding the indications and extent of lymphadenectomy. Most surgeons would do a hilar and immediate adjacent para-aortic or paracaval nodes during a routine radical nephrectomy. Some authors have reported risk factors for lymph node metastases in RCC viz. large tumor size more than 10 cm, T3–T4 tumors, high tumor grade, sarcomatoid component and histological tumor necrosis.[85,86] They recommended a complete regional lymphadenectomy in patients with two or more of these risk factors in whom the risk of lymph node metastases being about 10%, as opposed only hilar lymphadenectomy in those with less than two risk factors (risk of lymph node metastases 0.6%).

Radical nephrectomy can be done by a variety of surgical approaches (open, laparoscopic, robotic) and through various incisions, as decided by the size and location of the tumor and the body habitus of the patient. The choice of incision (transperitoneal vs. extraperitoneal vs. thoracoabdominal) has not shown to have any impact on patient outcome.

Laparoscopic Radical Nephrectomy

It has now emerged as a less morbid alternative to open radical nephrectomy in suitable patients with localized renal cell carcinoma with tumor size less than 10 cm, no local invasion, renal vein thrombus or lymph node metastases. It allows early control of the renal vessels prior to tumor manipulation and wide mobilization of the tumor due to excellent vision afforded by this approach. The postoperative pain is significantly less with this approach and the recovery from surgery as well as return to normal activity is significantly faster than the open approach. Although there are no randomized trials comparing open with laparoscopic approach, the surgical and oncological outcomes after laparoscopic surgery have been reported to be equivalent to those after open surgery, with equivalent cancer specific survival rates and postoperative morbidity rates. However, appropriate selection of patients as well as the experience and expertise of the surgeons remain vital factors for the success of the laparoscopic approach. A variety of approaches like transperitoneal, extraperitoneal or hand-assisted have been described, with equivalent results. Recently, many centers have reported their initial experience with robotic radical nephrectomy.

Nephron Sparing Surgery

Although the first nephron sparing surgery (NSS) for RCC was described by Czerney in 1890, it was Vermooten in 1950 who reported local excision of the renal tumor with surrounding normal renal tissue while preserving maximum functioning renal parenchyma.[87] Traditionally, the use of NSS in patients with RCC was limited to those patients with bilateral tumors or those with anatomically or functionally solitary kidney, where removal of the whole kidney would make the patient anephric with subsequent high risk of dialysis or transplant (absolute indications). Relative indications for this procedure are patients with unilateral cancer and the contralateral functioning kidney affected by a condition that might threaten its future function such as renal artery stenosis, nephrosclerosis, hydronephrosis, diabetes, calculus disease, ureteric reflux or hereditary forms of RCC with a high chance of developing a contralateral renal tumor.

Advances in renal imaging, better methods for preventing ischemic damage to the kidneys and more experience in renal vascular surgery along with the improved survival reported after NSS for RCC has stimulated interest in applying this procedure to patients with unilateral RCC with a normal contralateral kidney. With widespread use of imaging, more patients are being diagnosed with smaller tumors and the removal of the whole kidney to remove these small tumors is being questioned. Although radical nephrectomy has traditionally been the treatment of choice for such patients, a number of centers have reported excellent cancer specific survivals of 90–100% following NSS in this situation. Various studies have shown that the best results are obtained when the tumors were less than 4 cm in size, unilateral, unifocal and low pathological tumor stage. These studies suggest that NSS may be an acceptable alternative in patients with single small less than 4 cm RCC with a normal contralateral kidney. Comparative studies of NSS and radical nephrectomy for these patients have shown equivalent recurrence free and long-term cancer specific survivals.[66,88-90]

Hafez et al. compared the results of NSS in centrally versus peripherally located RCCs and also compared the results of NSS to radical nephrectomy. They found no differences in the overall cancer specific survival rates (100% vs. 97%), tumor recurrence rate (5.7% vs. 4.5%) or renal function. Moreover, there was no difference between results of NSS or radical nephrectomy irrespective of the location of the tumor.[91] The indications of NSS have been extended to include tumors up to 7 cm size. However, this remains controversial, with conflicting reports about its efficacy in larger tumors. However, many recent reports indicate that the overall and cancer-specific survival rates are not compromised and that the tumor recurrence rates as well as the renal function are not significantly different when NSS is done for renal cortical tumors 4–7 cm in size.[75,92-97] However, in order to obtain equivalent results, NSS should be offered to highly selected patients and must be done by surgeons experienced in these procedures. If RCC of larger size is treated with NSS, more rigorous follow-up is advocated in view of an increased risk of local intrarenal recurrence.

The minimum cancer-free surgical margin considered to be adequate is 1 mm all around and at the base of the tumor. So long as the margins are negative, the width of the margin does not correlate with the risk of recurrence.[98,99] Li et al. (2010) found no significant difference in overall survival and 1.6% local recurrence rate at a mean follow-up of 69 months for mini-margin NSS as compared to 1 cm margin NSS for patients with tumors 4 cm or less in size.

Laparoscopic partial nephrectomy can be a viable alternative to the open approach but for its success, it needs to be done by an experienced surgeon, due to the long warm ischemia time with the laparoscopic approach and the higher risk of intraoperative and postoperative complications including urological complications, especially for tumors more than 2 cm. Hence, the optimal indication for laparoscopic partial nephrectomy is a smaller, peripheral renal tumor, even though successful surgical and oncological outcome has been demonstrated for larger tumors as well as central or hilar tumors.[100,101] In recent times, numerous new techniques for laparoscopic renal hypothermia have been developed, which are likely to expand the scope of indications of laparoscopic partial nephrectomy to include larger and more complex tumors.[102] Although some recent studies have suggested equivalent oncological and functional outcomes, there are few large studies with long-term data available.[103-106]

The main advantages of NSS are potential preservation of renal function and not removing the whole kidney if the renal mass turns out to be benign. It is well known that nearly one-fourth to one-third of all renal masses less than 3.5 cm are benign.[107-109] Matched comparisons of radical nephrectomy versus NSS patients have shown that patients undergoing radical nephrectomy had significantly greater risk of chronic renal insufficiency, metabolic acidosis, proteinuria rates as well as need for dialysis than a well-matched group undergoing NSS.[93,110-113] This decline in renal function may not be evident for several years after surgery. Factors that predict renal insufficiency after radical nephrectomy include elevated preoperative serum creatinine, hypertension and proteinuria,[114] preoperative low glomerular filtration rate (GFR)[111] and nomograms to define the risk of renal insufficiency after radical nephrectomy have also been developed.[115] Patients with postoperative GFR less than 60 mL/m^2 had a 10% increased risk of hospitalization, 40% increased risk of cardiovascular events and a 20% increased risk of death as compared to those with GFR more than 60 mL/m^2.[116] A combined analysis of 39 studies found that the health related quality of life was better with partial nephrectomy.

NSS has been found to be associated with an improved overall survival in patients with renal masses less than 4 cm in size.[117] Thompson et al. (2008) found that radical nephrectomy was associated with a significantly higher risk of death than NSS [risk ratio (RR) 2.16, p=0.02] in patients less than 65 years of age.[118] A similar increase in risk of death was reported by Huang et al. (2009) in patients more than 65 years of age [hazard ratio (HR) 1.38, p=0.01] and 1.4 times higher number of cardiovascular events after surgery.[119] The preoperative aspects and dimensions used for anatomical classification (PADUA) score is a simple anatomical system that can be used to predict the risk of surgical and medical perioperative complications in patients undergoing open NSS.[120] This can help clinicians stratify patients suitable for NSS into subgroups with different complication rates and can help reasonably evaluate suitability of a surgical approach to an individual patient.

Ablative Surgical Procedures

Many ablative procedures e.g. radiofrequency ablation (RFA), cyrotherapy, microwave and high-intensity focused ultrasonic ablation (HIFU) have been recommended as alternatives to surgery.[121-126] They can be done by the open surgical route or by laparoscopic or even a percutaneous route. The potential advantages of these procedures are that they are less morbid, can be done at outpatient procedures and can be offered to patients unfit for radical nephrectomy.[127] They can be offered to selected patients with small, incidental renal tumors, patients with genetic predisposition to multiple tumors, patients with tumors in solitary kidney or with bilateral tumors; or elderly patients with significant comorbidities who are unfit for an open surgical approach etc. However, the main disadvantages of these procedures are that there is no tissue available for histological confirmation of the lesion and that there is no histological proof of completeness of ablation, which is indirectly assumed by CT criteria. Although small series demonstrate initial technical success and short-term benefit, long-term data from large or randomized studies are not available and hence these procedures are still investigational at present. In fact, a recent population-based comparison of survival after nephrectomy versus nonsurgical management for small renal masses showed inferiority of these nonsurgical modalities compared to nephrectomy.[128]

Observation

Many patients are presently being diagnosed with small incidental renal masses, which are histologically indeterminate by clinicoradiological features. Numerous studies have looked at the growth rate of RCCs by observing small renal masses in carefully selected patients who are not candidates for conventional surgery or ablative approaches. The mean growth rate in these studies has been low, ranging from 0.01 cm/year to 0.86 cm/year over a 2–5 years follow-up and the metastatic potential has also been low.[129] Hence, an initial time period of surveillance with close follow-up seems quite appealing. However, this data must be viewed with caution as most of these studies have studied growth rate retrospectively and have only included patients with small, homogeneous renal masses, many of which may have been benign. Besides, there is no discrete cut-off for proceeding to treatment, most urologists using a cut off value of 3–4 cm empirically. Nevertheless, based on these studies, there appears to be a place for close observation of small homogeneous well-defined renal masses and monitoring with serial renal imaging in elderly or moribund patients who are poor risk for surgery or ablative procedures. This approach is not advocated for young fit patients with small renal masses if the radiographic features suggest a RCC.

MANAGEMENT OF TUMOR EXTENSION TO RENAL VEIN OR INFERIOR VENA CAVA

Extension of tumor thrombus into the renal vein and inferior vena cava (IVC) is a unique feature of RCC and is seen in 4–10% of patients. It may extend cephalad in the IVC to reach the right atrium.

Venous tumor thrombus is suspected in patients with a renal tumor demonstrating one or more of the following features: lower extremity edema, unilateral right sided varicocoele or one which does not collapse on recumbency, dilated veins on anterior abdominal wall, nonfunctioning involved kidney, proteinuria, history of pulmonary embolism or a right atrial mass on imaging.

Accurate assessment of the presence and extent of thrombus, especially its cephalad limit is mandatory for planning treatment. MRI is probably the best modality for accurate demonstration of the thrombus and for differentiating between a tumor thrombus and a bland thrombus by demonstrating postcontrast enhancement of the thrombus. Inferior venacavography being an invasive procedure is generally reserved for patients in whom the MRI findings are equivocal or in whom MRI is contraindicated. Transesophageal USG and abdominal color flow Doppler may also be employed to accurately assess the cephalad extent of thrombus. The venous thrombus extension is classified as follows:

- I: Adjacent to renal vein ostium
- II: Extending up to lower border of liver (infrahepatic)
- III: Involving intrahepatic portion of IVC but below the diaphragm
- IV: Extending above the diaphragm

The prognostic impact of the cephalad extent of thrombus is controversial since many patients with type IV thrombus can be cured with surgery if the primary disease is otherwise confined to the kidney.[130-132] Many type III or IV thrombi are however associated with advanced locoregional disease and hence have a poorer prognosis.[130,133,134]

Since the prognosis in these patients is related to locoregional extent of disease and not to the tumor thrombus and because there are no effective nonsurgical management options in RCC, surgery remains the only hope of cure in these patients. Excellent survivals of 40–70% at 5 years have been reported with complete excision of the primary tumor and its extension into the renal vein or IVC.[135] The survival results are compromised in presence of gross perirenal spread, lymph node metastases or invasion of the wall of the IVC.[133,136,137] Type I and II thrombi can be managed by vascular control of IVC above and below the thrombus and of the contralateral renal vein and surgical removal of the thrombus (Fig. 9). Type III and IV thrombi however require partial or total cardiopulmonary bypass with hypothermic circulatory arrest. Since the surgery is associated with a significant mortality and morbidity, patient selection is extremely important and only patients with good performance status and with no gross extrarenal spread should be chosen for this surgery.[138,139]

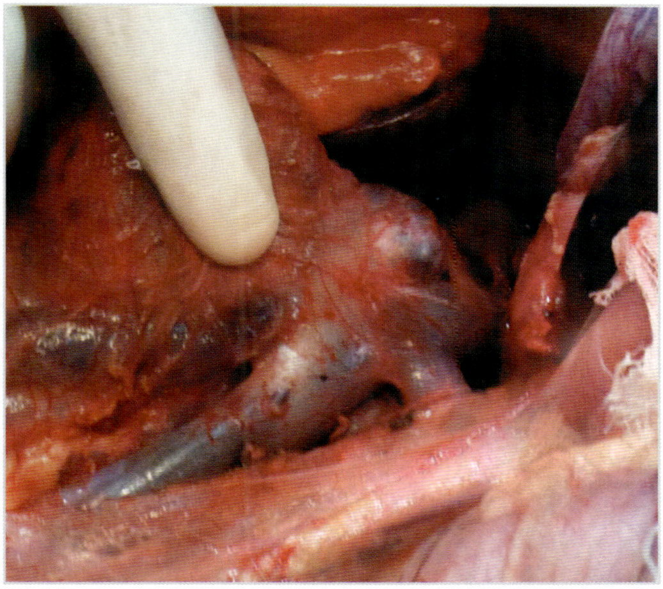

Fig. 9: Intraoperative photograph showing right renal vein and inferior vena cava tumor thrombus

Adjuvant Therapy

A significant number of patients relapse after radical nephrectomy. Various studies have tried to identify the high-risk factors for relapse and several different treatment modalities and approaches such as immunotherapy, radiation therapy; vaccine related strategies etc. have been investigated in the adjuvant setting in these high-risk patients.[140,141] To date, there is no conclusive evidence of survival benefit with any of these approaches. A trial with autologous tumor cell vaccine given in the adjuvant setting showed some improvement in progression free survival in patients with T3 disease but there was no impact on overall survival. Presently, adjuvant therapy after radical nephrectomy is not advocated outside of clinical trials. Targeted therapy agents are being investigated for their role as adjuvant therapy in patients undergoing radical nephrectomy at high risk of subsequent relapse.

Surveillance following Surgery for RCC

After definitive surgical treatment of RCC, monitoring of the patients from the points of local recurrence, recurrence in contralateral kidney, development of distant metastases and the functional status of the remaining renal units is mandatory. However, there are no evidence based surveillance guidelines. The patients may be classified into different risk groups according to one of the risk assignment systems based on clinicopathological factors and histological subtype and then the surveillance may be individualized depending on the risk of relapse.[142-144] The American Urological Association guidelines 2013 provides risk-stratified follow-up guidelines. Although identification of relapsed disease early is desirable and it appears logical that early treatment of relapse should improve survival, actually only a small percentage of patients with relapse—such as with solitary or limited metastatic disease, can be salvaged by curative therapy. In the remaining patients, there is presently no evidence that treating relapsed disease early improves survival.

Local Recurrence after Radical Nephrectomy or Nephron Sparing Surgery

Local recurrence after radical nephrectomy is rare, occurring in 1–4% of patients;[144-146] and are more common in patients with locally advanced or node positive disease (Fig. 10). Nearly two-thirds of these are associated with a systemic relapse and hence it is essential to rule out systemic disease before planning treatment. In the absence of distant metastatic disease, surgery may be offered to these patients. However, this surgery is more complex, often requires resection of adjacent organs and has significant morbidity associated with it. Hence, proper patient selection for surgery is mandatory and patients unsuitable for surgery may be managed with local radiation therapy or oral targeted therapy.

Local recurrence after NSS is uncommon, seen in 1–10% of patients and are usually seen in patients with higher T stage. The site of recurrence may be the same as the site of original tumor (true recurrence) or away from the site of original tumor (de novo occurrence due to multifocality of disease). In the absence of metastatic disease, these are treated with repeat partial nephrectomy if feasible, especially if the preservation of renal parenchyma is important; or total nephrectomy or ablative therapies.[147]

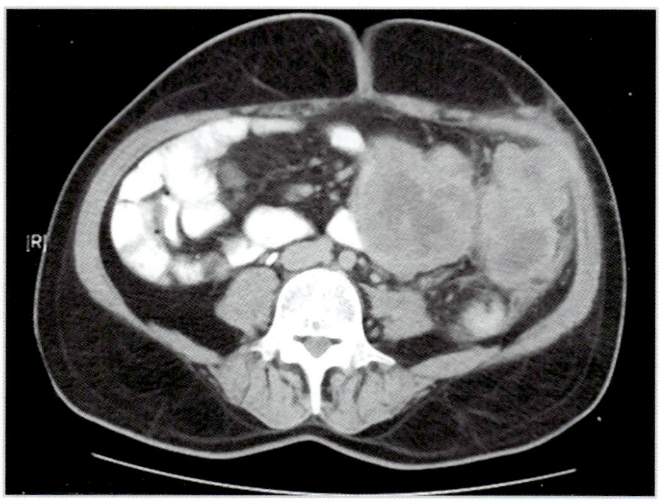

Fig. 10: Computed tomography (CT) scan picture showing recurrence in left renal fossa following radical nephrectomy

Local recurrences after local ablative therapies are usually at the site of the original tumor. They are suspected by persistent enhancement within the tumor bed or in rest of the kidney and usually treated by reablative therapy or total nephrectomy.

METASTATIC RENAL CELL CARCINOMA

Approximately one-third of patients with RCC have metastatic disease at presentation. Besides, another 40–50% will develop distant metastases some time during their natural history.[148] Patients with metastatic RCC have a dismal outlook, the majority of these patients dying of their disease within 12–24 months. However, there may be a small subset of patients with solitary metastasis, who may have a better biological behavior than those with multiple metastases and may benefit with an aggressive therapeutic approach with intent of cure.

Solitary metastases are seen in 1–4% of all patients with metastatic disease. It is mandatory to rule out a local recurrence in the renal fossa as well as metastatic disease elsewhere before contemplating aggressive treatment. Many centers have reported excellent 5-years survival rates of 33–60% after complete excision of the primary renal tumor and the metastatic disease. Patients with lung-only metastasis, those with metachronous metastases with a long relapse-free interval, those in whom the metastasis can be completely resected and those with a good performance status have a better prognosis than other patients.[149-151] In a study of 278 patients who underwent surgical resection of metastases at the Memorial Sloan Kettering Cancer Center, the prognostic factors affecting survival were a disease free survival of greater than 12 months (55% vs. 9% 5-year overall survival), solitary versus multiple sites of metastases (54% vs. 29% 5-year overall survival) and age less than 60 years (49% vs. 35% 5-year overall survival), solitary site of metastases lung versus brain (54% vs. 18% 5-year overall survival). The same authors also noticed that complete resection of all metastatic sites was more important than the number of metastatic nodules.[150] Metastasectomy can also be considered in patients with residual metastatic lesions responding to immunotherapy, provided the metastasis is resectable.

Patients with multiple metastases have been classified into different prognostic groups based on variables found to impact response to treatment and overall survival.[69,152] This substratification in different risk groups aids in planning optimum therapy and prognostication. The aim of treatment in patients with multiple metastases is palliative. In the presence of multiple metastases, the value of nephrectomy has traditionally been confined to palliation for bleeding, pain and paraneoplastic syndromes. Besides, nephrectomy in the setting of metastatic disease has been reported to induce spontaneous regression of lung metastases in 1–2% cases.[153] However, the impact of nephrectomy on survival was not conclusively shown. Two prospective randomized trials have examined the value of cytoreductive nephrectomy prior to immunotherapy.[154,155] Both these randomized patients to given cytokine therapy with or without prior nephrectomy. The results of both these trials as well as their combined analysis have shown improvement in survival in the nephrectomy arm (13.6 vs. 7.8 months).[156] In view of this, cytoreductive nephrectomy followed by systemic treatment should be considered in patients of metastatic RCC. The factors which indicate an improved survival are presence of lung-only metastases, absence of central nervous system (CNS) metastases, good performance status and more than 75% reduction in the total disease burden by nephrectomy. Proper selection of patients on these lines is important since it has been shown that 10–20% of patients undergoing cytoreductive nephrectomy are unable to take systemic treatment due to postoperative complications or rapid disease progression.

Since many patients are unable to take systemic therapy after cytoreductive nephrectomy, an approach of initial systemic treatment with delayed nephrectomy only in patients who demonstrate regression or stability of their metastatic lesions has been advocated. This may allow selection of betters with biologically more responsive tumors, reserving aggressive treatment for the patients most likely to benefit from it. A prospective randomized study is needed to better define the timing of nephrectomy.

Pantuck et al. recommended complete regional lymphadenectomy in patients undergoing cytoreductive nephrectomy for advanced disease and demonstrated a survival benefit in those undergoing lymphadenectomy in a retrospective analysis.[157] The role of cytoreductive nephrectomy for a nonclear cell histology is yet unproven.

Radiotherapy may be given for selected patients with brain metastases or painful skeletal metastases, for symptomatic relief.

Systemic Therapy for Metastatic RCC

Hormonal therapy in the form of progestational agents[158,159] and chemotherapy[160] have not been found to be effective in RCC. Both these approaches have been extensively tested in clinical trials and have not shown any significant anti-tumor activity in RCC. Chemotherapy may have a role in nonclear cell histology or in patients with sarcomatoid differentiation, the preferred agents being doxorubicin and gemcitabine.[161]

Immunotherapeutic approaches to RCC include treatment with alpha interferon (IFN-α) or interleukin (IL-2) or a combination of the two. Several randomized trials have been published to quantify the benefit of IFN-α in metastatic RCC, with an overall response rate of about 10–15%—the majority of responses being partial.[162] The Medical Research Council trial (1999) randomized 350 patients of metastatic RCC to IFN-α and medroxyprogesterone acetate and showed a statistically significant improvement in median survival in favor of the IFN-α arm (8.5 vs. 6.0 months). The optimum dose, schedule and route of administration of the drug is yet unknown. The recommended starting dose is 2 mIU subcutaneously thrice a week to be escalated to 9 mIU thrice a week if tolerated well. The best responses are seen in patients with good performance status, prior nephrectomy, clear cell histology and metastases limited to lungs.[59,163,164] The results of IFN-α monotherapy have been examined in several meta-analysis, with an overall response rate of 12.5% and survival benefit of 3.8 months.[165]

As a single agent, IL-2 has been evaluated in various doses and treatment schedules. It was approved by US Food and Drug Administration (FDA) on the basis of the data of 255 patients compiled from various phase II trials demonstrating a durable complete response rate of 5–7%.[166] A review of literature shows an objective response rate of 8–35% depending on the schedule and dose used. A randomized trial comparing intravenous high dose IL-2 to low dose IL-2 given either intravenously or subcutaneously showed higher response rates in the high dose arm but that did not translate into an improved survival. Besides, there was no difference in response rates whether the low dose IL-2 was given intravenously or subcutaneously.[167] The toxicity associated with high dose IL-2 is significantly higher than that with IFN or low dose IL-2 therapy, mainly fever, hypotension, respiratory distress, capillary leak syndrome, edema, neurocortical defects and liver dysfunction. In view of the high toxicity, the drug is advocated only for young patients with no comorbidities and a good performance status. There is no demonstrable superiority seen for treatment with either IL-2 or IFN or their combination. Negrier et al. (1998) reported a higher response rate but no survival benefit for combination of IL-2 and IFN-α compared to either agent alone.[168] Only those patients with a clear cell histology benefit clinically from IL-2 immunotherapy.

Targeted Therapy

Better understanding of the molecular pathways has led to the development of targeted agents with robust clinical benefits.

Various criteria are presently used to stratify patients with metastatic disease into good, intermediate and poor risk groups, with significant difference in survivals among the three risk groups. This has helped to individualize patient management and has allowed better prognostication.

Targeted therapy is basically of two broad subtypes: (1) Tyrosine kinase inhibitors (TKI), e.g. sunitinib, sorafenib, pazopanib, axitinib etc. and (2) Mammalian target of rapamycin (mTOR) inhibitors, e.g. temsirolimus, everolimus etc. All these drugs have been extensively tried in RCTs and have been recommended for clinical use in patients with metastatic RCC.[169-180] With the availability of several treatment options to the oncologist in the current era, it is important to use these agents judiciously and to minimize the risk to benefit ratio while treating patients with metastatic RCC. The suggested management algorithm for patients with metastatic RCC based on European Society for Medical Oncology (ESMO) evidence-based guidelines (2012) is given in Table 2.[181]

Although targeted therapy had a tremendous impact on the management of metastatic RCC, these are not curative approaches and optimum therapy yet and needs to be defined. Future efforts are directed towards use of combination therapy, optimum sequencing of agents, identifying predictive biomarkers (clinical, radiological and molecular) and use of novel agents.

Surgical resection of RCC after targeted therapy is feasible with low morbidity in most patients. However, significant complications can occur, raising concern for possible compromise of tissue and/or vascular integrity associated with surgery in this setting.[182]

TABLE 2: Management for patients with metastatic renal cell carcinoma based on European Society for Medical Oncology (ESMO) evidence-based guidelines (2012)

Setting	*Patients*	*Primary therapy (Level I evidence)*	*Other options (≥ Level 2 evidence)*
First line	Good or intermediate risk	Pazopanib Bevcizumab + IFN Sunitinib	HD IL-2 Sorafenib Observation
	Poor risk	Temsirolimus	Sunitinib, Pazopanib
Second line	Post-cytokine	Sorafenib Pazopanib Axitinib	Sunitinib Bevacizumab Temsirolimus
	Post-VEGF inhibitor	Everolimus Axitinib	Other VEGF inhibitors Temsirolimus
	Post-mTOR inhibitor		VEGF inhibitors
Third line	Post-TKI—TKI	Everolimus	
	Post-mTOR—TKI		Different TKI
	Post-TKI—mTOR		Rechallenge TKI

Abbreviations: TKI, tyrosine kinase inhibitor; mTOR, mammalian target of rapamycin; VEGF, vascular endothelial growth factor

REFERENCES

1. Pantuck AJ, Zisman A, Belldegrun AS. The changing natural history of renal cell carcinoma. J Urol. 2001;166(5):1611-23.
2. Landis SH, Murray T, Bo den S, et al. Cancer statistics, 1999. CA Cancer J Clin. 1999;49(1):8-31.
3. Novick AC, Campbell SC. Renal tumours. In: Walsh PC, Retik, AB, Vaughan ED, Wein AJ (Eds). Campbell's Urology. Philadelphia: WB Saunders; 2002. pp. 2672-731.
4. Luciani LG, Cestari R, Tallarigo C. Incidental renal cell carcinoma: age and stage characterization and clinical implications: study of 1,092 patients (1982–1997). Urology. 2000;56:58-62.
5. Lindblad P. Epidemiology of renal cell carcinoma. Scand J Surg. 2004;93(2):88-96.
6. Escudier B, Kataja V, ESMO Guidelines Working Group. Renal cell carcinoma: ESMO clinical recommendations for diagnosis, treatment and follow-up. Ann Oncol. 2009;20:81-2.
7. Parsons JK, Schoenberg MS, Carter HB. Incidental renal tumors: casting doubt on the efficacy of early intervention. Urology. 2001;57(6):1013-5.
8. Hock LM, Lynch J, Balaji CK. Increasing incidence of all stages of kidney cancer in the last 2 decades in the United States: an analysis of surveillance, epidemiology and end results program data. J Urol. 2002;167:57-60.
9. Asanuma H, Nakai H, Takeda M, et al. Renal cell carcinoma in children: experience at a single institution in Japan. J Urol. 1999;162(4):1402-5.
10. Broecker B. Non-Wilms' renal tumors in children. Urol Clin North Am. 2000;27(3):463-9.
11. Geller JI, Dome JS. Local lymph node involvement does not predict poor outcome in pediatric renal cell carcinoma. Cancer. 2004;101(7):1575-83.
12. Freedman AL, Vates TS, Stewart T, et al. Renal cell carcinoma in children: the Detroit experience. J Urol. 1996;155(5):1708-10.
13. Bergström A, Hsieh CC, Lindblad P, et al. Obesity and renal cell cancer-a quantitative review. Br J Cancer. 2001;85(7):984-90.
14. Pischon T, Lahmann PH, Boeing H, et al. Body size and risk of renal cell carcinoma in the European prospective investigation into cancer and nutrition (EPIC). Int J Cancer. 2006;118(3):728-38.
15. Lowrance WT, Thompson RH, Yee DS, et al. Obesity is associated with a higher risk of clear cell renal cell carcinoma than with other histologies. BJU Int. 2010;105(1):16.
16. Theis RP, Dolwick Grieb SM, Burr D, et al. Smoking, environmental tobacco smoke, and risk of renal cell cancer: a population-based case-control study. BMC Cancer. 2008;8:387.
17. Parker AS, Cerhan JR, Janney CA, et al. Smoking cessation and renal cell carcinoma. Ann Epidemiol. 2003;13(4):245-51.
18. Chow WH, Gridley G, Fraumeni JF, et al. Obesity, hypertension, and the risk of kidney cancer in men. N Engl J Med. 2000;343(18):1305-11.
19. Makay B, Ordonez NG, Khoursand J,et al. The ultrastructure and immunocytochemistry of renal cell carcinoma. Ultrastruct Pathol. 1987;11(5-6):483-502.
20. Holthöfer H. Immunohistology of renal carcinomas. Eur Urol. 1990;18:15-6.
21. Linehan WM, Walther MM, Zbar B. The genetic basis of cancer of the kidney. J Urol. 2003;170(6):2163-72.
22. Pavlovich CP, Schmidt LS. Searching for the hereditary causes of renal-cell carcinoma. Nat Rev Cancer. 2004;4(5):381-93.
23. Pantuck AJ, Zisman A, Belldegrun A. Biology of renal cell carcinoma: changing concepts in classification and staging. Semin Urol Oncol. 2001;19(2):72-9.
24. Oyasu B, Lloreta J, Gelabert-Mas A. Cystic renal cell carcinoma: pathological features, survival and implications for treatment. Br J Urol. 1998;82(1):16-20.
25. Imura J, Ichikawa K, Takeda J, et al. Multilocular cystic renal cell carcinoma: a clinicopathological, immuno- and lectin histochemical study of nine cases. APMIS. 2004;112(3):183-91.
26. Nassir A, Jollimore J, Gupta R, et al. Multilocular cystic renal cell carcinoma: a series of 12 cases and review of the literature. Urology. 2002;60(3):421-7.
27. Chow GK, Myles J, Novick AC. The Cleveland Clinic experience with papillary (chromophil) renal cell carcinoma: clinical outcome with histopathological correlation. Can J Urol. 2001;8(2):1223-8.
28. Blataci S, Orhan D, Soyupek S, et al. Influence of tumour stage, size, grade, vascular involvement, histological cell type and histological pattern on multifocality of renal cell carcinoma. J Urol. 2000;164(1):36-9.
29. Campbell SC, Fichtner J, Novick AC, et al. Intraoperative evaluation of renal cell carcinoma: a prospective study of the role of ultrasonography and histopathological frozen sections. J Urol. 1996;155(4):1191-5.
30. Thoenes W, Storkel S, Rumpelt HJ, et al. Chromophobe cell renal carcinoma and its variants—a report of 32 cases. J Pathol. 1988;155:277-87.
31. Srigley JR, Delahunt B. Uncommon and recently described renal carcinomas. Mod Pathol. 2009;22:S2-S23.
32. Sukov WR, Hodge JC, Lohse CM, et al. ALK alterations in adult renal cell carcinoma: frequency, clinicopathologic features and outcome in a large series of consecutively treated patients. Mod Pathol. 2012;25:1516-25.
33. Fuhrman SA, Lasky LC, Limas C. Prognostic significance of morphologic parameters in renal cell carcinoma. Am J Surg Pathol. 1982;6(7):655-63.
34. Delahunt B, McKenney JK, Lohse CM, et al. A novel grading system for clear cell renal cell carcinoma incorporating tumor necrosis. Am J Surg Pathol. 2013;37:311-22.
35. Linehan WM, Lerman MI, Zbar B. Identification of the von Hippel-Lindau (VHL) gene: its role in renal cancer. JAMA. 1995;272:564-70.
36. Zbar B. Von Hippel-Lindau disease and sporadic renal cell carcinoma. Cancer Surv. 1995;25:219-32.
37. Maher ER, Yates JR, Harries R, et al. Clinical features and natural history of von Hippel-Lindau disease. Q J Med. 1990:77(283):1151-63.
38. Neumann HP, Bender BU, Berger DP, et al. Prevalence, morphology and biology of renal cell carcinoma in Von Hippel-Lindau disease compared to sporadic renal cell carcinoma. J Urol. 1998;160(4):1248-54.

39. Richstone L, Scherr DS, Reuter VR, et al. Multifocal renal cortical tumors: frequency, associated clinicopathological features and impact on survival. J Urol. 2004;171(2):615-20.
40. Kletscher BA, Qian J, Bostwick DG, et al. Prospective analysis of multifocality in renal cell carcinoma: influence of histological pattern, grade, number, size, volume and deoxyribonucleic acid ploidy. J Urol. 1995;153:904-6.
41. Pantuck AJ, Zisman A, Rauch MK, et al. Incidental renal tumors. Urology. 2000;56(2):190-6.
42. Lee CT, Katz J, Fearn PA, et al. Mode of presentation of renal cell carcinoma provides prognostic information. Urol Oncol. 2002;7(4):135-40.
43. Patard JJ, Leray E, Rodriguez A, et al. Correlation between symptom gradation, tumor characteristics and survival in renal cell carcinoma. Eur Urol. 2003;44(2):226-32.
44. Jayson M, Sanders H. Increased incidence of serendipitously discovered renal cell carcinoma. Urology. 1998;51:203-5.
45. Rosenblum SL. Paraneoplastic syndromes associated with renal cell carcinoma. J Scand Med Assoc. 1987;83:347-78.
46. Magera JS, Leibovich BC, Lohse CM, et al. Association of abnormal preoperative laboratory values with survival after radical nephrectomy for clinically confined clear cell renal cell carcinoma. Urology. 2008;71(2):278-82.
47. Davidson AJ, Hartman DS, Choyke PL, et al. Radiologic assessment of renal masses: implications for patient care. Radiology. 1997;202:297-305.
48. Zagoria RJ. Imaging of small renal masses: a medical success story. Am J Roentgenol. 2000;175:945-55.
49. Nelson CP, Sanda MG. Contemporary diagnosis and management of renal angiomyolipoma. J Urol. 2002;168:1315-25.
50. Bosniak MA. Renal-cell carcinoma. N Engl J Med. 1997;336(11):810.
51. Silver DA, Morash A, Brenner P, et al. Pathologic findings at the time of nephrectomy for renal mass, Ann Surg Oncol. 1997;4:570-4.
52. Licht MR. Renal adenoma and oncocytoma. Semin Urol Oncol. 1995;13:262-6.
53. Kang DE, White RL, Zuger JH, et al. Clinical use of fluorodeoxyglucose F 18 positron emission tomography for detection of renal cell carcinoma. J Urol. 2004;171(5):1806-9.
54. Jadvar H, Kherbache HM, Pinski JK, et al. Diagnostic role of (F-18) FDG positron emission tomography in restaging renal cell carcinoma. Clin Nephrol. 2003;60(6):395-400.
55. Herts BR, Remer EM. Role of percutaneous biopsy in the evaluation of renal and adrenal mass. AUA Update Series. 2000;19(36):282-7.
56. Schatz SM, Lieber MM. Update on oncocytoma. Curr Urol Rep. 2003;4(1):30-5.
57. Li G, Culleron M, Gentil-Perret A, et al. Characteristics of image-detected small renal masses: Implications for optimal treatment. Int J Urol. 2004;11:63-7.
58. Vasudevan A, Davies RJ, Shannon BA, et al. Incidental renal tumours: the frequency of benign lesions and the role of preoperative core biopsy. BJU Int. 2006;97:946-9.
59. Stage Information for Breast Cancer. Edge SB, Byrd DR, Compton CC, Fritz AG, Greene FL, Trotti A (Eds). AJCC Cancer Staging Manual, 7th edition. New York: Springer; 2010.
60. Linehan WM, Rini BI, Yang JC. Cancer of the kidney. In: DeVita VT, Lawrence TS, Rosenberg SA (Eds). Cancer: Principles and Practice of Oncology, 8th edition. Philadelphia: Lippincott, Williams & Wilkins; 2008. pp. 1331-58.
61. Kattan MW, Reuter V, Motzer RJ, et al. A postoperative prognostic nomogram for renal cell carcinoma. J Urol. 2001;166:63-7.
62. Zisman A, Pantuck AJ, Wieder J, et al. Risk group assessment and clinical outcome algorithm to predict the natural history of patients with surgically resected renal cell carcinoma. J Clin Oncol. 2002;20:4559-66.
63. Kontak J, Campbell SC. Prognostic factors in renal cell carcinoma. Urol Clin North Am. 2003;30(3):467-80.
64. Patard JJ, Kim HL, Lam JS, et al. Use of the University of California Los Angeles integrated staging system to predict survival in renal cell carcinoma: an international multicenter study. J Clin Oncol. 2004;22(16):316-22.
65. Licht MR, Novick AC, Goormastic M. Nephron sparing surgery in incidental versus suspected renal cell carcinoma. J Urol. 1994;152:39-42.
66. Fergany AF, Hafez KS, Novick AC. Long-term results of nephron sparing surgery for localized renal cell carcinoma: 10 year follow-up. J Urol. 2000;163:442-5.
67. Patard JJ, Leray E, Rodriguez A, et al. Correlation between symptom graduation, tumor characteristics and survival in renal cell carcinoma. Eur Urol. 2003;44(2):226-32.
68. Patard JJ, Dorey FJ, Cindolo L, et al. Symptoms as well as tumour size provide prognostic information on patients with localized renal tumours. J Urol. 2004;172:2167-71.
69. Motzer RJ, Bacik J, Schwartz LH, et al. Prognostic factors for survival in previously treated patients with metastatic renal cell carcinoma. J Clin Oncol. 2004;22:454-63.
70. Leibovich BC, Blute ML, Cheville JC, et al. Prediction of progression after radical nephrectomy for patients with clear cell renal cell carcinoma: a stratification tool for prospective clinical trials. Cancer. 2003;97(7):1663-71.
71. Négrier S, Escudier B, Gomez F, et al. Prognostic factors of survival and rapid progression in 782 patients with metastatic renal carcinomas treated by cytokines: a report from the Groupe Français d'Immunothérapie. Ann Oncol. 2002;13(9):1460-8.
72. Guinan PD, Vogelzang NJ, Fremgen AM, et al. Renal cell carcinoma: tumor size, stage and survival. Members of the Cancer Incidence and End Results Committee. J Urol. 1995;153:901-3.
73. Frank I, Blute ML, Cheville JC, et al. Solid renal tumours: an analysis of pathological features related to tumour size. J Urol. 2003;170:2217-20.
74. Frank I, Blute ML, Cheville JC, et al. An outcome prediction model for patients with clear cell renal cell carcinoma treated with radical nephrectomy based on tumour stage, size, grade and necrosis: the SSIGN score. J Urol. 2002;168:2395-400.
75. Sorbellini M, Kattan MW, Snyder ME, et al. A postoperative prognostic nomogram predicting recurrence for patients with conventional clear cell renal cell carcinoma. J Urol. 2005;173(1):48-51.
76. Parker AS, Leibovich BC, Lohse CM, et al. Development and evaluation of BioScore: a biomarker panel to enhance prognostic algorithms for clear cell renal cell carcinoma. Cancer. 2009;115(10):2092-103.

77. Robson CJ, Churchill BM, Anderson W. The results of radical nephrectomy for renal cell carcinoma. J Urol. 1969;101:297-301.
78. Lam JS, Shvarts O, Pantuck AJ. Changing concepts in the surgical management of renal cell carcinoma. Eur Urol. 2004;45(6):692-705.
79. Siemer S, Lehmann J, Kamradt J, et al. Adrenal metastases in 1,635 patients with renal cell carcinoma: outcome and indication for adrenalectomy. J Urol. 2004;171(6):2155-9.
80. Paul R, Mordhorst J, Busch R, et al. Adrenal sparing surgery during radical nephrectomy in patients with renal cell cancer: a new algorithm. J Urol. 2001;166:59-62.
81. Tsui K, Shvarts O, Barbaric Z, et al. Is adrenalectomy a necessary component of radical nephrectomy? UCLA experience with 511 radical nephrectomies. J Urol. 2000;163:437-41.
82. O'Malley RL, Godoy G, Kanofsky JA, et al. The necessity of adrenalectomy at the time of radical nephrectomy: a systematic review. J Urol. 2009;181(5):2009-17.
83. Guiliani L, Gilberti C, Martorana G, et al. Radical extensive surgery for renal cell carcinoma: long term results and prognostic factors. J Urol. 1990;143:468-73.
84. Phillips CK, Taneja SS. The role of lymphadenectomy in the surgical management of renal cell carcinoma. Urol Oncol. 2004;22(3):214-23.
85. Blute ML, Leibovich BC, Cheville JC, et al. A protocol for performing extended lymph node dissection using primary tumor pathological features for patients treated with radical nephrectomy for clear cell renal cell carcinoma. J Urol. 2004;172(2):465-9.
86. Leibovich BC, Blute ML. Lymph node dissection in the management of renal cell carcinoma. UCNA. 2008;35:673-8.
87. Vermooten V. Indications for conservative surgery in certain renal tumors: a study based on the growth pattern of the cell carcinoma. J Urol. 1950;64(2):200-8.
88. Lau WK, Blute ML, Waver AL, et al. Matched comparison of radical nephrectomy versus nephron sparing surgery in patients with unilateral renal cell carcinoma and a normal contralateral kidney. Mayo Clin Proc. 2000;75:1236-42.
89. Nieder AM, Taneja SS. The role of partial nephrectomy for renal cell carcinoma in contemporary practice. Urol Clin North Am. 2003;30:529-42.
90. Lerner SE, Hawkins CA, Blute ML, et al. Disease outcome in patients with low stage renal cell carcinoma treated with nephron sparing or radical surgery. J Urol. 1996;155(6):1868-73.
91. Hafez KS, Novick AC, Butler BP. Management of small solitary unilateral renal cell carcinomas: impact of central versus peripheral tumour location. J Urol. 1998;159:1156-60.
92. Thompson RH, Siddiqui S, Lohse CM, et al. Partial versus radical nephrectomy for 4 to 7 cm renal cortical tumors. J Urol. 2009;182(6):2601-6.
93. Hafez KS, Fergnay AF, Novick AC. Nephron sparing surgery for localized renal cell carcinoma: impact of tumour size on patient survival, tumour recurrence and TNM staging. J Urol. 1999;162:1930-3.
94. Leibovich BC, Blute ML, Cheville JC, et al. Nephron sparing surgery for appropriately selected renal cell carcinoma between 4 and 7 cm results in outcome similar to radical nephrectomy. J Urol. 2004;171:1066-70.
95. Patard JJ, Shvarts O, Lam JS, et al. Safety and efficacy of partial nephrectomy for all T1 tumours based on an international multicenter experience. J Urol. 2004;171:2181-5.
96. Dash A, Vickers AJ, Schachter LR, et al. Comparison of outcomes in elective partial vs. radical nephrectomy for clear cell renal cell carcinoma of 4-7 cm. BJU Int. 2006;97:939-45.
97. Crépel M, Jeldres C, Perrotte P, et al. Nephron-sparing surgery is equally effective to radical nephrectomy for T1BN0M0 renal cell carcinoma: a population-based assessment. Urology. 2010;75(2):271-5.
98. Castilla EA, Liou LS, Abrahms NA, et al. Prognostic importance of resection margin width alter nephron sparing surgery for renal cell carcinoma. Urology. 2002;60:993-7.
99. Sutherland SE, Resnik MI, Maclenanan GT, et al. Does the size of the surgical margin in partial nephrectomy for renal cell carcinoma really matter? J Urol. 2002;167:61-4.
100. Richstone L, Montage S, Ost M, et al. Laparoscopic partial nephrectomy for hilar tumours: evaluation of short term oncologic outcome. Urology. 2008;71:36-40.
101. Permpongkosol S, Bagga HS, Romero FR, et al. Laparoscopic versus open partial nephrectomy for the treatment of pathological T1N0M0 renal cell carcinoma: a 5 year survival rate. J Urol. 2006;176(5):1984-8.
102. Aron M, Turna B. Laparoscopic partial nephrectomy: newer trends. Indian J Urol. 2009;25:516-22.
103. Gill IS, Kavoussi LR, Lane BR, et al. Comparison of 1,800 laparoscopic and open partial nephrectomies for single renal tumours. J Urol. 2007;178:41-6.
104. Lane BR, Gill IS. 5 year outcomes of laparoscopic partial nephrectomy. J Urol. 2007;177:70-4.
105. Guilloneau B, Bermudez H, Gholami S. et al. Laparoscopic partial nephrectomy for renal tumour: single centre experience comparing clamping and no clamping techniques of the renal vasculature. J Urol. 2003;169:483-6.
106. Gill IS, Matin SF, Desai MM, et al. Comparative analysis of laparoscopic versus open partial nephrectomy for renal tumours in 200 patients. J Urol. 2003;170:64-8.
107. Johannes J, Razdan S, Cox M, et al. Current practice patterns in urological management of upper tract transitional cell carcinoma. J Endourol. 2005;19:366-71.
108. Silver DA, Morash C, Brenner P, et al. Pathologic findings at the time of nephrectomy for renal mass. Ann Surg Oncol. 1997;4:570-4.
109. Snyder ME, Bach A, Kattan MW, et al. Incidence of benign lesions for clinically localized renal masses smaller than 7 cm in radiological diameter: influence of sex. J Urol. 2006;176:2391-5.
110. Matin SF, Gill IS, Worley S, et al. Outcome of laparoscopic radical and open partial nephrectomy for the sporadic 4 cm or less renal tumour with a normal contra ateral kidney. J Urol. 2002;168:1356-9.
111. Huang WC, Levy AS, Serio AM, et al. Chronic kidney disease after nephrectomy in patients with renal cortical tumours: a retrospective cohort study. Lancet Oncol. 2006;7:735-40.
112. McKiernan J, Simmons R, Russo P, et al. Natural history of chronic renal insufficiency after partial and radial nephrectomy. Urology. 2002;59:816-20.

113. Ito K, Nakashima J, Hanawa Y, et al. The prediction of renal function 6 years after unilateral nephrectomy using preoperative risk factors. J Urol. 2004;171(1):120-5.
114. Malcolm JB, Bagrodia A, Derweesh IH, et al. Comparison of rates and risk factors for developing chronic renal insufficiency, proteinuria and metabolic acidosis after radical or partial nephrectomy. BJU Int. 2009;104(4):476-81.
115. Sorbellini M, Kattan MW, Snyder ME, et al. Prognostic nomogram for renal insufficiency after radical or partial nephrectomy. J Urol. 2006;176(2):472-6.
116. Lesage K, Joniau S, fransis K et al. Comparison between open partial and radical nephrectomy for renal tumours: perioperative outcome and health-related quality of life. Eur Urol. 2007;51:614-20.
117. Zini L, Perrotte P, Capitanio U, et al. Radical versus partial nephrectomy: effect on overall and noncancer mortality. Cancer. 2009;115(7):1465-71.
118. Thompson RH, Boorjian SA, Lohse CM, et al. Radical nephrectomy for pT1a renal masses may be associated with decreased overall survival compared with partial nephrectomy. J Urol. 2008;179:468-71.
119. Huang WC, Elkin EB, Levy AS, et al. Partial nephrectomy versus radical nephrectomy in patients with small renal tumours–is there a difference in mortality and cardiovascular outcomes? J Urol. 2009;181:55-61.
120. Ficarra V, Novara G, Secco S, et al: Preoperative aspects and dimensions used for anatomical (PADUA) classification of renal tumours in patients who are candidates for nephron sparing surgery. Eur Urol. 2006;56:786-93.
121. Murphy DP, Gill IS. Energy-based renal tumor ablation: a review. Semin Urol Oncol. 2001;19(2):133-40.
122. Lowry PS, Nakada SY. Renal cyrotherapy 2003 clinical status. Curr Opin Urol. 2003;13(3);193-7.
123. Hinshaw JL, Lee FT. Image-guided ablation of renal cell carcinoma. Magn Reson Imaging Clin N Am. 2004;12(3):429-47.
124. Johnson DB, Solomon SB, Su LM, et al. Defining the complications of cryoablation and radiofrequency ablation of small renal tumours: a multiinstitutional review. J Urol. 2001;172:874-7.
125. Hegarty NJ, Gill IS, Desai MM, et al. Probe-ablative nephron sparing surgery: Cryoablation versus radiofrequency ablation. Urology. 2006;68:7-13.
126. Zagoria RJ, Traver MA, Werle DM, et al. Oncological efficacy of CT-guided percutaneous radiofrequency ablation of renal cell carcinomas. Am J Roentgenol. 2007;189:429-36.
127. Levinson AW, Su LM, Agarwal D, et al. Long-term oncological and overall outcomes of percutaneous radiofrequency ablation in high risk surgical patients with a solitary small renal mass. J Urol. 2008;180:499-504.
128. Zini L, Perrotte P, Jeldres C, et al. A population-based comparison of survival after nephrectomy vs. nonsurgical management for small renal masses. BJU Int. 2009;103(7):899-904.
129. Chawla SN, Crispen PL, Hanlon AI, et al. The natural history of observed enhancing renal masses: meta-analysis and review of world literature. J Urol. 2006;175:425-31.
130. Sweeney P, Wood CG, Pisters LL, et al. Surgical management of renal cell carcinoma associated with complex inferior vena caval thrombi. Urol Oncol. 2003;21(5):327-33.
131. Glazer AA, Novick AC. Long-term followup after surgical treatment for renal cell carcinoma extending into the right atrium. J Urol. 1996;155(2):448-50.
132. Zisman A, Wieder JA, Pantuck AJ, et al. Renal cell carcinoma with tumor thrombus extension: biology, role of nephrectomy and response to immunotherapy. J Urol. 2003;169(3):909-16.
133. Leibovich BC, Cheville JC, Lohse CM, et al. Cancer specific survival for patients with pT3 renal cell carcinoma-can the 2002 primary tumor classification be improved? J Urol. 2005;173(3):716-9.
134. Kim HL, Zisman A, Han KR, et al. Prognostic significance of venous thrombus in renal cell carcinoma. Are renal vein and inferior vena cava involvement different? J Urol. 2004;171(2):588-91.
135. Blute ML, Leibovich BC, Lohse CM, et al. The Mayo Clinic experience with surgical management, complications, and outcome for patients with renal cell carcinoma and venous tumour thrombus. BJU Int. 2004;94:33-41.
136. Montie JE, El Ammar R, Pontes JE, et al. Renal cell carcinoma with inferior vena cava tumour thrombi. Surg Gynecol Obstet. 1991;173:107-15.
137. Moinzadeh A, Libertino JA. Prognostic significance of tumor thrombus level in patients with renal cell carcinoma and venous tumor thrombus extension. Is all T3b the same? J Urol. 2004;171(2):598-601.
138. Parekh DJ, Cookson MS, Chapman W, et al: Renal cell carcinoma with renal vein and inferior vena cava involvement: clinicopathological features, surgical techniques and outcomes. J Urol, 2005;173:1897-902.
139. Boorjian SA, Blute ML. Surgery for vena caval tumor extension in renal cancer. Curr Opin Urol. 2009;19(5):473-7.
140. Lam JS, Belldegrun AS, Figlin RA. Adjuvant treatment for renal cell carcinoma. Expert Opin Pharmacother. 2006;7(6):705-20.
141. Messing EM, Manola J, Wilding G, et al. Phase III study of interferon alfa NL as adjuvant treatment for resectable renal cell carcinoma: an Eastern Cooperative Oncology Group/Intergroup trial. J CLin Oncol. 2003;21:1214-22.
142. Klatte T, Lam JS, Shuch B, et al. Surveillance for renal cell carcinoma: why and how? When and how often? Urol Oncol. 2008;26(5):550-4.
143. Siddiqui SA, Frank I, Cheville JC, et al. Postoperative surveillance for renal cell carcinoma: a multifactorial histological subtype specific protocol. BJU Int. 2009;104(6):778-85.
144. Stephenson AJ, Chetner MP, Rourke K, et al. Guidelines for the surveillance of localized renal cell carcinoma based on the patterns of relapse after nephrectomy. J Urol. 2004;172(1):58-62.
145. Dimarco DS, Lohse CM, Zincke H, et al. Long term survival of patients with unilateral sporadic multifocal renal cell carcinoma according to histological subtype compared with patients with solitary tumour after radical nephrectomy. Urology. 2004;64:462-7.
146. Levy DA, Slaton JW, Swanson DA, et al. Stage specific guidelines for surveillance after radical nephrectomy for local renal cell carcinoma. J Urol. 1998;159(4):1163-7.
147. Bruno JJ, Snyder ME, Motzer RJ, et al. Renal cell carcinoma local recurrences: impact of surgical treatment and concomitant metastasis on survival. BJU Int. 2006;97(5):933-8.
148. Bukowski RM. Natural history and therapy of metastatic renal cell carcinoma: the role of interleukin-2. Cancer. 1997;80(7):1198-220.

149. Friedel G, Hürtgen M, Penzenstadler M, et al. Resection of pulmonary metastases from renal cell carcinoma. Anticancer Res. 1999;19(2C):1593-6.

150. Kavolius JP, Mastorakos DP, Pavlovich C, et al. Resection of metastatic renal cell carcinoma. J Clin Oncol. 1998;16:2261-6.

151. Murthy SC, Kim K, Rice TW, et al. Can we predict long-term survival after pulmonary metastasectomy for renal cell carcinoma? Ann Thorac Surg. 2005;79(3):996-1003.

152. Staehler M, Rohrmann K, Bachmann A, et al. Therapeutic approaches in metastatic renal cell carcinoma. BJU Int. 2005;95:1153-61.

153. Walther MM, Yang JC, Pass HI, et al. Cytoreductive surgery before high dose interleukin-2 based therapy in patients with metastatic renal cell carcinoma. J Urol. 1997;158:1675-8.

154. Flanigan RC, Salmon SE, Blumenstein BA, et al. Nephrectomy followed by interferon alpha 2b compared with interferon alpha 2b alone fore metastatic renal cell carcinoma. N Engl J Med 2001:345:1655-9.

155. Mickish GH, von Popoel H, De Prijck L, et al. Radical nephrectomy plus interferon alpha based immunotherapy compared with interferon alpha alone in metastatic renal cell carcinoma: a randomized trial. Lancet. 2001;358:966-70.

156. Flanigan RC, Mickisch G, Sylevester R, et al. Cytoreductive nephrectomy in patients with metastatic renal cancer: a combined analysis. J Urol. 2004;171:1071-6.

157. Pantuck AJ, Zisman A, Dorey F, et al. Renal cell carcinoma with retroperitoneal lymph nodes: role of lymph node dissection. J Urol. 2003;169(6):2076-83.

158. MRC Renal Cancer Collaborators. Interferon alfa and survival in metastatic renal cell carcinoma: early results of a randomized controlled trial. Lancet. 1999;353(9146):14-7.

159. Negrier S, Perd D, Ravaud A, et al. Do cytokines improve survival in patients with metastatic renal cell carcinoma of intermediate prognosis? Results of prospective randomized PERCY Quattro trial. J Clin Oncol. 2005;23(165):380S.

160. Yagoda A, Petrylak D, Thompson S. Cytotoxic chemotherapy for advanced renal cell carcinoma. Urol Clin North Am. 1993;20(2): 303-21.

161. Nanus DM, Garino A, Milowsky MI, et al. Active chemotherapy for sarcomatoid and rapidly progressing renal cell carcinoma. Cancer. 2004;101(7):1545-51.

162. Rini BI, Campbell SC, Escudier B. Renal cell carcinoma. Lancet. 2009;373(9669):1119-32.

163. Motzer RJ, Basik J, Murphy BA, et al. Interferon alfa as a comparative treatment for clinical trials of new therapies against advanced renal cell carcinoma. J Clin Oncol. 2002;20:289-96.

164. Bukowski RM. Natural history and therapy of metastatic renal cell carcinoma. The role of interleukin-2. Cancer. 1997;80:1198-220.

165. Coppin C, Porzolt F, Awa A, et al. Immunotherapy for advanced renal cell carcinoma. Cochrane Database Syst Rev. 2005;(1):CD001425.

166. Fyfe G, Fisher RI, Rosenberg SA, et al. Results of treatment of 225 patients with metastatic renal cell carcinoma who received high dose recombinant interleukin-2 therapy. J Clin Oncol. 1995;13:688-96.

167. McDermott DF, Rean MM, Clark JI, et al. Randomized phase III trial of high dose interleukin-2 versus subcutaneous interleukin-2 and interferon in patients with metastatic renal cell carcinoma. J Clin Oncol. 2005;23(1):133-41.

168. Negrier S, Escudier B, Lasset C, et al. Recombinant human interleukin-2, recombinant human interferon alfa 2a or both in metastatic renal cell carcinoma. N Engl J Med. 1998;338:1273-8.

169. Motzer RJ, Hutson TE, Tomczak P, et al. Sunitinib versus interferon alfa in metastatic renal cell carcinoma. N Engl J Med. 2007;356(2):115-24.

170. Escudier B, Eisen T, Stadler WM, et al. TARGET Study Group. Sorafenib in advanced clear cell renal cell carcinoma. N Engl J Med. 2007;356(2):125-34.

171. Szczylik C, Demkow T, Staehler M, et al. Randomized phase III trial of first line treatment with sorafenib versus interferon in patients with advanced renal cell carcinoma: final results. J Clin Oncol (Meeting abstracts). 2007;25(18):241s.

172. Gollob JA, Rathmell WK, Richmond TM, et al. Phase II trial of sorafenib plus interferon alfa 2b as first or second line therapy in patients with metastatic renal cell cancer. J Clin Oncol. 2007;25(22):3288-95.

173. Escudier B, Pluzanska A, Koralewski P, et al. Bevacizumab plus interferon alfa 2a for treatment of metastatic renal cell carcinoma: a randomized double blind phase III trial. Lancet. 2007;370(9605):2103-11.

174. Rini BI, Halabi S, Rosenberg JE, et al. Bevacizumab plus interferon alfa compared with interferon alfa monotherapy in patients with metastatic renal cell carcinoma: CALGB 90206. J Clin Oncol. 2008;26:5422-8.

175. Sternberg CN, Davis ID, Mardiak J, et al. Pazopanib in locally advanced or metastatic renal cell carcinoma: results of a randomized phase III trial. J Clin Oncol. 2010;28(6):1061-8.

176. Motzer RJ, Hutson TE, Cella D, et al. Pazopanib versus sunitinib in metastatic renal-cell carcinoma. N Engl J Med. 2013;369:722-31.

177. Motzer RJ, Escudier B, Tomczak P, et al. Axitinib versus sorafenib as second-line treatment for advanced renal cell carcinoma: overall survival analysis and updated results from a randomized phase 3 trial. Lancet Oncol. 2013;14(6):552-62.

178. Turner KJ, Moore JW, Jones A, et al. Expression of hypoxia-inducible factors in human renal cancer: relationship to angiogenesis and to the von Hippel-Lindau gene mutation. Cancer Res. 2002;62:2957-61.

179. Hudes G, Carducci M, Tomczak P, et al. Temsirolimus, interferon alfa or both for advanced renal cell carcinoma. N Engl J Med. 2007;356(22):2271-81.

180. Motzer RJ, Escudier B, Oudard S, et al. Efficacy of everolimus in advanced renal cell carcinoma: a double blind randomized placebo controlled phase III trial. Lancet. 2008;372:449-56.

181. Escudier B, Eisen T, Porta C, et al. Renal cell carcinoma: ESMO clinical practice guidelines for diagnosis, treatment and follow-up. Ann Oncol. 2012:23(7):vii65-71.

182. Thomas AA, Rini BI, Stephenson AJ, et al. Surgical resection of renal cell carcinoma after targeted therapy. J Urol. 2009;182(3): 881-6.

44 Prostate Cancer

Jagdeesh Kulkarni, Varun Gunavanthe, Nasreen Gite, Abhijit Dhale, Devendra Choudhary

INTRODUCTION

The prostate gland is an ovoid accessory sex organ in the male, situated below the neck of the urinary bladder. It is composed of glandular (70%) and fibromuscular stromal (30%) tissue. Along with the seminal vesicles, it contributes in the secretion of seminal fluid.[1] The normal prostate weighs about 18–20 grams, has a base beneath the bladder and an apex towards the sphincter urethrae. It lies behind the pubic symphysis and anterior to the rectum and seminal vesicles (Fig. 1). Inferiorly, it rests on the levator ani muscle. It has a capsule composed of smooth muscles, collagen and elastin.[1]

It has been classified into zones (McNeal) (Fig. 2):

- Transitional zone: Five to ten percent of the glandular tissue, lying posterior and lateral to the proximal prostatic urethra. Most benign enlargements and 20% malignancies of the prostate arise here.
- Central Zone: Twenty five percent of the glandular tissue, lying around the ejaculatory ducts, and it is cone-shaped. One to five percent adenocarcinomas arise here.
- Peripheral zone: Constitutes about 70% of the glandular tissue, makes up the posterior and lateral parts of the gland. Chronic prostatitis and 70% cancers arise in this zone.

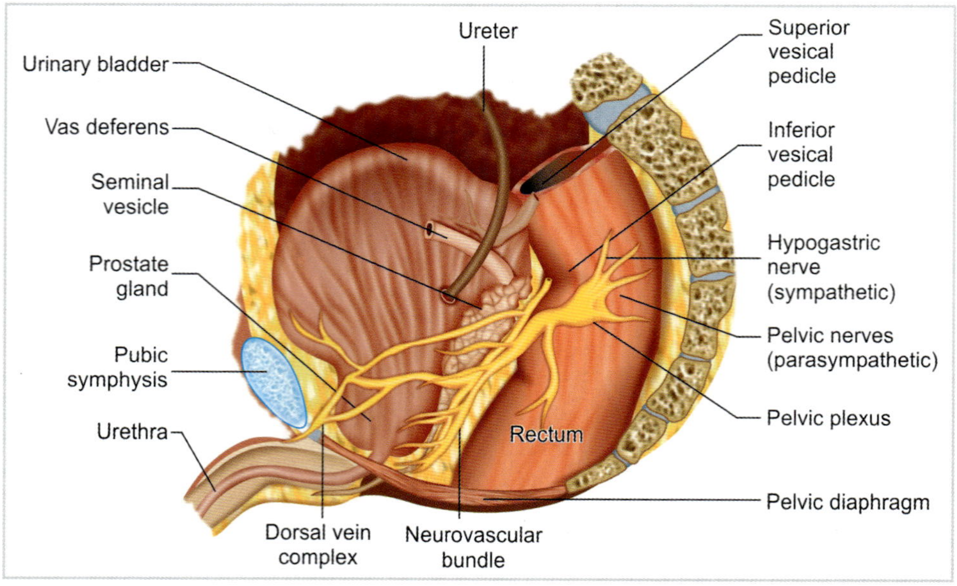

Fig. 1: Anatomy

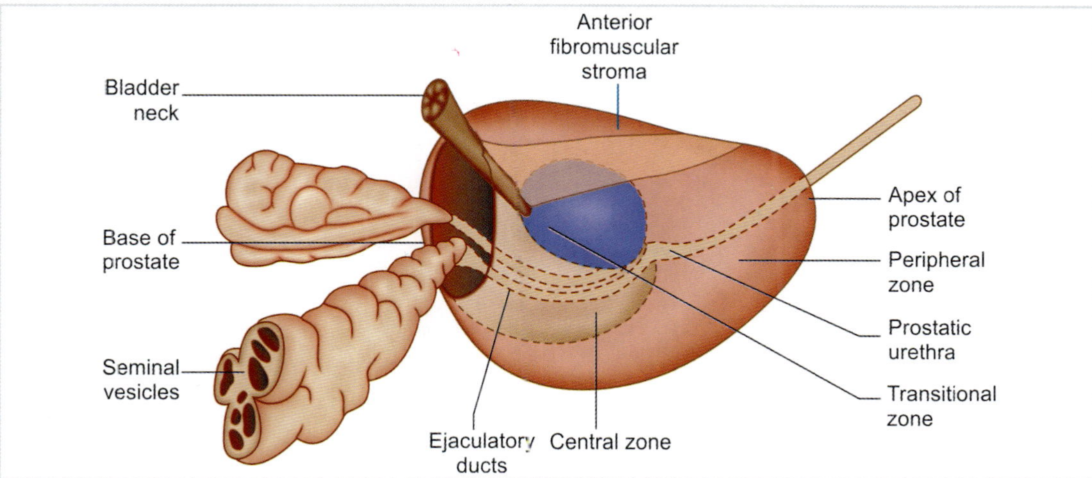

Fig. 2: Zonal anatomy of the prostate

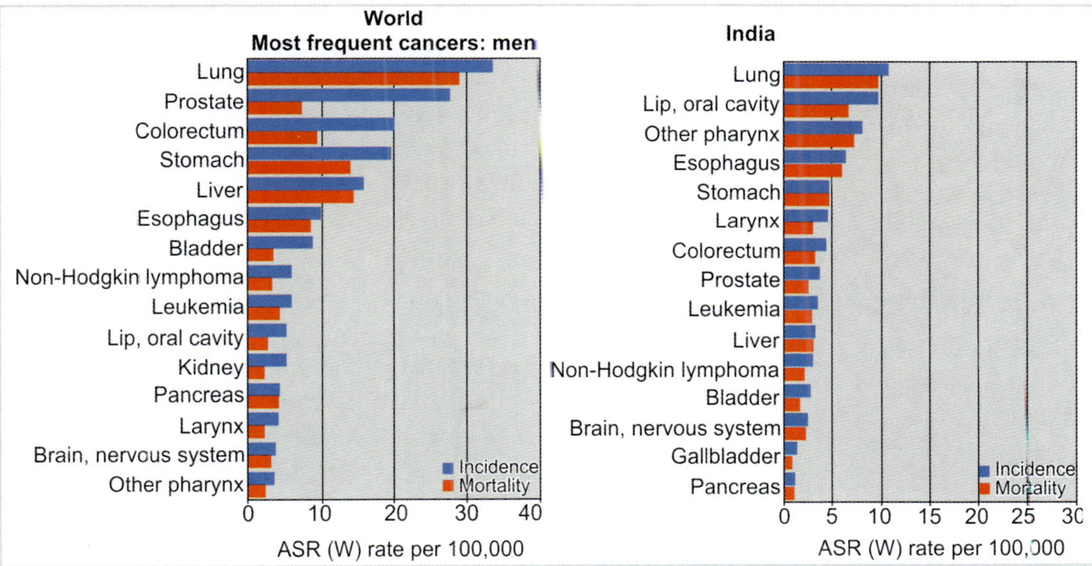

Fig. 3: Incidence and mortality statistics of cancers in men throughout the world and those specific for India

- Anterior fibromuscular stroma forms one-third of the prostatic mass—may get replaced by glandular tissue from benign prostatic hyperplasia (BPH).[1]

EPIDEMIOLOGY

Prostate cancer is the most common cancer in men in the Western world and second most common cause of cancer death. About 15% of male cancers in developed countries are prostate cancer, compared to 4% of male cancers in developing countries (Fig. 3). Further, prostate cancer incidence ranges: 161.4 cases per 100,000 white males (mortality of 25.6/lakh), 255.5 cases per 100,000 African-American males (mortality of 62.3/lakh) and 96.5 per lakh Asian males (mortality of 11.3/lakh) (American Cancer Society 2000-2004 statistics). These racial differences seem to be due to environmental exposure, diet, lifestyle and attitudes towards health care.[2] A lifetime estimated risk of developing the disease is 16.72% and lifetime risk of death from prostate cancer is 2.57%. Longer the life expectancy and lesser the mortality from smoking-related diseases, higher is the risk of developing prostate cancer (e.g. in Sweden, 37% of all new cases of cancer in 2004 were prostate cancer).[2]

Risk Factors (Fig. 4)

Age

Prostate cancer affects elderly men more often than young men (<50 years age). Sixty-three percent are diagnosed

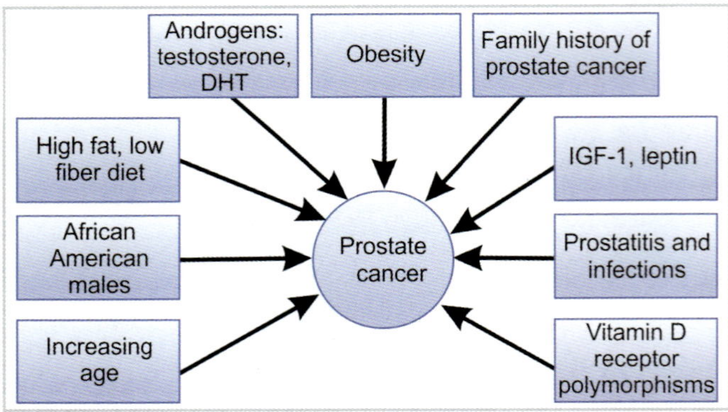

Fig. 4: Risk factors for prostate cancer

after the age of 65 years. Autopsy findings suggest that 50% men in their 50s and more than 75% men older than 85 years carry occult cancer.[2,3]

Stage

Impact of widespread use of prostate-specific antigen (PSA) has resulted in 60–75% newly diagnosed disease found to be nonpalpable cancers and hence more cases are detected early in the natural course and in organ-confined stage.[2,3]

Familial and Genetic Predisposition

In general, incidence of sporadic and familial cancers is about 85% and 15% respectively. The risk of cancer amongst the family members increases with the number, pedigree and the age at which they were affected. Paternal incidence predisposes an increase in the risk by 2.17 times and this increases to 3.37 times if a sibling is affected. Similarly with early onset of disease, the risk is higher (about 3.34 times) in the siblings. Further, it more than two first degree relatives were affected, the relative risk is 5.08. Lastly, 43% cases with early onset disease (55 years of age or younger) have hereditary prostate cancer and 9% of all cancers that occur by 85 years of age are hereditary.

There has been some evidence that carriers of BRCA 1(17q21) and BRCA 2(13q12) genes exhibit double and sixfold higher risk respectively of prostate cancer. Other genetic association has been HPC1 autosomal dominant gene, somatic mutation leading to tumor initiation and progression. Finally, there is a genetic pathway between prostatic inflammatory atrophy, high-grade prostatic intraepithelial neoplasia (PIN) and cancer.[2,3]

Diet and Obesity

Excessive polyunsaturated fat consumption and obesity have been correlated to higher incidence of prostate cancer.

Vasectomy, Smoking, Alcohol and Sexually Transmitted Diseases

These have all been implicated as factors associated with the development of prostate cancer, but none has been clearly found to be causative in recent studies.

PRIMARY CHEMOPREVENTION

There has been some discussion about primary prevention with the aim of decreasing the incidence of cancer and reducing both treatment-related side effects and mortality. The Prostate Cancer Prevention Trial (PCPT) demonstrated that finasteride reduces the period prevalence of prostate cancer by 25%. Further, Selenium and Vitamin E Cancer Prevention Trial (SELECT) demonstrated that neither selenium nor vitamin E could prevent prostate cancer. The 5-alfa-reductase inhibitors and other hormonal agents, antioxidants and statins are among the many agents currently being investigated in prostate cancer chemoprevention.[2] Serms, soy, lycopene, green tea, statins have all been suggested as having protective effect against carcinoma prostate, but evidence is lacking.[2]

PATHOLOGY

Proliferative inflammatory atrophy (Flow chart 1) is a condition where hyperproliferative lesions are formed following infection, inflammation and oxidant injury. These appear to be precursors of PIN and atypical small acinar proliferation (ASAP). PIN and ASAP have an intact basal cell layer, but are in turn precursor lesions for prostate cancer. This happens when the basal cell layers are lost and the lesion is more invasive. Most common histology of the prostate cancers is adenocarcinoma, while transitional and neuroendocrine variety is rare. The basis of its grading is glandular architecture, loss of basal cell layer by high molecular weight cytokeratin staining on low-power microscopy. Individual cellular changes are not as important as in other solid malignancies.[3,4]

Gleason scoring of prostate cancer (Fig. 5) is based on the patterns of differentiation. Well-differentiated is Gleason pattern 1 and poorly differentiated is pattern 5. Gleason scoring is done based on the predominant pattern and the next most widely seen pattern on low power microscopy, e.g. Gleason (3+4) represents a predominant (primary) Gleason pattern 3 of differentiation and the next most common (secondary) Gleason pattern 4. Some have suggested mentioning the tertiary pattern also. Higher Gleason score is associated with poorer outcome, owing to

Flow chart 1: Pathology of prostate cancer

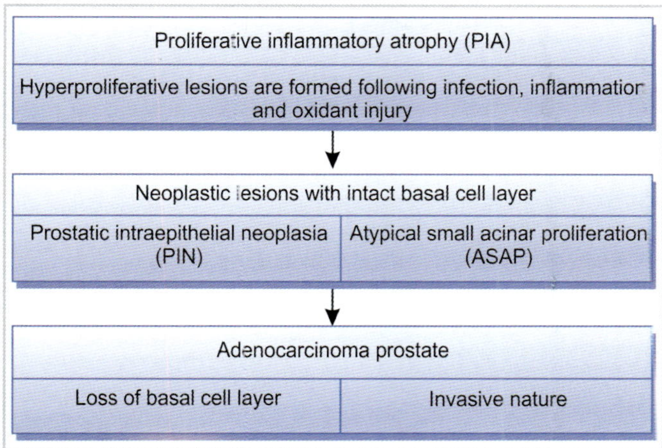

Flow chart 2: Biological progression of the disease

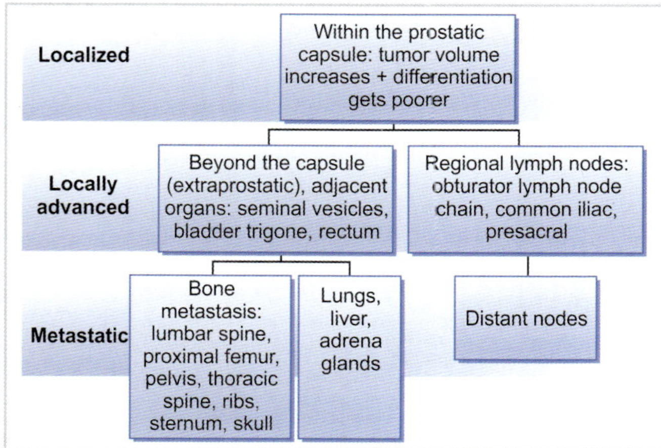

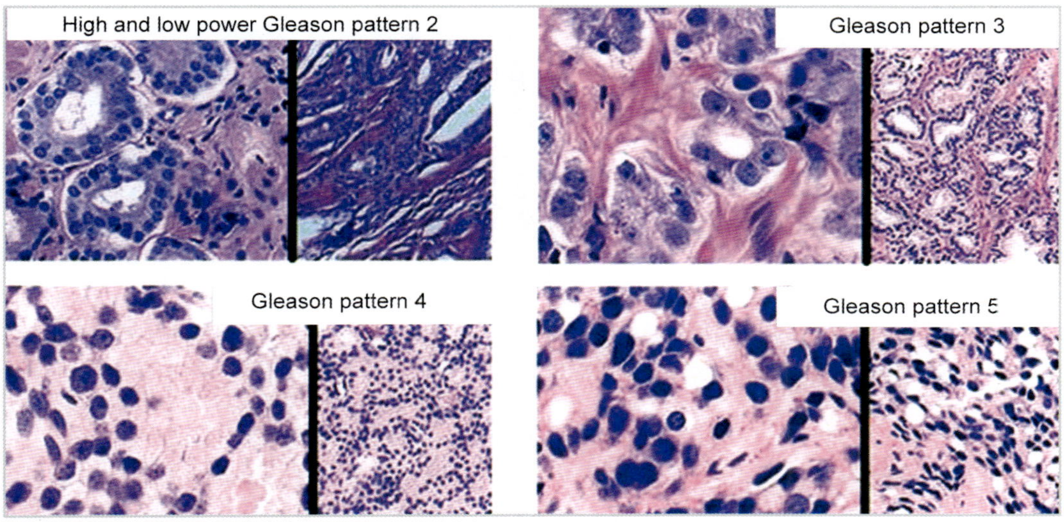

Fig. 5: Gleason patterns for grading prostate cancer

higher likelihood of extraprostatic extension, lymph nodal involvement and chances of metastasis.

Biologically, progression of cancer may follow the stepwise pattern (Flow chart 2) or may become aggressive depending on the Gleason grade.

DIAGNOSIS

One of the most important clinical presentations is the occult form (histological/latent form), seen in approximately 30% of men older than 50 years of age and may rise to 50–70% in men above 80 years of age. Further, early or localized cancer may be picked up by a histopathology report of prostatic tissue from transurethral resection specimen for benign prostatic enlargement, or by needle biopsy done for elevated serum PSA level. Locally advanced cancer may present with lower urinary tract symptoms, hematuria, bladder outlet or ureteral obstruction, hematospermia and even impotence. Metastatic disease presents with bone pain, pathological fractures, anemia and pedal edema, and sometimes even as paraneoplastic symptoms, malignant retroperitoneal fibrosis or disseminated intravascular coagulation. PSA and digital rectal examination (DRE) in combination increase the likelihood of early prostate cancer detection.[3,5-7]

Screening of patients with digital rectal examination (DRE) and PSA has been recommended for patients between 55 and 69 years of age as they will benefit most for treatment, in the event that clinically significant prostate cancer is diagnosed at an early stage.[9] Risks and benefits

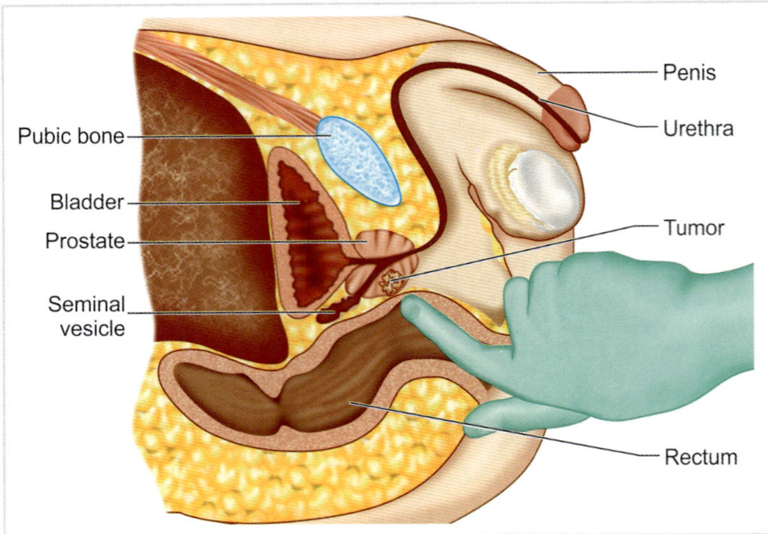

Fig. 6: Digital rectal examination

associated with screening (such as need for invasive TRUS guided biopsy) need to be explained to the patients prior to screening.[8]

Digital Rectal Examination (Fig. 6)

Digital rectal examination is done with the patient in left lateral decubitus position with hips and knees flexed up or in knee elbow position. Hard consistency of the prostate, nodular feel, fixity of rectal mucosa may be considered as abnormal DRE findings.[9]

Prostate-specific Antigen

As the name suggests, PSA is organ-specific but not disease-specific. It is a human kallikrein secreted by the prostatic cells into seminal fluid and circulates in complexed and free forms (together add up to total PSA). It is influenced by androgen levels, age, race (higher in blacks) and prostate size. Elevation of PSA is seen in prostate disease [BPH, prostatitis and urinary tract infection (UTI), prostate cancer]. Lower PSA levels are seen in patients on 5-alfa-reductase inhibitors for BPH (PSA levels decreased to half the true baseline values, after 6–12 months of therapy), post-surgery for BPH, during and after medical [luteinizing hormone-releasing hormone (LHRH) analogs] or surgical management (orchiectomy, radical prostatectomy) or radiation therapy for prostate cancer.[3,5,7]

For the purpose of prostatic needle biopsy, the normal threshold levels accepted are 2.5–4 ng/mL. However to increase the diagnostic accuracy in patients with PSA of intermediate levels of 4–10 ng/mL, volume-based parameters are popular and include:

- *Prostate-specific antigen density* (PSAD, PSA divided by prostate volume): A value greater than 0.15 is an indication for prostate biopsy
- Complexed PSA density (complexed PSA divided by prostate volume)
- Prostate-specific antigen transition zone density (PSA divided by transition zone volume): Most sensitive and specific marker for prostate cancer.

Some other estimations:

- *Prostate-specific antigen velocity* or PSAV (rate of change in PSA): More than 0.75 ng/mL per year is a marker for prostate cancer.
- Lower free PSA (fPSA) and higher complexed PSA (cPSA) are suggestive of prostate cancer. Percentage of fPSA cutoff of 25% detected 95% of cancers while avoiding 20% of unnecessary biopsies.
- Precursor PSA (proPSA), human kallikrein 2 (hK2) and prostate cancer gene 3 (PCA-3) mRNA overexpression have also been found to be useful markers.

Transrectal Ultrasound-guided Needle Biopsy (Fig. 7)

Transrectal ultrasound (TRUS) appearance per se is not used for diagnosis of prostate cancer which may reveal a hypoechoic lesion in the peripheral zone, but it is used to direct needle biopsies of the prostate. Color Doppler or power Doppler TRUS can show increased vascularity

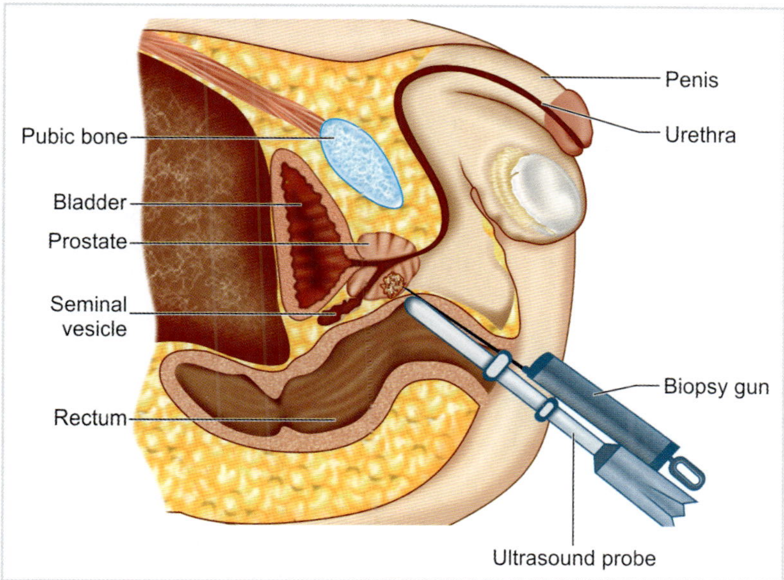

Fig. 7: Transrectal ultrasound-guided biopsy of prostate

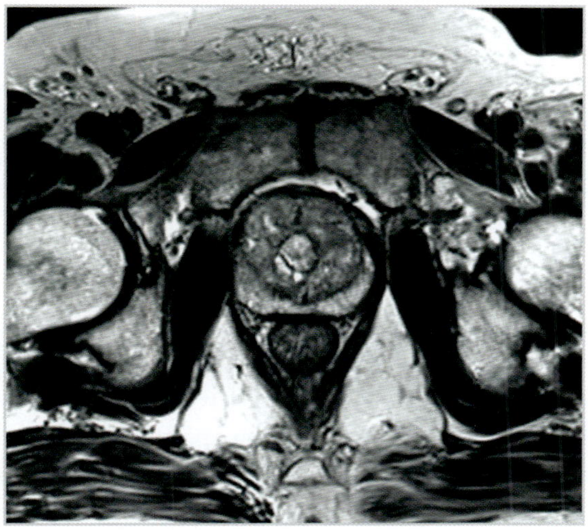

Fig. 8: Magnetic resonance imaging

of the prostate in the region of the suspicious nodule. The coagulation profile is done prior to the procedure and antibiotics are started. It is usually done under local anesthesia with the patient in left lateral decubitus. Typically, a 12-core systematic biopsy is taken under ultrasound guidance of the peripheral zone of both the lobes and any suspicious hypoechoic lesions. The biopsy cores are sent separately for histopathology. Post procedure, patient may sometimes have hematuria. Oral antibiotics are continued for another 2–3 days. In case of negative biopsies despite elevated PSA, abnormal DRE and previous histopathological diagnosis of malignancy, repeat biopsy may be done on individual basis but the yield generally tends to reduce with subsequent biopsies.[6]

Imaging

Magnetic resonance imaging (Fig. 8): Endorectal or axial MRI helps in detection of bilobar prostate involvement as well as seminal vesicle and extracapsular involvement of prostate cancer more accurately than DRE, TRUS and CT scan. Prostate cancer is hypointense on T2-weighted MR imaging, but this lacks specificity. Functional MRI (contrast-enhanced MRI, spectroscopy and diffusion-weighted imaging) can improve the accuracy of T2 imaging to localize cancer and estimate tumor.[7]

CT scan of abdomen and pelvis may be done for pelvic lymphadenopathy, despite its low sensitivity (as microscopic extent cannot be assessed). CT-guided biopsy of enlarged pelvic lymph nodes may be done prior to decision regarding treatment. Positive lymph nodes may lead to choice of alternative therapy.[7] X-ray or CT scan of chest should be done to rule out lung metastasis.

Radionuclide bone scan (bone scintigraphy): is done if the patient has clinical stage T3 or T4, bony symptoms, or an elevated serum alkaline phosphatase levels or a serum PSA greater than 20 ng/mL or a Gleason score of 8–10. Increased radiotracer uptake by lumbar vertebrae, ribs, pelvic bones, skull or long bones of limbs may be suggestive of metastatic disease.[7]

Fluorodeoxyglucose positron emission tomography (FDG-PET) scan and Choline PET scan may be useful in diagnosing and staging of primary tumors with a high Gleason score, in detecting metastatic disease in selected patients with biochemical failure (scan sensitivity increases with increasing PSA level), in assessing the extent of metabolically active castrate-resistant disease, in monitoring response to androgen deprivation and other therapies, and in prognostication.[10]

STAGING AND RISK STRATIFICATION

There are two types of staging followed in clinical practice, namely clinical and pathological staging.

Clinical Staging (Table 1)

Clinical staging [Tumor Node Metastasis (TNM)] requires a combination of the following: (1) DRE findings; (2) serum PSA level; (3) biopsy report; (4) imaging studies.

TNM staging has become the most popular staging and details of which are given in Table 1. Despite the newer advances in imaging studies, their accuracy to predict T staging is at best modest; however, the same is not true for prediction of the N+ve status (nodal involvement). Hence, pelvic lymph node dissection (PLND) still remains the best alternative. One may avoid the morbidity of lymph node dissection in patients with T stage less than 2, PSA less than 20 ng/mL and Gleason score less than 6 who have a less than 10% chance of having lymph node involvement and hence these patients can be spared the nodal dissection and ensuing morbidity. Further, in patients with organ confined disease (T1-2): 80% have PSA <4 ng/mL; 66% have PSA between 4 ng/mL and 10 ng/mL; less than 50% have PSA >10 ng/mL while in N+ve patients: >75% patients have PSA >50 ng/mL. Similarly in spite of refinements of techniques, biopsy Gleason score is upgraded in pathology specimen ranging from 30% to 60% (Kulkarni et al.).[11-14]

Pathological Staging (After Radical Prostatectomy)

Generally, this helps in better assessment of tumor burden and is more accurate to predict prognosis, compared to clinical staging. Histopathology of the excised specimen will reveal: tumor (Gleason) grade, percentage of prostate tissue involved and size of dominant nodule, if found surgical margin status, extracapsular disease, seminal vesicle invasion and pelvic lymph node involvement.[7]

In clinical practice, D'Amico's (1998) (Table 2) risk stratification has become the standard procedure to predict both pathological stage of the disease and prognosis with acceptable result.

TREATMENT OPTIONS AND OPTIMUM MANAGEMENT

Treatment options depend on the stage and risk stratification as discussed above.

Localized Prostate Cancer (T1 and T2)

In this clinical setting, there has been considerable debate regarding the best option. However, it is incumbent on the clinician, to discuss the various options with the patient, underlining their pros and cons, benefits and risks. Based on the grade, the stage, life expectancy, comorbidities and choice of the patient, the final decision may be made.

Active Surveillance and Watchful Waiting

It is suited for compliant patients, willing for regular follow-up, having early-stage and low-grade (no Gleason pattern 4 or 5) cancer. Treatment is offered at the first sign of progression (DRE findings, increasing PSA or progressive grade on prostate biopsy).

Surgery: Radical Prostatectomy and Our Experience

Standard indications are patients with a life expectancy of more than 10 years/young patients, those with comorbidities which do not preclude a major surgery (medical fitness) and organ-confined disease (T1-T2).

Retropubic radical prostatectomy (open): Retropubic radical prostatectomy (first described by Millin in 1945) can be performed by open, laparoscopic or robotic techniques, as per the availability, proper patient selection, patient's choice and the surgeon's expertise. We herein highlight some technical points:

- Vertical midline incision is made and the peritoneum is reflected upwards and the bladder is pushed downwards
- Bilateral pelvic lymphadenectomy is done and sent for histopathology (frozen section of the lymph nodes to be done if they are enlarged or appear to be involved and if the patient has decided that the procedure be stopped in case of lymph nodal involvement)

TABLE 1: **TNM classification of prostate cancer**

TNM		*Description*
TX		Primary tumor cannot be assessed
T0		No evidence of primary tumor
T1 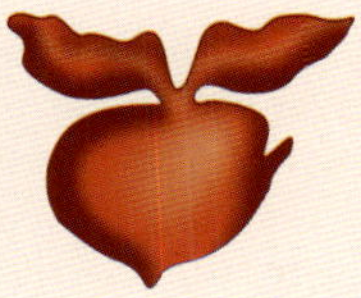		Clinically inapparent tumor not palpable or visible by imaging
	T1a	Tumor incidental histological finding in 5% or less of tissue resected
	T1b	Tumor incidental histological finding in more than 5% of tissue resected
	T1c	Tumor identified by needle biopsy (e.g. because of elevated prostate-specific antigen level)
T2		Tumor confined within the prostate
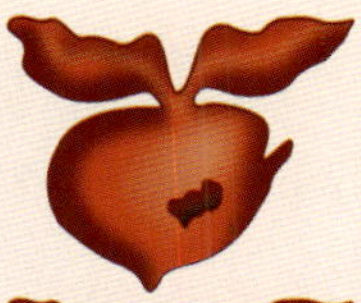	T2a	Tumor involves one half of one lobe or less
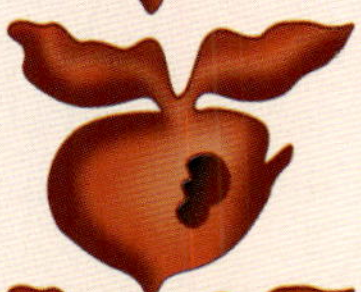	T2b	Tumor involves more than half of one lobe, but not both lobes
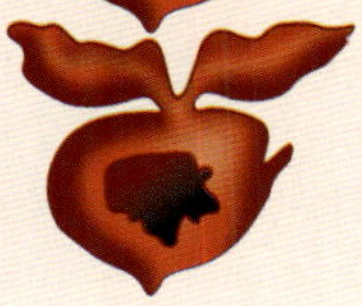	T2c	Tumor involves both lobes
T3		Tumor extends through the prostatic capsule
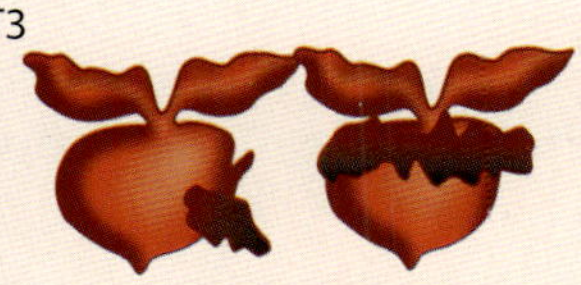	T3a	Extracapsular extension (unilateral or bilateral) including microscopic bladder neck involvement
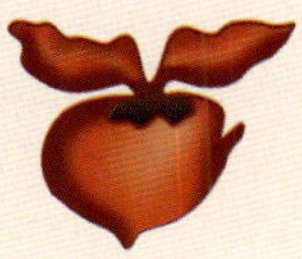	T3b	Tumor invades seminal vesicle(s)
T4 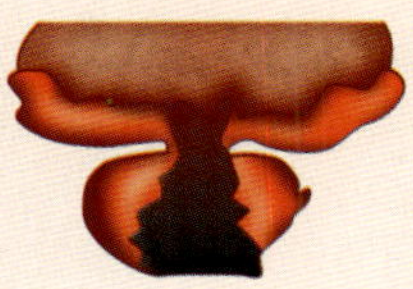		Tumor is fixed or invades adjacent structures other than seminal vesicles: external sphincter, rectum, levator muscles, and/or pelvic wall
NX	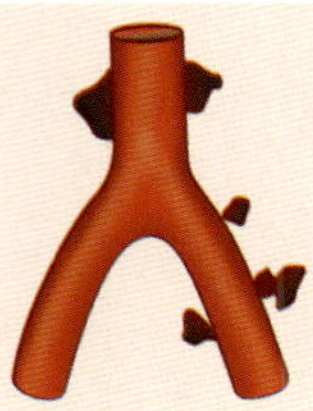	Regional lymph nodes cannot be assessed
N0		No regional lymph node metastasis
N1		Regional lymph node metastasis
MX		Distant metastasis cannot be assessed
M0		No distant metastasis
M1 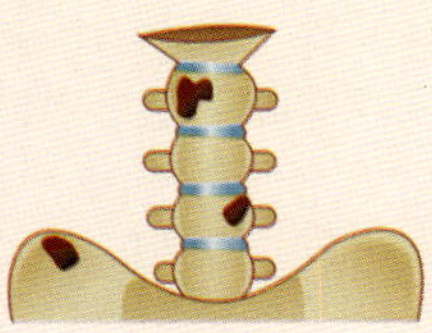		Distant metastasis
	M1a	Nonregional lymph node(s)
	M1b	Bone(s)
	M1c	Other sites

Abbreviation: TNM, tumor node metastasis

TABLE 2: D'Amico risk stratification of carcinoma prostate

Risk category	Clinical stage	PSA value	Gleason score	Disease free survival at 10 years post RP
Low risk	T1–T2a	10 ng/mL or less	6 or less	83%
Intermediate risk	T2b	>10 but <20 ng/mL	7	46%
High risk	T2c–3a	>20 ng/mL	8–10	29%

Abbreviations: PSA, prostate-specific antigen; RP, radical prostatectomy

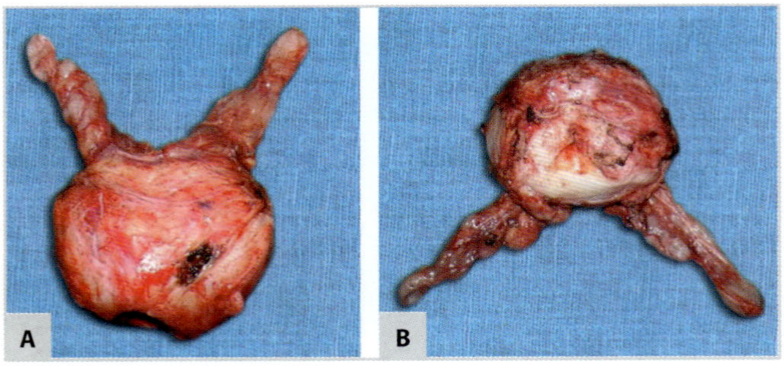

Figs 9A and B: Specimen of radical prostatectomy

- Endopelvic fascia is opened and puboprostatic ligaments are incised
- Santorini dorsal venous complex is suture ligated and transected
- Urethra at the apex of the prostate is dissected and transected
- Prostate is dissected off the neurovascular bundles (Figs 9A and B)
- Prostatic pedicles are secured and transected
- Bladder neck is transected and reconstructed
- Seminal vesicles and ampullary portion of the vas deferens are dissected
- Vesicourethral anastomosis is performed.

The detailed discussion about the preferred technique vis-a-vis advantages of the open versus minimal invasive technique is out of the scope of this chapter. Most authors believe that advantages of retropubic prostatectomy (RP) are that urologists are familiar with this approach; there is a wider field of exposure with lesser chances of rectal injury and fecal incontinence. Side effects of RP are: stress urinary incontinence (which usually improves over the period of 3–9 months and patients may benefit from pelvic floor exercises) and erectile dysfunction (which usually improves by 12 months and patients may benefit from early phosphodiesterase inhibitor therapy). Nerve sparing prostatectomy is dependent on the local factors and surgeon's expertise and should be offered whenever possible to preserve erectile function.

We initiated radical prostatectomy in mid-90s and standardized the technique by early 2000 since suitable cases were relatively less.[11,12] Recently, we published our experience of consecutive 428 open radical prostatectomy.[13] We noted that after year 2002, the incidence of organ-confined disease increased compared to the pre-2002 era with the advent of PSA being routinely available, in India. In this study, we observed that 7-year survival in patients with Gleason scores <4, 5–6, 7 and 8–10 was 95.8%, 89%, 75.9% and 56% respectively. Further, the same data when analyzed by pathological stagewise, i.e. in pT0-2, pT3a, pT3b and LN positive, it was 96.9%, 79%, 73% and 72% respectively. We compared the complications in our study with the literature and found that they were comparable (Table 3). Lastly, biopsy Gleason score was upgraded in pathology specimen of radical prostatectomy and had an impact on survival.[14] Table 4 gives brief outline of our current management protocol.

Pelvic lymphadenectomy: Pelvic lymphadenectomy is done for intermediate and high-risk groups and is not a routine in low-risk disease (Gleason score 6 or less). Traditionally, standard PLND includes clearance of the lymph nodes in the region between obturator nerve and external iliac vessels extending distally up to cloquet nodes and proximally up to common iliac bifurcation. However, some have advised extended PLND (ePLND) in high-risk patients which includes additional tissue clearance from common iliac region extending up to the ureteric crossing. This may lead to increased morbidity.[15]

Minimal invasive surgery: Laparoscopic prostatectomy offers the patient earlier recovery and a shorter hospital stay but at the cost of surgical margins and technical difficulty for the surgeon. Robotic-assisted laparoscopic radical prostatectomy (RALP) offers better three-dimensional vision, range of movement of the robotic endo-instruments, ergonomics and magnification to the surgeons as well as lesser blood loss and good final surgical outcome, but requires special training for the surgeon and is a much more expensive mode of therapy for the patient.[3,5,7,11,12,16]

TABLE 3: Complications of radical prostatectomy and review of literature

Complications	*Kulkarni et al.*[11]	*Literature (%)*[11]
Early complications		
Urinoma/urine leak	8 (2%)	0.2–17.3
Urinary retention	3 (0.7%)	0.6–2.0
Wound complications		
Major wound infection	4(1%)	2.3–13
Minor wound infection	10 (2.4%)	
Dehiscence	2 (0.5%)	0.03–1.4
Catheter expulsion	6 (1.5%)	
Lymphorrhea	6 (1.5%)	
Late complications		
Bladder neck contracture	10 (2.5%)	1.0–8.6
Urethral stricture	2 (0.5%)	0.4–1.7
Hernia	4 (1%)	1.5–17
Bladder calculus: suture/clip	4 (1%)	0.6–3.0
Lymphocele	8 (2%)	0.1–6.9

Perineal radical prostatectomy: (first performed by Hugh Hampton Young in 1904) reportedly had the advantages of lesser operative time and blood loss. However, lymphadenectomy requires separate approach, it is a non-nerve-sparing procedure and it has a higher chance of rectal problems. Perioperative complications include deep vein thrombosis, pulmonary embolism, and wound infection.

External Beam Radiotherapy

Radiation therapy for prostate cancer is an important primary modality of treatment offered to patients. With improvements in imaging and treatment planning (three-dimensional, conformational and intensity-modulation), better targeting and higher dose delivery to the prostate is now possible, without exceeding tolerance of adjacent normal tissues. Further, it has also decreased radiation-related toxicity and improved tumor control. Accurate delivery of higher doses of radiation (>72 cGy) result in improved biochemical outcomes. In summary, results of radiation therapy using modern techniques and neoadjuvant, concurrent or adjuvant androgen deprivation therapy (ADT) (especially in intermediate and high-risk groups) has produced favorable outcomes. However, side effects reported are obstructive/irritative voiding symptoms, bowel symptoms: diarrhea, rectal bleeding (radiation-induced proctitis), tenesmus, and delayed reduction of sexual function (may take about 18–24 months to manifest).[3,5,7,11,12,16]

Brachytherapy

It involves placement of radioactive seed implants (permanent: iodine 125 or palladium 103; or temporary: iridium 192) into the prostate by TRUS guidance and computer-aided preplanned dosing. It is useful in low-risk disease and can be complemented by external beam radiotherapy (EBRT) and androgen deprivation for high-risk cases.

High Intensity Focused Ultrasound and Cryotherapy

High intensity focused ultrasound (HIFU) delivered to the prostate by rectal probes, induces coagulative necrosis.

Cryotherapy by percutaneous or TRUS-guided probes causes destruction of prostatic tissue by freeze-thaw cycles. Extent of tissue destruction cannot be precisely monitored. Better imaging and smaller probes have led to reduction of side effects. Urinary retention is the commonest complication of these techniques.[3]

Locally Advanced Disease (T3a-T3b)

Conventionally, these tumors necessitate combined modality approach such as radiation and neoadjuvant,

adjuvant or concurrent hormone therapy or neoadjuvant hormone therapy followed by radical prostatectomy.

Metastatic Disease

Hormone (Endocrine) Therapy

Hormone therapy is based on the fact that prostate cancer depends on androgens. Further, androgen ablation or ADT is the main stay of treatment of metastatic cancer of prostate. Recently, there has been some discussion about androgen deprivation as monotherapy (bilateral orchiectomy or LHRH) or combined androgen blockade (CAB), i.e. orchi/LHRH+ antiandrogen therapy. Our experience of CAB during Urological Society of India trial (1998-2000) using orchiectomy alone versus orchi+flutamide in the metastatic setting has been far from satisfactory.[11,17] Further, patients who are on LHRH agonists/orchiectomy monotherapy, may benefit from addition of antiandrogens, i.e. secondary hormone therapy at relapse. Of interest is some patients do respond to pure estrogen (Honvan) or antiandrogen withdrawal at relapse or during progression.[7,9,17-19]

There has been some debate about standard practice of continuous ADT versus the recent modification, i.e. Intermittent ADT and the recent reports indicate the benefit of later in patients who respond initially to ADT.[19] Further, it results in less cost, inconvenience and potential toxicity. Lastly, there is unanimity of the opinion regarding early ADT even in asymptomatic scenario.[18]

The targeted sites are as follows:

- *Testes*: Bilateral scrotal *orchiectomy* eliminates the source of testosterone and castrate levels (<50 ng/mL) can be achieved within 24 hours. This usually is effective for about 2–3 years when eventually PSA starts rising due to increase in production of the weak adrenal androgens and changes in the androgen receptor. This is still most popular and economically viable operation in our country with minimum morbidity.
- *Hypothalamo-pituitary-gonadal axis:* (1) *Estrogens* (diethylstilbesterol) act by a negative feedback signaling to the hypothalamo-pituitary axis (thousand times stronger than testosterone in this action), causing down regulation of LHRH secretion. They also directly suppress Leydig cell function and cause direct prostate cancer cell cytotoxicity. These have been used for castration resistant prostate cancer (CRPC) and have good efficacy, but owing to their thromboembolic and cardiovascular complications, they are now used more sparingly; (2) *LHRH agonists* (goserelin, triptorelin, leuprolide, histrelin): desensitize the LH receptors causing transient rise followed by prolonged fall of testosterone levels, castrate levels being achieved by 2–4 weeks. These are administered as 1–6 monthly intramuscular or subcutaneous depot preparations. They have certain side effects such as "flare" phenomenon (during initial testosterone surge) and allergic reactions; (3) *LHRH antagonists* (abarelix, degarelix): directly block LH receptors, hence no flare phenomenon is seen. But severe allergic reactions occur to these drugs.[3,18]
- *Androgen receptor* on prostate cell: *Antiandrogens* (flutamide, bicalutamide, cyproterone) appear to act by competitively binding the receptor for dihydrotestosterone (DHT). These are available as oral tablets to be taken daily. The testosterone levels may be normal or increased, thus maintaining libido and erection, but androgen receptors on prostate cancer cells are blocked. These drugs can cause hepatotoxicity.
- *Adrenal androgen production*: Drugs are used to block the enzymes of the androgen synthesis pathway, thus leading to reduced production of androgens:
  - *Aminoglutethimide*: Cortisol and aldosterone supplementation is required
  - *Ketoconazole* has a rapid action and is an inexpensive antifungal agent
  - *Abiraterone*: Is known to block enzyme CYP17 leading to complete androgen synthesis blockade in adrenal gland and within tumor cells. It is used in combination with prednisolone in CRPC patients who had failed after docetaxel therapy.[18,20]

CASTRATION RESISTANT PROSTATE CANCER

Most patients on primary ADT eventually show rise in PSA in spite of postorchiectomy status or ongoing gonadotropin-releasing hormone (GnRH) therapy. The various etiological factors proposed are: (1) Androgen receptor mutation, causing it to respond to ligands other than androgens, like antiandrogens and steroids. It may be treated by withdrawing antiandrogens (30% will show secondary PSA response); (2) Increased androgen receptor sensitivity to residual androgens from extragonadal sources (like adrenals) and increased androgen receptor expression on tumor cells: It is treated by giving androgen synthesis inhibitors like ketoconazole, aminoglutethimide, abiraterone; (3) Outlaw pathway: Androgen receptor stimulation in absence of ligands, due to growth factors [insulin-like growth factor 1 (IGF-1), epithelial growth factor] and interleukin-6 (IL-6); (4) Prostatic stem cell reactivation with malignant progression. In this clinical situation, docetaxel-based chemotherapy has shown some promise and novel agents for targeted therapy are being investigated currently. Finally, hormone refractory prostate cancer (HRPC) is a term reserved for conditions where there is no secondary PSA response to any form of hormonal manipulation.[20]

Secondary Hormonal Management in Patients with Castration Resistant Prostate Cancer

- Antiandrogen withdrawal: Effect should become apparent 4–6 weeks after the discontinuation of flutamide or bicalutamide.
- Abiraterone and MDV3100 (enzalutamide) may also be tried to prolong survival.
- Chemotherapy for CRPC patients: In patients with metastatic CRPC and who are candidates for cytotoxic therapy, docetaxel at 75 mg/m^2 IV infusion over 1 hour, every 3 weeks is the drug of choice since it has shown survival benefit and causes significant pain relief. In patients with symptomatic osseous metastases due to CRPC, either docetaxel or mitoxantrone with prednisone or hydrocortisone are reasonable therapeutic options. In patients with relapse following first-line docetaxel chemotherapy, cabazitaxel and abiraterone can be used as second-line treatment.[3,20]

Follow-up

Post therapy, be it localized or metastatic prostate cancer, PSA level falls to nadir (early and sometimes undetectable levels after surgery), and low normal levels, i.e. about 0.5–1 ng/mL (after radiation therapy and hormone therapy), and needs to be monitored at regular intervals (3 monthly for 2 years, followed by 6 monthly) along with DRE for evidence of recurrent disease. Follow-up should be tailored to the individual patient, according to symptoms, prognostic factors and the treatment given. In patients with stage M0 disease with a good treatment response, follow-up is scheduled every 6 months, and should include at least a disease specific history, DRE and serum PSA measurement. In patients with M1 disease with a good treatment response, follow-up is scheduled for every 3–6 months. Where disease progression occurs, or if the patient does not respond to the treatment given, follow-up needs to be individualized. Routine imaging of stable patients is not recommended. Follow-up after hormonal treatment: at 3 and 6 months after treatment initiation: serum PSA measurement, DRE, serum testosterone and careful evaluation of symptoms are done in order to assess the treatment response and side effects. If patients undergo intermittent androgen deprivation, PSA and testosterone should be monitored at 3-month intervals during the treatment phase.[19]

Recurrent Disease

Abnormal DRE or three consecutive elevated levels of PSA during post-treatment follow-up (>0.2 ng/mL after surgery or >2 ng/mL after radiotherapy) is suggestive of recurrence. Post-treatment PSA doubling time <3 months is suggestive of high risk of metastatic disease (will require systemic therapy), and >10–12 months is suggestive of recurrent localized disease (may benefit from salvage radiation). Second-line therapy after curative treatments: (1) Presumed local failure after RP: Patients may be candidates for salvage radiotherapy or active surveillance (active monitoring), with possible hormonal therapy later on. Salvage radiotherapy should be given with at least 64 Gy and preferably before PSA rises above 0.5 ng/mL; (2) Presumed local failure after radiotherapy: Selected patients may be candidates for salvage RP or active surveillance (active monitoring), with possible hormonal therapy (ADT) later on, or brachytherapy or cryotherapy. Patients to undergo salvage RP should be informed about the high risk of complications, such as incontinence and erectile dysfunction; (3) Presumed distant failure: Early hormonal therapy may be of benefit in cases of metastasis with or without local failure. It delays progression, and may be more beneficial than delayed therapy. Local therapy is not recommended except for palliative reasons; (4) Systemic relapse or residual disease after surgery can cause persistently detectable PSA levels. Detection of local recurrence by TRUS and biopsy is only recommended if it will affect the treatment plan. In most cases TRUS and biopsy are not necessary before second-line therapy. Metastasis may be detected by pelvic CT/MRI or bone scan.

Flow chart 3: Clinical flow chart of events involving diagnosis and management of prostate cancer

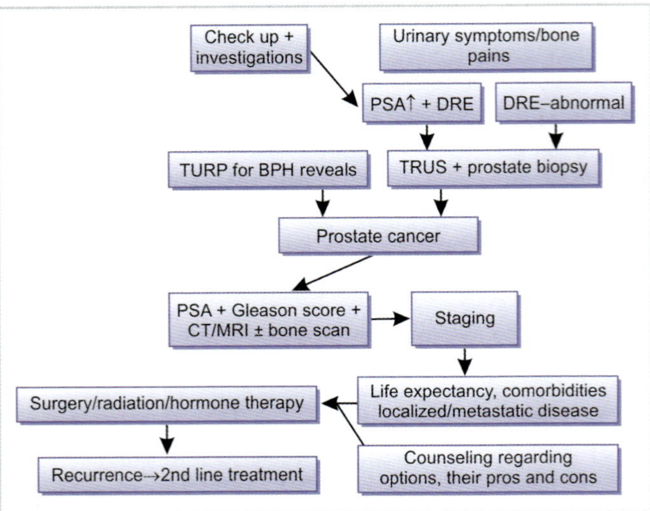

Palliation in Castration Resistant Prostate Cancer Patients

Patients with extensive and symptomatic bony metastases, improvement in quality of life and pain reduction, with minimal side effects is the goal of therapy, as no treatment modality confers any survival benefit. Bisphosphonates (e.g. zoledronic acid) should be offered to patients with bone metastasis to prevent osseous complications. Major side effect: jaw necrosis must be avoided. Palliative radionuclides, EBRT and analgesics must be considered for early management of painful bone metastases. Decompression spinal surgery or radiotherapy must be considered emergency procedures to palliate patients with neurological symptoms.[20]

Brief outline of diagnosis management of prostate cancer, stagewise (Flow chart 3 and Table 4).[5]

TABLE 4: Stagewise management of prostate cancer

Stage TNM	*Watchful waiting (WW)*	*Radical prostatectomy (RP)*	*Radiation therapy (RT)*	*Hormonal therapy (HT)*
T1a	Life expectancy (LE) <10 years, well/ moderately differentiated tumors. If LE >10 years → Restaging with TRUS and biopsy	Poorly differentiated tumors + long LE (young patients)	Poorly differentiated tumors + long LE (young patients)	Not standard
T1b, T2a, T2b	Asymptomatic patient Well/ moderately differentiated tumors. LE <10 years. Patient not wanting treatment related complications	LE >10 years Patient willing to accept treatment-related complications	LE >10 years Patient willing to accept treatment-related complications (if surgery is contraindicated) or patient is unfit for surgery, LE 5–10 years	Symptomatic patients who need palliation and are unfit for curative treatment. Neoadjuvant HT prior to RT may help better local control but has no survival benefit
T3-T4	Asymptomatic patients with T3 Well/moderately differentiated tumors. LE <10 years.	Selected patients of T3a with LE >10 years	T3 + LE >5–10 years (Dose escalation >70 Gy or combination with HT may be better)	Symptomatic patients, extensive T3-T4 disease. PSA >25 ng/mL Unfit patients
Nodes +	Asymptomatic patients Patient refuses treatment (will negatively influence survival)	Not recommended	Not recommended	Standard therapy
Metastasis+	Patient refuses treatment (will negatively influence survival)	Not recommended	Not recommended	Standard therapy

Abbreviations: TNM, tumor node metastasis; TRUS, transrectal ultrasound; PSA, prostate-specific antigen

REFERENCES

1. Chung BI, Sommer G. Anatomy of the Lower Urinary Tract and Male Genitalia. In: Alan J Wein (Ed). Campbell-Walsh Urology, 10th Edition. Elsevier Saunders. 2012;33-70.
2. Abouassaly R. Epidemiology, Etiology, and Prevention of Prostate Cancer. In: Alan J Wein (Ed). Campbell-Walsh Urology, 10th Edition. Elsevier Saunder. 2012;2704-25.
3. Presti JC. Neoplasms of the prostate gland. In: Emil A Tanagho (Ed). Smith's General Urology, 17th Edition. McGraw Hill. 2008;348-74.
4. Epstein J. Pathology of Prostate Neoplasia. In: Alan J Wein (Ed). Campbell-Walsh Urology, 10th Edition. Elsevier Saunders 2012;2726-34.
5. Heidenreich A. Guidelines on Prostate Cancer. European Association of Urology Guidelines 2012; Section 4. 132-295.
6. Trabulsi EJ. Ultrasonography and Biopsy of the prostate. In: Alan J Wein (Ed). Campbell-Walsh Urology, 10th Edition. Elsevier Saunders. 2012;2735-47.
7. Loeb S. Early Detection, Diagnosis, and Staging of Prostate Cancer. In: Alan J Wein (Ed). Campbell-Walsh Urology, 10th Edition. Elsevier Saunders. 2012;2763-70.
8. AUA releases new clinical guideline on prostate cancer. [online] Available from http://www.auanet.org/advnews/press_ releases/ article.cfm?articleNo=290.
9. Kulkarni JN. Early diagnosis of prostate cancer. Indian J Urol. 1998;14:1-3.
10. Jadvar H. Prostate cancer: PET with 18F – FDG, 18F – or 11C – Acetate and 18F – or 11C – Choline. J Nuclear Med. 2011;52(1):81- 9.
11. Kulkarni JN, Tongoankar HB, Kamat MR. Radical retropubic prostatectomy: initial experience: Radical retropubic prostatectomy. Ind J Urol. 1994;10:24-6.
12. Kulkarni JN. Prostate cancer. Indian J Surg. 1999;61(2):95-9.
13. Kulkarni JN, Dayal P, Bansal S, et al. Retropubic radical prostatectomy: Clinico pathological observations and outcome analysis of consecutive 428 cases. Indian J Urol. 2011;27:337-44.
14. Kulkarni JN, Valasangakar R, Jadhav Y, et al. Impact of Gleason pattern up gradation after radical prostatectomy for carcinoma prostate patients with low biopsy score (≤6). J Cancer Res Ther. 2011;7:473-8.
15. Briganti A, Chun FK, Salonia A, et al. Complications and surgical outcomes associated with extended pelvic lymph adenectomy in men with localized prostate cancer. Eur Urol. 2006;50:1006-13.
16. Catalona WJ. Definitive Therapy for Localized Prostate cancer: An Overview. In: Alan J Wein (Ed). Campbell-Walsh Urology, 10th Edition. Elsevier Saunders. 2012;2771-88.
17. Kulkarni JN, Guptal R. Early report of randomized double blind clinical trial of hormonal therapy of carcinoma prostate stage D2. Indian J Urol. 2003;19(2):135-9.
18. Nelson JB. Hormone Therapy for Prostate Cancer. In: Alan J Wein (Ed). Campbell-Walsh Urology, 10th Edition. Elsevier Saunders. 2012;2932-53.
19. Niraula S, Le LW, Tannock IF. Treatment of prostate cancer with intermittent versus continuous androgen deprivation: a systemic review of randomized trials. J Clin Oncol. 2013;31(16):2029-36.
20. Antonarakis ES. Treatment of Castration Resistant Prostate Cancer. In: Alan J Wein (Ed). Campbell-Walsh Urology, 10th Edition. Elsevier Saunders. 2012;2954-71.

45 Bladder Cancer

Jagdeesh Kulkarni, Varun Gunavanthe,
Nasreen Gite, Abhijit Dhale, Devendra Choudhary

INTRODUCTION

Urothelial cancers [transitional cell carcinoma (TCC)] account for 5.6% of male and 1.8% of female cancers in India.[1] Amongst them bladder cancer is the most common urological malignancy in India with median age of presentation being 6th–7th decades.[1] Interestingly, bladder cancer appearing before the age of 50 years is likely to be nonaggressive and well differentiated.[1,2] Occupational bladder cancers are known to have an aggressive biological potential.[2]

ETIOLOGY AND RISK FACTORS

Etiology of bladder cancer can be subcategorized into two groups: (1) external risk factors and (2) genetic factors. Amongst the various external factors, smoking and tobacco consumption tops the list with a fourfold increased risk.[3,4] Other factors like chemicals, e.g. aromatic amines used in dye, leather and rubber industries and certain drugs, e.g. phenacetin, cyclophosphamide are known carcinogenics. Some dietary habits like less of fluid, fried meat and low vitamin A have been shown to be associated with higher incidence of bladder cancer while diet rich in fruits and vegetables offers protection against bladder cancer. Other rare causes of bladder cancer include chronic urinary tract infection, schistosomiasis (endemic area) and pelvic irradiation. Over the years, some epidemiologic (population) studies have found an increase in risk of bladder cancer in hairdressers and barbers.[5,6] Recently there has been some data suggesting a correlation between genetic abnormalities (17p deletion, p53 expression, etc.) and risk of bladder cancer and aggressive biology.[7]

CLINICAL FEATURES

The most common clinical presentation is a gross painless hematuria occurring in about 85% patients. Remaining patients may present with irritative symptoms like frequency, urgency, dysuria especially in high grade disease and carcinoma in situ (CIS). Of interest is, some patients may be totally asymptomatic and may be incidentally detected during a health checkup. Prior history of urolithiasis helps to suspect bladder cancer in patients with chronic lower urinary tract symptoms.

PATHOLOGY

Some of the important conditions which need to be differentiated from the urothelial carcinoma (UC) are described below. Epithelial metaplasia is a condition when there are focal areas of transformed urothelium into either squamous (squamous metaplasia) or glandular (glandular metaplasia) cells. Leukoplakia is often premalignant but cytogenetically, it is innocuous and no active treatment is necessary.

Inverted Papilloma

An inverted papilloma is a benign proliferative lesion that is associated with chronic inflammation or bladder outlet obstruction, comprising less than 1% of all bladder tumors. Further these lesions show normal urothelial cells invaginating from the surface urothelium into the lamina propria but not into the muscularis propria. Inverted papillomas exhibit a benign course with only a 1% incidence of tumor recurrence.

Papilloma

Urothelial papilloma is proliferative growth composed of delicate stalks lined by normal-appearing urothelium. They rarely show mitotic figures and lack markers of aggressive growth such as TP53 or RB mutations. Lastly they may recur, but do not progress or invade.

Nephrogenic Adenoma

Nephrogenic adenoma is a rare tumor caused by chronic irritation of the urothelium; it arises from a variety of sources, including trauma, previous surgery, renal transplantation, intravesical chemotherapy, stones, catheters, and infection. The most frequent presenting symptom is gross hematuria, often in conjunction with a urinary tract infection. Treatment consists of transurethral resection (TUR) and elimination of the chronic irritation.

Cystitis Cystica and Glandularis

Cystitis cystica and/or glandularis is a common finding in normal bladders, usually associated with inflammation or chronic obstruction. Cystitis glandularis may be associated with pelvic lipomatosis and may occupy the majority of the bladder. Further cystitis glandularis can develop into or coexist with intestinal metaplasia, which are benign tumors characterized by goblet cells that are histologically similar to colonic epithelium. Based on few case reports of cystitis cystica or glandularis transforming into adenocarcinoma, regular endoscopic evaluation of patients with these entities is recommended. The most common presenting feature of cystitis cystica or glandularis is irritative voiding symptoms and hematuria. Treatment is TUR and relief of the obstruction or inflammatory condition.

Carcinoma In Situ

Carcinoma in situ is flat, noninvasive UC that is high grade by definition. Although it is confined to the urothelium in the same manner as stage Ta, CIS is regarded as a precursor for the development of invasive high-grade cancer. CIS lesions are composed of severely dysplastic urothelium showing disorderly histology with nuclear atypia characteristic of high-grade malignancy. A pathology report read as dysplasia or atypia can create confusion. Progression to invasive carcinoma occurs in 40–83% if untreated. CIS presents with irritative symptoms.

Urothelial or Transitional Carcinoma

Since urothelium is anatomically lined by transitional epithelium, 90% cancers are TCCs, others are squamous cell carcinoma (SCC), adenocarcinoma, etc. Clinicopathologically UCs are subgrouped into two types: (1) Non-muscle invasive carcinoma and (2) Muscle invasive carcinoma depending on the depth of invasion.

Non-muscle invasive bladder cancer (NMIBC)[8] includes CIS, papillary urothelial neoplasia of low-malignant potential (PUNLMP), and low and high-grade urothelial cancer that was previously called "superficial bladder cancer".

Papillary urothelial neoplasia of low-malignant potential is a papillary growth with minimal cytological atypia that is more than seven cells thick and is generally solitary and located on the trigone. PUNLMP is composed of thin papillary stalks, where the polarity of the cells is maintained and the nuclei are minimally enlarged. PUNLMP has a low proliferation rate and is not associated with invasion or metastases.

Low-grade UC is typically papillary in nature with a fibrovascular stalk and frequent papillary branching with increased cellular size, some nuclear atypia (more than in PUNLMP), and occasional mitotic figures. Low-grade papillary lesions are likely to recur in up to 60% of patients but invade in less than 10% of cases.

High-grade papillary urothelial cancer is composed of fused papillary stalks with high-grade cancer in the urothelial layer. There is a disordered growth pattern, with numerous mitotic figures present, and there are pleomorphic cells with exaggerated nuclei. Over 80% of high-grade cancers will invade the underlying stroma if left untreated. High-grade lesions also recur; however, invasion and subsequent stage progression can occur in 50% of tumors. This is particularly true if CIS is associated with a high-grade papillary lesion. Some of the rare but aggressive histological variants are micropapillary, sarcomatoid, small cell and nested, and are grouped under high-risk category.

Muscle-invasive UC is by definition a high-grade lesion and is composed of cancerous cells extending through the lamina propria into the deep muscle bundles.

STAGING

Pathological Staging[8]

Morphologically about 90–95% are UCs; the ones with unusual histologic appearance are called "UC with divergent differentiation". In 1972, WHO accepted Mostofi, et al. classification of TCC in three grades. Later years saw further modification in grading due to better understanding of the biology, and histological appearance. Mostofi et al.

(1997) and International Society of Urologic Pathologists (ISUP) (1998) proposed the concept of primary neoplastic and putative preneoplastic tumors. Finally WHO/ISUP combined classification recommended five histological types of tumors—papilloma, PUNLMP, TCC low grade corresponding to G1 and TCC high grade which includes G2 and G3.[8]

Historical Perspective[9,10]

Historically, the staging of TCC has been clinicopathological. In 1922, Broders created a landmark by formulating a grading system based on the percentage of undifferentiated urothelial cells, which was predictive of both behavior of the bladder urothelium over time and prognosis. In 1931, Aschner classified neoplasms of the bladder as papillary versus a solid configuration and in relation to the presence or absence of invasion where disease severity increased with solid tumors. In 1944, Jewett and Strong analyzed the relation of depth of penetration (stage) to the incidence of local extension and metastases and concluded that increasing depth caused widespread dissemination. In 1948, McDonald and Thompson discovered the concept of vascular and lymphatic invasion and showed that there was a direct relation to prognosis. In 1952, Jewett-Marshall-Strong redefined the staging based on bimanual palpation and biopsy into stage 0, A and B1 (superficial disease), B2 (deep muscle invasion) and C (perivesical invasion). Continuing his studies, in 1956 Marshall established the impact of gradation of tumor.

Tumor Node Metastasis Staging

Till 1967, the Jewett-Marshall-Strong classification was in vogue; however, later Jewett and his group under the aegis of American Joint Committee System formed the AJCC Task Force. This group recognized a need to broaden the staging to accommodate additional tumor characteristics and a common taxonomy. Continued efforts by this Task force led to further refinements and birth of TNM staging in 1983. TNM classification is currently (2010)[9] the standard staging procedure for bladder cancer universally and is based on clinicopathological findings (Table 1 and Fig. 1).[9,10]

INVESTIGATIONS AND STAGING TECHNIQUES

Routine hemogram, biochemistry and urine cytology form an important component of investigation package. Recently, there has been some interest generated in evaluating therapeutic potential of urinary markers in clinical practice.[11]

TABLE 1: Comparison of Jewett-Strong-Marshall and Tumor Node Metastasis classification 2010[9]

TNM	*TNM*	*Jewett*	*Characteristics*
Ta		0	Noninvasive papillary carcinoma
Tis			Carcinoma in situ: flat tumor
T1		A	Tumor invades subepithelial connective tissue (lamina propria)
T2		B	Tumor invades muscle
	T2a	B1	Tumor invades superficial muscle (inner half)
	T2b	B2	Tumor invades deep muscle (outer half)
T3		C	Tumor invades perivesical tissue
	T3a		Microscopically
	T3b		Macroscopically (extravesical mass)
T4		D1	Tumor invades any of prostate, uterus, vagina, pelvic wall, abdominal wall
	T4a		Tumor invades prostate or uterus or vagina
	T4b		Tumor invades pelvic wall or abdominal wall
N0			No regional lymph nodes metastasis
N1		D1	Metastasis in a single lymph node ≤ 2 cm in greatest dimension
N2		D1	Metastasis in a single lymph node > 2 cm but ≤ 5 cm in greatest dimension, or multiple lymph nodes none > 5 cm
N3		D1	Metastasis in a single lymph node > 5 cm in greatest dimension
M0			No distant metastasis
M1		D2	Distant metastasis

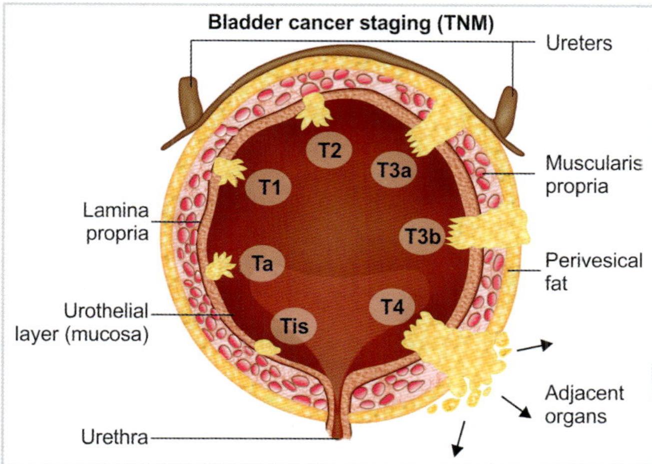

Fig. 1: Pictorial "T" staging (IJU 2008)
[Readapted from IJU 2008 (with permission)]

Imaging Modalities

The basic aim is to use noninvasive techniques like CT, MRI, and ultrasonography (US) to document T, N, and M status of the tumor (Figs 2A and B). Amongst them US is extremely popular as an initial work up but has limited accuracy in terms of T and N status. Further the timing of CT or MRI either pre-TUR or 2–3 weeks after TUR of bladder tumor (TURBT) is done to augment the positive predictive value.

T Status

Abdominal, transrectal, transvaginal and transurethral sonography have all been used to stage bladder cancer. At times, it is difficult to differentiate between clot and tumor and small tumors are missed on sonography especially those arising from the ureteric orifice. The most important concerns of urologists in addressing the issues of the depth of invasion and locoregional spread have been answered by newer techniques in CT like multislice imaging and have shown an accuracy of greater than 80%, with sensitivity of 94% and specificity of 62%.[12] Further "T" related sensitivity is 73%, 68.2%, 84% and 97.7% for T1, T2, T3 and T4 respectively. Lastly joining the race, technical nuances in MRI as well as contrast media highlight tumor by suppressing signals from surrounding normal structures. Thus, as per recent reports, it is thought that the submucosal layer is the one which enhances rather than the earlier thought mucosal layer. MRI has an accuracy of 73%; sensitivity, 82%; specificity, 62%.[12] Advantages MRI offers over CT include higher contrast resolution, multiplanar imaging, accuracy of staging with smaller tumors and imaging in patients with chronic kindney disease.

N Status

Regarding nodal disease, both CT and MRI can accurately predict nodal involvement if size is around 5–8 mm, while micrometastases are still undetectable. However, CT has a slight edge over MRI in detecting N status.

Cystourethroscopy and Transurethral resection (Figs 3A and B)

This includes a complete inspection of lower urinary tract from external urinary meatus to the bladder with ureteric orifices. A careful and accurate mapping of tumor/tumors vis a vis site, size, relation of bladder neck and ureteric orifices, and the intervening mucosa. Bimanual palpation

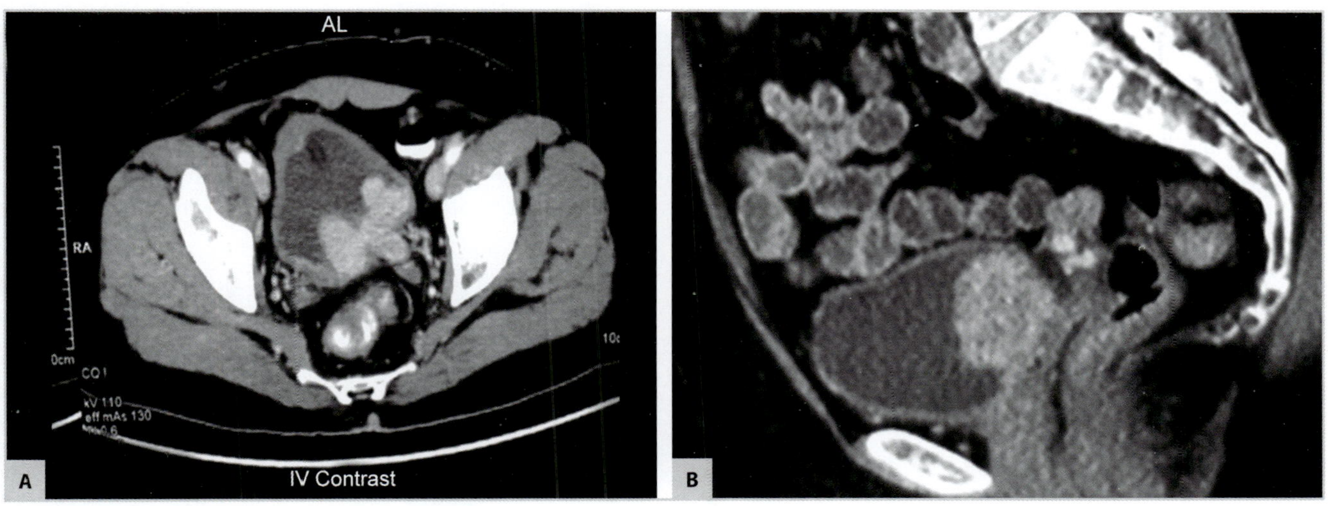

Figs 2A and B: CT scan showing tumor in male and female

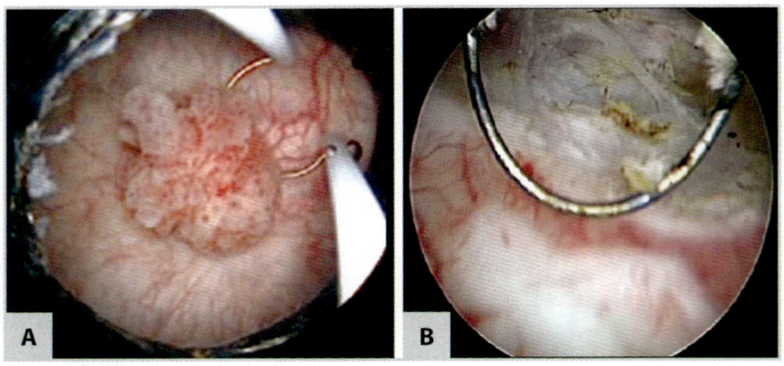

Figs 3A and B: Cystoscopy showing bladder tumor and transurethral resection bladder tumor

of the bladder is done to assess the invasion of the wall of the bladder and fixity. However, it has an error of 25–50% in staging.[9] TUR of the tumor or tumors is both diagnostic and therapeutic. Lastly, complete resection of tumor and a deep biopsy of the muscle is mandatory. Tumor in diverticulum is an important finding and due to absence of muscle coat, it may be treated like early muscle invasive disease.

Restaging TURBT

This is a recent useful concept towards improving the accuracy in staging. A deep biopsy can at times be false-negative due to technical reasons like charring or deeper tissue from peripheral area or with unreliable prior history. This also emphasizes the need of performing TUR with a thin loop and pure cutting current. A second TUR in cases of T1 G2 and G3 is aimed at unmasking the presence of TCC in muscle layer thus upstaging disease, which at times can be missed. This helps in identifying a subset of patients who require early aggressive therapy to improve survival. Second TUR in cases of G3 tumors help in achieving a "radical resection".[10]

CONTEMPORARY MANAGEMENT OF BLADDER CANCER

As described earlier, bladder cancer is categorized into two subgroups; non-muscle invasive (superficial) disease and muscle invasive (deep) disease. This stems from the fact that the biological behavior of the former is relatively less aggressive and therefore bladder conservation is possible without compromising the ultimate outcome and quality of life (QoL). The latter, however, necessitates radical and ablative therapy. The third category, CIS, is completely different when seen as primary pathology. CIS is characterized as nonpapillary, flat, high-grade tumors in which the surface epithelium contains cancer cells. There is severe nuclear atypia, loss of cellular polarity, and a noncohesive cellular structure. The cells are large, pleomorphic, chromatin clumping, and abnormal mitotic figures are common. Loss of umbrella cells is a characteristic, separating CIS from dysplasia. All CIS is high grade by definition. Currently intravesical Bacillus Calmette-Guérin (BCG) therapy is the most accepted therapy in this setting.

Non-muscle Invasive Bladder Cancer (Ta-T1)

Recently, the NMIBC has been stratified into three risk groups (low, intermediate and high) depending on grade, depth and number of tumors. Low-risk group is put on surveillance after complete TUR while the intermediate and high-risk groups are candidates for adjuvant intravesical therapy.

Transurethral Resection

This procedure as described above is aimed at excision of all visible tumor and to stage and grade the disease.[13] In some patients more than one sitting may be required. However, in some cases restaging TUR is an excellent option. Further management depends on post-TUR "risk stratification" and adjuvant therapy as per protocol given in Table 2.

Intravesical Therapy

Post TURBT adjuvant intravesical therapy is indicated depending on the risk stratification and staging. In literature various guidelines are available; however, we will describe the protocol followed by us and report our results with literature. There are two types of intravesical therapies in vogue: (1) chemotherapy and (2) BCG therapy.

Thiotepa was the first chemotherapeutic agent tried in early 80s with acceptable results. We reported our results in 1981.[14] Later, this was replaced by other agents like mitomycin and doxorubicin. Currently, mitomycin 40 mg is the most common chemotherapeutic agent used in intravesical instillation, others being epirubicin and doxorubicin.

Immediate postoperative instillation of chemotherapeutic agent (mitomycin C) is recommended for all patients with NMIBC after TURBT. In patients who are planned to be treated with BCG, the use of an immediate postoperative instillation of chemotherapy is optional as its benefit in this situation is less clear. The efficacy of postoperative intravesical instillation of chemotherapy is within 6 hours of TURBT, and after 24 hours it is of no use.[15]

TABLE 2: Risk group stratification and therapy for NMIBC

Risk group	*Pathology*	*Management*
Low	Grade 1 stage Ta	TUR with surveillance
	Grade 1 stage T1 single tumor	TUR with surveillance
	Size up to 1 cm	TUR with surveillance
Intermediate	Grade 1 stage T1 multiple tumor	TUR with intravesical adjuvant therapy with BCG
	Grade 2 stage Ta	TUR with intravesical adjuvant therapy with BCG
	Grade 2 stage T1 single tumor	TUR with intravesical adjuvant therapy with BCG
	Size 1–3 cm	TUR with intravesical adjuvant therapy with BCG
High	Grade 2 stage T1 multiple tumor	TUR with intravesical adjuvant therapy with BCG
	Grade 3 stage Ta	TUR with intravesical adjuvant therapy with BCG
	Grade 3 stage T1 single tumor	TUR with intravesical adjuvant therapy with BCG/early cystectomy
	CIS association	TUR with intravesical adjuvant therapy with BCG/early cystectomy
	Size > 3 cm	TUR with intravesical adjuvant therapy with BCG/early cystectomy

Abbreviations: TUR, transurethral resection; BCG, Bacillus Calmette-Guérin; CIS, carcinoma in situ

Intravesical BCG: Of the various intravesical strains available in the world we reported the successful results of Danish Strain 1331 (BCG) in 1994.[16] Later reports detailed outcome analysis of superficial bladder tumors treated with all chemotherapeutic and BCG results.[17,18] Thus, Danish Strain of BCG (available in India) is equally effective, nonexpensive and well-tolerated.[18] Further, it is given in all high-grade diseases including CIS, Ta G3, T1 diseases.[19-23] There are different schedules but we follow Southwest Oncology Group (SWOG) 24 protocol, i.e. induction—starting from 2–4 weeks from resection, weekly for 6 weeks 120 mg BCG. Check cystoscopy should be done at 3 months and if no recurrence is noted then weekly BCG for 3 weeks is advisable. Check cystoscopy is repeated at 6 months and weekly BCG for 3 weeks. Every 6 months BCG is instilled weekly for 3 weeks, for a total of 3 years after TUR.

BCG failure: Recurrent or persistent disease after induction course of BCG has been referred to as BCG failure. It is of three types: (1) BCG refractory where there is no improvement or worsening of the disease despite BCG; (2) BCG resistant where there is recurrence or persistence of lesser degree after initial course can resolve with a further course of BCG; (3) BCG relapsing where there is recurrence after initial resolution with BCG. These patients are high risk and should be considered for early cystectomy.[17,23]

Complications of BCG: Approach to management of BCG toxicity is as follows.

Grade 1: It includes mild irritative symptoms and fever less than 38.5°C which lasts for less than 48 hours. Urine culture is sent to rule out bacterial urinary tract infection. These patients are managed symptomatically using anticholinergics, analgesics and nonsteroidal anti-inflammatory drugs.

Grade 2: Severe symptoms and/or symptoms which last for more than 48 hours are seen. All maneuvers for Grade 1 are done along with urine culture, chest radiograph and liver function test. Dose reduction has to be considered to one-half to one-third of dose when instillations resume. Antituberculosis drug therapy is administered with isoniazid and rifampicin—300 mg/day and 600 mg/day—orally until symptom resolution.

Grade 3: It is defined as complications, e.g. hemodynamic changes, persistent high-grade fever and allergic reactions (joint pain, urticaria) which require immediate attention. Therapy described for grades 1 and 2 and isoniazid (300 mg/day) and rifampin (600 mg/day) for 3–6 months depending on response. If there is solid organ involvement, isoniazid (300 mg/day), rifampin (600 mg/day), ethambutol (15 mg/kg/day) single daily dose for 3–6 months is exhibited. Prednisone, 40 mg/day, should be considered when response is inadequate or for septic shock (never given without effective antibacterial therapy).

T1G3 Dilemma

Although included in the non-muscle invasive category, T1G3 bladder tumors have become a distinct entity because of their higher potential for recurrence and progression.[18] The aim of treatment in these patients is to retain a functioning bladder without compromising survival. Previously these patients were either treated by TURBT alone[19,20] or by radical cystectomy.[18,20-22] The T1G3 recurrences after BCG were treated with either a second course of BCG in a few or radical cystectomy in most patients. Intravesical BCG Danish 1331 is an effective adjuvant therapy for T1G3 tumors.[18]

Management of CIS: It can be managed with intravesical BCG instillation or early cystectomy in patients where follow-up is in doubt.

Summary of Post-therapy Surveillance Strategies in NMIBC (Table 2)

Low-risk (single TaG1): Cystoscopy at 3 months and if negative at 9 months, then yearly till 5 years.

Intermediate-risk (multiple TaG1, large tumor): Cystoscopy every 3 monthly for 2 years and annually thereafter.

High-risk: Cystoscopy and cytology at 3 months, if negative, then every 3 months cystoscopy and cytology for 2 years, every 4 months in the 3rd year, every 6 months thereafter until 5 years and then yearly. Yearly upper tract imaging is recommended.

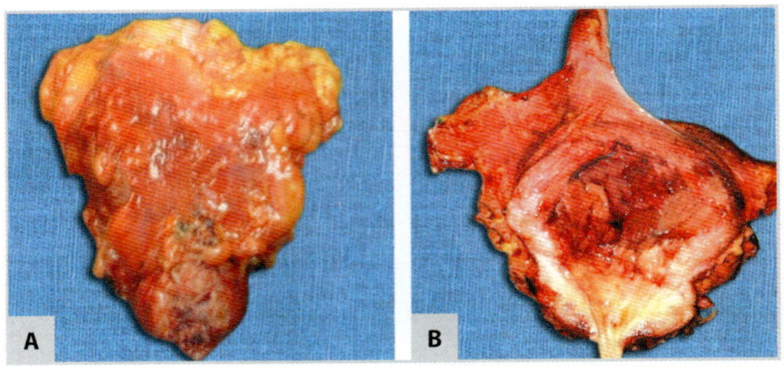

Figs 4A and B: Cystectomy in males

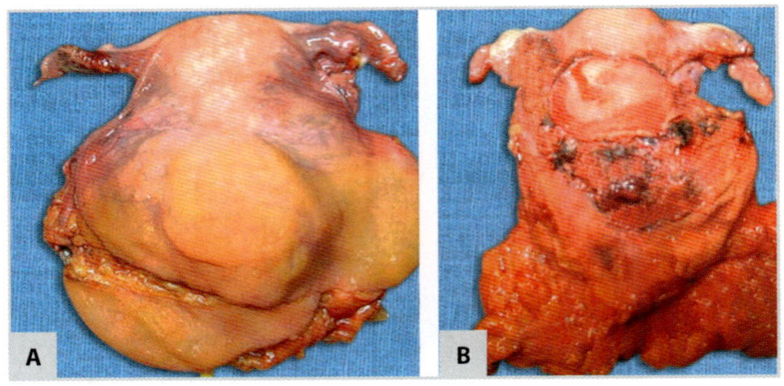

Figs 5A and B: Anterior exenteration in females

Management of Muscle Invasive Carcinoma Bladder (T2–4)

After histological confirmation of muscle invasion patient is counseled for radical cystectomy with urinary diversion. A routine evaluation includes complete hematocrit and biochemical profile, cardiac and pulmonary checkup in addition to the metastatic work up. Stoma counseling and marking of stoma is an important preoperative step. Antibiotic therapy may be required to control infection in the urinary tract. Adequate nutritional status goes a long way in reducing postoperative recovery.

Radical Cystectomy and Bilateral Pelvic and Iliac Lymphadenectomy

Radical cystectomy has two components: (1) excision of bladder with surrounding perivesical soft tissue, prostate, seminal vesicles and lower ureters and part of the urethra up to the levators is performed en bloc in males (Figs 4A and B). In females, surgical extent includes bladder and surrounding soft tissue, the ovaries, uterus/cervix, and anterior vagina (Figs 5A and B). Further regional lymphadenectomy includes bilateral pelvic nodes up to the common iliac nodes above, Cooper's ligament below, genitofemoral nerve as the lateral limit and obturator nerve as the medial limit.

Operative technique: There are two popular techniques: (1) conventional or intraperitoneal radical cystectomy, (2) extraperitoneal (EP) retrograde cystectomy.[24]

Conventional radical cystectomy: After exploring the abdominal cavity and operability is ascertained first. Urachus is ligated and cut at the origin. Ureters are cut at the pelvic brim and proximal ends are stented and put in iliac fossa on either side. Vasa deferentia are divided at the internal inguinal ring. Further obliterated hypogastric and vesical pedicles are ligated and cut. Bladder is mobilized on either side. Next, by incising the rectovesical peritoneum bladder dissected off the rectum down to the urethra. Care is taken to develop the plane between prostate and rectum. Radical cystectomy is completed after dividing the dorsal venous complex and urethra beyond the prostate. Left ureter is brought on right iliac region behind the sigmoid mesentery for urinary diversion either ileal conduit (IC) or neobladder.

Extraperitoneal retrograde cystectomy:[24] Initially like the steps of radical prostatectomy, dorsal venous channels and urethra are sectioned early after EP pelvic node dissection on either side. Later, the prostate with the seminal vesicles and bladder are dissected off the rectum and Denonvillier's fascia cranially without opening the peritoneum. All the vascular pedicles of the bladder are ligated and cut. Cystectomy is completed by incising the peritoneum after sectioning the ureters. The bowel segment with its vascular pedicle is isolated (both for conduit or neobladder) and the peritoneum is closed around the mesentery. This bowel segment lies extraperitoneally and can be reconstructed as a conduit or neobladder and the ureters are implanted. Left ureter does not cross the mesentery of the sigmoid. Thus, bowel anastomosis is intraperitoneal and urinary pouch or conduit is EP (Fig. 6). This EP approach has shown significant reduction in ileus, effective management of minor urinary leaks without intervention. Others have reported antegrade technique (extraperitoneal) with successful results in terms of reduction in morbidity. In women we have used this technique for sparing the gynecological tract effectively to reduce perioperative morbidity (POM) and to improve QoL (Fig. 7).[25]

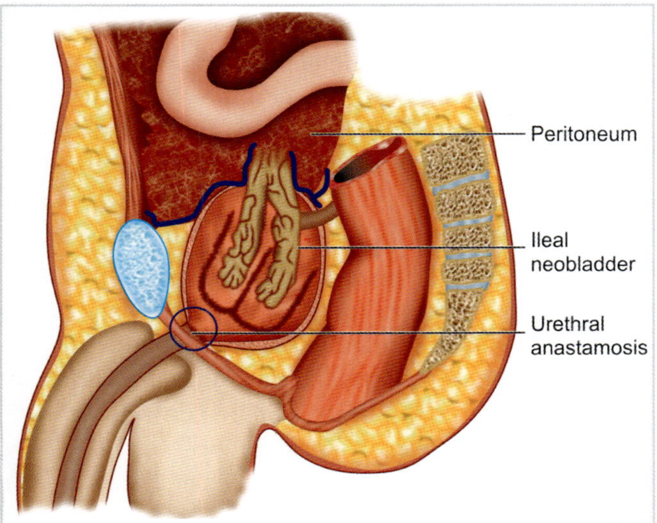

Fig. 6: Extraperitoneal radical cystectomy[25]

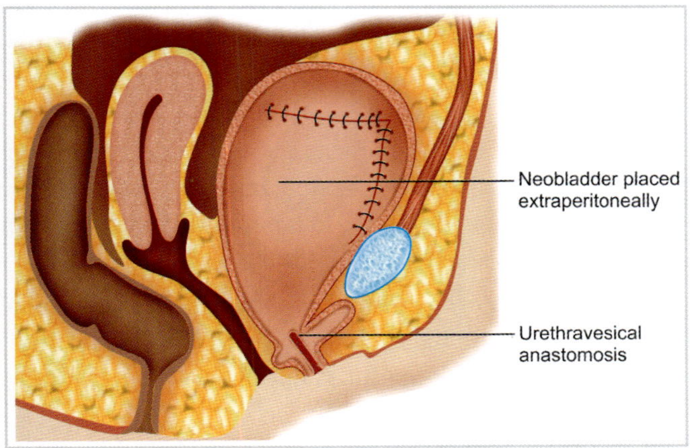

Fig. 7: Gynecological tract cystectomy with neobladder in females[26]

Post-cystectomy Urinary Diversion

There has been a long search for the ideal bladder substitute after radical cystoprostatectomy. In the last three decades, several attempts have been made to devise an operation to create neobladder that preserves continence, self-image and a better QoL, without compromising radical surgery. Further, the technical objectives to create low-pressure reservoirs which preserve the upper tracts, cause no biochemical derangements and ensure near-complete emptying on voiding have been met with some success. Hence, orthotopic neobladder substitution has emerged as the procedure of choice after radical cystectomy and has acceptable complication rates in properly selected patients.[26,27] However, every patient may not be a candidate for a neobladder and may require incontinent cutaneous stoma, e.g. IC. Described below are some of the common procedures done by us.

Bricker's ileal conduit: The IC can be considered an appropriate surgical solution after RC in most patients because of the relative simplicity of the surgical technique, the acceptable complication rate, and the satisfactory postoperative QoL. Till today this urinary diversion remains widely advisable for elderly patients and for those with compromised renal function, with severe comorbidities, or who are unfit to manage continent reservoirs (Figs 8A and B).[28]

Continent urinary diversion: We reported the experience of 30 continent urinary reservoirs after radical cystectomy elsewhere.[29] The first 20 patients had a standard CUR procedure and the last 10 had a modified CUR. The modifications were, use of appendicular stump instead of cecostomy, incision on anterior tenia to detubularize the colon which reduces the blood loss, the pull through technique of delivery of the ureters into colonic cavity has increased the ease of anastomosis. Complete continence was achieved in 25 patients—2 of them had revision

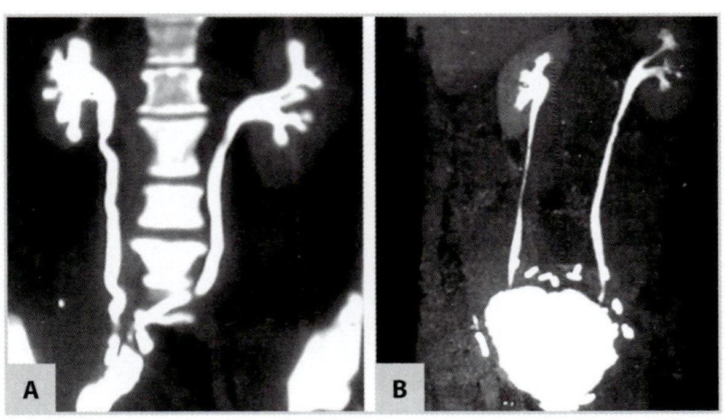

Figs 8A and B: (A) Postoperative intravenous pyelogram of standard RCIC; (B) Continent (Indiana) pouch

surgery, giving a success rate of 89% with a follow-up of 6–48 months (median 24). We believe continent urinary diversion is a better option than IC in selected patients and obviates the need of a stoma bag. It is economically more suitable and complication rates are comparable to IC.

Orthotopic neobladder: Orthotopic neobladder reconstruction is recommended for patients who satisfy the following criteria: those with muscle-invasive bladder cancer with no medical contraindications, those willing to comply with voiding re-education and follow-up, with no clinicoradiological evidence of spread to adjacent organs, no regional lymphadenopathy, no metastatic findings, negative pelvic lymph nodes on frozen-section analysis, and the prostatic urethra uninvolved by disease. Having used all three types of neobladder substitutes, we favor the ileal neobladder because it is completely detubularized, and is a high capacity, low-pressure and highly compliant urinary reservoir with the best continence rates (Figs 9A and B).[27] However, each reconstructive method is associated with specific problems and complications. It is our belief that the surgeon should be technically familiar with more than one procedure (to avoid undue reliance on any one) and customize the operation for each patient and disease (Figs 10A and B).[27]

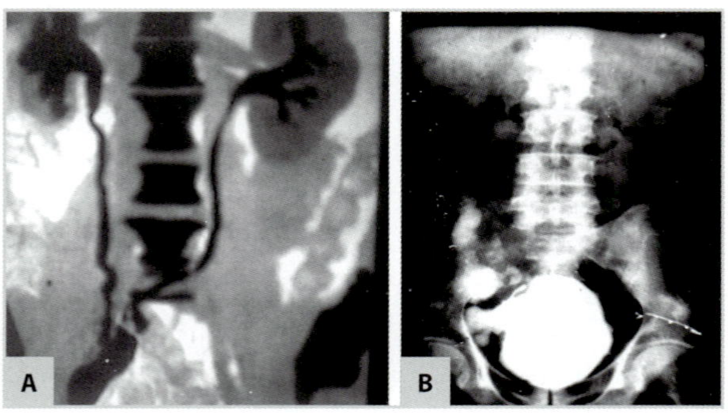

Figs 9A and B: (A) Intravenous pyelogram—conventional neobladder with left ureter crossing; (B) Extraperitoneal neobladder

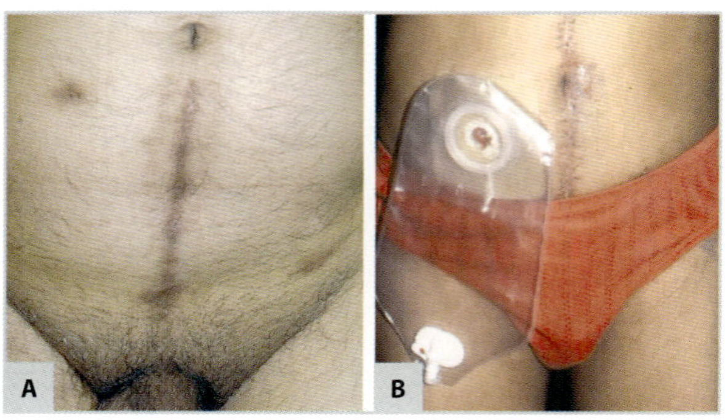

Figs 10A and B: Postoperative rehabilitation. (A) Neobladder; (B) Ileal conduit

Perioperative Morbidity (POM)

Radical cystectomy is a complex operation and has avoidable POM. Some authors have reported measures to help reduce or prevent them.[27-31] Various technical improvements in surgical and anesthesia techniques, multidisciplinary approach for correction/control of comorbidities and early postoperative rehabilitation have led to salutary effect in reducing the mortality but their impact on POM is at the best moderate.[32] There are few issues like patient selection criteria, surgical technique and its refinements, individual surgeon's preferences and skills and institutional volumes affecting the POM. Classification of the POM reporting is inconsistent in the majority of cohorts hence it is difficult to derive conclusions.[32-37]

Patient selection criteria: Age greater than 70 years particularly in females have been labeled as higher risk factors.[37-40] However, with proper selection and risk balancing there is a beneficial impact on reduction in morbidity.[39] Greater than two comorbidities are not a contraindication to surgery but will necessitate optimum correction (in ASA > 2) and preventive measures to reduce morbidity.[32] Prior pelvic surgery, radiotherapy (RT) (preoperative or radical) and neoadjuvant chemotherapy may produce some difficulties during surgery and postoperative period but with careful planning and modern technique these can be managed.[37-41]

Surgeon and Hospital Volume: An individual or institution which handles 10 radical cystectomy per year and has all facilities for major surgeries can continue to undertake radical cystectomy. However, orthotopic neobladder or continent pouches should be handled at larger volume centers. In the Indian context, we believe that all the teaching and large private hospitals can undertake radical cystectomy with acceptable results.

Surgical Issues: Impact of optimum surgical technique on reduction of POM of radical cystectomy depends on: (1) preoperative factors, (2) anesthesia and perioperative anesthetic management, (3) clinical care pathways and (4) operative technique.

Preoperative factors: Renal failure (serum creatinine > 2.5 g/dL) and poor nutritional status necessitate correction. In these patients urinary diversion with an IC is preferable than complex procedures.[41] Older patients with significant comorbidities are better suited for IC.

Anesthesia and perioperative management: Preanesthetic optimization of medical comorbidities (cardiac, pulmonary, diabetes) and epidural anesthesia has favorably affected perioperative complications.

Clinical care pathway: Clinical care pathways are referred to enhanced recovery protocols with standardized perioperative plan of care.[32,41,42] Generally, this pathway is directed toward the standardization of antibiotic and analgesic therapy, bowel preparation, nutrition, and surgical drain management. These pathways are used as a guide and minor deviation may be required in a given clinical scenario.

Perioperative complications: We describe some of the factors and measures to prevent or reduce these.[32]

Blood loss: Acute blood loss is common during or after RC and is difficult to predict.[37-41] In our setting, the majority of patients present with bulky disease and are nutritionally compromised and hence require replacement of either whole blood or blood products intraoperatively and/or postoperatively (Table 2). However, with the EP approach the blood loss has been reduced. Harmonic scalpel ligasure can be used to reduce blood loss.

Urinary leak: Meticulous dissection, proper hemostasis and attention to vascular supply are the key issues in construction of the conduit or pouch and urteroenteric anastomosis. An EP approach which separates the bowel anastomosis from the reconstructed urinary segment has helped in reducing the urinary leak spreading into the peritoneal cavity progressing to sepsis and can be diagnosed easily by noting the increased drainage.[24] Major leak can be managed by instituting measures like antibiotics, total parenteral nutrition, proper drainage of pelvic collection and percutaneous nephrostomy. We routinely use stents across the ureteroenteric anastomosis and a suprapubic catheter in the neobladders. Both stents are brought out in the stoma bag in conduits and with suprapubic cystostomy in pouches. Further, problem of mucus blockage is prevented by gentle irrigation of the stents and suprapubic cystostomy washes.

Postoperative ileus: It is the inability to tolerate solid food by fifth postoperative day, the need to place a nasogastric tube or the need to stop oral intake due to abdominal distention, nausea or emesis. Prolonged ileus could be due to a bowel or urinary leak and should be dealt with appropriately.

Bowel leak and fistulae: Our preference is a hand-sewn anastomosis with acceptable results and a cost benefit. Generally management of bowel fistulae revolves around nutrition, diversion or reoperation and treatment of sepsis.

Sepsis, pulmonary and peripheral vascular complication: Appropriate antibiotics, active pulmonary physiotherapy, low molecular weight heparin and intermittent pneumatic compression stocking (ICSI) reduce these complications. Early ambulation and frequent change of position during critical stages can prevent bed sores.

Wound dehiscence: Meticulous closure of the fascia and rectus sheath using non absorbable sutures, a subcutaneous suction drain, proper closure of skin and subcutaneous tissue, regular inspection of wound postoperatively reduces the complication of wound dehiscence. If it occurs early repair is warranted.

Lymphorrhea and lymphocele: Lymphorrhea needs patience and symptomatic treatment. Lymphoceles are generally detected after first and second follow up visit and may require percutaneous drainage.[42]

Chemotherapy

Neoadjuvant chemotherapy: Neoadjuvant chemotherapy has been used for patients with operable clinical stage T2 to T4a. Chemotherapy before surgery is given with the intent to treat micrometastasis. In the neoadjuvant setting it is better tolerated, a larger dose and more cycles can be given, and in vivo drug sensitivity can be assessed. The tumor can be downgraded.[43] However, a major disadvantage is that it delays local therapy. An interval longer than 12 weeks between the diagnosis of muscle invasion and cystectomy has even been associated with a poorer outcome. Meta-analysis of cisplatin-containing combination neoadjuvant chemotherapy trials reveal a 5% difference in favor of neoadjuvant chemotherapy. Unfortunately, the quality of life data are not available.

Adjuvant chemotherapy: Adjuvant chemotherapy has been advocated for high-risk patients to delay recurrence and prolong survival.[43] Adjuvant chemotherapy has potential advantages of selecting patients at highest risk of metastatic or recurrent disease on the basis of an accurate histopathologic evaluation and surgery is generally performed without delay. The major disadvantages are that the bladder is not preserved, there is a delay in starting systemic therapy for occult metastases, response cannot be easily evaluated, and the only clinical end point that can be assessed is the time to tumor recurrence.

Radiotherapy

Historically RT was used as a definitive therapy (60–70 cGY) in muscle invasive bladder cancer stage B–C disease.[44] Subsequently role of RT was evaluated as preoperative therapy (20–40 cGY) prior to cystectomy in early 1990s. However, postoperative morbidity and unsatisfactory outcome led to discontinuation of the combination of RT and cystectomy.[45-47] Later, with modern newer chemotherapy there has been increasing trend of combining systemic chemotherapy with RT to achieve bladder preservation by sensitizing the tumor to RT and perhaps also treating occult metastases. Thus, currently trimodality therapy for selected patients with clinical stages T2 to T4a includes maximal TURB of the bladder tumor, modern external beam RT with radiosensitizing chemotherapy given concurrently.

METASTATIC AND RECURRENT TUMORS

These tumors are generally treated with combined modalities, e.g. surgery/RT and or chemotherapy with an acceptable outcome. However, treatment has to be tailored to the patient's requirement. Post-cystectomy urethral tumors are treated with urethrectomy while upper tract relapse may need nephrectomy.

MINIMALLY INVASIVE SURGERY FOR BLADDER CANCER

Traditional open surgical approach for radical cystectomy and urinary diversion is being slowly challenged by laparoscopic or robotic techniques. The advantages of the later approaches are less blood loss, early recovery time, less pain and in an expert hand has an equal operative time as open surgery plus complication rates are comparable but it has long and steep learning curve.[48] Robotic radical cystectomy with intracorporial urinary diversion is the latest addition to the surgical armamentarium. Certainly, it is a further step in the development of minimally invasive techniques for cystectomy. Additionally, robotic surgery has distinct benefit of higher magnification and surgeon's comfort but the availability of robot and cost is a concern.[49]

REFERENCES

1. Kavarana NM, Kamat MR, Kurkure AP, et al. Cancer Morbidity and Mortality in Greater MumbaiMumbai Cancer Registry, National Cancer Registry Project. Indian Council of Medical Research; 2003.
2. Jemal A, Murray T, Ward E, et al. Cancer statistics, 2005. CA Cancer J Clin. 2005;55(1):10-30.
3. Morrison AS. Advances in the etiology of urothelial cancer. Urol Clin North Am. 1984;11(4):557-66.
4. Burch JD, Rohan TE, Howe GR, et al. Risk of bladder cancer by source and type of tobacco exposure: a case-control study. Int J Cancer. 1989;44(4):622-8.
5. Bolt HM, Golka K. The debate on carcinogenicity of permanent hair dyes: new insights. Crit Rev Toxicol. 2007;37(6):521-36.
6. Harling M, Schablon A, Schedlbauer G, et al. Bladder cancer among hairdressers: a meta-analysis. Occup Environ Med. 2010;67(5):351-8.
7. Uchida T, Wada C, Ishida H, et al. p53 mutations and prognosis in bladder tumors. J Urol. 1995;153(4):1097-104.
8. Amin MB, McKenney JK, Paner GP, et al. ICUD-EAU International Consultation on Bladder Cancer 2012: Pathology. Eur Urol. 2013;63(1):16-65.
9. American Joint Committee on Cancer. AJCC Cancer staging Manual, 7th edition. Chicago, IL, Springer; 2010. p. 1.650
10. Kulkarni JN, Bakshi GK. Staging of transitional cell carcinoma: Has anything changed? Indian J Urol. 2008;24(1):68-71.
11. van Rhijn BW, van der Poel HG, van der Kwast TH. Urine markers for bladder cancer surveillance: a systematic review. Eur Urol. 2005;47(6):736-48.
12. Husband JE, Olliff JF, Williams MP, et al. Bladder cancer: staging with CT and MR imaging. Radiology. 1989;173(2):435-40.
13. Saad Aldousari, Wassim Kassouf. Update on the management of non-muscle invasive bladder cancer. Can Urol Assoc J. 2010;4(1):56-64.
14. Kamat MR, Kulkarni JN. Use of intravesical thiotepa in bladder tumors. Indian J Cancer. 1981;18:223-34.
15. Kaasinen E, Rintala E, Hellström P, et al. Factors explaining recurrence in patients undergoing chemoimmunotherapy regimens for frequently recurring superficial bladder carcinoma. Eur Urol. 2002;42(2):167-74.
16. Kamat MR, Kulkarni JN, Tongaonkar HB, et al. Intravesical bacillus Calmette-Guerin for superficial bladder cancer: experience with Danish 1331 strain. J Urol. 1994;152(5 Pt 1):1424-8.
17. Tongaonkar HB, Kulkarni JN, Kamat MR. Superficial bladder cancer. A 10 year experience. Indian J Cancer. 1995;32(3):141-8.
18. Kulkarni JN, Gupta R. Recurrence and progression in stage T1G3 bladder tumour with intravesical bacille Calmette-Guérin (Danish 1331 strain). BJU Int. 2002;90(6):554-7.
19. Baniel J, Grauss D, Engelstein D, et al. Intravesical bacillus Calmette-Guerin treatment for stage T1 grade3 transitional cell carcinoma of the bladder. Urology. 1998;52(5):785-9.
20. Kaubisch S, Lum BL, Reese J, et al. Stage T1 bladder cancer: grade is the primary determinant for risk of muscle invasion. J Urol. 1991;146(1):28-31.
21. Jakse G, Loidl W, Seeber G, et al. Stage T1, grade 3 transitional cell carcinoma of the bladder: an unfavorable tumor? J Urol. 1987;137(1):39-43.

22. Malkowicz SB, Nichols P, Lieskovsky G, et al. The role of radical cystectomy in the management of high grade superficial bladder cancer (PA, P1, PIS and P2). J Urol. 1990;144(3): 641-5.
23. Lamm DL, Blumenstein BA, Crissman JD, et al. Maintenance bacillus Calmette-Guerin immunotherapy for recurrent TA, T1 and carcinoma in situ transitional cell carcinoma of the bladder: a randomized Southwest Oncology Group Study. J Urol. 2000;163(4):1124-9.
24. Kulkarni JN, Gulla RA, Tongoankar HB, et al. Radical cystoprostatectomy— an extraperitoneal retrograde approach. J Urol. 1999:161(2);545-8.
25. Kulkarni JN, Rizvi SJ, Acharya PU, et al. Gynecologic-Tract Sparing Extra Peritoneal Retrograde Radical Cystectomy with Neobladder. Int Braz J Urol. 2008;34(2):180-90.
26. Kamat MR, Kulkarni JN, Tongaonkar HB. Neobladder after cystectomy: an Indian experience. Br J Urol. 1993;71(6):700-4.
27. Kulkarni JN, Pramesh CS, Rathi S, et al. Long-term results of orthotopic neobladder reconstruction after radical cystectomy. BJU Int. 2003;91(6):485-8.
28. Johnson DE, Lamy SM. Complications of a single stage radical cystectomy and ileal conduit diversion: review of 214 cases. J Urol. 1977;117(2):171-3.
29. Kulkarni JN, Tongaonkar HB, Ravi R, et al. Continent Urinary Reservoirs. Br J Urol. 1992:69(5);513-7.
30. Skinner DG, Crawford ED, Kaufman JJ. Complications of radical cystectomy for carcinoma of the bladder. J Urol. 1980;123(5): 640-3.
31. Sullivan JW, Grabstald H, Whitmore WF. Complications of ureteroileal conduit with radical cystectomy: review of 336 cases. J Urol. 1980;124(6):797-801.
32. Kulkarni JN. Perioperative morbidity of radical cystectomy: A review. Indian J Urol. 2011;27(2):226-32.
33. Donat SM. Standards for surgical complication reporting in urologic oncology: time for a change. Urology. 2007;69(2):221-5.
34. Hautmann RE. Editorial comment on: Defining early morbidity of radical cystectomy for patients with bladder cancer using a standardized reporting methodology. Eur Urol. 2009;55(1):174.
35. Shabsigh A, Korets R, Vora KC, et al. Defining early morbidity of radical cystectomy for patients with bladder cancer using a standardized reporting methodology. Eur Urol. 2009;55(1):164-76.
36. Dmochowski R, Scarpero H. Surgical outcomes reporting-closer to reality. Eur Urol. 2007;52(5):1306-8.
37. Lawrentschuk N, Colombo R, Hakenberg OW, et al. Prevention and management of complications following radical cystectomy for bladder cancer. Eur Urol. 2010;57(6):991-1001.
38. Hollenbeck BK, Taub DA, Miller DC, et al. The regionalization of radical cystectomy to specific medical centers. J Urol. 2005;174(4 Pt 1):1385-9.
39. Gamé X, Soulié M, Seguin P, et al. Radical cystectomy in patients older than 75 years: assessment of Kulkarni: Perioperative morbidity of radical cystectomy morbidity and mortality. Eur Urol. 2001;39(5):525-9.
40. Lee KL, Freiha F, Presti JC, et al. Gender differences in radical cystectomy: complications and blood loss. Urology. 2004;63(6):1095-9.
41. Mills RD, Studer UE. Metabolic consequences of continent urinary diversion. J Urol. 1999;161(4):1057-66.
42. Chang SS, Cookson MS, Baumgartner RG, et al. Analysis of early complications after radical cystectomy: results of collaborative care pathway. J Urol. 2002;167(5):2012-6.
43. Calabrò F, Sternberg CN. Neoadjuvant and adjuvant chemotherapy in muscle-invasive bladder cancer. Eur Urol. 2009;55(2):348-58.
44. Duncan W, Quilty PM. The results of a series of 963 patients withtransitional cell carcinoma of the urinary bladder primarily treated by radical megavoltage X-ray therapy. Radiother Oncol. 1986;7(4):299-310.
45. Barbiere JM, Saeb-Parsy K, Greenberg DC, et al. Trends in the use of radiotherapy and radical surgery for patients with bladder urothelial cell carcinoma in East Anglia, 1995-2006. BJU Int. 2011;108(7):1106-14.
46. Kotwal S, Choudhury A, Johnston C, et al. Similar treatment outcomes for radical cystectomy and radical radiotherapy in invasive bladder cancer treated at a United Kingdom specialist treatment center. Int J Radiat Oncol Biol Phys. 2008;70(2):456-63.
47. Kiltie AE, Efstathiou JA, Choudhury A, et al. Radiotherapy for bladder cancer. BJU Int. 2011:Virtual edition. Nov 28,2011
48. Haber GP, Campbell SC, Colombo JR, et al. Perioperative outcomes with laparoscopic radical cystectomy: 'pure laparoscopic' and 'open assisted laparoscopic' approaches. Urology. 2007;70(5):910-5.
49. Nix J, Smith A, Kurpad R, et al. Prospective randomized controlled trial of robotic versus open radical cystectomy for bladder cancer: perioperative and pathologic results. Eur Urol. 2010;57(2):196-201.

46 Testicular Tumors

Jagdeesh Kulkarni, Abhijit Dhale, Devendra Choudhary, Nasreen Gite, Varun Gunavanthe

INTRODUCTION

Testicular cancer is an uncommon neoplasm, however, it is the most common solid tumor in young adults, highest being in the age group of 20–34 years.[1] There are various histological types of testicular tumors, but the most common are germ cell tumors (GCT). Recent advances in management strategies including aggressive surgery and newer chemotherapeutic agents have led testicular tumor as a potentially curative tumor model. After having achieved cures in majority, current emphasis is on early diagnosis, reduction in treatment related morbidity and fertility preservation.

EPIDEMIOLOGY AND RISK FACTORS

The incidence of testicular tumors is reported as 5–10/100,000 males per year. These tumors form about 5% of urological tumors in males in the West.[2,3] In India, incidence of testicular tumors varies from 100–150 new cases per year at Tata Memorial Hospital, Mumbai, India.[4]

Although the exact etiology and risk factors are not known, however, some of the congenital and acquired factors are: (a) cryptorchidism/undescended testis; (b) family history of cryptorchidism/undescended testis;[5,6] (c) Klinefelter's syndrome; (d) family history of testicular intraepithelial neoplasia (TIN) in first degree relative (father/brother); (e) presence of contralateral tumor or TIN and infertility. A specific genetic marker has been described in all types of histology (Bosl)[7] plus TIN shows same chromosomal anomalies. Other factors, for example, trauma and infection related atrophy (mumps) have shown a weak association.

CLASSIFICATION

Table 1 gives the pathological classification of the testicular tumors. Broadly, testicular tumors are sub classified as: (a) germ cell tumors; (b) non-germ cell tumors.

GERM CELL TUMORS

Pathogenesis

These are the most common testicular tumors compromising 90–95% while the remaining are non-GCT. About 2% GCT occur bilaterally either as a synchronous[4] or metachronous presentation. Current accepted model of development of GCT development is that totipotent germ cells follow abnormal pathways of differentiation resulting in either seminoma or embryonal carcinoma (EC). Embryonal cells give rise to teratoma by intraembryonic differentiation while yolk sac tumor or choriocarcinoma are produced by extraembryonic differentiation.[8,9]

Virtually all GCT develop from the intratubular germ cell neoplasia (ITGCN) or carcinoma in-situ (CIS) except spermatocytic seminoma and a few rare prepubertal tumors. Being diffuse in nature, ITGCN can be diagnosed by random testicular biopsy. In approximately 50% ITGCN may end up in invasive GCT in 5 years.

Only 40% GCT belong to one histologic type while remaining exhibit mixed variety. Further combination of seminoma and one or more nonseminomatous elements are considered as nonseminomatous germ cell tumors (NSGCT). Moreover, pure seminoma with abnormal alpha-fetoprotein (AFP) (above 10–20 ng/mL) and/or highly elevated human chorionic gonadotropin (hCG) (above 200 mIU/mL) are treated like NSGCT. Pure

TABLE 1: Histopathological classification of testicular tumors

1A) Germ cell tumors
Precursor lesion—Intratubular germ cell neoplasm (ITGCN)
1A.1) Tumors with one histology
1. Seminoma a. Classical seminoma b. Spermatocytic seminoma
2. Nonseminomatous germ cell tumors (NSGST) a. Embryonal carcinoma b. Yolk sac tumor c. Teratoma d. Polyembryoma e. Trophoblastic tumor
1A.2) Mixed tumors
1B) Non-germ cell tumors /Sex cord/Gonadal stromal tumors
1. Leydig cell tumors
2. Sertoli cell tumors
3. Granulosa cell tumor
4. Thecoma /fibroma
5. Mixed tumors
1C) Tumors with both germ cell and stromal elements
1. Gonadoblastoma
2. Mixed tumors/unclassified
1D) Other tumors
1. Lymphoma
2. Leukemia
3. Metastasis

seminomas spread by lymphatics (hematogenous spread is rare) and are extremely sensitive to radiotherapy. Nonseminomatous germ cell tumors spread by lymphatic and hematogenous route.

Cryptorchidism[6,10]

The relative risk of malignancy in a cryptorchid testis is six times that of a normally descended one. This is thought to be due to transplacental damage to fetal gonads by maternal estrogens. Orchidopexy done before puberty reduces the risk to 2–3 times. Further in a unilateral undescended testis, the normal testis is also at an increased risk for malignancy. First degree relative with testicular malignancy significantly increases the chances for GCT with a relative risk being 2–4 for affected father to 8–12 times for affected brother. Past testicular malignancy increases chances of tumor in contralateral testis by 12 times. While ITGCN is found in up to 80% of GCT, it independently has a 50% risk of causing invasive tumors over 5 years.

CLASSIFICATION OF GERM CELL TUMORS OF TESTIS[9,10]

Germ cell tumors are subclassified as seminomas (52–56%) and NSGCT (44–48%).

Intratubular Germ Cell Neoplasm

This consists of undifferentiated germ cells located basally within seminiferous tubules. This is the precursor lesion for all tumors, but spermatocytic seminoma.

Seminoma

This is the most common GCT and has two variants; the classical and the spermatocytic seminoma. On gross examination, seminoma is a tan to white, diffuse or multinodular mass (Figs 1A and B). Histological

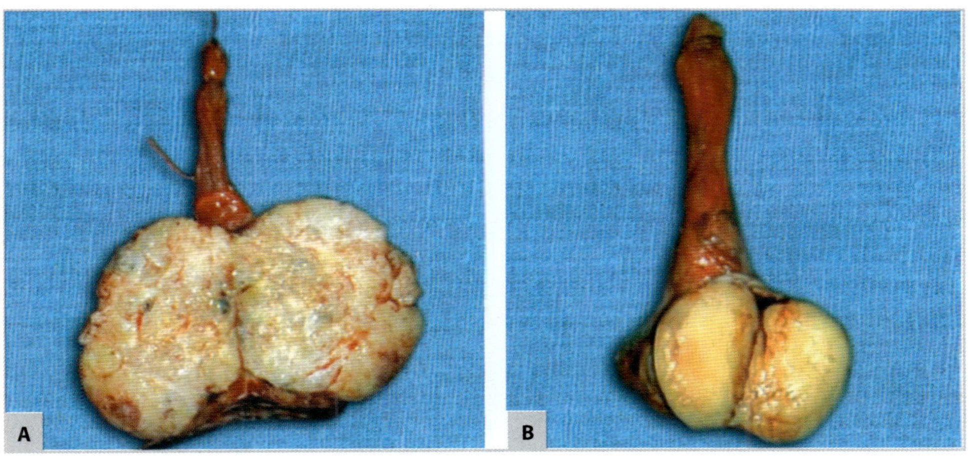

Figs 1A and B: (A) Nonseminoma; (B) Seminoma

examination shows sheet-like cell arrangement with polygonal nuclei and clear cytoplasm with the presence of lymphocytes in fibrovascular septa. Pure seminomas are highly sensitive to chemotherapy and radiotherapy and carry an excellent prognosis.

Embryonal Carcinoma

It is a highly malignant undifferentiated tumor with totipotent capacity to differentiate into other NSGCT. It shows areas of necrosis and hemorrhages on gross examination and may show solid, papillary or tubular pattern on microscopy.

Choriocarcinoma

It is an hCG producing tumor with syncytiotrophoblasts and cytotrophoblasts. Hematogenous spread and metastasis are common.

Yolk Sac Tumor

This tumor is also called endodermal sinus tumor and produces AFP. A characteristic feature is presence of Schiller–Duval bodies which mimic endodermal sinuses.

Teratomas

These tumors are derived from one or more germ cell lines. They are classified based on differentiation of the tissues within, into mature and immature types. Mature teratomas also called dermoid cysts contain tissues like cartilage, bone, hair, teeth, are slow growing and rarely metastasize. Immature teratomas are malignant tumors and contain undifferentiated tissue. In general, teratomas are resistant to chemotherapy and require surgery for primary and metastatic sites.

CLINICAL FEATURES[5]

The standard presentation is a unilateral painless enlargement of the testis, however some may complain dragging pain or heaviness in the scrotum. Interestingly about 10–20% patients present with retroperitoneal disease, e.g. an abdominal mass, pain in abdomen, neck nodes, or with gastrointestinal upset while dyspnea, cough, chest pain or hemoptysis are seen with lung metastasis. After investigations 60% of NSGCT and 15% of seminomas reveal asymptomatic metastasis. Occasionally, bone metastasis and pain could be the only symptom at presentation.[11] A tumor in third testis in a patient with polyorchidism has been reported.[12]

On examination patients present with a nontender, firm to hard testicular swelling. Diminished testicular sensation is the finding in majority of patients. Systematic survey of the chest, abdomen and neck may give clues to their involvement with metastatic disease.

INVESTIGATIONS

Scrotal Ultrasound with Doppler

Scrotal ultrasound is the primary modality of investigation in testicular tumors. It can easily detect tumors few millimeters in size and can also detect increased vascularity within the mass or microcalcification. Young men who present with abdominal masses or raised AFP or hCG and infertility must have scrotal sonography to detect impalpable lesion in the testis. Seminomas are typically homogenous and hypoechoic, whereas NSGCT are heterogeneous. Additionally, ultrasound is also helpful in screening the contralateral testis for incidental masses.

Computed Tomography/Magnetic Resonance Imaging/Positron Emission Tomography Scan

A computed tomography (CT) scan of the abdomen and chest is recommended for assessing retroperitoneal and mediastinal nodes and the lungs. At a 10-mm cut-off for lymph nodes the false-negative rate is as high as 63% and CT fails to detect 25–35% of pathologically proven retroperitoneal metastasis.[13] Magnetic resonance imaging (MRI) is currently optional[14] and fluorodeoxyglucose positron emission tomography (FDG-PET scan) is currently recommended for staging and in follow-up.[15]

Tumor Markers

Serum tumor markers like AFP, beta-hCG (β-hCG) and lactate dehydrogenase (LDH) levels reliably contribute to the diagnosis and staging of the tumors and has great prognostic significance[15,16] as it is used for follow up.

Alpha-fetoprotein[17]

Alpha-fetoprotein is normally produced by the fetal liver and is secreted by embryonal and yolk sac tumors. In clinical practice, these are elevated in 50–70% of low stage NSGCT and 60–80% of advanced NSGCT. Seminomas with raised AFP indicates nonseminoma element and should be investigated. Half-life of AFP is 5–7 days.

Beta-Human Chorionic Gonadotropin

Beta-hCG is secreted by trophoblastic cells and is elevated in 20–40% of low stage NSGCT and 40–60% of advanced NSGCT and 15% of seminomas. Higher levels are in favor of NSGCTs. Raised β-hCG in pure seminomas could be due to nonseminomatous component or syncytiotrophoblasts. Half-life of β-hCG is 2–3 days.

Lactate Dehydrogenase

Being a nonspecific marker, it reflects tissue damage and destruction and is elevated in 20% of low stage NSGCT and 20–60% of advanced NSGCT.

It is important to obtain baseline levels of tumor markers before orchiectomy so that postoperatively the levels can be monitored for staging and prognosticating the disease. A rising or a persistently high tumor marker level is in favor of recurrent or residual disease respectively.

TREATMENT OF PRIMARY TUMOR—ORCHIECTOMY

Testicular masses need to be explored by inguinal approach and exteriorization of testis with its tunics and division of the spermatic cord at the inguinal region.[4] In doubtful cases, Chevassu's maneuver (Figs 2A to E) and frozen section can be done. In disseminated cases with life-threatening situations, e.g. lung metastases with respiratory insufficiency orchiectomy can be deferred. In these patients after obtaining marker study, and if possible, fine-needle aspiration cytology/fine-needle aspiration biopsy (FNAC/FNAB) from the testis or abdominal mass, chemotherapy can be started. Later once the patient is stabilized orchiectomy can be performed.

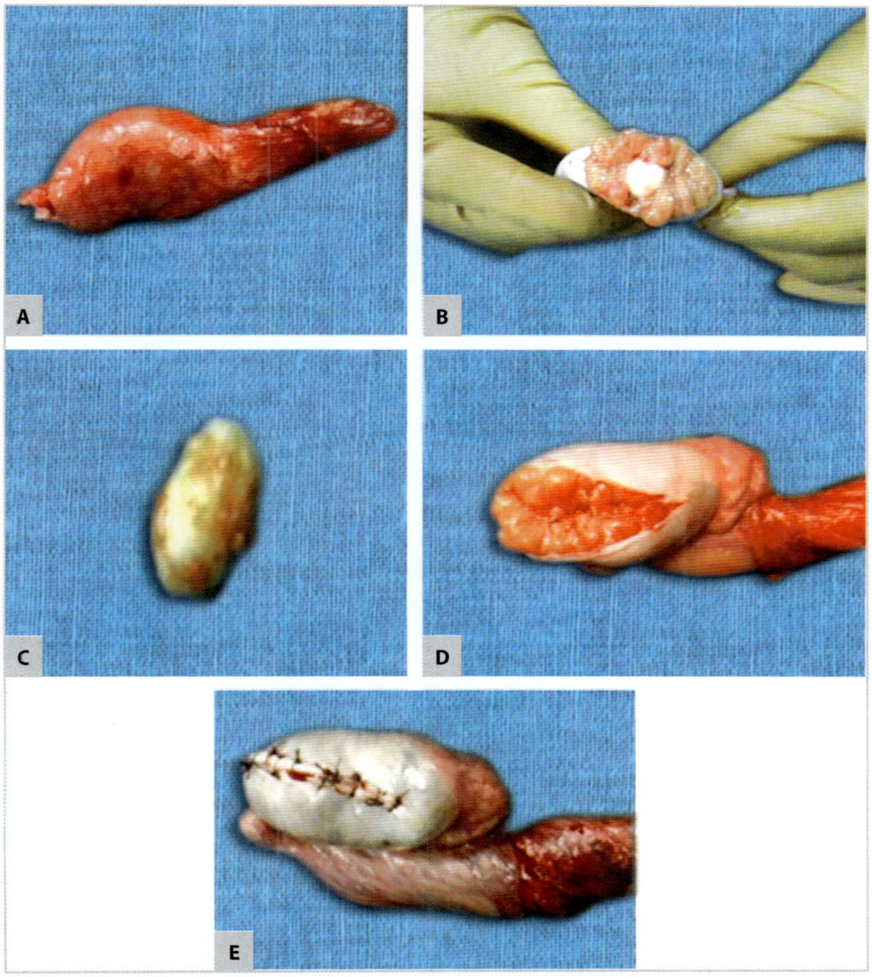

Figs 2A and E: Chevassu's maneuver with testis sparing surgery

TESTES SPARING SURGERY

Recently, there has been some discussion about organ sparing approach in patients with bilateral synchronous tumors, metachronous contralateral tumors or tumors in solitary testis with normal testosterone levels. However, tumor volume should be less than 30% and sonography on table may be required. This option must be discussed with patient and preferably done in experienced centers.[18] Post-orchiectomy staging imaging studies and tumor markers are done to make a treatment plan.[19] Figures 2A to E show the authors' patient who had small seminoma, which was treated by testis sparing surgery.

STAGING, STAGE GROUPING AND RISK STRATIFICATION[20,21]

Classification system recommended by the Union for International Cancer Control (UICC)[20] is given in Table 2. This TNM system is aimed at anatomical extent of disease, assessment of tumor markers after orchiectomy, node status and metastasis.[20] Broadly, in population-based patient series stage-wise distribution for seminomas is 85%, 10% and 5% in stages I, II and III while 33% each in stages I, II, III in NSGCT. Further in 1997, the IGCCCG (International Germ Cell Cancer Collaborative Group)[21] defined staging system for metastatic GCT based on identification of some clinically adverse factors. Prognostic risk factors for Stage I seminomas are tumors bigger than 4 cm and invasion of rete testis. Lympho/vascular invasion (LVI)[22] is the most important factor for stage I NSGCT, while proliferation rate and more than 50% of embryonal carcinoma are added to improve predictive value of LVI.

TABLE 2: TNM staging of testicular tumors 2009[20]

TNM	*Description*
pTX	Primary tumor cannot be assessed
pT0	No evidence of primary tumor
pTis	Intratubular germ cell neoplasm in situ
pT1	Tumor limited to testis and epididymis without vascular/ lymphatic invasion, tumor may invade into tunica albuginea but not tunica vaginalis
pT2	Tumor limited to testis and epididymis with vascular/ lymphatic invasion, or tumor extending through the tunica albuginea with involvement of tunica vaginalis
pT3	Tumor invades the spermatic cord with/without vascular/ lymphatic invasion
pT4	Tumor invades the scrotum with/without vascular/ lymphatic invasion
Regional Lymph Nodes	
Clinical Staging	
NX	Regional lymph nodes cannot be assessed
N0	No regional lymph node metastasis
N1	Metastasis with a lymph node mass 2 cm or less in greatest dimension, or multiple lymph node masses none more than 2 cm in greatest dimension
N2	Metastasis with a lymph node mass, more than 2 cm but not more than 5 cm in greatest dimension , or multiple lymph node masses any one mass more than 2 cm but not more than 5 cm in greatest dimension
N3	Metastasis with a lymph node mass more than 5 cm in greatest dimension
Distant Metastasis	
MX	Distant metastasis cannot be assessed
M0	Distant metastasis cannot be assessed
M1	Distant metastasis
M1a	Nonregional nodal or pulmonary metastasis
M1b	Distant metastasis at other sites

MANAGEMENT OF GERM CELL TUMORS OF THE TESTIS

Testicular Intraepithelial Neoplasia (TIN) or Carcinoma In Situ

Generally, this is a noninvasive precursor of GCT and contralateral testis biopsy is advised in high-risk patients with testicular volume of less than 12 cc, history of cryptorchidism and poor spermatogenesis. Once TIN is diagnosed, local radiotherapy (20 Gy in 20 fractions) is recommended after counseling.[23]

Seminoma

Stage I and II

In the past, adjuvant radiotherapy was a standard treatment for stage I seminoma, however, since 1990 there has been a considerable debate about the increased late side-effects of radiotherapy including second non-germ cell malignancy and cardiovascular disease. Additionally, the success of surveillance strategy in stage I NSGCT and improved imaging has led to considering "surveillance" after orchiectomy for stage I seminoma and reserve therapy for relapse.[23] Thirdly, carboplatin chemotherapy has shown comparable results to radiotherapy. Hence, there are three therapeutic approaches available for stage I seminoma, i.e. adjuvant radiotherapy, chemotherapy and surveillance. Surveillance is used in a compliant patient after counseling. Seminoma is exquisitely radiosensitive and sensitive to carboplatin based chemotherapy. Standard radiation therapy (20 Gy) is given to retroperitoneal nodes and upper pelvic nodes. Lastly, carboplatin if chosen, includes 1–2 courses. Adjuvant radiotherapy is the treatment of choice for low volume stage II A/B, with chemotherapy in advanced disease. Long-term follow-up is indicated to screen the side-effects of therapy, treatment induced second malignancy and cardiac problems. Data of the 81 stage I seminomas with radiotherapy (71 patients) or surveillance (10 patients) show long-term disease-free and total survival in seminomas as 92.6% and 100% respectively.[24]

Nonseminomatous Germ Cell Tumor

Clinical Stage I

Optimal management of stage I NSGCT is controversial, except stage IS [only serum tumor markers (STM) elevated] is treated like stage IIC NSGCT (Table 3). Surveillance, retroperitoneal node dissection and primary chemotherapy are established treatment options in this setting of stage I NSGCT with 97% long-term survival.[23] Important risk factors for occult metastasis in this stage are LVI, predominant EC component. Further, the reported occult metastasis in patients with these two factors range from 30% to 80%.[25] Finally, retroperitoneal lymph nodes on imaging greater than 5–9 mm in primary drainage zone are viewed with suspicion for regional lymph node (LN) metastasis.[26]

Surveillance: Surveillance is based on the fact that occult metastasis in stage I (in patients with no LVI and EC in orchiectomy specimen) is noted in only 20–30%.[26] Hence, morbidity and overtreatment for 70–80% is a concern. Therefore, it is logical to believe that almost 70–80% of clinical stage I NSGCT are cured by orchidectomy alone. In them mean relapse risk is 28%; greater than 90% relapse occur within first 2 years with late relapse greater than 5 years in up to 1% patients.[27] Further, virtually all relapsing patients can be salvaged with modern chemotherapy. Amongst the patients who present with bulky (> 3 cm) retroperitoneal relapse, elevated tumor markers are treated with induction chemotherapy. Others with relapse limited to nonbulky (< 3 cm) retroperitoneal LN with normal tumor markers may be managed initially with retroperitoneal lymph node dissection (RPLND). No schedule for surveillance is standard, but should be intense in first 2 years with abdominopelvic CT.[26,27]

TABLE 3: Treatment algorithm for clinical stage I nonseminomatous germ cell tumors (NSGCT)[23]

NSGCT

↓

Negative chest, abdomen and pelvic imaging

↓

Rising post-orchidectomy AFP or hCG

↓

Category	*YES*	*NO*			
		High risk of occult metastasis based on histopathological and CT parameters			
		YES			*NO*
Treatment	Chemotherapy False positive STM elevations should be considered in patients with slightly elevated and stable AFP or hCG levels	BEP* x 2	Surveillance*	NS-RPLND** +/– Adjuvant BEP x 2 or EP x 2 For PS II	Surveillance BEP x 2 may be considered in regions without expertise in diagnosis and treatment of GCT

* -Treatment based on patient preference and physician-hospital expertise

** RPLND – Retroperitoneal lymph node dissection

Abbreviations: AFP, alpha-fetoprotein; hCG, human chorionic gonadotropin; STM, serum tumor markers; BEP, bleomycin, etoposide, cisplatin; EP, etoposide plus cisplatin; GCT, germ cell tumors

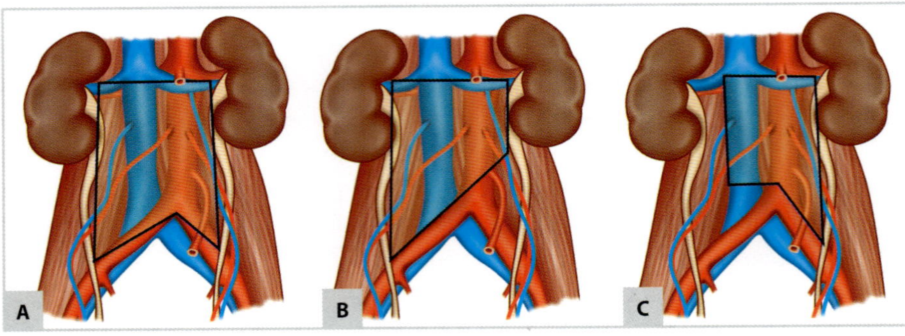

Figs 3A to C: Retroperitoneal lymph node dissection (RPLND) templates: (A) Standard; (B and C) Right and left modified RPLND

Retroperitoneal node dissection: The basis of primary RPLND is to excise occult metastasis which range from 15% to 25% and majority of these are teratoma (chemoresistant).[2,23,28] High cure rates with RPLND alone can obviate the need of surveillance and chemotherapy.

The standard RPLND (Fig. 3A) includes removal of all nodal tissue from the level of both renal hila proximally to the distal level of common iliac bifurcation on either side or to the level of the ureters crossing the iliac vessels. Additionally, the tissue between and behind the aorta and vena cava is removed. Since this necessitates removal of L1 sympathetic ganglion there is a risk of retrograde ejaculation. Hence, Donohue et al.[28] after describing the detailed anatomical studies of the lymphatic spread reported the modified RPLND (Figs 3B and C) with preservation of ejaculation in 95% patients. Since a negative RPLND patients have less than 5% chance of relapse in the retroperitoneum, follow-up studies including marker studies and X-ray chest are enough.[19,28] Other important issues are experience of the surgical team and volume of patients especially for ejaculation preservation.[27] Conversely, positive nodes on RPLNDs are likely to relapse outside retroperitoneum in about 25% patients; they are advised strict follow-up or given two cycles bleomycin, etoposide, cisplatin (BEP). After counseling with this approach the cure rates in stage I NSGCTs are reported to be around 90–100%.[28] The authors reported their short series of 75 patients of stage I NSGCT treated with either RPLND and surveillance in nonrandomized setting with long-term survival of 100% and 93%.[24] Recently, there is a trend towards the use of minimally invasive (laparoscopic or robotic) technique for RPLND with reduced morbidity and hospitalization.[23,27]

Primary chemotherapy: For stage I NSGCT after orchiectomy, BEP × 2 is the usual regimen. Recently, population-based study and randomized clinical trial (RCT) showed equal efficacy of BEP x 1 course as primary chemotherapy;[29] however, this regimen is still under study. Lastly, chemotherapy can be given at a community-based institution with a high chance of relapse-free survival. The only concern is late relapses in these patients which are chemoresistant teratomas and require aggressive surgery as a salvage measure with ensuing morbidity and failure.[27]

Clinical stage IS NSGCT is characterized by elevated post-orchiectomy serum markers without clinical or radiographic evidence of metastatic disease. These tumors are generally treated with induction chemotherapy with over 90% cancer-specific survival.[7,24]

Clinical Stage IIA and IIB NSGCT (Any T N1–2 M0)[23]

The risk of systemic disease is higher in this group of patients. Hence, patients with elevated AFP, hCG post-orchiectomy should receive induction chemotherapy which yields complete response in 60–80% patients. On the other hand, RPLND is preferred initially in patients with risk of retroperitoneal teratoma, who are otherwise at low risk of systemic disease (stage IIA), i.e. normal tumor markers, lymphadenopathy less than 3 cm. For patients with stage IIB and normal markers, induction chemotherapy is better while primary RPLND can be considered in select cases in whom teratoma is suspected. Further post chemotherapy residual masses should undergo RPLND.

Advanced Germ Cell Tumors

Clinical stage IIc and III seminomas and NSGCT (IIc: N3) (III: M1/N1-3 with S2-3): International Germ Cell Cancer Collaborative Group (IGCCCG, 1997)[21] described new risk group stratification for advanced testicular tumors (Flow chart 1) depending on histology, primary site, site of metastasis and serum tumor marker elevation into: good, intermediate and poor risk to predict the outcome to cis-platinum combination chemotherapy. Further, advanced

Flow chart 1: Treatment algorithm for clinical stage IIA and IIB nonseminomatous germ cell tumors (NSGCT)[23]

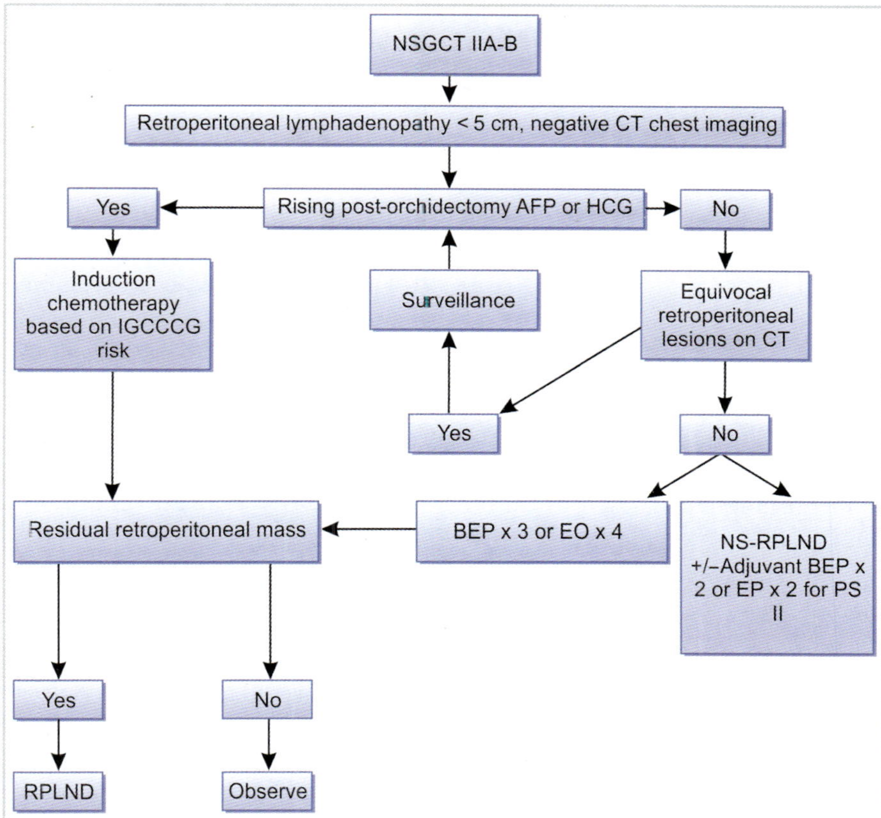

Abbreviations: AFP, alpha-fetoprotein; hCG, human chorionic gonadotropin; IGCCCG, International Germ Cell Cancer Collaborative Group; BEP, bleomycin, etoposide, cisplatin; EP, etoposide plus cisplatin; CT, computed tomography; RPLND, retroperitoneal lymph node dissection

GCT are subcategorized into pure seminoma and non-seminoma which may consist of mixture of seminoma and nonseminoma.

Initial management of advanced GCT: Standard treatment for Stage IIc and III GCT is induction chemotherapy with cisplatin based multi-agent regimen: BEP × 4 cycles (Table 4). However, for *good risk* GCT: (As per IGCCCG risk stratification) BEP × 3 cycles is also found to be equally effective and is the current standard of care.[30] It has been shown that omission of cisplatin to reduce toxicity of the regimen may yield inferior results.[23] Bleomycin can cause pulmonary fibrosis and Raynaud's phenomenon and hence EP × 4 is an acceptable alternative regimen (to BEP × 3) for good risk patients. However, many trials have shown superiority of the bleomycin containing regimen[23] including the vinblastine, actinomycin D, bleomycin (VAB 6) regimen from Memorial Sloan-Kettering Cancer Center (MSKCC).[7]

For *intermediate and poor risk GCT***:** Williams et al. in 1987[31] established BEP × 4 as the standard regimen as the initial therapy based on a randomized trial which included

TABLE 4: Standard chemotherapy regimens for patients with advanced germ cell tumors[23]

Drug combination	*Dosage and schedule*
BEP	
Bleomycin	30 IUS-P IV bolus days 2, 9 and 16
Etoposide	100 mg/m^2 IV (30–60 min), days 1–5
Cisplatin	20 mg/m^2 IV (30–60 min), days 1–5 plus hydration
Repeat cycle every 21 days for 3–4 cycles*	
EP	
Etoposide	100 mg/m^2 IV (30–60 min), days 1–5
Cisplatin	20 mg/m^2 IV (30–60 min), days 1–5 plus hydration
Repeat cycle every 21 days for 4 cycles*	
VIP	
Ifosfamide	1.2 g/m^2 IV days 1–5
Etoposide	75 mg/m^2 IV (30–60 min), days 1–5
Cisplatin	20 mg/m^2 IV (30–60 min), days 1–5 plus hydration
Mesna	400 mg IV bolus prior to first Ifosfamide dose then 1.2 g/m^2 IV infused continuously on days 1–5
Repeat cycle every 21 days for 4 cycles*	

*Therapy should preferably be given every 21 days on schedule without reduction of the doses. There is no role of prophylactic administration of hematopoietic growth factors such as, granulocyte colony-stimulating factor (G-CSF). However, if infectious complications have occurred during chemotherapy, prophylactic administration of G-CSF is recommended for the remaining cycles.

72 patients of poor risk NSGCT. Etoposide, ifosfamide, cisplatin (EIP) × 4 regimen may be substituted in patients with compromised pulmonary function and in whom extensive chest surgery for residual disease is likely.[32] EIP has a high chance of hematological and genitourinary toxicity. The role of high-dose chemotherapy (HDCT) with autologous stem cell support was evaluated and reported by Einhorn et al.[33] In spite of various studies reporting results of HDCT, there is no clear benefit of this regimen hence BEP × 4 still remains the first line of therapy.[23]

Postchemotherapy management: Majority of advanced GCT patients will achieve complete remission (CR) following initial chemotherapy in the form of normalization of markers and regression of metastases (≤ 1 cm) on imaging. These patients need to be followed. However, other 30% may continue to show elevated markers and/or persistent disease on imaging and graded as partial response (PR). Remaining patients with marker positive and disease progression form a minority (15%) group and need salvage chemotherapy.[23,31]

Advanced Seminoma (Table 5)

Post-chemotherapy surgical resection of seminoma is technically challenging due to desmoplastic reaction and carries high morbidity.[34] Currently, these are treated with surveillance or with excision as per need.[23]

Advanced Nonseminoma (Table 6)

Partial responders with normal markers and residual disease need RPLND to achieve a cure.[23,28-30] Pathology of these masses may show fibrosis or necrosis in 40–50% mature or 30–40% in immature teratoma and active or viable cancer in remaining 10–20%.[23] In contrast, in partial responders, with elevated markers viable cancer is reported in 40–80%. In patients with residual disease less than or equal to 1 cm RPLND is advised if teratoma was present in orchiectomy histology. The rationale for this approach lies in their unpredictable growth and malignant transformation in future. Figures 4A to D show post-chemotherapy residual mass and a full bilateral RPLND. Patients with well-defined small masses less than or equal to 5 cm can be treated by local excision to reduce morbidity.[23-30,31] Occasionally, excision of multiple diseased sites may be required, e.g. retroperitoneum, lung nodules and soft tissue metastasis.

Postsurgery chemotherapy is required in patients who had viable disease in the specimen.

GROWING TERATOMA SYNDROME

Rarely (1.9–7.6%), in NSGCTs, some metastatic masses enlarge despite appropriate systemic chemotherapy and normalized serum markers (Logothetis et al.).[35] Histology of these mass lesions reveals benign mature teratomatous elements with no components of viable GCT. Full, bilateral template (nerve sparing, if possible) dissection is recommended as treatment for this condition, so that no residual mass is left behind.[36] Four cases of growing teratoma syndrome has been reported.[37] All had enlarging retroperitoneal masses in the presence of normal serum biomarkers following chemotherapy for

TABLE 5: Treatment algorithm for advanced seminoma IIC/ III[23]

IGCCCG Prognosis	*Good*				*Intermediate*		
Treatment received	3 cycles of BEP (3 or 5 days schedule)*				4 cycles of BEP#		
Status after chemotherapy	CR	Residual tumor < 3 cm			Residual tumor > 3 cm		
Recommendation	Follow- up	PET optional			PET recommended		
		PET done			PET done		
		No	Yes		No	Yes	
			Negative	Positive		Negative	Positive
		Follow-up	Follow-up	Consider resection or alternatively follow-up	Resection or follow-up	Follow-up	Consider resection or alternatively follow-up

*-If bleomycin contraindicated then 3 cycles of VIP or (PEI)
#- If bleomycin contraindicated then 4 cycles of VIP or (PEI)
Abbreviations: IGCCCG, International Germ Cell Cancer Collaborative Group; BEP, bleomycin, etoposide, cisplatin; PET, positron emission tomography; CR, complete remission/response; VIP, ifosfamide, etoposide,cisplatin

TABLE 6: Treatment algorithm for advanced nonseminoma IIC-III (GCT)[23]

IGCCCG Prognosis	*Good*	*Intermediate or poor*
Treatment received	3 cycles of BEP (3 or 5 days schedule)*	4 cycles of BEP#

↓

Result

Result	*Further Treatment*	*Result*	*Further Treatment*
Markers normalized and no residual tumor			Follow-up
Markers normalized and residual but resectable tumor	Resection	R 1/2	Salvage CT
		R0, no viable tumor	Follow-up
		R0, viable tumor < 10 %	Follow-up
		R0, teratoma	Follow-up
		R0, viable tumor > 10%	Consolidation CT (ex VIP 2 cycles)
		R ?, unclear resection margins	
Markers not normalized and residual tumor but potentially resectable	Follow up q 6–12 weeks	Markers normalized or plateau	Resection
		Markers increased	Salvage CT
Markers normalized but irresectable and/or multiple residual tumors	Follow up q 8 weeks	In case of progression	Salvage CT

*-If bleomycin contraindicated then 3 cycles of VIP or (PEI)
#- If bleomycin contraindicated then 4 cycles of VIP or (PEI)
Abbreviations: IGCCCG, International Germ Cell Cancer Collaborative Group. BEP, bleomycin, etoposide, cisplatin; VIP, ifosfamide, etoposide, cisplatin; CT, computed tomography

nonseminomatous tumors. Surgical excision was carried out in all four patients, with long-term survival in all.

SALVAGE THERAPY

At present, it is unclear whether in salvage setting conventional cisplatin therapy is sufficient or should be replaced by HDCT with stem cell rescue.[23] It is therefore important that these patients are treated within clinical trials at higher centers especially when they had initial poor risk disease.

FERTILITY IN TESTICULAR TUMORS

Approximately, 40–70% patients are believed to be at least temporarily hypofertile post orchiectomy prior to further treatment. The exact etiology of this state is unknown however, a cryptorchid state, stress due to diagnosis and high volume cancer are important factors.[38] Further, chemotherapy has profound effect on fertility (azoospermia) and takes almost 2 years to recover spermatogenesis. All patients who desire fertility are advised cryopreservation prior to orchiectomy.[39]

TUMORS IN UNDESCENDED TESTIS

Tumors in undescended testis are seen in about 13% with GCT of the testis in India. Further, by the time these patients present for therapy they are advanced with confluent metastasis in significant numbers of patients. Some of them are so large in size with infiltration of bowel or bladder; primary resection may be difficult, incomplete and may lead to unacceptable morbidity. The authors, therefore, modified their management approach and the outcome analysis is reported elsewhere.[40]

As per the authors' modified approach, after a primary diagnosis based on marker, imaging and FNAC/trucut biopsy, induction chemotherapy (platinum-based) is given followed by delayed orchiectomy and excision of residual masses. It appears logical to believe that initial chemotherapy followed by one-stage surgical removal of the primary and residual metastasis is a favorable option to improve the ultimate outcome, compliance and decrease the incidence of "lost to follow-up".[40]

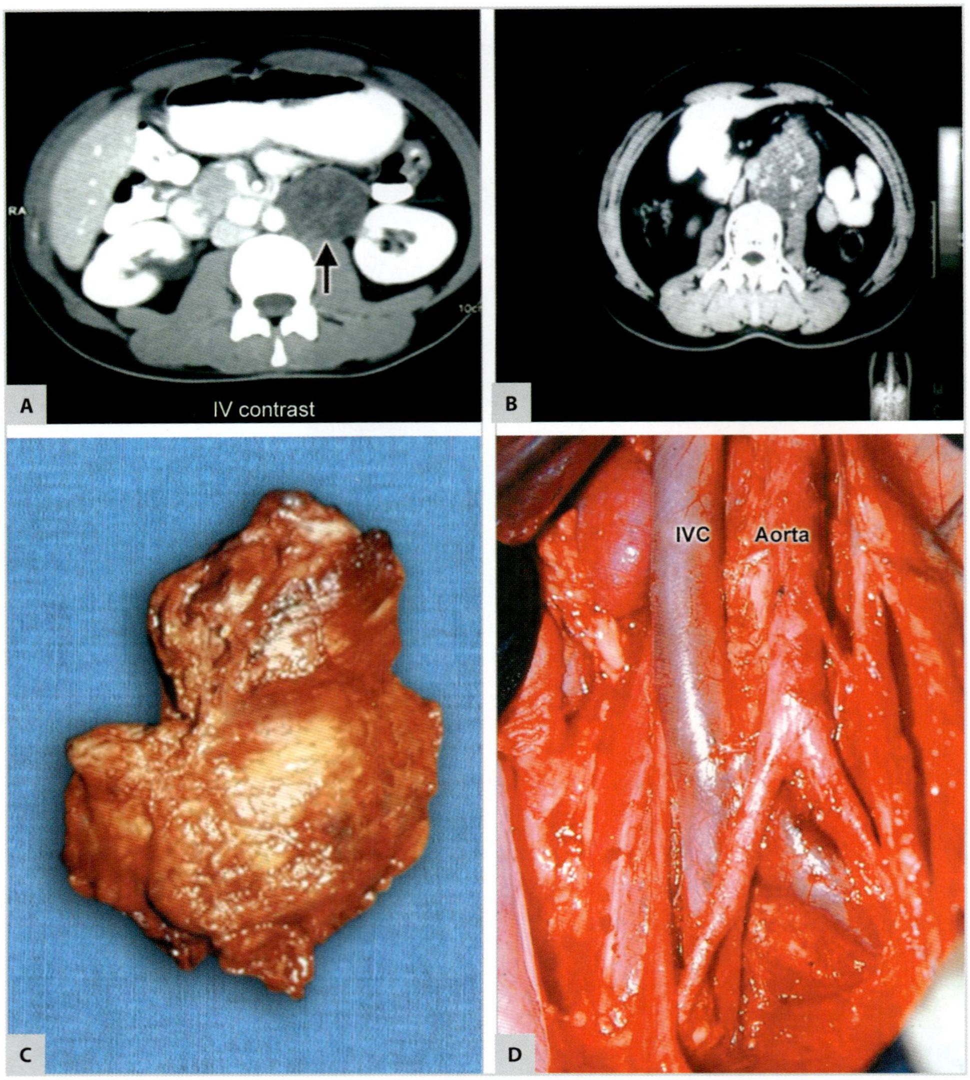

Figs 4A to D: (A) Prechemotherapy mass; (B) Post-chemotherapy mass; (C) Postchemotherapy mass; (D) Full retroperitoneal lymph node dissection (RPLND)

REFERENCES

1. Stephenson AJ, Gilligan TD. Neoplasms of the testis. In: McDougal WS (Ed). Campbell Walsh Urology, Tenth Edition Review. Philadelphia, PA: Elsevier Saunders; 2012. Chapter 31: pp.837-70.
2. Sheinfeld J, Bosl GJ. Surgery of testicular tumors. Campbell Walsh Urology, tenth edition. Elsevier Saunders; 2012. Chapter 32: pp.871-92.
3. Anderson JK, Cadeddu JA. Surgical anatomy of the retroperitoneum, adrenals, kidneys, and ureters. Campbell Walsh Urology, tenth edition. Elsevier Saunders; 2012. Chapter 1: pp.3-32.
4. Kulkarni JN. Cancer of the testes. Indian Journal of Surgery. 1991;52:545-51.
5. Kulkarni JN, Kamat MR, Borges AM. Bilateral synchronous tumors in tests in a previously unrecognized mixed gonadal dysgenesis: a case report and review of literature. Journal of Urology. 1990;143:362-4.
6. Kulkarni JN, Kamat MR. Tumour in undescended testis. Journal of Surgical Oncology. 1991;46:257-60.
7. Bosl GJ, Motzer RJ. Testicular germ-cell cancer. N Engl J Med. 1997;337(4):242-53.
8. Dixon FH, Moore RA. Tumors of the male sex organs. In: Atlas of Tumour Pathology. Washington DC: AFIP; 1952.
9. Mostofi FK. Proceedings: Testicular tumors. Epidemiologic, etiologic and pathologic features. Cancer.1973;32(5):1186-201.

10. Møller H, Prener A, Skakkebaek NE. Testicular cancer, cryptorchidism, inguinal hernia, testicular atrophy, genital malformations: case control studies in Denmark. Cancer Causes Control. 1996;7(2):264-74.

11. Kulkarni JN, Kamat MR. Solitary metastasis to pubic bone from germ cell tumor of the testis: a case report. Tumori. 1991;77(3):271-2.

12. Kulkarni JN, Bhansali MS, Tongoankar HB, et al. Carcinoma in the third testis in a case of poly orchidism and persistent Müllerian structure syndrome. Eur Urol. 1992,22:174-6.

13. Jing B, Wallace S, Zornoza J. Metastases to retroperitoneal and pelvic lymph nodes: computed tomography and lymphangiography. Radiol Clin North Am. 1982:20(3):511-30.

14. Ellis JH, Bies JR, Kopecky KK, et al. Comparison of NMR and CT imaging in the evaluation of metastatic retroperitoneal lymphadenopathy from testicular carcinoma. J Comput Assist Tomogr. 1984;8:709-19.

15. de Wit M, Brenner W, Hartmann M, et al. [18F]-FDG-PET in clinical stage I/II nonseminomatous germ cell tumours: results of the German multicentre trial. Ann Oncol. 2008;19(9):1619-23.

16. Javadpour N. The role of biologic tumor markers in testicular cancer. Cancer. 1980; 45:1755-61.

17. Kulkarni JN, et al. Value of tumour markers in NSGCT of testis. European Urology. 1993;24:168-72.

18. Heidenreich A, Holtl W, Albrecht W, et al. Testis-preserving surgery in bilateral testicular germ cell tumours. Br J Urol.1997;79(2):253-7.

19. Kashyapi BD, Kulkarni JN. Testicular Cancer: Current Management. Bombay Hospital Journal. 1999;41(3):437-45.

20. Sobin LH, Gospodarowicz MK, Wittenkind C (Eds). UICC: International Union Against Cancer TNM Classification of Malignant Tumours, 7th edition. Willey-Blackwell, Oxford;2009. pp. 249-54.

21. International Germ Cell Cancer Collaborative Group. International Germ Cell Consensus Classification: a prognostic factor-based staging system for metastatic germ cell cancers. J Clin Oncol.1997;15:594-603.

22. Bokemeyer C, Kuczyk MA, Serth J, et al. Treatment of clinical stage I testicular cancer and a possible role for new biological prognostic parameters. J Cancer Res Clin Oncol. 1996; 122:575-84.

23. Oscanto S, Richie JP (Eds). Testicular Cancer – International Consultation on Testicular Cancer; 2009. pp.12-3.

24. Tongaonkar HB, Dalal AV, Kelkar DS, et al. Stage I testicular tumours: the Tata Memorial Hospital experience. J Surg Oncol. 1993;54(2):114-8.

25. Vergouwe Y, Steyerberg EW, Eijkemans MJ, et al. Predictors of occult metastasis in clinical stage I nonseminoma: a systematic review. J Clin Oncol. 2003;21:4092-9.

26. Leibovitch L, Foster RS, Kopecky KK, et al. Improved accuracy of computerized tomography based clinical staging in low stage nonseminomatous germ cell cancer: assessment of size criteria of retroperitoneal nodes. J Urol. 1995;154:1759-63.

27. Sogani PC, Perrotti M, Herr HW, et al. Clinical stage I testis cancer: long-term outcome of patients on surveillance. J Urol. 1998;159:855-8.

28. Donohue JP, Foster RS, Rowland RG, et al. Nerve sparing retroperitoneal lymphadenectomy with preservation of ejaculation. J Urol. 1997;15:594-603.

29. Albers P, Siener R, Krege S, et al. Randomized phase III trial comparing retroperitoneal lymph node dissection with one course of bleomycin and etoposide plus cisplatin chemotherapy in the adjuvant treatment of clinical stage I nonseminomatous testicular germ cell tumors: AUO trial AH 01/94 by the German Testicular Cancer Study Group. J Clin Oncol. 2008;26:2966-72.

30. Einhorn LH, Williams SD, Loehrer PJ, et al. Evaluation of optimal duration of chemotherapy in favorable prognosis disseminated germ cell tumors: a Southeastern Cancer Study Group protocol. J Clin Oncol.1989;7:387-91.

31. Williams SD, Birch R, Einhorn LH, et al. Treatment of disseminated germ-cell tumors with cisplatin, bleomycin, and either vinblastine or etoposide. N Engl J Med. 1987;316:1435-40.

32. Nichols CR, Catalano PJ, Crawford ED, et al. Randomized comparison of cisplatin and etoposide and either bleomycin or ifosfamide in treatment of advanced disseminated germ cell tumors: an Eastern Cooperative Oncology Group, Southwest Oncology Group, and Cancer Leukemia Group B Study. J Clin Oncol. 1998;16:1287-93.

33. Einhorn LH, Williams SD, Chamness A, et al. High-dose chemotherapy and stem-cell rescue for metastatic germ-cell tumors. N Engl J Med. 2007;357:340-8.

34. Kamat MR, Kulkarni JN, Tongaonkar HB, et al. Value of retroperitoneal lymph node dissection in advanced testicular seminoma. J Surg Oncol. 1992;51(1):65-7.

35. Logothetis CJ, Samuels ML, Trindade A, et al. The growing teratoma syndrome. Cancer. 1982;50:1629-35.

36. Gorbatiy V, Spiess PE, Pisters LL. The growing teratoma syndrome: Current review of the literature. Indian J Uro . 2009;25(2):186-9.

37. Tongaonkar HB, Deshmane VH, Dalal AV, et al. Growing teratoma syndrome. J Surg Oncol. 1994;55(1):56-60.

38. Foster RS, Donohue JP. Fertility in testicular cancer patients-AUA update series, Lesson19, Volume XIV;1995.

39. Spermon JR, Kiemeney LA, Meuleman EJ, et al. Fertility in men with testicular germ cell tumors. Fertil Steril. 2003;79:1543-9.

40. Kulkarni JN, Desai SM, Phadke GK, et al. Improved management of abdominal undescended testicular tumors with bulky confluent retroperitoneal nodal metastases. J Urol. 1996; 156(4):1341-4.

47 Stoma Care

Harikesh Buch, Carlo Pezcoller, Louise Forest Lalande

INTRODUCTION

Word "stoma" means mouth or opening in the Greek language. Most ostomy surgery means an artificial opening created by surgeons for voiding of stool or urine for various indications. Broadly speaking, diversion stomas are: (a) fecal stoma (colostomy or ileostomy) and (b) urinary stoma are known as urostomy. Preoperative preparation for a stoma creation includes the selection of the most optimal site for the stoma, while preoperative counseling prepares the patient mentally for life with a stoma. The surgeon and the enterostomal therapist should emphasize that a stoma does not hinder a normal lifestyle.

DEVELOPMENT OF STOMA APPLIANCE AND STOMA CARE

Although creating a collecting system for patients who had undergone stoma surgery was first investigated in 1824, production of stoma appliances did not occur until the 1930s and 1940s. Until 1934, there was no real stoma appliance to collect urine that was diverted to skin; but in 1944, the invention of the rubber bag for collecting waste products from the body created a new era for the care of patients with a stoma. The American surgeon Dr Rupert Turnbull from the Cleveland Clinic in Ohio was the first to realize that people with a stoma needed specialized care. In 1958, he trained one of his patients, Ms Norma Gill to be a stoma therapist and in 1961, he established the first stoma training program. In England, the first training program for stoma therapy was established in 1972 in London, and Scandinavia followed in 1980 with the first school founded in Gothenburg, Sweden. Similar schools exist today in many countries of the world except in Africa.

INCIDENCE OF STOMAS

Among the ostomies created, most common stoma is the colostomy. Ileostomy and urostomy surgery is less commonly performed. Estimated figures of members of ostomy associations in India reveals among their members about 65–70% are colostomates, 20–25% are ileostomates and less than 5% are urostomates.

MARKING THE STOMA SITE AND CREATION OF IDEAL STOMA

Marking the Stoma Site

This procedure represents the most important preoperative phase. The surgeons must remember that stoma can be created by them in 20 minutes but patients have to live with a stoma for the rest of his/her life; therefore, a properly created stoma at the correct site is absolutely a must. A badly sited stoma may give rise to situations that are sometimes impossible to manage and may require a further operation to be performed immediately or some time later. Adaptation in life of patients with a stoma depends to a great extent on how easily they can manage the stoma appliance and avoid leakage. The stoma should be adapted to the patient not the other way around. Among other things, this means that the stoma must be sited where the person will find it easiest to care for, i.e. the person must be able to see the stoma and be able to reach it to change appliance. At least half of the patients seen in the stoma clinic with peristomal skin problems, leaks or difficulty in appliance adhesion, suffer from a surgeon induced complication that could have been prevented by appropriate preoperative location of the stoma.

In planned surgical procedures, the stoma site should be marked 2 days prior to surgery. This is especially important if the patient is very thin, since the abdomen may change shape with preoperative bowel preparation. The marking is done jointly by the enterostomal therapist (ET) or stoma care trained nurse, surgeon and patient. In routine situations, marking begins with identifying the "ostomy triangle" bounded by the anterior superior iliac spine, the pubic tubercle and the umbilicus. The stoma, ileostomy traditionally on the right and colostomy on the left, is placed in the center of this triangle, through the rectus muscle slightly below the umbilicus. Ideally, after determining the appropriate site for stoma (Figs 1A and B), the patient should wear a water-filled ostomy bag under his/her clothing to assess the comfort level. The patient will need to lie down, stand, sit, crouch and bend forward and sideways so that all postures are taken into consideration for the comfort of the patient and reliable adhesion of the appliance. Patients undergoing pelvic exenteration require two stomas. The urinary stoma should be placed higher than the fecal stoma if a belt needs to be worn with the stoma bag. Keeping the stomas on different horizontal planes will avoid the possibility of the ostomy belt traumatizing the other stoma. Only in emergency surgical cases when there is a possibility of creating stomas as a part of surgical procedure, surgeons must mark the stoma site on abdomen prior to laparotomy. On the operating table when the abdomen has been opened, trying to select a proper stoma site is at best, hit or miss and often leads to a bad placement of the stoma that jeopardizes a good stoma care.

The correct sitting should permit: (1) a reduction in stoma complications; (2) easier management of the stoma by the patient; (3) correct and effective adhesion and application of the bag; and (4) effective irrigation later on if required. Therefore, the following must be avoided:

- Bone protuberances
- Folds of skin (in the obese, watch out for adipose apron)
- The belt line
- Any previous scars
- The laparotomy incision, any areas of the abdomen damaged in any way.

The following factors should be kept in mind while deciding the stoma site:

Physiological Factors

The stoma should transects (come out through) the rectus abdominis muscle. This will provide muscle fibers to keep the intestinal loop in place and might help to prevent it from prolapse and forming a sliding hernia.

The Patient's Body Contours

For the adhesive to adhere around a stoma, it should have at least 10 cm of smooth surface around it. This means that the stoma should not be sited in immediate proximity to natural body contours (folds) and skin creases, scars and bony prominences. The distance to the umbilicus must be sufficient to ensure that the adhesive does not cover the umbilicus. In women with large, heavy breasts, the stoma should not be sited where the breasts will cover it. In obese patients, the stoma should be sited on the upper part of the abdomen to ensure that the patient can see the stoma. In most patients who have lost weight in the period prior to surgery (commonly seen in cancer patients) it must be taken into account that the patient will typically regain weight after surgery, so the stoma should not be sited too low. The stoma should not be formed near old hernias as these may increase the risk of complications.

Any Disability

If the patient has a physical disability requiring the use of disability aids, like for example a wheelchair, the stoma should be marked while the patient is seated in

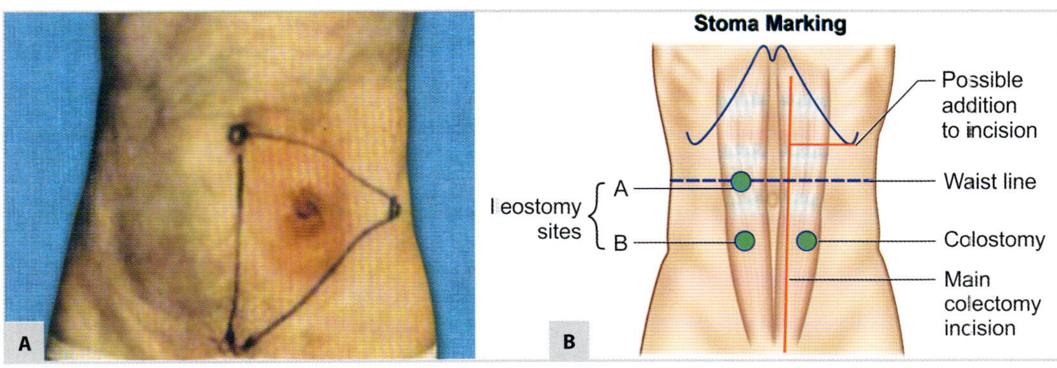

Figs 1A and B: (A) Correctly placed stoma which has served the patient well for many years; (B) Stoma marking

the wheelchair. The stoma should be sited anywhere on the abdomen that will make it easy to see and manage. If the patient already has one stoma, the second stoma, if required, must not be positioned along the same vertical or horizontal line as the existing stoma, as this will make it impossible to use ostomy products (pouch) without disturbing the others

The Operative Scar

In the past, the stoma was often created on the laparotomy incision. Today it is always sited laterally with respect to the incision in order to avoid the risk of contamination and to permit the immediate application of ostomy appliance and make it easy to use stoma pouches in the future. The distance from the operative scar (and old scars) must be sufficient to allow the base plate to be attached without the scar getting in the way. If the stoma is sited too close to the operative scar itself, the skin around the stoma (peristomal skin) will be uneven and the adhesive will not adhere properly to the skin. This increases the risk of leakage under the base plate. Any leakage is generally regarded as being a major inconvenience as it will cause peristomal skin complications

Occupational Factors

Working posture and the actual work duties can influence stoma sitting which should be done at the site where patient will have good comfort level and will have a good adhesion of the stoma bag

Vision

Ability to see the stoma is an important consideration in patients with poor vision because this will make it difficult to apply stoma appliance. They will need a special training and should be taught to use a simple to use appliance

Clothing

The stoma must be sited so as not to interfere in the type of clothing usually worn by the patient. In the majority of cases, this means that it needs to be sited below the waistline where it would otherwise be exposed to friction from the waistband or belt. In people from certain cultures who wear leggings or saris for example, where most of the garment is concentrated around the waist, the stoma should ideally be sited away from this area

Cultural Background

Muslims pray about five times a day. This is done kneeling with the trunk bent forward. For Muslims it will, therefore, be more appropriate to position the stoma above the navel in order to avoid leakage.

Stoma Site will be Different Depending on the Type of Ostomy

- Ileostomy: The ideal position is located approximately in the middle of the line joining the umbilicus to the right anterior superior iliac spine
- Right transverse colostomy: The ideal position is located approximately in the middle of the line joining the umbilicus to the outer edge of the right costal arch
- Left transverse colostomy: The ideal position is located approximately in the middle of the line joining the umbilicus to the outer edge of the left costal arch
- Left colostomy: The ideal position is located approximately in the middle of the line joining the umbilicus to the left anterior superior iliac spine
- Urostomy (Bricker technique): the ideal position is located approximately in the middle of the line joining the umbilicus to the right anterior superior iliac spine.

Creation of a Good Stoma

Intestinal stomas are created by surgeons in a few minutes as compared to the main surgical procedure; but it always leaves behind the most lasting impact upon the patient's life. When the patient has been discharged from the hospital and has fully recovered from surgery the predominant memory and change in the patient's lifestyle will be directly caused by the stoma. Whether temporary or permanent, and the type of stoma like ileostomy, colostomy or urostomy, it will require more of the patient's attention than any other aspects brought about by surgery. The process not only involves the surgical steps of making the stoma, but also involves choosing the correct stoma site and identifying the appropriate intestinal segment. Therefore, attention to details during the preoperative planning and construction of a stoma will help reduce postoperative difficulties and complications from stomas.

Unfortunately, stoma creation is often regarded as the least important part of an operation, which may be delegated to the most junior member of the operating team. "Delegating stoma creation to an unsupervised junior surgical resident, who has minimal experience of creating a stoma, is never appropriate;" but this happens very often. This vastly underscores its importance when considering the multitude of complications; a poorly constructed stoma has major impact on the patient's quality of life. This delegation of responsibility to junior resident implies that the surgeon is only concerned about "saving the patient's life," but not the "quality of patient's life." The creation of a good stoma requires a team approach including the operating surgeon, surgical trainees, an enterostomal therapist and surgical support staff. It is an excellent opportunity for education and if well done, will be a learning experience for the surgical team and will reduce the impact of the stoma on the future of the ostomate's quality of life. This should be remembered and emphasized throughout the entire process of stoma creation.

INDICATION FOR INTESTINAL STOMA SURGERY

Stoma for fecal diversion is created either in emergency or elective surgery and may be temporary or permanent.

Elective indications for creation of colostomy are most commonly due to low rectal cancers, which require an "abdominoperineal resection" (APR). Other indications for an elective colostomy include protection of a low colorectal or coloanal anastomosis, rectovaginal fistula, incontinence, radiation proctitis, perianal sepsis, etc. Indications for emergency creation of an ileostomy are generally due to conditions requiring small bowel or proximal colon resection, in which the integrity of a primary anastomosis would be compromised. This may be due to a long-standing peritonitis or obstruction, radiation injury to small bowel or Crohn's disease. Other emergency indications for an ileostomy are hemorrhage, ischemia, perforation or sepsis. This includes neonates who develop intestinal perforation due to necrotizing enterocolitis with resection of the involved segment and ileostomy.

An elective ileostomy is commonly used for patients undergoing surgery for rectal cancer, inflammatory bowel disease or familial polyposis. These patients require the removal of the rectum and possibly the entire colon as well. The ileostomy may be used as an alternative to a colostomy for fecal diversion, proximal to a low colorectal or coloanal anastomosis, or proximal to an ileal pouch and anal anastomosis. In cases where a total proctocolectomy is necessary and the anal sphincter cannot be salvaged, an ileostomy is the only option for fecal diversion. A cecostomy is only indicated as an emergency measure to decompress the distal colon. This is done for the critically ill patient with massive colonic dilatation with impending colonic perforation. It may be due to an obstructing cancer or a pseudo-obstruction seen in elderly and immunocompromized patients. It can also be used for cecal and right-sided colon injuries.

PREOPERATIVE PREPARATIONS

Preoperative counseling, stoma marking and informed consent is very important for stoma surgery. In elective surgery a meeting with another ostomate (according to type of stoma, age, sex and occupation match ostomate who is also called visitor) will resolve most of the issues that patient might have, when patient has to face the possibility of having a stoma. The goal of the meeting is to reinforce the information given by the surgeon and provide real-life experiences of patients with a stoma. Correct stoma placement and its creation increase the ability to care for the stoma and maintain a secure pouch without leakage for few days.

Selecting the Stoma Type

Following factors should be considered when selecting which type of stoma should be created for a particular patient and condition:

- The indication for the stoma (fecal diversion, intestinal decompression or urinary diversion)
- The site of intestinal pathology
- Available stoma sites
- Patient body contours (obesity)
- Complications related to specific stoma configurations
- Ease of caring for the stoma
- If required, difficulty of subsequent stoma reversal.

Ileostomy patients are more prone to metabolic problems such as chronic dehydration, electrolyte imbalance, cholelithiasis and nephrolithiasis. This is an even greater concern in patients with short bowel due to prior resection and patients receiving chemotherapy. In these cases, a colostomy is a better option if available. It is generally easier to care for an ileostomy than a loop colostomy. An ileostomy requires more frequent appliance changes than a colostomy, and the odor of the ileostomy effluent is much less offensive than a colostomy. Ileostomy effluent is also more damaging to a patient's skin because it has active digestive enzymes. Colostomies are also more prone to prolapse than ileostomies, especially transverse loop colostomies. Although colostomies have several disadvantages in caring for them, end colostomy irrigation can eliminate the output from the stoma for as much as 24–48 hours. During this period, the patient may elect to cover the colostomy with a gauze dressing rather than wear an appliance, which would require emptying several times each day.

Although many stomas are intended to be temporary, nearly half of all stomas are not reversed. Therefore, it is important to create the most appropriate stoma with the fewest complications and difficulties in management to optimize patient satisfaction and quality of life.

TECHNIQUE OF CREATION OF STOMA

Ideally stoma should be a protruding, tension free and well-vascularized (pink). Common initial surgical steps for most types of stomas are showing in Figure 2. The abdomen should be opened in the midline to have options to make a stoma at a suitable place. The segment of intestine to be brought out as a stoma is adequately mobilized with the mesentery with utmost care to preserve the blood supply of the end of the intestinal segment.

The layers of the abdominal wall are oriented together by placing a clamp on the dermis and the fascia and pulling them medially. A folded big sponge is placed under the proposed stoma site to protect the viscera. The skin, both clamps and sponge are all held in the non-dominant hand throughout the creation of the aperture.

A small circular incision, about 2 cm in diameter, is made at the designated site. The epidermis and dermis are removed, and the subcutaneous fat is preserved and divided with diathermy (electrocautery) in a vertical direction. Preservation of the subcutaneous fat provides support for the stoma and helps to maintain it in an everted position. The vertical incision is continued through the subcutaneous fat down to the anterior rectus sheath. Exposure is provided with two right angle retractors, which are frequently repositioned as the incision is deepened.

A cruciate incision is made in the anterior rectus sheath with each limb being about 3 cm. The rectus muscle is split in the direction of its fibers using a curved clamp to expose the posterior rectus sheath. This is done to avoid injury to the inferior epigastric vessels and unnecessary bleeding.

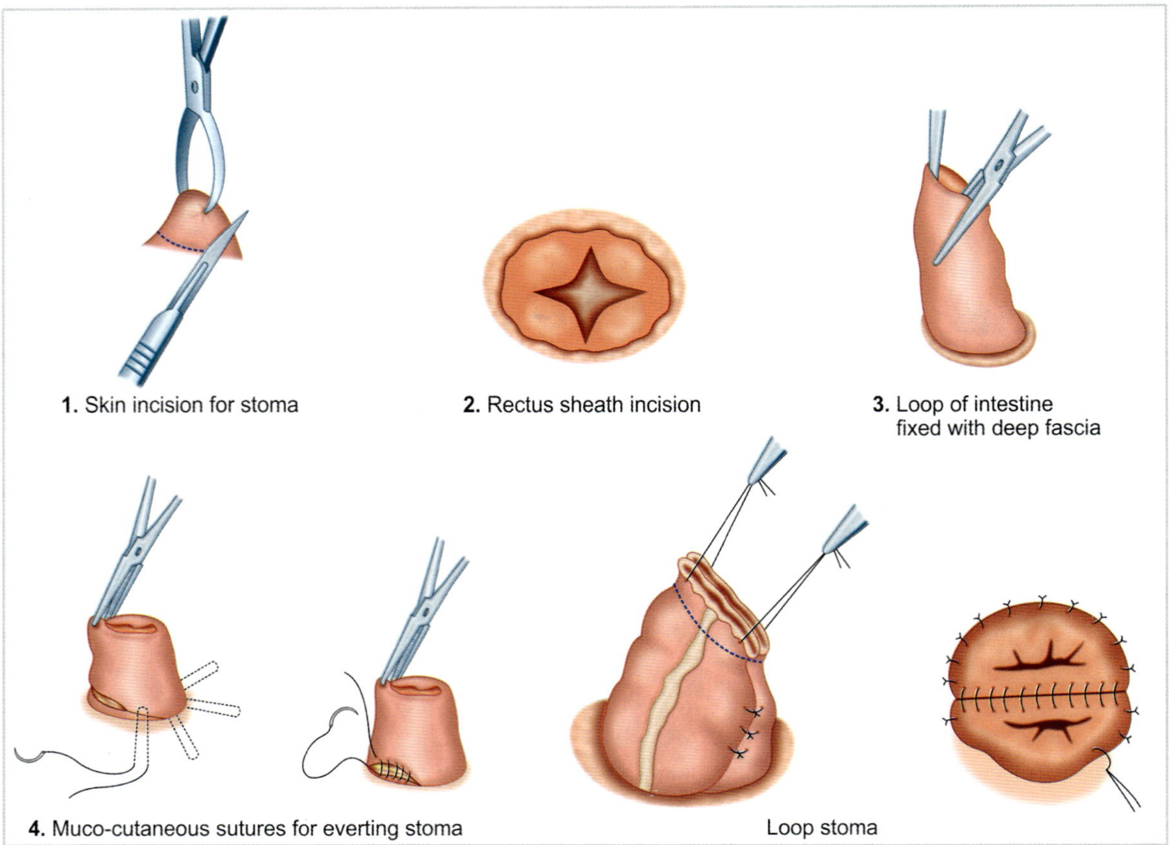

Fig. 2: Surgical steps for creation of stomas

Once the posterior rectus sheath is identified, a longitudinal incision is made through this layer and the peritoneum. The folded laparotomy sponge protects the viscera. The opening in the abdominal wall should allow operating surgeon's two fingers to pass easily. The aperture is then inspected from both the internal and external surfaces for bleeding, especially from the rectus muscle. Placing the curved clamp through the aperture and using it as a handle to expose the internal surface of the aperture facilitates inspection. Prior to removing the clamp, the laparotomy sponge should be pulled through the aperture and clamped to itself to maintain the path for the bowel. This type of opening, in the rectus sheath inferior to the umbilicus, allows the stoma to be passed through the strongest portion of the abdominal musculature and the strongest fascia. This will help reduce postoperative complications such as parastomal hernia and stomal prolapse.

The bowel selected for the stoma is then delivered through the aperture, avoiding tension or torsion of the bowel. Care must be taken when delivering the bowel through the aperture. Excessive external pulling with clamps or drains may damage the bowel wall or tear the mesentery and cause bleeding. This is most often encountered with narrow apertures, obese patients, and large appendices epiploicae. Reducing the size of the appendices, pushing the bowel up from within the abdomen, and increasing aperture size may help.

End Colostomy

An end colostomy is usually located in the left lower quadrant. An end colostomy is typically created during an abdominoperineal resection for low rectal cancer or with a sigmoid colectomy, with a closure of rectum which is left behind in the abdomen, for diverticulitis (Hartmann's procedure). For an adequate length of the colon to be brought through the abdominal wall without tension, the left colon and sigmoid colon should be mobilized on its mesentery and detached from its lateral peritoneal reflection. This may include mobilization of the splenic flexure in special circumstances like obese patient or short sigmoid mesentery. Obese patients have larger abdominal wall depth and require the additional length obtained from detaching the splenic flexure. If the inferior mesenteric artery requires ligation, the entire sigmoid colon must be removed because its arterial blood flow has been divided. The end of the descending colon is used for the stoma because its blood supply is not compromised as its blood supply is through the marginal artery which is based on the middle colic artery. It is extremely important to confirm that the distal end of the colon bleeds with a well pulsatile arterial blood flow by removing the clamp applied on its end or the colon should be transected more proximally; this may be affected by an excessively narrow aperture, atherosclerosis or tension on the bowel.

After the aperture has been made in the abdominal wall as described previously, the closed end of the colon is grasped with Babcock clamps and brought through it gently, without rotation or tension. The colon should protrude about 3–4 cm from the skin. Some surgeons take tacking sutures between the fascia and colonic wall, but these are not necessary. Small defects between the colonic mesentery and the lateral abdominal wall should be closed to prevent internal hernia; large defects can be left open. After completing the intraabdominal portion of the operation and closing and covering the abdominal incision, the colostomy is matured. The end of the colostomy is opened and matured by using approximately eight absorbable sutures between the full-thickness colon and the dermis of the abdominal wall; it is helpful to create a nipple type colostomy.

Loop Colostomy

A loop colostomy is usually made using the transverse or sigmoid colon. The transverse loop colostomy tends to be placed in the right or left upper quadrants through an adequate transverse incision. Only if required the colon may be mobilized, by detaching the adjacent flexure. The greater omentum is divided over the transverse colon to allow the colon to be brought through the aperture without the omentum. A small opening is made in the mesentery of the colon near the edge of the bowel wall with a curved hemostat. An umbilical tape or red rubber catheter is passed through this defect. The tape or catheter and colon are passed through the abdominal wall carefully ensuring that there is no tension on the colon. After the colon has been delivered, a T-shaped or straight glass rod is placed through the mesentery. As with an end colostomy, the remainder of the operation is completed and the abdominal wound is closed and protected.

The loop colostomy is then matured, by opening it longitudinally along one of the taenia coli. Fecal diversion can be enhanced by the use of the stoma rod and creating the colostomy mostly in the bowel proximal to the rod. This results in a very small eccentrically placed opening over the distal bowel. The end of the rod can be tacked to the skin so that it does not slip out from under the colon prematurely. Full-thickness bowel is then sutured to the dermis using absorbable sutures. The transparent drainable one piece colostomy appliance is placed hanging to the side to avoid wound contamination. The rod can be removed after three days providing the rod is loose. It may be necessary to leave the rod in place longer for obese or malnourished patients.

Cecostomy

A cecostomy is created for the critically ill patient with massive colonic distention due to an obstructing cancer or a pseudo-obstruction. These operations are typically done urgently and the anatomy is distorted due to the distention. The incision is made directly over the dilated cecum, and this location can be determined preoperatively by placing a radiopaque marker on the umbilicus and obtaining an abdominal film. The incision is carried through the fascia and peritoneum. Once the cecum is identified, a series of interrupted peritoneal-seromuscular sutures are placed at appropriate locations, which will allow the cecum to reach the skin when opened. Once the cecum is sealed off from the rest of the abdominal cavity, it is needle decompressed to reduce the tension on the intestinal wall. The cecum is then incised and opened, and its full-thickness bowel wall is sutured to the dermis. The disadvantage of this approach is that it does not allow for full abdominal exploration to assess for bowel viability.

An alternative to a formal cecostomy is a tube cecostomy. A tube cecostomy can be constructed using a large-bore Foley or Malecot catheter. The catheter is secured within the cecum using two purse-string sutures and brought out through a separate stab incision. The cecum is also tacked to the abdominal wall at this location. A formal cecostomy does not close spontaneously and requires an operation to close the colocutaneous fistula. The advantage of a tube cecostomy is that it will frequently close spontaneously. However, the tube needs to be irrigated often to maintain patency because the tube tends to clog with feces and will occasionally leak around the drain.

End Ileostomy

The surgical steps to create an end ileostomy should be followed up meticulously as the ileal effluent is a high-volume liquid containing active digestive enzymes. The stoma location should be determined preoperatively, and it should be of a nipple type to allow for precise appliance placement and the stomal opening will be above skin level to minimize the chances of the leakage of effluent. The abdominal opening is made in the right lower quadrant with the technique previously described as in end colostomy. The distal ileum is brought gently through the opening while assuring that there is no rotation or tension. The end of the ileum should protrude 6 cm from the skin. The mesentery should be sutured to the peritoneum to close the right paracolic space to prevent volvulus of the prestomal bowel, and reduce the possibility of internal herniation. The remainder of the intraabdominal operation is completed and the incision is closed and protected. The staple line is removed from the end of the ileum and an adequate blood supply is confirmed. At the base of the ileal loop where it comes out of skin aperture, the seromuscular coat should be tacked with subcutaneous and dermis layer with sutures in four quadrants. Next, a protruding, everting ileostomy is created by suturing full-thickness ileum at the cut end to the seromuscular coat at the stomal base and then to the dermis in four quadrants (Figs 3A to C). The mesenteric fat should not be removed because this may compromise the stoma's blood supply. An additional four sutures are placed between the first four, excluding the seromuscular bite. Sutures through the epidermis should be avoided because this may result in the formation of mucosal islands in the skin beneath the appliance and prevent proper appliance adherence due to the moisture placed between the appliance and skin. After completing the stoma, the transparent drainable one piece appliance is placed (to observe the status of stoma initially) with the pouch hanging to the side to prevent wound contamination and ease of emptying.

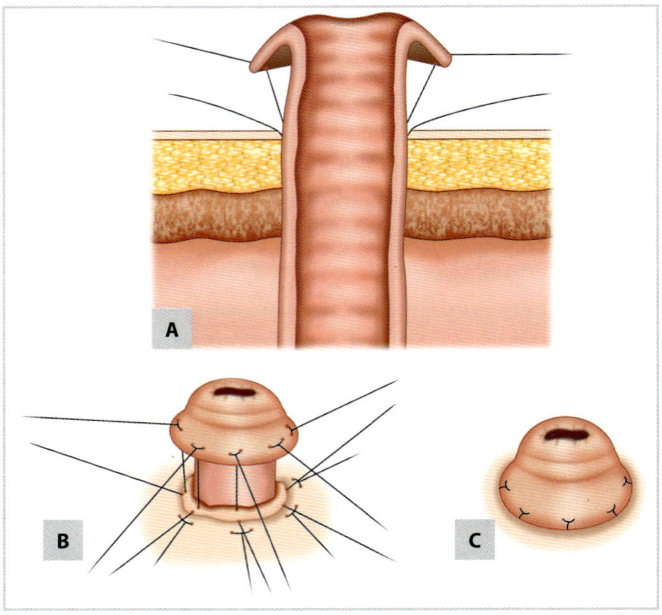

Figs 3A to C: Everted end ileostomy creation

Loop Ileostomy

The loop ileostomy is indicated when both fecal diversion and distal decompression are required. It has the additional advantage of being able to be reversed without a reexploration. The location is the same as that for an end ileostomy. First, orienting sutures are placed on the proximal and distal end of the ileum. One can use a different colored dyed suture proximal to the proposed ostomy site and distal to the site. A small mesenteric opening is created with a curved hemostat through which an umbilical tape is passed. The tape and ileum are delivered through the abdominal opening. Normally if a total proctocolectomy and pelvic pouch has been performed, the proximal (functional) end is placed in the superior position, while the distal end is placed inferiorly. If the IC junction is still present, the loop is better oriented with the functional end in the inferior position.

A rod is placed through the mesenteric opening and it is sutured in place with absorbable suture. The remainder of the intraabdominal operation is completed and the abdominal incision is closed and protected. The ileostomy is opened transversely (Figs 4A to C), making a four-fifths circumferential opening 1 cm from the skin margin on the recessive limb. The recessive limb is matured first, using three interrupted sutures between the full-thickness cut edge and the dermis. The lateral and medial sutures in the recessive limb are placed eccentrically in the inferior half of the stoma aperture to narrow the opening. The functional limb is then matured with five sutures between the full-thickness cut edge of bowel and the dermis. The central stitch is placed first, the medial and lateral sutures near the stoma rod are next, and medial and lateral sutures between central and "rod" sutures are placed last. The blunt end of a short forceps is used to evert the bowel by placing it between the two opposed serosal surfaces of the functional limb and pushing gently away from the skin. The sutures are tied in the same order as they were placed. A transparent drainable appliance is placed, hanging to the side, on the stoma and the rod is removed in a few days.

Urostomy (Bricker Technique)

The procedure is just like the end ileostomy done in right iliac fossa.

After completing the radical resection of the bladder, involving a section of the bowel as an outlet duct, the ureters are detached from the bladder and stitched to a 20–25 cm section taken from the small or large intestine. One end of the section is sutured, while the other end is brought out to the abdominal skin, where this will form a nipple type stoma. The section of intestine is too small to act as a reservoir, and there is no muscle like in Caffey's procedure or valve as in Kock's reservoir to retain urine.

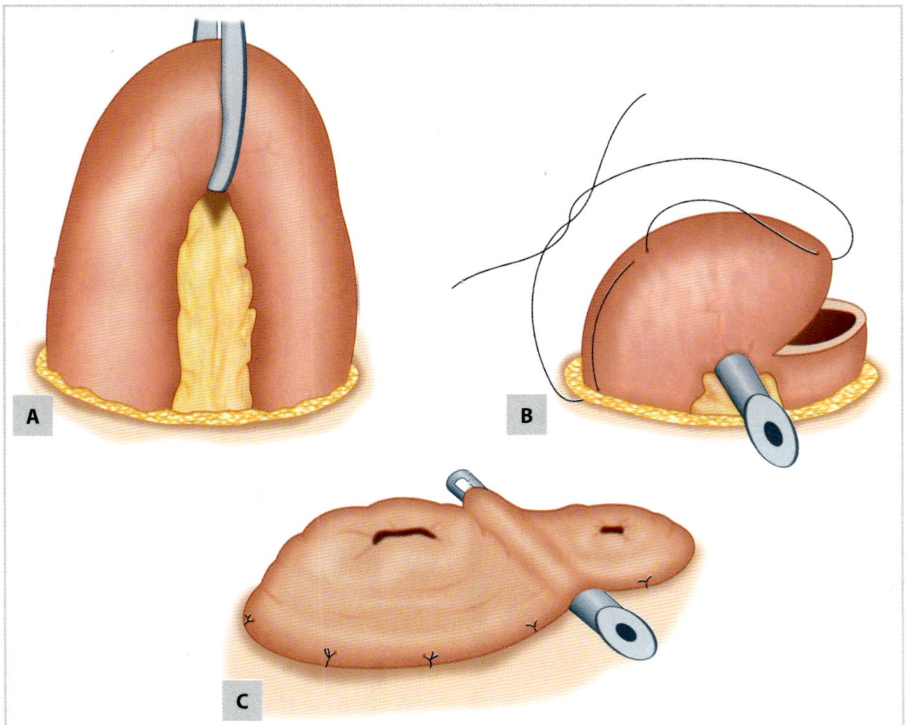

Figs 4A to C: Creation of loop ileostomy

Therefore, urine will flow out as fast as it is produced in the kidneys. Because of this, the patient will need to wear a bag constantly to collect urine from the stoma. In the majority of cases, a Bricker bladder will start working immediately after the operation, the urine will flow through urostomic stents, passing through the ileal conduit to the outside surface of the abdomen protecting the ureteric intestinal anastomoses. The ideal height of the stoma is 2 cm in order to make the bag easier to attach, so that urine does not seep under the adhesive, causing it to fall off. Anatomically, the ureters are positioned in such a way that there are fewer complications if the Bricker bladder is sited on the right-hand side, which is usually also the most convenient for right-handed patients.

Use of Appliances in Urostomy

To ensure proper healing of ureteric anastomosis with the intestinal loop used for construction of urostomy, ureteric stents are placed in each ureters for the first 10 days or so. The catheters will extend from the kidneys out through the stoma and down into the bag. About 4–5 days after the operation, the catheters will typically be cut off so that they protrude just 4–5 cm from the stoma. This will make it easier for the patient to start learning to change the bag and baseplate. Postoperatively, these stents are removed after 10–15 days.

PREOPERATIVE AND POSTOPERATIVE COUNSELING

It is extremely important for the surgeon and an ET nurse to do preoperative and postoperative counseling of the patient who is likely to have a stoma after surgery. By doing this, they can facilitate early acceptance of stoma by the patient which in turn will enhance the early rehabilitation process of the patient. The best way to build up the confidence of the patient, about the living with a stoma and answer all the questions that the patient will have would be to arrange a meeting with another ostomate (also called a visitor, preferably age, sex and occupation match). During preoperative counseling, the diagnosis of the disease, its surgical management and the necessity of creation of stoma should be explained to the patient and family members by the surgeon in presence of the stoma nurse.

When the patient has recovered from surgery and discharge is planned, counseling by the stoma nurse and surgeon is mandatory. Patient and care givers should be taught about how to change a stoma appliance and details of stoma care must be given. We should make sure that patient and care givers are familiar with different types of stoma appliances and ostomy products and where to get them. They should also get information about ostomy support groups locally and nationally.

COMMON STOMA COMPLICATIONS AND ITS MANAGEMENT

Stoma complications can present early, after a few days or later. Early stoma complications are malposition, edema, ischemia, retraction, peristomal suppuration and fistulas. Late complications are stenosis, prolapse, parastomal hernia, granulomas, skin lesions, etc.

Improper Stoma Sitting

Malpositioning of the stoma is a rather frequent problem and demonstrates haste on the part of the surgeon or a lack of collaboration between the surgeon and the ET. The creation of a stoma in a surgical incision, near costal cartilage or iliac crest makes it difficult to apply a stoma appliance properly leading to leakage between the stoma adhesive surface and skin which will result in peristomal skin erosions. This will lead to further problems of improper adhesion of ostomy bags with the peristomal skin because of oozing from peristomal skin surface (wet surface). Therefore, it is important to have stoma marking at proper site prior to planned surgery or preoperatively by surgeon prior to emergency laparotomy which may require a creation of stoma. It is also important to mobilize sufficient length of corresponding intestinal loop with adequate blood supply to create a stoma at a proper site.

Ischemia of Stoma

Commonly, this happens in the immediate postoperative period. If it happens the following changes in stoma are observed: from the first hours the stoma appears cyanotic, then becomes blackish, then light brown-greenish in color and finally mucocutaneous separation occurs. This phenomenon can involve the entire loop or only a part. Most common causes of these complications are ligation of main artery to the loop of intestine forming a stoma, excessive skeletonization of this loop or inadequate mobilization of the intestine resulting into excessive tension on the stoma. If the necrosis involves the entire stoma below the fascial plane, the patient must be operated on immediately to avoid a perforative peritonitis. This involves surgical interventions that are laborious and often performed urgently. The surgeon, faced with the impossibility of considering the optimal position, is forced to rebuild the stoma where he can. But if the necrosis is partial, the treatment will be conservative. It is important to gently clean the lesion with mild disinfectant and to use appropriate collecting bags. Often it is possible to perform limited resections of the necrotic parts, carrying out small touch-ups on the stoma, under local anesthesia.

Stoma Retraction

The process of retraction of the stoma starts in the operating room. It is because of an inadequate mobilization of the corresponding intestinal loop resulting into excessive tension on the stoma or inadequate blood supply to the stoma. This can lead to improper fitting of the stoma appliance resulting in a leakage of stoma output and all the complication related to leakage. In the past, this required redoing of the stoma which was a major surgical procedure in itself. But now a day, because of the availability of stoma paste or stoma strips and convex ostomy bags, the resultant retraction can be managed easily, but it increases the cost of stoma management.

Peristomal Suppuration

This can be primary due to intraoperative contamination or secondary to stomal dehiscence. Management is conservative if possible by drainage of pus, cleaning of suppurated area, use of disinfectants, removal of necrotic parts, use of gauze plug and the use of cutaneous protective barriers.

Stomal Stenosis

There can be early stenosis or late stenosis of the stoma. It can be at skin level or at the level of deep fascia or inside the abdomen. It can present many different symptoms like painful and difficult evacuation, difficulty in irrigation, abdominal distension and difficulty in doing endoscopy or fecal impaction. Treatment of mild stenosis can be repeated dilation with finger or with dilators. Severe cases will require step wise surgical correction as shown in pictures.

Stomal Prolapse

Incidence of stomal prolapse is 1–16%. Defunctioning loop stoma has high incidence of prolapse. It can be partial mucosal or can be full-thickness large prolapse. It can produce problems like unsightful (cosmetic), bleeding, ulceration of mucosa, difficulty in pouch application and difficult to maintain hygiene due to continuous discharge of serous fluid. The most serious complication it can produce, though uncommon, is strangulation of prolapsed part. This will commonly occur when two piece system is used with a rigid ring on the base plate. Therefore, the use of this type of stoma appliance should be avoided. In most cases, strangulation can be resolved with delicate reduction maneuvers, squeezing the prolapsed loop with two hands. It is best to teach this procedure to the patient or family members so that it can be applied immediately when it occurs.

Parastomal Hernia

A parastomal hernia develops when there is a total or partial detachment of the stomal loop from the fascial plane. Intestinal loops and/or the omentum protrude through this breach, forming a subcutaneous bulge that can obstruct the correct fit of the appliance. It is more like a sliding hernia. Incidence in ileostomy is low and is between 2–10% where in colostomy it is between 5–15%. If all the patients are followed up for a long time, almost 70% of patients will develop some sort of parastomal hernia. Most common symptoms are parastomal bulge, bowel movement disturbances, colicky abdominal pain, difficulty in irrigation in large hernias, difficulty in wearing a stoma appliance. Strangulation almost never occurs and most of the patients with parastomal hernia managed well and are asymptomatic.

After surgical repair of parastomal hernia, recurrence rate is very high (63% reported recurrence rate in the largest review of parastomal hernia repair by Rubin et al.), therefore, unless it is absolutely necessary surgical repair should be avoided. Surgical options are simple repair of defect around the stoma, mesh repair using Prolene® mesh placed in intraperitoneal or extraperitoneal plane or using it in extrafascial plane. In some cases relocation of stoma with repair of the defects may be most suitable especially in very large hernias. If surgery has to be done then Prolene® mesh repair is the best choice (Figs 5A and B). Hernia belt, specially designed for ostomates, can help to manage this without surgery. It is mandatory that the patient, with a parastomal hernia, be told to contact his surgeon if the stoma is not functional for few hours. In short: (1) no technique of parastomal repair gives satisfactory long-term results; (2) all repair techniques are associated with significant morbidity; (3) there is no consensus as to the best technique of repair; (4) parastomal hernias are generally well-tolerated, rarely cause life-threatening complications and repair should be avoided if possible.

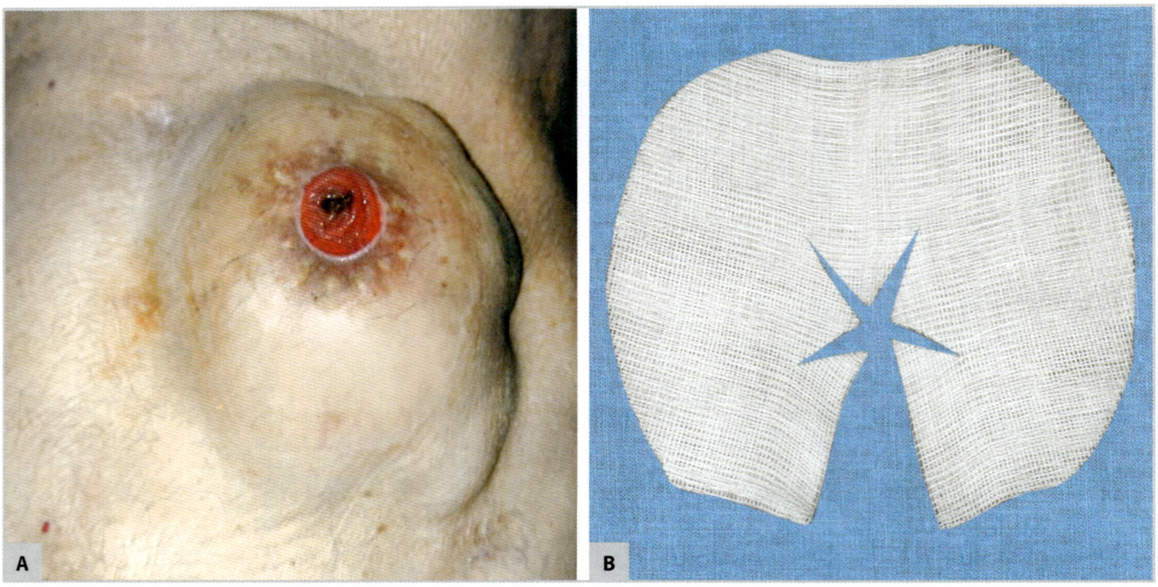

Figs 5A and B: Parastomal hernia and mesh repair

Peristomal Skin Lesions

Incidence of peristomal skin problems are as much as 20–30% and must be dealt with aggressively otherwise it progresses very rapidly and produce very difficult and expensive after care. Most common cause of peristomal skin lesions is the ill-fitting of stoma appliances resulting in a leakage of stoma effluent especially in ileostomy and urostomy. Output from ileostomy has active digestive enzymes and in urine, from urostomy, contains chemicals which will cause damage to the skin (Figs 6A to D).

COMPLICATIONS RELATED TO UROSTOMY

Peristomal Skin Related Problems

Skin maceration due to leakage, stripping, friction, folliculitis, contact dermatitis, allergic contact dermatitis, warts, granulomata and fungal infections.

Problems Involving the Stoma

Retraction, bleeding, sliding hernia, prolapse, stomal stenosis, fistulae, edema and ischemia. Above mentioned complications and their management is same as discussed with gastrointestinal (GI) stomas.

Special Complications with Urostomy

Mucous shreds, odor, urinary tract infections, ureteral stenosis, stones, metabolic acidosis, inadequate absorption of vitamin B_{12}, phosphate or urate precipitation, kidney disorders.

Mucous Shreds

The loop of the intestine used to construct the urinary diversion having its blood supply intact, therefore, will continue to produce the mucous. When mixed with urine, this mucous secretion produces thread-like structures commonly called mucous shreds. The production of mucous shreds is greatest during the first 2–3 weeks after the operation, and is initially brownish in color. Later they become yellow and decrease in volume because the cells that produce the mucous reduce in number. However, the shreds never completely disappear. If there are many mucous shreds in the urine they can obstruct the drainage of urine. Problems with excessive mucous shreds in the urine can be solved by increasing fluid intake, ideally by drinking cranberry juice or taking vitamin C, which makes the urine acidic and this is thought to reduce the quantity of mucous shreds.

Odor

Alkaline urine has the smell of ammonia (fishy), which is an offensive odor. Any odor of this kind, or the fear of odor from the ostomy bag, is a familiar concern to the majority of the patient with a urostomy. The most common causes of odor are not drinking enough, a high volume of mucous shreds in the urine (typical in continent stomas), the wearer neglecting to wipe the outlet of the bag thoroughly after emptying or failure to change the bag often enough.

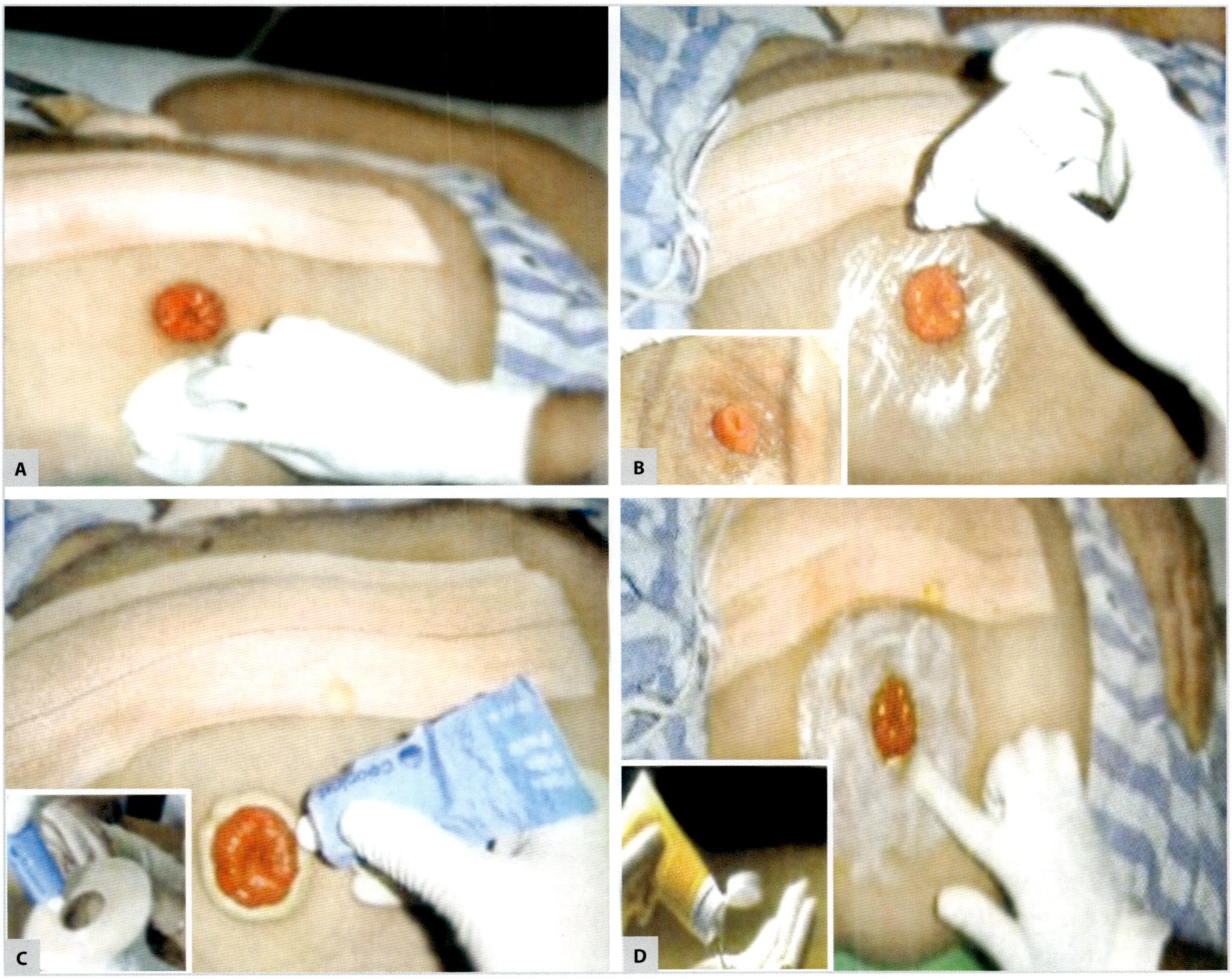

Figs 6A to D: Peristomal skin protection. Use of ostomy powder and stoma-adhesive paste

Any odor from the night drainage bag can be counteracted by cleaning it with water and white vinegar which is acidic in nature.

Urinary Tract Infections

Since the bacteria have easier access to the urinary tract than normal urinary tract infections are commonly seen in people with a urostomy. In the case of a reservoir, the risk of infection is especially high because a catheter is inserted into the stoma several times a day. This can introduce bacteria into the bag if the stoma is not cleansed carefully. Constriction, ineffective one-way valves, or stones can also cause urinary tract infections.

People with a urostomy are advised to have daily fluid intake of 2–3 L to thoroughly flush out the stoma and prevent bacteria from causing an infection. Ideally, urine output should be at 1–2 L a day. It is also a good idea to change the bag daily, so that bacteria do not accumulate and migrate to the stoma.

Urinary tract infections are commonly caused by *Escherichia coli* bacteria. The binding properties of *E. Coli* bacteria are inhibited by fructose, which is found in all types of fruit juice and by substances found in blueberry and cranberry juice. Therefore, cranberry juice is likely in helping urinary tract infections. A urine sample should be taken by washing the stoma thoroughly and inserting a sterile catheter into the base of the stoma. This procedure prevents bacteria from the skin or from the urine in the ostomy bag from contaminating the sample. It is very important for any urinary tract infection to be treated immediately, as infections can be spread to the kidneys and ultimately lead to kidney infection and stones.

Ureteral Stenosis

This is a narrowing of the ureters that is most commonly seen in patients with a Bricker bladder. Normally a Bricker bladder is sited, whenever possible, on the patient's right iliac fossa. This means that the left ureter has to be stretched quite a distance to reach the Bricker bladder. Stretching the ureter in this way narrows it and impairs urine flow. Narrowing thus causes poor drainage from the kidney and leads to impaired kidney function. Treatment consists of introducing a catheter into the ureter from the kidney to the Bricker bladder in order to keep the ureter open. Alternatively, the percutaneous nephrostomy can be done on that side.

Stones

At some stage, approximately 20% of people with a urostomy will develop stones (mineral concretions) in the urinary tract. Most common causes of the stones are the change in the urine pH, increased calcium excretion and recurrent urinary tract infections. As clips are used to create the Kock's reservoir, patients with this type of urostomy will have an increased tendency for stones because of encrustation of calcium on the clips which will result in stones formation.

Stones may be removed with least damage by first crushing them with forceps inserted into the stoma and then flushing out the debris. If this is not possible, surgery will be required.

Metabolic Acidosis

About 10–20% of all people with a urostomy will suffer some degree of metabolic acidosis. The reason is that the loop of intestine used for a urinary diversion, will absorb hydrogen ions from the urine, which leads to the development of chronic hyperchloremic acidosis.

Typical symptoms are weight loss, fatigue, weak appetite and intense thirst. The treatment is simple and consists of a dietary supplement of bicarbonate tablets and possibly electrolyte therapy if the condition is very severe.

Malabsorption of Vitamin B_{12}

Vitamin B_{12} is absorbed by a relatively small area of the terminal ileum. Since mostly this is used to form the urostomy, vitamin B_{12} is not adequately absorbed resulting in development of pernicious anemia.

The symptoms of this are fatigue, pallor, palpitations, tinnitus and paralysis of the tongue, which becomes smooth and glistening. The treatment is a course of injections of vitamin B_{12}. This condition is rarely seen now because surgeons use only the section of the terminal ileum that is located more than 15 cm away from the ileocecal (IC) junction, thereby maintaining the absorption of vitamin B_{12}.

Phosphate and/or Urate Precipitation

A urinary tract infection caused by the strains Proteus, *E. Coli, Klebsiella, Pseudomonas* or *Staphylococcus* will make the urine more alkaline, and phosphate or urate will precipitate as crystals. The crystals may be seen as a grayish-brown area around the stoma or as white flakes on the stoma itself. The stoma will also bleed slightly, and the urine will be bloodstained and have a strong odor. As a rule, the patient will have no pain. The condition is seen relatively rarely, as the one-way valve on the bag should prevent it.

The condition is treated by maintaining a high fluid intake, and by applying vinegar (acetic acid) on the skin around the stoma to reestablish the pH balance. Vinegar or vitamin C added to the bag will also counteract the alkaline environment. Use of a bag with a one-way valve and a night drainage bag to prevent bacterial access to the stoma should be recommended. The patient must also be educated to cut the appliance not too large to prevent peristomal skin exposure to urine.

Kidney Disorders

Within 20 years of having a urostomy, the majority of people will have suffered from some form of kidney diseases, possibly due to frequent, recurrent urinary tract infections.

PSYCHOSOCIAL ISSUES OF OSTOMATES

All the patients and their family members go through the five phases of recovery or adaptation as described by Dr Kubler Ross in 1969. These are denial and shock, anxiety and anger, depression, bargaining and last one is acceptance. It may take from 3 months to 2 years from stage of denial to stage of acceptance depending up on the mental, emotional and physical makeup of the patient. Next of kin or family members also go through the same process. But both go through at a different time frame. When the patient accepts the stoma and its consequences, rehabilitation starts and this is a continuous process throughout the life of an ostomate to live as normal a life as prior to surgery.

OTHER COMMON PROBLEMS THAT PATIENT WILL HAVE

Clothing: Almost all ostomates will be able to wear normal clothes, but some of them prefer to wear little loose clothes for comfort. In India, women wearing sari will have to adapt to new stoma life and might have to wear little higher than normal or will have to change to a dress. Therefore, while doing preoperative stoma marking this fact should be considered.

Dietary advice for ostomates: Ostomates have to find which food will suit them by trial and error. They can have almost every item of diet that they are used to in daily life prior to surgery. They must chew their food very well, more than prior to surgery. They must drink lots of liquids, but avoid aerated drinks as these can give rise to more gas formation. Very heavy spices and garlic will produce more odors in their stool. The patients with an ileostomy must avoid eating high fiber diet like cabbage, corn, lots of raw salads and peels of fruit and vegetables as these can result in blockage of their stoma. Patients with urostomy should drink cranberry juice if they have to acidify their urine on medical advice.

Joining work: Ostomates have to use restroom facilities more often and they take more time using this facility as well. Employers and colleagues of ostomates will notice this as well and wonder why. But this is because of lack of knowledge and awareness amongst the society in general about the ostomates' lives and their needs.

Travel and hobbies: Ostomates can travel as usual prior to surgery in any transport they like as well as pursue their hobbies or sports as before. Ostomates who travel by air must have their ostomy products supplies in their hand luggage and in their check in luggage. This is because their check in luggage can get lost or get delayed in reaching its destination. They must have doctor's certificate mentioning type of surgery done and kind of ostomy products they will be carrying with them.

Religious practices: Ostomates can pray and visit their place of worship as prior to stoma surgery. Ostomates should try to clean their bags prior to doing this as they will feel clean themselves while praying. There is a "Fatwa" from religious leaders for Muslims following Islam so that they can do their prayers as long as they take ablution prior to their prayer time.

Sexuality in ostomates: This is common concern especially in young and sexually active adult Ostomates. Most issues between partners are because of lack of knowledge about elimination of body waste, its collecting systems which ostomates use in daily life and sex. Communicating between partners on the above subjects and help from fellow ostomates or expert healthcare professionals will make ostomates and their partners overcome their problems to enjoy their sex life.

Amongst most ostomates, the stoma appliance coming off or leakage of the stoma bag during sexual intimacy is a common fear. Therefore, all ostomates must empty their pouch and wash the pouch or put on a new one piece pouch before physical intimacy with their partners. Studies have shown that patients with end sigmoid colostomy who use colonic irrigation, gives them tremendous sense of security during physical intimacy.

Amongst male patients with stoma, most common problems are erectile dysfunction and dry orgasm. The former is because of damage to pelvic nerves during surgery while dissecting rectum or because of chemotherapy or radiotherapy (hormonal imbalance). Later is because of retrograde ejaculation or removal of seminal vesicles which may be required for complete clearance of cancer.

Erectile dysfunction can be treated by specific drugs or penile implants as suggested by andrologists /urologists, but there is no specific treatment for dry orgasm.

Amongst the female patients with a stoma, most common problem is painful intercourse. This may be because of fibrosis around vagina due to surgery or radiotherapy. Simplest solution is to advocate use of local anesthetic jelly few minutes before sexual relationship.

Fertility in most women ostomates is not affected. There are enough examples of woman ostomates who have become pregnant after their stoma surgery and have children. The majority of these pregnancies will have cesarean section rather than normal delivery as these are precious children.

Children with stoma: Children adapt to stoma life more easily than adults. Most ostomies in children are temporary. Children's skin is very sensitive to adhesives especially in newborn and premature babies. Smaller ostomy bags with colorful outer coverings are available nowadays. Most importantly, parents of child with a stoma needs counseling and it is always better for them to talk to other parents who have a child with stoma.

Stoma Appliances and Finances

In India, ostomy products are expensive and we do not get any subsidy from the government nor do insurance companies cover the expenses of ostomates care including ostomy products. We have a lack of adequate numbers of health care professionals with expertise in stoma care. We have very few fully trained nurses (ETs) and few nurses with limited knowledge on stoma care to look after approximately more than 100,000 ostomates in India. This expert care when available is in major metro cities only. Therefore, there are ostomates in provincial places who have no awareness about how to use ostomy products nor many can afford to buy these products. The use of cotton or newspaper or cloth to cover their stoma is a common occurrence. Therefore, ostomates get complications of skin surrounding the stoma. Because they do not use stoma appliances they smell of urine and stool. Therefore, children with stomas do not go to school or have friends or mix with people among society. Children like these will grow up illiterate and become recluse and will not have a bright future. Some ostomates use innovation and make their own appliances. However, these are not leak proof nor they are odor proof. But something is better than nothing to collect either stool or urine in a bag.

MANAGEMENT OF DIFFERENT TYPES OF STOMA

Colostomy

End colostomy can be managed by using one piece bag with closed end (will need frequent changing of bag which can become expensive) or a drainable end. Two piece drainable bag can also be used (Figs 7A and B).

Irrigation

Very effective and economical way to manage left iliac end colostomy is use of irrigation on daily basis. Irrigation is nothing but a bowel wash with the use of an irrigator and an irrigation sleeve. Clean warm water needs to be used. Quantity of water to be used will vary for different individuals starting with 1 L increasing to 1.5 L depending on the need to remain stool free in stoma bag for next 24 hours. Many such ostomates after irrigation use either just a gauze piece or a stoma cap to cover their stoma (Fig. 8). Irrigation keeps the ostomates stool free for next 24 hours and problems of passing gas and bad odor are minimized to a large extent. It improves self-confidences and self-esteem of the patient thereby improving the quality of life of an ostomate. This results in improving their sex life as well.

Contraindications to colostomy irrigation are:

- Right-sided colostomy
- Temporary colostomy
- Disease of remaining colon
- Irritable bowel syndrome
- Colostomy in an infant or child
- Physical or mental limitations in an adult
- Parastomal hernia
- Stomal prolapse
- Inadequate sanitary facilities
- Potential fluid overload complicating cardiac or renal disease
- Radiation enteritis
- Patient lack of interest or desire in doing the procedure.

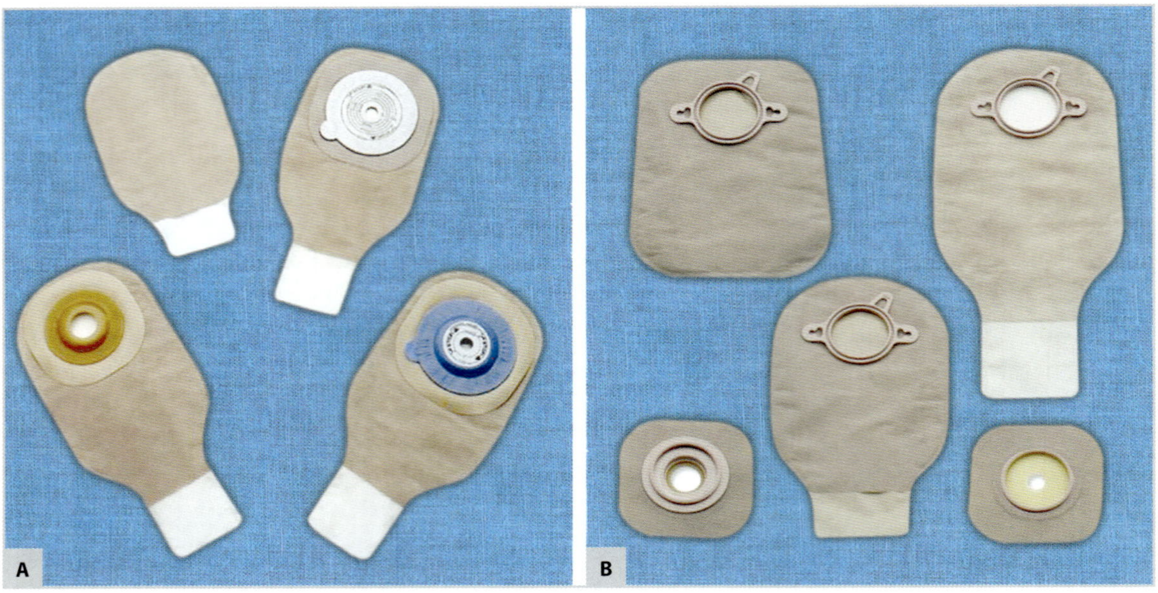

Figs 7A and B: Pouching system. (A) One piece system; (B) Two piece system

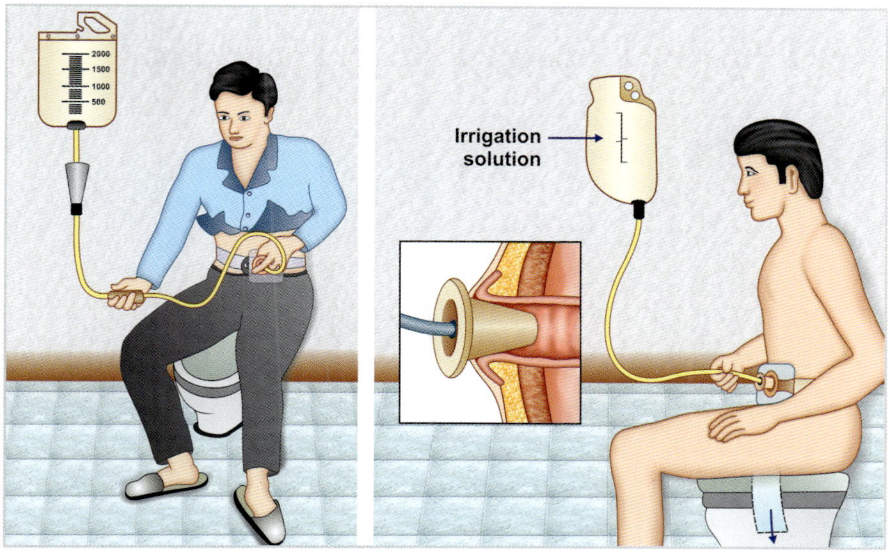

Fig. 8: Irrigation

Transverse or Sigmoid Loop Colostomy

This is best managed by the use of one piece drainable bag. The use of a rigid base plate of two piece system can damage the periphery of stoma and if a very tight rigid ring around stoma is used it can cause strangulation of stoma. Irrigation cannot be used to manage this type of stoma.

End or Loop Ileostomy

Management options are only drainable one piece or two piece system. The size of the aperture of the adhesive surface of the bag should be very fitting to stoma to avoid exposing any skin surface around stoma to come in contact with effluent from the ileostomy. Ileostomy effluent has active digestive enzymes therefore if peristomal skin comes in contact with the effluent, it will get eroded and this will make it difficult to manage the stoma. Use of stoma paste around stoma and the aperture of the bag diminish such problems.

Urostomy

This stoma also has options of using drainable one or two piece urostomy bag which has a nozzle at the bottom end with a lock to drain the urine. It has nonreturnable valve to stop reflux of urine from the bag back in to stoma. Attachment of a night large volume urine bag to urostomy appliance will make it easier for the patient to manage because patient will not have to get up frequently at night to empty the urostomy bag.

STOMA SUPPORT GROUPS

In India we have two main stoma support groups or Ostomy associations. One is Mumbai based, called "Ostomy Association of India" which is located at ground floor of Indian Cancer Society building, in Bhoiwada, Parel, Mumbai. The second is in Bangalore known as "Ostomates India." Both associations are more than 30-year-old. The main activity of both groups is to procure and distribute ostomy products to their members at a concessional rates, arrange group meetings to share new information related to stoma life and share each-others life experiences, organize an educational sessions with surgeons and other related experts on topics of stoma care, have a stoma clinics in premises with attending ET nurse to solve the issues related to stoma of the ostomates and most importantly to give hope to new or would be ostomates, who come to the center by fully rehabilitated ostomates visiting the association center. They also participate in World Ostomy Day (WOD) celebrations to create awareness about ostomates' rights and needs among the society. This is held on first Saturday of October every 3 years. The role of regional and international ostomy associations is to promote and help establish new ostomy support groups in different countries of the world, where one does not exists. They also promote and create awareness in society in general about ostomates rights and needs in different countries and deal with issues of ostomates with governments of different countries.

BIBLIOGRAPHY

1. Abcarian H, Pearl RK. Stomas. Surg Clin North Am. 1988;68(6): 1295-305.
2. Bass EM, Del Pino A, Tan A, et al. Does preoperative stoma marking and education by the enterostomal therapist affect outcome? Dis Colon Rectum.1997;40(4):440-2.
3. Berry J, Black P, Smith R, et al. Assessing the value of silicone and hydrocolloid products in stoma care. Br J Nurs. 16(13):778-88.
4. Bradley M, Pupiales M. Essential elements of ostomy care. Am J Nurs. 1997;97(7):38-45.
5. Brand MI, Dujovny N. Preoperative consideration and creation of normal ostomies. Clin Colon Rectal Surg. 2008;21(1): 5-16.
6. Carne PW, Robertson GM, Frizelle FA, et al. Parastomal hernia. Br J Surg. 2003;90(7):784-93.
7. Cataldo PA. History of stomas. In: MacKeigan JM, Cataldo PA (Eds). Intestinal Stomas: Principles, Techniques, and Management. St Louis: Quality Medical Publishing; 1993.
8. Cataldo PA. Intestinal stomas: 200 years of digging. Dis Colon Rectum. 1999;42(2):137-42.
9. Cataldo PA. Technical tips for stoma creation in the challenging patient. Clin Colon Rectal Surg. 2008;21(1):17-22.
10. Cheung MT. Complications of an abdominal stoma: an analysis of 322 stomas. Aust N Z J Surg. 1995;65(11):808-11.
11. Cohen A, Zierstein R. Drawing your body image. World Council of Enterostomal Therapists Journal. 1995;15(3):30-1.
12. Cohen A. The stoma as a dominant symbol in the transition from sickness to health; WCET Journal. 1993;13(3):23-26.
13. Colostomy Background and Consequences, Dialogue Education series from Coloplast; 2nd edition. 2006.
14. Comb J. Role of the stoma care nurse: Patient with cancer and colostomy. Br J Nurs. 12(14):852-6.
15. Corman ML. Intestinal stomas. Corman ML (Ed). Colon and Rectal Surgery, 4th edition. Philadelphia: Lippincott-Raven; 1998. pp. 1265-315.
16. Dimond B. Generalist and specialist nurses: caring for a patient with a stoma. Br J Nurs. 15(14):769-70.
17. Doughty D. Principles of ostomy management in the oncology patient. J Support Oncol. 2005;3(1):59-69.
18. Doughty DB. History of ostomy surgery. J Wound Ostomy Continence Nurs. 2008;35(1):34-8.
19. Duchesne JC, Wang YZ, Weintraub SL, et al. Stoma complications: a multivariate analysis. Am Surg. 2002;68(11):961-6.
20. Flesch L. Care of stomas. In: Nyhus LM, Baker RJ, Fischer JE (Eds). Mastery of Surgery, 3rd edition. Boston: Little, Brown and Company; 1997. pp. 1431-6.
21. Gorfine SR, Gelernt IM, Bauer JJ. In: Operative Colorectal Surgery. Philadelphia: WB Saunders; 1994. Intestinal stomas: construction and care. pp. 447-87.
22. Jänes A, Cengiz Y, Israelsson LA, et al. Preventing parastomal hernia with a prosthetic mesh: a 5-year follow-up of a randomized study. World J Surg. 2009;33(1):118-21.
23. Kodner IJ. Intestinal stomas. In: Zinner MJ, Schwartz SI, Ellis H (Eds). Maingot's Abdominal Operations, 10th edition. Stamford: Appleton and Lange; 1997. pp. 427-60.
24. Lavery IC. Techniques of colostomy construction and closure. In: Nyhus LM, Baker RJ, Fischer JE (Eds). Mastery of Surgery, 3rd edition. Boston: Little, Brown and Company; 1997. pp. 1420-30.
25. Lee J. Common stoma problems: a brief guide for community nurses. Br J Community Nurs. 2001;6(8):407-13.
26. MacKeigan JM. Stomas. In: Nicholls RJ, Dozois RR (Eds). Surgery of Colon and Rectum. New York: Churchill Livingstone; 1997. pp. 879-94.
27. Martin L, Foster G. Parastomal hernia. Ann R Coll Surg Engl. 1996;78(2):81-4.
28. McLeod SR, Cohen Z. Quality of life with a stoma. In: MacKeigan JM, Cataldo PA, (Eds). Intestinal Stomas: Principles, Techniques, and Management. St Louis: Quality Medical Publishing; 1993.
29. Nicholls RJ. Surgical procedures. In: Myers C (Ed). Stoma Care Nursing: A Patient-Centred Approach. London: Arnold; 1996.
30. Ofek I, Goldhar J, Zafriri D, et al. Anti-Escherichia Coli adhesion activity of cranberry and blueberry juices. N Engl J Med. 1991;324(22):1599.
31. Ostomy and Sexuality. The Document from Dutch Ostomy Association, Content advisers Pieternel Haspels (health care psychologist), Rik van Lunsen (physician-sexologist NVVS), Bianca van Moorst (psychotherapist-sexologist NVVS).
32. Paula MAB, Takahashi RF, Paula PR. Experiencing sexuality after intestinal stoma. J Coloproctol. 2012;32(2):163-74.
33. Pearl RK, Prasad ML, Orsay CP, et al. Early local complications from intestinal stomas. Arch Surg. 1985;120(10):1145-7.
34. Pearl RK. Parastomal hernias. World J Surg. 1989;13(5):569-72.
35. Ratliff CR, Donovan AM. Frequency of peristomal complications. Ostomy Wound Manage. 2001;47(8):26-9.
36. Reasbeck PG, Smithers BM, Blackley P, et al. Construction and management of ileostomies and colostomies. Dig Dis. 1989;7(5):265-80.
37. Robb BW, Rafferty JF. Pregnancy and the Ostomate. Ostomy Quarterly. 2003;40(3).
38. Robertson I, Leung E, Hughes D, et al. Prospective analysis of stoma-related complications. Colorectal Dis. 2005;7(3):279-85.
39. Rubin MS, Schoetz DJ, Matthews JB. Parastomal hernia. Is stoma relocation superior to fascial repair? Arch Surg. 1994;129(4):413-8.
40. Saghir JH, McKenzie FD, Leckie DM, et al. Factors that predict complications after construction of a stoma: a retrospective study. Eur J Surg. 2001;167(7):531-4.
41. Shabbir J, Britton DC. Stoma complications: a literature overview. Colorectal Dis. 2010;12(10):958-64.
42. Stephenson BM, Myers C, Phillips RKS. Minimally raised end colostomy. Int J Colorectal Dis. 1995;10(4):232-3.
43. United Ostomy Associations of America, Inc. (2014). Sex and the male ostomate fact sheet. [online] Available from http://www.ostomy.org/ostomy_info/factsheets/facts_man_en.shtml [Accessed January, 2014].
44. Urostomy Association, Great Britain and Ireland. The Urostomates Handbook; 2003.
45. Urostomy Background and Consequences, Dialogue Education series from Coloplast; 2nd edition. 2008.
46. Walsh BA. Urostomy and urinary pH. J ET Nurs. 1992;19(4):110-3.
47. Williams JG, Etherington R, Hayward MW. Paraileostomy hernia: a clinical and radiological study. Br J Surg. 1990;77(12):1355-7.

48 Neuroendocrine Tumors (Carcinoids)

Praful Desai, Keyuri Patel

INTRODUCTION

Neuroendocrine tumors (NETs—Carcinoids) are a comparatively rare group of tumors, earlier believed to account for only 1% of all neoplasms.[1] Recent studies indicate that NET is not nearly as rare as it was believed to be and there is, in fact, a ten-fold increase in its incidence and now believed to be 10% of all neoplasms.[2,3] Seer program data reports an increase from 1.09/100,000 in 1973 to 5.25/100,000 in 2004. Autopsy data from Mayo Clinic reports 6,500 cases per million population.[4] Though NETs are uncommon, they generally occur in the gastrointestinal (GI) tract and respiratory system. Earlier described as carcinoids, NET better describes and encompasses these group of lesions as they share the various cytochemical features of pheochromocytoma, medullary cancer of the thyroid and pancreatic NET.[5] Neuroendocrine tumors originate from actively secreting enterochromaffin cells of the entire endocrine system which can produce histamine and are also known to produce active peptides like serotonin, somatostatin, prostaglandins and various other amines responsible for a biochemical syndrome which can produce dyspnea, flushing, diarrhea, conjunctival suffusion and facial edema. Apart from anatomical location of the tumor, this symptom component requires urgent and appropriate therapy. The most common site is the GI tract with the highest incidence in the small intestine, stomach (often at the cardia),[6] appendix and rarely in the colorectal region. Nearly 75% of lesions occur in the GI tract, followed by the lung and bronchus (20%). It is also known to occur in the pancreas and rarely in the biliary tract. Very rare cases of skeletal NETs have been reported (Figs 1A to C).

The reported recent increase in the incidence is probably due to common and widespread use of proton-pump inhibitors for hyperacidity leading to prolonged hypochlorydia due to acid suppression. Long standing hypergastrinemia is also a complementary cause.[7,8] The resulting chronic atrophic gastritis appears to be a major etiological factor in the increasing incidence of NET.[6] A major recent study by Yao et al.[4] on epidemiology and prognostic factors of 35,825 cases of NET in 2008 strongly support the above causative factors.

PATHOLOGY

Diffuse neuroendocrine system consists of variety of cells present in central and peripheral nervous systems and endocrine organs. They share the ability to produce biologically-active amines, peptides and hormones. Neuroendocrine neoplasms can arise in most organs of the body. Many neoplasms have distinct clinical and pathologic features. Precise diagnosis and classification by ancillary techniques is necessary for optimal clinical management as specific targeted therapies are being developed for specific neoplasms. The current neuroendocrine classification of cells and tumors uses morphologic, immunohistochemical, ultrastructural and molecular biologic features to define members of neuroendocrine system.[9,10]

"Morphologic features" suggestive of well-differentiated neuroendocrine neoplasms are generally uniform polyhedral or cuboidal cells; nesting and/or broad trabeculae with nuclear palisading; rosettes and rosette-like structures. Small cell undifferentiated neuroendocrine carcinoma (NEC), is composed of cells with scanty

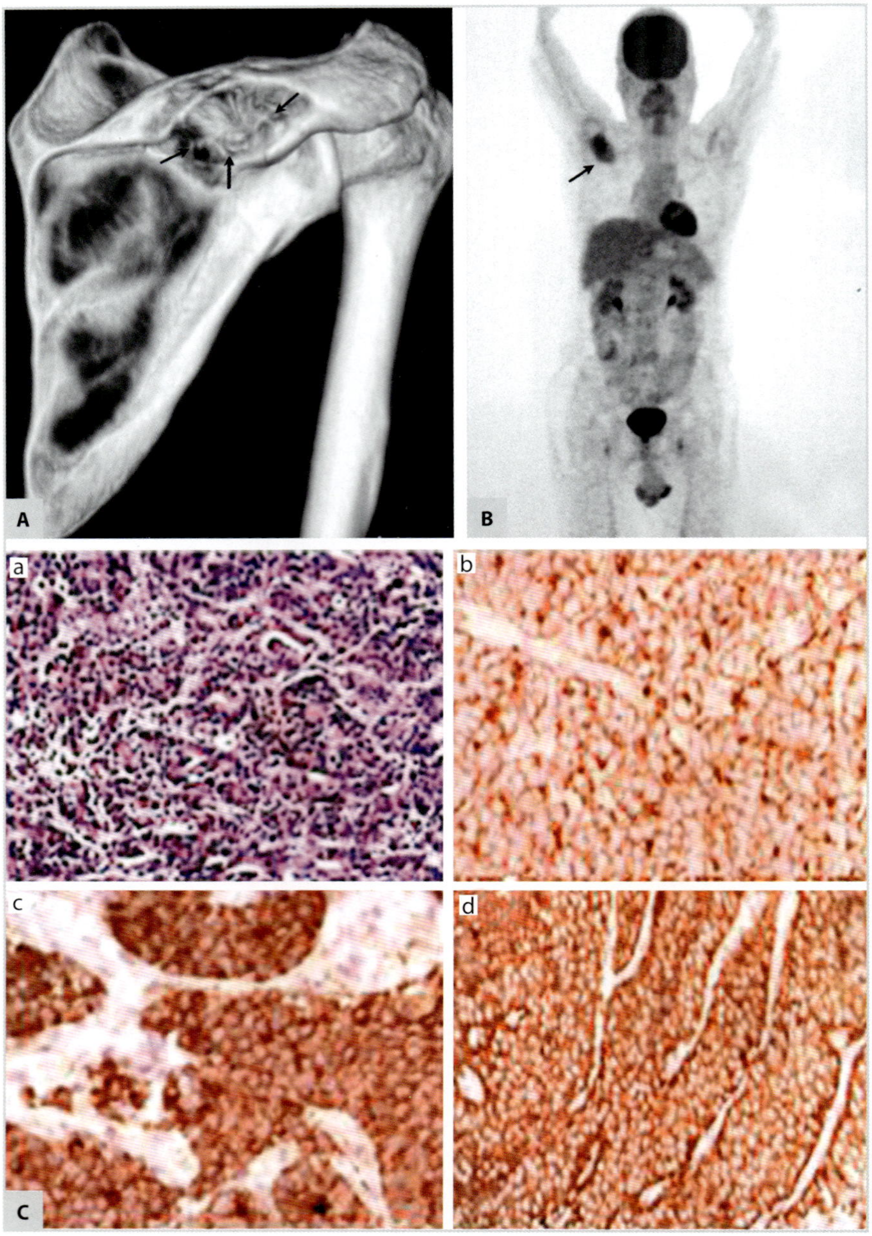

Figs 1A to C: (A) Scan showing destructive lesion of the spine of the scapula. Histopathology proved a neuroendocrine tumor. Positron emission tomography-computed tomography (PET-CT) scan showed only a localized lesion; (B) PET-CT scan showing only a localized lesion in the spine of the scapula: upper and lower endoscopies were normal; (C) H&E 20x. Cellular epithelial tumor, the cells are fairly monomorphic and arranged in a nested pattern (a). Immunohistochemically, the cells showed positivity for cytokeratin (b), and diffuse strong immunopositivity for neuroendocrine markers, chromogranin and synaptophysin (c and d).

cytoplasm, exhibiting very high nuclear-cytoplasmic (N:C) ratio, finely granular stippled chromatin, small to absent nucleoli, nuclear molding and frequent mitotic activity.

"Immunohistochemical markers" need to be used as a panel since no single antibody has perfect specificity and sensitivity. A few neuroendocrine cells can be seen with immunohistochemistry in a variety of non-neuroendocrine carcinomas. Chromogranin A and synaptophysin are the two commonly used neuroendocrine markers (Fig. 1C). Chromogranin A has a specificity of 100% but sensitivity of 75%. Intensity of staining is reduced in poorly differentiated tumors. Synaptophysin is a broad-spectrum neuroendocrine marker with increased sensitivity but lower specificity, compared to chromogranin A.

"Ultrastructural characteristics" of neuroendocrine cells in the form of cytoplasmic secretory granules ranging from 50 nm to 400 nm with central or eccentric core of variable density, can help establish the diagnosis of NETs in undifferentiated neoplasms.

"Molecular biologic techniques" may be useful for characterization of neuroendocrine neoplasms in some cases which contain mainly the messenger ribonucleic acid (mRNA) and not the translated product for specific hormones. This includes localization of mRNA for specific peptides and other neuroendocrine markers by in situ hybridization (ISH).[11] Neuroendocrine tumors associated with inherited syndromes [multiple endocrine neoplasia 1 and 2 (MEN 1 and 2), von Hippel–Lindau disease, tuberous sclerosis],[12] may be responsive to novel therapies targeting the underlying genetic defect. Hence, analysis of molecular aberrations in NETs will be increasingly relevant as additional molecular targeted therapies are developed.

Neoplasms with Multidirectional or Divergent Differentiation

Presence of endocrine cells in non-endocrine tumors is well-documented in many organs. Percentage of neuroendocrine cells in neoplasms with divergent differentiation may be important in determining prognosis such as seen in carcinoma of the colon and rectum. Molecular studies show that poorly differentiated neuroendocrine carcinoma and associated adenocarcinoma of the colon appear to be derived from the same cell of origin. In these mixed endocrine-exocrine carcinomas, it is usually the most aggressive cell population that drives the clinical behavior of the tumor.

Pathologic Classification of Neuroendocrine Tumors

Standardization of pathologic classification of all NETs irrespective of primary site is important for prediction of outcome and determination of therapy (Tables 1 and 2).

Neuroendocrine Tumors of the Gastrointestinal Tract

Gastrointestinal tract NETs are divided into foregut (stomach, duodenum, upper jejunum, pancreas), midgut (lower jejunum, ileum, appendix, cecum) and hindgut (colon and rectum) tumors based on differences in

TABLE 1: Systems of nomenclature for neuroendocrine tumors

Grade	*GIT-NETs (WHO-2010)[13]*	*Lung and Thymus (WHO)[14]*	*Lung and Thymus (Moran et al.)[15]*	*Pancreas (Hochwald et al.)[16]*
Low grade	Neuroendocrine neoplasm, grade 1	Carcinoid tumor	Neuroendocrine carcinoma, grade 1 (Fig. 1)	Well-differentiated pancreatic endocrine neoplasm, low grade
Intermediate grade	Neuroendocrine neoplasm, grade 2	Atypical carcinoid tumor	Neuroendocrine carcinoma, grade 2 (Fig. 1C)	Well-differentiated pancreatic endocrine neoplasm, intermediate grade
High grade	Neuroendocrine carcinoma, grade 3, small cell carcinoma	Small cell carcinoma	Neuroendocrine carcinoma, grade 3, small cell carcinoma (Fig. 3)	Poorly-differentiated pancreatic endocrine carcinoma, small cell carcinoma
	Neuroendocrine carcinoma, grade 3, large cell neuroendocrine carcinoma	Large cell neuroendocrine carcinoma	Neuroendocrine carcinoma, grade 3, large cell neuroendocrine carcinoma (Fig. 2)	Poorly-differentiated pancreatic endocrine carcinoma, large cell neuroendocrine carcinoma

Abbreviations: GIT, gastrointestinal tract; NETs, neuroendocrine tumors

TABLE 2: Grading systems for neuroendocrine tumors

Grade	*GIT-NETs (WHO)[13]*	*Lung and Thymus (WHO)[14]*	*Lung and Thymus (Moran et al.)[15]*	*Pancreas (Hochwald et al.)[16]*
Low grade	< 2 mitoses/10 hpf and/or ≤ 2% Ki67 index	< 2 mitoses/10 hpf and no necrosis	≤ 3 mitoses/10 hpf and no necrosis	< 2 mitosis/50 hpf and no necrosis
Intermediate grade	2–20 mitoses/10 hpf and/or 3–20% Ki67 index	2–10 mitoses/10 hpf or foci of necrosis	4–10 mitoses/10 hpf or foci of necrosis	2–50 mitoses/50 hpf or foci of necrosis
High grade	> 20 mitoses/10 hpf and/or > 20% Ki67 index	> 10 mitoses/10 hpf	> 10 mitoses/10 hpf, necrosis present	> 50 mitoses/50 hpf

Abbreviations: GIT, gastrointestinal tract; NETs, neuroendocrine tumors biology and behavior. All GI NETs should be considered potentially malignant since they can metastasize.

Esophageal NETs

These are typically high grade, poorly-differentiated neuroendocrine carcinomas, often large cell type; may have a component of adenocarcinoma.

Gastric NETs

Three types; cell of origin for types I, II and most III, is the enterochromaffin-like (ECL) cell within oxyntic mucosa. Type I—arises in the setting of autoimmune gastritis. No metastatic risk. Type II—associated with MEN 1 or 2E syndrome. Type III—sporadic and much more aggressive than types I and II.

Small Bowel NETs

These have different etiologies and prognosis depending on the site and are thus divided into: proximal (duodenum and proximal jejunum) tumors with less aggressive behavior and distal (terminal ileal) tumors which are more aggressive and often present with lymph node and hepatic metastasis.

Appendix NETs

Most are well-differentiated tumors (<1 cm in size), incidentally found at the tip, with little or no chance of metastasis. Goblet cell carcinoids show both neuroendocrine and glandular differentiation and only focal staining for synaptophysin and chromogranin.

Colonic and Rectal NETs

Rectum is the most common site for well-differentiated NET of colorectum. Rectal NETs express synaptophysin and prostatic acid phosphatase and are negative for chromogranin.

High Grade (Poorly-differentiated) Neuroendocrine Carcinoma

It occurs throughout the gastrointestinal tract (GIT) but is rare. It may occur as a primary neoplasm or in association with adenocarcinoma. By definition, it needs to have morphologic features of neuroendocrine carcinoma and stain with neuroendocrine markers such as synaptophysin or chromogranin. Pancreatic NETs, though rare, are known and can be aggressive. They are more common in the body and tail and are avid to metastasize in the liver (Fig. 2). Appropriate surgery depending on the site and size of the lesion, if resectable, is feasible (local-excision, Whipple's procedure, distal pancreatectomy as indicated).

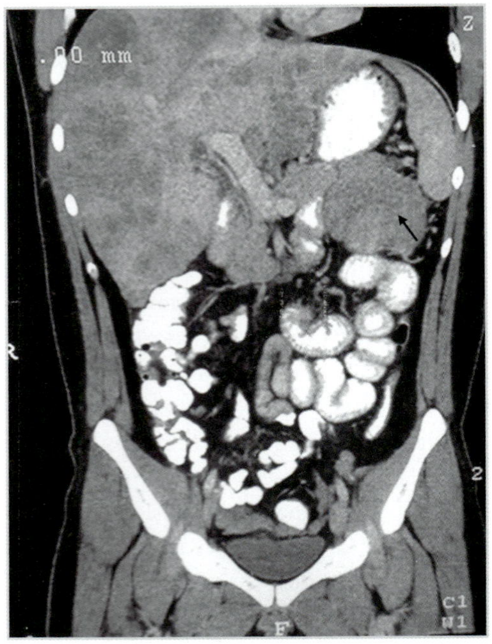

Fig. 2: Neuroendocrine tumor arising from the tail of the pancreas. Extensive metastasis in both the lobes of the liver

Neuroendocrine Tumors of the Lung

Neuroendocrine tumors of the lung represent a spectrum of clinical behavior ranging from indolent to highly aggressive with striking differences in prognosis, survival and treatment strategies.[17] The 2004 WHO classification[14] recognizes four types of neuroendocrine tumors of lung based on morphologic features, including mitotic rate and presence or absence of necrosis. Ki67 (MIB1) is useful, particularly in small biopsies and cytology specimens) (Figs 3A to C).

INVESTIGATIONS

In about 25% of patients, asymptomatic NETs are diagnosed incidentally by endoscopy for other reasons. In symptomatic patients, apart from routine blood chemistry and cardiovascular and hepatorenal profiles, a CT (or PET-CT) scan of the chest and abdomen are mandatory. Upper and lower GI endoscopy is essential. Estimation of gastrin, 5-HIAA (in relevant cases) and chromogranin A (CGA) will help confirm the diagnosis. The latter will show an increase in more than 90% of patients. Localization can be achieved apart from imaging by MIBG (**metaiodobenzylguanidine**) scans labeled with I^{131} when routine investigations fail to localize the lesion.

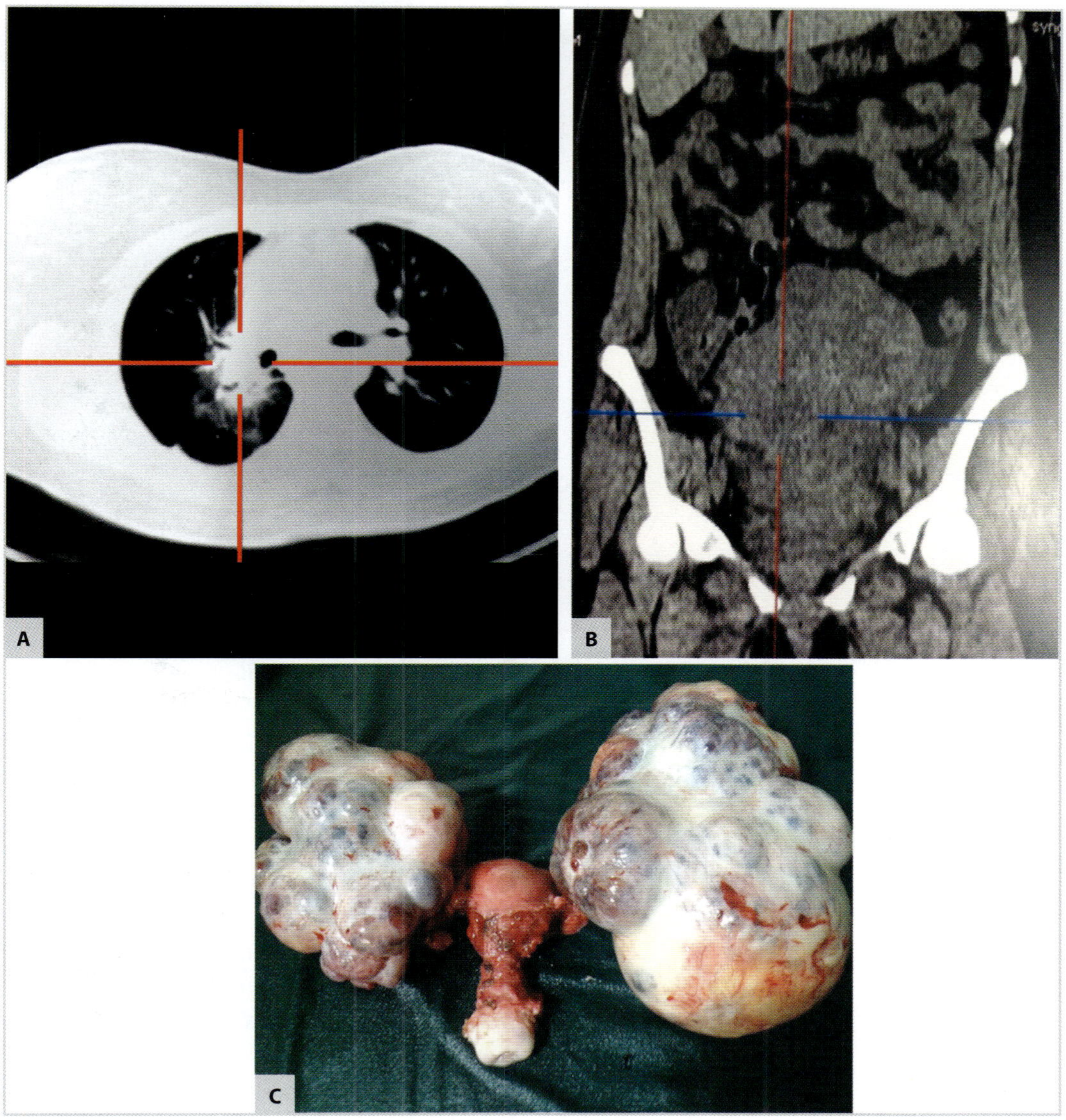

Figs 3A to C: (A) Primary neuroendocrine tumor (initially diagnosed as small cell carcinoma) of the right lung (hilar lesion); 2 years later developed bilateral metastasis in the ovary; (B) Magnetic resonance imaging (MRI) of the same patient showing a mass in the pelvis; (C) Exploratory laparotomy showed bilateral ovarian masses. A total hysterectomy and bilateral salpingo-oophorectomy was performed. Histopathology showed metastatic neuroendocrine tumor of the ovary from the lung primary NET

GASTROINTESTINAL CARCINOIDS (NETs)

The small bowel is the most frequent site followed by appendix and stomach. Colorectum is a rare site and often remains an incidental finding as a small button or a nodule of less than 1 or 2 cm on a routine per-rectal clinical examination or a sigmoidocolonoscopy. A biopsy will reveal the histology of a carcinoid. Transanal endoscopy can excise small lesions less than 2 cm.

Actively secreting lesions often secrete 5-HIAA (hydroxyindoleacetic acid), 5 hydroxytryptamine, gastrin, ACTH (Cushing's syndrome) and rarely even growth hormone. A classic carcinoid syndrome can occur in secretory lesions with symptoms of flushing, diarrhea, brochospasm, itching, urticaria, hypertension, facial edema and conjunctival suffusion. The symptoms may vary in severity and may be absent in nonsecretory lesions. Mild symptoms can be controlled by medical therapy like 150 µg of subcutaneous inj. octreotide three times daily, which can even reduce the rate of growth of the lesion in nearly 75% of patients.[18]

Appendicular carcinoids are generally small, around 1 to 1.5 cm. Smaller lesions can be managed by appendicectomy. For larger lesions, a wide resection with ileocolic anastomosis is worthwhile.

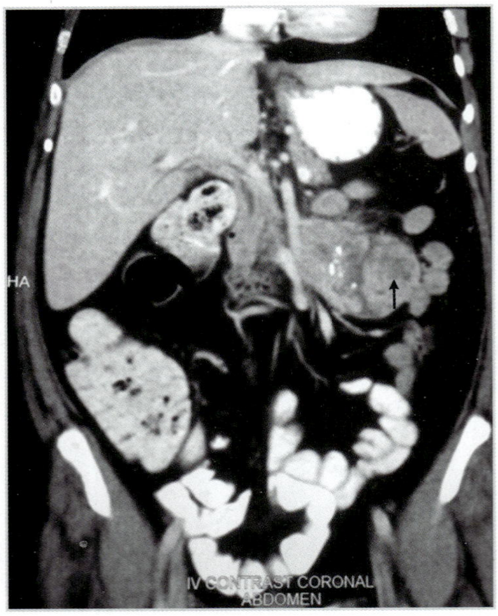

Fig. 4: Neuroendocrine tumor of the jejunum. Patient presented with episodes of subacute intestinal obstruction. Intraoperatively, there was a large mass arising from the jejunum and extending into the mesentery encasing the superior mesenteric vessels

Small Bowel Carcinoids

Mid and lower ileum is a frequent site for carcinoids and on occasions may be multicentric in the ileum. It can grow to a large size (Fig. 4) as they remain asymptomatic for a long time and may present with a large asymptomatic mass or with vague abdominal symptoms which may produce recurrent subacute type of intestinal obstruction or recurrent pain after meals. They are apt to metastasize and often produce symptoms of a carcinoid syndrome. The therapy of choice is a complete surgical excision with lymph nodes and will involve bowel resections. Larger lesions may be nonresectable as it may involve mesenteric vessels around its origin. Partial resection and by-pass anastomosis may occasionally palliate. Adjuvant injectable octreotide and appropriate chemotherapy will be needed to prolong a remission. Staging carcinoids (primary lesions) between T1 to T4 will depend on upon the size, invasion of submucosa, muscularis propria (T2) and serosa and other organs (T4). T2 lesions are bigger than 1 cm.

Gastric Carcinoids

Generally these are classified as type I, II and III based on histologic differentiation.[19] Well-differentiated are type I and II and a poorly-differentiated (type III) lesion.[20] These (small lesions—asymptomatic)—type I are often detected incidentally on upper GI endoscopy for other reasons. They are well-differentiated and may represent an autoimmune disorder. It may produce hypergastrinemia. The survival rates in type I lesion is 96% five-year survival and nearly 75% at 10 years almost similar to a general population.[20] Lesions are generally small (1–3 cm) and endoscopic resections for the primary lesion and repeat endoscopies for recurrences may be required. Medical therapy with octreotide may control the lesion to avoid repeated endoscopies or surgery to avoid potential morbidities. Somatostatin analogs inhibit enterochromaffin cell proliferation and is a useful therapeutic intervention. Conservative therapy to reduce gastrinemia and proliferation is an effective intervention. Types I and II are generally hypergastrinemia dependent[20] and are known to be associated with hypothyroidism (39%), diabetes (19%) and Addison's disease (6%). Type III gastric NETs are normogastrinemic and sporadic in nature and may be well or a poorly differentiated type. They often behave like a gastric adenocarcinoma and can avidly metastasize in the liver. The therapy of choice is a surgical resection like a gastric adenocarcinoma. Removal of the source of hypergastrinemia is the major aim of surgery for NET.[19,20] Large tumors can be down-staged by neoadjuvant chemotherapy (NACT). The drugs preferred are cisplatinum, etoposide, streptozotocin and adriamycin either as mono- or polychemotherapy. Adjuvant chemotherapy is useful in palliation for advanced non-resectable primary lesions or metastatic liver lesions. After a controlled primary stomach lesion, liver metastasis should be aggressively treated by surgery if feasible and may result in a significant palliation.

Carcinoid Crisis

Carcinoid crisis can occur during surgery or in the postoperative phase and it is advisable to administer octreotide preoperatively to prevent a carcinoid crisis. Chemoembolization for large liver metastasis can be considered in suitable patients but significant morbidities are known to occur. Even radiofrequency ablation (RFA) can provide temporary palliation. A typical carcinoid syndrome can be controlled by 150 µg octreotide, three times daily to reduce the growth rate which can occur in around 70–75% of patients. A typical Zollinger-Ellison syndrome may occur as a part of multiple endocrine neoplasia/syndrome (MEN) in lesions of the stomach. Long acting release (LAR) octreotide, 20–30 mg intramuscular (IM) injections monthly are recommended to suppress tumor growth. LAR may not significantly control or reduce the lesion itself; however, it is effective in controlling the biochemical symptoms of the carcinoid syndrome. Palliative radiotherapy may be considered for a non-resectable lesions. Renal dysfunction/failure, liver metastasis and bowel ischemia are known complications.

A complete resection of the primary lesion may result in 100% five-year survival and complete resection of metastatic lesion may accrue a 65–70% survival. Even an unresectable lesion with proper medical management can achieve a 35–40% of five-year survival.[18] Systemic chemotherapy is generally ineffective for NET; however, when left without any options, SUTENT (sorfenib), everolimus have been used for palliation.

MOLECULAR BASED THERAPY

Vascular endothelial growth factor (VEGF) monoclonal antibodies, bevacizumab (Avastin) have been tried as a biologic targeted therapy has no significant role in NET.[19] Tumor biology insights at a clinical level and in terms of basic cell biology and the role of epigenome in neuroendocrine cell proliferation can lead to consideration of other targets that are known candidates for molecular based therapies in other cancers.

REFERENCES

1. Modlin IM, Lye KD, Kidd M. A 5-decade analysis of 13,175 carcinoid tumors. Cancer. 2003;97(4):934-59.
2. Modlin IM, Lye KD, Kidd M. A 50-year analysis of 562 gastric carcinoids: small tumor or larger problem? Am J Gastroenterol. 2004;99(1):23-32.
3. Godwin JD. Carcinoid tumors. An analysis of 2,837 cases. Cancer. 1975;36(2):560-9.
4. Yao JC, Hassan M, Phan A, et al. One hundred years after "carcinoid": epidemiology of and prognostic factors for neuroendocrine tumors in 35,825 cases in United States. J Clin Oncol. 2008;26(18):3063-72.
5. Ferolla P, Faggiano A, Mansueto G, et al. The biological characterization of neuroendocrine tumors: the role of neuroendocrine markers. J Endocrinol Invest. 2008;31(3):277-86.
6. Thomas D, Tsolakis AV, Grozinsky-Glasberg S, et al. Long-term follow-up of a large series of patients with type 1 gastric carcinoid tumors: data from a multicenter study. Eur J Endocrinol. 2013;168(2):185-93.
7. Gough DB, Thompson GB, Crotty TB, et al. Diverse clinco-pathologic features of gastric carcinoid and the relevance of hypergastrinemia. World J Surg. 1994;18(4):473-9.
8. Jordan PH, Barrosso A, Sweeney J. Gastric carcinoids in patients with hypergastrinemia. J Am Coll Surg. 2004;199(4):552-5.
9. Lloyd RV. Overview of neuroendocrine cells and tumors. Endocr Pathol. 1996;7(4):323-8.
10. Lloyd RV. Use of molecular probes in the study of endocrine diseases. Hum Pathol. 1987;18(12):1199-211.
11. Hamid Q, Corrin B, Sheppard MN, et al. Expression of chromogranin A mRNA in small-cell carcinoma of the lung. J Pathol. 1991;163(4):293-7.
12. Leotlela PD, Jauch A, Holtgreve-Grez H, et al. Genetics of neuroendocrine and carcinoid tumours. Endocr Relat Cancer. 2003;10(4):437-50.
13. Bosman F, Carneiro F, Hruban R, Theise N (Eds). WHO Classification of Tumours of the Digestive System. Lyon, France: IARC Press; 2010.
14. Travis WD. The concept of pulmonary neuroendocrine tumours. In: Travis WD, Brambilla E, Muller-Hermelink HK, Harris CC (Eds). Pathology and Genetics: Tumours of the Lung, Pleura, Thymus and Heart. Lyon, France: IARC Press; 2004. pp. 19-20.
15. Moran CA, Suster S, Coppola D, et al. Neuroendocrine carcinomas of the lung: a critical analysis. Am J Clin Pathol. 2009;131(2): 206-21.
16. Hochwald SN, Zee S, Conlon KC, et al. Prognostic factors in pancreatic endocrine neoplasms: an analysis of 136 cases with a proposal for low-grade and intermediate-grade groups. J Clin Oncol. 2002;20(11):2633-42.
17. Rekhtman N. Neuroendocrine tumors of the lung: an update. Arch Pathol Lab Med. 2010;134(11):1628-38.
18. Thompson GB, van Heerden JA, Martin JK, et al. Carcinoid tumors of the gastrointestinal tract: presentation, management, and prognosis. Surgery. 1985;98(6):1054-63.
19. Rindi G, Luinetti O, Cornaggia M, et al. Three subtypes of gastric argyrophil carcinoid and gastric neuroendocrine carcinoma: a clinicopathologic study. Gastroenterology. 1993;104(4): 994-1006.
20. Borch K, Ahren B, Ahlman H, et al. Gastric carcinoids, biologic behavior and prognosis after differentiated treatment in relation to type. Ann Surg. 2005;242(1):64-73.

49 Bone Tumors and Soft Tissue Sarcomas

Ajay Puri, Nirmala Jambhekar

INTRODUCTION

Bone and soft tissue sarcomas are malignant tumors arising from the connective tissue. These tumors account for less than 1% of all cancers. They constitute less than 20% of all orthopedic biopsies and only 1.7% of orthopedic disorders.[1,2] According to the surveillance, epidemiology and end results database, it was estimated that 2,570 new cases of bone and joint cancer would be diagnosed in the year 2009 in United States and one-fourth of them would be in the population under the age of 20 years. The data base also estimated that during the same year 10,660 new cases of soft tissue cancer would be diagnosed. It predicted that 1,470 people would die of bone and joint cancer and 3,820 of soft tissue cancers. Bone cancers are relatively more common in males and in white races. The peak incidence of osteosarcoma and Ewing sarcoma is seen in the second decade and chondrosarcomas are more common in the population above 35 years of age.

Soft tissue sarcomas account for about 1% of all malignancies and the incidence rates range between 1.8 cases per million population per year and 5.0 cases per million population per year. Approximately 55–60% of soft tissue sarcomas develop in the appendicular system. Other sites of involvement are trunk (15–20%), head and neck region (10%), internal organs and the retroperitoneum (15%).

There is no comprehensive epidemiological database for bone and soft tissue sarcomas in India however despite the bias inherent in referral to a tertiary cancer hospital a survey conducted at Tata Memorial Hospital, Mumbai over a period of one year from 01/01/2010 to 31/12/2010 does shed some light on the case spectrum of these tumors in our scenario.[3] Of the 31,951 new patients registered at the Tata Memorial Hospital, 1,627 (5%) were registered primarily in the Bone and Soft Tissue (BST) Service. Out of the total 2,007 patients seen by the BST Service (including 380 referred cases), 60% (n = 1,203) were bone tumors, 36% (n = 723) were soft tissue tumors and details of primary site of affection were not known in 4% (n = 81) patients. Of the total 794 malignant bone tumors, 70% (n = 553) were primary bone sarcomas and 30% (n = 241) metastatic lesions. Primary malignant bone tumors (n = 553) were most common in the second decade (42%) of life. Males were predominantly affected (67%). Osteogenic sarcoma was the most common histopathological diagnosis in 43% (n = 243) of patients, followed by primitive neuroectodermal tumor (PNET)/ Ewing's 27% (n = 147) tumor and chondrosarcoma in 11% (n = 61). About 24.6% of osteosarcoma, 35% of Ewing sarcoma and 11% of chondrosarcoma were metastatic at presentation. The most common site of metastasis was lung (84% in osteosarcoma, 74% in Ewing sarcoma and 83% in chondrosarcoma).

There were 413 malignant soft tissue tumors of mesenchymal origin (soft tissue sarcoma) with synovial sarcoma 22.5% (n = 93) being the most common. Spindle cell sarcoma was seen in 18.5% (n = 76), soft tissue PNET/ Ewing's sarcoma in 12% (n = 51), pleomorphic sarcoma in 8% (n = 32), leiomyosarcoma in 7% (n = 31), liposarcoma in 6% (n = 25), rhabdomyosarcoma and dermatofibrosarcoma protuberans in 5% each followed by epithelioid sarcoma in 3% patients.

PRIMARY BONE TUMORS

By virtue of their rarity and their complex presentations clinically, radiologically and histologically, malignant tumors of bone and cartilage often pose diagnostic and therapeutic dilemmas. They present an enormous challenge to the orthopedic surgeon, radiologist and the pathologist. An integrated multispecialty approach to the diagnosis and treatment of these intriguing lesions helps to formulate a rational and logical management pathway with the best chance of obtaining an optimal result.

The last few decades have seen tremendous advances in the management of bone sarcomas. Besides improving survival, an increased incidence of limb salvage has enabled preservation of function in extremity sarcomas without jeopardizing local control. Various factors have contributed to this encouraging change. The advent of better imaging modalities, more effective chemotherapy, improved radiotherapy techniques, a better understanding of anatomy with continuous refinement in surgical techniques and advances in prosthesis design and materials have all played a part in achieving this goal. In order to ensure that the patient management is optimized, it is imperative for the treating clinician to be aware of the various definitive treatment modalities and formulate a diagnostic strategy that would provide maximum functional benefits without compromising local control options and overall survival.

The etiology of bone tumors still belongs to the realm of the unknown, even though a large body of work has come up suggesting various etiological factors. Osteosarcoma is especially seen during the accelerated growth which occurs at puberty. An increased risk for the development of osteosarcoma is seen in the following settings: Post-radiation (at site of previous radiotherapy, i.e. ribs in case of radiotherapy for breast), Paget's disease, bone infarcts, fibrous dysphasia, familial retinoblastoma.[4] The genetic basis for some tumors has for long been suggested by the increased incidence of bone sarcomas in patients with hereditary retinoblastoma or patients with Li-Fraumeni syndrome. Gross chromosomal rearrangements can result in duplication, deletion, translocation of amplification of large segments of the genome. For example, the characteristic genetic abnormality in Ewing Sarcoma is the t (11:22) translocation which occurs in 85% of cases. Osteosarcomas are known to show abnormalities of p-53 gene and the retinoblastoma gene.

A complete list of the types of bone tumors is published in the WHO classification of 2013.[5] The classification (Table 1) is essentially based on the type of matrix which the tumor produces (osseous, or cartilage) or the possible cell of origin (fibroblasts, nerve cells); finally some tumors, however, such as Ewing's sarcoma, do not have a cell counterpart in the normal setting.

The commonest symptom of a primary bone sarcoma is nonmechanical pain. The presence of pain or a palpable mass arising from any bone should be viewed with suspicion. A plain X-ray in two planes is the first investigation of choice. The presence of any of the following on the X-ray is suggestive, but not diagnostic of a bone sarcoma: (1) bone destruction, (2) new bone formation, (3) periosteal swelling, (4) soft tissue swelling.

Though histopathological analysis is vital in establishing a diagnosis in the majority of these tumors, a biopsy should be the final step in a systematic approach to arriving at a diagnosis. Correlation of clinical data such as the age of the patient, site of the disease combined with its clinical course and the radiological imaging helps to narrow the prospective diagnosis prior to obtaining a tissue sample. Additional ancillary investigations can be performed depending on the differential diagnosis obtained after clinicoradiologic correlation.

Magnetic resonance imaging (MRI), because of its excellent soft tissue contrast, its sensitivity to bone marrow and soft tissue edema, and its multiple imaging planes adds valuable information in the evaluation of musculoskeletal tumors. It helps to determine whether the tumor has breached normal anatomical boundaries and also illustrates its relation with the adjacent neurovascular

TABLE 1: A simplified classification system for the common bone tumors

Tissue of origin	*Benign*	*Malignant*
Cartilage	Osteochondroma, chondroma, chondroblastoma, chondromyxoid fibroma	Chondrosarcoma
Osteoid	Osteoid osteoma, osteoblastoma	Osteosarcoma
Fibroblastic	Fibroma, desmoplastic fibroma	Fibrosarcoma
Unknown	Giant cell tumor, benign fibrous histiocytoma, aneurysmal bone cyst	Ewing sarcoma, malignant fibrous histiocytoma, adamantinoma
Hematopoietic tissue		Myeloma, lymphoma
Notochord		Chordoma

structures. MRI also helps to detect skip lesions and is useful in helping the surgeon decide on the extent and planes of resection.

A surgeon must be constantly aware of the fact that other commoner lesions such as trauma, metabolic bone disease and infection, especially tuberculosis mimic tumors and can be a pitfall for the unsuspecting clinician.

Serologic and biochemical tests are of limited value in primary bone sarcomas. The alkaline phosphatase level is high in about half the cases of osteosarcoma. Currently there is an absence of consensus regarding the prognostic value of this test prior to initiating treatment or its value in monitoring the course of the disease. A wide variation in values can occur because of growth spurts during adolescence when these neoplasms most commonly occur. Similarly, LDH levels are of doubtful prognostic value in patients with Ewing sarcoma.

The lung is the most common site for metastasis in bone and soft tissue sarcomas and metastatic spread to the lung via the hematogenous route may be seen in approximately 20% of patients at presentation. A CT scan of the chest at initial evaluation can help in the detection of disseminated disease. A Tc-99 bone scan while documenting the extent of local pathology also helps to rule out multifocal disease or skeletal metastasis. Newer modalities like positron emission transmission scan are evolving to further help in early identification of metastatic or multifocal disease.

Besides the *TNM staging system* the other common staging system followed is the simpler *Musculoskeletal Tumor Society* staging system as devised by Enneking (Table 2).[6] This system was designed for sarcomas arising from the mesenchymal connective tissue of the musculoskeletal system. Lesions derived from the marrow, reticuloendothelial tissue and mesenchymal soft tissue are excluded. Thus, it is not applicable to leukemias, plasmacytoma, lymphomas, Ewing sarcoma, undifferentiated round cell lesions, and metastatic carcinomas.

TABLE 2: Enneking system for malignant tumors

Stage	Grade	Site	Metastasis
IA	Low (G1)	Intracompartmental (T1)	No regional or distant metastasis
IB	Low (G1)	Extracompartmental (T2)	No regional or distant metastasis
IIA	High (G2)	Intracompartmental (T1)	No regional or distant metastasis
IIB	High (G2)	Extracompartmental (T2)	No regional or distant metastasis
III	Any (G)	Any (T)	Regional or distant metastasis

It is based on histological grade, local tumor extent (whether confined to an anatomical compartment or not) and the presence or absence of metastasis.

Biopsy of Bone Tumors

Biopsy plays a very vital part in the diagnostic workup of bone tumors. The importance of obtaining representative tissue adequate for a definitive diagnosis and that too in the least traumatic way, without jeopardizing subsequent local control of the tumor cannot be overemphasized. A poorly placed biopsy incision, a poorly performed biopsy, or the complications of a biopsy make it difficult to salvage an extremity and, in some instances, may affect the survival of the patient. A casual approach to the biopsy is known to lead to an almost 60% discrepancy between the primary report and the final outcome.[7] *Ideally, the biopsy must be performed by or under the supervision of the surgeon who will be carrying out the final treatment.*

Though the material obtained by an open biopsy is generally adequate in quantity and less challenging to the skills of the pathologist, it is a more traumatic procedure. An open biopsy is less forgiving and a correct technique is of utmost importance if limb salvage is considered. Hence, a core needle biopsy with its inherent advantages is preferred nowadays.[8] In areas which are difficult to access such as the spine or pelvis, using an image intensifier or CT guidance ensures accurate targeting.[9]

A surgical pathologist faces many challenges while interpreting the biopsy material, such as lack of familiarity due to overall rarity of bone tumors, nonavailability of the radiologic images and their interpretation, a wide array of morphological appearances of individual tumors and biopsies or excision of reparative tissue which has been clinically and radiologically mistaken for a tumor which is known to occur with myositis ossificans and florid periostitis.[10]

The commonest primary bone tumors are osteosarcoma, Ewing sarcoma and chondrosarcoma. However, in clinical practice metastatic bone tumors and myelomas are far more common bone malignancies especially in elderly patients.[11]

OSTEOSARCOMA

Osteogenic sarcoma (osteosarcoma) is defined as a primary malignant tumor in which the malignant mesenchymal cells produce osteoid and/or immature bone. It is the most common primary malignant tumor of bone, excluding those of hemopoietic origin with an incidence of 0.2–0.3 per 100,000/year.

Osteosarcomas can be broadly classified into intramedullary, surface and extraskeletal. Osteosarcomas are divided into high and low grade tumors. High grade osteosarcomas include conventional osteosarcoma, telangiectatic osteosarcoma, small cell osteosarcoma and high grade surface osteosarcomas. Low grade osteosarcomas include low grade central and parosteal osteosarcoma. Periosteal chondrogenic type of osteosarcoma is an intermediate grade osteosarcoma. Conventional intramedullary osteosarcoma accounts for 80–90% of all osteosarcomas.

Etiology

Previous radiation therapy, Paget's disease of the bone and germ cell abnormalities [such as the Li-Fraumeni syndrome (germ line mutation of the p53 gene), Werner syndrome, Rothmund-Thomson syndrome, Bloom syndrome, hereditary retinoblastoma] predispose to occurrence of osteosarcoma.[4]

Age: Peak incidence is during second decade in the adolescent years and a second peak is seen in advanced age in the fifth decade.

Sex: Males are more affected with a ratio of about 3:2.

Site: The metaphysis of long bones is involved in more than 90% of cases with a predilection for bones around the knee (distal femur and proximal tibia) followed by the upper humerus.

Radiology

The roentgenographic findings of osteosarcoma may include a variable mixture of radio opacities of osteogenesis and the radiolucencies due to destructive changes and replacement with osteoid tissue. One or the other may dominate the picture so that there is great variation in the radiographic shadows. As the periosteum is elevated, a triangle of reactive periosteal ossification produces triangular radio opacity at the upper and lower angles (Codman's triangle) (Fig. 1). Non-neoplastic bone may also be deposited in layers by the periosteum, producing a lamellated appearance. The radiograph may also show presence of a pathological fracture or skip metastasis.

Pathology

Histologically, osteosarcomas have over 20 histological patterns, the better known patterns being osteoblastic, chondroblastic, fibroblastic, telangiectatic and small cell types amongst others. Grading of osteosarcoma is linked to location and histology (parosteal osteosarcoma and low grade intraosseous osteosarcoma is usually Grade 1, periosteal osteosarcoma is Grade 2 or 3 and the conventional osteosarcoma, high grade surface osteosarcoma and dedifferentiated parosteal osteosarcoma is grade 3 or 4

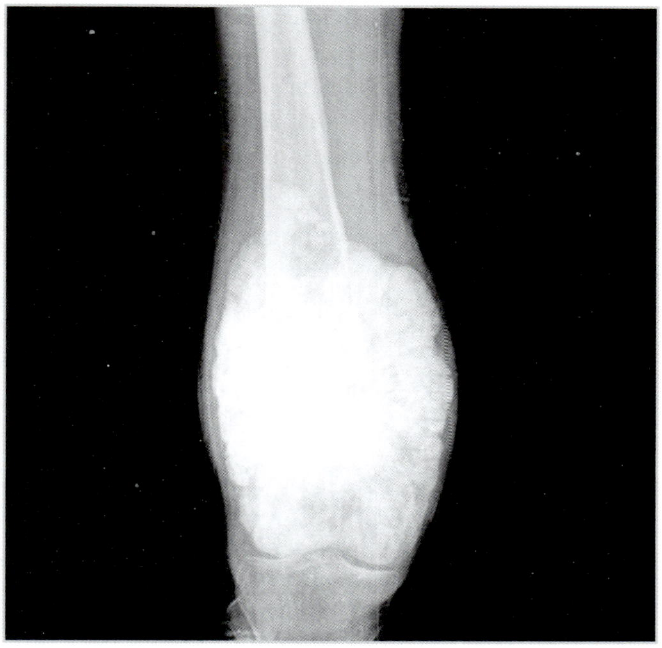

Fig. 1: Osteosarcoma. Elevation of the periosteum produces triangular radio opacity at the upper angles (Codman's triangle)

The excised specimen needs to be elaborately grossed for evaluation of the amount of necrosis, since this is the single most important prognostic factor.[12]

Treatment

For high grade osteogenic sarcoma, it is crucial to combine surgical excision of the primary tumor with chemotherapy.[13] Multiagent chemotherapy is the standard of care in osteosarcoma. Doxorubicin, cisplatin, high-dose methotrexate, etoposide and ifosfamide have demonstrated antitumor activity in osteosarcoma. Most current protocols incorporate these agents in three or four drug combinations.[14]

Chemotherapy for osteogenic sarcoma usually includes a preoperative, neoadjuvant phase (for 3–4 cycles), followed by surgery and subsequent postoperative or adjuvant chemotherapy. Preoperative chemotherapy is thought to have many advantages: it could immediately treat micrometastatic disease; it provides a safety margin for resection and may permit potentially less resection of normal tissue if there is a significant response; it allows time for surgical planning, manufacture of custom prostheses and procurement of allografts. Nevertheless, there is no study which demonstrates a clear survival benefit for neoadjuvant therapy.

Importantly, preoperative chemotherapy enables us to analyze the histologic response to chemotherapy in the surgical specimen.[12] There are various scoring systems for the histologic response. Huvo's system includes four grades:

Grade I: 0–50% necrosis

Grade II: 51–90% necrosis

Grade III: 91–99% necrosis

Grade IV: 100% necrosis.

Patients with a grade III or IV response demonstrate significantly higher disease-free survival at 5 years than patients with grade I or II response. Though theoretically the idea seems attractive to administer different agents postoperatively when a patient shows poor response to the preoperative agents, altering postoperative chemotherapy in poor responders has not been shown to improve outcomes.

Radiation therapy though once commonly used before the emergence of modern chemotherapy no longer plays a part in the standard treatment for primary tumors. Palliative radiotherapy may be useful in incurable or metastatic patients for alleviation of local symptoms like pain, bleeding, fungation or metastatic symptoms like dyspnea, spinal cord compression, brain metastases, etc.

Parosteal osteogenic sarcomas are usually low grade and have a favorable prognosis. They arise directly adjacent to but distinct from the external surface of a bone.[15] The most frequent site for the tumor is on the posterior aspect of the distal femur with the proximal end of the humerus being the next most favored site (Figs 2A and B). Treatment entails wide surgical excision. Chemotherapy is not employed in the treatment of these low grade tumors.[16] If a high grade component is identified in the excised specimen then the patient should receive postoperative chemotherapy, similar to a conventional high grade osteosarcoma.

Low grade intramedullary osteosarcoma: The treatment is essentially similar to parosteal osteosarcoma, requiring only surgery without systemic chemotherapy.

Periosteal osteogenic sarcoma arises from the diaphyseal cortex or periosteum, frequently located in the diaphysis of long bones mainly the femur and tibia. The tumor has a particular feature that it contains a remarkable cartilaginous component which occasionally makes it difficult to distinguish from chondrosarcoma. Though there is debate regarding the use of chemotherapy in these lesions, currently these tumors are treated similar to conventional high grade osteosarcomas but the prognosis is better than conventional high grade osteogenic sarcoma.[17]

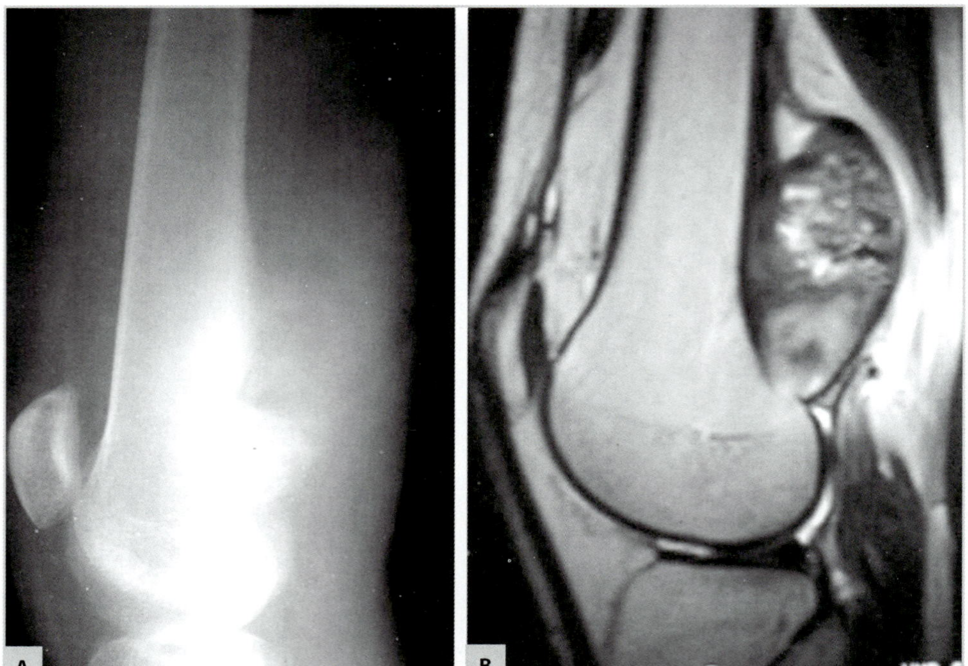

Figs 2A and B: Parosteal osteogenic sarcoma on the posterior aspect of the distal femur

Secondary osteogenic sarcoma arises on the background of a previous bone disorder such as Paget's disease, bone infarct, fibrous dysplasia, or prior radiation. Secondary osteogenic sarcoma is uncommon in young patients but accounts for more than half of the patients over 60 years of age. These are treated like conventional high grade osteosarcoma. They show a poor prognosis and do not respond well to adjuvant therapy.

EWING SARCOMA

Ewing sarcoma is the third most common primary tumor of bone overall, but the second most common malignant bone tumor of late childhood and early adulthood accounting for approximately 1% of childhood cancers. The incidence of Ewing sarcoma is around 0.3 per 100,000/year. Although the precise cell of origin is unclear, this small round blue cell tumor is thought to arise from primitive mesenchymal cells. Molecular biology studies have shown that all these tumors share a common gene rearrangement involving the EWS gene on chromosome 22, most commonly a reciprocal translocation with FLI1 gene on chromosome 11 t(11; 22) (q24; q12) in 85% of cases but other translocations do occur. When prominent neurogenic differentiation is observed, the term PNET of bone tumor is applied.

Etiology

Ewing sarcoma is much commoner in the white population as compared to the African and Asian population.

Age: The peak incidence of Ewing sarcoma is in the first 2 decades of life

Sex: Slight preponderance in males, with a ratio of 1.4: 1.

Site: The tumor occurs throughout the skeleton but the most frequent sites of involvement are the pelvis, long bones, ribs and the vertebral column.

Radiology

Radiographs generally show a nonmatrix producing destructive lesion in the metadiaphysis and diaphysis of the long bones with an aggressive periosteal reaction that is described as "onion-peel", though the classical Codman's triangle may also be occasionally seen (Figs 3A and B). Often a large circumferential soft tissue mass is also present. In axial locations such as the sacrum and pelvis, radiographic changes can be subtle and often missed on initial examination. A rare form of periosteal-based Ewing sarcoma has also been reported that arises on the periosteum of long bones with saucerization of the cortex but without underlying medullary extension.

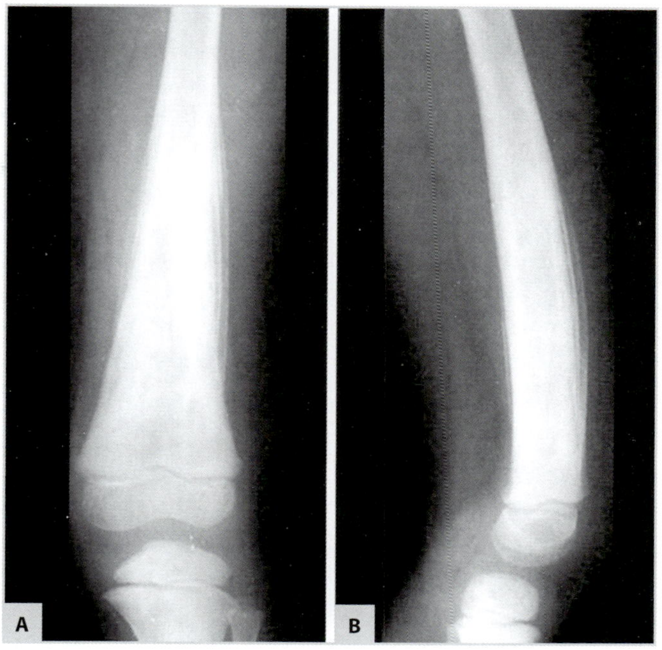

Figs 3A and B: Ewing sarcoma of the femur demonstrating an "onion-peel", periosteal reaction

Pathology

It is a tumor composed of small round cells and hence histologically mimics other malignant round cell tumors namely, lymphoma, leukemias, metastatic neuroblastoma, rhabdomyosarcomas, mesenchymal chondrosarcoma and small cell osteosarcoma, all of which can figure in the differential diagnosis. Good morphological preservation showing the monotonously uniform round cells with vacant looking nuclei and lack of nucleoli or significant cytoplasm help to suspect this tumor.[18] Further confirmation can be obtained with immunoreactivity to the antibody Mic2/ CD99 or the more "specific" molecular methods utilizing PCR, FISH techniques and the fusion of EWS-FI gene. Ewing's sarcoma treated with neoadjuvant chemotherapy is evaluated on lines similar to osteosarcoma but the tumor response is graded as per the criteria of Picci.

Treatment

Treatment for patients with Ewing sarcoma requires a multidisciplinary approach amongst surgeons, radiologists, pathologists, and medical and radiation oncologists. Systemic multiagent chemotherapy is essential in all patients and surgery, radiation or a combination of the two is important for local disease control. All current regimes employ 3-6 cycles of initial chemotherapy after biopsy followed by local therapy and another 6-10 cycles of chemotherapy usually applied at 3 week intervals. The total duration of treatment is about 10-12 months. Chemotherapeutic agents considered most active in Ewing sarcoma include doxorubicin, cyclophosphamide, ifosfamide, vincristine, dactinomycin and etoposide. Most current protocols incorporate these agents in 4-6 drug combinations. Myeloablative therapy and stem cell transplantation is of uncertain value in the treatment of patients with aggressive or advanced Ewing sarcoma.

Surgery and radiotherapy have been the principle modes of local disease control in patients with Ewing sarcoma.[19] Over the years, the role of radiotherapy as a primary means of local control has diminished for a number of reasons, the most significant being the apparent survival benefit seen in patients with nonmetastatic Ewing sarcoma treated with surgery. There also exists a risk of secondary malignancy following radiotherapy. Though radiotherapy in combination with chemotherapy can achieve local control, definitive surgery when feasible has to be regarded as the first choice of local therapy.[20] Incomplete surgery even when followed by postoperative radiotherapy is not superior to radiotherapy alone and should be avoided. However, postoperative radiotherapy should be given in cases of inadequate surgical margins. The choice of modalities for local disease control depends on the age of the patient, the extent of the disease at the time of presentation, tumor site, functional consideration and concern for delayed or late effects of therapy.

CHONDROSARCOMA

Chondrosarcoma is a malignant tumor of cartilage producing cells. The term chondrosarcoma is used to describe a heterogeneous group of lesions with diverse morphologic features and clinical behavior. Chondrosarcoma is the most common sarcoma of bone in patients over 20 years of age and represents about 25% of all sarcomas.

Primary Chondrosarcoma

A malignant cartilage tumor arising centrally in a previously normal bone is known as primary chondrosarcoma. It is also known as central or conventional chondrosarcoma. After myeloma and osteosarcoma it is the third most common primary malignancy of bone. Of the chondrosarcomas, more than 90% are of primary (conventional) type.

Etiology

Age: This is a tumor of adulthood and old age, usually beyond the third decade of life. Peak incidence is in the fifth to seventh decades of life.

Sex: Males are affected more often than females in a ratio of approximately 3: 2.

Site: Pelvis is the most common site of skeletal involvement (the ilium is the most frequently involved bone) followed by the proximal femur, proximal humerus, distal femur and ribs. Primary chondrosarcoma is uncommon in the small bones of the hands and feet accounting for less than 1% of all chondrosarcomas. The spine and craniofacial bones are rarer sites for chondrosarcoma.

Radiology

The typical findings are expansion of the medullary portion of the bone and thickening of the cortex, but periosteal reaction is scant or absent. It also shows endosteal scalloping as well as annular, punctate or comma-shaped stippled calcifications (rings and arcs appearance) (Figs 4A and B). Rarely a soft tissue mass may be present.

Computed tomography may be particularly helpful in detection and characterization of lesions located in anatomically complex areas like sacrum and spine. MRI depicts a high water content of the lesions and exhibits low intensity on T1 and very high signal intensity with T2-weighted images. The lesions appear lobulated at margins and intramedullary extent is best demonstrated with MRI. Evaluation of features like intramedullary extent, endosteal scalloping, entrapment of normal marrow within the lesion, cortical thickening or break, soft tissue extension and reactionary edema are well-appreciated on MRI which help in differentiating enchondromas from chondrosarcomas.[21]

Pathology

Chondrosarcoma is a cartilage producing malignant tumor which has four distinct histological subtypes: conventional chondrosarcoma which affects flat bones, or small bones of hands and feet; mesenchymal chondrosarcoma which involves any bone including bones of the head and neck as also extraosseous sites such as meninges; clear cell chondrosarcoma seen particularly in the epiphysis of long bones and dedifferentiated chondrosarcoma which is a low grade conventional tumor accompanied with rhabdomyosarcomatous, or liposarcomatous

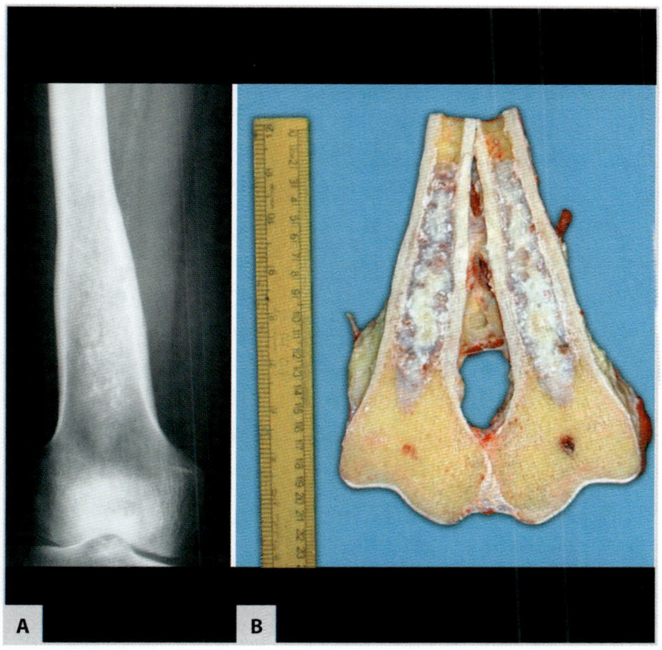

Figs 4A and B: Chondrosarcoma—radiology demonstrates punctate or comma-shaped stippled calcifications (rings and arcs appearance). Gross c/s of the specimen demonstrating calcific matrix

differentiation. The conventional chondrosarcoma is grade 1 in more than two-thirds of the cases whereas grade 3 tumors are rare to the extent that in a young patient this diagnosis should be viewed skeptically as this could very well be a chondroblastic osteosarcoma. Since most chondrosarcomas are low grade (grade 1) well-differentiated lesions composed of hyaline cartilage, the major challenge faced by the pathologist is distinguishing it from a benign chondroma. Since the cytological features of grade I chondosarcomas overlap with those of benign chondromas radiologic features (outlined above) can help make a differentiation. In the small bones of the hands and feet the criteria for diagnosing, a chondrosarcoma are more stringent. In fact all cartilage lesions of such small bones should be considered benign unless they show overwhelming features of malignancy accompanied with soft tissue involvement. Mesenchymal, clear cell and dedifferentiated chondrosarcomas are all high grade sarcomas

Treatment

These tumors are generally not sensitive to chemotherapy and radiotherapy and therefore do not respond to these modalities of treatment. Thus, surgery is the only reliable treatment for these tumors.[22] A wide resection observing oncologic principles is recommended for grade 2 and grade 3 chondrosarcomas of long bones. In the case of grade 1 chondrosarcomas in long bones with aggressive radiological findings a wide resection is preferable for adequate margins. Recent reports suggest that there may be a role for safely treating extremity grade I chondrosarcoma with extended intralesional curettage without increasing the risk for local recurrence or metastatic disease. Case selection is critical and should be based on imaging characteristics. Cartilaginous lesions in the pelvis and sacrum frequently recur after intralesional excision even if the histologic appearance is benign or suggestive of a low grade neoplasm. Therefore, wide excisions are recommended for nearly all cartilaginous lesions of the pelvis and sacrum.

The role of radiotherapy in chondrosarcoma is limited. Though not the first choice for local control in these lesions, the advent of newer techniques of delivery has resulted in radiation playing an increasing role in unresectable lesions or after incomplete resection especially in the skull base and the spine. It may also be useful for palliation.

Secondary Chondrosarcoma

Chondrosarcoma arising in a known benign precursor lesion is known as a secondary chondrosarcoma. This precursor lesion may either be an osteochondroma or an enchondroma. The risk of chondrosarcoma arising in a solitary osteochondroma has been reported to be less than 1%. However, in osteochondromatosis, this risk increases to 5%. Secondary chondrosarcomas develop at a somewhat earlier age than primary chondrosarcoma. They are usually of low grade malignancy and have a favorable prognosis.

The principles of treatment of periosteal chondrosarcoma, dedifferentiated chondrosarcoma, mesenchymal chondrosarcoma and clear cell chondrosarcoma are essentially similar to conventional chondrosarcomas.

PRINCIPLES OF SURGICAL TREATMENT AND RECONSTRUCTION AFTER WIDE EXCISION IN BONE TUMORS

Surgical ablation of the diseased bone with oncologically safe margins is the best means of local control in malignant bone tumors. For decades, amputation and ablative surgery were widely practiced in an attempt to remove the tumor with safe margins and the least chance of local relapse. From an era where amputation was the only option to the current day function preserving resections and complex reconstructions has been a major advance. While the number of limb salvage surgeries undertaken for malignant bone tumors of the extremity has increased, the principles that govern surgical resection of bone tumors remain unchanged. The surgeon must ensure adequate resection of involved bone and soft tissue so as to minimize the chance of local recurrence. If after achieving this goal he is still able to preserve adequate function of the limb after reconstruction then the patient is a suitable candidate for limb salvage. At no stage must adequate disease clearance be compromised in an attempt to achieve limb salvage.

The advent of computer-assisted tumor surgery in malignant bone tumors has increased the accuracy of intended bone resection and may be beneficial in resection and reconstruction of pelvic, sacral and difficult joint-preserving tumor surgery. It provides a useful tool in achieving a better balance between disease resection and preservation of function in anatomically challenging locations.

Reconstruction after excision of bone tumors requires restoration of both, skeletal and soft tissue elements. Most bone sarcomas occur in the metaphyseal portion of the bone. The articular cartilage serves as a barrier to extension of the tumor and the joint itself is rarely involved but in order to achieve adequate margins resection usually involves the articulating or joint surface. At the metadiaphyseal end a marrow margin of 3 cm as evaluated on the T1-weighted MRI image is usually considered adequate. The gap remaining needs reconstruction with either metal or bone. Metallic prostheses (megaprostheses) which span the resection gap and allow for movement of the joint form the mainstay in limb salvage surgery for reconstruction after tumor resection, providing both mobility and stability (Fig. 5).[23] Biological means of reconstruction using autografts, allografts and re-implantation of sterilized tumor bone (after autoclaving/pasteurization/irradiation) offer an attractive alternative biological option in certain scenarios (Figs 6A and B).[24,25] Rotationplasty is essentially an intercalary limb resection preserving the continuity of the neurovascular bundle.[26] The most common site where rotationplasty is used is for tumors of the distal femur and proximal tibia (Figs 7A and B). Patients undergo an en bloc excision of the distal femur and proximal tibia including skin and all surrounding soft tissues. The limb continuity is then re-established by fusing the tibia with the proximal femoral remnant after 180° external limb rotation. Once rotated, the ankle now becomes the knee and the foot becomes a useful attachment for a below knee prosthesis. Ankle movements simulate knee movements and the patient has the equivalent of a functioning below knee amputation rather than a high above knee one.

Because of the dynamic nature of growing bones, children pose a unique challenge. The issue of ultimate limb length discrepancy also influences the choice of reconstruction especially in the lower limb. Vascularized epiphyseal transfers (proximal fibular epiphysis, iliac crest, lateral scapular crest) may provide a solution to this

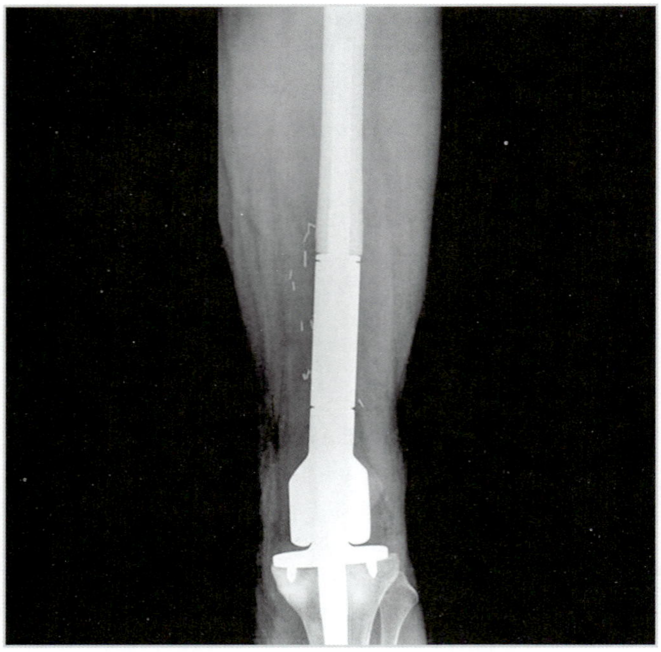

Fig. 5: Megaprosthesis reconstruction after excision of a distal femur tumor

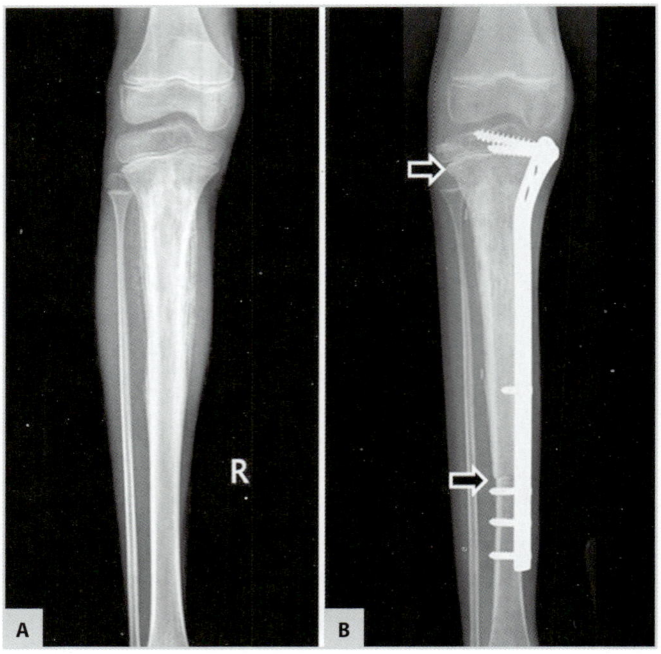

Figs 6A and B: Pre- and postoperative radiograph of a tibial diaphyseal osteosarcoma treated with excision and reimplantation of the irradiated "tumor" bone. The arrows demonstrate the osteotomy/resection cuts

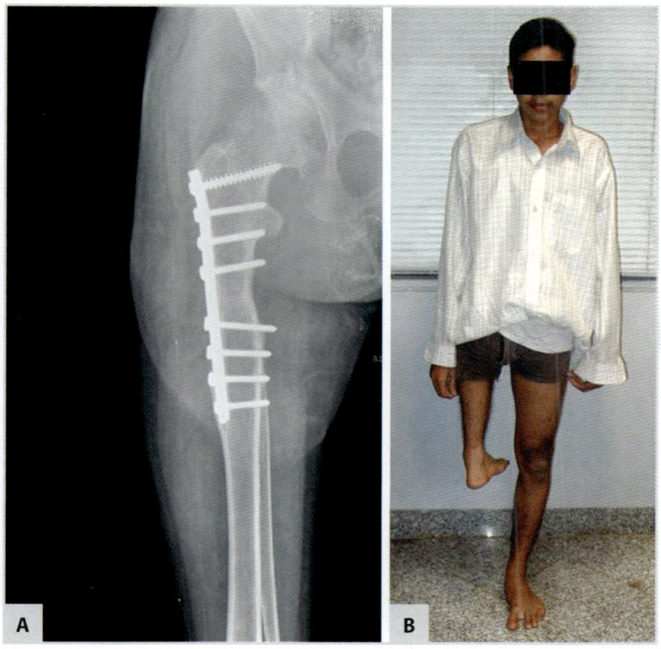

Figs 7A and B: Rotationplasty for a distal femur tumor. Osteosynthesis of the residual femur with the rotated tibia (note that the fibula now lies on the medial side in the radiograph)

complex problem. A properly planned rotationplasty can help ensure that the opposite knee and the repositioned rotated ankle of the operated limb lie at the same level at skeletal maturity thus limiting the cosmetic deformity after prosthetic fitting. An expandable prosthesis is another solution to the problem of limb length discrepancy that would result in young children offered salvage with a megaprosthesis.[23]

Limb salvage entails a well-orchestrated effort involving various specialties and better outcomes are likely to be achieved with centralization of expertise at regional centers, so that surgeons and their teams can offer a full range of surgical options to their patients, based upon experience and knowledge.

Though properly indicated and executed limb salvage offers the advantage of better function and psychological benefits resulting in an overall improvement in quality of life it does have its limitations. It requires a well-coordinated experienced multidisciplinary team. The cost of treatment can be expensive and the postoperative rehabilitation is prolonged often requiring increased inpatient hospital care. Limb salvage procedures have a high complication rate and patients and their families need to be counseled regarding the potential setbacks that may occur in the course of their road to recovery.

SOFT TISSUE SARCOMAS

The extremities are the commonest site with about 60% of soft tissue sarcomas arising in the extremities. Approximately, half of all patients with intermediate or high grade soft tissue sarcomas develop metastatic disease and the overall survival is approximately 50% at 5 years.[27]

Though, no specific etiology can be identified, in most patients the risk factors for soft tissue sarcomas include previous radiation therapy, exposure to chemicals (e.g. vinyl chloride, arsenic), immunodeficiency, prior injury (scars, burns), chronic tissue irritation (foreign-body implants, lymphedema), neurofibromatosis and certain germ line mutations like Li-Fraumeni syndrome (*p53* mutations).[28,29]

The presenting symptoms and signs of soft-tissue sarcomas are nonspecific. They commonly present as a painless, slow-growing mass. While sarcomas in the extremities may present earlier, diagnosis of sarcomas involving the pelvic cavity may be delayed. Their location deep within the body precludes palpation of the tumor mass early in the course of the disease. Consequently, these tumors often reach tremendous size prior to diagnosis without causing overt symptoms. Any soft tissue lump exhibiting any of the following clinical features should be considered to be malignant until proved otherwise: (1) increasing size, (2) size more than 5 cm, (3) deep to the deep fascia, (4) painful.[27] The risk of malignancy is high with increasing size being the best individual indicator. An important dictum may be that "*any tumor found deep to the deep fascia or larger than 5 cm should be regarded as a soft tissue sarcoma until proven otherwise.*"

The principles of biopsy are essentially similar to those of bone sarcomas. Imaging studies should be completed prior to biopsy (contrast-enhanced MRI is the preferred method for limb lesions). Core needle biopsies are usually accomplished as an outpatient procedure under local anesthesia.[30] Excision biopsies are not routinely recommended; however, an excisional biopsy may be a practical option for less than 5 cm superficial lesions.[31] An open biopsy may be an option in selected cases where repeated core biopsies have failed to achieve a diagnosis. Soft tissue sarcomas are classified histologically according to the soft tissue cell of origin, though the cell type is not a part of the prognostic staging system. Additional studies, including electron microscopy, histochemistry, flow cytometry, cytogenetics and tissue culture studies may allow identification of particular subtypes within the major histologic categories.[29] Malignant fibrous histiocytoma is the most common histologic type (28%). Others are leiomyosarcoma (12%), liposarcoma (15%), synovial sarcoma (10%), and malignant peripheral nerve sheath tumors (6%). Pathologists assign grade based on number of mitoses per high-powered field, presence of necrosis, cellular and nuclear morphology and the degree of cellularity. The metastatic potential of soft tissue tumors is better reflected by their histologic grade rather than the cellular classification.

The major staging system used is the one formed by the International Union against Cancer and American Joint Committee on Cancer. This TNM system incorporates histologic grade, tumor size, depth, regional lymph node involvement and distant metastasis.[29] The lungs are the most common site for metastasis of soft tissue sarcomas. Approximately, 10% of patients have pulmonary metastasis at presentation. Additional imaging to complete staging will include an X-ray or a computed tomographic (CT) scan of the chest and an ultrasound or CT scan of the pelvis to identify involved lymph nodes if present. CT scan of the chest is recommended for sarcomas larger than 5 cm or with moderate to poor differentiation. Nodal involvement is rare, occurring in less than 3% of patients with sarcoma.[32] It is more likely in epitheloid sarcomas, clear cell sarcomas, rhabdomyosarcomas, angiosarcomas and synovial sarcomas.

The prognosis for patients with adult soft tissue sarcomas depends on several factors, including age, size, histologic grade, and stage of the tumor. Factors associated with a poorer prognosis include age older than 60 years, tumors larger than 5 cm, or high grade histology.[33]

When feasible, function-sparing surgical excision with wide margins is the cornerstone of effective treatment, with the goal of preservation of a functional extremity (Fig. 8). This may be facilitated by soft tissue reconstructive surgery including the use of local or free flaps and occasionally vascular and nerve resection with suitable graft reconstruction, when indicated. Generally 2 cm beyond the tumor is used as a cut-off to ensure adequate clearance, but the margin can be quantitatively less in the case of resistant anatomic barriers, such as muscular fasciae, periosteum and perineurium as described by Kawaguchi's concept of "barrier effects".[34,35]

In the case of inadequately excised tumors, reoperation should be considered if adequate margins can be achieved without major morbidity.

Radiotherapy complements adequate surgery as standard treatment of intermediate and high grade, deep

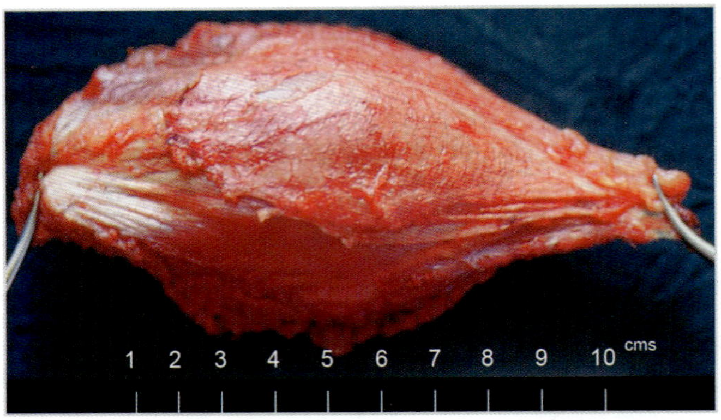

Fig. 8: Excised specimen of soft tissue sarcoma of the thigh. Remove the growth, the growth as a whole and the growing ends of the growth

(*Courtesy:* Dr Praful Desai)

tumors with a diameter of more than 5 cm. It can consist of preoperative or postoperative radiation depending on institution protocols. Preoperative radiotherapy can occasionally permit limb conservation of extremity sarcomas which otherwise would be inoperable or require amputation. Reports suggest that preoperative radiotherapy is associated with a greater risk of wound complications than postoperative radiotherapy. Intraoperative brachytherapy either exclusively or in combination with postoperative radiation is an option that is often employed. Radical brachytherapy alone, when used judiciously has demonstrated a good local control and functional outcomes with reduced treatment-related morbidity.[36] Intensity-modulated radiation therapy has the potential to better target the delivered radiation dose with decreased morbidity, and is under investigation.

The role of chemotherapy in soft tissue sarcomas is still debatable. The histological type may play a role in the decision making to offer chemotherapy, since some types are felt to be more chemosensitive, whereas others are less so. Patients with high grade tumors larger than 5 cm in diameter have the greatest tendency for disease to metastasize and are likely candidates for prospective clinical trials of adjuvant chemotherapy.[29] Commonly used drugs are cisplatin, adriamycin and ifosfamide in an adjuvant fashion after resection of a high grade sarcoma and as a therapeutic measures after the onset of nonresectable metastasis or in a neoadjuvant fashion in a disseminated sarcoma at initial clinical presentation. There is no robust evidence of significant benefit of chemotherapy, though partial responses are known with variable periods of remission.

Patients with localized tumors that, despite multimodality treatments, cannot be resected completely should be considered for amputation to minimize the risk of distant site relapse. In addition, patients with multiple relapses, untreatable pain, bleeding or fungation may also benefit from an amputation of a limb.

MANAGEMENT OF METASTATIC DISEASE FROM BONE AND SOFT TISSUE SARCOMAS

Praful Desai

Bone and soft tissue sarcomas are avid in dissemination particularly to the lungs and liver. A locally advanced lesion at initial presentation (stage IV) will obviously have to be treated initially by chemotherapy to see the response and then manage the primary lesion by surgery, if so indicated. Lung and liver metastasis often develop a few years later with a long latent period after the primary lesion remains controlled. Since majority of bone and soft tissue malignancies do not respond favorably with cytotoxic therapy, consideration must be given to a surgical excision of lesion in the lung or liver or at any other site particularly when they are localized. Depending on the extent of the lesion, segmental resections or a lobectomy should be considered. Long-term remissions have been recorded and a 5-year-disease-free survival can achieved in more than 30%. Multiple metastasectomy of more than one or more lesions in the lungs (particularly from osteogenic sarcoma) is feasible. For bilateral spread even staged thoracotomy can be considered when indicated, when the primary tumor is under control. A similar aggressive surgical approach for liver metastasis is also feasible and can lead to a significant DFS with a good quality of life. Often, in osteogenic sarcoma metastatic lesions in the lungs are superficial and subpleural and easy to excise. They are also more differentiated histologically than the primary lesion, which may be an effect of chemotherapy. Metastatic disease from a solid tumor (bone tumors, soft tissue sarcomas) kidney, colorectum, pancreas, stomach is not an end point in treatment and appropriate therapy by a multidisciplinary team can result in a satisfactory outcome.

Metastatic disease in the lungs and occasionally liver should be carefully evaluated by the following criteria:

- Whether the primary lesion is controlled
- The latent period between control of the primary lesion and onset of metastasis. The longer the period, better are the chances of longer survival even in presence of metastasis
- Whether metastases are unilateral or bilateral in the lungs
- Resectability—metastatectomy (pulmonary), segmental resection or lobectomy
- Staged thoracotomy—feasibility exists in suitable cases
- Proper imaging studies of the lungs
- One stage or two stage thoracotomies—preferably staged (Figs 9 and 10).

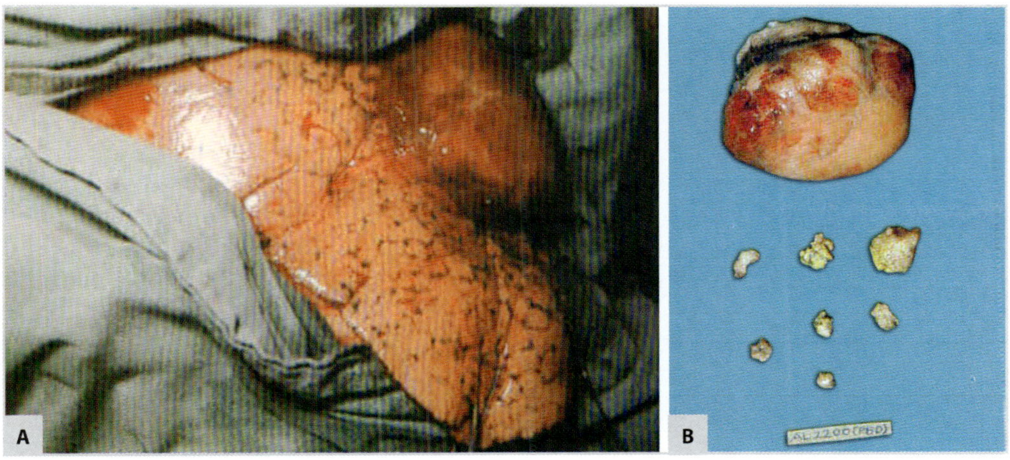

Figs 9A and B: Most metastatic deposits in the lung are subpleural in situation and are of varying size. Maximum nodules (42) removed at one thoracotomy. Conservative enucleation usually possible

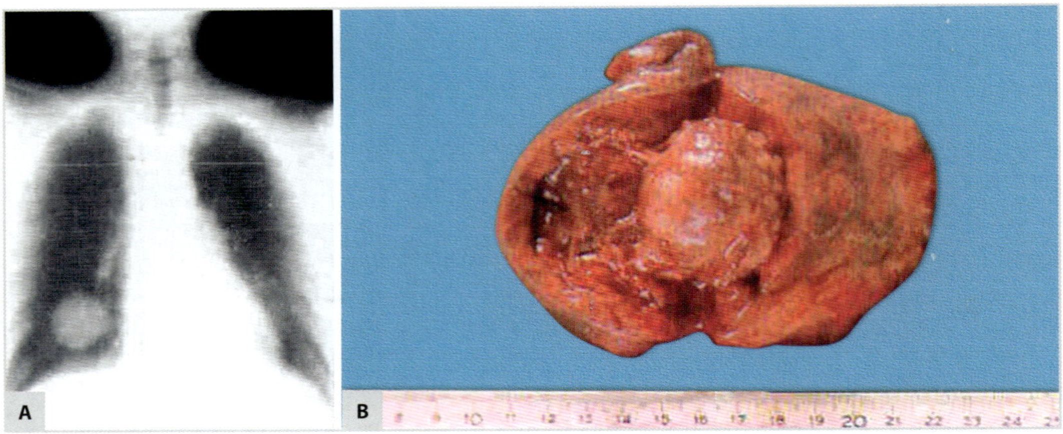

Figs 10A and B: A 14-year-old-male adolescent with osteogenic sarcoma. Adjuvant chemotherapy given after amputation. Eighteen months later chest X-ray and tomogram shows a solitary metastasis. Lobectomy had to be done as the metastasis was deeply situated within the parenchyma

REFERENCES

1. Chitale AR, Jambhekar NA. Report of bone registry, 1970-1982 (a twelve year study). Indian J Pathol Microbiol. 1987;30(2):201-18.
2. Tuli SM. The art and science of orthopaedics in developing countries. J Bone Joint Surg Br. 1985;67(5):840-2.
3. Puri A, Gulia A. Multimodality management of extremity soft tissue sarcomas-an Indian perspective. Indian J Surg Oncol. 2011;2(4):291-7.
4. Ritter J, Bielack SS. Osteosarcoma. Ann Oncol. 2010;21(Suppl 7): vii320-5.
5. WHO Classification of Tumours of Soft Tissue and Bone. Fourth Edition IARC. WHO Classification of Tumours, No 5. Fletcher CDM, Bridge JA, Hogendoorn P, Mertens F (Eds); 2013.
6. Enneking WF, Spanier SS, Goodman MA. A system for the surgical staging of musculoskeletal sarcoma. Clin Orthop Relat Res. 1980;153:106-20.
7. Mankin HJ, Lange TA, Spanier SS. The hazards of biopsy in patients with malignant primary bone and soft-tissue tumors. J Bone Joint Surg Am. 1982;64(8):1121-7.
8. Pramesh CS, Deshpande MS, Pardiwala DN, et al. Core needle biopsy for bone tumours. Eur J Surg Oncol. 2001;27(7):668-71.
9. Puri A, Shingade VU, Agarwal MG, et al. CT-guided percutaneous core needle biopsy in deep seated musculoskeletal lesions: a prospective study of 128 cases. Skeletal Radiol. 2006;35(3):138-43.
10. Jambhekar NA, Desai SS, Puri A, et al. Florid reactive periostitis of the hands. Skeletal Radiol. 2004;33(11):663-5.
11. Desai S, Jambhekar N. Clinicopathological evaluation of metastatic carcinomas of bone: a retrospective analysis of 114 cases over 10 years. Indian J Pathol Microbiol. 1995;38(1):49-54.
12. Pakos EE, Nearchou AD, Grimer RJ, et al. Prognostic factors and outcomes for osteosarcoma: an international collaboration. Eur J Cancer. 2009;45(13):2367-75.
13. Agarwal M, Anchan C, Shah M, et al. Limb salvage surgery for osteosarcoma: effective low-cost treatment. Clin Orthop Relat Res. 2007;459:82-91.
14. Jaffe N, Puri A, Gelderblom H. Osteosarcoma: evolution of treatment paradigms. Sarcoma. 2013;2013:203531.
15. Okada K, Frassica FJ, Sim FH, et al. Parosteal osteosarcoma. A clinicopathological study. J Bone Joint Surg Am. 1994;76(3): 366-78.
16. Agarwal M, Puri A, Anchan C, et al. Hemicortical excision for low-grade selected surface sarcomas of bone. Clin Orthop Relat Res. 2007;459:161-6.
17. Cesari M, Alberghini M, Vanel D, et al. Periosteal osteosarcoma: a single-institution experience. Cancer. 2011;117(8):1731-5.
18. Desai SS, Jambhekar NA. Pathology of Ewing's sarcoma/PNET: Current opinion and emerging concepts. Indian J Orthop. 2010;44(4):363-8.
19. Weber KL. Current concepts in the treatment of Ewing's sarcoma. Expert Rev Anticancer Ther. 2002;2(6):687-94.
20. Puri A, Gulia A, Jambhekar NA, et al. Results of surgical resection in pelvic Ewing's sarcoma. J Surg Oncol. 2012;106(4):417-22.
21. Murphey MD, Flemming DJ, Boyea SR, et al. Enchondroma versus chondrosarcoma in the appendicular skeleton: differentiating features. Radiographics. 1998;18(5):1213-37; quiz 44-5.
22. Marco RA, Gitelis S, Brebach GT, et al. Cartilage tumors: evaluation and treatment. J Am Acad Orthop Surg. 2000;8(5):292-304.
23. Abed R, Grimer R. Surgical modalities in the treatment of bone sarcoma in children. Cancer Treat Rev. 2010;36(4):342-7.
24. Puri A, Subin BS, Agarwal MG. Fibular centralisation for the reconstruction of defects of the tibial diaphysis and distal metaphysis after excision of bone tumours. J Bone Joint Surg Br. 2009;91(2):234-9.
25. Puri A, Gulia A, Jambhekar N, et al. The outcome of the treatment of diaphyseal primary bone sarcoma by resection, irradiation and re-implantation of the host bone: extracorporeal irradiation as an option for reconstruction in diaphyseal bone sarcomas. J Bone Joint Surg Br. 2012;94(7):982-8.

26. Agarwal M, Puri A, Anchan C, et al. Rotationplasty for bone tumors: is there still a role? Clin Orthop Relat Res. 2007;459: 76-81.
27. Grimer R, Judson I, Peake D, et al. Guidelines for the management of soft tissue sarcomas. Sarcoma. 2010;2010:506182.
28. Kasper B, Gil T, D'Hondt V, et al. Novel treatment strategies for soft tissue sarcoma. Crit Rev Oncol Hematol. 2007;62(1): 9-15.
29. Institute NC. Adult Soft Tissue Sarcoma Treatment (PDQ®) National Cancer Institute; 2011.
30. Narvani AA, Tsiridis E, Saifuddin A, et al. Does image guidance improve accuracy of core needle biopsy in diagnosis of soft tissue tumours? Acta Orthop Belg. 2009;75(2):239-44.
31. Casali PG, Jost L, Sleijfer S, et al. Soft tissue sarcomas: ESMO clinical recommendations for diagnosis, treatment and follow-up. Ann Oncol. 2009;20(Suppl 4):132-6.
32. Fong Y, Coit DG, Woodruff JM, et al. Lymph node metastasis from soft tissue sarcoma in adults. Analysis of data from a prospective database of 1772 sarcoma patients. Ann Surg. 1993;217(1):72-7.
33. Vraa S, Keller J, Nielsen OS, et al. Prognostic factors in soft tissue sarcomas: the Aarhus experience. Eur J Cancer. 1998;34(12): 1876-82.
34. Novais EN, Demiralp B, Alderete J, et al. Do surgical margin and local recurrence influence survival in soft tissue sarcomas? Clin Orthop Relat Res. 2010;468(11):3003-11.
35. Kawaguchi N, Ahmed AR, Matsumoto S, et al. The concept of curative margin in surgery for bone and soft tissue sarcoma. Clin Orthop Relat Res. 2004;419:165-72.
36. Laskar S, Bahl G, Puri A, et al. Perioperative interstitial brachytherapy for soft tissue sarcomas: prognostic factors and long-term results of 155 patients. Ann Surg Oncol. 2007;14(2):560-7.

50 Retroperitoneal Sarcomas

Praful Desai

INTRODUCTION

Retroperitoneum is a potential space between the posterior parietal peritoneum and the posterior musculoskeletal frame. Though uncommon, retroperitoneal sarcomas (RPS) account for 12–15% of all soft tissue sarcomas.[1]

ETIOLOGY

No definite cause is known to initiate a RPS; trauma, postradiotherapy sequalae after 10–15 years and rarely a genetic predisposition may be responsible. No robust evidence exists for any of these factors. Its histogenensis is not entirely definable.

PATHOLOGY

Almost all subtypes occur, the most common is a liposarcoma or a fibrous histiocytoma (malignant variant) which accounts for almost 25–30%, nearly one-third of RPS.[2] Synovial sarcomas, myxofibrosarcomas, alveolar soft part sarcoma, dermatofibrosarcomas, leiomyosarcoma and even rhabdomyosarcomas are known to occur in the retroperitoneal space. Occasionally Ewing's hemangiopericytoma and peripheral nerve sheath (neurilemmoma) tumors have been reported. Even a round cell sarcoma can arise in the retroperitoneal space. As in other sarcomas, the pathologic grading is classified as low, intermediate and high-grade tumors.

CLINICAL FEATURES

Generally asymptomatic to begin with RPS attain a large size before producing any significant symptoms and since the retroperitoneum is a potential space the lesion increases in size and pushes the bowel to the opposite side. The presenting symptoms are vague abdominal pain and often an abdominal mass when it reaches a significant size. Rarely, radiating pain in the lower extremities may be present if there is nerve irritation due to involvement. It is quite uncommon to have bowel symptoms unless there is significant pressure on the small or large bowel or the rectum.

INVESTIGATIONS

Routine imaging techniques, blood chemistry and cardiopulmonary, renal and hepatic status needs to be evaluated as most RPS when resectable, may require surgery which may involve organal resections of the kidney, stomach and major large or small bowel. A CT and/or MRI scans and rarely a PET-CT study to see any dissemination beyond the abdomen particularly in the lungs should be obtained. An appropriate core biopsy of the lesion is mandatory prior to final treatment planning. An unsatisfactory core may mandate an open biopsy and frozen section study before the actual surgical procedure. Infiltration or involvement of important vascular structures (IVC, the aorta or its bifurcations) is uncommon but known to occur and relevant vascular studies (venous and arterial) and investigations are imperative before final treatment decisions.

TREATMENT

Retroperitoneal sarcomas are rare but are a fascinating group of soft tissue sarcomas, mostly diagnosed after the lesion reaches a significant size due to paucity of symptoms in its early genesis. A team of surgical, medical and radiation oncologists should carefully evaluate the lesion in its entirety and carefully plan the best therapeutic approach by surgery or combination therapies based on a given clinical setting. Long-term satisfactory results can be achieved in many patients. Chemoradiotherapy are essentially palliative as only occasional responses occur.

Surgery

The therapy of choice for all soft tissue sarcomas is a good surgical excision with a wide margin (when possible) (Figs 1 to C). Depending on the lesion an incision providing a generous exposure of the lesion is the first and most important step. RPS are usually quite large in size and often occupies a major portion of the retroperitoneal space. Adjacent organal excisions, when involved and infiltrated by the lesion needs to be excised in continuity. This may involve the kidney, the bowel, a part of the pancreas, duodenum, the stomach and on occasion even a portion of the infiltrated liver. Incisions which provides good exposure depending on the site of the lesion includes a large midline incision with a T extension, a bilateral Kocher's incision with a midline extension, a thoraco-abdominal incision or a transverse Pfannenstiel incision with midline proximal incision will provide a good pelvic exposure.

Vascular Involvement

One of the major technical issues is the presence of vascular invasion of the inferior vena cava (IVC), involvement of the superior mesenteric artery, lower reaches of the aortic region and its bifurcation. Primary leiomyosarcoma of the IVC is a known histologic entity and may entail excision of the IVC.[3] Ligation below the renal veins is generally safe though troublesome lower limb edema could result which generally settles within a year. Vena caval grafts are

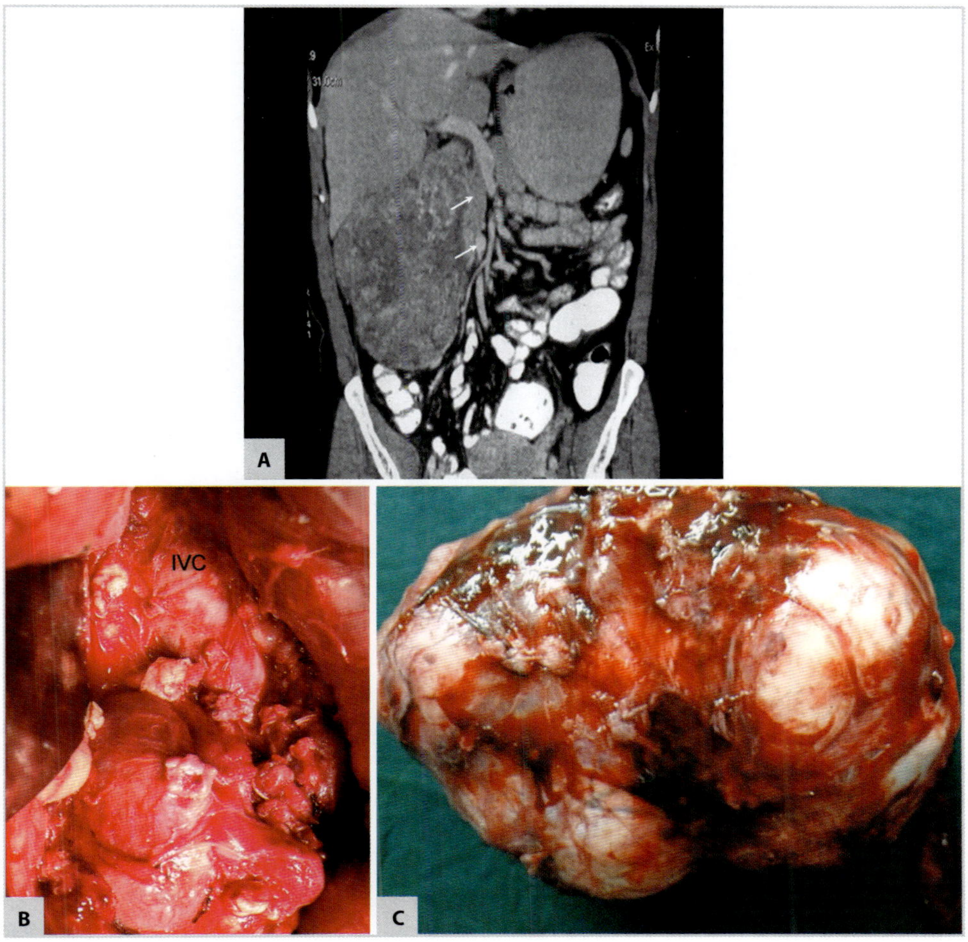

Figs 1A to C: (A) Retroperitoneal sarcoma closely abutting the liver, duodenum and inferior vena cava; (B and C) Intraoperative photograph of retroperitoneal sarcoma view after complete surgical excision showing the dissected vena cava; Excised specimen. Final h stopathology—leiomyosarcoma

used after a complete segment excision of the IVC. Partial resection of IVC with a fascio-peritoneal graft is a useful and simple procedure.[4] Resection of lower aorta with or without the bifurcation is a more complicated issue and compatible with serious complication. Venous bypass (femoral vein to axillary vein) during the procedure often results in complications and should be undertaken only if competent vascular team acts in cohort. Long-term results in few such cases are difficult to comment upon. These procedures are very rarely performed.

In a large study from the Memorial Sloan Kettering indicate that a complete resection results in a 10-year disease free survival (DFS) rate of 53% and an incomplete resection yields around 18% DFS.[5,6] The latter group often benefits if adjuvant radiotherapy (30–40 Gy) and chemotherapy are administered and may result in prolonged survival.[7] Routine adjuvant chemoradiotherapy has no significant role after a complete excision has been achieved. Intraoperative radiotherapy (IORT) by electron beam therapy has been used (up to 20 Gy) but is compatible with significant morbidity due to bowel obstruction and fistula.[8] No increase in overall survival has been reported. Postoperative radiotherapy over large areas is difficult to handle.

Chemotherapy

The drugs generally used are cisplatin, adriamycin, ifosfamide and methotrexate. The feasibility of using neoadjuvant chemotherapy for a large lesion is still debated; however, regression has been reported and helps to determine sensitivity and efficacy of the drug based on response.

Chemoradiotherapy, therefore, should be used carefully and selectively to increase palliation when a complete excision is unlikely before surgery and in an adjuvant fashion to control a grade III large lesion after complete or R_1/R_2 resection (presence of microscopic or macroscopic disease).

REFERENCES

1. Feig BW, Ching CD. The MD Anderson Surgical Oncology Handbook, 5th Edition. Texas: Lippincott Williams & Wilkins; 2011. pp. 196-219.
2. Dalal KM, Kattan MW, Antonescu CR, et al. Subtype specific monogram for patients with primary liposarcoma of the retroperitoneum, extremity, or trunk. Ann Surg. 2006;244:381-91.
3. Hollenback ST, Grobmyer SR, Kent KC, et al. Surgical treatment outcome of patients with primary inferior vena cava leiomyosarcoma. J Am Coll Surg. 2003;197:575-9.
4. Suzman MS, Smith AJ, Brennan MF. Fascio-peritoneal patch repair of the IVC: a workhorse in search of work? J Am Coll Surg. 2000;191:218-20.
5. Lewis JJ, Lewing D, Brennan MF. Retroperitoneal soft-tissue sarcoma: analysis of 500 patients treated and followed at a single institution. Ann Surg. 1998;228:355-65.
6. Shibata D, Lewis JJ, Leung DH, et al. Is there a role for incomplete resection in the management of retroperitoneal liposarcomas? J Am Coll Surg. 2001;193:373-9.
7. Glenn J, Sindelar WF, Kinsella T, et al. Results of multimodality therapy of resectable soft-tissue sarcomas of the retroperitoneum. Surgery. 1985;97:316-25.
8. Gronchi A, Casali PG, Fiore M, et al. Retroperitoneal soft tissue sarcomas: patterns of recurrence in 167 patients treated at a single institution. Cancer. 2004;100:2448-55.

51 Management of Skeletal Metastases

Jai Prakash Agarwal, Nikhil Kalyani

INTRODUCTION

Skeletal metastasis is a common and adverse complication in advanced malignant diseases. It occurs in about 14–70% of cancer patients and is known in 70–85% patients at autopsy.[1,2] Certain cancers like breast, prostate, lung, thyroid, kidney and myeloma have higher incidence of skeletal metastases. The scale of the clinical problem is substantial, as breast, lung and prostate cancer are the three most common cancers globally.[3] It develops in up to 70% of patients with prostate and breast cancer and about 30–40% of patients with cancers of the lung, bladder and thyroid.[4]

The incidence of bone metastases is expected to increase as improvements in diagnosis and therapy allow patients to live longer.[5] Patients with predominantly bone metastases show almost twice longer survival than those with predominantly visceral metastases, seen best in metastatic breast cancer patients.[6,7] Life expectancy of patients with bone metastases has been estimated to be from 3.5 months to 30 months, with a wide range among different primary tumor types. As expected survival rates are low in patients with disseminated and symptomatic osseous metastases.

CLINICAL PRESENTATION AND DIAGNOSIS

Bone metastasis frequently causes pain (50%).[8] Cancer patients with bone metastases experience more disabling symptoms and become symptomatic earlier in the clinical course of the disease than patients with visceral metastases.[9] The complications include severe pain, spinal cord compression, pathological fractures and hypercalcemia. These may restrict mobility or cause insomnia and lead to poor quality of life. More than 70% of patients with bone metastases will experience symptoms at some point of time.

The etiopathogenesis of pain include stretching of the periosteum by tumor expansion, mechanical stress of the weakened bone, nerve entrapment by the tumor, release of cytokines or direct destruction of the bone with a consequent collapse.[10-12] Pain increases gradually over a period of weeks or months. Initially, it is localized in a particular area and is often felt at night or on weight bearing. Pain is characteristically described as a dull ache, constant and gradually increasing in intensity. Continuous pain may get exacerbated by different movements or change in positions. There may be referred pain, muscle spasm or paroxysms of stabbing pain, particularly if accompanied by nerve compression.

Complications like pathological fractures and spinal cord compression can occur in patients with bone metastasis; these occur due to increased bone fragility. It is reported to occur in 8–30% of patients with bone metastases and is commonly seen in patients of myeloma and breast cancer. The long bones and vertebrae are more frequently involved.[13] Spinal cord compression occurs as a result of bone fragment or metastatic deposit compressing the cord with progressive neurological deficits and worsening of pain at the local site.

Hypercalcemia is associated with pain, nausea, vomiting, anorexia, constipation, weakness, dehydration, polyuria, mental disturbances and confusion. Gastrointestinal symptoms are often mistaken for opioid effects or potentiated by opioid-related symptoms.

Neurologic symptoms are seen in about 10–20% of patients, commonly with lung and breast cancers due to hypercalcemia and are mistakenly attributed to cerebral metastases.

On clinical examination, there may be tenderness over the involved sites. Patients may have restriction of movements at involved joints due to disease involvement or muscle spasms. Neurological deficits may be present in patients having spinal cord compression. Fracture of the site may cause limb deformity, restriction of movement and uncommonly neurovascular deficit. On biochemical examination, serum alkaline phosphatase is usually elevated. The most frequently involved sites are the vertebrae, pelvis, ribs, femur and skull.[13] Skeletal metastases may be diagnosed by conventional radiography, bone scintigraphy, CT scan and/or MRI. Recently, fluorodeoxyglucose positron emission tomography (FDG-PET) CT scan is being done frequently which helps to identify if the lesion is localized or disseminated (Figs 1A to D). Plain X-ray films are a useful screening procedure and readily available. However, in case of high clinical suspicion, a negative X-ray should be investigated with modern imaging techniques. With conventional radiography, a change of about 40% in bone density is required before bone metastases may be identified. Small or early lesions may remain undetected.

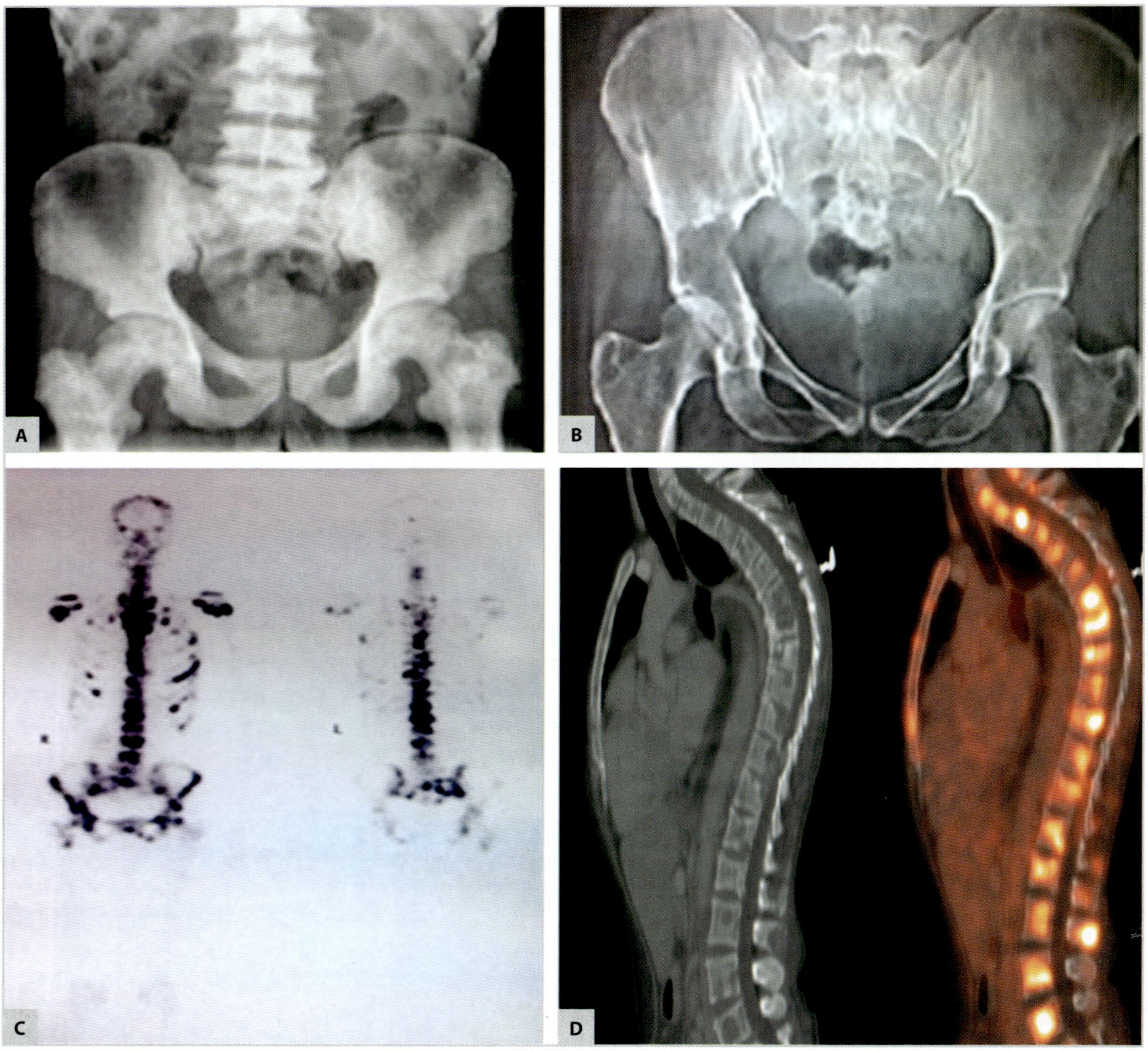

Figs 1A to D: Imaging modalities for skeletal metastases. (A) Conventional X-ray showing osteoblastic metastases; (B) Osteolytic metastases; (C) Bone scintigraphy with disseminated increased uptake at bones "hot spots"; (D) Positron emission tomography-computed tomography—fused images showing increased uptake at vertebrae

TABLE 1: Comparison between diagnostic imaging modalities

Imaging modality	*Anatomic detail*	*Causes of false-negative findings*	*Causes of false positive findings*	*Diagnostic sensitivity*	*Diagnostic specificity*
Conventional X-ray	Yes	Bone marrow only Lysis/sclerosis not at threshold for detection osteopenia	Trauma, inflammation, benign tumor healing	Low 44–50%	Low
Bone scan	No	Rapid/pure osteolytic progression	Trauma, inflammation, benign tumor healing	Varies 62–100%	Varies 78–100%
CT	Yes	Lysis/sclerosis not at threshold for detection	Trauma, inflammation, benign tumor healing	High 71–100%	Moderate
MRI	Yes	Lesion only in the cortex	Edema	High 82–100%	High 73–100%
PET	No	Lesion only in the cortex	After chemotherapy	Varies 62–100%	High 95–100%
PET-CT	Yes	Lesions only in cortex, below threshold for detection	Trauma, post-chemotherapy, flare, necrosis	High 95–100%	High 95–100%

(*Source*: Adopted from Hamakoa T, Madewell JE, Podoloff DA, et al. Bone imaging in metastatic breast cancer. J Clin Oncol. 2004;22(14):2942-53)

Bone scan/scintigraphy is the most common investigation used in work up for bone metastasis. The patient is injected with a small amount of radioactive material such as technetium-99m-MDP and then scanned with a gamma camera, a device to detect the radiation emitted by the injected material. Two-dimensional projections of scintigraphy may be enough, but in order to view small lesions (less than 1 cm) especially in the spine, single photon emission computed tomography (SPECT) imaging technique is useful. Five percent to 10% change in bone density is required to get a positive bone scan. It is positive in 14–34% of patients who have no radiographic evidence of bone metastases even though the images seen are biplanar. However, sensitivity is much less for detection of purely osteolytic metastases like in multiple myeloma. Since abnormalities seen are nonspecific, physicians should note that several benign conditions may also give rise to false positive results.[13]

A CT scan allows the identification of the type of metastases and results are more sensitive than the above two methods. Myelography though invasive, can accurately identify the site and extent of lesion(s) throughout the whole spine. It is rarely performed as MRI use has increased. MRI delineates the whole spine and identifies multiple sites of vertebral involvement, the paravertebral epidural extension and integrity of the spinal cord. Since increasingly available and being a noninvasive procedure, it has nearly replaced CT scan imaging for vertebral metastases. It allows differentiation between traumatic, osteoporotic or pathological fractures and compressions without the need of invasive techniques. The disadvantages of MRI include its relatively higher cost.[14] All the data derived from these radiological studies should always be correlated with the clinical findings.

Use of FDG-PET CT is rapidly increasing as initial investigation for metastatic work up for advanced breast and lung cancer. The sensitivity of FDG-PET CT is high and is comparable to MRI for detection of bone metastases. The lytic bone lesions are better detected by PET scan than bone scan and three dimensional images decreases the likelihood of missing the findings.

To understand better a brief comparative table between the different diagnostic modalities is given in Table 1.

TREATMENT

Treatment of painful bone metastasis requires multimodality approach. This includes use of analgesics, radiotherapy, surgery, endocrine therapy, nerve blocks, bisphosphonates, chemotherapy and radiopharmaceuticals; either alone or in combination (Table 2).

Analgesics

The skillful use of analgesic drugs is the most important aspect of cancer pain treatment. According to the World Health Organization (WHO) guidelines on cancer pain management, nonsteroidal anti-inflammatory drugs (NSAIDs) like paracetamol (650 mg thrice a day), ibuprofen (400 mg thrice a day) are recommended as the first step of the analgesic ladder.[15] Even in the presence of severe pain, NSAIDs should be given due to additive or synergic analgesia given by them. The specific effect is presumably attributed to a reduction of the edema and prostaglandins-

TABLE 2: Dose schedules for commonly used drugs during the treatment of skeletal metastases

Drug	Dosage
Paracetamol	Oral: 650 mg thrice a day
Ibuprofen	Oral: 400 mg thrice a day
Diclofenec	Oral: 50 mg twice a day
Codeine	Oral: 30 mg three to four times a day
Tramadol	Oral: 50 mg twice/thrice a day
Morphine	Oral: 5-10 mg six times a day
Fentanyl	Transdermal: 25–100 µg/hour, transdermal patch to be changed after 72 hours
Zoledronic acid	Intravenous: 4 mg in 100 mL normal saline over 20 minute, once a month
Pramidronate	Intravenous: 60–90 mg in 250 mL normal saline over 4 hour, once a month
Alendronate	Oral: 70 mg once a week
Denosumab	Subcutaneous: 120 mg subcutaneous injection once a month

induced pain sensitization. Centrally mediated analgesia is achieved by additional mechanisms.

The opioids like morphine or codeine are very useful in pain management. They should be added if pain is not controlled by NSAIDs. Initially weak opioids like codeine (30 mg 3–4 times per day), tramadol (50 mg twice a day) are added. If still uncontrolled then weak opioids are replaced by stronger opioids like morphine (5–10 mg six times per day) or fentanyl (transdermal patch, 25–100 µg/hour). However, one should be using them very judiciously as per WHO guidelines. Corticosteroids are well-established co-analgesics. They have beneficial effects in reducing metastatic bone pain due to their anti-inflammatory properties of blocking the synthesis of cytokines. However, there are no controlled studies supporting this view. The duration of pain relief is generally short.

Radiotherapy

The role of radiotherapy in the palliation of symptomatic bone metastases is well established. External beam radiotherapy is the most commonly used modality for the treatment of uncomplicated bone metastases. Palliative radiotherapy improves quality of life of patients by rapidly relieving bone pain. For patients with widespread metastases, hemi-body irradiation (HBI) or bone seeking radiopharmaceuticals provide good and sustained pain relief.

Radiotherapy includes treatment with high energy X-rays/gamma rays. Radiation provides pain relief in bone metastases by killing tumor cells and inhibiting cytokine secreting cells. It is a simple procedure and is given on outpatient basis. Local site radiation is well tolerated and side effects are minimum.

A wide range of single and multifraction radiation dose regimens have been used for treatment of bone metastasis. Various studies have shown that single fraction treatments (8–10 Gy) are equivalent to multifraction regimens (20–30 Gy in 5–10 daily treatments, over period of 1–2 weeks) in achieving pain relief. Additionally, three meta-analyses have confirmed the same findings.[16-21] Single fraction treatment is advantageous for patient, as the treatment is completed in single visit to hospital. Among various single dose fraction schedules, 8 Gy gives higher probability of pain relief. It is the most common fractionation in the routine clinical practice.[22,23]

In spite of this, there is wide use of various multifraction schedules due to individual practices. In recent years, use of single fraction radiotherapy has been increasing. In HBI, radiation is given to approximately half of body surface, i.e. above umbilicus (upper hemi-body) or below umbilicus (lower hemi-body). The commonly used radiation fractionation is 6 Gy single fraction for upper hemi-body and 8 Gy single fraction for lower hemi-body. Side effects with such radiation are higher than localized radiation and includes nausea, vomiting, loose motions and in few cases myelosuppression. Chemotherapy is deferred for about 4–6 weeks after HBI.

A proportion of patients treated with radiotherapy either relapses or do not show response after the first treatment at all. These patients may be suitable for retreatment. Retreatment using both single-fraction and multifraction regimens are effective in this setting. Only a few proportion of total patients receive re-treatment .

American Society For Radiation Oncology (ASRTO) in coordination with Third International Consensus Conference on Palliative Radiotherapy has given guidelines for radiotherapy in bone metastases.[24] They concluded that radiotherapy is the mainstay for treatment of pain and prevention of morbidity due to bone metastases. Use of other modalities like radiopharmaceuticals, surgical decompression or stabilization or bisphosphonates for treatment of bone metastases does not obviate the need for radiotherapy. Recently published review article has also concluded that based on published studies, palliative radiotherapy for bone metastasis is cost effective as compared to other palliative treatments.[25]

There are clinical situations where bone metastasis remains asymptomatic. There is no clear consensus for treatment of asymptomatic bone metastases. The different characteristics to be taken into consideration for favoring treatment includes the site of metastasis, proportion of bone destruction, weight bearing areas, etc.

Radiopharmaceuticals

Radiopharmaceuticals have been used to treat metastatic bone pain. They can be systematically administered to deliver radiation within the body. Bone specific isotopes such as phosphorus-32, strontium-89 and samarium-153 are the most recognized radiopharmaceuticals used. Strontium-89 is chemically similar to calcium and has significant advantages. The uptake is greatest in areas with marked osteoblastic activity. Uptake is more selective and bone marrow depression is less likely. Hence, it is more useful in primarily sclerotic bone metastases as in prostate cancer. Patients achieve good pain relief within a median of 15 days with a duration of effect of up to 6 months in the majority of patients.[26] The response rate is 70–80% after a single intravenous doses. Compared to external beam irradiation, precision is less in delivering specific doses of radiation. The dose of radiation is delivered over a continuous period of time, at a relatively low dose-rate. Advantages include easy administration and effectiveness in subclinical sites of metastases. Toxicity from marrow suppression is higher in patients with wide spread bone marrow metastases and post multiples cycles of chemotherapy and/or radiotherapy. The major drawbacks include cost, storage, dispensing and requirement of protection, storage and disposal of urine. These may limit widespread use of this technique.

Surgical Interventions

Surgical interventions in cases of bone metastasis are reserved for pathological fracture or spinal cord compression. Surgical techniques range from palliative decompression by laminectomy, to more extensive procedures, such as radical en-bloc resection and stabilization with internal fixation. The choice of surgical technique depends on expected survival, treatment-related morbidity and outcome after treatment.

In cases of impending fractures, commonly used criteria for prophylactic surgical intervention include the size of a lesion (> 25 mm), proximally located lesions, a radiographic osteolytic appearance, more than 50% circumferential or axial cortical involvement greater than 50% and increasing local pain. In 1989, Mirel[27] proposed a scoring system for fracture prediction. Several radiographic and clinical factors were combined to derive a single score (Table 3). The surgical intervention is recommended in patients with scores more than 7.

TABLE 3: Mirel's scoring system

Variable	*1*	*2*	*3*
Site	Upper limb	Lower limb	Peritrochanteric
Pain	Mild	Moderate	Functional
X-ray	Osteoblastic	Mixed	Osteolytic
Size	< 1/3	1/3 to 2/3	> 2/3

TABLE 4: Harrington's classification for spinal metastases

Class type	*Extent of involvement*
Class I	No significant neurological involvement
Class II	Involvement of bone without collapse or instability
Class III	Major neurological impairment (sensory or motor) without significant involvement of bone
Class IV	Vertebral collapse with pain due to mechanical causes or instability but without significant neurological compromise
Class V	Vertebral collapse with pain due to mechanical causes or instability combined with major neurological impairment

For spinal lesions with or without impending or actual fracture, the choice of palliative treatment depends upon the Harrington's classification[28] (Table 4). Harrington divided patients into five classes depending on the extent of neurological compromise or bone destruction. Primary radiotherapy was recommended for classes I to III and primary surgical intervention for classes IV and V. Surgical intervention should be considered in patients with refractory pain or neurological symptoms or when spinal cord tolerance to radiation had been reached.

Vertebroplasty/cementoplasty comprises of instillation of acrylic material into vertebral cavity or in lytic cavity of bone. This provides mechanical strength to the diseased bone. The advantage includes rapid pain relief, good biomechanical strength and is minimally invasive. Postoperative radiotherapy can be given without any additional complications.

The patient may be inoperable because of comorbidity, deteriorating condition or because of a complicated fracture. For such patients, palliative radiotherapy is indicated for pain relief and may enable healing in a considerable percentage of patients. Steroids may be helpful if no contraindication exists.

In general, the choice between surgery alone, surgery plus radiotherapy or radiotherapy alone depends on the clinical setting of the patient, the time in which the motor and sensory deficits have developed and the availability of appropriate surgical expertise.

Chemotherapy and Hormonal Therapy

Potential indications for palliative chemotherapy include symptoms due to metastatic disease, hypercalcemia and marrow infiltration. It may be useful in patients with responsive tumors like breast, lung, etc. Pain relief is due to action on tumor cells. The response evaluation in the bone is more difficult to assess than at any other metastatic sites.

Hormonal therapy is based on the principle of depriving the growth stimulus to tumor cells induced by hormones. Hormone dependent tumors presenting with bone metastases are usually associated with a slow progression of disease and a longer survival. Hormonal therapy is of proven benefit in breast, prostate and endometrial cancers.[29] Because of lower toxicity compared to chemotherapy, endocrine therapy should be the first therapeutic modality in appropriately selected metastatic breast and prostate cancer patients.

Bisphosphonates

Bisphosphonates are structural analogues of pyrophosphates, a naturally occurring component of bone crystal deposition. The mechanism of action includes physicochemical protection by absorbing calcium phosphate, suppression of osteoclast function and prevention of maturation of osteoclast precursors. With all this action it strengthens the bones and decreases morbidity related to bone metastases. They are also extremely effective in the management of patients with hypercalcemia along with hydration and alkalization.

Zoledronic acid is the most common bisphosphonate used in oncology. It is given in a dose of 4 mg in 100 mL normal saline over 15 minutes infusion. The dose is repeated every month till 6–24 cycles as per primary tumor site.

Bisphosphonates are well-tolerated. The most common adverse events include flu-like symptoms (fever, arthralgia, myalgia, bone pain and weakness), nausea, dyspnea and peripheral edema. These events are mild to moderate and self-limiting. Their administration may result in elevated serum creatinine levels. Renal function should be closely monitored in patients receiving bisphosphonates. In case of renal derangement, further doses should be withheld till renal function returns to normal.

The systematic review by Wong et al. has concluded that there is evidence to support the effectiveness of bisphosphonates in providing some pain relief for bone metastases.[30] However, there is insufficient evidence to recommend bisphosphonates for pain relief as first line therapy. It is necessary to define the most effective bisphosphonates or their relative effectiveness for different primary neoplasms.

Denosumab

Denosumab is a newer agent approved for patients with bone metastasis. It is a monoclonal antibody and acts by inhibiting receptor activator of nuclear factor-kappa B ligand (RANK-L). By inhibiting RANK-L, it prevents maturation of osteoclasts and decreases bone demineralization. It is well tolerated and common side effects include constipation, skin rashes, etc. It can be safely used in renal impairment without any dose modification.

Psychological Support

As expected the incidence of depression and anxiety increases with higher levels of disability, advanced illness and pain. Patients with bone metastasis represent a particularly vulnerable group.

Depression is managed using a combination of supportive psychotherapy and cognitive, behavioral techniques. Antidepressant medications are vital for management in patients with major depressive episodes. Tricyclic antidepressants are the most common drugs used. Side effects are often distressing. The second generation antidepressants, including trazodone, maprotiline and fluoxetine, are less cardiotoxic than tricyclics. The benzodiazepines may also be used.

CONCLUSION

Bone is a common metastatic site for advanced cancer. Incidence of bone metastases is increasing along with increasing survival of cancer patients. Bone metastasis is common in patients with breast, lung and prostate cancer. FDG-PET CT and MRI is increasingly used for diagnosis of bone metastasis. Aim of treatment is to provide adequate pain relief and maintain quality of life. Treatment includes supportive care and adequate analgesics. Systemic chemotherapy or hormonal therapy along with bisphosphonates is given to further strengthen the bones and contain the primary cancer. Radiotherapy and radiopharmaceuticals provide long lasting pain relief to patients. Surgical intervention is indicated in cases of skeletal related events like pathological fracture or spinal cord compression. Prophylactic surgical fixation is done in cases of impending fracture.

KEY SUMMARY

- Skeletal metastasis is seen commonly in advanced cancers of breast, lung, and prostate with pain being the first symptom
- MRI and PET-CT are most sensitive and specific investigations; however, conventional X-ray and bone scintigraphy is commonly done
- Severe complications include hypercalcemia, fracture of bones and spinal cord compression
- General care—analgesics, bisphosphonates and anxiolytics
- Specific treatments include radiotherapy or use of radiopharmaceuticals for sustained pain relief.
- Surgical interventions—for complicated bone metastasis or for impending fracture sites.
- Systemic chemotherapy/hormonal therapy also help in containing the primary cancer.

REFERENCES

1. JD S. Radiation therapy for bone metastasis: the Hanemman Experience. GK Hall Medical Publishers; 1981. pp. 436-42.
2. Stoll BA. Natural History, Prognosis and Staging of Bone Metastasis. In: Stolla BA, Parbhoo S (Eds). Bone Metastasis: Monitoring and Treatment. 1983. pp. 1-20.
3. Ferlay J, Shin HR, Bray F, et al. Estimates of worldwide burden of cancer in 2008: GLOBOCAN 2008. Int J Cancer. 2010;127(12):2893-917.
4. Coleman RE. Skeletal complications of malignancy. Cancer. 1997;80(8 Suppl):1588-94.
5. Moore RE, Lackman RD. Metastatic bone disease. U Penn Orthopaed J. 2010;20:117-20.
6. Leone BA, Romero A, Rabinovich MG, et al. Stage IV breast cancer: clinical course and survival of patients with osseous versus extraosseous metastases at initial diagnosis. The GOCS (Grupo Oncologico Cooperativo del Sur) experience. Am J Clin Oncol. 1988;11(6):618-22.
7. Sherry MM, Greco FA, Johnson DH, et al. Metastatic breast cancer confined to the skeletal system. An indolent disease. Am J Med. 1986;81(3):381-6.
8. Namer M. Clinical consequences of osteolytic bone metastases. Bone. 1991;12 Suppl 1:S7.
9. Sim FH, Frassica FJ, Frassica DA. Metastatic bone disease: current concepts of clinicopathophysiology and modern surgical treatment. Ann Acad Med Singapore. 1992;21(2):274-9.
10. Bjurholm A, Kreicbergs A, Brodin E, et al. Substance P- and CGRP-immunoreactive nerves in bone. Peptides. 1988;9(1):165-71.
11. Campa JA, Payne R. The management of intractable bone pain: a clinician's perspective. Semin Nucl Med. 1992;22(1):3-10.
12. Foley KM. Pain assessment and cancer pain syndromes. In: D Doyle, GW Hanks, N Macdonald (Eds). Oxford Textbook of Palliative Medicine. Oxford: Oxford Medical Publications; 1993. pp. 148-65.
13. Tubiana-Hulin M. Incidence, prevalence and distribution of bone metastases. Bone. 1991;12 Suppl 1:S9-10.
14. Smoker WR, Godersky JC, Knutzon RK, et al. The role of MR imaging in evaluating metastatic spinal disease. AJR Am J Roentgenol. 1987;149(6):1241-8.
15. World Health Organisation. Cancer pain relief. Geneva; 1984.
16. Hartsell WF, Scott CB, Bruner DW, et al. Randomized trial of short- versus long-course radiotherapy for palliation of painful bone metastases. J Natl Cancer Inst. 2005;97(11):798-804.
17. Roos DE, Turner SL, O'Brien PC, et al. Randomized trial of 8 Gy in 1 versus 20 Gy in 5 fractions of radiotherapy for neuropathic pain due to bone metastases (Trans-Tasman Radiation Oncology Group, TROG 96.05). Radiother Oncol. 2005;75(1):54-63.
18. Kaasa S, Brenne E, Lund JA, et al. Prospective randomised multicenter trial on single fraction radiotherapy (8 Gy x 1) versus multiple fractions (3 Gy x 10) in the treatment of painful bone metastases. Radiother Oncol. 2006;79(3):278-84.
19. McQuay HJ, Carroll D, Moore RA. Radiotherapy for painful bone metastases: a systematic review. Clin Oncol (R Coll Radiol). 1997;9(3):150-4.
20. Wu JS, Wong R, Johnston M, et al. Meta-analysis of dose-fractionation radiotherapy trials for the palliation of painful bone metastases. Int J Radiat Oncol Biol Phys. 2003;55(3):594-605.
21. Sze WM, Shelley MD, Held I, et al. Palliation of metastatic bone pain: single fraction versus multifraction radiotherapy—a systematic review of randomised trials. Clin Oncol (R Coll Radiol). 2003;15(6):345-52.
22. Hoskin PJ, Price P, Easton D, et al. A prospective randomised trial of 4 Gy or 8 Gy single doses in the treatment of metastatic bone pain. Radiother Oncol. 1992;23(2):74-8.
23. Jeremic B, Shibamoto Y, Acimovic L, et al. A randomized trial of three single-dose radiation therapy regimens in the treatment of metastatic bone pain. Int J Radiat Oncol Biol Phys. 1998;42(1):161-7.
24. Lutz S, Berk L, Chang E, et al. Palliative radiotherapy for bone metastases: an ASTRO evidence based guideline. Int J Radiat Oncol Biol Phys. 2011;79(4):965-76.
25. Agarwal JP, Swangsilpa T, van der Linden Y, et al. The role of external beam radiotherapy in the management of bone metastases. Clin Oncol (R Coll Radiol). 2006;18(10):747-60.
26. Laing AH, Ackery DM, Bayly RJ, et al. Strontium-89 chloride for pain palliation in prostatic skeletal malignancy. Br J Radiol. 1991;64(765):816-22.
27. Mirels H. Metastatic disease in long bones. A proposed scoring system for diagnosing impending pathologic fractures. Clin Orthop Relat Res. 1989;(249):256-64.
28. Harrington KD. Orthopedic surgical management of skeletal complications of malignancy. Cancer. 1997;80(8 Suppl):1614-27.
29. Wood BC. Hormone treatments in the common 'hormone-dependent' carcinomas. Palliat Med. 1993;7(4):257-72.
30. Wong R, Wiffen PJ. Bisphosphonates for the relief of pain secondary to bone metastases. Cochrane Database Syst Rev. 2002;(2): CD002068.

52 Management of Primary Brain Tumors

Rakesh Jalali, Uday Krishna

INTRODUCTION

Tumors of the central nervous system (CNS) are rare constituting 1–2% of all neoplasms. They are the second most common overall and the most common solid tumors in the pediatric population. Approximately, 25% of all cancer related deaths in pediatric population occur due to CNS tumors. CNS is among the few sites where a significant number of patients with benign tumors are managed in the neuro-oncology practice. With the advances in the diagnosis, neuro-surgery, radiotherapy, chemotherapy and a greater understanding of biology, the outcomes of these tumors have improved over a period of time. There is also a greater recognition of incorporating ancillary expertise in the form of physiotherapy, occupational therapy and rehabilitation in the management paradigm for these patients.

EPIDEMIOLOGY

Statistics of brain tumors in the world is defined by two major data sources namely, the Surveillance, Epidemiology and End results (SEER) program of the National Cancer Institute and the Central Brain Tumor Registry of United States (CBTRUS). According to the SEER registry, the incidence of primary CNS tumors is between 2.2 and 8.3 per 100,000 people per year while the CBTRUS incidence of new CNS tumors in the United States is 43,800 cases per year that includes both benign and malignant histologies.[1]

Indian Data

Central nervous system tumors constitute about 3.5% of all cancers in Indian subcontinent (4.34% in males and 3% in females). It is seen in the adult population age 35–64 years with an increasing percentage with advancing age. Epidemiology and descriptive statistics from Tata Memorial Hospital neuro-oncology group database showed that the age of presentation of high-grade gliomas in the Indian population was a decade earlier than the Western population. A retrospective data collected from the major neuro-oncology facilities in India showed that 15% of the new primary brain tumors constituted of high-grade gliomas.[2] The Delhi Population Based Cancer Registry showed that the age adjusted (world population) incidence rates were 3.9 per 100,000 for males and 2.4 per 100,000 for females. Gliomas were the most frequently reported histology both in males (26.6%) and females (23.2%). A male predominance in incidence was observed for all histological classifications. The rates in Delhi are low compared to the incidences reported from developed countries.[3]

The analyses of a large retrospective study showed the histological spectrum of pediatric age group brain tumors in seven tertiary care hospitals in India. It has reported that the most common primary pediatric brain tumors were astrocytic tumors (34.7%), followed by medulloblastoma and supratentorial primitive neuro-ectodermal tumors (22.4%), craniopharyngioma (10.2%) and ependymal tumors (9.8%). The most common astrocytic tumor was pilocytic astrocytoma.[4] In comparison to adults, oligodendrogliomas (ODG) and lymphomas were rare in children. The histological profile of pediatric brain tumors in India is similar to that reported in the Western literature.

IMAGING OF PRIMARY BRAIN TUMORS

Imaging in neuro-oncology practice is necessary for diagnostic assessment, characterization of the grade of the tumor, tumor localization for surgery and radiation therapy and response assessment. Computed tomography (CT) aids in rapid acquisition of images, especially in an unstable patient, but lacks the soft tissue resolution capability of magnetic resonance imaging (MRI). Gadolinium enhanced MRI is the standard imaging of choice for primary brain tumors.[5] The various imaging modalities and imaging characteristics of various tumors are enumerated in Table 1. The postoperative imaging of primary brain tumors with gadolinium-enhanced MRI is necessary for assessing gross residual tumor and is performed ideally within 24 hours of resection of a preoperatively enhancing high-grade glioma. This timing avoids postoperative changes in the postoperative bed and minimizes difficulty in interpretation.

HISTOLOGY OF CNS TUMORS

The current 4th edition of classification was published in 2007.[6] Histological characteristics of certain primary brain tumors are described below.

"Pilocytic astrocytoma" shows a biphasic pattern of dense and loose regions and they commonly spread along the Virchow robin spaces and subarachnoid spaces. The classical rosenthal fibers and eosinophilic bodies might be present. "Pleomorphic xanthoastrocytoma" has a mixture of spindled to epitheloid astrocytes together with large, often multinucleate giant cells, sometimes with xanthogranulomatous intracytoplasmic lipid accumulations. "Diffuse fibrillary astrocytomas" are characterized by increased cellularity and nuclear atypia. The gemistocytic variant contains cells with plump eosinophillic cytoplasm and eccentric nuclei. "Anaplastic ODG" have clear cells with central spherical nuclei and well-defined cell borders, the so-called honeycomb appearance. They demonstrate a typical vascularization pattern consisting of dense network of branching capillaries resembling chicken wire pattern. "Anaplastic oligoastrocytoma (AOA)" shows a diffusely infiltrating oligoastrocytoma (OA) with focal or diffuse histological signs of anaplasia, such as high cellularity, nuclear atypia, cellular pleomorphism, obvious mitotic activity and microvascular proliferation. "Anaplastic astrocytoma" have nuclear atypia and mitotic activity, without necrosis or neovascularization. They are glial fibrillary acidic protein (GFAP) positive and positive for protein S-100. Nuclear p53 staining is found in about 60% of the cases.

Glioblastoma: Gross pathology is characterized by nuclear atypia, mitotic activity, vascular proliferation and necrosis (Figs 1A and B). They are positive for GFAP and S-100. Nuclear reactivity for P53 is seen in 30–40% of all glioblastomas and MIB labelling index is usually high (> 10%) (Figs 2A and B). Microvascular proliferation with a

TABLE 1: Contemporary imaging modalities

Imaging modality	*Remarks*	*Advantages*	*Disadvantages*
CT scan	First line imaging modality	• More widely available • Image acquisition faster • Relatively cheaper • Good anatomic visualization • Can be used with metal objects • Preferred in an unstable patient	• Exposure to ionizing radiation • Limited reconstruction ability • Poor resolution • Contrast reaction
MRI	Gold standard imaging modality	• Unparalleled resolution • Multiplanar imaging • No exposure to ionizing radiation	• Susceptible to motion artifacts • Cannot be used with metal objects • Claustrophobic, noisy, long times • Relatively expensive
MR spectroscopy	Assesses tumor metabolites	Useful for discriminating radiation necrosis from tumor	• Limited utility near bone, vessels or air spaces • Wide variability in interpretation
MR perfusion	Assesses blood flow and volume	• Generally correlates with grade • Useful to distinguish radiation necrosis from tumor progression	Limited utility near bone, vessels

Abbreviation: MRI, magnetic resonance imaging

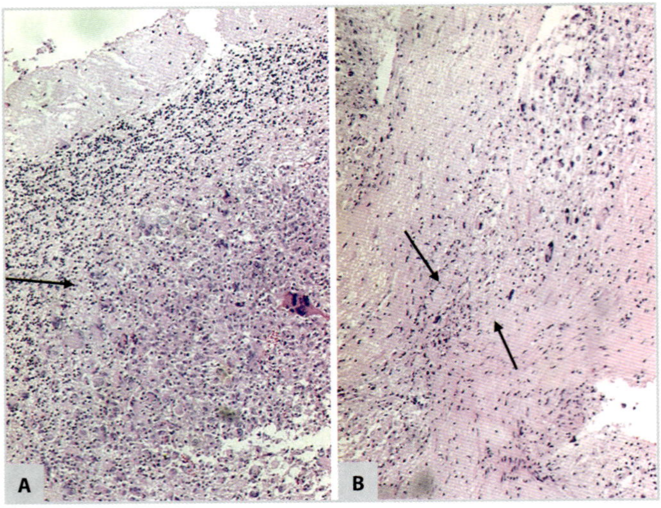

Figs 1A and B: (A) It shows high-grade infiltrating glial tumor with atypical cellularity and mitotic activity; (B) It shows the microvascular proliferation and areas of confluent necrosis

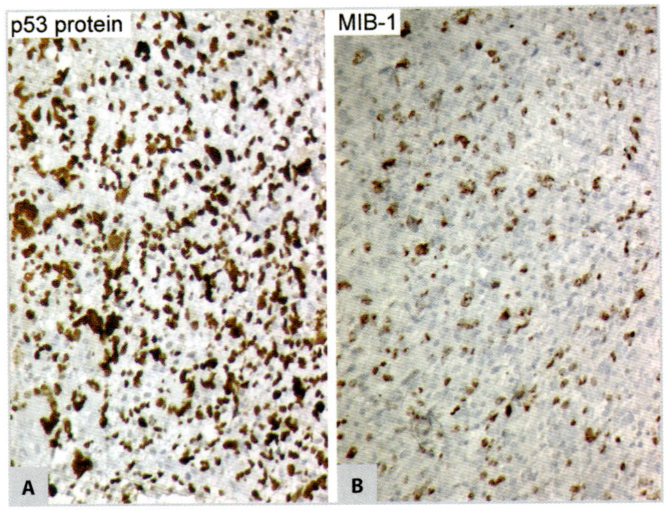

Figs 2A and B: Immunohistochemistry of glioblastoma multiforme (GBM) with P53 and MIB-1

glomerulum- or garland-like capillary structure is seen. Necroses with pseudopalisading pattern are characteristics of glioblastoma multiforme (GBM).

Molecular Biology of Glioma and Process of Progression to High-grade Glioma

Gliomagenesis is characterized by normal astrocytes undergoing transformation with the loss of tumor suppressor genes critical for cell growth, differentiation, and function, including TP53, the retinoblastoma (RB) gene, the INK4a (inhibitor of cyclin-dependent kinase 4) gene, and the phosphatase and tensin homolog (PTEN) gene.[7] TP53 gene mutation or gene deletion is seen in 60% of low-grade gliomas, leading to transformation to anaplastic astrocytoma and GBM. The so-called secondary GBM is also associated with RB and PTEN mutations with cell aneuploidy and overexpression of cyclin-dependent kinase 4 (CDK4). Forty percent of GBM are secondary GBM and the average patient age is younger, while 60% of GBM are primary and show amplification of epidermal growth factor receptor (EGFR), deletions in the INK4a gene with loss of p14 and p16, and diploid cells. The loss of heterozygosity (LOH) in chromosome 10q causes inactivation of PTEN and has been shown in several studies to have a highly significant and independent impact on prognosis. Recently a molecular subclassification of glioblastoma has been defined into proneural, neural, classical and mesenchymal subtypes based on genetic aberrations and gene expression of EGFR, NF1, platelet-derived growth factor receptor (PDGFR) and isocitrate dehydrogenase 1 (IDH1) genes. A subset of glioblastoma tumors harbor characteristic promoter DNA methylation alterations referred to as gliomas CpG island methylator phenotype (G-CIMP). These have distinct molecular features including a high frequency of IDH1 mutation. The patients with G-CIMP tumors are younger at diagnosis and have improved survival times.[8] Hypoxia plays a central role in the pathobiology of glioblastoma with the transcription factor, hypoxia inducible factor 1 (HIF-1) stabilized under hypoxic conditions. This causes physiologic changes including regulation of glycolytic pathway, blood vessel formation, and induction of genes encoding chemotactic molecules such as IL-8 and vascular endothelial growth factor (VEGF). This also leads to recruitment of macrophages that in turn lead to mitogenic, angiogenic and migration and invasion. These also affect host driven changes implicated in resistance to chemoradiation.[9]

O6-methylguanine-methyl-transferase (MGMT) gene promoter methylation has emerged as a promising molecular biomarker in glioblastoma. MGMT is a repair protein that removes alkyl groups from the O6 position of guanine and thus counteracts the effect of alkylating drugs like nitrosoureas or temozolomide (TMZ). MGMT protein expression is repressed by epigenetic methylation of the MGMT gene promoter. Methylation of the MGMT promoter can be demonstrated in 30–60% of glioblastoma patients and is associated with favorable outcome in patients treated with alkylating agents.[10] Mutations of unidentified tumor suppressor genes located on 1p/19q contribute to pathogenesis of ODG in adults whereas the genes involved in pediatric population is different. This is evidenced by presence of LOH of chromosomes 1p and 19q in adults while this is absent in children. Combined LOH is seen in 83%, 63%, 56%, 52% of pure ODG, anaplstic ODG, OA and AOA, respectively. Recent phase III prospective trials, Radiation Therapy Oncology Group (RTOG) 9402 and European Organization for Research and Treatment of Cancer (EORTC) 26951 have shown that LOH for either 1p or 19q was a significant independent prognostic variable correlating with outcome and survival.[11]

IDH1 and 2 mutations in gliomas: A genome wide study of mutational analysis of glioblastomas revealed somatic mutations of the IDH1 gene mutations in those tumors that have evolved from lower grade to glioblastoma. This is seen in stem cells that lead to both astrocytomas and ODG. It is seen in ODG as well as OA. Those with a wild type IDH had progressed to GBM. IDH1 mutation was characteristically not seen in pilocytic astrocytomas, which shows that the mechanism of origin is from a different pathway and that pilocytics very rarely transform to malignant gliomas.[9] Very recently it was shown that pilocytic astrocytomas demonstrate duplication at 7q34 producing a B-RAF fusion gene but not in high-grade gliomas. They are usually associated with NF1. They demonstrate KIAA1549-BRAF fusion protein having activated BRAF kinase activity, which establishes these gene alterations as being oncogenic.[12]

Molecular Biology of Medulloblastoma

Current classification schemes for medulloblastoma are based primarily on morphology (histopathology), and include variants such as desmoplastic/nodular, medulloblastoma with extensive nodularity (MBEN), classic medulloblastoma, large cell, and anaplastic medulloblastoma. With advancement in genomics and in particular with the ability to monitor transcription across the genome, a new subclassification of medulloblastoma is described based on the differences in the transcriptome. Tumors with similar transcriptomes behave in a biologically similar manner, and this subgroup classification serves as a guide to successful anti-neoplastic therapy. They are WNT, SHH, Group 3 and Group 4.[13]

Prognostic Factors for Survival in High-grade Gliomas

A recursive partitioning analysis (RPA) undertaken by the RTOG identified six prognostic classes of anaplastic gliomas based on clinical factors, in which classes III–VI are applicable to glioblastomas based on patients' ages, Karnofsky performance status, neurological function, mental status and extent of surgery.[14] It was developed and validated in the early 1990s. It is described in Table 2. Since then, there have been dramatic changes in diagnostic methods, radiotherapy planning, treatment techniques and revision of histopathological classification systems, with identification of molecular factors relevant for outcome. A companion study of the large EORTC/National Cancer Institute of Canada (NCIC) study has identified few more important prognostic factors as more relevant for the outcome of these patients.[15] This includes treatment with radiotherapy and concomitant adjuvant treatment with TMZ, age, extent of surgical resection, MGMT promoter

TABLE 2: Recursive partitioning analysis (RPA)

Class	*Age (years)*	*Histology*	*KPS*	*Mental status*	*Symptom duration*	*Surgery*	*Neuro-deficit*	*Total RT dose (Gy)*	*Median survival (months)*
I	< 50	AA		Normal					58.6
II	> 50	AA	70–100		> 3 months				37.4
III	< 50	AA		Normal					17.9
	< 50	GBM	90–100						
IV	< 50	GBM	< 90						11.1
	> 50	AA	70–100		> 3 months				
	> 50	GBM	70–100			PR/CR	No		
V	> 50	GBM	70–100			PR/CR	Yes		8.9
	> 50	GBM	70–100			Biopsy		> 54.4	
	> 50	GBM	< 70	Normal					
VI	> 50	GBM	70–100						4.6
	> 50	GBM	< 70	Abnormal		Biopsy		> 54.4	

Abbreviations: KPS, Karnofsky performance score; AA, anaplastic astrocytoma; GBM, glioblastoma multiforme; PR, partial response; CR, complete response methylation status, World Health Organization (WHO) performance status, neurological function expressed by the mini-mental state examination (MMSE), and the need for corticosteroids administration after surgery or biopsy. Use of corticosteroids might identify patients with more severe clinical signs and symptoms before surgery, or those with larger tumors or tumors that were amenable to biopsy only. This recent EORTC/RPA stratification nomogram predictions are more accurate than those based on the RPA classification.

MANAGEMENT OF COMMON SYMPTOMS AND COMPLICATIONS OF CNS TUMORS

Seizures: Up to 30–40% of malignant glioma patients have seizures at presentation or experience seizures during their disease course.[16] Approximately 80–90% of ODG and gangliogliomas present with seizures. Younger age group, cortical location of the tumor and multifocal or bihemispheric tumors are other risk factors for development of seizures. Tumor associated seizures originate from an intact, noninfiltrated neural tissue adjacent to the tumor tissue and not from the tumor itself. Increased glutamine and reduced gamma-aminobutyric acid (GABA) due to high alkalinity in the peritumoral tissue can lead to seizures. Monotherapy with phenytoin, valproate or carbamazepine is the initial management approach in most patients. Older antiepileptic drugs (AEDs) induce hepatic cytochrome P450-mediated metabolism and thus substantially increase the metabolism of most antineoplastic drugs (except nitrosoureas and TMZ). Hence, non-enzyme-inducing AEDs like levetiracetam are now increasingly used.[17]

Brain edema: Brain edema in gliomas is primarily the result of leakage of plasma into the tissue through dysfunctional cerebral capillaries (vasogenic edema) and is detectable on T2-W or fluid-attenuated inversion recovery (FLAIR) images. Brain edema is associated with increased intracranial pressure with headache, vertigo, and nausea/vomiting and can lead to life-threatening brainstem compression and herniation. Dexamethasone is usually the drug of choice.[16] This long-acting corticosteroid can be administered orally or intravenously at equal efficacy. Initial doses are typically 12–16 mg per day; doses more than 16 mg per day have not been shown to increase efficacy. Steroid dosage should be rapidly reduced and tapered to individual needs. In emergency situations, intravenous dexamethasone may be combined with osmotic agents such as mannitol or glycerol. In case of obstructive hydrocephalus secondary to the tumor diversion of the cerebrospinal fluid (CSF), using a shunt may be required to palliate the symptoms of raised intracranial pressure.

Venous thromboembolism: Up to 30% of malignant glioma patients develop deep venous thromboembolism (DVTE) at some point in the course of their disease. Risk factors include neurological deficits associated with reduced mobility, large and incompletely resected tumors, frontal tumor location, age greater than 60 years and the use of corticosteroids.[18] Compression stockings beginning 12–24 hours after neurosurgery together with prophylactic low-molecular-weight heparin (LMWH) are recommended. No data are available for prolonged thrombosis prophylaxis. However, beyond postoperatie period there is no data to show benefit of prophylactic anticonvulsants and active physiotherapy plays a significant role in reducing chances of venous thromboembolic phenomena.

Principles of Neurosurgery

Maximum cytoreduction of malignant gliomas confers an overall survival (OS) advantage. Most neurosurgeons attempt to remove contrast-enhancing tumor as completely as possible. However, this aim is achieved only in few patients, partly because of the difficulty in identifying marginal, contrast-enhancing tumor intraoperatively. Recently, a large randomized study was conducted to analyze fluorescence guided surgery with 5-aminolevulinic acid (5-ALA) for resection of malignant gliomas. Contrast-enhancing tumor was resected completely in 65% patients assigned to 5-ALA compared with 36% in patients assigned to white light.[19] It was postulated that by this new technique, there can potentially be doubling of the number of patients without residual, contrast-enhancing tumor on early postoperative MRI.

Principles of Radiotherapy

Radiotherapy is an intergral component of management of all types of CNS tumors. Most of the glial tumors are highly invasive in nature and are not always amenable for complete excision. Types of radiation used with therapeutic intent are photons (Gamma rays or X-rays), electrons, heavy particles such as protons and neutrons. Rationale of radiotherapy is to achieve a therapeutic ratio which is to maximize tumor control and minimize normal tissue complications.

In the context of gliomas, early part of the 20th century saw various cooperative groups across the world practicing only whole brain radiotherapy (WBRT), with the notion that the whole brain beyond surgical cavity was at risk of recurrence. Later with large number of autopsy studies and clinical studies it was shown that majority of recurrences occurred at an area of 2 cm beyond the surgical resection cavity. Subsequently, focal radiation to surgical resection cavity plus a 2 cm margin was found to be adequate and studies comparing results of this with the historical WBRT demonstrated no survival difference. On similar grounds, dose escalation beyond 60 Gy by using various techniques has not shown any survival advantage.

Recently with advances in radiation technology and delivery systems, 3D conformal radiotherapy (3DCRT), intensity modulated radiotherapy (IMRT) and image guided radiotherapy (IGRT) have been utilized to improve the therapeutic ratio. The latest technology includes the tomotherapy, cyberknife, novalis and more recently the truebeam. These techniques are utilized more in benign and low-grade tumors and especially the pediatric tumors with the intent to reduce late normal tissue toxicity.

Principles of Chemotherapy and Targeted Therapy

Temozolomide, an oral alkylating agent is rapidly absorbed and spontaneously converts to the active metabolite 3-methyl-(triazen-1-yl) imidazole-4-carboxamide (MTIC). Maximum plasma concentrations are observed 30–90 minutes after oral intake, and the plasma half-life is approximately 2 hours, with some delayed absorption when taken with food. Multiple potential therapeutic targets have been identified as a consequence of improved insight into molecular mechanisms and pathogenesis of malignant gliomas. As descrided previously, EGFR is amplified and overexpressed in approximately 50% of GBM. The EGFR tyrosine kinase inhibitors like gefitinib and erlotinib have been investigated in several studies in recurrent malignant glioma but did not demonstrate any survival advantage. Malignant gliomas are highly vascularized and infiltrative tumors that are strongly dependent on endothelial cell proliferation regulated by proangiogenic cytokines (e.g. VEGF) and integrins. In lieu of encouraging results in the recurrent setting, survival advantage conferred by Bevacizumab was tested in a randomized manner by addition of the drug to present standard of care. In a recent update, however, there is no added survival advantage.

MANAGEMENT OF INDIVIDUAL TUMORS

Glioblastoma

This most challenging form of primary brain tumor carries a dismal prognosis (Figs 3A and B) and tumors tend to be diffusely infiltrative beyond the gross tumor and recur locally. In the mid-1990s, the Brain Tumor Study Group (BTSG) conducted various protocols for assessing the use of radiation and chemotherapy in malignant gliomas. They concluded that radiation in combination with chemotherapy (nitrosoureas) improved the survival, compared to radiation or chemotherapy alone or best supportive care. These studies formed the basis of upfront treatment of malignant gliomas with radiation therapy. Furthermore, dose escalation studies employing IMRT, brachytherapy, gliadel wafer, etc. have not demonstrated additional survival benefit.

In a randomized trial by the EORTC and NCIC, it was shown that the addition of TMZ to RT as initial treatment prolongs the survival of patients with GBM. RT consists of 30 fractions of 2 Gy each, administered Monday to Friday for 6–7 weeks. TMZ chemotherapy, at a low dose of 75 mg/m^2, was administered daily, including weekends, from the first to the last day of RT, for up to maximum of 49 days. After a 4-week break, patients receive up to six cycles of maintenance TMZ (150–200 mg/m^2) daily for 5 days every 4 weeks. At tumor progression, treatment was at the physician's discretion.[20] This study demonstrated a survival advantage of 24% versus 11% with use of concurrent and

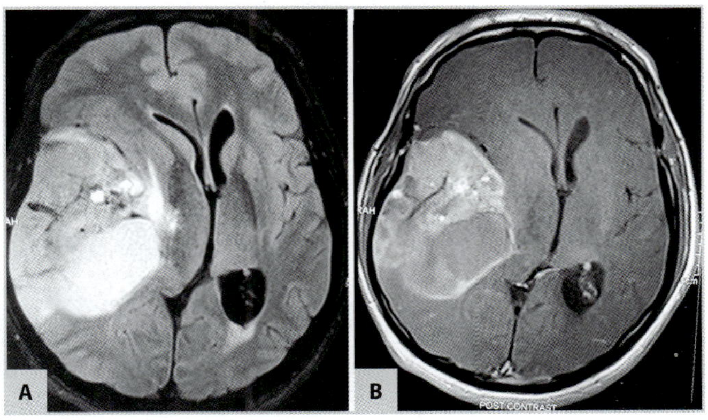

Figs 3A and B: (A) It shows a fluid-attenuated inversion recovery (FLAIR) sequence MRI with a large hyperintense lesion with mass effect and surrounding edema; (B) It shows a postcontrast axial section with a heterogeneously enhancing lesion with rim enhancement

adjuvant TMZ along with radiotherapy. Long-term results of this study showed an OS of 12% at 5 years. A companion study showed that in patients with MGMT methylation, the 2-year survival was 47% compared to those with an unmethylated MGMT.[21] Indian experience with same protocol for patients with GBM reported 1- and 2-year survival was 67% and 29%, respectively.[22] Toxicity profiles of a large cohort of patients showed a clinically significant neutropenia and thrombocytopenia was 7% and 12% respectively. TMZ was well tolerated by our patient population.[23]

Since the introduction of chemoradiotherapy with TMZ as the new standard of care for patients with glioblastoma, there has been an increasing awareness of progressive and enhancing lesions on MRI, noted immediately after the end of treatment, which are not related to tumor progression, but which are a treatment effect. This so-called pseudoprogression can occur in up to 20% and can explain about half of all cases of increasing lesions after the end of this treatment (Figs 4A and B). These lesions decrease in size or stabilize without additional treatments and often remain clinically asymptomatic.[24] There is evidence that treatment-related necrosis occurs more frequently and earlier after TMZ chemotherapy than after radiotherapy alone. The mechanism behind these events is likely to be due to a higher degree of tumor-cell and endothelial-cell killing. This increased cell kill might lead to secondary reactions, such as edema and abnormal vessel permeability in the tumor area, mimicking tumor progression, in addition to subsequent early treatment-related necrosis in some patients and milder subacute radiotherapy reactions in others. In patients managed with TMZ chemoradiotherapy who have clinically asymptomatic progressive lesions at the end of treatment, adjuvant TMZ should be continued; in clinically symptomatic patients, surgery should be considered.

With the standard MRI modalities (e.g. T2, T1 with gadolinium, and FLAIR), a reliable distinction between tumor recurrence and pseudoprogression or treatment related necrosis is not possible. Magnetic resonance spectroscopy (MRS) can distinguish residual or recurrent tumors from pure treatment-related necrosis, but not from mixed necrosis and tumor tissue. Diffusion weighted imaging (DWI) has also been assessed as an instrument for differentiating between tumor and necrosis after radiotherapy. The apparent diffusion coefficient was noted to be higher in necrotic tissue than in recurrent tumor tissue in several studies. However, available evidence for

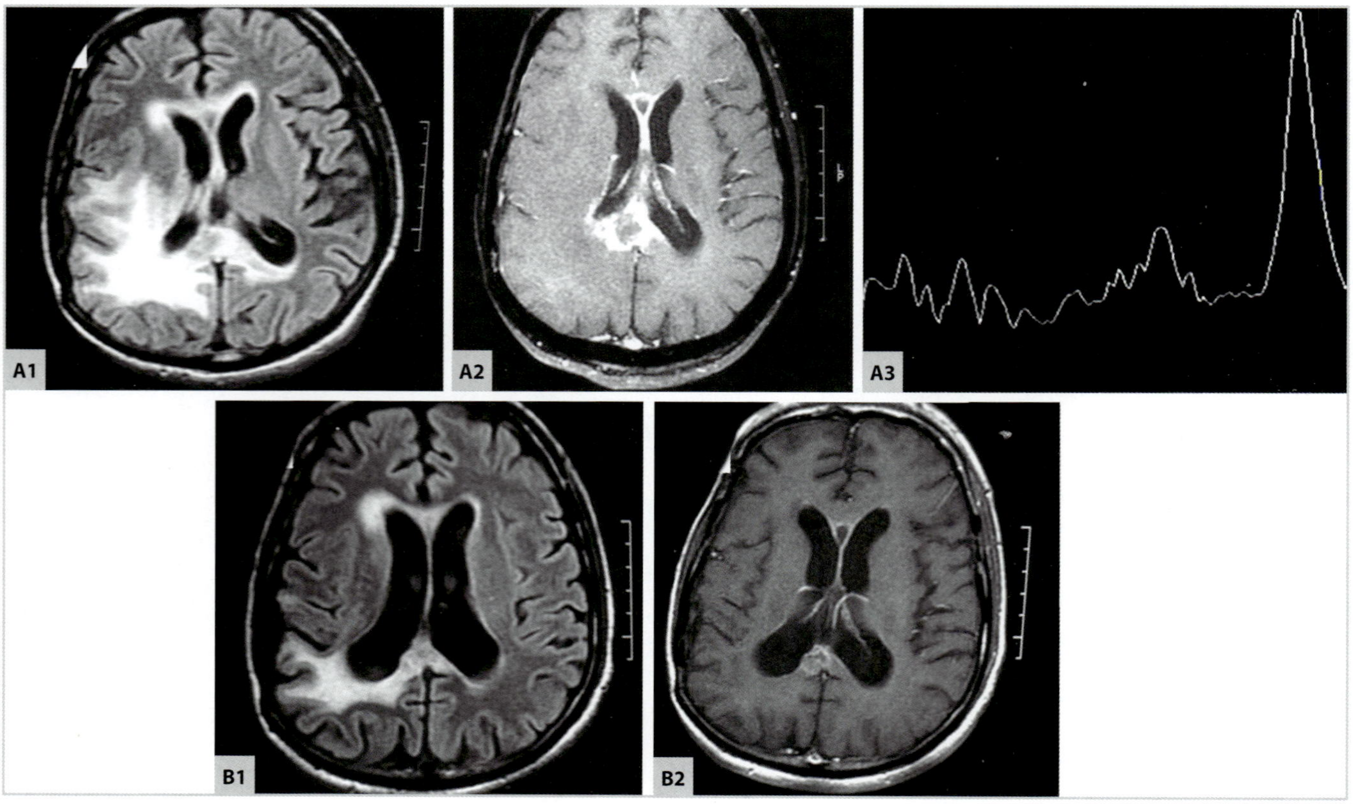

Figs 4A and B: (A) A1 shows the fluid-attenuated inversion recovery (FLAIR) abnormality; A2 shows an enhancing lesion away from the postoperative cavity; A3 shows MR spectroscopy shows tall lipid peak; (B) B1 and B2 show reduction in the FLAIR and enhancing abnormality after a course of steroids this imaging modality is still limited and the specificity of DWI might be less than with MRS. A combination of DWI and MRS can improve the differentiation of recurrent glioma and radiation injury.[25]

Anaplastic Astrocytoma

Anaplastic astrocytoma is an uncommon disease in the adult population. A complete resection is generally not possible and recurrence in the surgical cavity is common.[26] Based on randomized data available, chemotherapy has consistently failed to improve the outcome of patients with anaplastic astrocytoma, while a meta-analysis showed a small, but significant improvement in survival favoring the use of chemotherapy. Outside a clinical trial, postoperative radiotherapy (30 × 2 Gy) remains the standard adjuvant therapy for most patients. The conclusions are based on extrapolation and rational interference from high-grade glioma in general.

Anaplastic Oligoastrocytoma and Oligodendroglioma

In 1988, oligodendroglioma was identified as a subtype of malignant glioma that is more likely to respond to chemotherapy. Cairncross and Macdonald and their colleagues were the first to report on a high response rate of 75% to PCV chemotherapy for patients with enhancing recurrent oligodendroglioma. They subsequently demonstrated that responses were associated with loss of genetic information on chromosomes 1p and 19q [(LOH) 1p/19q], usually associated with pure oligodendroglioma. Based on these observations, the RTOG in the United States and the EORTC in Europe conducted separate randomized trials for patients with AOA and oligodendroglioma.[27] In the RTOG trial, four cycles of intensive procarbazine lomustine and vincristine (PCV) chemotherapy were administered prior to RT, while in the European trial, six cycles of adjuvant PCV were planned after completion of RT. While both trials confirmed a more favorable prognosis for patients with pure oligodendroglioma with LOH 1p/19q, early chemotherapy administration surprisingly did not translate into longer OS. Nevertheless, chemotherapy did significantly prolong disease-free survival, and in the EORTC study, a statistically nonsignificant prolongation, by 10 months, of the median OS time was noted.[28,29] In a recent update of both the RTOG 9402 as well as the EORTC showed that, OS in the patients who received RT/PCV arm was significantly longer (42.3 vs 30.6 months in the RT arm) and in patients with 1p/19q codeletion, OS was increased, with a trend toward more benefit from adjuvant PCV (OS not reached in the RT/PCV group vs 112 months in the RT). IDH mutational status was also of prognostic significance.[30,31] AOAs can be further classified into two subgroups depending on presence of 1p/19q deletion and IDH1 deletion status into Group I and II respectively. A recent study has shown that the progression-free survival (PFS) and OS rates in those patients with deletion is comparable with anaplastic oligodendroglioma, while those in group II have similar survival as these patients with anaplastic astrocytomas. This difference in survival was found to be statistically significant.[32]

Gliomatosis Cerebri

Gliomatosis cerebri is defined as a diffuse glial tumor, extensively infiltrating the normal brain, involving at least two lobes. It frequently extends bilaterally and has been assigned a WHO grade III. In symptomatic patients, treatment with RT would require large radiation fields. Addition of chemotherapy leads to clinical and radiological improvement. A recent study shows a PFS and OS times of 16 and 29 months, respectively. Patients with oligodendroglial gliomatosis have a significantly better prognosis.[33] A recent Indian study shows that inital WBRT followed by local boost, with concurrent TMZ, followed by adjuvant TMZ for a total of 12 cycles shows excellent radiological response.[34] Longer follow-up is required to assess the survival advantage. Patients with pure or mixed oligodendroglialtumors show better radiological response rates compared to those patients with pure astrocytomas.

Low-grade Gliomas

The optimal management of low-grade gliomas remains controversial with variations in clinical practice observed in different centers. The variability of natural history as well as the long-term survival is a challenge for clinical investigations and does not allow easy comparisons between trials. Large randomized studies have shown that a dose in excess of 45–50 Gy provides no additional benefit in terms of disease control and survival.[35] An EORTC trial evaluated the usefulness of radiotherapy immediately after initial diagnosis (e.g. after presentation with seizures) versus radiotherapy administered only with a progressive disease. There was no improvement in OS.[36] Age over 40 years, tumor size over 6 cm, and tumor crossing the midline, as well as the presence of a neurological deficit, were identified as negative prognostic factors. Radiotherapy could be considered at clinical and radiological progression. This strategy allows to delay the indication of treatment averaged about 2–3 years. At present, a maximum resection at initial diagnosis or during growth and an active surveillance should be considered as a recommendation for patients with low-grade astrocytoma. For patients with progressive or uncontrollable symptoms (for example, poorly controlled epilepsy) or considered high risk, focal radiation to 54 Gy is recommended.

Glioblastoma in Elderly Patients

Age is an important prognostic factor for survival in glioblastoma. Because of the overall poor outcome of elderly patients with glioblastoma, it was suggested that patients over the age of 70 years or even 60 years should be managed with supportive care only. In the EORTC/NCIC trial described above, patients up to the age of 70 years were included. Patients over 50 years of age treated with TMZ/RT had a median survival time of 13.6 months, compared with 17.4 months for patients younger than 50 years. However, the benefit afforded by TMZ/RT persisted across all age groups.

Two recent trials have evaluated the role of RT in elderly patients with glioblastoma. A French randomized trial compared RT (28 × 1.8 Gy, 50.4 Gy) with best supportive care in 84 patients over the age of 70 years (median, 73 years). RT produced a longer PFS time, 14 vs 7 weeks, while the OS time in patients receiving RT was 6.5 months, compared with 4.0 months with best supportive care only. These trials demonstrate that RT is also beneficial in the elderly and that the overall treatment time can be considerably shortened without a detrimental effect on outcome.[37] The overall short survival time justifies hypofractionated RT schedules. Shorter treatment duration is clearly justified based on the overall short survival time. Treatment should not be withheld based on age alone. The Nordic randomized, phase 3 trial was designed to look at appropriate treatment options in elderly with glioblastoma. The analysis showed that, in patients more than age of 60 years, hypofractionated RT or TMZ alone showed better OS rates compared to standard radiotherapy. In patients more than age of 70 years, TMZ and hypofractionated radiotherapy should be considered as standard treatment options. MGMT promoter methylation status might be a useful predictive marker for benefit from TMZ but not for radiotherapy alone.[38]

Treatment of Recurrent Glioblastoma

Recommendations for the treatment of recurrent gliomas are based almost exclusively on noncontrolled phase II studies and treatment decisions have to be made on a case-by-case evaluation, depending on prior therapy, time to relapse, tumor grade, and performance status. Given the low response rate in this situation, in recent years, the rate of patients alive at 6 months without progression (PFS rate at 6 months or PFS6) has been established as a measure of efficiency. A PFS6 beyond 20% is considered potentially promising. TMZ is used upfront for high-grade gliomas and hence for patients after a free interval of several months, a new treatment of TMZ may be considered. There is phase II data available for using bevacizumab along with iriniotecan. The BRAIN study evaluated the role of bevacizumab (alone or in combination with irinotecan) in GBM in a Phase II trial with recurrent disease. The PFS-6 was 42.6% and 50.3%, objective response rate was 28.2% and 37.8% and median OS was 9.2 months and 8.7 months in the monotherapy and combination arms respectively.[39] Similar results were found in NCI initiated study and with this, Food and Drug Administration (FDA) approved use of bevacizumab in recurrent glioblastoma. With these promising results of bevacizumab, it was intended to add the drug along with the present of standard of care. The results were presented in the recently concluded American Society of Clinical Oncology meeting. There was no additional survival benefit by addition of upfront bevacizumab to RT + TMZ compared to RT + TMZ alone.[40]

MANAGEMENT OF PEDIATRIC CNS TUMORS

Medulloblastoma

Medulloblastoma is the infratentorial embryonal tumor of childhood (Figs 5A to E). The median age of presentation is 5–7 years with a slight male preponderance.[41] It is the most common of all the childhood tumors and demonstrates unique biological and clinical heterogeneity.[42] Between the ages 0 and 14 years, it constitutes 15% whereas only 4.3% in ages 15–19 years of all the histologies in Brain and CNS tumors in childhood.[1] Suboccipital craniotomy and maximal resection of the primary tumor to restore normal CSF outflow is the initial therapeutic intervention.[43] The timing of adjuvant radiotherapy is very vital and should be ideally initiated within 4 weeks of surgery.[44,45]

The current risk classification system in place is modified Chang classification which has been used for many years to stage the disease[46] and solely based on clinical features, which includes age at diagnosis, extent of surgical resection and metastatic status. Accordingly, infants (≤ 3 years of age), patients with residual tumor (≥ 1.5 sq cm in size) after a radical excision and leptomengeal disease are considered to be high risk and

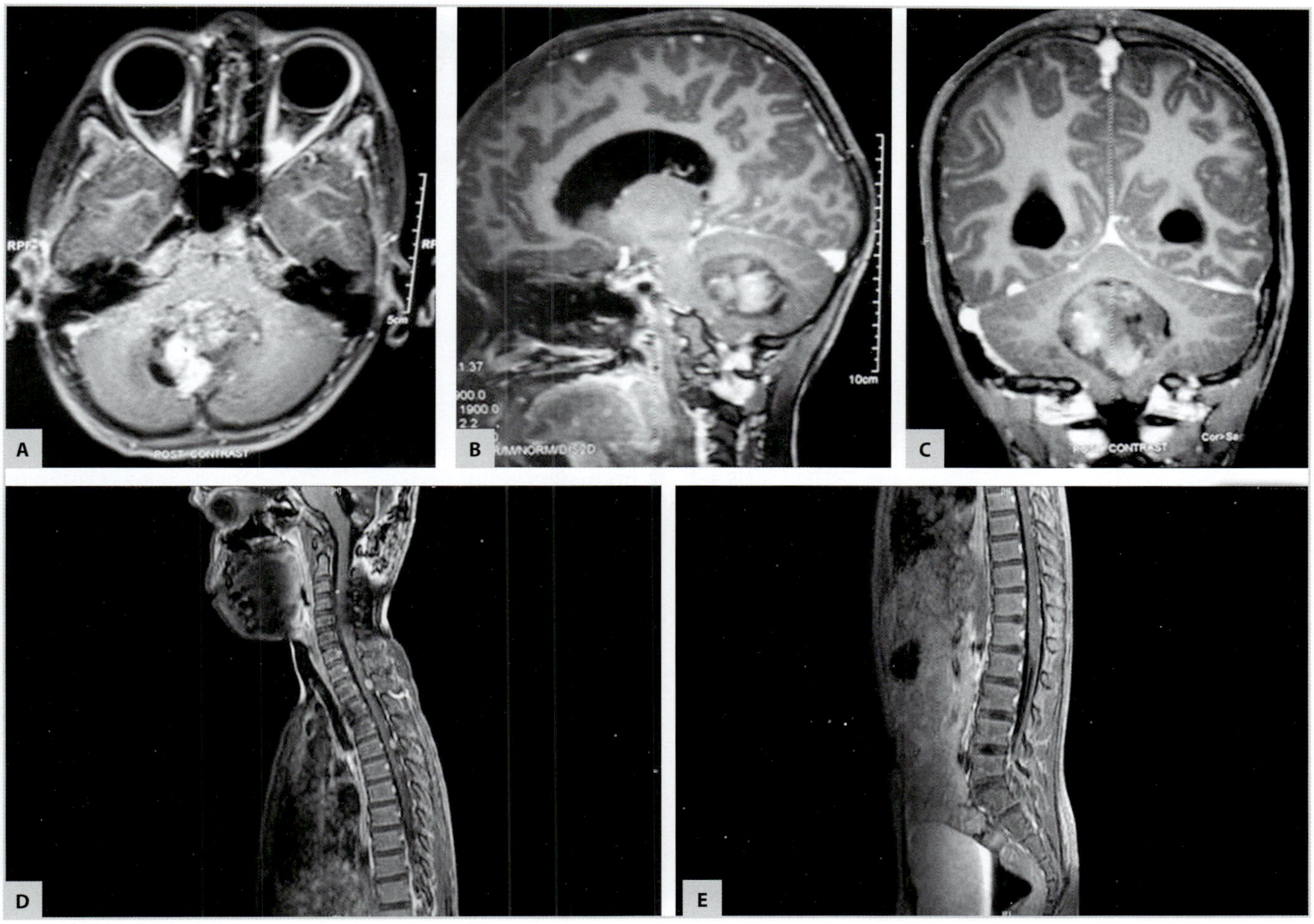

Figs 5A to E: (A to C) Show postcontrast MRI sequences with heterogeneously enhancing lesion in the posterior fossa; (D and E) Show cerebrospinal fluid (CSF) deposits along the spinal cord

rest all as average risk. Occasionally, even histology has been considered for the risk classification and studies have shown that desmoplastic variant is the most common in the childhood and confers very good prognosis whereas large cell and anaplastic histology have very bad prognosis and hence are attributed as high-risk disease.[47]

Northcott et al.[48] new approach of classifying medulloblastoma into various subgroups by integrative genomics approach (microarray expression profiling-SHH, WNT, Group C and Group D) is a new landmark. They have shown that Group C patients (NPR3-positive tumors) exhibit a significantly diminished PFS and OS irrespective of their metastatic status. Integration of this subgroup classification for risk stratification of medulloblastoma alongside with clinical and radiological outcome indicators is necessary to refine the classification and individualizing therapy.[49] A large Indian study demonstrates microRNAs as useful markers for molecular sub-grouping of medulloblastomas from archived FFPE stains.

Packer et al.[50] have demonstrated that there was a significant difference in the 5-year survival rate for poor-risk patients treated prior to 1982 without chemoradiotherapy (35%) compared to those treated later with craniospinal irradiation (CSI) followed by posterior fossa (PF) boost and chemotherapy (87%). The current standard of care for average risk disease is CSI to a dose of 35 Gy followed by whole PF boost to 55.8 Gy. A phase III randomized trial, CCG A9961 has shown that by reducing the CSI to 23.4 Gy along with concurrent vincristine chemotherapy and PF boost to 55.8 Gy followed by adjuvant chemotherapy showed event-free survival (EFS) of 81% at 5 years and OS of 86%.[51]

In order to reduce the radiation related late toxicity, few studies have shown that by delivering CSI to 23.4 Gy followed by PF boost to 35 Gy and primary site radiotherapy to 55.8 Gy, the 5-year EFS rate was 83% and there was a 13% reduction in the volume of PF receiving 55.8 Gy and a statistically significant reduction in dose to the temporal lobes, cochleae and hypothalamus.[52] Although use of chemotherapy along with reduced dose CSI is more or less the standard of care worldwide, our institution experience has shown that with hyperfractionated radiotherapy, 3-year relapse free survival and OS of 83.5% and 83.2%, respectively and there was no cognitive decline in children with average risk medulloblastoma.[53] The standard of care for high-risk group is CSI to a dose of 36 Gy with concurrent chemotherapy followed by PF boost to a dose of 55.8 Gy followed by adjuvant chemotherapy. Although various chemotherapy schedules have been used by various groups, our institution experience has been promising with use of carboplatin in the concurrent setting and a combination of cyclophosphamide, etoposide and carboplatin (or cisplatin) in the adjuvant setting.

Extraneural metastasis occurs in 5–10% of patients and the most common mode of extraneuraxial metastasis has been through the ventriculoperitoneal shunt causing intra-abdominal dissemination.[54]

Atypical Teratoid Rhabdoid Tumor

Atypical teratoid rhabdoid tumors (ATRTs) are rare comprising 1–2% of all pediatric brain tumors; however, in patients less than 3 years of age this tumor accounts for up to 20% of cases. It is characterized by loss of the long arm of chromosome 22 which results in loss of the *hSNF5/INI-1* gene. OS in ATRT is poor with median survival around 17 months. Radiation is an effective component of therapy but is avoided in patients younger than 3 years of age due to long-term neurocognitive sequelae. Studies have shown better survival rates with addition of RT early in the course compared to those with delayed RT or alkylator chemotherapy alone.[55] Various chemotherapy schedules have been tried.[56] A modified IRS III was followed by few groups with addition of TMZ showed a significant improvement in survival, although in a very small groups. But this benefit and improved survival could not be translated in a large patient population. Due to the rarity of this tumor and the lack of controlled trials it has been challenging to define optimal therapy and advance treatment.

Ependymomas

Surgery remains an extremely important component of management of ependymomas and the best survival rates have been reported in patients whose tumors have been gross totally resected. Over 75% of patients with infratentorial tumors after gross total resection and focal, primarily conformal, radiotherapy can be expected to survive without evidence of recurrent disease 5 years from diagnosis. Tumor location, patient age, and degree of histological anaplasia are important prognostic factors.[57] Most of the progress in the treatment of childhood ependymomas has been to the result of more aggressive surgery and earlier use of conformal radiotherapy. To date, new approaches for childhood ependymomas have not been biologically based, although there is new information concerning the cellular origin of these tumors.

Brainstem Gliomas

Progress in the management of high-grade gliomas, including brainstem gliomas, has been minimal over the past two decades. Other than the recognition that some brainstem gliomas (e.g. tectal tumors and exophytic cervicomedullary lesions) are more likely to be low-grade pilocytic lesions and should be treated differently than diffuse intrinsic brainstem gliomas. Treatment approaches for diffuse intrinsic brainstem tumors, including those involving preradiation chemotherapy and postradiation chemotherapy or those that have increased the total dose of radiotherapy by means of different radiation fractionation schedules (primarily hyperfractionated radiation therapy), have not resulted in improved survival and often have caused increased morbidity. A prospective evaluation of children with brainstem gliomas from India, did not show any statistically significant survival advantage by addition of TMZ to radiation in children with BSTG.[58] At present, a host of biologic agents are under study and are primarily being used concomitant with radiotherapy, to act as both radiosensitizers and antineoplastic agents. A major limitation in discovering new directions for the therapy of brainstem gliomas is the lack of tissue available for biologic study.

MANAGEMENT OF BENIGN TUMORS AND INTRACRANIAL EXTRA-AXIAL TUMORS

Meningiomas

Meningiomas can be found throughout the CNS, from the optic nerve sheath to the spinal cord, but tend to cluster along sites where arachnoid granulations return CSF to the venous system, that is, the convexity and basal venous sinuses. The extent of excision has significant impact on the need for further adjuvant therapy, local control and survival. It has been analyzed that in patients with Simpsons I, II, III or termed as total excision (TE), has significantly better local control and survival at 15-years of 80% versus 30% when compared to those patients with Grade IV or subtotal excision (SE).[59] However, in petroclival meningiomas in which TE can cause significant morbidity, SE followed by adjuvant radiation has shown good results.[55] Radiotherapy has been found to be a significant factor in long-term local control and survival of both benign and malignant meningiomas.[60]

Indications of radiotherapy in meningioma: Optic nerve sheath meningioma arises from the dura encompassing the optic nerve, and account for 1–2% of meningiomas.[61] Observation alone can cause gradual loss of vision. Surgery can lead to immediate blindness due to injury to the nerve or gradually due to vascular injury of the nerve. In these situations, RT forms an integral part of the treatment. With a dose prescription of 46–50 Gy, there is improved or stable visual acuity (86%), excellent overall disease control (95%), early visual improvement (within 3 months of radiotherapy in about 55% of children) and complications are relatively uncommon.[62]

Adjuvant radiotherapy after subtotal excision: Meningiomas exhibit a dose response relationship and it has been shown in various studies that 10-year PFS is significantly better with doses more than 53 Gy (63% vs 17%).[63] There is lack of a prospective randomized trial to analyze the benefit of radiotherapy after subtotal excision. Recently a large retrospective analysis showed benefit of local control and PFS with radiotherapy. Patients who received radiotherapy after a STR had a significant difference in 5-year PFS of 91% versus 38% in those without adjuvant RT.[64] CT/MRI registration based volume delineation and high precision or stereotactic conformal radiotherapy (SCRT) is found to significantly improve local control and PFS. For meningiomas located at the skull base, MRI based volume delineation and stereotactic conformal fractionated radiotherapy to a dose of 50–55 Gy in 30–33 fractions, showed 100% local control at 3 years and PFS at 5 years of 91%.[65]

Vestibular Schwannoma

Although initially there was initial enthusiasm for radiosurgery in these tumors and with claims of higher efficacy without toxicity, there has been better understanding of the disease and a more reasoned approach and clear indication for treatment and what treatment can achieve. An untreated schwannoma grows at a very slow rate—an average of 1.2–1.9 mm in diameter a year. Main symptom in these tumors is progressive hearing loss and intermittent vestibular dysfunction. The principal concern is compression of the PF structures by an enlarging mass in the cerebello-pontine angle causing hydrocephalus, brainstem or cranial nerve deficit.[66] RT is ideally delivered as a fractionated regimen with conventional or adapted linac either by IMRT or SCRT. The dose prescription is to 80% or 90% isodose covering the target plus a margin. The prescription dose varies from 45 Gy to 56 Gy at less than 2 Gy per fraction. Various studies have demonstrated that 10-year locoregional control with SCRT is about 93%,[67] while the results are deleterious with stereotactic radiosurgery (SRS) and hypofractionated RT in which nearly 30% of the patients showed radiological progression at 5 years.[68]

Pituitary Adenomas

First line of management of functioning pituitary adenomas is medical management such as, cabergoline and bromocriptine in prolactinoma and octreotide in growth hormone (GH) secreting adenoma. External beam radiotherapy is generally used in patients with resistant functioning pituitary adenoma as second-line treatment after failure of surgery and medical therapy and in nonfunctioning adenomas.[69] The intent of radiotherapy in pituitary adenomas is for normalization of hormonal levels in secreting tumors, while for locoregional control in aggressive nonfunctioning adenomas. Various techniques have been described in literature. The long-term local control of conventional RT is 10-year PFS of 94% and 20-year PFS of 88%. The hormone normalization rate is GH—normalization in 60% after 5–10 years of treatment and in Cushing's disease—normalization in 70–100% by 2 years post-treatment.[70] However, the major toxicity is pan hypopituitarism, and about 30–40% of patients with normal pituitary function require replacement at 10-years after RT. Although the risk of radiation related optic neuropathy is 1–2%, radiation is related to late onset decline in neurocognition due to radiation damage to the temporal lobes and hippocampus.[71]

In order to reduce the dose to these organs, various advances have been made in radiation delivery techniques and one of this is SCRT. The aim of stereotactically guided conformal radiotherapy is to deliver a uniform, therapeutic dose to the target region with maximum sparing of normal tissues.[72] Evaluation of dosimetric data from a prospective study in India in benign tumors showed that younger age and radiotherapy doses to the left temporal lobe were strong predictors of neurocognitive decline in children with benign and low-grade brain tumors treated with stereotactic radiotherapy.[73]

Craniopharyngioma

Craniopharyngioma is a histologically benign, extra-axial, slow-growing tumor that predominately involves the sella and suprasellar space.[74] They are dysodontogenic epithelial tumors derived from the Rathke cleft, which is the embryonal precursor to the adenohypophysis. Three distinct subtypes primarily based on histologic appearance have been described which include adamantinomatous, papillary and mixed. The most common type is the adamantinomatous tumor which is partly solid, partly cystic with characteristic machine oil fluid. A bimodal age distribution is seen, with the first peak occurring in childhood and early adolescence, predominately at age 5–10 years. The second peak (for papillary types) occurs at age 40–60 years. The most common presenting symptoms are headache, nausea, vomiting and visual disturbances and hydrocephalus due to obstruction of the third ventricle.

Craniopharyngiomas have been surgically divided into three groups: (1) sellar, (2) prechiasmatic, and (3) retrochiasmatic. The primary treatment of choice is complete surgical excision. Local recurrence is common after surgical excision alone, with reported recurrence rates of 25–40% without adjuvant radiation.[75] The size of the tumor at presentation also impacts upon local recurrence (70% for tumors greater than 5 cm and 20% for tumors less than 5 cm). Cystic degeneration and enlargement is a common finding on follow-up scans and needs intervention in almost 20% of patients. In recent times conservative surgery (maximal safe resection) followed by adjuvant radiation therapy is preferred to aggressive radical excision to improve outcome.[76] A 5-year survival rate of 70–80% is achieved with contemporary microsurgery and adjuvant radiation therapy. The 10-year OS is 60–75%.

PALLIATIVE AND SUPPORTIVE CARE

Majority of symptomatology in patients with glial tumors, like headache, nausea and vomiting, drowsiness are due to raised intracranial pressure. Other neurological manifestations like motor or sensory deficits, personality changes (mood fluctuations, depression) are due to local tumor effects. These manifestations can be strongly affected by the disease laterality. Over this, interventions like surgery, radiation and chemotherapy can lead to significant morbidity and further aggravation of already preexisting neurological deficits.[77] In particular, neurological toxicity of radiotherapy is well documented. Late radiation effects are irreversible and can become increasingly problematic in patients who live for several years after therapy. The deleterious psychosocial effect of high-grade glioma and its treatments on patients and their families is profound.

In 2006, NICE, UK, published guidelines for health professionals for treatment of malignant CNS tumors.[78] It also provided guidelines for psychological support, rehabilitation services, palliative care, social support and continuing care. Cognitive impairment interferes with communication, understanding and decision-making. Lack of information and uncertainty about treatment and prognosis lead to anxiety. Recently a systematic review has shown the importance of effective communication between physicians and caregivers and therefore caregivers have to be involved in decision-making with the palliative team.[79] Cognitive decline in patients with primary malignant brain tumors has been linked to tumor progression. Indeed, the evidence suggested that cognitive deterioration may be an early marker of disease progression. In addition, systematic evaluation of cognitive status or deterioration would not only help clinicians deliver information appropriately but may also give an early indication of tumor progression. Communication style of the physician with the caregivers must take into account potential cognitive deficits, mental health issues, the dynamics of shifting personal identity, and the importance of caregivers inpatient decision-making. Therefore, communication skills training tailored to address these issues would be beneficial and should be a primary focus of new research in this area.

HOSPICE/END OF LIFE CARE

Despite aggressive multimodal therapy, most glioblastoma patients eventually die from their disease. In the terminal disease phase, patients present severe symptoms that need appropriate palliative care to allow the patient to experience a peaceful death. Early involvement of palliative care services is important to ensure that the needs of patients and their caregivers are met. However, there is lack of data to guide psychosocial and supportive care. The interface between community healthcare services and specialists is essential to ensure that patients receive optimal palliative care, avoiding useless emergency rehospitalization in the terminal phase.[80]

The most frequent symptoms in the last month of life are seizures, headache, drowsiness, dysphagia, and eventually death rattle, agitation and delirium. The most commonly used drugs in this phase are AEDs, corticosteroids and analgesics, including opioids and sedatives. Owing to unconsciousness or difficulties in swallowing, drugs may need to be given intramuscularly, subcutaneously or intravenously. The indication for artificial nutrition and hydration needs to be considered individually, as the benefits and burdens are unclear, and no evidence-based guidelines exist. If possible, end-of-life preferences should be discussed with patients and their families early in the disease course.

QUALITY OF LIFE

Improvements in treatment approaches especially in the field of surgical resection, radiation therapy delivery methods, and newer systemic agents for primary brain tumors, have demonstrated improved survival of these patients. There have been tremendous advances in the understanding of the molecular biology of these tumors and newer agents that target these molecular pathways. With the advancement in technology of radiation delivery and newer systemic agents, it is very essential to address quality of life (QOL). Preservation of normal daily activities and neurological function is increasingly being taken into consideration in the present day neuro-oncology practice and QOL is considered an important end point.

Quality of life depends on various patient, tumor and treatment-related factors. The tumor related factors are the major factors influencing cognitive function and QOL domain scores and particularly the site, laterality, size, hypothalamic involvement, hormonal deficiencies and epilepsy. Among the treatment related factors, anticonvulsants, corticosteroids, higher dose of radiation therapy and chemotherapy all have detrimental effects on QOL. In benign tumors like craniopharyngiomas and pituitary tumors, hydrocephalus, GH deficiency and hypothalamic involvement have been shown to impair cognitive function.

There are various QOL and neurocognitive function assessment tools being used in clinical trials and clinical practice. Functional evaluations are either with objective assessment (e.g. clinical examination by physician or nurse) or subjective assessment through questionnaire-based evaluation of well-being and QOL. Commonly used objective evaluation tools are Karnofsky performance score (KPS), neurological performance score (NPS) and Barthel's activity of daily living. Objective questionnaire-based QOL evaluation tools are mainly EORTC Core Quality of Life Questionnaire (QLQ-C30), brain-specific module (BN-20), and Functional Assessment of Cancer Therapy (FACT) cancer-specific scales.[81] Neurocognitive function is assessed using a various battery of tests. The extensive MD Anderson Symptom Inventory-Brain Tumor Module (MDASI-BT) has 22 symptom items that measures affective, cognitive, focal neurologic deficit, constitutional, generalized symptom and gastrointestinal related factor. As described previously, QOL scores depend on various tumor and treatment-related factors.

An Indian study on QOL showed that patients with brain tumors in developing countries have a different demographic profile, compared with patients from developed countries. The malignant gliomas occur one decade earlier than in developed countries, and the proportion of patients with benign tumors was relatively lower.[82] Tumor type (high grade or low grade) and neurological function status (KPS and NPS) influenced baseline QOL domain scores. An important analysis however was that economic status and literacy status did not have a significant influence on QOL scores.

REFERENCES

1. Dolecek TA, Propp JM, Stroup NE, et al. CBTRUS statistical report: primary brain and central nervous system tumors diagnosed in the United States in 2005-2009. Neuro Oncol. 2012;(Suppl 5): v1-49.
2. Jalali R, Datta D. Prospective analysis of incidence of central nervous tumors presenting in a tertiary cancer hospital from India. J Neurooncol. 2008;87(1):111-4.
3. Manoharan N, Julka PK, Rath GK. Descriptive epidemiology of primary brain and CNS tumours in Delhi, 2003-2007. Asian Pac J Cancer Prev. 2012;13(2):637-40.
4. Asirvatham JR, Deepti AN, Chyne R, et al. Pediatric tumors of the central nervous system: a retrospective study of 1,043 cases from a tertiary care center in South India. Childs Nerv Syst Chns Off. 2011;27(8):1257-63.
5. Chang SM, Clarke JL. Neuroimaging: diagnosis and response assessment in Glioblastoma. Cancer J. 2012;18(1):26-31.
6. Louis DN, Ohgaki H, Wiestler OD, et al. The 2007 WHO classification of tumours of the central nervous system. Acta Neuropathol. 2007;114(2):97-109.
7. Preusser M, de Ribaupierre S, Wöhrer A, et al. Current concepts and management of glioblastoma. Ann Neurol. 2011;70(1):9-21.
8. Stupp R, Hegi ME. Brain cancer in 2012: molecular characterization leads the way. Nat Rev Clin Oncol. 2013;10(2):69-70.
9. Weller M, Stupp R. Prime time for molecular marker diagnostics in neuro-oncology. Curr Opin Neurol. 2012;25(6):743-4.
10. Hegi ME, Diserens AC, Gorlia T, et al. MGMT gene silencing and benefit from temozolomide in glioblastoma. N Engl J Med. 2005;352(10):997-1003.
11. Van den Bent MJ, Hegi ME, Stupp R. Recent developments in the use of chemotherapy in brain tumours. Eur J Cancer. 2006;42(5):582-8.

12. Hawkins C, Walker E, Mohamed N, et al. BRAF-KIAA1549 fusion predicts better clinical outcome in pediatric low-grade astrocytoma. Clin Cancer Res. 2011;17(14):4790-8.
13. Northcott PA, Dubuc AM, Pfister S, et al. Molecular subgroups of medulloblastoma. Expert Rev Neurother. 2012;12(7):871-84.
14. Gaspar LE, Scott C, Murray K, et al. Validation of the RTOG recursive partitioning analysis (RPA) classification for brain metastases. Int J Radiat Oncol Biol Phys. 2000;47(4):1001-6.
15. Gorlia T, van den Bent MJ, Hegi ME, et al. Nomograms for predicting survival of patients with newly diagnosed glioblastoma: prognostic factor analysis of EORTC and NCIC trial 26981-22981/CE.3. Lancet Oncol. 2008;9(1):29-38.
16. Chang SM, Parney IF, Huang W, et al. Patterns of care for adults with newly diagnosed malignant glioma. JAMA. 2005;293(5):557-64.
17. Weller M, Stupp R, Wick W. Epilepsy meets cancer: when, why, and what to do about it? Lancet Oncol. 2012;13(9):e375-82.
18. Perry JR. Anti-coagulation of malignant glioma patients in the era of novel anti-angiogenic agents. Curr Opin Neurol. 2010;23(6):592-6
19. Stummer W, Pichlmeier U, Meinel T, et al. Fluorescence-guided surgery with 5-aminolevulinic acid for resection of malignant glioma: a randomised controlled multicentre phase III trial. Lancet Oncol. 2006;7(5):392-401.
20. Stupp R, Mason WP, van den Bent MJ, et al. Radiotherapy plus concomitant and adjuvant temozolomide for glioblastoma. N Engl J Med. 2005;352(10):987-96.
21. Stupp R, Hegi ME, Mason WP, et al. Effects of radiotherapy with concomitant and adjuvant temozolomide versus radiotherapy alone on survival in glioblastoma in a randomised phase III study: 5-year analysis of the EORTC-NCIC trial. Lancet Oncol. 2009;10(5):459-66.
22. Jalali R, Basu A, Gupta T, et al. Encouraging experience of concomitant temozolomide with radiotherapy followed by adjuvant temozolomide in newly diagnosed glioblastomamultiforme: single institution experience. Br J Neurosurg. 2007;21(6):583-7.
23. Gupta T, Mohanty S, Moiyadi A, et al. Factors predicting temozolomide induced clinically significant acute hematologic toxicity in patients with high-grade gliomas: A clinical audit. Clin Neurol Neurosurg. 2013;115(9):1814-9.
24. Brandsma D, van den Bent MJ. Pseudoprogression and pseudoresponse in the treatment of gliomas. Curr Opin Neurol. 2009;22(6):633-8.
25. Agarwal A, Kumar S, Narang J, et al. Morphologic MRI features, diffusion tensor imaging and radiation dosimetric analysis to differentiate pseudo-progression from early tumor progression. J Neurooncol. 2013;112(3):413-20.
26. Stupp R, Reni M, Gatta G, et al. Anaplastic astrocytoma in adults. Crit Rev Oncol Hematol. 2007;63(1):72-80.
27. Van den Bent M, Chinot OL, Cairncross JG. Recent developments in the molecular characterization and treatment of oligodendroglial tumors. Neuro Oncol. 2003;5(2):128-38.
28. Intergroup Radiation Therapy Oncology Group Trial 9402, Cairncross G, Berkey B, et al. Phase III trial of chemotherapy plus radiotherapy compared with radiotherapy alone for pure and mixed anaplastic oligodendroglioma: Intergroup Radiation Therapy Oncology Group Trial 9402. J Clin Oncol. 2006;24(18):2707-14.
29. Van den Bent MJ, Carpentier AF, Brandes AA, et al. Adjuvant procarbazine, lomustine, and vincristine improves progression-free survival but not overall survival in newly diagnosed anaplastic oligodendrogliomas and oligoastrocytomas: a randomized European Organisation for Research and Treatment of Cancer phase III trial. J Clin Oncol. 2006;24(18):2715-22.
30. Cairncross G, Wang M, Shaw E, et al. Phase III trial of chemoradiotherapy for anaplastic oligodendroglioma: long-term results of RTOG 9402. J Clin Oncol. 2013;31(3):337-43.
31. Van den Bent MJ, Brandes AA, Taphoorn MJ, et al. Adjuvant procarbazine, lomustine, and vincristine chemotherapy in newly diagnosed anaplastic oligodendroglioma: long-term follow-up of EORTC brain tumor group study 26951. J Clin Oncol. 2013;31(3):344-50.
32. Jiang H, Ren X, Cui X, et al. 1p/19q codeletion and IDH1/2 mutation identified a subtype of anaplastic oligoastrocytomas with prognosis as favorable as anaplastic oligodendrogliomas. Neuro Oncol. 2013;15(6):775-82.
33. D'Urso PI, D'Urso OF, Marsigliante S, et al. Gliomatosiscerebri type II: two case reports. J Med Case Rep. 2009;3:7225.
34. Pungavkar S, Tanawde P, Epari S, et al. Gliomatosis cerebri: assessment of clinical and radiological response to temozolomide and radiation in 20 patients. RA-046. Abstract No. R14; ASNO 2013.
35. Shaw E, Arusell R, Scheithauer B, et al. Prospective randomized trial of low versus high dose radiation therapy in adults with low supratentorial low grade glioma: results of north central cancer treatment group/RTOG study. J Clin Oncol. 2002;20(9):2267-76.
36. Van den Bent MJ, Afra D, de Witte O, et al. Long-term efficacy of early versus delayed radiotherapy for low-grade astrocytoma and oligodendroglioma in adults: the EORTC 22845 randomised trial. Lancet. 2005;366:985-90.
37. Laperriere N, Weller M, Stupp R, et al. Optimal management of elderly patients with glioblastoma. Cancer Treat Rev. 2013;39(4):350-7.
38. Malmström A, Grønberg BH, Marosi C, et al. Temozolomide versus standard 6-week radiotherapy versus hypofractionated radiotherapy in patients older than 60 years with glioblastoma: the Nordic randomised, phase 3 trial. Lancet Oncol. 2012;13(9):916-26.
39. Møller S, Grunnet K, Hansen S, et al. A phase II trial with bevacizumab and irinotecan for patients with primary brain tumors and progression after standard therapy. Acta Oncol Stockh Swed. 2012;51(6):797-804.
40. Gilbert MR, Dignam J, Won M, et al. RTOG 0825: Phase III double blind placebo-controlled trial evaluating bevacizumab (Bev) in patients (Pts) with newly diagnosed glioblastoma (GBM). J Clin Oncol. 2013;31(suppl 1):18.
41. Roberts RO, Lynch CF, Jones MP, et al. Medulloblastoma: a population-based study of 532 cases. J Neuropathol Exp Neurol. 1991;50(2):134-44.

42. Louis DN, Ohgaki H, Wiestler OD, et al. The 2007 WHO classification of tumours of the central nervous system. Acta Neuropathol (Berl). 2007;114(2):97-109.
43. Gnanalingham KK, Lafuente J, Thompson D, et al. Surgical procedures for posterior fossa tumors in children: does craniotomy lead to fewer complications than craniectomy? J Neurosurg. 2002;97(4):821-6.
44. Del Charco JO, Bolek TW, McCollough WM, et al. Medulloblastoma: time-dose relationship based on a 30-year review. Int J Radiat Oncol Biol Phys. 1998;42(1):147-54.
45. Taylor RE, Bailey CC, Robinson KJ, et al. Impact of radiotherapy parameters on outcome in the International Society of Paediatric Oncology/United Kingdom Children's Cancer Study Group PNET-3 study of preradiotherapy chemotherapy for M0-M1 medulloblastoma. Int J Radiat Oncol Biol Phys. 2004;58(4): 1184-93.
46. Chang CH, Housepian EM, Herbert C. An operative staging system and a megavoltage radiotherapeutic technic for cerebellar medulloblastomas. Radiology. 1969;93(6):1351-9.
47. Rutkowski S, von Bueren A, von Hoff K, et al. Prognostic relevance of clinical and biological risk factors in childhood medulloblastoma: results of patients treated in the prospective multicenter trial HIT'91. Clin Cancer Res. 2007;13(9):2651-7.
48. Remke M, Hielscher T, Northcott PA, et al. Adult medulloblastoma comprises three major molecular variants. J Clin Oncol. 2011;29(19):2717-23.
49. Kunder R, Jalali R, et al. Real time PCR assay based on the differential expression of microRNAs and protein coding genes for molecular classification of formalin fixed paraffin-embedded medulloblsatomas. Neuro Oncol. 2013;12:1644-51.
50. Packer RJ, Sutton LN, Goldwein JW, et al. Improved survival with the use of adjuvant chemotherapy in the treatment of medulloblastoma. J Neurosurg. 1991;74(3):433-40.
51. Packer RJ, Gajjar A, Vezina G, et al. Phase III study of craniospinal radiation therapy followed by adjuvant chemotherapy for newly diagnosed average-risk medulloblastoma. J Clin Oncol. 2006;24(25):4202-8.
52. Merchant TE, Kun LE, Krasin MJ, et al. Multi-institution prospective trial of reduced-dose craniospinal irradiation (23.4 Gy) followed by conformal posterior fossa (36 Gy) and primary site irradiation (55.8 Gy) and dose-intensive chemotherapy for average-risk medulloblastoma. Int J Radiat Oncol Biol Phys. 2008;70(3):782-7.
53. Gupta T, Jalali R, Goswami S, et al. Early clinical outcomes demonstrate preserved cognitive function in children with average-risk medulloblastoma when treated with hyperfractionated radiation therapy. Int J Radiat Oncol Biol Phys. 2012;83(5):1534-40.
54. Rutkowski S, von Hoff K, Emser A, et al. Survival and prognostic factors of early childhood medulloblastoma: an international meta-analysis. J Clin Oncol. 2010;28(33):4961-8.
55. Tekautz TM, Fuller CE, Blaney S, et al. Atypical teratoid/rhabdoid tumors (ATRT): improved survival in children 3 years of age and older with radiation therapy and high-dose alkylator-based chemotherapy. J Clin Oncol. 2005;23(7):1491-9.
56. Chi SN, Zimmerman MA, Yao X, et al. Intensive multimodality treatment for children with newly diagnosed CNS atypical teratoid rhabdoid tumor. J Clin Oncol. 2009;27(3):385-9.
57. Vaidya K, Smee R, Williams JR. Prognostic factors and treatment options for paediatricependymomas. J Clin Neuro Sci. 2012;19(9):1228-35.
58. Jalali R, Raut N, Arora B, et al. Prospective evaluation of radiotherapy with concurrent and adjuvant temozolomide in children with newly diagnosed diffuse intrinsic pontineglioma. Int J Radiat Oncol Biol Phys. 2010;77(1):113-8.
59. McCarthy BJ, Davis FG, Freels S, et al. Factors associated with survival in patients with meningioma. J Neurosurg. 1998;88(5):831-9.
60. Jung HW, Yoo H, Paek SH, et al. Long-term outcome and growth rate of subtotally resected petroclival meningiomas: experience with 38 cases. Neurosurgery. 2000;46(3):567-74.
61. Rogers L, Mehta M. Role of radiation therapy in treating intracranial meningiomas. Neurosurg Focus. 2007;23(4):E4.
62. Turbin RE, Thompson CR, Kennerdell JS, et al. A long-term visual outcome comparison in patients with optic nerve sheath meningioma managed with observation, surgery, radiotherapy, or surgery and radiotherapy. Ophthalmology. 2002;109(5):890-9.
63. Goldsmith BJ, Wara WM, Wilson CB, et al. Postoperative irradiation for subtotally resected meningiomas. A retrospective analysis of 140 patients treated from 1967 to 1990. J Neurosurg. 1994;80(2):195-201.
64. Soyuer S, Chang EL, Selek U, et al. Radiotherapy after surgery for benign cerebral meningioma. Radiother Oncol J Eur Soc Ther Radiol Oncol. 2004;71(1):85-90.
65. Jalali R, Loughrey C, Baumert B, et al. High precision focused irradiation in the form of fractionated stereotactic conformal radiotherapy (SCRT) for benign meningiomas predominantly in the skull base location. Clin Oncol R Coll Radiol Gt Br. 2002;14(2):103-9.
66. Brada M. Radiotherapy for benign brain tumours coming of age; example of vestibular schwannoma. Radiother Oncol J Eur Soc Ther Radiol Oncol. 2013;106(2):157-60.
67. Combs SE, Adeberg S, Dittmar JO, et al. Skull base meningiomas: Long-term results and patient self-reported outcome in 507 patients treated with fractionated stereotactic radiotherapy (FSRT) or intensity modulated radiotherapy (IMRT). Radiother Oncol. 2013;106(2):186-91.
68 Brada M, Ford D, Ashley S, et al. Risk of second brain tumour after conservative surgery and radiotherapy for pituitary adenoma. BMJ. 1992;304(6838):1343-6.
69. Brada M, Jankowska P. Radiotherapy for pituitary adenomas. Endocrinol Metab Clin North Am. 2008;37(1):263-75, xi.
70. Shah NS, George J, Acharya SV, et al. Cushing disease in children and adolescents: twenty years' experience in a tertiary care center in India. Am Assoc Clin Endocrinol. 2011;17(3):369-76.
71. Fernandez A, Brada M, Zabuliene L, et al. Radiation-induced hypopituitarism. Endocr Relat Cancer. 2009;16(3):733-72.

72. Jalali R, Brada M, Perks JR, et al. Stereotactic conformal radiotherapy for pituitary adenomas: technique and preliminary experience. Clin Endocrinol (Oxf.). 2000;52(6):695-702.

73. Jalali R, Mallick I, Dutta D, et al. Factors influencing neuro cognitive outcomes in young patients with benign and low-grade tumours treated with stereotactic conformal radiotherapy. Int J Radiat Oncol Biol Phys. 2010;77(4):974-9.

74. Brada M, Thomas DG. Craniopharyngioma revisited. Int J Radiat Oncol Biol Phys. 1993;27(2):471-5.

75. Rajan B, Ashley S, Thomas DG, et al. Craniopharyngioma: improving outcome by early recognition and treatment of acute complications. Int J Radiat Oncol Biol Phys. 1997;37(3):517-21.

76. Aggarwal A, Fersht N, Brada M. Radiotherapy for craniopharyngioma. Pituitary. 2013;16(1):26-33.

77. Catt S, Chalmers A, Fallowfield L. Psychosocial and supportive-care needs in high-grade glioma. Lancet Oncol. 2008;9(9):884-91.

78. Guilfoyle MR, Weerakkody RA, Oswal A, et al. Implementation of neuro-oncology service reconfiguration in accordance with NICE guidance provides enhanced clinical care for patients with glioblastoma multiforme. Br J Cancer. 2011;104(12):1810-5.

79. Ford E, Catt S, Chalmers A, et al. Systematic review of supportive care needs in patients with primary malignant brain tumors. Neuro Oncol. 2012;14(4):392-404.

80. Pace A, Di Lorenzo C, Lorenzo CD, et al. End of life issues in brain tumor patients. J Neurooncol. 2009;91(1):39-43.

81. Budrukkar A, Jalali R, Dutta D, et al. Prospective assessment of quality of life in adult patients with primary brain tumours in routine neuro oncology practice. J Neurooncol. 2009;95(3):413-9.

82. Jalali R, Dutta D. Factors influencing quality of life in adult patients with primary brain tumors. Neuro-Oncol. 2012;14(Suppl 4):iv8-16.

53 Management of Brain Metastasis

Rakesh Jalali, Uday Krishna

EPIDEMIOLOGY

Metastatic brain tumors represent the most common neurological complication of systemic cancer.[1] Brain metastases are the considered to be the most common intracranial tumors, outnumbering primary brain tumors by a ratio of 10:1 in the published Western data.[2] The worldwide incidence of brain metastasis has been reported to be 9–17% in neuro-oncology practice, although the exact incidence is thought to be higher[3] and about 11% in the Indian context.[4] Between 60% and 80% of all brain metastases in adults are comprised of tumors arising from lung, breast, melanoma, colon and kidney primary sites. The most common primary site is the lungs, comprising approximately 40–60% of all brain metastases, followed by breast, melanoma, and, less frequently, colon and kidneys, with relative incidences of 10%, 3.5%, 2.8% and 1.2%, respectively. Lung metastases predominate in men, whereas breast metastases predominate in women. Primaries of unknown origin may constitute 5–10% of the cases. Overall risk of brain metastasis has been found to be relatively higher in the series reported based on autopsy, where as high as 20% and 40% of all patients with metastatic cancer are found to have brain metastases. In a recent review of multiple autopsy series, the probability of developing brain metastases from a specific primary tumor site in patients dying from lung, breast, melanoma, gastrointestinal (GI) and renal cell primaries was calculated to be 32%, 21%, 48%, 6% and 11%, respectively.[5]

The incidence of brain metastases appears to be rising, and has been variably attributed to improvements in systemic therapy leading to longer survival, and the ability of magnetic resonance imaging (MRI) to detect small metastases.[6]

CLINICAL PRESENTATION

- Features related to cerebral edema and/or increased intracranial pressure like headache, nausea/vomiting and impaired cognition[6]
- Compression effects manifesting as weakness, numbness, speech disturbance or seizures.

About 50% of patients with brain metastasis present with features of increased intracranial pressure. Altered mental status, personality change and impaired cognition may be present in approximately 30% of patients and is more prevalent with multiple metastases. Between 5% and 10% of patients have sudden onset focal neurological symptoms associated with intratumoral hemorrhage, particularly from metastases originating from melanoma, choriocarcinoma or renal cell carcinoma (RCC).

Seizure as the first sign of brain metastasis is seen in only approximately 10–20% of patients. Tumors that involve cerebral hemispheres present as seizures, causes being cerebral edema, ischemia and mechanical traction of the cerebral cortex may also play important roles in epileptogenesis.

DIAGNOSIS AND EVALUATION

Up to 30% of patients presenting with brain metastases do not have a prior diagnosis of cancer.[6] In these patients, a thorough evaluation to look for the site of primary cancer is essential. On the other hand, onset of neurological symptoms in a patient with systemic cancer guides to a high suspicion of brain metastasis and warrants further systemic evaluation. As explained previously, majority of primary cancers that metastasize to the brain are from lung primaries, and hence a plain chest radiograph and chest computed tomography (CT) are always recommended as the preliminary investigations, following which it should be followed by systemic evaluation that includes whole body positron emission tomography (PET)-CT scan.

Most brain metastases grow as spherical, well-demarcated, solid masses that displace rather than destroy adjacent tissue and may be surrounded by minimal to extensive edema. Some rapidly growing metastases undergo central necrosis or cystic change, and others, especially those from melanoma, choriocarcinoma and testicular carcinoma may be hemorrhagic.

Computed tomography scan is the usual first diagnostic tool to be performed for evaluation of location, number of lesions and other features. CT scan is an ideal tool for rapid assessment of an unstable patient. It is also indicated in a patient with contraindications for a MRI evaluation. MRI with gadolinium enhancement is the most sensitive imaging modality for both diagnosis and follow-up of patients with brain metastases.[7] Metastatic tumors are generally well enhancing (Fig. 1A) relatively dark on T2-weighted images and classically located at the gray-white matter junction. Almost all of them are associated with significant peritumoral edema (Fig. 1B). The appearance of blood products on T1-weighted images depends on the "age" of bleeding, and ranges from isointense in the first 24 hours to hyperintense after 24–72 hours. Metastatic melanomas often have both components (blood and melanin), which appear bright on noncontrast T1-weighted scans. Common differential diagnosis with similar MRI features includes lymphoma, meningiomas and high-grade gliomas. MR spectroscopy in brain metastasis usually exhibits high choline and relatively high lipid-lactate in view of necrosis and absent creatine/N-acetyl aspartate (NAA) (Fig. 1C).

PATHOGENESIS AND SPREAD OF METASTASES TO THE BRAIN

The most common route for metastasis to the brain is by hematogenous spread via internal carotid and vertebrobasilar arteries or via Batson's venous plexus. The postulated mechanism suggests metastatic cells get trapped at the gray-white junction, due to the change in the size of the blood vessels in this zone.[6]

Studies have shown that once tumor emboli reach 1 mm in size, they lead to angiogenesis, increases vascular permeability and disrupt the blood-brain barrier (BBB). Capillary endothelial cells of the brain metastatic cells acquire morphologic and functional characteristics of vasculature of systemic neoplasm, in terms of having gap junctions and membrane fenestrations. In view of this disruption of BBB, molecular pathways in systemic metastasis also apply to brain metastasis.[8]

PROGNOSTIC FACTORS AND STAGING

Retrospective recursive partitioning analysis (RPA) of prognostic factors was performed by Gaspar, et al., who studied over 1,000 patients receiving external beam radiotherapy as a part of various Radiation Therapy Oncology Group (RTOG) trials during 1979 to 1993.[9] They

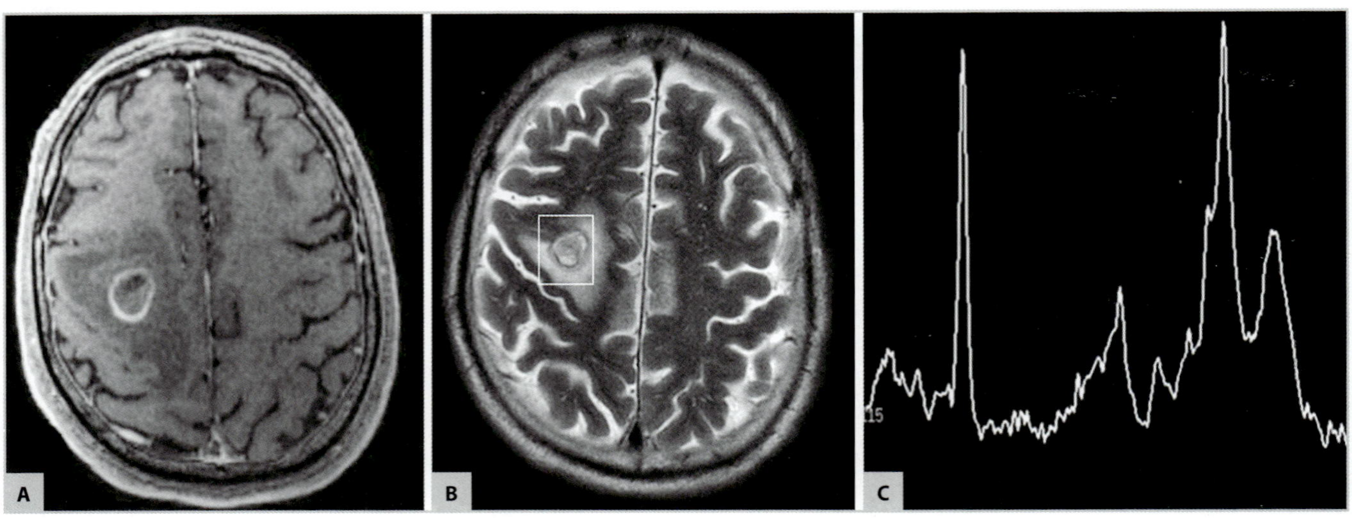

Figs 1A to C: (A) The T1 plain magnetic resonance (MR) imaging of a patient with brain metastasis; (B) The T2-weighted heterogeneously hyperintense lesion in the left temporal region; (C) The characteristic MR spectroscopic pattern of brain metastasis with high choline and lipid peak

TABLE 1: Prognostic indices for brain metastasis

A: Recursive partitioning analysis (RPA)[9]			
Prognostic index	*Variables*	*Score or class*	*Median survival*
RPA	Age, Karnofsky performance scale (KPS) and status of primary cancer	Class I: Age < 65 years, KPS ≥ 70 Controlled primary No extracranial disease Class II: All others Class III: KPS < 70	7.1 months 4.2 months 2.3 months

B: Graded prognostic assessment (GPA)[10] *Score 3.5–4.0 = Median survival is 11 months; 3.0 = 6.9 months; 1.5–2.5= 3.8 months*			
Variable	*Score 0*	*Score 0.5*	*Score 1.0*
Age	> 60 years	50–59 years	< 50 years
KPS	< 70	70–80	90–100
No. of central nervous system (CNS) metastases	> 3	2–3	1
Extracranial metastases	Present	-	None

found that patients fell into three well-defined prognostic groups, with significantly different median survivals. Since then, various classification systems have been defined such as the *graded prognostic assessment* (GPA). GPA was found to be least subjective, most quantitative and easiest of all the scales. It had few advantages—number of metastases included; which has been found to be prognostic, eliminates treatment factors and eliminates components that are difficult to quantify and/or are subjective.[10] These are enumerated in Table 1.

MEDICAL MANAGEMENT OF BRAIN METASTASIS

Role of Steroids

A systematic review on role of steroids in brain metastasis has drawn the following conclusions:[11]

- Asymptomatic brain metastases patients without mass effect: corticosteroids are recommended to provide temporary symptomatic relief of symptoms related to increased intracranial pressure and edema secondary to brain metastases, although there is lack of evidence
- It is recommended for patients who are symptomatic from metastatic disease to the brain that a starting dose of 4–8 mg/day of dexamethasone be considered
- Brain metastases patients with moderate to severe symptoms related to mass effect: corticosteroids are recommended to provide temporary symptomatic relief of symptoms related to increased intracranial pressure and edema secondary to brain metastases. If patients exhibit severe symptoms consistent with increased intracranial pressure, it is recommended that higher doses such as 16 mg/day or more be considered
- Choice of steroid: dexamethasone is the most optimal drug choice
- Duration of corticosteroid administration: corticosteroids, if given, should be tapered slowly over a 2-week time period, or longer in symptomatic patients, based upon an individualized treatment regimen and a full understanding of the long-term sequelae of corticosteroid therapy.

The role of prophylactic anticonvulsants has been extensively studied. For adults with brain metastases who have not experienced a seizure due to their metastatic brain disease, routine prophylactic use of anticonvulsants is not recommended.[12]

Role of Chemotherapy

The impermeability of the BBB to ionized water-soluble compounds greater than 180 Da (dalton) and the presence of the P-glycoprotein efflux pump at the luminal surface of the brain capillaries result in lack of penetration of the chemotherapeutic drugs. Though breast cancer is a chemosensitive disease, there is limited data on the use of chemotherapy for breast cancer metastatic to brain. Most commonly used are cyclophosphamide-based regimens [along with methotrexate, 5-fluorouracil (5-FU), prednisolone, etc.) and high-dose intravenous methotrexate. The HER2 targeted dual tyrosine kinase inhibitor (TKI) lapatinib has been found to have significant activity in metastatic breast tumors.[7]

The use of chemotherapy for brain metastases has been in four primary contexts:[13]

1. Whole brain radiotherapy (WBRT) versus WBRT plus chemotherapy
2. Chemotherapy versus chemotherapy plus WBRT
3. Chemotherapy plus concurrent WBRT versus chemotherapy plus delayed WBRT
4. Chemotherapy first, followed by WBRT versus WBRT first, followed by chemotherapy.

Role of Targeted Therapy in Brain Metastasis[14]

Advances in understanding the molecular pathways and discovery of new molecular compounds that mediate brain metastasis have led to an increase in use of these compounds. Various targets include the definite activity of epidermal growth factor receptor (EGFR) inhibitors gefitinib and erlotinib in brain metastases from non-small cell lung cancer (NSCLC) with activating EGFR mutations, lapatinib (small molecule TKI) in HER2-positive breast cancer patients, particularly in association with capecitabine, bevacizumab in NSCLC, breast cancer and melanoma. Sunitinib, a multitarget small molecule TKI, is a promising agent in brain metastases from renal cell cancer. Brain metastases from melanoma with BRAF V600E mutations respond to a specific inhibitor such as vemurafenib. The immunomodulator ipilimumab is also active on brain metastases from melanoma.

RADIOTHERAPY

Whole brain radiotherapy for patients with unresected brain metastases results in symptomatic response in about 50% of patients and improvement in median survival to 3–6 months. Historically, various fractionation schedules have been practiced for WBRT. Patients with single brain metastasis and with controlled or absent extracranial tumor activity should be treated with surgery and radiotherapy, especially when they are younger than 60 years. For patients with progressive extracranial disease, radiotherapy alone seems to be sufficient.[15] Most patients with brain metastases are treated with a protracted palliative course of 30 Gy in 10 fractions over 2 weeks.[16] Recently, it was demonstrated by Rades, et al. that a short-course WBRT with 20 Gy in five fractions is preferable for most patients with brain metastases as 30 Gy in 10 fractions.[17] Although the biological effective dose of short-course accelerated radiotherapy (SCAR) of 20 Gy in 5 fractions is lower as compared with the more commonly used protracted fractionation schedule of 30 Gy in 10 fractions, it has been shown to result in equivalent survival, especially for patients with multiple brain metastases from different histological subtypes. Expecting limited survival as compared with other histologies, NSCLC patients particularly benefit from SCAR. The short-course schedule is convenient for patients who have to make fewer visits to the hospital and also to pay less for palliative radiotherapy. SCAR also benefits the hospital in terms of increasing the patient throughput, thus enabling more patients to be treated on a priority basis. Thus, SCAR is definitely a resource-sparing measure in a busy Indian setup.[5]

Whole Brain Radiotherapy for Multiple Metastases

Median survival of patients with symptomatic multiple brain metastases is 1 month when left untreated and 2 months with steroid use. Whole brain radiotherapy (WBRT) with a standard dose fractionation of 3,000 cGy in 10 fractions has been used for decades in the management of patients with brain metastases. Initial nonrandomized studies showed an improvement of median survival up to 6 months[18] that was later confirmed in large randomized studies. WBRT has been shown to improve neurological symptoms and function with minimal morbidity and this was initially shown on nonrandomized studies and later proven by large randomized studies.[19,20] Despite WBRT, 50% of patients die of intracranial progression. In order to improve the survival of these patients with multiple metastases, various altered fractionation schedules, addition of radiosensitizers and chemotherapy with WBRT have been tried. In a recent systematic review, none of the randomized trials showed survival benefit with altered fractionation schedules as compared to standard (3,000 cGy in 10 fractions or 2,000 cGy in 5 fractions). There was no survival benefit with addition of radiosensitizers (e.g. Motexafin gadolinium) or chemotherapy agents with WBRT.[21]

Management of Oligo Brain Metastasis

A large randomized study showed that in patients with completely excised single brain metastasis, addition of WBRT significantly improved the overall length of survival.[22] This study showed that in patients with single metastasis and controlled extracranial disease has longer survival by addition of surgery to radiotherapy compared to WBRT alone (40 weeks vs 15 weeks). Further randomized studies were conducted to assess the effectiveness of postoperative WBRT when compared to surgery alone, to see if addition of WBRT improved neurological control of disease and increased survival. Postoperative WBRT resulted in reduced recurrent rates at initial sites (10% vs 46%) as well as distant recurrence (14% vs 37%). Death due to neurologic causes was significantly less in RT arm versus surgery only arm (14% vs 44%). However, there was no statistically significant difference in overall length of survival between the two groups.[23]

Local Therapy for Oligo Brain Metastases

Stereotactic radiosurgery (SRS) was found to be very effective in controlling solitary brain metastasis with reduced morbidity. It has an acceptable, less complication rate, and is easily applicable to surgically inaccessible lesions or multiple lesions.[24] In light of this evidence, a large randomized study, RTOG 95-08 showed that addition of SRS boost after WBRT added a significant survival benefit compared to WBRT alone (median survival 6.5 months vs 4.9 months) and also that the survival benefit was seen maximum in patients with RPA class I.[25] A retrospective review of patients who received S+WBRT in Patchell, et al. study was compared with patients who received SRS+WBRT and found that median survival and functional independence of SRS+WBRT was better than S+WBRT in patients with single metastasis (56 weeks and 44 weeks vs 40 weeks and 38 weeks).[26]

Timing of WBRT with Respect to SRS

Efficacy of SRS was further tested by addition WBRT in patients with one to four metastases and found that compared with SRS alone, use of WBRT plus SRS did not improve survival for patients with one to four metastases but the intracranial relapse occurred considerably more frequently in those who did not receive WBRT.[27] In these patients, WBRT could be considered at the time of recurrence.

Radiosurgery Alone versus SRS with WBRT for Oligo Metastases

As evidenced by earlier studies, WBRT is needed in patients with multiple metastases, to reduce distant recurrence. It was also found that in patients with one to four metastases, WBRT can be deferred till recurrence.

A large retrospective study found that there were two major shortcomings of WBRT—long-term survivors developed neurocognitive deficits and that local control may be inadequate, in patients who live longer than a few months.[28] It was found that omission of WBRT in the initial management of patients treated with radiosurgery (RS) for up to four brain metastases did not compromise survival or intracranial control allowing for salvage therapy as indicated.

The neurocognitive outcome after WBRT was further studied in a randomized manner and found that patients treated with SRS plus WBRT were at a greater risk of a significant decline in learning and memory function by 4 months compared with the group that received SRS alone.[29] They found that the Hopkins Verbal Learning Test-Revised (HVLT-R) total recall was impaired in patients who received WBRT compared to those who received SRS alone. The results of the other neurocognitive function tests mirrored those of the HVLT-R tests, but were not as robust.

The major drawback of the study, however, is that the neurocognitive outcomes are studied very early when the actual drop in intelligence quotient (IQ) and cognition impairment after radiotherapy, ideally starts between 6 months and 1 year post-RT. The effect was mostly seen in those patients who had lesions close to hippocampus.

Recent Advances in the Delivery of WBRT

In order to spare hippocampus during cranial irradiation, advances have been made in the intensity-modulated radiotherapy (IMRT) delivery techniques, to reduce radiation-induced neurotoxicity. RTOG 0933, a phase II study was designed to look for WBRT techniques that spare hippocampus and thereby lead to reduction in radiation-induced neurocognitive decline. As a part of this study, it was estimated that perihippocampal risk of metastasis risk was 8.6%.[30] Mehta, et al. have compared hippocampal dosimetry by helical tomotherapy and linear accelerator (LINAC)-based IMRT and found that, on a per fraction basis, mean dose to the hippocampus (normalized to 2 Gy fractions) was reduced by 87% to 0.49 Gy_2 using helical tomotherapy and by 81% to 0.73 Gy_2 using LINAC-based IMRT. Target coverage and homogeneity was acceptable with both IMRT modalities, with differences largely attributed to more rapid dose fall off with helical tomotherapy.[31]

Neurocognition and Quality of Life Measures in Patients with Brain Metastasis

Patients with brain metastasis present with neurocognitive impairment due to various reasons, and many at times this goes unnoticed. Disease location, extent, low performance status, treatment modalities like radiation, chemotherapy and various other factors are known to cause a significant neurocognitive impairment. A decline in neurocognition caused by treatment induced factors, even in these patients with relatively short life span have to addressed as this can have significant negative impact on quality of life (QOL) and recently it was shown that patients with poor overall QOL have shortened length of survival.[32]

Quality of life is a complicated, multidimensional variable with three domains—which include (1) physical, (2) psychological and (3) social domains. Physical domain is the ability to perform activities of daily living (ADL) and specific disease symptom control. Psychological domain includes emotional and neurocognitive components. Social domain involves interpersonal relationships and individual's roles and functions.[33] "Health-related" QOL (HRQOL) refers to the measurement of functional outcomes in which these dimensions are manifested as they relate to the disease.[34] HRQOL is a concept referring to the effect of an illness and its therapy upon a patient's physical, psychological and social well-being as perceived by the patient himself. The four factors which contribute to HRQOL are physical and occupational function, psychological state, social interaction and somatic sensation.

The premise of incorporating HRQOL in oncologic trials has been given serious attention only in recent times when it was realized that standard end points do not measure effects of cancer or its treatment on the emotional, spiritual and social dimensions of patient's lives and that upcoming treatments may not necessarily be superior to standard treatments with respect to standard end points as much. Because majority of patients with brain metastases still cannot be cured and treatments are directed toward the palliation of symptoms; maintenance of HRQOL becomes an important end point in trials of brain metastases.

Health-related QOL can be measured either by generic instruments or more recently, by specific instruments, which mainly focus on aspects of health that are specific to area of primary interest. QLQ-C30 is EORTC's core HRQOL questionnaire that assesses a range of functional outcomes and symptoms relevant to a wide range of cancer populations. The QLQ-BN20 was developed as a site-specific supplement to the QLQ-C30 for use amongst brain cancer patients undergoing chemotherapy or radiotherapy. It addresses symptoms that are specific to brain cancer or its treatment. EORTC QLQ-30 comprises five function scales—physical role (i.e. daily life), emotional, cognitive and social; three symptom scales—fatigue, nausea and vomiting, and pain; six single-item scales—dyspnea, insomnia, appetite loss, constipation, diarrhea, financial effect of tumor and treatment and overall quality of life. EORTC QLQ-BN20 has 20 items that assess visual disorder, motor dysfunction, communication deficit, various disease symptoms (e.g. headaches and seizures), toxic effects of treatment (e.g. hair loss) and future uncertainty. The QLQ-BN20 questionnaire was recently validated for use in primary brain tumors by Taphoorn, et al.[35] after it demonstrated adequate psychometric properties when used on diverse sample of patients with primary brain tumors participating in large scale international clinical trials. (This instrument has also been translated into Hindi and the Hindi version has been validated by Budrukkar and Jalali, et al.).[36] They also encouraged the use of this tool in patients with brain metastases. The BN-20 has henceforth been applied in HRQOL studies of patients with brain metastases and a systematic review by Hird, et al.[37] shows that the EORTC QLQ-C30-BN20 is the instrument most frequently used for measuring HRQOL in patients with brain metastases. It also reports fair rates of compliance with questionnaire filling and that addition of WBRT had a negative impact on HRQOL even while improving disease control.

Very recently (2013) Soffietti, et al. have reviewed the HRQOL results of the EORTC trial 22952-26001.[38] HRQOL was assessed at baseline, 8 weeks after, and then every 3 months for 3 years with the EORTC QLQ-C30 and BN20 module. They showed that addition of WBRT may negatively impact some aspects of HRQOL (global health, physical functioning, cognitive functioning and fatigue) even if these effects are transitory. Consequently observation with close monitoring with MRI imaging is not detrimental for HRQOL. Determining the minimal clinically important difference (MCID) for HRQOL scores from cancer clinical trials is useful to clinicians, patients and researchers as a benchmark for assessing the effectiveness of a health care intervention and for determining the sample size in a clinical trial. It is important to determine the MCID for HRQOL outcomes because statistical significance based on, e.g. P value, does not provide information about the clinical meaningfulness. Investigators have relied on two distinct approaches for identifying the MCID: (1) the anchor-based and (2) distribution-based.[39] Anchor-based methods link HRQOL measures to external criteria, either to a known indicator that has clinical relevance (e.g. progression of disease, performance status, etc.) or to patient-derived ratings of change in health. Distribution-based approaches hinge on the statistical features of the HRQOL data. Commonly used approaches include fractions of the standard deviation (SD) of HRQOL scores, the effect size and standard error of measurement (SEM). Based on the works of Osoba[40] and King[41] mean differences of 10 points or more were widely viewed as being clinically significant when interpreting the results of the randomized clinical trials that use the QLQ-C30. A recent study to determine the change in selected QLQ-C30 and QLQ-BN20 scales, which corresponds to the MCID for improvement and deterioration in HRQOL for brain cancer patients, was carried out by Maringwa, et al.[39] Their findings support the following integer estimates of the MCID for improvement and deterioration, respectively: physical (6, 9), role (14, 12) and cognitive functioning (8, 8); global health status (7, 4), fatigue (12, 9) and motor dysfunction (4, 5).

A detailed prospective evaluation of clinical outcomes and QOL in patients with oligo brain metastases (1–3) treated with image-guided frameless SRS is ongoing at a tertiary care center in India (Jalali and Bose, unpublished work). At an initial analysis of the study, it was found that at a follow-up of 6 weeks, there were improvements in global heath scores, domains of headache, seizures and communication deficit. No appreciable differences were seen in functional scales. Maximum MCID improvements in global health scores and communication deficits were seen, with 60% and 40% patients showing meaningful differences respectively. It was also found that there was a decline in cognitive function and motor dysfunction after treatment whereas global health score and communication deficit markedly improved with treatment. The study showed that there was a 10-point improvement in median global health scores which was also clinically meaningful in 60% of patients. There was no change in the functionality scores. Among the symptom scores, there was a meaningful decline in the domains of fatigue and motor weakness in 20% and 50% of patients respectively whereas communication deficit improved in 40% patients.

REFERENCES

1. Posner JB. Brain metastases: 1995. A brief review. J Neurooncol. 1996;27(3):287-93.
2. Sawaya R, Ligon BL, Bindal RK. Management of metastatic brain tumors. Ann Surg Oncol. 1994;1(2):169-78.
3. Nayak L, Lee EQ, Wen PY. Epidemiology of brain metastases. Curr Oncol Rep. 2012;14(1):48-54.
4. Jalali R, Datta D. Prospective analysis of incidence of central nervous tumors presenting in a tertiary cancer hospital from India. J Neurooncol. 2008;87(1):111-4.
5. Agarwal JP, Wadasadawala T, Munshi A, et al. Validation of recursive partitioning analysis classification in patients with brain metastases from non-small cell lung cancer treated with short-course accelerated radiotherapy. Clin Oncol. 2010;22(10):837-43.
6. Biswas G, Bhagwat R, Khurana R, et al. Brain metastasis: evidence-based management. J Cancer Res Ther. 2006;2(1):5-13.
7. Wadasadawala T, Gupta S, Bagul V, et al. Brain metastases from breast cancer: management approach. J Cancer Res Ther. 2007;3(3):157-65.
8. Hasegawa H, Ushio Y, Hayakawa T, et al. Changes of the blood-brain barrier in experimental metastatic brain tumors. J Neurosurg. 1983;59(2):304-10.
9. Gaspar L, Scott C, Rotman M, et al. Recursive partitioning analysis (RPA) of prognostic factors in three Radiation Therapy Oncology Group (RTOG) brain metastases trials. Int J Radiat Oncol Biol Phys. 1997;37(4):745-51.
10. Sperduto PW, Berkey B, Gaspar LE, et al. A new prognostic index and comparison to three other indices for patients with brain metastases: an analysis of 1,960 patients in the RTOG database. Int J Radiat Oncol Biol Phys. 2008;70(2):510-4.
11. Ryken TC, McDermott M, Robinson PD, et al. The role of steroids in the management of brain metastases: a systematic review and evidence-based clinical practice guideline. J Neurooncol. 2010;96(1):103-14.
12. Mikkelsen T, Paleologos NA, Robinson PD, et al. The role of prophylactic anticonvulsants in the management of brain metastases: a systematic review and evidence-based clinical practice guideline. J Neurooncol. 2010;96(1):97-102.
13. Mehta MP, Paleologos NA, Mikkelsen T, et al. The role of chemotherapy in the management of newly diagnosed brain metastases: a systematic review and evidence-based clinical practice guideline. J Neurooncol. 2010;96(1):71-83.
14. Soffietti R, Trevisan E, Rudà R. Targeted therapy in brain metastasis. Curr Opin Oncol. 2012;24(6):679-86.
15. Noordijk EM, Vecht CJ, Haaxma-Reiche H, et al. The choice of treatment of single brain metastasis should be based on extracranial tumor activity and age. Int J Radiat Oncol Biol Phys. 1994;29(4):711-7.
16. Sneed PK, Suh JH, Goetsch SJ, et al. A multi-institutional review of radiosurgery alone vs radiosurgery with whole brain radiotherapy as the initial management of brain metastases. Int J Radiat Oncol Biol Phys. 2002;53(3):519-26.
17. Rades D, Bohlen G, Dunst J, et al. Comparison of short-course versus long-course whole-brain radiotherapy in the treatment of brain metastases. Strahlenther Onkol. 2008;184(1):30-5.
18. Posner JB. Management of brain metastases. Rev Neurol (Paris). 1992;148(6-7):477-87.
19. Sneed PK, Larson DA, Wara WM. Radiotherapy for cerebral metastases. Neurosurg Clin N Am. 1996;7(3):505-15.
20. Borgelt B, Gelber R, Kramer S, et al. The palliation of brain metastases: final results of the first two studies by the Radiation Therapy Oncology Group. Int J Radiat Oncol Biol Phys. 1980;6(1):1-9.
21. Tsao MN, Lloyd N, Wong RK, et al. Whole brain radiotherapy for the treatment of newly diagnosed multiple brain metastases. Cochrane Database Syst Rev. 2012;4:CD003869.
22. Patchell RA, Tibbs PA, Walsh JW, et al. A randomized trial of surgery in the treatment of single metastases to the brain. N Engl J Med. 1990;322(8):494-500.

23. Patchell RA, Tibbs PA, Regine WF, et al. Postoperative radiotherapy in the treatment of single metastases to the brain: a randomized trial. JAMA. 1998;280(17):1485-9.
24. Flickinger JC, Kondziolka D, Lunsford LD, et al. A multi-institutional experience with stereotactic radiosurgery for solitary brain metastasis. Int J Radiat Oncol Biol Phys. 1994;28(4):797-802.
25. Andrews DW, Scott CB, Sperduto PW, et al. Whole brain radiation therapy with or without stereotactic radiosurgery boost for patients with one to three brain metastases: phase III results of the RTOG 9508 randomised trial. Lancet. 2004;363(9422): 1665-72.
26. Auchter RM, Lamond JP, Alexander E, et al. A multi-institutional outcome and prognostic factor analysis of radiosurgery for resectable single brain metastasis. Int J Radiat Oncol Biol Phys. 1996;35(1):27-35.
27. Aoyama H, Shirato H, Tago M, et al. Stereotactic radiosurgery plus whole-brain radiation therapy vs stereotactic radiosurgery alone for treatment of brain metastases: a randomized controlled trial. JAMA. 2006;295(21):2483-91.
28. Sneed PK, Lamborn KR, Forstner JM, et al. Radiosurgery for brain metastases: is whole brain radiotherapy necessary? Int J Radiat Oncol Biol Phys. 1999;43(3):549-58.
29. Chang EL, Wefel JS, Hess KR, et al. Neurocognition in patients with brain metastases treated with radiosurgery or radiosurgery plus whole-brain irradiation: a randomised controlled trial. Lancet Oncol. 2009;10(11):1037-44.
30. Gondi V, Tome WA, Marsh J, et al. Estimated risk of perihippocampal disease progression after hippocampal avoidance during whole-brain radiotherapy: safety profile for RTOG 0933. Radiother Oncol. 2010;95(3):327-31.
31. Gondi V, Tolakanahalli R, Mehta MP, et al. Hippocampal-sparing whole-brain radiotherapy: a "how-to" technique using helical tomotherapy and linear accelerator-based intensity-modulated radiotherapy. Int J Radiat Oncol Biol Phys. 2010;78(4):1244-52.
32. Sehlen S, Lenk M, Hollenhorst H, et al. Quality of life (QoL) as predictive mediator variable for survival in patients with intracerebral neoplasma during radiotherapy. Onkologie. 2003;26(1):38-43.
33. Lovely MP. Quality of life of brain tumor patients. Semin Oncol Nurs. 1998;14(1):73-80.
34. Osoba D, Brada M, Prados MD, et al. Effect of disease burden on health-related quality of life in patients with malignant gliomas. Neuro Oncol. 2000;2(4):221-8.
35. Taphoorn MJ, Claassens L, Aaronson NK, et al. An international validation study of the EORTC brain cancer module (EORTC QLQ-BN20) for assessing health-related quality of life and symptoms in brain cancer patients. Eur J Cancer. 2010;46(6):1033-40.
36. Budrukkar A, Jalali R, Kamble R, et al. Translation and pilot validation of Hindi translation of assessing quality of life in patients with primary brain tumors using EORTC brain module (BN-20). J Cancer Res Ther. 2006;2(4):166-70.
37. Lydick E, Epstein RS. Interpretation of quality of life changes. Qual Life Res. 1993;2(3):221-6.
38. Soffietti R, Kocher M, Abacioglu UM, et al. A European Organisation for Research and Treatment of Cancer phase III trial of adjuvant whole-brain radiotherapy versus observation in patients with one to three brain metastases from solid tumors after surgical resection or radiosurgery: quality-of-life results. J Clin Oncol. 2013;31(1):65-72.
39. Maringwa J, Quinten C, King M, et al. Minimal clinically meaningful differences for the EORTC QLQ-C30 and EORTC QLQ-BN20 scales in brain cancer patients. Ann Oncol. 2011;22(9):2107-12.
40. Osoba D, Rodrigues G, Myles J, et al. Interpreting the significance of changes in health-related quality-of-life scores. J Clin Oncol. 1998;16(1):139-44.
41. King MT. The interpretation of scores from the EORTC quality of life questionnaire QLQ-C30. Qual Life Res. 1996;5(6):555-67.

54 Cancers from an Unknown Primary Site

Praful Desai

INTRODUCTION

Despite our current capacity to adequately investigate and histologically prove and treat a given cancer, in a minority group of patients (5% or less) it becomes difficult to identify the primary site of origin in a metastatic setting mainly in the lymph nodes, skeleton and the brain. According to moderate estimates, nearly 4,000 (5%) patients in the United States fall into this category. Surveillance, epidemiology, and end results (SEER) reports indicate this volume to be about 2% and other reported series between 2.3% and 7.8%.[1] No data is available from India; however, any busy oncologist will face this clinical setting, though rarely.

CLINICAL PRESENTATION

Most patients will present with a lymph node enlargement (neck, axilla, inguinal region, chest or the retroperitoneal region). The next common group will present with skeletal metastasis (spine, pelvis or axial skeleton) and some others with pleural effusion or ascites. Rarely neurological symptoms with headaches, palsy or a frank paralytic stroke can be due to a metastatic lesion from the lung or breast.

CLINICAL APPROACH AND INVESTIGATIONS INCLUDING HISTOLOGIC STUDIES OF THE METASTATIC LESION

A good clinical examination will often indicate the primary site which may be clinically overt or covert. Often, the primary site may be less than a centimeter or microscopic which is difficult to identify despite all investigations. A metastatic neck node (squamous carcinoma) has generally primary disease in the naso-oro- or laryngopharynx, oral cavity, base tongue or rarely in the esophagus or lung, if the node is in the supraclavicular or mid-neck region. Hoarseness due to vocal cord palsy is often due to locally advanced cancers of the lung or esophagus or the mediastinum. Metastatic axillary lymph nodes point towards the breast in the females or rarely a lymphoma, just as inguinal nodes point towards the anorectal region, uterus, ovary or the prostate gland as the primary site of disease.

Apart from a good clinical examination depending on the anatomic region, appropriate regional endoscopies and imaging studies are mandatory with a positron emission tomography (PET)/computed tomography (CT) or a magnetic resonance imaging (MRI). It is imperative that besides appropriate investigation, special attention must be directed towards a good family history. Cancers of the breast, colon, ovary, uterus, kidney and even lung have strong genetic and familial predisposition. This is particularly true in pleural and peritoneal effusions due to carcinomatosis. The therapy decisions will often depend on a summation of clinical, investigative and laboratory findings.

In a clinical setting where no primary is discernible, a node biopsy (excision) rather than a needle aspiration is mandatory, which will enable the pathologist to study the type of lesion and its histopathology and molecular biopathology. Effusions will have to be tapped (significant amount—not merely 10 or 20 mL) to identify the cytologic pattern of the lesion (lung, ovary, mesothelioma).

Appropriate investigations based on location are indicated as mammogram for an axillary metastatic node or a sonography and scans of the abdomen and pelvis for a metastatic node in the inguinal region.

Tumor Markers

Appropriate biomarker studies often indicate the primary site of lesion, though not always. Carcinoembryonic antigen (CEA), prostate-specific antigen (PSA), cancer antigen (CA)-125, β-human chorionic gonadotropin (β-hCG), CA-19.9 are commonly studied to locate a possible primary site. Appropriate endoscopies have been alluded to. Despite all the above and more in less than 5% of patients the primary site of disease will remain undetected. The most difficult to pinpoint and locate are lymphomatous and neuroendocrine tumors. The next logical step after routine histopathology is to study the immunohistochemistry (IHC), cytogenetic analysis and molecular or gene expression profiling. Deoxyribonucleic acid (DNA) microanalysis are the other more advanced biologic studies available to pinpoint the primary site. In majority of cases these advanced studies are not necessary, and IHC and cytogenetic studies will reveal the site of the primary disease.

Such clinical settings are often disconcerting to patients, clinical oncologists and histopathologists as it raises the important issues of appropriate therapy. One of the major reasons for inability to make an adequate diagnosis on simple hematoxylin and eosin (H and E) light microscopy is poorly handled tissue biopsy or cytology due to inadequate or crushed tissue and poor fixation. The common histologic types are adenocarcinoma (well, moderate and poorly differentiated types), squamous carcinoma, lymphoma, sarcomatous lesions and rarely neuroendocrine carcinoma. The most common histologic type associated with an unknown primary is an adenocarcinoma-forming nearly 60% of all lesions. Immunohistochemical staining (studies) is frequently performed when the simple H and E light microscopy staging is inconclusive. Formalin-fixed and paraffin-embedded tissues are adequate enough for IHC staining which helps to identify the correct lineage of poorly differentiated neoplasms in most instances,[2] e.g. presence of thyroid transcription factor 1 (TTF-1), chromogranin and synaptophysin staining in neuroendocrine tumors. Most of the common malignancies are appropriately diagnosed by IHC tumor staining.

The pathologist, when unable to designate a definitive histologic diagnosis will, report the lesion as a "poorly differentiated neoplasm". Precise diagnosis is mandatory as some of these untyped lesions can be effectively treated. In a reported series, 35–65% of poorly differentiated neoplasms were found to be lymphomas after further studies. Most of the remaining tumors in this group are carcinomas including poorly differentiated neuroendocrine tumors.[3]

Electron Microscopy

This may be helpful in some poorly differentiated neoplasms. Electron microscopy (EM) studies are useful if a simple light microscopy and IHC are non contributory in certain types of undifferentiated sarcomas. EM is not useful in differentiating various types of adenocarcinomas.

Molecular Profiling and Cytogenetic Analysis

Light H and E microscopy and IHC staining will be able to pinpoint the primary site in most cases; if the origin of a tumor is still unidentified only then cytogenetic analysis and molecular profiling would be the next step in tracing the origin.[4] Chromosomal rearrangements and specific chromosomal analysis can indicate the diagnosis of B-cell/T-cell lymphomas with high accuracy including hematopoietic neoplasms. Further search for the origin of an unknown primary is gene expression profiling, DNA microanalysis, reverse-transcriptase polymerase chain reaction (RT-PCR) assays.[5] These are rarely used, though it is now in vogue in tertiary centers for nearly 15 years. Genetic studies involving BRCA-2 may be considered in appropriate in patients.

TREATMENT

Therapeutic approach will pose problems if the primary site of disease still remains elusive. Empirical approach then becomes necessary essentially by chemotherapy as solid localized lesions can always be surgically resected or controlled by radiotherapy. In a study of 1,515 patients (45 trials) Greco and Hainsworth[2] recorded overall responses of 19% with cisplatin, 0–16% with 5-fluorouracil (5-FU) and 8–39% overall responses. Various combinations of cisplatin or carboplatin, taxanes, 5-FU, gemcitabine and cyclophosphamide in doublets or triple combinations may provide an extended remission from 6 months to 3 years depending on the patient's general condition and response to therapy. Supportive and symptomatic care is vital. In many situations, best supportive care, particularly in very advanced disseminated disease, may be the best and only option.

REFERENCES

1. Pavlidis N, Briasoulis E, Hainsworth J, et al. Diagnostic and therapeutic management of unknown primary. Eur J Cancer. 2003:39(14):1990-2005.
2. Greco FA, Hainsworth JD. Cup site. In: DeVita VT, Hellman S, Rosenberg SA (Eds). Cancer: Principles and Practice of Oncology, 7th edition. Philadelphia: Lippincott Williams and Wilkins; 2005. p. 2213.
3. Horning SJ, Carrier EK, Rouse RV, et al. Lymphoma presenting as histologically unclassified neoplasms: characteristics and response to treatment. J Clin Oncol. 1989;7(9):1281-7.
4. Greco FA, Erlander MG. Molecular classification of unknown primary site. Mol Diagn Ther. 2009;13(6):367-73.
5. Varadhachary G, Talantov D, Raber MN, et al. Molecular profiling of carcinoma of unknown primary and correlation with clinical evaluation. J Clin Oncol. 2008;26(27):4442-8.

55 Paraneoplastic Syndromes in Cancer

Praful Desai

Almost all cancers produce symptoms due to anatomic and physiologic disturbances in and around their site of origin by their proximity or infiltration of the organs or tissues around the site. The ability of some tumors to produce substances, hormones and fluids, though infrequent, results in distinctive symptomatic clinical syndromes which are known as paraneoplastic syndromes (PNPSs). Not all cancers produce PNPS. The syndrome can involve and impact almost any system or tissues in the body. It is important for the clinician to be aware of these unusual and protean clinical manifestations to be able to pinpoint the likely reason for the symptom complex so as to obtain appropriate investigations to reach a diagnosis of the primary disease site for adequate therapy. The symptom complex may affect and produce abnormalities far away from the primary site of cancer. Essentially, it is the host response which results in the syndrome known as PNPS.

Appropriate diagnosis, location and treatment of the primary lesion will result in the disappearance of the PNPS. In some clinical settings, the primary cancer may be difficult to control or cure; nevertheless, therapy of symptoms will help palliate or ameliorate the distressing symptoms. Rarely cancers can metabolize steroids to biologically active forms which results in PNPS. As mentioned, PNPS can be the first sign and symptom of an underlying malignant disease.

Endocrine manifestations are among the more common presenting symptoms particularly in lung cancer. Production and hypersecretion of ectopic adrenocorticotrophic hormone (ACTH) frequently will result in a clinical picture of Cushing's syndrome with truncal obesity, hypertension, pigmentation, facial swelling and edema, myopathy and weakness. Appropriate investigations of imaging the chest and abdomen will reveal the presence of a lung lesion. Almost 60–70% of patients of sporadic Cushing's syndrome are caused by adrenal lesions and the diagnosis of this condition can be easily confirmed by urine free cortisol levels and dexamethasone suppression tests.[1]

Among the other reasons, besides lung cancer, Cushing's syndrome is known to arise from cancers of the thyroid, thymus, pancreas, carcinoids and even a pheochromocytoma. Lung cancer is the most common cause of ectopic ACTH secretion resulting in PNPS producing a clinical picture of Cushing's syndrome. Successful therapy of lung cancer with a surgical excision will result in disappearance of the syndrome. More often, small cell lung cancer is the reason for this clinical spectrum. The syndrome of inappropriate secretion of antidiuretic hormone (SIADH), though uncommon, is a distinct clinical entity which is also known to occur in small cell cancer of the lung. Seventy five percent of SIADH are due to small cell lung cancer. Occasionally, head and neck cancers are known to produce SIADH. The major features are loss of water and sodium resulting in hyponatremia of varying intensity. Other causes of hyponatremia needs to be excluded like renal dysfunction, Addison's disease, hypothyroidism, pulmonary or central nervous system (CNS) disorders and rarely iatrogenic causes due to liberal use of opiates. Symptoms of CNS toxicity like fatigue, anorexia, headaches, mental changes, delirium can occur in severe cases.

Therapy essentially consists of trying to identify the likely primary disease, (small cell lung cancer or head and neck cancers). Correction of sodium levels is the key feature in the symptomatic therapy of SIADH. Hyponatremia should be very gradually corrected often over a week.

Life-threatening complications can occur when sodium levels drop below 125–130 mg/mL. A 3% hypertonic saline infusion is indicated in severe hyponatremia and the sodium levels should be raised in a very gradual fashion. Rapid attempts to increase sodium levels can result in central pontine damage. Renal function needs to be monitored carefully.

Hypoglycemia is a cardinal feature in insulinoma, which has the classic Whipple's triad and is not an unknown problem. It is easy to diagnose with modern imaging techniques and appropriate biochemistry estimation of sugar levels. Apart from insulinoma, large liver tumors, fibromas and other mesenchymal tumors, gastrointestinal stromal tumor (GIST), lymphomas and adrenal cancers are known to produce hypoglycemia.

Thrombotic manifestations (thrombophlebitis/thrombocytosis): A fairly frequent clinical manifestation in PNPS is the recurrent vascular thrombotic manifestation often in the lower extremities known to occur in many cancers. Often it preceeds[2] the presence of cancer and unexplained lower limb deep vein thrombosis (DVT) or thrombophlebitis should initiate search for a lesion of the pancreas, stomach, liver, lung, ovary and lymphoproliferative disorders including chronic myeloid leukemia. The main reason for thrombotic manifestations is an over production of thrombopoietin or interleukin. Patients with existing cancer or metastatic lesions can be treated with anticoagulants for a long period if there is no contraindication.[3]

Renal nephropathies: Derangements and dysfunction of the kidneys can be one of the PNPS for malignancy and must be adequately investigated for any associated cancer. Lymphomas, colon and stomach cancer should be excluded in the investigation of an idiopathic renal dysfunction. Hypertension, proteinuria and hematuria can occur.

Tumor-induced osteomalacia is common with metastatic osteolytic lesions and the common causes are lung, breast and myeloma, which may precede the cancer. Patients often present with a spontaneous fracture with minimal trauma.

Polycythemia with increased hemoglobin and erythrocytosis are known to be associated or precede a liver, kidney or Wilm's tumor. Pheochromocytoma can occasionally produce polycythemia. Very high levels of hemoglobin may occasionally require phlebotomy.

Cutaneous manifestations: The skin is very often a reflection of the entire system, particularly in latent malignancies (lymphomas). Erythematous patches, exfoliative dermatitis, dermatomyositis, generalized dry itchy skin (acquired ichthyosis), hyperpigmentation, clubbing are all different manifestations in occult malignant lesion.[4]

Mycosis fungoides is a cutaneous manifestation and a dermatologic form of various lymphomas or occasionally a primary skin lymphoma.

Neuromuscular disorders: Various forms of myopathies, myasthenia gravis (thymoma), peripheral polyneuritis, motor neuron disease, encephalomyelitis, movement disorders, visual loss and personality changes are rare but important variants of the protean manifestations of a large clinical spectrum of PNPS. The clinician must be aware of this symptom syndrome in the search for a latent malignancy (Also see Chapter 62).

REFERENCES

1. Neiman LK, Billen BM, Findling JW, et al. The diagnosis of Cushing's syndrome: an Endocrine Society Clinical Practice Guidelines. J Clin Endocrinol Metab. 2008;93(5):1526-40.
2. Sørensen HT, Mellemkjaer L, Steffensen FH, et al. The risk of diagnosis of cancer after deep venous thrombosis or pulmonary embolism. N Engl J Med. 1998;338(17):1169-73.
3. Noble SI, Shelly MD, Coles B, et al. Management of thromboembolism in patients with advanced cancer: a systemic review and meta-analysis. Lancet Oncol. 2008;9(6):577-84.
4. DeVita VT, Lawrence TS, Rosenberg SA (eds). Cancer: Principles and Practice of Oncology, 9th edition. Philadelphia, PA: Lippincott Williams & Wilkins; 2011. pp. 2393-410.

56 Reconstructive Surgery in Oncology

Dhairyasheel Savant, Mridula Kuchekar

INTRODUCTION

Major oncologic surgery, on occasion, requires appropriate reconstructive surgery in order to restore form and for total rehabilitation to restore normal anatomy and physiologic function. In addition to these means of rehabilitation, psychosocial, vocational and emotional counseling is necessary for a total recovery. The extent of tissues loss from ablative surgery relates to the loss of soft tissue and bone. The soft-tissue loss may be due to loss of the cutaneous or mucosal lining or bulk of underlying soft tissues. Ideally, all bone losses should be replaced with bone reconstruction; however, the need for bony reconstruction depends on the site and the extent of bone resection whether it is in the mandible, maxilla, or calvarium or the chest wall. In addition to this, the planning of reconstructive surgery requires assessment of tissue loss, which may be from mobile parts of the anatomy of the head and neck region, or it may be from immobile tissues. Special consideration is necessary for reconstruction of resected nerves, blood vessels, cartilage, etc. The surgical defect created by resection of either a primary or a metastatic tumor in the body region can usually be repaired by primary closure if the loss of tissue is modest in nature and the site has not been previously irradiated. However, if primary closure is not feasible, then viable tissue should be brought over to repair the surgical defect. This may be done by mobilization of local tissues, or transfer of adjacent tissues from the neighboring region, or by bringing in tissues from distant sites by microvascular free tissue transfer. The tissue flaps available for reconstruction of defect in the body may be local regional or distant.

The viability of a cutaneous flap depends on its blood supply, which may be axial or random. In general, axial flaps are more reliable due to adequate perfusion from its identifiable vascular pedicle. The width-to-length ratio of an axial skin flap may be as much as 1:5 or more depending on the particular flap chosen and its blood supply. In contrast, random flaps are less reliable due to the absence of an identifiable vessels supplying blood to the flap. A random flap is generally less reliable when the width-to-length ratio exceeds 1:2. Thus, the applicability of random flaps is somewhat limited. The identification of myocutaneous circulation has resulted in the availability of a number of myocutaneous flaps, which are currently very popular, and has a wide range of application in reconstruction of various defects, not only in the head and neck region but also elsewhere in the body. The myocutaneous flaps are axial since there is an identifiable vascular pedicle perfusing the flap, providing the blood supply to the underlying muscle and through perpendicular perforators to the overlying skin. The availability of the operating microscope and development of vascular surgery the earlier past of this century led to the development of microsutures and opened up the whole new field of microvascular tissue transfer. Microvascular free flaps are also axial since this is an identifiable vascular pedicle perfusing the flap. The reliability of the myocutaneous flaps and microvascular free flaps is comparable to axial regional cutaneous flaps. Preoperative planning of reconstructive surgery influences surgical approach for resection of the tumor including the planning of the incisions and the availability of the desired tissue reconstruct the anticipated defect. Ideally, the reconstructive surgeon should have sufficient training and familiarity with application and techniques of local, regional and myocutaneous flaps in postoncologic reconstructive surgery. Microvascular surgery requires special expertise by additional training and is best performed by a separate reconstructive surgical team. Several special considerations come into the picture during planning reconstructive surgery in various regions of the body, namely the head and neck region, breast, chest and abdominal wall reconstruction and are discussed individually in the following chapters.

RECONSTRUCTION TECHNIQUES IN HEAD AND NECK CANCERS

Reconstructive techniques have revolutionized the extent of extirpative surgery in the head and neck region. The pectoralis major myocutaneous (PMMC) flap; its variations and the use of microvascular free flaps have broadened the armamentarium of the plastic surgeon for treatment of major defects. The surgical concept of "en bloc" resection dates back in Kocher in the 1980s. Later, Crile and others advocated the combined approach wherein the primary tumor and the regional lymph nodes were excised in a single operation which was known as a composite resection or heroically a "Commando" or what is now called a composite resection. Although surgery for head and neck malignancies were for curative purposes only, there was a definite hesitancy in undertaking large excisions because initial reconstructive techniques were restricted to primary closure, skin grafts and local flaps. In the 1950s, the development of two important regional flaps, the forehead flap and the deltopectoral (DP) flap (Fig. 1), made a major impact. Subsequent progress resulted in development of myocutaneous flaps.

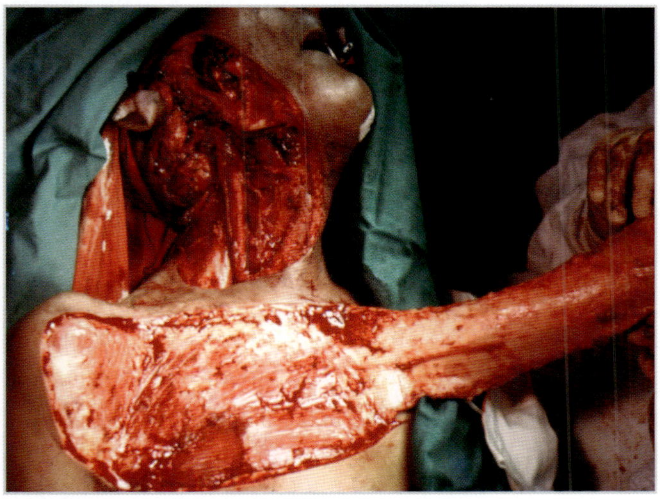

Fig. 1: Deltopectoral flap: extremely simple to raise and can cover major defects in the neck and up to the temporal region

Courtesy: Dr P B Desai

Commonly Used Flaps

Historically, the DP flap is one of the most widely used flaps and was developed by Bakamjian in 1965. It is an axial pattern flap based on the perforating branches of the internal mammary artery. Its advantages are that it provides a large amount of thin cutaneous tissue while its major disadvantages are that it is a two-stage procedure and requires a split-thickness skin graft for the donor defect. This flap is used mainly in conjunction with a PMMC flap or as outer cover for neck or parotid defects. The forehead flap introduced by McGregor in 1963, is a reliable axial pattern flap based on the superficial temporal artery. This flap was used infrequently but exclusively in cases where there is an internal lining and outer cover would give a greater bulk. But the disadvantage is in leaving an esthetic deformity at the donor site, which is very visible. The visor forehead flap is also used to reconstruct the upper or lower lips.

The PMMC flap was described by Ariyan (Figs 2A to D) and coworkers, who showed that the dominant blood supply was a large segmental vessel, the thoracoacromial artery. The PMMC flap is workhorse of all the types of head and neck reconstructions.[1] This is a type V musculocutaneous flap as per Mathes and Nahai's classification, i.e. it has a dominant pedicle at the insertion and the secondary vessel at the origin.

The blood supply of the PMMC flap is derived from the descending branch of the acromiothoracic artery which runs directly on the under surface of the pectoralis major muscle. So, a line joining the midclavicular point to the nipple is recommended for the surface marking of the vessel. The PMMC flap may be elevated in a variety of ways. It can be elevated in the manner of a full paddle with the dimensions of the skin matching the dimensions of the underlying pectoralis major muscle. It can be elevated with two islands of skin), positioned medial to the nipple or the flap may be elevated with two islands of skin to provide an inner and outer lining with a longer muscle paddle and an island inferior to the nipple to form a bipaddled flap and it can also be raised as a myofascial flap with no skin paddle. This flap can be combined with a DP flap to raise a dual flap for cover and lining of extensive defects. Finally, the PMMC flap may be elevated and the vascular pedicle divided for the transfer of the whole unit with free microvascular anastomosis at the recipient site. It may also be used as a muscle flap to protect the carotid artery or to provide bulk. A pectoralis osteomyocutaneous flap with the fourth or fifth rib can be elevated for mandibular reconstruction.

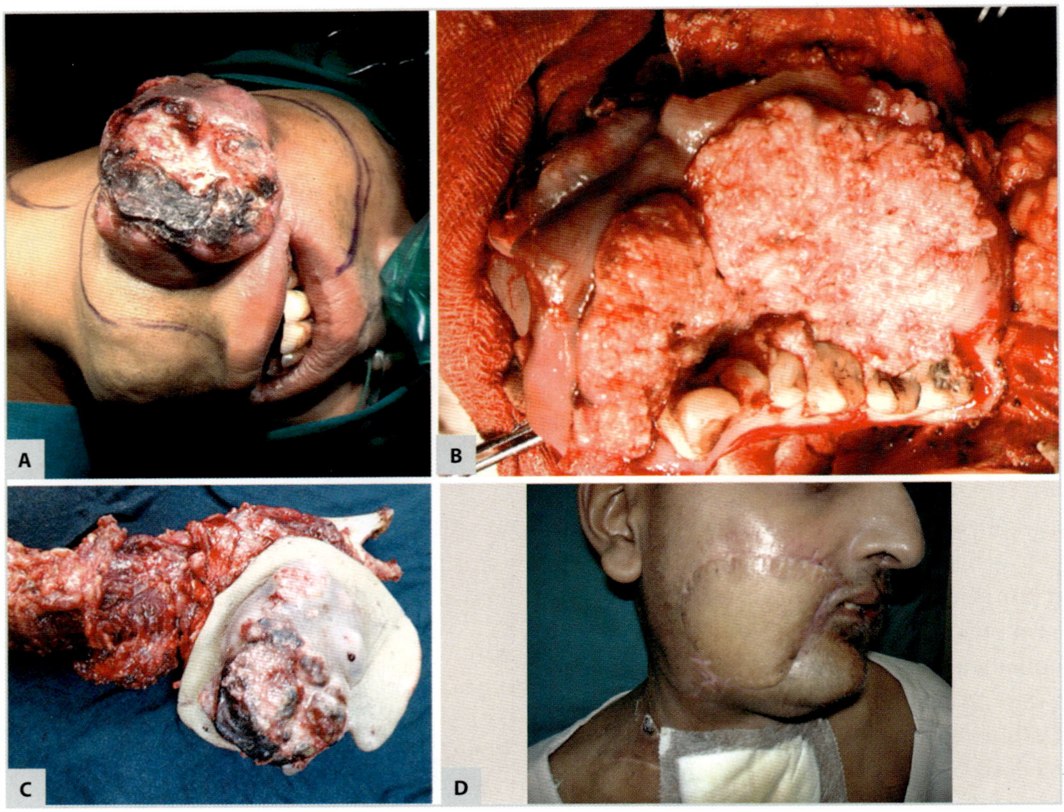

Figs 2A to D: (A) Fungating mass on the skin from an advanced infiltrating carcinoma of buccal mucosa; (B) Lesion in the buccal mucosa seen during surgery; (C) Operative specimen with neck dissection (composite resection); (D) Final result using PMMC flap

While raising the flap, the following points should be noted. The outline of the flap is drawn on the skin. The length and width of the skin island of myocutaneous flap as well as the length of its pedicle are determined by the site, size and shape of the surgical defect. The point of pivot for the flap is the midclavicular point. A tape or string is used to measure the distance from this point up to the most distal portion of the surgical defect. The flap should never be elevated prior to resection of the tumor and assessment of the surgical defect. Elevation of the flap begins on its medial aspect first. The incision is deepened through the subcutaneous tissue and fat up to the underlying pectoralis major muscle and no attempt is made to retract the skin and subcutaneous tissue overlying the muscle in the area of the flap since it may produce undue traction on and avulsion of the perforating vessels. At this point, 8–10 interrupted chromic catgut sutures are placed between the transected edge of muscle and the subcutaneous tissue of overlying skin. These sutures maintain the entire myocutaneous unit as one block of tissue, avoiding any undue tension, traction or laceration of the perforating vessels to the skin. The subcutaneous vascular plexus is thus preserved providing the blood supply to the skin of the distal part of the flap. The pectoralis major is easily separated from pectoralis minor muscle by blunt dissection. The undersurface of the pectoralis major muscle is mobilized up to the clavicle freeing up its entire posterior surface. This enables identification of the acromiothoracic vessels at about the midclavicular point viewed from the right hand side of the patient. Once the location and the course of the vessels are noted, the pectoralis major muscle is divided medial to the vessels. At this point, flap is rotated by 180° and is ready for its transfer to the neck for the repair of the defects.[2] If the skin surface of the flap is to be used for pharyngeal repair or for the surface cover then the flap is flipped 180° in a radial plane. Regardless of the plane of rotation, utmost care should be taken to avoid kinking or excessive stretch on the vascular pedicle.

The disadvantages of the PMMC flap however are:

- It can be too bulky, particularly when used in the oral cavity
- Its arc of rotation is limited for upper facial and oromaxillary defects
- There is distortion of symmetry at the donor site more apparent in the females

- Impairment of shoulder function due to loss of pectoralis major muscle

Other Flaps

The vascular anatomy of circulation of trapezius myocutaneous flap is similar to that described in PMMC flap. However, the vascular pedicle is from the transverse cervical artery and its accompanying veins. Two types of this flap are available. The lateral trapezius myocutaneous flap overlying the acromioclavicular region has very limited application. The island in this flap is limited in its surface extent and the arc of rotation is very short. Hence, application of this flap is limited to small pharyngeal defects. The posterior or vertical trapezius myocutaneous flap however is more versatile for scalp defects.[3] This flap is dependent on descending branch of transverse cervical artery deep to the trapezius muscle. One disadvantage is that the patient has to be positioned laterally to elevate the flap. This flap provides a generous amount of soft tissue and a large portion of skin island for repair of major surgical defects particularly on the lateral aspect of face, parotid region, mastoid region and the temporoparietal region of the scalp. This flap is ideally suitable for repair of postparotidectomy defect or as cover with other flaps.

A latissimus dorsi myocutaneous flap is also available for coverage of large soft tissue and skin defects in the head and neck region. However, elevation of this flap requires repositioning of the patient and often will unduly increase the length of the operative procedure. Therefore, if other means of repair of the surgical defect are available, a latissimus dorsi myocutaneous flap is not preferred.

RECONSTRUCTIVE OPTIONS FOR VARIOUS SITES IN THE HEAD AND NECK REGION

Lips

Small malignant lesions of the lip may be excised by a wedge excision requiring only a primary closure. Lesions involving only the vermilion border can be covered after excisions with a mucosal out-roll. Medium-sized malignant lesions of the upper or lower lip including the angle may be excised widely and reconstructed with an Abbe Estlander flap. Larger lesions involving almost the whole of either the upper or lower lip can be conveniently reconstructed with bilateral Gillies fan-flaps. If the oral commissure becomes too small with these procedures, a secondary commissuroplasty is performed usually after 2–3 weeks.

Paranasal Sinuses, Orbit and Skull Base

Repair of bony, soft tissue and skin defects created by major resections of tumors from the paranasal sinuses, orbit and skull base requires the need for the repair of the bony defect at skull base to separate the dura from the nasal cavity, support to the globe if the orbital floor is resected, and the provision of the soft-tissue bulk and overlying skin for major three-dimensional composite defects. Repairs of the skull base can be performed without bone, using galeal pericranial flap or microvascular composite free flap.[4,5] Reconstruction of the floor of the orbit is best undertaken using a microvascular free flap of scapula with bone, soft tissue and skin when appropriate. If alloplastic material is used to repair the floor of orbit, then adequate soft tissue coverage should be provided to avoid exposure and extrusion of alloplastic material. Preoperative planning requires consultation with maxilla-fascial orthodontist for appropriate prosthetic support.

Submucous Fibrosis

This condition has been described as a peculiar oral disease seen mainly amongst Indians.[6] The condition is chronic and clinically characterized by blanching and stiffness of oral mucosa. The indiscriminate use of irritants predisposes this condition. The nasolabial flap based on terminal branch of fascial artery is preferred method of reconstruction for relief of submucous fibrosis.[7] Under general anesthesia, the mucosa is incised from the angle of the mouth to the anterior pillar on both sides; down to the muscle. This releases trismus. The resultant defects are filled with two inferiorly based nasolabial flaps, each approximately 5 cm × 1.5–2 cm. The pedicles of the flaps are divided after 3 weeks and the insetting is performed as to ensure that the divided bases of the flaps come up to the vermilion border at the commissure. This results in an average open bite of 3 cm. The postoperative rehabilitation is far superior as compared to other methods and this technique is recommended for all cases of submucous fibrosis requiring correction of severe trismus (Figs 3A to C).

Laryngopharynx

The goals of reconstructive surgery of the oral cavity are related in functional restoration and esthetic appearance. The factors to be considered in functional reconstruction are oral competency, speech, mobility of tongue, mastication, bolus transportation. Reconstruction using regional myocutaneous flap or a microvascular free flap, should be performed keeping in mind that the eventual

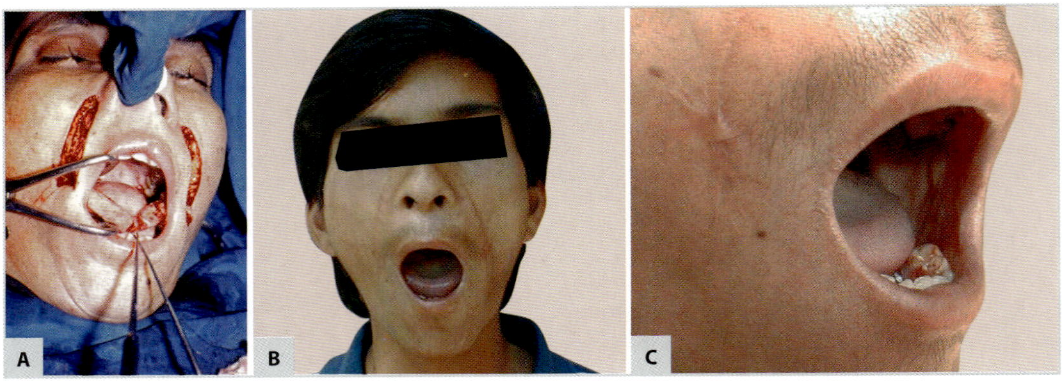

Figs 3A to C: (A) Standard bilateral nasolabial flap for submucous fibrosis. Premalignant condition; significant resolution of submucous fibrosis possible; (B) Post nasolabial flap; (C) Intraoral showing good opening and flap mucosalisation
Courtesy: Dr P B Desai

goal of such a reconstructive effort should be to restore the ability to swallow without aspiration or obstruction to the airway. When a laryngectomy is done in addition to pharyngectomy, the reconstructive choices are dependent on partial or total loss of the circumference of the pharynx. Partial defects can be repaired with PMMC flap or microvascular radial forearm free flap.[8] Clearly, the goals of reconstructive surgery in this setting are to create a satisfactory conduit, prevent stricture formation and avoid redundant soft tissue producing functional obstruction. When circumferential resection of the pharynx is undertaken, the choice of reconstruction depends on the length of the resected segment. A short segment loss limited to cervical region is best repaired using a microvascular free segment of jejunum.[9] However, when pharyngeal resection extends to involve upper esophagus, then the optimal means or restoration of esophageal continuity is gastric transposition. Hence, it is recommended that the defect up to 35% of the circumference should be closed primarily; the defect between 35% and 70% of the circumference should be reconstructed with a patch pharyngoplasty. Ideally, a DP flap, PMMC flap or microvascular jejunal transfer is indicated if the lower margin of the jejunum or the jejunoesophageal anastomosis is above the tracheostoma. If it is lower, then a gastric transposition should be performed. Other authors also used the colon, either pedicled or as a supercharged free flap.

Microvascular Free Tissue Transfer

The increasing application of microvascular surgery for free tissue transfer over the last 20 years has produced new dimensions in reconstructive techniques in head and neck surgery. Microvascular free tissue transfer can repair all types of defects created by resection of tumors in the head and neck area. Although the applicability of microvascular techniques is universal, some degree of discretion, restraint and wisdom should be employed before microvascular free tissue transfer is chosen for reconstruction. The success of microvascular free tissue transfer depends upon the technical perfection of the surgeon. The type of tissue necessary for the reconstruction of defect depends on the type of tissue loss. Thus, major resection of tumor in the head and neck region may result in loss of skin, soft tissues, mucosa, bone, cartilage or any combinations of these tissues. The microvascular free flap essential for reconstruction of a particular defect may therefore consist either of skin alone, skin and soft tissue such as muscle, skin, soft tissue and bone, soft tissue alone, bone alone or bone and skin. A variety of different combinations of tissues are available in several microvascular free flaps. The most commonly used free flaps in the head and neck region are the radial forearm, rectus abdominis, fibula, jejunum, scapula, latissimus dorsi and iliac crest with or without skin of groin.[10]

In the selection, design and the fabrication of a microvascular free flap, the reconstructive surgeon needs to remember that merely closing the defect is not enough, as replacing bone for bone loss or providing skin coverage for a large skin defect is not sufficient. Preoperative assessment is essential for understanding the nature of the anticipated surgical defect and an appropriate plan for the reconstructive effort should be developed before proceeding with the surgery.

Mucosa should be replaced with mucosa, bone with bone and skin with skin; however, if this is not feasible, then certain compromises may have to be made to achieve the most desired result. It is therefore essential that the surgeon has a proper understanding of the functional and esthetic effect of resectional surgery with its oncologic implications, so that the most appropriate flap is designed based on a given clinical sitting.[11,12]

Summary

Head and neck cancers form the major bulk of reconstruction in the schedule of reconstructive surgeon, ranging from simplest local rotation flaps to the most complex composite osteomyocutaneous flap with microvascular anastomosis. It covers the entire reconstructive ladder. It is up to the discretion of the reconstructive surgeon to choose the best option based on the age, general condition of the patient and most importantly on the stage of the disease.[13] If the objective is palliation, a simpler option should be exercised to rehabilitate the patient faster so that early adjunctive therapy (chemotherapy or radiotherapy) can be exhibited.[14,15] In early lesions with a good prognosis, it is a viable option to consider a major microvascular procedure to deliver optimum function as well as cosmesis.

MANDIBULAR RECONSTRUCTIONS

The mandible contributes to airway stability, is important in speech, deglutition and mastication, and largely determines the shape of the lower face. Functional and esthetic goals are therefore equally important considerations in mandible reconstruction.[16] Specific functional goals include preservation of tandem temporomandibular joint action with maximal opening ability and maintenance of occlusion. In more severe cases in which many teeth are missing, restoration of normal interarch distance and alignment is critical in order to facilitate subsequent dental rehabilitation. Key esthetic goals include symmetry, preservation of lower facial height and anterior chin projection, and correction of submandibular soft tissue neck defects. Squamous cell carcinoma is the etiology in the majority of cases with osteogenic sarcoma is the second most common cause overall and the most common bone tumor. A small number of segmental mandibular defects result from extensive benign cystic or fibrotic bone disease. Mandible defects requiring reconstruction are sometimes due to segmental bone loss alone. However, the majority of the reconstructions are sometimes due to segmental bone loss alone usually with adjacent intraoral soft tissue as well as submandibular neck soft tissue. Some bone defects include external skin loss instead of mucosa, and the most complex bone, mucosa, and skin. Various classification schemes have been proposed for mandible defects. The more practical one describes the bone loss in terms of symphysis (designated S and defined and lying between the two canine teeth), body (B), and hemimandible segments (H) ramus (R) and condyle (C). Hemimandible and body segments are similar except that the former includes the condyle whereas the latter segments do not. A defect commonly is a combination of more than one segment. Although this description may appear tedious, it is actually useful as a common media to standardize the variable reconstructive problems.

Methods of Reconstruction

Mandible reconstruction can be accomplished by a variety of means, which include nonvascularized bone grafts, metal plates, pedicled flaps, and free flaps. Nonvascularized grafts such as an iliac crest segment can be used for a short bone gap (less than 3 cm) in a setting of benign disease but this is a rare application. Although conceptually and technically simple, this method relies on creeping substitution for long-term mandible stability. Pedicled flaps include the trapezius and pectoralis osteomyocutaneous flaps. The primary attraction of these donor sites is the fact that they lie adjacent to the head, thus permitting their movement into this area without disconnection of their blood supple. Although this is an attractive concept, there are several important drawbacks. First, use of these flaps enlarges the size of the primary wound considerably compared to harvesting tissue from a distant donor site. This increases the potential for morbidity at the site of the reconstruction. More importantly, a significant portion of flap volume is used up just to reach the recipient site. The disproportion of the flap, which is used for the actual reconstruction, often has a marginal blood supply and is at risk for ischemic necrosis. The bone available with the pectoralis major muscle (rib) and the trapezius (spine of the scapula) is limited compared to free flap alternatives. Excellent results can be obtained with carefully reconstructed rib pectoralis major osteomyocutaneous flap which is a similar flap to raise except that fourth or the fifth rib is incorporated in it.[17] These flaps have a place where microvascular reconstructions are either not feasible or no skilled reconstructive microsurgeon is available.

Prosthetic mandible replacement has evolved as an alternate method of reconstruction that still has legitimate but limited applications today. Mesh trays made of Dacron or metal were introduced in the 1970s as scaffolds that were filled with bone graft chips and used for segmental bone defects. Silastic mandibles for extended defects have been used with greater efficacy especially in secondary reconstructive procedures where mucosa is intact. Long-term follow-up has shown this method to beneficial but problems with extrusion and bone graft dissolution commonly occurred. Metal reconstruction plates developed as a result of orthopedic hardware advances in other areas which offer advantages of decreased operating time and avoidance of a bone graft donor site. They have important disadvantages: risk of plate fracture; preclusion of dental reconstruction; and a thin shape that does not provide adequate bulk for reconstruction. Another important drawback is the functional limitation seen with the use of metal plates for hemimandible defects that include the condyle as the prosthetic condyle is a poor substitute for the native structure. Reconstruction plates require adequate soft-tissue leverage and plates that are not supplemented with a soft-tissue flap are prone to failure.[18] The PMMC flap is commonly used to provide soft-tissue coverage. However, plate exposure still occurs, particularly with anterior reconstruction, in which the tension on the flap is greatest. The most reliable soft-tissue coverage is provided by a combination of a soft-tissue free flap and a reconstruction plate best reserved for the elderly patient, for lateral defects, and for those with bad prognosis. Osteomyocutaneous flap reconstruction either pedicled or as a microvascular free flap is often the most effective method of mandible repair. These flaps have both soft tissue and bone components, which are available in a configuration for solving specific composite tissue problems.[19] Fortunately, the favored donor sites all have excellent flap pedicle qualities (vessel diameter and length), and the head and neck area generally has excellent recipient vessels available, even previous surgical treatment and radiation. Free-flap survival rates are generally about 95%.

Flap Donor Site Selection

Early in the development of free-flap mandible reconstruction there have been multiple donor sites from which rib, metatarsal, and ilium were among the first to be used. The ilium has been the most popular among the three owing to its abundant bone, which even resembles a hemimandible when harvested specifically. This has been the workhorse free flap for the first decade in free-flap mandible reconstruction. Further solution has led to the development of the radius, scapula and fibula donor sites. These additional sites have increased the flexibility and precision of the techniques the specific assets and limitations of each donor site have become clearer. Currently, the fibula is the donor site of choice for most patients but the radius, the scapula, and the ilium are better choices in a few for most patients but the radius, the scapula, and the ilium are better choices in a few specific settings. Each has unique advantages and disadvantages. A comparison of the donor site is helpful in selecting the proper one for a particular problem. Some have better bone qualities. Some have better skin, and some have significant disadvantages that make them seldom the flap of choice despite their good qualities.

Ilium

The ilium has abundant bone but has a predetermined shape that makes graft shaping inherently less precise than in other donor site options. It may be ideal in some hemimandible reconstructions because its shape resembles most closely this portion of the mandible. The blood supply is by the deep circumflex iliac artery and its vena commitans which are smaller caliber vessels with a short stump which makes this flap unacceptable to some reconstructive surgeons. The skin island available with the ilium does not have a reliable circulation in many patients. In addition, the soft tissue component of the flap is often bulky and lacks mobility with respect to the bone. This makes insetting sometimes difficult and limits the usefulness of the soft tissue component of the flap. The muscle may be covered with a skin graft when used inside the oral cavity. Closure of the ilium donor site is arduous and there is a possibility of hernia formation or late attenuation of the lateral abdominal wall. Perhaps the best indication is a short lateral segment not requiring mucosal lining replacement or short anterior segments with a skin paddle if properly aligned. Osteointegration is possible as this has a good bone stock (Fig. 4).[20]

Radius

The radius has the best quality skin island compared to other donor site alternatives. The vascular pedicle is also ideal, with long, large-diameter vessels capable of reaching the opposite side of the neck for difficult recipient vessel problems. The bone, in contrast, is the worst compared to other choices. The radius must be carefully split during harvest in order to prevent postoperative fracture at the donor site. Length is generally limited. The bone thickness is marginal for later placement of osteointegrated implants for dental rehabilitation. The radius is contraindicated for most anterior defects because adequate soft tissue and bony volume are essential in this area for the best functional and esthetic reconstruction. The forearm

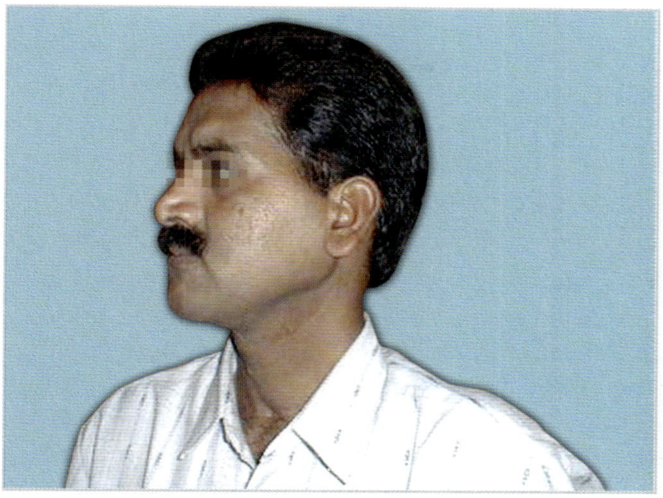

Fig. 4: Mandibular reconstruction using iliac crest deep circumflex iliac artery microvascular transfer

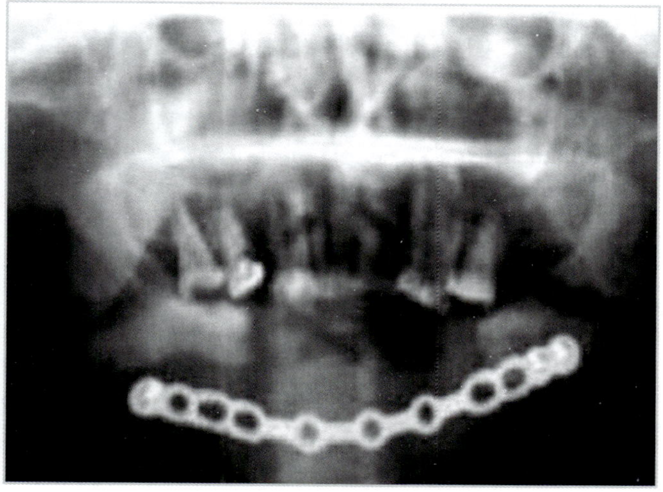

Fig. 5: Orthopantomogram of fibular reconstruction for mandibular defect

donor site is probably most useful as a soft-tissue free flap without bone for coverage of a metal plate when this method is chosen for reconstruction.[21]

Scapula

The scapula offers the greatest amount of soft tissue compared to other donor sites. Approximately 14 cm of bone is available from the lateral scapula. The bone does not have a segmental blood supply, and therefore multiple osteotomies can be hazardous to the viability.[22] The primary disadvantage of this flap is its donor site location, requiring delay in flap harvest until the resection is complete. Although rarely indicated, a combined scapula and latissimus dorsi flap is useful for large defects, includes that resulting from a radical neck dissection. The latissimus dorsi can restore neck contour and protect the exposed vessels and this entire complex of flaps can be raised on a single pedicle, the thoracodorsal artery.

Fibula

The donor site has many advantages, as the bone is available with enough length to reconstruct any mandible defect. There are no shape constraints that limit the graft contouring process, unlike the ilium. The periosteal blood supply is functionally of a segmental type, unlike the other donor sites. Osteotomies can be planned wherever necessary and can be placed as close as one centimeter apart without concern for bone viability. The vascular pedicle has sufficient length and is of large diameter. The skin island available with the fibula is reliable in approximately 91% of patients. A large skin paddle can be harvested for complex defects, but the donor site may require a skin graft closure.[23] Of all potential donor sites, the fibula is the most convenient because it is located farthest from the head and neck area. The fibula is indicated for all anterior defects and most lateral defects. It is the flap of choice for the majority of mandible defects except for a few special situations in which the ilium radius and scapula may constitute a better choice. It is particularly well suited to anterior defects because the skin paddle can be situated perfectly (Fig. 5).

Surgical Technique

All patients should have a tracheostomy for safety. Graft shaping can be done while ablation is in progress with the aid of the templates described previously. The surgical specimen is also a valuable visual aid. Measurements of total graft length can be obtained, as well as measurements to identify where osteotomies are best made in order to duplicate mandible shape. Bony fixation is best accomplished with the use of miniplate fixation. This is efficient, safe, and strong. Intermaxillary fixation is used only as an adjunctive form of fixation. Its primary role is to maintain occlusion during the insetting of lateral grafts. The angle of the mandible is generally planned where the vascular pedicle follows the bone in the case of the fibula, ilium, and scapula, which will ultimately provide maximum pedicle length to reach the recipient vessels in the neck. The condyle can often be harvested from the surgical specimen and then mounted directly onto the shaft as this is not often involved. The recipient site is prepared prior to dividing the flap pedicle. Recipient vessels are identified, and the intraoral wound closed as much as possible. Intermaxillary fixation is placed in the case of lateral grafts and the inner lining portion of the mandible placed in fixation in order to maintain occlusion during graft insetting. Anterior grafts are more difficult to inset correctly. Often the only visual guides are the maxillary arch and the midline. The lateral segments usually cannot be stabilized owing a lack of dentition. It is easy to make errors that can result in prognathism, retrognathia (Andy Gump effect), increased or decreased lower facial height, asymmetry after the bone is inset; the microvascular anastomoses are performed. The facial artery is usually selected as a recipient although the external carotid (end-to-side) and the superior thyroid artery are also good choices. The lingual artery is not preferred, particularly if partial glossectomy has been performed. The internal jugular vein is used as an end-to-side anastomosis. Watertight closure of the intraoral wound is absolutely mandatory. A leak will often lead to contamination of the miniplates. This often develops into an orocutaneous fistula and results in considerable morbidity. The wound is closed over suction drains.

Early patient mobilization is encouraged. Free flap monitoring is not precise in most cases of free flap mandible reconstruction because the bone is buried and the skin island (if present) usually lies within the oral cavity. A conventional Doppler often can be used to monitor the vascular pedicle of the flap. A clear arterial signal usually can be obtained over the mandible away from the neck vessels. Frequently, a venous hum also can be heard. Skin island bleeding response to pinprick is a useful confirmatory test to perform when there is some doubt as to flap viability. Follow-up studies of the mandible are limited to periodic orthopantomograms and radionuclide scans are not always necessary but can be used for documentation.

Complications

Pulmonary and cardiac problems are the most common source of general medical complications. Free-flap failure is the single most important complication pertaining to the head and neck area.[24] Fortunately, most failing flaps can be salvaged, and the actual incidence of total flap loss ranges from 37% to 5%. Reconstruction plate exposure and intraoral wound dehiscence (which may lead to orocutaneous fistula formation) constitute other serious problems. Donor site complications are uncommon and rarely require additional surgery. They include abdominal wall attenuation (ilium donor site), seroma (scapula), exposed tendons or fracture (radius), and delayed skin graft healing (fibula). Cellulitis can occur at site or in the head and neck area. Despite the complexity of mandible reconstruction cases, the incidence and severity of postoperative complications is low. Postoperative radiotherapy has no impact on these flaps as they are abundantly vascularized but the use of miniplates may cause some diffraction and dose delivery problems.

Postoperative Dental Rehabilitation

Mandible reconstruction is ideally, functionally not complete with osteointegration. Osteointegration implant reconstruction is the method of choice for dental restoration when conventional dentures are not feasible. These implants are placed into the bone cradle and serve as a permanent foundation upon which a dental prosthesis is aligned with screws.[25] These implants are usually no sooner than 6 months and more appropriately 1 year after mandible reconstruction. Three to four implants are usually sufficient for a long dental defect. Implant placement is usually an office procedure. Preparation of the site of implantation usually requires a preliminary procedure to remove bone graft miniplates, which may interfere with implant placement. Sometimes, the skin island overlying the bone must be thinned at the same time and the implants must be correctly aligned during placement. They are uncovered after osteointegration has taken place, usually about 4 months later. The dental bridge hooked on to a tooth can also suffice.

Summary

Mandible reconstruction is most commonly performed for tumors, of which epidermoid carcinoma and osteogenic sarcomas are the most common types. Lateral and mid-third defects constitute two distinct types of reconstructive problems. Reconstruction is most commonly performed either with reconstruction plates and regional flaps or with microvascular free flaps. Free flaps usually provide the best functional and esthetic results in anterior defects while in lateral segmental defects a pedicled flap or even prosthetic silastic mandibles can provide similar results.

CHEST WALL RECONSTRUCTION

Penetrating chest injuries resulting from wars and accidents necessitated the earliest surgical experiences with the chest wall. Around the turn of the century, with the introduction of general anesthesia, more aggressive surgery became possible. Surgeons began to resect tumors of the chest wall. Initially, when such surgery was attempted, every effort was made to avoid entering the pleura to avoid the potentially fatal situation of an open pneumothorax. In fact, many ingenious methods were devised to avoid collapse of the lungs at the time of resection by preliminary procedures to create adhesions between the lung and rib cage.

Flap Requirements

The semirigid skeletal frame of the chest renders the surrounding soft tissues less mobile for use in closure, as compared with the abdomen.[26] A large soft-tissue defect, therefore, requires addition of tissue from a distance. The rigidity makes the chances less likely of a chronic chest activity closing spontaneously by gradual contraction; therefore, any residual dead space must be filled with a leak-free technique to avoid the development of a pneumothorax. A secure closure of the surface and the dead space, which can withstand the repetitive and forceful respiratory movement of the ribs, must also be tension-free. Finally, the flap should be well vascularized to offer the best chance for uncomplicated primary wound healing. In chest-wall reconstruction any minor wound healing problems are likely to evolve into a major complication associated with significant morbidity and possible mortality.

Skeletal Reconstruction

There is usually some loss of disruption of the sternum-rib complex is seen following tumor resection. Optimal skeletal restoration should always being the goal. Failure to stabilize the semirigid skeletal framework results in paradoxical movement with ventilatory compromise. The importance of minimizing further loss of vital capacity cannot be overemphasized. Unless compromised by other associated factors, most patients can tolerate the loss of segments of up to four ribs without skeletal replacement.[27] When a thick flap, such as a latissimus dorsi musculocutaneous flap, covers the defect the amount of flailing is also reduced compared with that of a thin skin flap. In most massive chest-wall resection, some form of skeletal stabilization should be considered. This goal may be accomplished with autogenous bone grafts, rigid synthetic materials, such as acrylic, or a semirigid replacement (fascia or synthetic mesh). When the sternum is removed, however, the instability results in a more serious paradoxical movement of the entire chest necessitating proper stabilization.

Muscle and Musculocutaneous Flaps

Tansini described the use of latissimus dorsi muscle for chest-wall reconstruction. Olivari and others improved the understanding of the latissmus dorsi flap and popularized its uses for breast and chest-wall reconstructions as compared with random-pattern skin flaps. The pectoralis major and the rectus abdominis muscle flaps came a bit later to provide three reliable techniques for chest-wall reconstruction. The serratus anterior muscle is also useful but is limited in size. The trapezius muscle is of satisfactory size, but it reaches only the upper chest and its functional loss is not always well tolerated. The latissmus dorsi, pectoralis major, and rectus abdominus muscles are excellent donor muscles for chest-wall reconstruction because of their large mass, length, and consistent vascular pedicle and functional expendability. A complete understanding of the muscle anatomy, arc of rotation, and reconstructive capability is essential.

Latissimus Dorsi Muscle

This is a type V flap with a dual supply at the origin and insertion. The functional loss at the donor site is minimal, except, perhaps, in mountain climbers, gymnasts, or paraplegics when forceful upward pull of the body weight by the arms is important. Several anatomic features deserve special consideration. The anteriorly located vascular pedicle makes it highly efficient for transfer to the anterior chest wall. On the back, the latissimus dorsi flap can reach most of the upper back, shoulder, and neck. If skin is carried with the muscle, it becomes particularly important to plan its location properly on the muscle. Although the major skin perforators follow the course of the two main branches of the thoracodorsal artery along the anterior and the superior border, any skin island over the muscle should be more than adequately supplied. When needed, the skin island may extend beyond the muscle as a fasciocutaneous component. Primary skin closure may be accomplished for up to 7–10 cm and is easier when the skin island is oriented transversely. The subscapular artery supplies three reliable microvascular free flap donor sites: the latissimus dorsi muscle, the serratus anterior muscle, and the skin of the parascapular region. When needed, two or three of the components can be taken together on the same pedicle to cover a large defect.[28]

Flap Elevation

When a skin island is taken with the flap, the incision is made completely and the skin flaps are elevated in both directions to reveal, the superior and the anterior borders of the muscle. The broad expansion of the muscle's origin from the posterior ribs is detached by sharp and blunt dissection. The body of the muscle is lifted away from the chest, leaving it attached by its humeral insertion and the vascular pedicle. The pedicle runs through the axillary fat to become adherent to the undersurface of the muscle at approximately 10 cm from the humerus. The posterosuperior border of the muscle needs to be separated from the skin to allow comfortable anterior transposition of the muscle through a subcutaneous tunnel or a direct skin incision.

Pectoralis Major Muscle

Sisson, and Johnson described a flap from the medial aspect of the pectoralis major muscle, based on the medial perforators from the internal mammary vessels; it was used to close a midline sternal defect. The secondary supply to this muscle is by a row of perforators from the internal mammary vessels along its sternal origin. With the humeral insertion and the medial ribs origins detached, the muscle can be easily moved medially and superiorly to fill defects in the superior mediastinum, laterally to resurface the shoulder and through a window in the anterior ribs to fill the upper chest cavity. When the lateral humeral insertion is detached, the muscle can be turned on itself, based on the medial perforators, and used to fill mediastinal defects. The pectoralis major flap is generally as highly reliable and technically easy to raise. In the head and neck region, a 10–20 percent flap loss of some degree has been noted.[29]

Microvascular Free Flaps

Although the availability of musculocutaneous flaps and muscles has greatly expanded our ability to reconstruct many previously difficult defects, free flaps remain useful in certain special situations as the defect may be sufficiently large, so that it cannot be reconstructed with the available regional flaps. In most cases, a significant part of a muscle flap may be wasted in the transfer to the defect, so that the useful part of the flap is limited. Microvascular free flaps, on the other hand, can be harvested from any part of the body with relatively little wastage of their pedicles. During the past decade, with improving results and a survival rate of 95 percent, the indications for free flaps have broadened. As in other parts of the body, the technique is no longer indicated only when no other choices area available. Free flaps are chosen over regional flaps because of convenience, less functional loss, versatility of reconstruction, and better esthetic results.[30] An ideal free flap recipient vessel should be of reasonable caliber (1.5 mm to 2.5 mm), outside of the zone of injury, easily accessible, anatomically consistent, potentially dispensable, and conveniently located near the defect. Because of the large area of the chest and the paucity of the large trunk vessels in the anterior chest, the selection of proper recipient vessels must come from the axilla, neck, or mediastinum. At times, long vein grafts area also required. The subscapular and thoracodorsal system may be utilized at any convenient point.

Donor Sites

The most common requisite in chest wall reconstruction is usually for large surface coverage. Bone or fascia as a part of a microvascular free flap may be an additional feature when structural support is needed. The contralateral latissimus dorsi, lower rectus abdominis or tensor fascia musculocutaneous free flaps are the most commonly considered donor flaps has the advantage of being located at a distance away from the chest, therefore, allowing for simultaneous dissection while the chest is excised. The flap also does not further compromise the postoperative respiratory care, as may be the case with abdominal or back flaps. When a very large flap is needed, one can also incorporate the rectus femoris or the vastus lateralis muscles in the flap.

Technical Considerations

Aside from basic principles applicable to all microvascular free flap surgery and chest wall reconstructions, certain problems merit special attention. The exposure for microvascular anastomoses around the chest is generally much more awkward than in the extremities. Often the surgeon or the assistant may have difficulty sitting comfortably, and the anastomoses may even need to be done with the surgeon in the standing position. During the critical period of the anastomoses, it may be necessary to reduce the tidal volume and to use more frequent but smaller chest excursions. The need for rigid support may be more important for free flaps than regions flaps.

Grafts and Synthetic Materials for Structural Support

Indications for Skeletal Support

Not all skeletal components of chest-wall defects need to be specifically replaced. The semirigid frame of ribs, sternum, cartilage joints, and muscles cannot be fully submitted by either rigid materials or by fascia. Small defects in healthy patients with satisfactory functional reserves are extremely well tolerated. Patients with compromised pulmonary functional reserve from emphysema or other causes are more vulnerable to any loss of skeletal support. This is usually manifested by diminished exercise capacity. The functional loss is proportional to the size of the defect. Surgical loss of the sternum may be poorly tolerated and skeletal reconstruction should be considered.[31]

Methods of Skeletal Stabilization

A wide variety of methods have been used for chest wall stabilization. Autogenous sources include pedicled ribs, free rib grafts, iliac bone, irradiated tissue bank fascia/dura or fascia lata.[32] Synthetic materials include Marlex, Goretex patch or bone cement.

Silicone Implant Reconstruction

Experience with silicone implants for breast augmentation stimulated the choice of this material for correction of purely cosmetic deformities in adults. Although standard breast implants may be helpful to fill out well-localized depressions, they are rarely used today because of variations in deformity and the unpredictable development of implant contractures. As with the use of all prosthetic materials, possible complications of bleeding, infection, and extrusion of the implant must be anticipated.[33] It is generally preferable to slightly under correct in order to avoid protrusion of the implant. Such implants should also be made of moderately firm silastic material behind the previously expanded thin skin.

The Irradiated Chest Wall

There are certain fundamental principles for surgery involving irradiated tissues such as excision as much of the irradiated tissue as possible to minimize the presence of compromised tissue vulnerable to chronic infection and reconstruction with healthy, well-vascularized tissue to maximize the chances of primary wound healing, avoiding foreign material, poorly vascularized tissue, or closure under tension. In practice, this means wide excision of the necrotic center along with adjacent irradiated margins and reconstruction with a large regional musculocutaneous flap or microvascular free flap.[34]

Summary

The flaps available for reconstruction of chest defects have improved significantly. Laterally or medial based abdominal flaps provided the first the more reliable flaps followed by the omentum became popular because of its availability and familiarity to the general surgeon. The latissimus dorsi, pectoralis major, and rectus abdominis muscle and musculocutaneous flap are currently most commonly used and available. Finally, microvascular free flaps can provide, consistently the largest coverage and have the additional advantage of not borrowing from the adjacent area. Skeletal stability is required with either mesh, fascia lata or Goretex® (Figs 6A and B) meshes which will provide for a smooth inner lining and bridge the gap. The newer and larger flaps have reduced the complication rate of reconstruction probably because of the more adequate resection of the margin along with the more vigorous blood supply supplied by the flaps.

ABDOMINAL WALL RECONSTRUCTION

Defects of the abdominal wall result from tumor resection, radiotherapy, postoperative incisional hernia, and con-

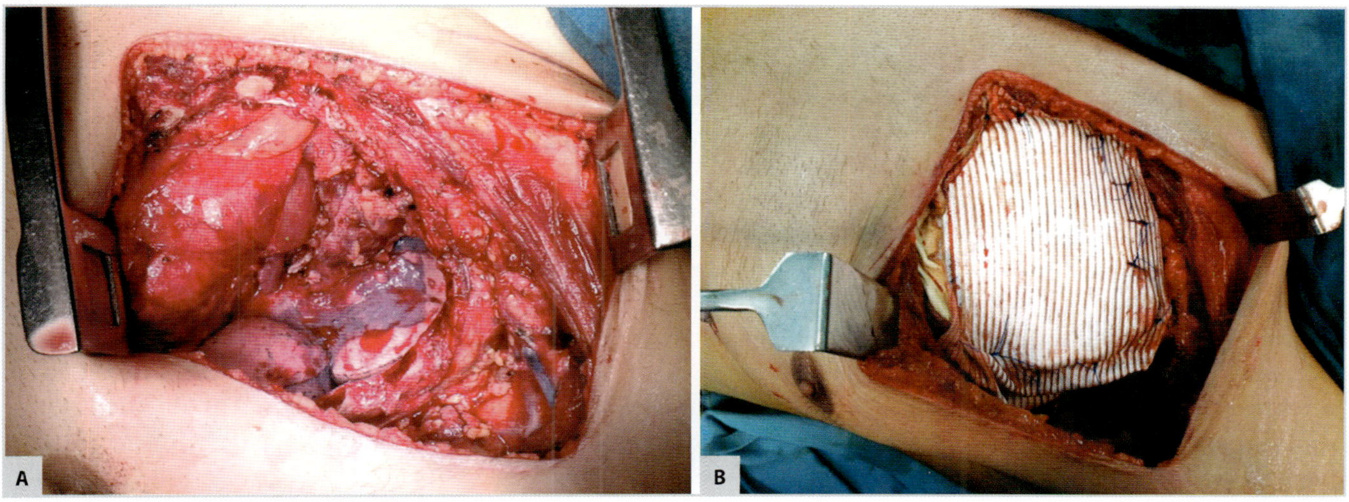

Figs 6A and B: Chest wall postexcision reconstruction with a Goretex mesh repair genital anomalies. The usual priorities in abdominal wall reconstruction are wound coverage or closure, protection of the visceral organs, fascial support, muscle function, and esthetics. Immediate closure or reconstruction of abdominal wall defects is always preferred to minimize the problems of massive fluid and protein loss, the likelihood of intraperitoneal infection, and the chances of undesirable scarring. Occasionally, primary closure may not be feasible because of uncertain tumor margins, established residual local infection, and excessive bulk of the bowels from edema or meconium, lack of available regional flaps, or the physiologic status of the patient. In such situations, the exposed bowels may be treated with sterile wet dressings for a few days until the conditions have improved sufficiently for closure. If closure is not possible, one can wait a few more days for granulation tissue to develop over the surface of the bowels and the communication of the peritoneal cavity to become sealed. This delay ensures the absence of deep-seated infection and reduces the urgency of the reconstructive procedures. If a flap is not available or suitable at this time, skin grafts may be sufficient to achieve the most important goal of wound closure, leaving the task of definitive reconstruction to a later and more opportune time.

Skin Grafts

Although the application of skin grafts is a relatively simple method for the closure of abdominal wall defects, the associated problems are that the skin grafts are adherent to the surface of the gastrointestinal tract, the potential for massive adhesion formation is present. Subsequent surgery under such conditions is obviously risky. In cases of massive fasciitis or enormous abdominal wounds, closure with normal tissue cannot be achieved. Skin grafts provide the only means of coverage.

Flaps

Defects requiring full-thickness reconstructions were traditionally managed by multiple local flap delays, waltzing tube flaps, or even jumps flaps carried via the wrist. Instead of thinking of the abdomen as a large randomly supplied skin area, surgeons should be aware of the multiple specific sources of blood supply to the abdomen. This concept has provided abundant options in terms of the regional skin flaps, muscles with skin graft, or musculocutaneous flaps. Many of the flaps previously described for chest reconstruction are also suitable for upper abdomen reconstruction and are therefore not repeated. The omentum with a skin graft over it is also readily available in most of these cases to cover large surface areas.

Skin Flaps

Full-thickness skin flaps may be elevated based medially on perforators from the rectus abdominis, laterally from the intercostal perforators, superiorly from the superficial superior epigastric vessels, or inferolaterally from the inferior epigastric vessels. Either rotation or transposition flaps may be used. The flap dissection should include the entire subcutaneous layer above the deep fascia, consistent with the concepts of fasciocutaneous flaps. Laterally, it may be convenient to include the thin fascia over the external oblique esthetic result. A large area of the lower and lateral abdominal wall is suitable for design of the groin flap that can be extended and rotated upwards.

De-epithelized Skin Flaps

De-epithelized skin flaps were described by Poulard to correct scar craters in as manner similar to the technique of reduction mammoplasty. The obvious primary advantage of flaps over free transplants is that they carry their own blood supply, making survival more certain. Studies of the fate of skin placed in a subcutaneous position in this manner showed that epithelium, hair follicles, and sebaceous glands disappear but sweat glands are preserved.

Musculofascial Flaps

The earliest and most hard closure of large musculofascial defects of the abdominal wall by using the iliotibial tract of fascia lata as a flap.[35] The fascia, suspended by the tensor fasciae femoris muscle with its nerve and blood supply intact, can provide closure of the abdominal-wall defects below the umbilicus.

Rectus Abdominis Muscle and Myocutaneous Flap

The anatomy and variations of the long and paired muscles have been previously described in detail in the chest-wall reconstruction section. Based either superiorly or inferiorly, they have the widest arc of rotation of any regional muscle for abdominal reconstruction. Bostwick et al. used an inferiorly based rectus abdominis muscle to reconstruct the pelvic floor in a case of abdominoperineal resection.

Extra-abdominal Muscles and Musculocutaneous Flaps

The latissimus dorsi flap in certain circumstances can be rotated or used as a free tissue transfer.[36] Muscle from the proximal thigh provides a ready source of large mass and wide skin territories for lower abdominal reconstruction. The morbidity is lower because the technique does not interfere with postoperative respiratory care. Such muscle can also potentially be dynamic substitutes for the lost abdominal muscle function in posture, can prevent hernia, and can assist in the expulsive efforts of bowel function. The most common muscles used are the rectus femoris, the tensor fasciae latae, and the vastus lateralis. The gracilis muscle medially is useful mainly for perineum reconstruction, but its muscle mass and width are limited. For large abdominal wall cover even an anterolateral thigh flap used with microvascular transfer can be used.[37]

Summary

Abdominal-wall reconstruction following extirpative oncologic surgery requires muscle and skin cover and unlike chest wall no rigid supports. The size of the defects however severely limits the use of the most regional flaps and may require microvascular intervention.

BREAST RECONSTRUCTION

In 20th century, when radical mastectomy was developed for local treatment of breast cancer by W S Halsted, plastic repair of the defect was never advised. Later, breast sharing (Rhienhard, 1932) and local and distant sharing flaps (Gilles and Millard, 1957) was developed which required multiple stages with a far from pleasing result. During last 25–30 years, breast reconstruction has evolved significantly. The esthetic quality of these reconstructions has emerged from that of amorphous blobs appearing as breast mound to nearly normal appearing breast. Symmetry, which was hardly possible and seldom achieved, is now standard. Modern reconstruction is fostered by developments like shifting trend towards modified radical mastectomy (MRM) from radical mastectomy, improvement in prosthesis and tissue expanders and description of various musculocutaneous flaps.

Why Reconstruction

Psychologically, post-mastectomy, there is alteration of mood, body image, sexuality, feminity, social and occupational adjustments. There is also a sense of mutilation and a fear of recurrence, spread and postoperative therapy.[38,39] The reaction to diagnosis of cancer quotient (RDCQ) is significantly different (p = 0.037) in patients post-mastectomy immediate breast reconstruction (MIBR) versus only MRM (Gross, et al. from MSKCC). The mastectomy awareness score (MAS) is also different (p = 0.001) in MIBR versus external prostheses as reported by reading and there was significantly betterment of physical activities (p = 0.01), anger, depression, sexual desire (p = 0.001) as reported by Franchelli.

Breast reconstruction therefore plays major role in rehabilitation after mastectomy.

Types of Surgery

The various types of reconstructive procedures available in breast cancer patients are:

Oncoplastic surgery: This combines latest plastic surgical techniques with breast surgical techniques. It is well known that local tumor control is better if more glandular tissue around tumor is excised. But breast conservation therapy (BCT) is worthwhile only if conserved breast is without major deficiencies. Hence, in volume reduction surgery in patients with large breasts and tumors that require reconfiguration after tumor specific resection, BCT is combined with standard or modified mastopexy techniques. In volume replacement surgery, small breasts that may be deformed after lumpectomy or segmentectomy, may be reconstructed with rotation, bilobed or customized regional flaps may be utilized.

Reconstructive Surgery after Failed Breast Conservative Surgery

In spite of fact that as many as 90% patients have good esthetic results after partial mastectomy and radiotherapy; several patients still require reconstructive procedures after a failed BCT. Deficient volume of breast parenchyma, constricted and fibrotic overlying skin and resultant distorted of the nipple areola complex are main areas requiring reconstructive procedures. Irradiated tissue being susceptible to infection due to impaired vascularity, use of local flaps and implants are contraindicated for replacement of skin and parenchymal loss and also for correction of nipple-areola complex. In such patients, probably use of the latissimus dorsi flap is ideal. The use of transverse rectus abdominis myocutaneous (TRAM) flap is usually kept reserved for severe deformities.

Breast Reconstruction Following Mastectomy

This is the most important and biggest group. Two options here are MIBR[40] or mastectomy with delayed reconstruction. Both must be understood by the oncologist and the reconstructive surgeon. In both these methods are options of either autologous reconstruction or of use of implants or a third choice of flap with an implant.

Patient Selection

Selection of the patient for breast reconstruction is very important and the basic criteria that need evaluation are previous psychiatric treatment and patients' and surgeons' concept of a successful result. Current techniques make successful breast reconstruction possible in virtually all women regardless of extent of surgery or RT. Cooperation with oncologic surgeon is essential in planning and offering this modality to almost all patients. A suitable candidate should have a realistic understanding of the possibilities and limitations of any procedure. All the women who are about to undergo or have already undergone mastectomy are potential candidates to be informed of breast reconstruction, however, not every woman elects, and therefore must not be pushed or to pursue it. There is perhaps no other area of reconstructive surgery where patient individualization is more important.[41]

The reconstructive surgeon must listen carefully to each patient's expressed needs and desires and juxtapose them with her emotional status, clinical staging and technical reconstructive possibilities. Lengthy initial consultation with surgeon to assess their goals and to explain the alternatives with the reasonable expectations and possible complications of each is required. Photographs and diagrams are especially helpful as are educational brochures.

Selection of Techniques

Many techniques for breast reconstruction have been described and that factors that help decide which method can be best used in an individual patient include the patient's overall health and body habitus, the mastectomy site, the contralateral breast, and the patient's preference with the option of primary reconstruction to delayed one.

Mastectomy Site

The type of mastectomy performed has major role in selection of the procedure. A radical mastectomy may have left an infraclavicular depression, loss of anterior axillary fold with inadequate soft tissue cover, whereas a MRM may have left ample soft tissue, and a conservative quadrantectomy would have only skewed breast. Evaluation of amount of pectoralis muscle present, the amount of skin present, quality of these tissues, and the quality of the mastectomy scar is must. Based on this evaluation, one can decide if an implant alone is satisfactory, if the skin and muscle present can be adequately expanded, or if flap is required.

Patient's Health and Body Habitus

Healthy patients may be candidates for any type of reconstruction, whereas elderly patients or those with compromised health are probably best suited for the simpler procedures, submuscular implants or tissue expansion. Healthy patients with a flabby abdomen may be suitable for TRAM flap. Previous subcostal incisions dividing rectus muscle, paramedian incisions injuring perforators and midline and lower quadrant incisions that may alter TRAM flap viability should be considered. Heavy smoking and diabetes are also considered as contraindications to TRAM by many surgeons. Innervation of latissimus dorsi muscle must be clinically evaluated if latissimus flap is in consideration. The texture and color of the back skin should also be observed. Tendency to develop keloids or hypertrophic scars may render the new scars, from rectus or latissimus procedures, nondesirable.

Contralateral Breast

Symmetry being the goal of the reconstruction, the size and shape of the contralateral breast must be evaluated and the appropriate reconstruction procedure should be planned accordingly. Alteration of contralateral breast in form of reduction, augmentation or mastopexy can be considered for better match. It must be always kept in mind that the opposite breast is at increased risk to develop cancer.[42] If a contralateral prophylactic procedure (total mastectomy or subcutaneous mastectomy) is planned, it may alter the reconstruction technique.

Timing and Indications

Improved operative techniques, flap designs, and prosthetic biomaterials have made breast reconstructive surgery a natural adjunct and a positive step for the patients recuperating from breast cancer. Historically, there have been many objections and concerns regarding the timing of the reconstructions in the management of issues like potential delay in detection of recurrence. However, a recent review of literature showed no evidence that any form of reconstruction caused any appreciable delay in recurrent disease detection. In fact, there is additional significant reduction in psychological trauma. A common belief was that if a patient underwent mastectomy, then there is better acceptance in these patients after a period of several months and many do not opt for a second surgery. Mustoe has shown conclusively that there is significantly larger acceptance if this procedure is added as the desire for reconstruction cuts across all socioeconomic, educational, rural/urban barriers once the procedure has been clearly explained to the patients. There have been several studies showing that MIBR does not compromise the tumor ablative procedures, alter survival or delay diagnosis or treatment of recurrences.[43,44] The postoperative complication rate is low and not significantly different than patients undergoing mastectomy alone. Immediate breast reconstruction may reduce the number of operations with potential cost savings and a combined recovery period. The difference between complication rates for MIBR versus delayed reconstructions is not significant even in our series (approximately 5-9%).

Breast Implants

Since the advent of tissue expansion, implants have been the most common type of breast reconstruction all over the globe. Types of alternative procedures are: (1) a permanent implant; or (2) a permanent expandable implant or (3) a serial expander with a permanent implant exchange. Relative ease of the procedure and quick postoperative recovery are the advantages. One of the most common complications of alloplastic materials is rejection phenomenon and formation of capsule. Mostly, this capsule is insignificant but in 10% of the patients, the capsule hardens and becomes symptomatic requiring intervention. Placement of implant in the submuscular compartments either subpectoral or under latissimus dorsi flap reduces the incidence of capsular contracture.[45] Smooth-walled and textured both implants are available, of which textured ones are less prone to capsular contracture.

Implants used may be:

Silicone Implants

Silicone implants had been popular since 1970. These implants are used widely, because of their consistency which closely resembled that of natural breast and their relatively natural shape. Because of their alleged association with connective tissue disorders and a possible increased risk of malignancy, they became controversial. However, now at least two new prospective studies have shown no such relationship.

Saline Implants

Saline implants have been a very good option for breast augmentation and after the learning curve has been overcome, are also good option for MIBR. The problem with saline implants have a tendency to cause fullness and waviness in the upper half, less natural contour in the erect position and a harder feel to touch. Newer implants have corrected most of these difficulties.

Autogenous Reconstructions

With the rise in controversies in the use of implants, there has been a concomitant rise in the request for autogenous reconstructions. Additional advantages are replacing the skin envelope, which has been removed during mastectomy, and filling the glandular tissue with tissue of similar feel; which results in better contour and symmetry. Unfortunately, there can be patch like appearance on the breast. This problem can be minimized with skin sparing mastectomy. Apart from patient preference, there are specific indications for breast reconstruction namely patients who have undergone chest wall irradiation or those requiring coverage for areas of radiation necrosis. Patients, who had capsular contracture, periprosthetic infections or autoimmune disorders and wish for reconstruction, would benefit from autogenous reconstruction.

Since the description of the latissimus dorsi flaps in 1977, a growing number of flaps have been in use.[46]

Latissimus Dorsi Myocutaneous Flap

Schnieder and Olbrisch first used the LD flap using the thoracodorsal pedicle in 1977 for breast reconstruction. This flap has been used in various modifications ranging from using only the flap with all its soft tissue or along with an implant. The use of this flap is now nearly exclusive with a submuscular implant as the flap has usually insufficient bulk to form the breast mound. Modification using a three-cornered skin paddle, the Fleur-de-lis design can also be used with more favorable scar. In immediate reconstruction with this flap, the advantages are same as those of TRAM flap. The skin island can replace the skin that was excised during mastectomy and it allows an opportunity to operate on a nonscarred bed. The muscle can be sutured with lateral border of pectoralis muscle to provide complete coverage for the implant. This can be combined with skin sparing mastectomy and de-epithelized LD flap used for contour around the implant. Shape in this procedure is more normal and problems of waviness have been decreased with better projection. Raising of the flap however requires a change in position and draping. The scar can be modified to make its lie transverse, along the line of brassiere and the entire muscle is raised and transferred anteriorly. There is comparatively

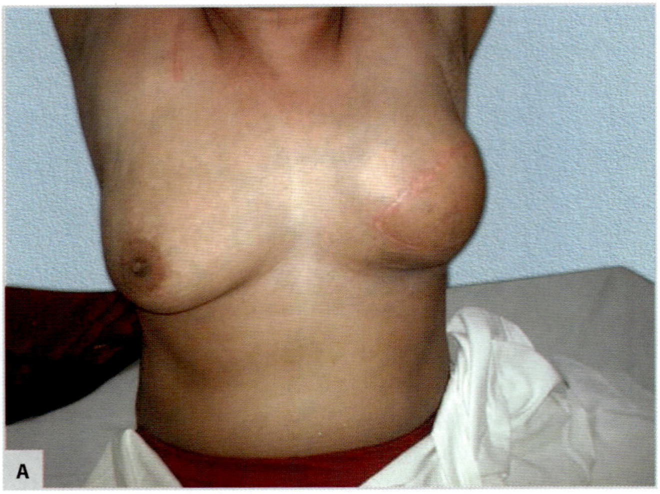

Fig. 7: Primary breast reconstruction using latissimus dorsi flap and implant

less blood loss and lesser complication rates. The donor site functional deficit is minimal to abundance of muscle in the area but a persistent complaint is that the patient has to change to a front hooking brassiere as the movement of hooking behind is hampered. When using for delayed reconstruction, results of LD flap can be improved with use of tissue expanders; especially suitable for patients with irradiated defects. In a large series from Tata Memorial Hospital, 73 cases were reconstructed using only LD flap and 50% of these had more than 50–60% reduction in final size of the breast mound over the period of one year. The second set of 23 patients had submuscular implants, which resulted in excellent results. Patients in this series also received chemotherapy postoperatively (n = 47) and none had any delay in their adjuvant treatment schedules (Fig. 7).

Transverse Rectus Abdominis Myocutaneous Flap

The TRAM flap as it is popularly known was introduced by Hartrampf.[47] The aim of the surgery is to transfer skin and subcutaneous fat from middle or lower abdomen to thoracic region and form a symmetrical breast. TRAM flap can be performed as immediate reconstruction with appropriate coordination with the oncosurgeon so that the reconstructive surgeon can elevate the abdominal flap during mastectomy in a two-team approach in an effort to reduce the operating time and blood loss.[48]

Anatomically, TRAM flap is based on the rectus muscle with transversely situated skin paddle. The predominant blood supply to the abdominal wall skin is periumbilical perforators. The deep superior and inferior epigastric vessels are the supplying arteries. The superior epigastric artery has a predictable watershed distribution extending below the umbilicus. Therefore, a pedicled flap based on superior vessels must be based around the umbilicus either 1/4th above and rest below or an equal distribution. The only problem with a single pedicled flap is that no more than 60–70% of the abdominal tissue can be safely transferred to breast. The flap is divided in four zones based on the side of rectus. Zone 1 and 2 are on the same side and are extremely safe. Zone 3 and 4 are on the opposite side and are relatively random. We hence use only the first and second zones and third and fourth zones are used only as lipid filler to give shape and contour to the breast. The inferior epigastric pedicle can be anastomosed to increase circulation of an otherwise compromised flap, in effect of supercharging the flap. Resultant abdominal wall defect is repaired by using mesh and umbilicus is then resited to lie on the upper part of abdominal incision. A Tummy Tuck procedure is an added bonus in these patients. All flaps in our series were single pedicled flaps.

Bipedicled TRAM flaps are used to improve the blood supply more than 70% but in that case, it causes more abdominal muscle weakness and a free flap would then be more appropriate. A Fleur-de-Lis pattern incorporating a vertical rectus and TRAM flap can be used for patients with large size breasts or those requiring a large amount of skin cover.

Microsurgical Breast Reconstruction

Since its inception, TRAM flap has been plagued by two specific complications: partial flap loss due to marginal blood supply and abdominal wall weakness caused by abdominal wall sacrifice. These two problems with conventional TRAM flap are related in that the amount of blood supply is determined by number of musculocutaneous perforators included in the flap; thus an increase in flap blood supply is obtained at the expanse of more abdominal wall sacrifice. The problem with the conventional TRAM flap is design, in which the lower abdominal skin island is carried on the superior epigastric system, which is nondominant blood supply to that skin territory. The free TRAM, however, utilizes the inferior epigastric system, which is dominant blood supply. Thus, use of free TRAM flap allows for maximally perfused flap with a minimum of abdominal wall sacrifice.[49] Here, issue is risk of thrombosis of the microanastomoses and subsequent total loss of flap, something that is not a problem of conventional TRAM. For the free TRAM to be acceptable, the flap failure rates have to be lower than those for the other free flaps available for breast reconstruction including two flaps based on gluteus maximus muscle: one utilizing the superior gluteal vessels and one using inferior gluteal vessels, and the transverse lateral thigh or "saddlebag" flap based on tensor fasciae latae muscle. Use of all three of these flaps is limited due to excessive donor site deformity. Another flap consisting of the flank ("love handle") area supplied by the deep circumflex iliac vessels has recently been described. The donor site deformity is minimal and harvest can actually improve the contour in some patients, as in case of the TRAM flap. Best second choice for autogenous tissue breast reconstruction after free TRAM flap is christened the Rubens' flap, after the painting style of the artist of the same name. An added benefit of this flap is its availability even after abdominoplasty or previous TRAM transfer. Despite the success of the above flaps, the free TRAM flap is by far the most common free flap used for breast reconstruction.

The only absolute indication for the free TRAM flap is previous upper abdominal surgery that has divided the superior muscle pedicle, so that the conventional TRAM using pedicle is not possible and similarly previous lower abdominal surgery like inguinal hernia or paramedian incision that has interrupted inferior epigastric blood supply. Most abdominal scars, either upper or lower, do not preclude use of the free TRAM flap but may dictate how much flap is available for use. A Pfannensteil's incision is not a contraindication for use of free TRAM flap. Tobacco smoking and obesity are relative contraindications to both of these operations, increasing the chances for partial flap loss and hernia formation. Another important relative indication for use of free TRAM is immediate breast reconstruction. The transfer of the flap is facilitated by axillary dissection, which exposes the thoracodorsal vessels, making them readily available for use as recipient vessels. The improved blood supply of the flap helps to lower the complication rate, which is especially important reconstruction due to frequent need for postoperative adjuvant chemotherapy.

Nipple-Areola Reconstruction

Nipple-areola reconstruction is usually performed as a second operative procedure, although it can be deferred to a third procedure. Either local or general anesthesia can be used and it can be done on an in- or outpatient basis. Several techniques have been described for creation of nipple and areola. The method selected depends on the size and color of the opposite nipple and areola, the type of breast mount on which it is placed and the patient's and surgeon's preference.[50]

Nipple Creation

When the contralateral nipple is of adequate size and the patient is accepting, a composite graft can be taken from opposite nipple. Alternatively, a bat-shaped flap can be raised on the operated site and a nipple mound created, this can then be tattooed as per requirements.

Summary

Breast reconstruction has come a long way from external breast prosthesis to oncoplastic surgery, reconstructions following BCT and reconstructions following MRM with autologous and implant based reconstructions. Most Indian patients are however not demanding the final nipple creation stage and wish only a creation of a mound which looks adequate in normal Indian attire.

REFERENCES

1. El-Marakby HH. The reliability of pectoralis major myocutaneous flap in head and neck reconstruction. J Egypt Natl Canc Inst. 2006;18(1):41-50.
2. McLean JN, Carlson GW, Losken A. The pectoralis major myocutaneous flap revisited: a reliable technique for head and neck reconstruction. Ann Plast Surg. 2010;64(5):570-3.
3. Ozbek MR, Kutlu N. Vertical trapezius myocutaneous flap for covering wide scalp defects. Handchir Mikrochir Plast Chir. 1990;22(6):326-9.
4. Gullane PJ, Lipa JE, Novak CB, et al. Reconstruction of skull base defects. Clin Plast Surg. 2005;32(3):391-9.
5. Valentini V, Fabiani F, Nicolai G, et al. Use of microvascular free flaps in the reconstruction of the anterior and middle skull base. J Craniofac Surg. 2006;17(4):790-6.
6. Agarwal M, Gupta DK, Tiwari AD. Extended nasolabial flaps in the management of oral submucous fibrosis. J Maxillofac Oral Surg. 2011;10:216-9.
7. Cunha-Gomes D, Kavarana NM, Choudhari C, et al. Total oral reconstruction for cancers associated with advanced oral submucous fibrosis. Ann Plast Surg. 2003;51(3):283-9.
8. de Bree R, Rinaldo A, Genden EM, et al. Modern reconstruction techniques for oral and pharyngeal defects after tumor resection. Eur Arch Otorhinolaryngol. 2008;265(1):1-9.
9. Disa JJ, Pusic AL, Mehrara BJ. Reconstruction of the hypopharynx with the free jejunum transfer. J Surg Oncol. 2006;94(6):466-70.
10. Bianchi B, Ferri A, Ferrari S, et al. Free and locoregional flap associations in the reconstruction of extensive head and neck defects. Int J Oral Maxillofac Surg. 2008;37(8):723-9.

11. George RK, Krishnamurthy A. Microsurgical free flaps: Controversies in maxillofacial reconstruction. Ann Maxillofac Surg. 2013;3(1):72-9.
12. Patel SG, Deshmukh SP, Savant DN, et al. Comparative evaluation of function after surgery for cancer of the alveolobuccal complex. J Oral Maxillofac Surg. 1996;54(6):698-703.
13. McLean JN, Carlson GW, Losken A. The pectoralis major myocutaneous flap revisited: a reliable technique for head and neck reconstruction. Ann Plast Surg. 2010;64(5):570-3.
14. Bhathena HM, Savant DN, Kavarana NM, et al. Reconstruction with different free flaps in oro-facial cancer patients. Acta Chir Plast. 1996;38(2):43-9.
15. Savant DN, Patel SG, Deshmukh SP, et al. Folded free radial forearm flap for reconstruction of full-thickness defects of the cheek. Head Neck. 1995;17(4):293-6.
16. Urken ML, Buchbinder D, Weinberg MD, et al. Functional evaluation following microvascular reconstruction of the oral cancer patient: a comparative study of the reconstructed and non-reconstructed patients. Laryngoscope. 1991;101:935-42.
17. Savant DN, Bhathena HM, Kavarana NM, et al. Osteomyocutaneous flap reconstructions for major mandibular defects. J Surg Oncol. 1994;55:122-5.
18. Cordeiro PG, Hidalgo DA. Soft tissue coverage of mandibular reconstruction plates. Head and Neck. 1994;16:112-6.
19. Rosen IB, Mankletow RT, Zuker RM, et al. Application of microvascular free osteocutaneous flaps in the management of post-radiation recurrent oral cancer. Am J Surg. 1985;150:474-8.
20. Savant DN, Patel SG, Verghese T, et al. Reconstruction of the mandible with vascularized iliac crest free flap. Acta Chir Plast. 1995;37:35-9.
21. Boyd JB, Rosen I, Rotstein LE, et al. The iliac crest and the radial forearm flap in vascularized oromandibular reconstruction. Am J Surg. 1990;159:301-9.
22. Swartz WM, Banis JC, Newton ED, et al. The osteocutaneous scapular flap for mandible and maxillary reconstruction. Plast Reconst Surg. 1986;77:531-6.
23. Hidalgo DA. Fibular free flap: a new method of mandible reconstruction. Plast Reconst Surg. 1989;84:71-6.
24. Schusterman MA, Horndeski G. Analysis of the morbidity associated with immediate microvascular reconstruction in head and neck cancer patients. Head Neck. 1991;13:51-5.
25. Frodel JL, Funk GF, Capper DT, et al. Ossteointegrated implants: a comparative study of bone thickness in four vascularized bone flaps. Plast Reconst Surg. 1993;92:449-58.
26. Boyd AD, Shaw WW, McCarthy JG, et al. Immediate reconstruction of full thickness chest wall defects. Ann Thorac Surg. 1981;32:337-43.
27. Arnold PG, Pairolero PC. Chest-wall reconstruction: an account of 500 consecutive patients. Plast Reconstr Surg. 1996;98:804-10.
28. Capanna R, Manfrini M, Briccoli A, et al. Latissimus dorsi pedicled flap applications in shoulder and chest wall reconstructions after extracompartmental sarcoma resections. Tumori. 1995;81:56-62.
29. Candiani P, Campiflio GL, Saccheri S, et al. The versatality of pectoralis major muscle and musculocutaneous flaps in the reconstruction of the oral cavity and of the anterior chest wall. Int Surg. 1994;79:130-4.
30. Sekido M, Yamamoto Y, Sugihara T, et al. Microsurgical reconstruction of chest-and abdominal wall defects associated with intraperitoneal vessels. J Reconstr Microsurg. 1996;12:425-30.
31. Cohen M, Ramasastry SS. Reconstruction of complex chest wall defects. Am J Surg. 1996;172:35-40.
32. Savant DN, Patel SG, Bokil KP, et al. Reconstruction of chest wall defects following extirpative surgery. J Surg Oncol. 1994;55:186-9.
33. Deschamps C, Tirnaksiz BM, Darbandi R, Trastek VF, Allen MS, Miller DL, Arnold PG, Pairolero PC. 1999. Early and long-term results of prosthetic chest wall reconstruction. J Thorac Cardiovasc Surg 117:588-91; discussion 591-2.
34. Samuels L, Granick MS, Ramasastry S, et al. Reconstruction of radiation-induced chest wall lesions. Ann Plast Surg. 1993;31:399-405.
35. Wiliams JK, Carlson GW, deChalain T, et al. Role of tensor fasciae latae in abdominal wall reconstruction. Plast Reconstr Surg. 1998;101:713-6.
36. Ninkovic M, Kronberger P, Harpf C, et al. Free innervated latissimus dorsi muscle flap for reconstruction of full-thickness abdominal wall defects. Plast Reconstr Surg. 1998;101:971-8.
37. Cunha-Gomes D, Choudhari C, Bhathena HM, et al. The hemithigh microvascular transfer (combined anterolateral thigh flap and tensor fasciae latae flap for a full thickness abdominal wall reconstruction: a case report. Acta Chir Plast. 1999;41:71-3.
38. Nissen MJ, Swenson KK, Ritz LJ, et al. Quality of life after breast carcinoma surgery. Cancer. 2001;91:1238-46.
39. Rowland JH, Desmond KA, Meyerowitz BE, et al. Role of breast reconstructive surgery in physical and emotional outcomes among breast cancer survivors. J Natl Cancer Inst. 2000;92(17):1422-9.
40. Feller WF, Holt R, Spear S, et al. Modified radical mastectomy with MIBR. Am Surg. 1986;52:129-32.
41. Fung KW, Lau Y, Fielding R, et al. The impact of mastectomy, breast-conserving treatment and immediate breast reconstructions on the quality of life of Chinese women. ANZ J Surg. 2001;71:202-6.
42. Slavin SA, Lover SM, Goldwyn MD. Recurrent breast cancer following immediate reconstruction with myocutaneous flaps. Plast Reconst Surg. 1984;73:619-26.
43. Vinton AL, Travezo WT, Zehring RD. Immediate breast reconstruction following mastectomy is as safe as mastectomy alone. Arch Surg. 1990;125:1303-11.
44. Jarret JR, Cutler RG, Teal DF. Aesthetic refinements in prophylactic subcutaneous reconstruction with submuscular reconstruction. Plast Reconst Surg. 1982;69:624-9.
45. Hartrampf CR, Scheflan M, Black PW. Breast reconstruction with transverse abdominis island flap. Plast Reconst Surg. 1982;69:216-21.
46. Trabulsy PP, Anthony JP, Mathes SJ. Changing trends in post-mastectomy breast reconstruction: a 13 year experience. Plast Reconst Surg. 1993;93:1418-25.
47. Elliot LF, Eskenazi L, Beegle Jr. MIBR with Tram flap: 128 consecutive cases. Plast Reconst Surg. 1993;92:217-25.
48. Johnson CH, van Heerden JA, Donohue JH, et al. Oncologic aspects of MIBR. Arch Surg. 1985;124:819-27.
49. Carlson GW, Moore B, Thornton JF, et al. Breast cancer after augmentation mammaplasty: treatment by skin-sparing mastectomy and immediate reconstruction. Plast Reconstr Surg. 2001;107:687-9.
50. Hudson DA, Dent DM, Lazarus D. One-stage immediate breast and nipple-areolar reconstruction with autologous tissue I: a preliminary report. Ann Plast Surg. 2000;45:417-6.

57 Emergencies in Oncology

Vijaya Patil, Kailash Sharma

INTRODUCTION

Cancer is generally a slowly growing disease which can, even if untreated, reside in the human system without producing major pathophysiologic upheavals; even untreated breast cancer patients, at least 20–25% of them often survive for 5 years or more; contrary wise, there could be cancers which can grow at a fast pace in an aggressive manner, metastasize rapidly and can produce an emergency. Small cell lung cancer (SCLC), anaplastic cancers at any site are few of the examples. Most oncologic emergencies are same as general emergencies such as severe bleeding, bowel or respiratory obstructions, acute cerebral or intracranial pathologies etc. In addition certain emergencies can also results due to therapeutic interventions like acute neutropenic sepis thrombocytopenia with bleeding and tumor lysis syndrome. By virtue of its ability to secrete hormones some cancers can produce emergency clinical situations. The following text summarizes the etiology, symptomatology, the basic pathophysiology and therapy of oncologic emergencies of which all practicing oncologists should be familiar with.

NEUTROPENIC SEPSIS

Pathophysiology

- Neutropenia due to bone marrow suppression following chemotherapy
- Infection risk increases as neutrophil count falls below 500/cumm
- Patients with hematologic malignancies, allogeneic bone marrow transplantation (BMT), neutropenia of more than 7–14 days duration are at high-risk
- Commonest cause of sepsis is bacterial infections (70–90%).

Symptoms

- Fever, malaise, mucositis, respiratory distress, loose motions
- May present directly in circulatory shock
- May be difficult to find site of infection clinically as classical signs of infection are absent.

Treatment

- Empiric broad spectrum antibiotics to cover Gram-negative organisms
- Gram positive cover in high-risk patients
- Fluid resuscitation and ionotropes in case of hypotension
- Isolate in positive pressure room
- Send peripheral blood culture and central line blood culture (if present)
- Removal of central venous catheter, if no response to antibiotics in 2–3 days.

TUMOR LYSIS SYNDROME

Pathophysiology

- More likely in highly chemotherapy responsive lesions (like lymphoma)
- Rapid destruction of large number of malignant cells lead to release of intracellular contents in blood
- Release of potassium, phosphorus, nucleic acids and their metabolites hypoxanthine, xanthine and uric acid
- Overwhelms renal and other buffering system in body and leads to metabolic derangements

- Systemic inflammatory response syndrome (SIRS) and multiorgan dysfunction due to release of cytokines due to tumor lysis syndrome (TLS)
- Generally seen 48–72 hours after initiation of chemotherapy in hematolymphoid malignancies due to large tumor load
- Sometimes seen with solid tumors-like hepatoblastomas or germ cell tumors
- Can occur spontaneously.

Symptoms

- Hyperkalemia
- Hyperuricemia
- Hyperphosphatemia
- Hypocalcemia
- Hyponatremia
- Renal failure
- Echocardiography (ECG)—arrhythmias and conduction defects.

Treatment

- Aggressive hydration: 200–300 mL/hour to maintain urine 80–100 mL/mt^2/hour
- Diuretics, if signs of fluid overload
- Urine alkalinization is not indicated especially, if using allopurinol or rasburicase
- Allopurinol 600–900 mg/day
- Febuxostat can be used for patients hypersensitive to allopurinol
- Rasburicase 0.2 mg/kg intravenous (IV) oral dose (OD) as single dose but can be given upto 5 days
- Treat hyperkalemia with $NaHCO_3$ and glucose insulin infusion
- Hemodialysis for volume overload, uncontrolled hyperkalemia, hyperphosphatemia and patients in renal failure
- Treat hypocalcemia only in symptomatic patients
- Restrict phosphate intake and use phosphate binders like aluminum hydroxide or calcium carbonate orally.

HYPERCALCEMIA

Pathophysiology

- Increased release of calcium from bone due to metastasis commonly seen with Ca breast, lungs and kidney
- Release of parathyroid hormone related; leads to increased bone resorption seen in squamous Ca from head and neck region
- Release of calcitriol causing increased absorption of calcium from gut seen with lymphomas
- Primary hyperparathyroidism with cancer.

Symptoms

- Constipation
- Vague abdominal pain, anorexia
- Rarely may present with pancreatitis
- Nephrolithiasis
- Nephrogenic diabetes insipidus
- Neuropsychiatric problems like anxiety and depression
- Cognitive dysfunctions like delirium, hallucination, somnolence and even coma
- Echocardiography may show short QT interval and ventricular and supraventricular arrhythmias.

Treatment

- Measure ionized calcium
- Fluid resuscitation with 0.9% normal saline (NS) as patients are often hypovolemic
- Also expansion of extracellular fluid volume helps in calciuresis
- Closed hemodynamic monitoring for patients with renal and cardiac dysfunction
- After adequate fluid resuscitation consider loop diuretics but avoid thiazide diuretics
- Bisphosphonates; pamidronate 60–90 mg over 2–3 hours or zolandronic acid 4mg over 15 minutes
- Calcitonin 4–8 intrauterine(IU)/kg subcutaneous (SC) or IV every 12 hours
- Glucocorticoids only in lymphomas; hydrocortisone 100 mg 6 hourly or predinisolone 60 mg orally daily
- Dialysis in case of acute renal failure or cardiac dysfunction
- End of life care in case of advanced malignancy.

ANAPHYLACTIC REACTIONS DUE TO CHEMOTHERAPEUTIC AGENTS

Pathophysiology

- Massive histamine release
- Seen with intravenous infusions and fast infusion rates.

Symptoms

- Angioedema
- Urticarial
- Chest tightness

- Laryngeal edema
- Bronchospasm
- Hypotension
- Commonly seen with L-Asparginase, Taxanes and platinum derivatives.

Treatment

- Airway management
- Fluid resuscitation
- Adrenaline SC or IV
- Glucocorticoids
- Antihistamines.

PHEOCHROMOCYTOMA

Pathophysiology

- Excessive catecholamine secretion by tumor
- Secretion can be intermittent or continuous
- Increased catecholamine levels induce rise in blood pressure, heart rate, cardiac contractility, hyperglycemia.

Symptoms

- Episodic or sustained resistant hypertension
- Arrhythmia, severe headache, perspiration
- May present with hypertensive emergencies like encephalopathy and cardiac failure.

Treatment

- Adrenergic blocking drugs like labetalol, phentolamine, phenoxybenzamine, prazocin
- Labetalol, sodium nitroprusside or nitroglycerine in hypertensive emergency
- Surgical excision.

TUMOR-INDUCED HYPOGLYCEMIA

Pathophysiology

- Excess insulin production as by insulinoma
- Production of insulin-like growth factors by certain mesenchymal tumors like sarcomas
- Excessive consumption of glucose by rapidly growing tumors with poor intake by patient.

Symptoms

- Symptoms due to adrenergic counter-regulation
- Tachycardia, palpitations, diaphoresis, mydriasis
- Symptoms due to neuroglycopenia
- Confusion, blurred vision, seizures and coma.

Treatment

- Surgical removal of underlying tumor, chemotherapy or radiotherapy
- Intravenous glucagon at dose of 1 mg
- Intravenous dextrose
- Diazoxide 3 mg/kg/day
- Frequent carbohydrate intake.

SUPERIOR VENA CAVA SYNDROME

Pathophysiology

- Common causes bronchogenic carcinomas (SCLC), non-Hodgkin lymphoma, etc. Benign conditions like teratoma, thymoma, aortic aneurysm can cause superior vena cava (SVC) obstruction
- Pathophysiology involves direct tumor compression, thrombosis, fibrosis.

Symptoms

- Dyspnea is commonest presentation
- Facial, conjunctival, arm edema, nasal stuffiness, hoarseness
- May present with signs of raised intracranial pressure
- Prominent collaterals may be seen on anterior chest wall and abdomen
- Respiratory distress in presence of respiratory tract compression.

Treatment

- Head elevation and oxygen supplementation
- Obtain biopsy (not always possible) preferably before starting any definitive treatment
- Steroids and chemotherapy for chemosensitive tumors
- Radiotherapy for small cell and non-small cell lung cancer
- Thrombolysis for SVC thrombosis
- Superior vena cava stenting in selected cases.

AIRWAY OBSTRUCTION

Pathophysiology

- May result from intraluminal growth or extrinsic compression
- Can occur at upper airway , trachea or main bronchial level

- Angioedema also can be cause of acute airway obstruction.

Symptoms

- Dyspnea on exercise or rest
- Stridor
- Asymptomatic patient can present in acute airway obstruction with sudden increase in tumor size as may occur with intra-tumor hemorrhage.

Treatment

- Tracheostomy, if obstruction is at proximal level
- For distal obstruction, bronchoscopy with laser or debulking with microdebrider
- External radiation and steroids in radiosensitive tumors
- Airway stenting for extrinsic compression.

CARDIAC TAMPONADE

Pathophysiology

- Primary cardiac tumor (rare)
- Metastatic tumor
- Radiation pericarditis and tamponade.

Symptoms

- Tachypnea, decreased exercise tolerance, shock and rarely cardiac arrest
- Muffled heart sounds, pulsus paradoxus
- Low voltage ECG
- Diastolic collapse of right atrium and right ventricle on 2-D echocardiogram (ECHO).

Treatment

- Fluid resuscitation
- Emergency pericardiocentesis preferably under ultrasonography (USG) guidance followed by pigtail catheter insertion or creation of pericardial window.

CARDIAC FAILURE

Pathophysiology

- Chemotherapy induced cardiomyopathies seen with anthracyclines, taxol, cyclophosphamide

Symptoms

- Poor effort tolerance, decreased appetite, tachypnea, low voltage ECG, ST-T wave changes, generalized anasarca
- Generalized hypokinesia and low left ventricular ejection fraction
- Dilated cardiomyopathy

Treatment

- Inotropic agents
- Diuretics
- Angiotensin-converting enzyme (ACE) inhibitors
- Mechanical assist devices in select cases.

SPINAL CORD COMPRESSION

Pathophysiology

- Compression due to extradural metastasis
- Bony metastasis to vertebrae.

Symptoms

- Localized backache and tenderness are early signs
- Motor weakness
- Sensory deficit
- Autonomic disturbances.

Treatment

- High level of suspicion and early diagnosis
- Adequate analgesia
- Imaging–magnetic resonance imaging (MRI) is gold standard, however computed tomography (CT) scan can be done
- When motor deficit or radiological evidence of cord compression present start steroids; dexamethasone 10–16 mg IV stat followed by 4 mg every 4 hours
- Appropriate chemotherapy
- Radiotherapy
- Surgery with spine stabilization (at appropriate moment)
- Hormone therapy and zolandronic acid for sensitive tumors like Ca Prostate, testicular tumor or lymphoma.

HYPERVISCOSITY SYNDROME

Pathophysiology

- Increased serum viscosity due to excess proteins
- Excess blood viscosity due to cellular component as in acute leukemia or polycythemia vera
- Excess blood viscosity lead to resistance to blood flow and decreased organ blood flow and increase thrombogenic potential
- Decreased cerebral perfusion
- Decreased tissue perfusion and cellular damage.

Symptoms

- Headache, altered mental status
- Blurred vision
- Vertigo, ataxia
- Paresthesia
- Seizure, coma
- Mucosal bleeding, purpura
- Congestive heart failure
- Renal failure
- Pulmonary edema.

Treatment

- Plasmapheresis on daily basis till symptoms resolve.

HYPONATREMIA

Pathophysiology

- Syndrome of inappropriate antidiuretic hormone (SIADH) due to ectopic antidiuretic hormone (ADH) secretion commonly seen with malignancies of lungs, pleura thymus or brain
- Excess ADH secretion leads to free water uptake by distal tubules which lead to dilutional hyponatremia
- Drugs like cisplatin, cyclophosphamide, vinca alkaloids and imatinib give rise to hyponatremia due to sodium loss by nephrons.

Symptoms

- With chronic hyponatremia patients may be asymptomatic
- Anorexia, nausea, vomiting, headache, agitation
- Lethargy, delirium, seizures, coma.

Treatment

- Asymptomatic euvolemic patients major cause of excess ADH secretions; control nausea, pain
- Restrict intake to 1,000–1,500 mL/day and avoid hypotonic fluids
- Consider V_2 receptor blockers like tolvaptan starting 15 mg/day
- Hypovolemic patients should be resuscitated with 0.9% saline
- Symptomatic patients: airway control if mentally obtunded, hypertonic saline (3%) to control symptoms, however rate of rise of sodium should not be more than 8 meq/24 hours for acute hyponatremia and 10–12 meq/24 hours for chronic hyponatremia to avoid central pontine myelinosis.
- Monitor serum electrolytes frequently to check for correction.

58 Pediatric Oncology: A Journey from Nihilism to Cautious Optimism

Purna Kurkure

INTRODUCTION

The recent understanding and advances in the total management of pediatric cancers form one of the most exciting chapters in the entire field of oncology. With increasing control of infectious disease, eradication of malnutrition and the rapid strides of pediatric surgeons in correcting benign surgical problems, more children are now going to be affected by cancer. In the US cancer is second to accidents as a cause of mortality in children beyond the first year of life.[1] Even in developing countries like India, cancer is gradually assuming an important place as a cause of childhood mortality.[2,3]

Cancer in children as compared to adults is clinico-biologically distinct. "Child is not a miniature adult". The types of childhood cancers and response to therapy totally differ from those in adults as shown in Table 1.

All pediatric cancers are considered as potentially curable. Also its sociologic impact in terms of disruption of family life, loss of productive years and sympathy for its victims is far greater than cancer in adults. There has been a phenomenal progress in the field of pediatric oncology over last 4 decades. A disease with an invariably fatal outcome in the past now enjoys a 5-year survival (equivalent to cure) of more than 70% and is one of the most gratifying illnesses to treat[1,4] and is indeed the major success story in current oncology.

BURDEN OF CHILDHOOD CANCERS

Globally, it is estimated that 10–12 children (less than 15 years) per 100,000 population per year develop cancer.[5] The age-adjusted incidence of childhood cancer in India varies from 3.2/100,000 in Barshi to 14.1/100,000 in Delhi Population-based cancer registry (PBCR)[6,7] (Table 2). In India, 36% of the population is in the pediatric group and approximately 30,000–40,000 new cases of cancer would occur in children annually. The risk of cancer appears to be slightly higher in males.[7]

The relative frequency of various childhood malignancies in India is shown in Table 3. Leukemias and lymphomas comprise nearly half of pediatric cancers followed by tumors of the central nervous system, sympathetic nervous system, soft tissues, kidney, bone, eye, liver and germ cells. The incidence of most pediatric hematological malignancies as well as solid tumors in India seems to be lower than most of developed countries. Compared to Western countries, India has a higher frequency of retinoblastoma, T-cell lymphoma/leukemia, and mixed cellularity Hodgkin's disease.[6,7]

Pediatric hematolymphoid malignancies, central nervous system tumors and bone and soft tissue sarcomas are discussed in the respective chapters. In ensuing paragraphs, the principles of management of pediatric solid tumors along with salient features of commonly occurring extracranial embryonal pediatric solid tumors will be highlighted.

Clinical Aspects

Solid tumors account for approximately 45% of all malignant diseases in children. They may present: (1) as localized mass or (2) as consequence of pressure from the mass on adjacent structures/tissues; or (3) as a consequence of disseminated disease causing systemic symptoms. The frequency of diagnosis varies with age, location and ethnic groups. In most cases, the exact etiology of childhood cancer is unclear, but it is likely to

TABLE 1: Differences in cancer characteristics for childhood and adult cancers

	Childhood cancer	*Adult cancer*
1.	Incidence patterns are similar between countries, suggesting a lower proportion of childhood cancers are related to exogenous exposures	Incidence patterns are vastly different between countries, suggesting a higher proportion of adult cancers are related to exogenous exposures
2.	For a given level of exogenous exposure (e.g. radiation) there is less variability in incidence rates	For a given level of exogenous exposure (e.g. Tobacco), these is more variability in incidence rates
3.	Higher proportion of incidence is related to inherited susceptibility	Higher proportion is tied to exogenous exposures
4.	Primary sites Involves tissues (i.e. hematopoietic lymphatic CNS, muscle, bone)	Primary sites Involves organs (e.g. breast, lung, colon, prostate, uterus)
5.	Malignancies involve neuroectodermal and mesoderm derived tumors	Malignancies involve epithelial tissues
6.	80% are disseminated at diagnosis	Most are local or regional at diagnosis
7.	Early detection mostly accidental during routine examination	Early detection improves with education and screening
8.	Less opportunity for development of new, more aggressive clones; tumors are more genetically homogeneous	Tumors are more heterogeneous, reflec ting the long time and multiple steps in the development of cancer
9.	Greater effectiveness of cytotoxic therapies	Less effective cytotoxic therapies
10.	Few risk factors are known and there is less opportunity for primary prevention	Many risk factors are known, and there is a greater opportunity for primary prevention

TABLE 2: Average age-adjusted (world population) incidence rates of childhood cancer by gender per 100,000 persons

PBCR	*Male*	*Female*
Bangalore	7.0	4.7
Bhopal	4.8	5.2
Barshi	3.2	3.6
Chennai	10.9	9.2
Delhi	14.1	8.3
Mumbai	10.2	6.4

Source: ICMR, 1997-1998.

TABLE 3: Frequency of types of cancer: hospital-based data*

Type of cancer	*% of all pediatric cancers*
Leukemia	28.6%
Lymphoma	13.2%
CNS	12.4%
Wilm's tumor	10.1%
Neuroblastoma	5.7%
Gonadal tumors	5.6%
Retinoblastoma	5.9%
Soft tissue tumors	5.3%
Bone	6.1%
Others	6.9%

*Computed from data from six cancer units/centers from India

represent an interaction between environmental factors (e.g. radiation; parental occupation and socioeconomic status; infections) and host genetic susceptibility (e.g. gene mutation). Most cancers occur as a result of mutations in cellular genes (tumor suppressor genes and oncogenes) which may either be inherited or sporadic or may occur as a result of epigenetic factors. The most talked about inherited cancer is bilateral retinoblastoma which is associated with a deletion on chromosome 13. Increasingly, modern molecular techniques are being used in clinical practice to identify characteristics which may be useful either to confirm diagnosis [e.g. t(11;22) (q24;q12) in Ewing's sarcoma] or to predict prognosis (e.g. amplification of the "N-myc" oncogene associated with a poor prognosis in neuroblastoma) or to study the biology of the disease (using micro array technique to study thousands of genes at the same time).

Solid tumors are evaluated using X-rays, ultrasound, CT and MRI scans. The functional PET scan is a new addition in this armamentarium and is useful for localizing primary disease, for evaluation of metastatic spread and for evaluating response to chemotherapy. Other nuclear medicine imaging [e.g. radiolabeled technetium bone scan, functional metaiodobenzyl guanidine (MIBG) scan] may also be useful to map primary and metastatic disease at presentation and monitor response to therapy. Tumor marker studies are helpful for germ cell tumors [alpha-fetoprotein (AFP) and β-human chorionic gonadotropin (β-hCG)]; hepatoblastoma (AFP) and neuroblastoma (urinary VMA). However, diagnosis, if possible, must be confirmed by biopsy. The differentiation between some solid tumors (especially small round blue cell tumors) may be difficult using standard microscopy, and further differentiation usually requires specialized pathology techniques such as immunohistochemistry (Table 4) and sometimes, electron microscopy. Modern molecular and imaging techniques add to the accuracy and precision of diagnosis and also recognition of residual disease.

Management

We started with Nihilism; the denial of the existence of any basis for curability of childhood cancers 50 years ago; we have now come a long way to a state of cautious optimism wherein nearly 50% of all children with cancer who manage to get optimum therapy can expect a cure. The success rate of 75% cures in developed countries can be reached if we optimize therapy with appropriate supportive care and infrastructure.

The journey from nihilism to cautious optimism has been a long one with incremental advances made by multidisciplinary approach executed through carefully orchestrated combined modality team comprising of a pediatric medical oncologist, pediatric surgeon, radiation oncologist, diagnostic specialists and supportive care services. Burchenal succinctly characterized the basic tenet of multidisciplinary approach by stating that "the pride of discipline must be put aside". All the experts should work together, keeping well-being of the child as the central issue.

The general guidelines in the management of the child with solid tumors are as follows:

- The general clinical status of the child (performance status) should be evaluated first to determine the child's ability to undergo various diagnostic and therapeutic procedures
- Systematic assessment of extent of disease (clinical staging)

TABLE 4: Small round cell tumors of childhood

Type	*NB*[1]	*RMS*[2]	*EWS*[3]	*Small cell OS*[4]	*NHL*[5]
Age in years	< 5	< 6	10–20	10–20	5–15
Sites of Presentation	Abdomen, thorax, neural crest	Skeletal muscle	Diaphysis of extremity and central axis bones; ST	Metaphysis of extremity bones	Lymph node liver, spleen; extranodal
Pathology	Rosette formation, cytoplasmic granules, dendritic process	Z-band formation	Small round cell	Osteoid formation	Small round cell
IHC[6]: MIC-2	-	–	+	-	-
NSE[7]	+	-	+	-	-
Desmin	-	+	-	-	-
Actin	-	+	-	-	-
Myosin	-	+	-	-	-
LCA[8]	-	-	-	-	+
Cytogenetics	1p-, n-myc	t(2;13) (95%) t(1;13) (5%)	t (11;22) (95%) t (21;22) (2%) t(7;22) (2%)	p53	t (8;22) t (8;14) t (2;8)
Treatment	[9]Sx + RT[10] + CT[11]	Sx + RT + CT	CT + Sx + RT	CT + Sx	CT
Prognosis	Low risk 85–95% High risk < 40%	60–70%	60–70%	60–70%	80–90%

Keywords: [1]Neuroblastoma, [2]Rhabdomyosarcoma, [3]Ewing's sarcoma, [4]Osteosarcoma, [5]Non-Hodgkin's lymphoma, [6]Immunohistochemistry, [7]Neuron specific esterase, [8]Leukcocyte common antigen, [9]Surgery, [10]Radiotherapy; [11]Chemotherapy.

- Histopathological confirmation of diagnosis with reference to known prognostic factors
- Risk stratification based on clinical, pathological and ancillary laboratory parameters
- Complete therapeutic strategy planning in multidisciplinary joint clinics including time and modality of locoregional treatment based on prevailing protocols
- Institution of risk-based therapy in sequence as per plan
- Monitoring the progress of treatment, acute toxicities of therapy and results regularly by pediatric oncologist
- Supportive services in form of rehabilitation, psychosocial support to the child and the parents
- Long-term follow-up with respect to disease activity as well as late effects of therapy.

Initial therapeutic effort offers the best chance and optimal therapy at the outset is the most important factor for a favorable outcome. Any advances in healthcare are only as valuable as it is available and accessible to those who need it. It has been well-documented that organized and co-ordinated treatment program carried out by experienced pediatric oncologist in well-staffed and well-equipped pediatric cancer unit is most effective; however, at the same time early referral for prompt diagnosis, therapy and ensuring efficient follow-up, the role of the community pediatrician is crucial. With this purpose, the "National Training Project in Practical Pediatric Oncology" has been initiated since 1998 under the auspices of Pediatric Hematology Oncology Chapter of Indian Academy of Pediatrics in collaboration with International Society of Pediatric Oncology (SIOP) with an aim to train, educate and encourage pediatricians to participate in shared care of childhood cancer patients.[8]

NEUROBLASTOMA[9-12]

Neuroblastoma (NB) is the most common extracranial solid tumor of childhood. The median age at presentation is 2 years. It arises from neural crest tissue which differentiates in cells of the sympathetic ganglia and adrenal medulla. It remains a complex medical challenge with spontaneous regression at one end to an unpredictable clinical course and dismal outcome at the other end of spectrum.

Most children present with an abdominal mass, typically of adrenal (medulla) origin, but the primary lesion can be anywhere along the sympathetic chain from the neck to the pelvis. It may cross the midline and para-vertebral tumors may even cause spinal cord compression. In older children, clinical symptoms are mostly from metastatic disease, particularly bone pain and bone marrow suppression. Diagnosis is made by clinical and radiological features (calcification), CT/MRI, raised urinary catecholamine (vanillylmandelic acid) levels, MIBG scan, bone marrow studies and biopsy of primary mass.

The most important prognostic features are age, stage of disease, histology. The biological characteristics [n-myc amplification, deletion of material of chromosome 1 (1p-) and gain of material on chromosome 17 (17p+)] are associated with poorer prognosis. Unfortunately, the majority of children over 1 year present with advanced disease, have unfavorable biology and histology and thus have poor prognosis (Figs 1 and 2).

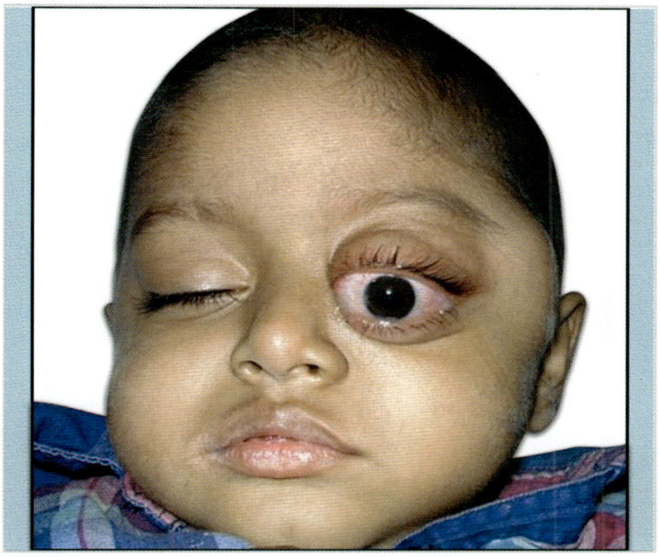

Fig. 1: A typical picture of metastatic neuroblastoma with proptosis. Bone marrow and bones are the most common metastatic sites

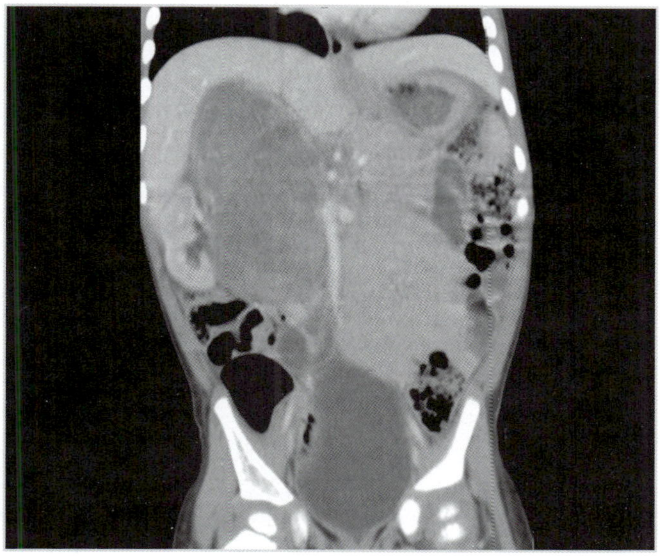

Fig. 2: CT scan showing a typical large neuroblastoma in a 2-year-old male child

Risk Stratification

- Risk stratification should be done at a tertiary center before initiation of therapy.
- In unresectable lesions generous core biopsy (image guided) should be performed for histopathology and molecular studies (Table 4).

Simplified version of risk stratification of NB based on complex matrix is shown in Table 5.

Risk-adapted treatment algorithm is shown in Figure 3.

Unfortunately, even with aggressive treatment the risk of relapse remains high and the prospect for cure of children with metastatic disease is around 40% in the developed countries and less than 20% in India. Attempts to reduce the relapse rate with the use of 13-cis-retinoic acid as a differentiating agent and immunotherapy with Anti-GD2 antibody to tackle minimal residual disease are being explored in all major treatment protocols.

TABLE 5: Risk stratification in neuroblastoma

Risk	*Age*	*Stage*	*MYCN status*
Low	< 547 days	1, 2A/B,4S	NA
	≥ 547 days	1, 2A/B	NA
Intermediate	< 547 days	3, 4	NA
	≥ 547 days	3	NA
High	< 547 days	1, 2, 3, 4, 4S	Amp
	≥ 547 days	1, 2, 3	Amp
	≥ 547 days	4	Any

Abbreviations: NA, not amplified; Amp, amplified

The clinical behavior of NB in infants is different from that in older children and the prognosis is very good (> 90% cure rate). A subgroup of infants present with stage 4s disease with a localized primary tumor but evidence of skin, liver and/or bone marrow disease has very good

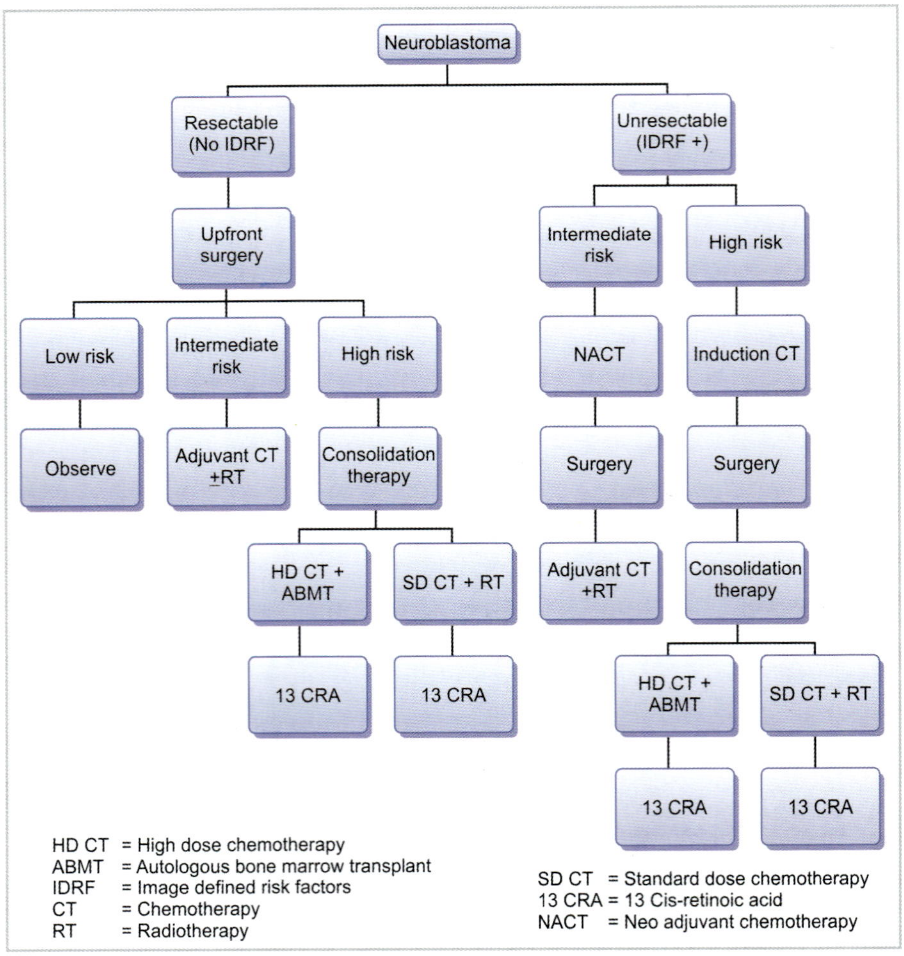

Fig. 3: Risk-adapted management algorithm in neuroblastoma

prognosis. Spontaneous regression can occur and cure is often possible even without any intervention or with minimal therapy.

WILM'S TUMOR[13-16]

Wilm's tumor (WT) is the commonest kidney tumor in children. Over 80% of children with WT present before 5 years of age and the peak incidence are before the age of 3 years. Most children present with large abdominal mass, often found incidentally in an otherwise well child. Hemorrhage into the mass may cause abdominal pain and pallor; occasionally the child may present with macroscopic hematuria. Hypertension is common at diagnosis. Radiological diagnosis from ultrasound or CT/MRI scan is characteristic (Fig. 4). These images also give information about tumor resectability, function of contralateral kidney and also the presence of bilateral (in 5%) WT. CT lung should be routinely done to evaluate for presence of pulmonary metastasis. A small number of children with WT may have congenital malformation syndromes like aniridia, genital abnormalities, Denys-Drash and WAGR syndrome, hemihypertrophy, and Beckwith-Wiedemann syndrome.

Differential diagnosis of intra-abdominal mass in children includes WT, neuroblastoma, lymphoma, hepatoblastoma, soft tissue sarcoma and sometimes nonmalignant conditions like tuberculosis, etc. Prognostic factors for WT include stage and pathology. Classical WT is a triphasic structure showing epithelial, blastemal and stromal elements. Features of diffuse anaplasia represent a high risk subtype, as also the persistence of blastemal component after initial chemotherapy. Clear cell sarcoma and renal rhabdoid tumors are now considered separate entities and convey poor prognosis.

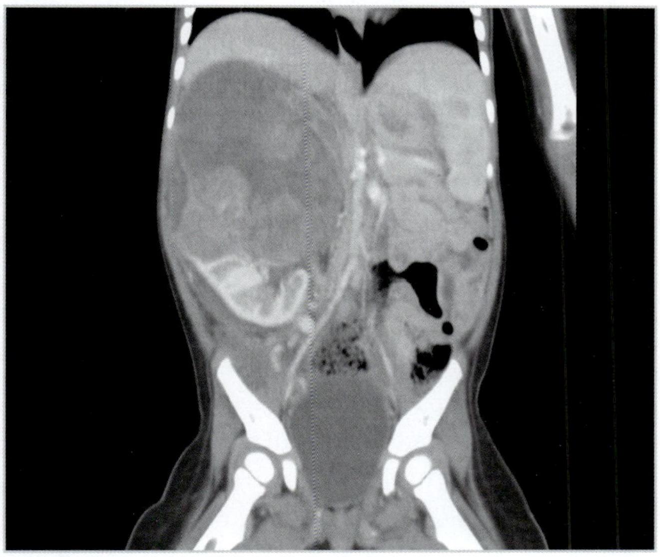

Fig. 4: Typical scan showing a right Wilm's tumor

Treatment involves surgery and chemotherapy (vincristine, actinomycin-D +/- doxorubicin). Radiotherapy is required only in a minority of patients including those with lung metastasis and a few with locally extensive intra-abdominal disease. Contemporary treatment of WT has led to an overall survival of over 85% and the emphasis is now shifting from successful treatment to reducing treatment-associated morbidity without loss of efficacy.

A long-standing difference of opinion about the optimal initial management for children with unilateral WT remains unresolved which is the timing of nephrectomy. Early nephrectomy, undertaken before commencing any other therapy, has been a long-standing policy in the United States (National Wilm's Tumor Study Group—NWTSG approach) whereas the use of prenephrectomy chemotherapy has been practiced in Europe (International Society of Pediatric Oncology—SIOP approach) for many years. Both approaches result in similar tumor control rates but a different overall burden of treatment. In NWTSG studies, approximately 30% of patients have stage III tumors and therefore receive treatment with both anthracycline and abdominal radiotherapy. Using the SIOP preoperative chemotherapy approach, tumors are "down staged" so that only 15% of patients have stage III disease and 50% have stage I. However, with a modification in chemotherapy protocol as a result of high incidence of abdominal relapses in SIOP studies anthracyclines are also added in stage II patients. Consequently 50% of children in SIOP studies receive an anthracycline whereas approximately 50% North American patients would be treated with abdominal irradiation.

The concept of the "total burden of therapy" (selection of components of neoadjuvant and adjuvant treatment) needs to be considered and quantified.

Using an intermediary approach, early nephrectomy for patients with operable tumors (NWTSG approach) and prenephrectomy chemotherapy (SIOP approach) in patients with borderline or inoperable tumors (as depicted in Figure 5) will be the best practical way forward in India which merits further studies. Even stage IV patients (15%) have a cure rate of nearly 60%. Treatment for children with bilateral disease is preoperative chemotherapy followed by "nephron sparing" surgery if possible once maximal response is achieved.

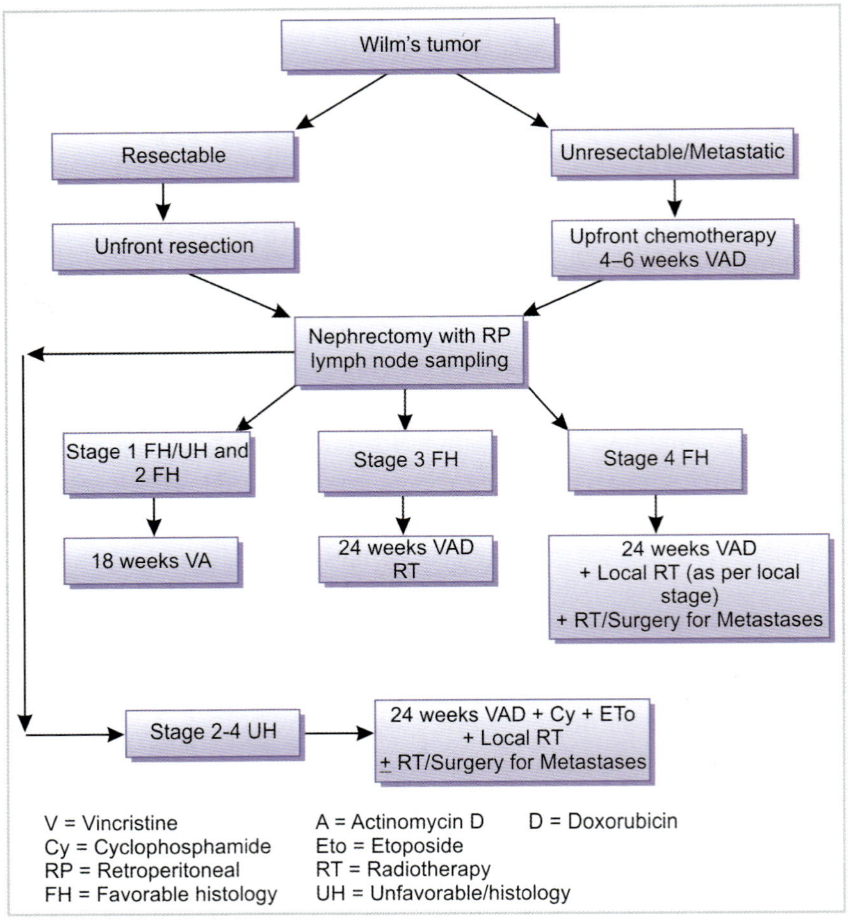

Fig. 5: Management algorithm in Wilm's Tumor

Since WT is one of the most curable malignancies of childhood, special emphasis needs to be laid on the need for surveillance for late effects of therapy in terms of cardiotoxicity, musculoskeletal development, fertility and second malignant neoplasm.

RETINOBLASTOMA[17,18]

Retinoblastoma (RB), a malignant tumor of the embryonic neural retina, is the most common primary malignant intraocular tumor of childhood and its incidence is high in India as compared to developed countries. The average age at diagnosis for bilateral tumor is 12 months and for unilateral tumors is 21 months. In trilateral RB syndrome, pineal tumors develop in approximately 1 in 100 patients with bilateral ocular disease. Characteristically, the diagnosis is made by ophthalmoscopic, radiographic and ultrasonographic appearance, without pathologic confirmation. This tumor which usually arises from the posterior portion of the retina, may appear as a single tumor in the retina, but typically has multiple foci. The most frequent extraocular sites of involvement are the optic nerve, orbit and periorbital tissues, cranial tissue, bone and bone marrow.

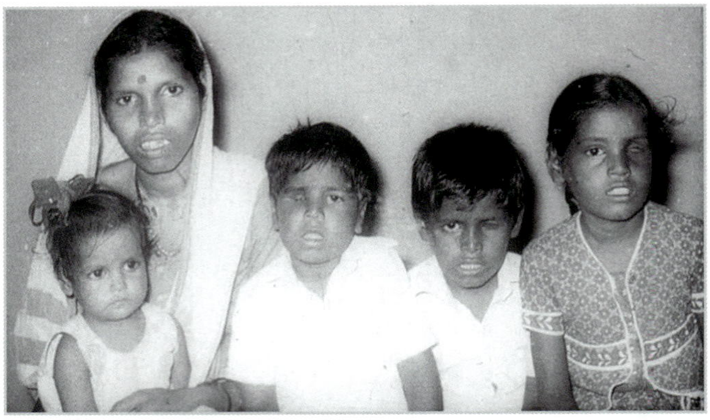

Fig. 6: Retinoblastoma—an inherited disorder (autosomal dominant)—out of four siblings three of them had retinoblastoma

Courtesy: Dr PB Desai

It occurs either spontaneously or as an inherited disorder. RB shows an autosomal dominant inheritance pattern with high penetrance (Fig. 6). Approximately, 55%

occur as nonhereditary, unifocal, unilateral tumors. An additional 15% are unilateral, but are hereditary with a family history. Thirty percent occur as heritable bilateral unifocal or multifocal tumors. The RB gene is a tumor suppresser gene and RB tumors are homozygous for chromosome 13q14 abnormalities with either deletions or alterations of genetic material at that locus.

The most common sign of RB is the white or cat's eye reflex (leukokoria). Other signs associated with RB are visual impairment, strabismus, pseudohypopyon, and vitreous hemorrhage. Proptosis, signs of increased intracranial pressure and bone pain may occur with very advanced or metastatic disease. A fundoscopic examination under anesthesia should be done. MRI scan of the orbit is performed to evaluate extent of tumor and to assess whether optic nerve, bony structures or pineal gland are involved. Ultrasound may aid in the differential diagnosis (other causes of leukokoria such as retinal detachment or dysplasia, retinopathy of prematurity, persistent hyperplastic vitreous, nematode endophthalmitis, cataract, coloboma of the choroids). Radionuclide bone scan and examination of bone marrow and CSF for tumor cells are necessary only if there is evidence of trans-scleral extension or extension beyond the cut end of optic nerve.

Treatment is highly individualized. Every effort is being made to save the child's life with preservation of eye and sight, if possible. Over the past decade, there has been a trend away from enucleation and external beam radiotherapy and toward chemoreduction followed by focal therapies. Chemotherapy may be useful in all three clinical settings: in intraocular RB, in cases of micrometastatic spread, and when there are overt extraocular metastases. Tumor shrinkage with chemoreduction may allow treatment with less invasive measures such as cryotherapy, laser photocoagulation, thermotherapy or plaque radiotherapy, thereby, avoiding enucleation and radiotherapy. The most commonly used chemotherapeutic agents are vincristine, etoposide and carboplatin.

The prognosis for patients with RB is directly related to the size and extension of the tumor. Most tumors that are confined to the eye can be cured. Cures are infrequent when extensive orbital or optic nerve extension has occurred or patient has CNS or distant metastasis. RB leads to metastatic disease and death in 50% of children worldwide but in less than 5% of children in the United States and other developed nations because of diagnosis and advanced medical care. Overall 5 years disease free survival with enucleation and external beam irradiation has been reported as 88–94%. Subsequent 10-year survival decreases in bilateral cases due to higher incidence of second malignant tumors in these patients.

BARRIERS TO OPTIMAL TREATMENT OF CHILDHOOD CANCERS IN INDIA

The optimal delivery of care to pediatric oncology patients in our country is fraught with many obstacles. Barriers to access Pediatric Oncology Services resulting in suboptimal outcome in childhood cancers in India are depicted in Figure 7.

It has been proposed that, the best way of capacity building for India is to optimize utility of the existing infrastructure. This can be accomplished by creation of pediatric cancer units (PCU) at tertiary care centers including university hospitals and regional cancer centers which collaborate with primary care providers for "shared care" (Fig. 8).[19] An ideal PCU should have a full time pediatric oncology specialist and other allied specialists such as pediatric surgeon.[20] Other needs like radiation oncologist and anesthesiologist, availability of good hematological, microbiological and histopathology laboratories, good surgical, radiation facilities, dedicated onco nursing personnel, blood components, data management and follow-up facilities are common needs for all cancer patients (including adults) and should be available. However, social workers, psychologist must be specifically trained to play a crucial role in pediatric oncology.[21] The mandate of such units would be to create infrastructure, train manpower, conduct research, develop indigenous protocols tailored for the local population and follow standards of care with respect to diagnosis, treatment and supportive care. There

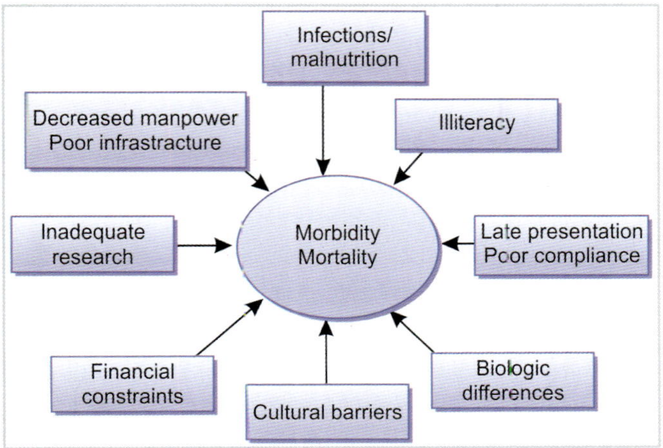

Fig. 7: Barriers to optimal outcome in childhood cancers

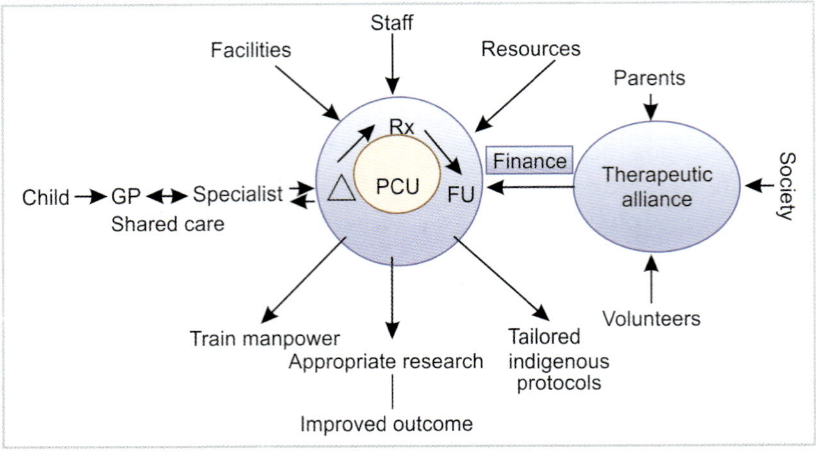

Fig. 8: Pediatric cancer unit model of care for childhood cancers in India

Source: Modified and reproduced with permission[19]

should also be an inbuilt mechanism for internal audit and step-wise improvement.

Biological cure is not the end of journey:[22-27] Presently more than 70% of children diagnosed with cancers are expected to survive at 5 years from diagnosis and beyond. Most of these survivors are potentially cured. The optimism of curability of childhood cancer is shared with a note of caution. Clinicians have learnt to appreciate that this success has come at cost of both short- and long-term morbidity of treatment.

It has been estimated that in USA, the prevalence of childhood cancer survivors is expected to increase from 1 in 900 among young adults in society to 1 in 250 by 2020. Similar figures are not available from India. Approximately 30,000–40,000 cases of childhood cancer occur in our country annually. Even with conservative estimates of 10–20% long-term cure, approximately 3.5–7,000 survivors are added to our population each year. This is expected to increase exponentially as we strive to improve patient care and survival. Two-third of survivors are known to have at least one chronic or late occurring complications of their cancer therapy and of these, one-third have serious or life-threatening complications. The incidence of most late effects increases with age, often becoming clinically apparent decades after therapy. Consequent to this success arise challenges inherent in co-coordinating life-long healthcare for a high risk group of patients predisposed to a variety of cancer-related complications.

As there is a burgeoning population of vulnerable aging adult survivors, there is a pressing need to study the delayed effects of childhood cancer therapy and adverse health outcomes in the context of organ senescence. An awareness of the potential long-term complications is important not only for optimizing healthcare of the current survivors but also for modifying future treatment protocols to avoid therapies that are associated with unacceptable morbidity and mortality. Many of the potential late effects can be ameliorated by prevention or by early diagnosis with therapeutic intervention. Hence a specialized and structured plan for lifelong surveillance and prevention based on risks inherent to primary cancer, cancer therapy, genetics, lifestyle and comorbidities is required for each survivor. Creation of nationwide after completion of therapy clinics for long-term follow-up of childhood cancer survivors with tight linkage to primary care providers would be the right beginning.

The need to predict the future impact of current therapeutic strategies is a major challenge for the pediatric oncologist. A balance of reassurance to the survivor and vigilance in monitoring for relapse, second malignancies and other sequel is required. Recent concept of a truly "cured child" in pediatric oncology envisages not only a biological cure of the disease but a child on par with peers in growth and development physically and in achievements and aspirations, both mentally and emotionally.

It is time; all healthcare workers involved in the care of pediatric oncology patients realize that "biological cure is not enough". We should all strive toward meaningful cure, i.e. complete restoration of physical, mental and social well-being and not merely the absence of disease.

REFERENCES

1. Coleman MP, Estève J, Damiecki P, et al. Trends in cancer incidence and mortality. IARC Sci Publ. 1993;(121):1-806.
2. Arya LS. Childhood cancer: Where do we stand? Indian Pediatr. 1997;34(7):583-7.
3. Health profile of Kerala. Ministry of Health and Family Welfare. Government of Kerala, Trivandrum, 1989.
4. Levi F, La Vecchia C, Lucchini F, et al. Patterns of childhood cancer mortality: America, Asia and Oceania. Eur J cancer. 1995;31A(5):771-82.
5. Parkin DM, Kramarova E, Draper GJ, Masuyer E, Michaelis J, Neglia J, et al (Eds). International incidence of childhood cancer. IARC scientific publication No. 144; 1998.
6. Indian Council of Medical Research, (2001). National Cancer Registry Programme. Consolidated Report of the Population Based Cancer Registries 1990-1996: Incidence and distribution of cancer. Indian Council of Medical Research, New Delhi.
7. Indian Council of Medical Research, (2004). National Cancer Registry Programme. Consolidated Report of the Population Based Cancer Registries 1997-1998: Incidence and distribution of cancer. Indian Council of Medical Research, New Delhi
8. Agarwal B, Marwaha R, Kurkure P, et al. Indian National training project in practical pediatric oncology (INTPPO): Evaluation of progress and lessons for the future. SIOP XXXIII meeting Abstracts O 1. Med Pediatr Oncol. 2001;37:163.
9. Davidoff AM. Neuroblastoma. Semin Pediatr Surg. 2012;21(1): 2-14.
10. Matthay KK, Villablanca JG, Seeger RC, et al. Treatment of high-risk neuroblastoma with intensive chemotherapy, radiotherapy, autologous bone marrow transplantation, and 13-cis-retinoic acid. Children's Cancer Group. N Engl J Med. 1999;341(16): 1165-73.
11. Rao SR, Iyer RS, Nair CN, et al. Infantile neuroblastoma: 10 year TMH experience. Indian J Cancer. 1993;30(3):85-7
12. Biswas G, Kurkure P, Banavali SD, et al. Challenges in the management of advanced neuroblastoma: experience at Tata Memorial hospital, Mumbai, India. J Clin Oncol. 2004;22(14S):8562.
13. Kalapurakal JA, Dome JS, Perlman EJ, et al. Management of Wilms' tumour: current practice and future goals. Lancet Oncol. 2004;5:37-46.
14. Tongaonkar HB, Qureshi SS, Kurkure Pa, et al. Wilm's tumour: An update. Indian J Urol. 2007;23(4):458-66.
15. Hamilton TE, Shamberger RC. Wilms tumor: recent advances in clinical care and biology. Semin Pediatr Surg. 2012;21(1): 15-20.
16. Kurkure P, Vora A, Potdar M, et al. Can three drug chemotherapy for all stages of WILMS' tumor (WT) be practical compromise for lacunae in the optimum therapeutic planning in developing countries? SIOP XXXII meeting Abstracts O- 45. Med Pediatr Oncol. 2000;35:180.
17. Chantada G, Luna-Fineman S, Sitorus RS, et al. SIOP-PODC Graduated-Intensity Retinoblastoma Guidelines Writing Committee SIOP-PCDC recommendations for graduated-intensity treatment of retinoblastoma in developing countries. Pediatr Blood Cancer. 2013;60(5):719-27. doi: 10.1002/pbc.24468. Epub 2013 Jan 17.
18. Chantada GL, Qaddoumi I, Canturk S, et al. Strategies to manage retinoblastoma in developing countries. Pediatr Blood Cancer. 2011;56(3):341-8. doi: 10.1002/pbc.22843. Epub. 2010 Nov 11.
19. Agarwal B, Dalvi R. Treatment of childhood leukemias in underprivileged countries. In: Pui CH (Ed) Current Clinical Oncolgy: Treatment of acute leukemias: New directions for clinical research. Totowa; Humana Press Inc. NJ; 2004. pp. 321-9.
20. SIOP committee on standards of care and training in Pediatric Oncolgy. Requirements for the training of a pediatric hematologist-oncologist and recommendations for the organisation of a pediatric cancer unit (PCU). Amsterdam: SIOP; 1991.
21. Masera G, Spinetta JJ, Jankovic M, et al. Guidelines for a therapeutic alliance between families and staff: a report of the SIOP Working Committee on Psychosocial Issues in Pediatric Oncology. Med Pediatr Oncol. 1998;30(3):183-6.
22. Li FP, Myers MH, Heise HW, et al. The course of five-year survivors of cancer in childhood. J Pediatr. 1978;93(2):185-7.
23. Wallace WH, Blacklay A, Eiser C, et al. Late Effects Committee of the United Kingdom Children's Cancer Study Group (UKCCSG). Developing strategies for long term follow up of survivors of childhood cancer. BMJ. 2001;323:271-4.
24. Oeffinger KC, Hudson MM. Long-term complications following childhood and adolescent cancer: foundations for providing risk-based health care for survivors. CA Cancer J Clin. 2004;54(4): 208-36.
25. Hudson MM, Mertens AC, Yasui Y, et al. Health status of adult long-term survivors of childhood cancer: a report from the Childhood Cancer Survivor Study. JAMA. 2003;290:1583-92.
26. Kurkure PA, Achrekar S, Uparkar U, et al. Surviving Childhood Cancer: What next? Issue under consideration at the After Completion of Therapy (ACT) Clinic in India. Med Pediatric Oncology. 2003;41:588-9.
27. Kurkure P, Achrekar S, Dalvi N, et al. Childhood Cancer Survivors – Living Beyond Cure Indian J Pediatr. 2003;70(10):825-8.

59 Lymphomas in Children

Brijesh Arora, Vishal Sondhi

LYMPHOMAS IN CHILDREN

Lymphomas are the third most common group of cancers in children and adolescents after leukemias and brain tumors in west, accounting for 10–15% of newly diagnosed cancers in this age group. In India, lymphomas are the second most common malignancies in children ahead of central nervous system (CNS) tumors especially in males. Lymphomas are neoplasms of lymphocytes or their precursors which arise as a consequence of genetic aberrations that influence their proliferation, differentiation and ability to undergo apoptosis (or cell death). They usually present with distinct clinical syndromes reflecting the histological subtype. In the west, 60% of all childhood lymphomas are non-Hodgkin lymphomas (NHL) representing 3% of all childhood malignancies for children younger than 5 years and 8–9% in children and adolescents between 5 years and 19 years of age. Hodgkin lymphoma (HL) comprises approximately 5–7% of childhood cancers and 1% of all deaths.[1] However, HL exceeds NHL in India in contrast to west due to significantly higher incidence of HL in males in India. Both these major lymphoma subtypes have distinct origins, clinical presentations, biology, treatment approaches and outcome (Table 1) and hence are discussed separately in the following sections.

TABLE 1: Comparative clinical features of Hodgkin and non-Hodgkin lymphoma

Clinical feature	*Hodgkin's disease*	*Non-Hodgkin's lymphoma*
Nodal spread	Contiguous	Discontiguous
Localized	Yes	Rare
Extranodal disease	Rare	Common
Central nervous system (CNS) disease	Rare	Common
Bone marrow	Rare	Common
B-symptoms	Common	Uncommon
Abdominal disease	Uncommon	Common
Subtype based therapy	Not important	Crucial
Cure rates	85–95%	70–80%

Pediatric Hodgkin Lymphoma

Hodgkin lymphoma (formerly called Hodgkin's disease) is one of the few pediatric malignancies that shares aspects of its biology and natural history with its adult counterpart. With the currently available treatment modalities and the use of risk-adapted therapy, over 90% of children diagnosed with HL are long-term survivors. Hence, management designed to achieve maximal cure rates with the fewest late-effects of therapy is the current paradigm for HL in children (Fig. 1).

Epidemiology

In industrialized countries, HL presents with a bimodal distribution with regard to age, with a rise in incidence in young adults (20–34 years) and in the elderly (55–74 years).[2] In contrast, in low-income countries, there is trimodal distribution. There is an inverse relationship between the incidence of the HL in children and young adults within countries according to their economic development.[3] As many as 20–30% of childhood HL cases in developing countries occur before 5 years of age[4,5] against 5% in industrialized countries. Overall, there are three distinct forms of HL:

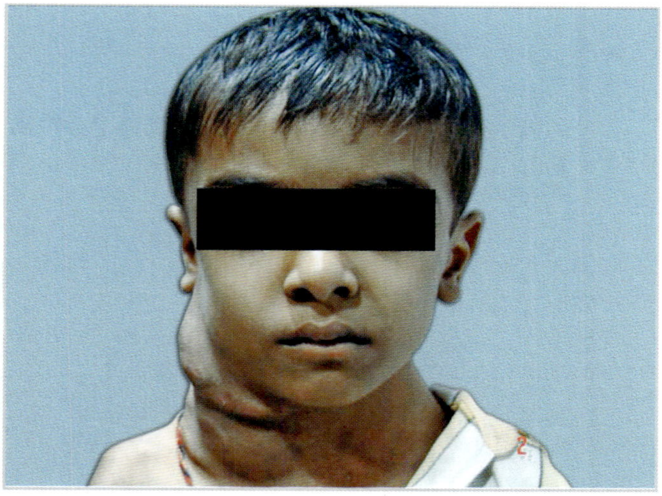

Fig. 1: Child with cervical lymphadenopathy, one of the several presentations of childhood lymphoma. The biopsy was suggestive of Hodgkin lymphoma

1. *Childhood form* (ages 14 years and younger): This type increases in prevalence in association with larger family size and lower socioeconomic status. Early exposure to common infections in early childhood infection appears to decrease the risk of HL, most likely by maturation of cellular immunity.[2]
2. *Young adult form* (ages 15–34 years): This is associated with a higher socioeconomic status in industrialized countries, increased number of siblings, and earlier birth order. Delayed EBV infection, particularly when associated with infectious mononucleosis, is a risk factor for the young adult form. It has been proposed that delayed exposure to a common infectious agent may also play a role in EBV-negative young-adult cases, although the identity of the agent has not been established.[6]
3. *Older adult form*: Most commonly presents in individuals aged 55–70 years.

The age standardized incidence of HL in Indian children ranges from 8.2 to 19.6 per million children per year compared to 5.7 in United States of America (USA) and 6.4 in Britain. Furthermore, mixed cellularity is most common phenotype in India (likely related to early childhood EBV exposure) leading to much younger age peak (median age 8–9 years) compared to 16–30 years in west where nodular sclerosis is most common.[7] Pediatric HL shows a significant male predominance in low-income countries including India (male: female ratios being 2.5:1 to 8:1) compared to ratio of about 1.5:1 in west.[8,9]

Etiology

The etiology of HL is believed to be multifactorial and may include the following:

Infectious agents: Several studies have documented a link between HL and EBV. EBV deoxyribonucleic acid (DNA) can be identified in tumor cells in approximately 50% of patients in the west and in more than 90% of patients in developing countries.[10] EBV positivity is most commonly observed in tumors with mixed-cellularity histology and in children younger than 10 years compared with adolescents and young adults. Patients with a prior history of infectious mononucleosis have a fourfold increased risk of developing EBV-positive HL.[11]

Genetic Predisposition: Clustering in families suggests a genetic predisposition, with an increased incidence observed among same-gender siblings, monozygotic twins, and parent-child pairs. Familial HL has been associated with specific human leukocyte antigens and accounts for 4.5% of all cases.

Immune Dysregulation: The increased susceptibility to HL in patients with T-cell immunodeficiency, human immunodeficiency virus (HIV) infection, or congenital immunodeficiency syndromes suggests a role for immune dysregulation in its development.

Environment: Clustering of cases in families or racial groups supports the idea of a common environmental link. At present, no conclusive association is recognized with common environmental factors other than EBV infection.

Biology

Hodgkin lymphoma is a B-lineage lymphoma. The malignant cells of HL are clonal Hodgkin/Reed-Sternberg (HRS) cells or lymphocytic and histiocytic (L and H) cells and their morphologic variants, which usually constitute less than 1% of the cells in involved lymph nodes. Characteristic Reed-Sternberg (RS) cells are binucleate or multinucleate giant cells with prominent nucleoli and abundant cytoplasm. The rest of the lymph node contains a variable cellular infiltrate consisting of lymphocytes, eosinophils, macrophages, plasma cells, and fibroblasts. These infiltrating cells secrete an array of cytokines and chemokines, which are important for HRS cell survival and maintenance of the characteristic cellular infiltrate. These malignant cells have three distinct origins. In nodular lymphocyte predominant HL, the tumors cells (L and H) derive from germinal center (GC) or post-GC B-cells and retain expression of all B-cell specific antigens. In classical HL, HRS cells are GC B-cells but have crippling mutations that destroy the coding capacity of their functional IGV gene rearrangements. In a minority (2%) of classical HL cases, HRS cells display a cytotoxic T-lymphoid phenotype.

In EBV-positive HL, EBV-encoding genes play a role in preventing apoptosis. Latent membrane protein-1 (LMP-1) expressed in EBV-positive HRS cells mimics an activated CD40 receptor, activating the antiapoptotic nuclear factor-kappa-B (NF-κB) pathway. A paracrine activation of NF-κB in HL is observed; both HRS cells and the surrounding supporting cells produce cytokines that upregulate several members of the tumor necrosis factor (TNF) receptor superfamily, including CD30, CD40, or EBV LMP-1. The production of the ligand for these receptors is responsible for the phosphorylation and translocation to the nucleus of NF-κB. The constitutive translocation of NF-κB to the nucleus of HRS cells is essential for the malignant transformation of HRS cells. It leads to inhibition of apoptosis, proliferation, and secretion of proinflammatory cytokines.[12]

Pathologic Classification

The current World Health Organization (WHO) classification classifies HL in two broad types based on both morphologic appearance as well as immunophenotypic characterization including type of neoplastic cells, inflammatory milieu and overall growth pattern as detailed below.[13]

Classical Hodgkin Lymphoma

The hallmark of classic HL is the RS cells and their mononuclear (Hodgkin cells) and multinucleate variants which lack the immunophenotypic evidence of B-cell differentiation. RS cells almost always express CD30, and approximately 70% of patients express CD15. CD20 is expressed in approximately 6–10% of cases, and generally RS cells do not express B-cell antigens such as CD45, CD19 and CD79A.

The classical HL is subclassified into four subtypes according to the number of RS cells, characteristics of the inflammatory milieu, and the presence or absence of fibrosis. The histologic features and clinical symptoms of HL have been attributed to the numerous cytokines secreted by the RS cells, which include interleukin-1, interleukin-6, and tumor necrosis factor. Classical HL subtypes as detailed in the Table 2.

Nodular Lymphocyte-Predominant Hodgkin Lymphoma

This pathologic class of HL is characterized by large cells with multilobed nuclei, referred to as popcorn cells. These cells express B-cell antigens, such as CD19, CD20, CD22 and CD79A, are negative for CD15 and may or may not express CD30. The OCT-2 and BOB-1 oncogenes are both expressed unlike classical HL. Nodular lymphocyte-predominant HL (NLPHL) is most common in males younger than 10 years and constitutes 5–10% of all HL cases. Patients with NLPHL generally present with slow growing, localized, nonbulky disease usually in axilla and inguinal regions without any B symptoms.

Presenting Symptoms and Signs

Huntington's disease (HD) has an insidious onset. The most frequent presentation in up to 80% of patients is painless cervical or supraclavicular lymphadenopathy, of which 60% have asymptomatic involvement of the mediastinum. Enlarged nodes are generally firm and have a rubbery texture. Constitutional or class "B" symptoms such as fever, night sweats, and weight loss are more common with advanced disease (stage I-5%, stage IV-81%) and are associated with a poorer outcome. Approximately,

TABLE 2: Histopathologic classification of classical Hodgkin lymphoma

	WHO subgroups	*Distinctive features*	*Relative frequency (%)*
1.	Lymphocyte rich (LR)	Benign appearing lymphocytes with or without histiocytes. Few Reed-Sternberg (RS) cells No fibrosis	10–15
2.	Nodular sclerosis (NS)	Thickened capsule with proliferation of orderly collagenous bands that divide lymphoid tissue in nodules: lacunar variant of RS cells	20–50
3.	Mixed cellularity* (MC)	5–15 RS cells per high power field. Fine fibrosis in interstitium. Focal necrosis may be present	20–40
4.	Lymphocyte depletion (LD)	Abnormal cells with relative paucity of lymphocytes. Fibrosis and necrosis common but diffuse	5–16

*Most common in developing countries and in children.

20% of patients have bulky adenopathy. Fifteen to twenty percent of patients have noncontiguous extranodal involvement (stage IV) of lung, liver, bones, and bone marrow. A reduced cell mediated immunity results in an increase susceptibility to infections (See Fig. 2).[14-19]

Evaluation of a Patient

- History and physical examination.
- Complete blood count.
- Liver and renal function tests, serum lactic dehydrogenase (LDH), serum albumin.
- *Lymph node biopsy*: The least invasive procedure should be used to establish the diagnosis of lymphoma by biopsy of one or more peripheral lymph nodes. Fine needle aspiration cytology alone is not recommended because of the lack of stromal tissue, the small number of cells present in the specimen, and the difficulty of classifying HL into one of the subtypes.
- *Bone marrow aspiration and biopsy*: This is done in patients with advanced disease (III/IV), B-symptoms, bony involvement or abnormal counts. Recently, with the advent of positron emission tomography-computed tomography (PET-CT) scans, which is highly sensitive for bone marrow involvement, bone marrow biopsy is considered mandatory only in ambiguous cases.
- *Radiological studies*: Chest X-ray, CT scan of neck, chest and abdomen and pelvis, should be obtained. Contiguous nodal clustering or matting, focal mass lesion in a visceral organ, size on long axis of 2 cm or greater or between 1 cm and 2 cm with other suggestive clinical features favors lymphomatous involvement. Bulky peripheral (nonmediastinal) lymphadenopathy is generally accepted as aggregate nodal masses exceeding 5–6 cm and bulky mediastinal mass as a transverse mediastinal diameter over one-third of the maximum intrathoracic diameter on an upright posterior-anterior (PA) chest radiograph.
- *Positron emission tomography (PET) scan of the whole body*: PET scanning may identify more sites of initial disease than conventional imaging and is more accurate in detecting viable HL in post-therapy residual masses. In recent studies, PET findings resulted in a change in staging in more than 50% of patients and subsequent adjustments in involved-field radiation therapy (RT) treatment volumes in 70% of patients. Concordance between PET and CT is generally high for nodal regions, but lower for extranodal sites such as spleen, lung nodules, bone/bone marrow, and pleural and pericardial effusions. Rapid early response documented by significant reduction in disease volume and PET negativity at an early stage (after one or two cycles of chemotherapy) is associated with a favorable outcome. PET scanning should be performed at baseline and a minimum of 3 weeks postchemotherapy completion and 8–12 after radiotherapy.[20-22]

Staging, prognostic factors and risk stratification: Current HL staging is based on Cotswolds modification of Ann Arbor staging proposed in 1998 (Table 3). Studies have attempted to use prognostic factors to delineate a group of

TABLE 3: Modified Ann Arbor classification of Hodgkin lymphoma

Stage	*Description*
I	Involvement of single lymph node region (I) or of a single extralymphatic organ or site (I_E) by direct extention
II	Involvement of two or more lymph node regions on the same side of diaphragm or localized involvement of an extra-lymphatic organ or site and of one or more lymph node regions on the same side of the diaphragm (IIE)
III_1	Involvement of lymph node regions on both sides of the diaphragm Abdominal disease is limited to the upper abdomen (i.e. spleen, splenic hilum nodes, celiac nodes, porta hepatis nodes)
III_2	Involvement of lymph node regions on both sides of the diaphragm Abdominal disease includes para-aortic, mesenteric, and iliac involvement with or without disease in the upper abdomen
IV	Disseminated involvement of one or more extralymphatic organs or tissues with or without associated lymph node disease
A	No symptoms
B	Fever, night sweats, or weight loss of more than 10% of body weight in the previous 6 months
X	Bulky disease (greater than 10 cm in maximum dimension; greater than one-third of the internal transverse diameter of the thorax at the level T5/T6
E	Limited involvement of a single extranodal site
CS	Clinical stage: When based solely on physical examination and imaging technique
PS	Pathologic stage: When based on biopsies

patients at high risk for first relapse, who may benefit from more intensive initial therapy. Similarly, such factors may be able to identify a group of patients with an extremely low risk of relapse for whom therapy may be minimized. Different clinical trial groups have established various risk categorizations as outlined in Table 4. In general, these incorporate stage of disease, disease bulk, and systemic (B) symptoms.[23-26]

Treatment

The treatment of HL in children requires a careful balance to maximize treatment efficacy and minimize risks for late toxicity associated with both RT and chemotherapy. The treatment paradigm for childhood HL is risk, gender and response adapted use of non-cross-resistant combination chemotherapy with or without low-dose involved field RT.

Combined Modality Therapy in Children with Hodgkin Lymphoma

A number of randomized clinical trials have investigated the benefit of adding chemotherapy to RT in the treatment of HL. While the RT acts to control known sites of tumor, the chemotherapy is aimed at occult disease outside the radiation field. The judicious combination of the two modalities allows for a decrease in the dose and size of the radiation field used and a reduction in the intensity or duration of chemotherapy below toxicity thresholds that would not be possible if single modality chemotherapy or RT were used, thus decreasing overall acute and late toxicities. The use of RT in pediatric HL permits reduction in dose-related toxicity of anthracyclines, alkylating agents, and bleomycin that may preserve cardiopulmonary as well as gonadal function and reduce the risk of secondary leukemia. Combined modality therapy, compared with chemotherapy alone, produces a superior event-free survival (EFS) and has become the preferred initial therapy for children with HL.[27]

Chemotherapy Regimens in Children with Hodgkin Lymphoma

Contemporary chemotherapy regimens in HL combine non-cross-resistant agents wherein each agent is individually active against tumor but targets different cellular events to prevent drug-resistance and have nonoverlapping toxicities, which allow delivery of each agent at full dose which are detailed in Table 5. All of the agents in original MOPP [mechlorethamine, oncovin (vincristine), procarbazine and prednisone] and ABVD (adriamycin, bleomycin, vinblastine and dacarbazine) regimens continue to be used in contemporary pediatric treatment regimens. However, COPP (cyclophosphamide, vincristine, procarbazine and prednisone) with less

TABLE 4: Prognostic factors and risk stratification in pediatric Hodgkin lymphoma

Study group/trial	*Low risk*	*Intermediate risk*	*High risk*
Children's oncology group	• IA/IIA no bulk or extranodal extension	• IA bulk or "E" extension • IB • IIA bulk or "E" extension • IIB • IIIA • IVA	• IIIB, IVB
German studies/Euronet PHL	• IA/B • IIA	• IIB • IIEA • IIIA	• IIEB • IIIEA/B • IIIB • IV
St Jude/Stanford/Dana Farber†	• IA/IIA no bulk	• IA bulk • IB • IIA bulk • IIB • III • IV	
Children's Cancer Group 5942	• IA/B patients no adverse features* • IIA patients no adverse features*	• IA/B patients with adverse features* • IIA patients with adverse features* • IIB • IIIA/B	• IV

*Adverse factors include hilar lymphadenopathy, more than four sites of nodal disease, or bulky disease.

†Patients categorized as favorable or unfavorable risk.

TABLE 5: Contemporary chemotherapy regimens for children with Hodgkin lymphoma

Name	Drugs
COPP	Cyclophosphamide, vincristine (oncovin), procarbazine, prednisone
COPDAC	Dacarbazine substituted for procarbazine in COPP
OPPA	Vincristine (oncovin), procarbazine, prednisone, doxorubicin (adriamycin)
OEPA	Vincristine (oncovin), etoposide, prednisone, doxorubicin (adriamycin)
ABVD	Doxorubicin (adriamycin), bleomycin, vinblastine, dacarbazine
COPP/ ABV	Cyclophosphamide, vincristine (oncovin), procarbazine, prednisone, doxorubicin (adriamycin), bleomycin, vinblastine
VAMP	Vinblastine, doxorubicin (adriamycin), methotrexate, prednisone
DBVE	Doxorubicin, bleomycin, vincristine (oncovin), etoposide
ABVE-PC	Doxorubicin (adriamycin), bleomycin, vincristine (oncovin), etoposide-prednisone, cyclophosphamide
BEACOPP	Bleomycin, etoposide, doxorubicin (adriamycin), cyclophosphamide, vincristine (oncovin), prednisone, procarbazine

leukemogenic and gonadotoxic potential (substituting cyclophosphamide for mechlorethamine) has replaced MOPP as the preferred alkylator regimen. In contrast to adult HL, pediatric chemotherapy approaches have focused on two unique strategies:

Avoidance of late toxicity: Non-cross-resistant regimen like ABVD has demonstrated superior efficacy (i.e. freedom from progression) and less toxicity when compared with MOPP in adults with HL.[28] However, due to cardiac and pulmonary toxicity of ABVD in children, many investigators have evaluated regimens either devoid of anthracyclines, alkylators and/or bleomycin such as VAMP (vinblastine, adriamycin, methotrexate, prednisone) (St. Jude), VBVP (vinblastine, bleomycin, etoposide (VP16) and prednisone) (French MDH-90 study) or hybrid regimens that utilize lower total cumulative doses of alkylators, doxorubicin, and bleomycin such as COPP/ABV (adriamycin, bleomycin, vinblastine) [Children's Cancer Group (CCG)] or ABVE-PC (adriamycin, bleomycin, vinblastine, etoposide-prednisone, cyclophosphamide) [Pediatric Oncology Group (POG)]. VAMP like less-toxic regimens can be safely used in favorable risk HL but not in intermediate or high risk HL.[29]

Gender adaptation: In an effort to decrease risk for male infertility, etoposide has been substituted for procarbazine in the initial courses of therapy in studies of the German pediatric HL group (OEPA) and POG [doxorubicin, bleomycin, vincristine and etoposide (DBVE) and DBVE-PC (prednisone, cyclophosphamide)][30] and dacarbazine [COPDAC (Dacarbazine substituted for procarbazine in COPP] has been used to replace procarbazine (COPP) with preservation of efficacy and minimization of infertility.[31]

Radiotherapy

Consolidative RT after risk-adapted chemotherapy is an integral part of treatment of children with HL.[27] Radiation has been used as an adjunct to multiagent chemotherapy in intermediate/high-risk pediatric HL with the goal of reducing risk of relapse in initially involved sites and preventing toxicity associated with second-line therapy. Compared with chemotherapy alone, adjuvant radiation produces superior EFS for children with intermediate/high-risk HL who achieve a complete remission (CR) to multiagent chemotherapy, but it does not affect overall survival (OS) because of the success of second-line therapy.[29,30] Since, adjuvant RT may be associated with excess late effects or mortality; there has been a movement to decrease the field of radiation as well as dose of RT in order to limit toxicities while maintaining survival rates.

Radiation Dose and Volume

Doses of 15–25 Gy are typically used with modifications based on patient age, the presence of bulky or residual (postchemotherapy) disease, and normal tissue concerns.[26] Some protocols prescribe a boost of 5 Gy in regions with suboptimal response to chemotherapy. Involved field RT (IFRT) is the current standard of care in children in place of total nodal RT. IFRT treats the clinically involved region(s), with coverage of the whole nodal region but accounts for tumor regression with chemotherapy and avoids extensive inclusion of uninvolved regions. While CT-based two-dimensional RT remains the standard technique for radiation delivery, three-dimensional conformal RT (3-D CRT) or intensity-modulated RT (IMRT) are often used in situations where the more conformal techniques would reduce dose to surrounding normal critical structures.

Response-Adapted Therapy

Response to therapy is one of the most robust prognostic factors in HL as in many other pediatric tumors. The concept of tailoring the extent as well as dose of radiotherapy and duration of chemotherapy based on response to therapy in HL is the focus of many recent and future trials. In patients with early stage favorable risk HL, recent studies[32,33] [COG-9542, German Society of Pediatric Oncology and Hematology-Hodgkin Lymphoma Trial 95 (GPOH-HD95) and EuroNet Pediatric Hodgkin's Lymphoma (PHL) C-1] have shown that RT can be safely avoided in patients who achieve complete response (CR) after initial chemotherapy. However, omission of RT was found to be detrimental in intermediate and high-risk subgroups except in a recent North American Study (COG AHOD0031) which showed that RT can be avoided in intermediate risk patients with rapid early response.[34]

In advanced HL, a recent POG study (P9425) has shown that in rapid early responders to a dose dense chemotherapy, further chemotherapy can be safely curtailed. In this study, 216 children with intermediate or high-risk HL received ABVE-PC every 21 days. Rapid early responders [(RERs), 63% of patients)] to three cycles received 21 Gy RT to involved regions. Slow early responders received two additional cycles before 21 Gy radiation.[35] Five-year EFS was 86% for the RER and 83% for the slow early responders (P = 0.85). Five-year OS was 95%. Similarly, CCG evaluated response-adapted therapy featuring four cycles of the dose-intensive BEACOPP [bleomycin, etoposide, doxorubicin (adriamycin), cyclophosphamide, vincristine (oncovin), prednisone, procarbazine] regimen followed by a gender-tailored consolidation for pediatric patients with high-risk HL. For rapid early responding girls, an additional four courses of COPP/ABV (without IFRT) was given in an effort to reduce breast cancer risk. RER boys received two cycles of ABVD followed by IFRT. Slow early responders received four additional courses of BEACOPP and IFRT. RER was achieved by 74% of patients after four BEACOPP cycles and 5-year EFS among the cohort was 94%.[36]

Recommendations for Treatment of Pediatric Hodgkin Lymphoma

Treatment of low-risk classical Hodgkin lymphoma: The preferred treatment option for early stage, favorable prognosis HL (stages I–IIA; no bulky disease; no B symptoms, less than four sites of disease) is combined modality treatment including hybrid chemotherapy with less or no alkylators and anthracyclines (VAMP/VBVP/OPPA OEPA or equivalent) for two to four cycles with or without low-dose IFRT of 15–25 Gy. IFRT can be safely avoided in children who achieve CR after initial chemotherapy in some regimens (Table 6).[29-31]

Treatment of intermediate-risk classical Hodgkin lymphoma: Patients with intermediate risk HL (all stage I and stage II patients not classified as early stage; stage IIIA) children require 3–6 cycles of dose-intense alkylator based chemotherapy followed by low-dose IFRT. In some studies, chemotherapy is given to maximal tumor response on imaging followed by two additional cycles of consolidation chemotherapy and limited RT (Table 6). The patients with RER may be treated with less number of chemotherapy cycles as shown in the recent studies (POG 9425)[35] or may not require RT (COG-AHOD0031).[34]

Treatment of high-risk classical Hodgkin lymphoma: Children with high-risk (Stages IIIB, IV) HL require 6–8 cycles of dose-intense alkylator based chemotherapy regimens followed by low-dose IFRT (Table 6).[26] Current trials for patients with intermediate/high-risk HL are testing if chemotherapy and RT can be limited in patients who achieve a rapid early response to dose-intensive chemotherapy regimens.

Treatment of nodular lymphocyte-predominant Hodgkin lymphoma: NLPHL, an uncommon subtype, represents a more indolent disease than classical HL, and is therefore managed differently. Generally, patients with stage I/II NLPHL without B symptoms are treated with less intensive therapy than patients with classical HL. Recent studies are evaluating chemotherapy alone or observation without treatment following excision in children with stage I NLPHL. The OS in most series is 100%, with lower progression-free survival (PFS) and EFS in series with surgery alone (67–82%)[37,38] or with CVP (cyclophosphamide, vincristine, prednisone) chemotherapy (74%).[39] In contrast, patients with stage III/IV are treated in a similar fashion to patients with classical HL with modest intensity chemotherapy regimens, some without anthracyclines, with or without IFRT. Given the indolent nature of NLPHL and substantial deaths observed related to complications from cytotoxic therapy, several pediatric study groups are examining treatment de-escalation.[37,40,41]

Relapsed or refractory disease: Most relapses in children with HL occur in first 3 years. Treatment and prognosis after relapse depends upon the timing of relapse, the initial stage of disease, and the initial treatment given. Also, presence of B symptoms, extranodal disease and inadequate response to second-line therapy portend poor prognosis. Relapsed patients may be classified in two groups for prognostication and treatment planning:

Low-risk (favorable) group: Children with localized late relapse (≥12 months after completing therapy) after limited risk-adapted therapy or with chemotherapy alone and/or IFRT have a high likelihood of achieving long-term survival following treatment with more intensive conventional chemotherapy alone. Intensive non-cross-

TABLE 6: Risk-adapted treatment of newly diagnosed Hodgkin lymphoma in children

Risk group	*5 years EFS*	*5 years OS*
Low risk disease		
Four cycles of VAMP with LD-IFRT (if not in CR after two cycles) or without IFRT (if in CR post two cycles)	92%	98%
Four cycles of COP/ABV plus LD-IFRT		
ABVE, administered for two to four courses depending on response, followed by LD-IFRT		
Two cycles of OEPA or OPPA with LD-IFRT (if not in CR after two cycles) or without IFRT (if in CR post two cycles)		
Intermediate risk disease		
Six cycles of COPP/ABV plus LD-IFRT	85%	95%
ABVE-PC, administered for three to five courses depending upon response, with or without LD-IFRT		
Two cycles of OPPA (for males) or OEPA (for females), followed by two cycles of COPP (for females) or COPDAC (for males) plus LD-IFRT		
High-risk disease		
ABVE-PC, administered for three to five courses depending upon response, followed by LD-IFRT	83%	94%
Two cycles of OPPA (for males) or OEPA (for females), followed by four cycles of COPP (for females) or COPDAC (for males) plus LD-IFRT		
Two cycles of cytarabine/etoposide, COPP/ABV, and CHOP plus LD-IFRT		
Four cycles of BEACOPP with subsequent dependent upon response; rapid responders: four cycles of COPP/ABV without IFRT (for females) or two cycles ABVD with IFRT (for males); slow responders: four additional cycles of BEACOPP plus IFRT		

Abbreviations: EFS: event-free survival; OS: overall survival; VAMP: vinblastine, adriamycin, methotrexate, prednisone; LD-IFRT: low-dose-involved-field radiation therapy; CR: complete remission; COP: cyclophosphamide, vincristine (oncovin), procarbazine; ABV: adriamycin, bleomycin, vinblastine; ABVE: adriamycin, bleomycin, vinblastine, etoposide; OEPA: vincristine (oncovin), etoposide, prednisone, doxorubicin (adriamycin); OPPA: vincristine (oncovin), procarbazine, prednisone, doxorubicin (adriamycin); COPP: cyclophosphamide, vincristine (oncovin), procarbazine, prednisone; ABVE-PC: doxorubicin (adriamycin), bleomycin, vincristine (oncovin), etoposide-prednisone, cyclophosphamide; COPDAC: dacarbazine substituted for procarbazine in COPP; CHOP: cyclophosphamide, hydroxydaunorubicin, oncovin, prednisone; DEACOPP: bleomycin, etoposide, doxorubicin (adriamycin), cyclophosphamide, vincristine (oncovin), prednisone, procarbazine.

resistant regimens using agents not part of initial treatment such as cytarabine at moderate or high doses, carboplatin and cisplatin, ifosfamide, etoposide, vinorelbine, gemcitabine, and vinblastine are used. Approximately, two-thirds of these patients may be salvaged with second line chemotherapy.

High-risk group: Children who develop relapse within 1 year after completing therapy require aggressive salvage chemotherapy and consolidation with autologous hematopoietic cell transplantation (HSCT) with survival rates ranging between 45% and 70%.[42,43] Salvage rates for patients with primary refractory HL are poor even with autologous HCT and range from 20% to 40%. Patients who fail autologous HCT or for patients with chemoresistant disease, allogeneic HCT has been used with encouraging results. Brentuximab vedotin (Anti-CD30 monoclonal antibody) has been evaluated in adults with relapsed/refractory HL and has shown promising response rates of 50–70% in recent phase-I/II studies.

Follow-Up and Late Effects

Current 5-year relative survival for HL is approximately 90% with higher rates reported in younger populations.[44] However, emergence of late toxicity among survivors can limit long-term survival and affect quality of life. Mortality in the first 15 years after diagnosis relates to the primary disease and following that to second cancers [second malignant neoplasms (SMNs)] and cardiovascular disease (CVD).[45] Hence, children treated with HL should be closely followed for relapse as well as late effects. Imaging is not recommended for routine follow-up, as recent studies have shown that most relapses can be detected based on symptoms, laboratory, or physical findings without any incremental value of imaging.[46]

Hodgkin lymphoma survivors continue to be at risk of treatment related mortality for decades beyond their initial disease. In a recent study of morbidity and mortality risks among 2,742 survivors of HL in the USA, substantial excess absolute risk of mortality per 10,000 person-years was identified: overall 95.5; death due to HL-38.3, SMNs-23.9, and CVD-13.1.[47] Commonly, adverse treatment effects may impact musculoskeletal development, endocrine, reproductive, cardiovascular and pulmonary function and risk of secondary carcinogenesis. Adverse effects have reduced over time with use of risk-adapted less toxic chemotherapy and low-dose radiotherapy.

Conclusion

Pediatric HL is currently one of the most curable childhood malignancies with more than 90% cure rates in recent studies. Risk and response-adapted combined modality therapy is the current standard of care and is stratified based on disease stage and the presence of adverse prognostic factors. Long-term follow-up of pediatric HL patients should take place in a comprehensive pediatric oncology center, where late complications can be anticipated, monitored, and treated. Recent trials are exploring to reduce toxicities of treatment with the selective elimination of radiotherapy, devising less toxic chemotherapy regimens and assessing the role of functional imaging with PET in assessing response and predicting outcome.

Pediatric Non-Hodgkin Lymphoma

Non-Hodgkin lymphoma is neoplasm of a wide range of cell types that comprise the immune system. NHL are generalized diseases from the outset and have patterns of spread that mimic the migration patterns of their normal cellular counterparts. NHL accounts for approximately 7% of cancers in children less than 20 years of age. Approximately 2,500 cases of childhood NHL are estimated to occur annually in India. NHL occurs most commonly in the second decade of life, and occurs less frequently in children younger than 3 years. Immunodeficiency, both congenital (e.g. Ataxia-telangiectasia, Wiskott-Aldrich syndrome) and acquired (HIV infection or post-transplant), increases the risk of NHL. EBV been shown to transform human B-cells in immunocompromised hosts. Indeed, NHL is the most frequent malignancy in children with acquired immunodeficiency syndrome (AIDS). With current treatments, about 80% of children and adolescents with NHL will survive at least 5 years.[48-49]

Classification and Clinical Presentation (Table 7)

In children, NHL is distinct from the more common forms of lymphoma observed in adults. While lymphomas in adults are more commonly low or intermediate grade, are dominantly nodal, have variable growth fraction and poor long-term outcome; almost all NHL that occurs in children is high grade, extranodal, has higher growth fraction and good outcome.

Non-Hodgkin lymphomas of childhood currently fall into three therapeutically relevant categories: (1) B-cell NHL [Burkitt lymphoma/leukemia (BLL) and diffuse large B-cell lymphoma (DLBCL)]; (2) lymphoblastic lymphoma (LL); primarily precursor T-cell lymphoma and less frequently, precursor B-cell lymphoma); and (3) anaplastic large cell lymphoma (ALCL); T-cell or null-cell lymphomas. Each type of childhood NHL is associated with distinctive clinical presentation, immunophenotype and molecular biological characteristics (Table 7). In India, the estimated incidence is between 6 and 10/million/year with an almost equal distribution of B- and T-cell tumors. Distribution of NHL subtypes among children and adolescents in India differs from the rest of the world,

TABLE 7: Major biologic subgroups in childhood non-Hodgkin lymphomas (NHL)

Histology	*Immunology*	*Clinical features*	*Cytogenetics*
Burkitt and Burkitt-like	B-cell	Abdominal masses, gastrointestinal stromal (GIT) tumors, Waldeyer's ring	t(8;14)(q24;q32) t(2;8)(p11;q24) t(8;22)(q24;q11)
Diffuse large B-cell lymphoma (DLBCL) Primary mediastinal DLBCL	B-cells (germinal center or postgerminal center) B-cells (medullary thymus)	Abdominal masses, GIT tumors, Waldeyer's ring Mediastinum	t(8;14)(q24;q32) t(2;17)(p23;q23)
Anaplastic large cell	T-cell, null cell or natural killer (NK) cell (CD30$^+$)	Skin, nodes, bone, lung	t (2;5) (p23;q35) t (1;2) (q21;p23) t (2;3) (p23;q21)
Precursor T-lymphoblastic	T-cell	Anterior mediastinal mass	t (1;14) (p32;q11) t (11;14) (p13;q11) t (10;14) (q24;q11) t (7;19) (q35;p13)
Precursor B-lymphoblastic	B-cell precursors	Skin, lymph node	

namely a higher prevalence of DLBCL and LL and a lower frequency of BLL.[50]

Clinical Features

Burkitt Lymphoma

Burkitt lymphoma accounts for about 50% of childhood NHL and exhibits consistent, aggressive clinical behavior. The malignant cells show a mature B-cell phenotype and tumor has "starry sky" appearance. Burkitt lymphoma expresses a characteristic chromosomal translocation, usually t(8;14) and more rarely t(8;22) or t(2;8). Each of these translocations juxtaposes the c-Myc gene to immunoglobulin locus regulatory elements, resulting in the inappropriate expression of c-Myc, the gene involved in cellular proliferation. The two most common primary sites of disease are the abdomen and head-neck region. In India, these patients usually present with abdominal pain, vomiting, abdominal distension, palpable mass, intussusception, ascites, obstructive jaundice or hepatosplenomegaly (sporadic presentation). Endemic Burkitt lymphoma is common in Africa, presents as jaw mass in majority of cases and is usually associated with EBV infection. Other sites of involvement include testes, bone, peripheral lymph nodes, skin, bone marrow, and CNS (Figs 2 to 4).[48,51]

Diffuse Large B-Cell Lymphoma

It is a mature B-cell neoplasm that represents 10% to 20% of pediatric NHL. DLBCL occurs more frequently during the second decade of life than during the first. Pediatric DLBCL may present clinically similar to Burkitt, though it is more often localized and less often involves the bone marrow or CNS. Outcomes for children with DLBCL are more favorable than those observed in adults, with overall 5-year EFS rates of approximately 90% at 5 years. About 20% of pediatric DLBCL present as primary mediastinal disease [primary mediastinal B-cell lymphoma (PMBCL)]. This presentation is more common in older children and adolescents and is associated with an inferior outcome compared with other pediatric DLBCL (Fig. 5).[48,51]

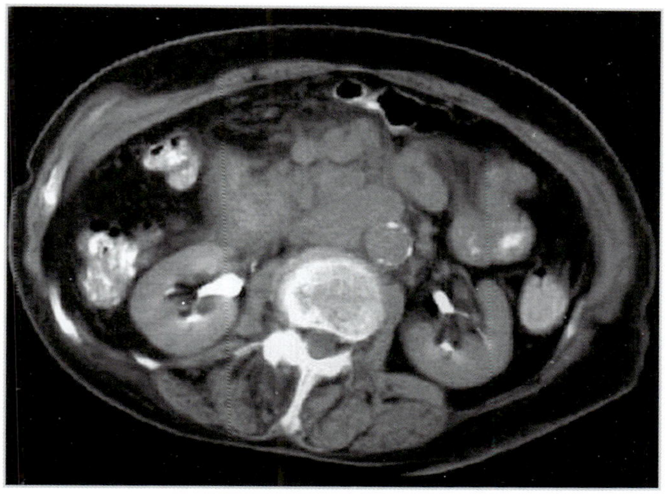

Fig. 3: Computed tomography (CT) scan of the abdomen and pelvis showing a retroperitoneal mass. The final diagnosis was Burkitt's lymphoma

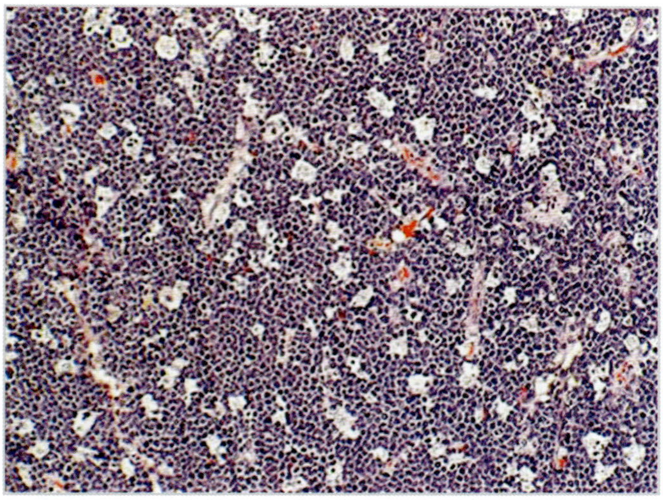

Fig. 2: Burkitt's lymphoma: Diffuse pattern comprising of immature, intermediate size round cells with high nuclear cytoplasmic ratio and prominent cytoplasmic vacuoles with many scattered histiocytes giving a classic "starry sky" appearance

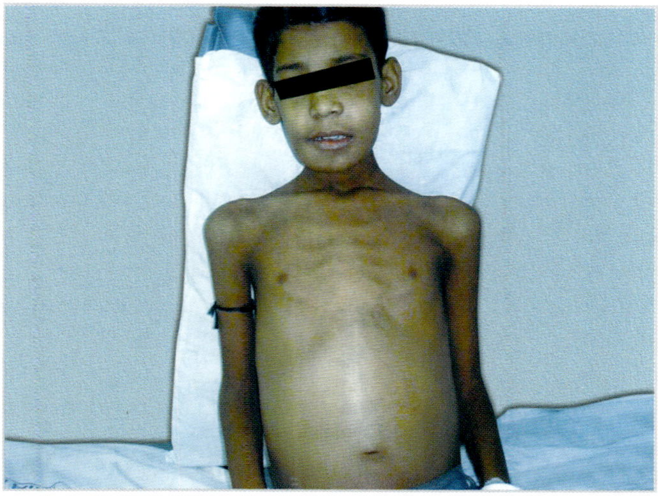

Fig. 4: Burkitt's lymphoma: A 10-year-old malnourished child with right jaw as well as abdominal lymph node and mesentric masses with ascites

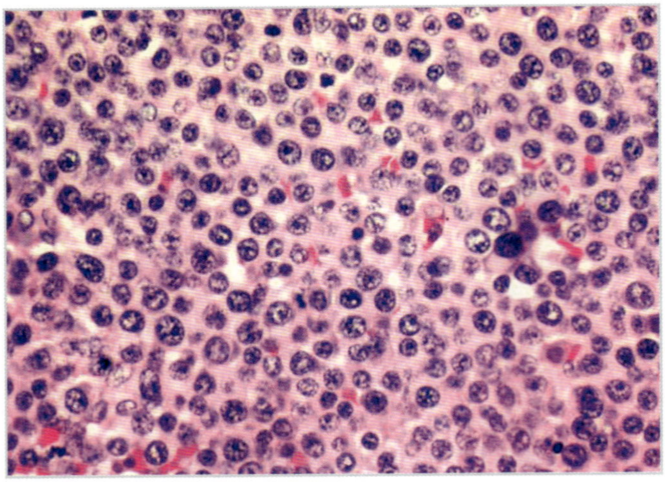

Fig. 5: Diffuse large cell lymphoma: Scattered large cells seen amidst a population of normal looking lymphocytes

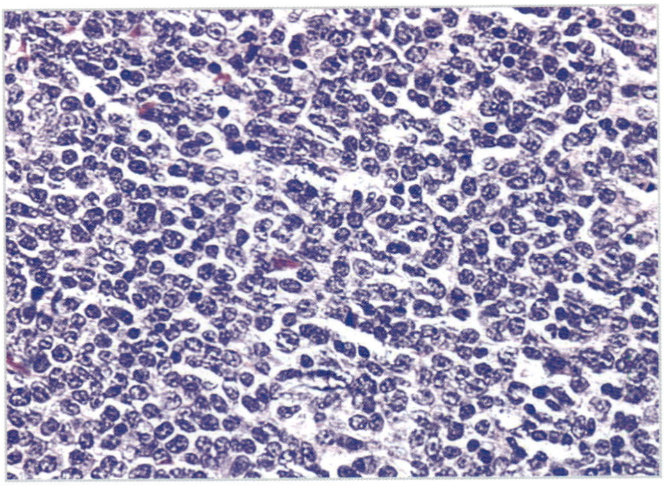

Fig. 6: Lymphoblastic lymphoma: Diffuse pattern with lymphoid blasts having a large nucleus, scanty cytoplasm and fine nuclear chromatin

Lymphoblastic Lymphoma

Lymphoblastic lymphoma makes up approximately 20% of childhood NHL. More than 75% of LLs have a T-cell immunophenotype and the remainder has a precursor B-cell phenotype.

Nearly 75% of patients with LL present with anterior mediastinal mass, and symptoms of dyspnea, wheezing, stridor, dysphagia, or swelling of the head and neck suggestive of superior vena cava syndrome (SVCS). Pleural effusions may be present, and the involvement of lymph nodes, usually above the diaphragm, may be a prominent feature. There may also be involvement of bone, skin, bone marrow, CNS, abdominal organs (but rarely bowel), and occasionally other sites such as lymphoid tissue of Waldeyer ring and testes. Patients with more than 25% marrow blasts are considered to have leukemia, and those with fewer than 25% marrow blasts are considered to have lymphoma (Figs 6 and 7).[48,51]

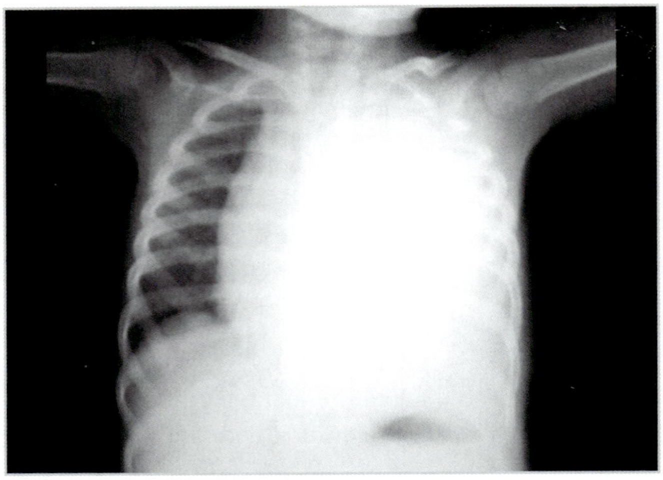

Fig. 7: Chest X-ray posterior-anterior (PA) view showing a large mediastinal mass in a child with superior vena cava (SVC) syndrome. The final diagnosis was lymphoblastic lymphoma

Anaplastic Large Cell Lymphoma

Anaplastic large cell lymphoma accounts for approximately 10% of childhood NHL. While the predominant immunophenotype of ALCL is mature T-cell; null-cell disease (i.e. no T-cell, B-cell, or NK-cell surface antigen expression) does occur. More than 90% of ALCL cases have the translocation t(2;5)(p23;q35) leading to the expression of the fusion protein nucleophosmin (NPM)/anaplastic lymphoma kinase (ALK). Clinically, ALCL has a broad range of presentations, including involvement of lymph nodes and a variety of extranodal sites, particularly skin, bone, gastrointestinal tract, lung, pleura, and muscle. Involvement of the CNS and bone marrow is uncommon. ALCL is often associated with systemic symptoms (e.g. fever, weight loss) and a prolonged waxing and waning course, making diagnosis difficult and often delayed (Fig. 8).[48,51]

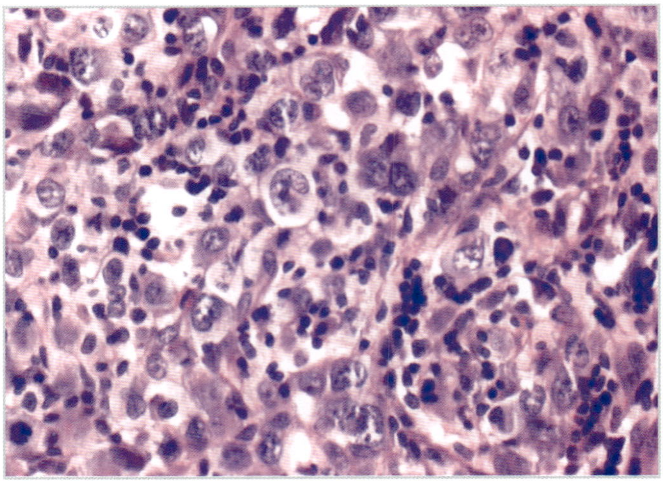

Fig. 8: Anaplastic large cell lymphoma: Large pleomorphic cells with horse shoe shaped and multiple nuclei

Rare Lymphomas in Children

Indolent mature B-cell lymphomas are rare in children but follicular lymphoma (FL) and nodal marginal zone lymphoma [or mucosa-associated lymphoid tissue (MALT)] have been described and accepted by WHO as unique entities. Pediatric FL predominantly occurs as cervical adenopathy and tonsillar enlargement generally in males, and is more likely to be localized disease. It can rarely involve extranodal sites such as the testis, kidney, gastrointestinal tract, and parotid. The outcome of pediatric FL is excellent. MALT lymphomas present as low-stage (stage I or II) disease both in nodal and extranodal sites such as stomach (associated with *Helicobacter pylori* infection) and conjunctiva (associated with *Chlamydia, psittaci* infections).[51-53]

Evaluation of Children with Non-Hodgkin Lymphoma

Pediatric NHL is a high grade and a very rapidly growing tumor; hence rapid diagnosis is imperative to prevent complications. Table 8 lists the diagnostic tests required in the evaluation of NHL. Determination of the histologic subtype and immunophenotype on lymph node/tissue guides therapy. Patients with large mediastinal masses and SVCS are at risk of cardiac or respiratory arrest during general anesthesia or heavy sedation. Due to these risks, the least invasive available procedure to establish the diagnosis of lymphoma such as bone marrow examination, thoracocentesis, a lymph node biopsy under local anesthesia or a computed tomography-guided core needle biopsy should be contemplated. PET-CT scan of whole body for staging and response evaluation in children is currently investigational. PET-CT appears to have a higher level of sensitivity than bone marrow biopsy in the detection of bone marrow infiltration and hence may be useful as a non-invasive modality for detecting bone marrow involvement. Similarly, PET may be potentially useful for assessing the speed of response and confirmation of post-therapy remission (CR).[54]

Staging, Prognostication and Risk Stratification

The modified Ann Arbor staging classification does not adequately reflect prognosis in childhood NHL. The most widely used staging scheme for childhood NHL is that of the St Jude Children's Research Hospital (Murphy's Staging), which is outlined in Table 9. In general, treatment for childhood NHL depends on localized versus disseminated disease. Localized disease is usually defined as stage I or II disease, while stage III or IV disease is generally considered disseminated. Currently, B-NHL is risk stratified further for treatment planning which incorporates stage, lactate dehydrogenase (LDH), extent of surgical resection and extent of bone marrow or CNS involvement (Table 10).[55-60]

Recent studies have suggested that involvement of mediastinal, lung, spleen and/or hepatic disease and skin lesions is associated with a significantly poorer outcome in ALCL[61]. Similarly, in B-NHL, adolescent age, PMBCL subtype, involvement of CNS with bone marrow, high LDH, and poor response to COP prophase (< 20% reduction in tumor burden) are associated with poor prognosis.[62] Also, secondary cytogenetic abnormalities, other than c-Myc rearrangement including gain of 7q or deletion of 13q have been shown to be strong adverse factors in BL.[63,64]

TABLE 8: Evaluation of child with non-Hodgkin lymphoma

• History and physical examination
• Complete blood count with peripheral smear for blasts
• Biochemistry: Blood urea, uric acid, creatinine, liver function tests, serum electrolytes, serum lactate dehydrogenase, calcium, phosphorous
• Imaging: X-rays, ultrasound, computed tomography (CT) scan or magnetic resonance imaging (MRI) of primary site and for staging, positron emission tomography (PET) scan (optional)
• Adequate surgical biopsy for immunophenotyping, cytogenetics/molecular studies
• Bone marrow aspiration and biopsy
• Cerebrospinal fluid (CSF) for cytology

TABLE 9: St. Jude's staging system for childhood non-Hodgkin lymphoma (NHL)

Stage	*Definition*
I	• Single tumor (extranodal) • Single anatomic area (nodal) excluding mediastinum or abdomen
II	• Single tumor (extranodal) with regional node involvement • Primary gastrointestinal tumor with or without involvement of mesenteric node only • On same side of diaphragm: - Two or more nodal areas - Two single extranodal tumors with or without regional node involvement
III	• All primary intrathoracic tumors • All extensive primary intra-abdominal disease • Two or more nodal or extranodal areas on both sides of diaphragm
IV	• Any of the above with CNS or bone marrow involvement

TABLE 10: Pediatric B-cell non-Hodgkin lymphoma (B-NHL): current risk grouping

Protocol	Group	Definition	5 years EFS
B-NHL (LMB89)	A	Completely resected stage I and abdominal stage-II	98%
	B	Unresected stage I nonabdominal stage-II	92%
		All stages III and IV	
	C	B-ALL < 25% blasts, CNS –ve	84%
		B-ALL > 25% blast or CNS +ve	
B-NHL (BFM)	R1	Stage I, II Initial complete resection	94%
	R2	Stage I, II unresected, stage III with LDH < 500 U/L	94%
	R3	Stage III with LDH < 500–999U/L,	85%
		BM +ve and LDH < 1,000 U/L	
	R4	LDH > 1,000U/L and/or CNS +ve	81%

Abbreviations: EFS, event-free survival; CNS, central nervous system; LDH, lactate dehydrogenase; BFM, Berlin-Frankfurt-Munster.

Monitoring of residual clonal lymphoma cells in the blood and/or bone marrow (BM) by means of aberrant immunophenotype or polymerase chain reaction (PCR)-based identification of specific fusion gene products is an emerging tool for evaluating the disease extent as well as kinetics of treatment response in childhood ALCL and BL.[64-65]

Management

Childhood NHL is an extremely chemosensitive disease. Surgery plays a very limited role, mainly for arriving at a diagnosis or for emergency management of obstruction or perforation. Radiation of primary sites is used very rarely in emergency situations. Hence, multiagent chemotherapy directed to the histologic subtype and stage of the disease remains the cornerstone of therapy.

Emergency Management

Pediatric NHL has very high growth fraction and short doubling time, sometimes as short as 24 hours seen with Burkitt lymphoma. Life threatening complications may develop as a result of physical compression of tumor masses on vital structures or because of high cell turnover in a large tumor with resultant biochemical disturbances. The following complications can occur and which must be anticipated early and addressed immediately:

- Superior vena cava obstruction and esophageal compression from mediastinal masses seen with LL
- Tumor lysis syndrome (TLS) due to metabolic disturbances seen with LL and BL
- Airway obstruction from pharyngeal or intrathoracic masses
- Respiratory or cardiac compromise from massive serous effusions related to involvement of pleura/peritoneum or pericardium
- Paraplegia from epidural tumor or raised intracranial pressure and neurological deficits from intracranial lymphoma/CNS involvement
- Obstructive jaundice and pancreatitis from compression of bile/pancreatic ducts
- Gastrointestinal bleeding, obstruction of bowel and rarely perforation from intestinal involvement.

Patients with large mediastinal masses are at risk of cardiac or respiratory arrest. These children should be closely monitored in intensive care units in propped-up lateral position and may be started on steroids if it is unsafe to perform a diagnostic biopsy because of the risk of anesthesia or sedation. Biopsy should be obtained as soon as patient is able to undergo the procedure safely.[48,51] TLS results from rapid breakdown of malignant cells resulting in a number of metabolic abnormalities, most notably hyperuricemia, hyperkalemia and hyperphosphatemia. Hyperhydration, allopurinol and rasburicase (urate oxidase) are essential components of therapy. Rasburicase, a recombinant urate oxidase rapidly lowers serum uric acid levels, and allows early administration of planned therapy. The use of rasburicase has dramatically reduced the requirement for dialysis in this population.[66]

Definitive Therapy of Pediatric Non-Hodgkin Lymphoma

Many studies including the seminal COG trial that randomized all children with NHL to be treated with short duration pulse intensive COMP (cyclophosphamide, vincristine, methotrexate and prednisone) regimen or to a long duration modified LSA_2L_2 regimen [used for acute lymphoblastic leukemia (ALL)] have shown that LL fare better when treated with long duration LSA_2L_2 leukemia regimen and short duration COMP was better for patients with B-cell NHL.[67,68]

Diffuse large B-cell lymphoma has a similar pattern of initial disease distribution and the same rapid response to chemotherapy as Burkitt lymphoma. Results from the large studies such as LMB and BFM suggest that with similar therapy, there is no difference in outcome between Burkitt lymphoma and DLBCL and these should be treated with the same approach. In B-NHL, in view of high growth fraction and short doubling time; short, pulse-intensive, multiagent chemotherapy is given in courses of 3–5 days with a schedule characterized by fractionation or continuous infusion of drugs. To prevent rapid re-growth, courses are administrated at shortest intervals. Treatment intensity is adapted to tumor burden (Stage, LDH level, BM involvement CNS involvement) and response to COP prephase. In addition, intensive CNS directed therapy using high-dose methotrexate or cytosine-arabinoside and intrathecal therapy (single agent methotrexate ± ara-c or triple intrathecal) is usually necessary. Cranial radiotherapy is not necessary.[55-60]

Management of T-cell Lymphomas (Table 11)

Precursor T-Lymphoblastic Lymphoma

Localized LL: For localized LL patients (stage I/II disease), induction therapy with short, pulsed chemotherapy (CHOP: cyclophosphamide, hydroxydaunorubicin, oncovin, prednisone) results in a 95% CR rate. However, only 60% can achieve long-term disease-free survival (DFS) due to late relapses in bone marrow. Using a leukemia approach with induction, consolidation, and maintenance therapy for a total of 24 months, most studies

TABLE 11: Treatment and outcome of T-cell non-Hodgkin lymphoma (T-NHL)

ALCL (T-cell type approach)				
Protocol	*Number*	*Stage*	*EFS%*	*Duration/number of cycles*
LSA2L2	19	III/IV	56	14–36 months
CCG5941	86	III/IV	78	12 months
POG9315	86	III/IV	72	12 months
AIEOP (LNH92)	34	II/III/IV	65	24 months
ALCL(B-cell type approach)				
BFM90	8 20 55 6	I II III IV	100 79 74 50	Stage I/II (completely resected): Three cycles Stage II (unresected)/stage III: Six cycles Stage IV/bone disease: Six intensified cycles
SFOP-HM 89/91	82	I/II III/IV	94 55	7–8 months
UKCCSG	72	III/IV	59	Stage III/IV (CNS –ve): Five cycles CNS positive: Intensified five cycles
MCP842	27	I/II III/IV	67 40	Six to eight (alternating A and B) cycles
Lymphoblastic lymphoma				
LSA2L2	281	I/II III/IV	84 64	18 months
POG8704	218	III/IV	67	24 months
LMT81	76 8	I/II III/IV	76 73	12 months
UKCCSG	59	III/IV	65	24 months
BFM90	82 19	III IV	90 95	24 months
BFM95	22 169	I/II III/IV	95 78	24 months

Abbreviations: EFS, event-free survival; CNS, central nervous system; LDH, lactate dehydrogenase; ALCL, anaplastic large cell lymphoma; AIEOP, Italian Association for Pediatric Hematology and Oncology; CCG, Children's Cancer Group; POG, Pediatric Oncology Group; SFOP, French Society of Pediatric Oncology; UKCCSG, United Kingdom Children's Cancer Study Group; MCP, macrophage chemotactic protein; BFM, Berlin-Frankfurt-Munster.

have shown more than 90% DFS for localized LL. No reinduction therapy or local or cranial radiation is given for stage I and II patients.[68-69]

Advanced Stage Lymphoblastic Lymphoma

Advanced LL have EFS rates higher than 80% with protocols designed for high-risk ALL consisting of a four-drug induction, consolidation incorporating high-dose methotrexate, cyclophosphamide, cytarabine, CNS directed therapy including intrathecal therapy and long maintenance with total 24 months of therapy.[21-26] Some recent studies have shown that patients receiving high-dose asparaginase regimen had a superior outcome.[23] Several studies also suggest that high dose methotrexate results in survival advantage. The results of the various chemotherapeutic regimens are shown in Table 11.[68-73]

Until recently, CNS directed therapy included the combined use of cranial irradiation and intrathecal chemotherapy. However, recent studies have demonstrated that cranial irradiation can be safely omitted if systemic high-dose methotrexate combined with intrathecal chemotherapy is administered. However, cranial irradiation may be necessary for children who present with CNS disease (fewer than 5% of children).[73] Irradiation of primary sites such as mediastinum has not been shown to improve outcome when added to chemotherapy. Even in patients with testicular disease at diagnosis, testicular radiation is only indicated for residual disease after systemic therapy incorporating high-dose methotrexate.[68-73]

Anaplastic Large Cell Lymphoma (Table 11)

Localized ALCL: For localized ALCL (grossly resected, i.e. >90% stage I/II disease), the best results have come from using pulsed chemotherapy similar to B-NHL therapy. Berlin-Frankfurt-Munster (BFM) group has shown results similar to those obtained with the BFM-90 regimen for B-NHL with use of three cycles after cytoreduction. In POG studies, stage I and II disease was very effectively treated with CHOP for three cycles without RT. The recent ALCL-99 trial used three cycles of chemotherapy following prophase for patients with stage I completely resected disease with good results. Overall, children with standard risk disease (Stage I/II completely resected with no high-risk features such as involvement of skin, mediastinum, viscera, CNS or BM) can be managed with three cycles (10–12 weeks) of B-cell type regimen and intrathecal therapy.[74-78]

Disseminated ALCL: Children with disseminated ALCL have EFS of approximately 60–75%. Majority of European studies [BFM, French Society of Pediatric Oncology (SFOP), United Kingdom Children's Cancer Study Group (UKCCSG), ALCL-99] have used short duration (5–8 months) pulse intensive B-cell type approach with good results while American (CCG, POG) and Italian groups [Associazione Italiana di Ematologia e Oncologia Pediatrica (AIEOP)] have used leukemia type long duration (12–24 months) less intensive approach with almost equivalent survival but increased hematological toxicity. Cranial prophylaxis using high or intermediate dose methotrexate with (BFM) or without intrathecal (SFOP) or only intrathecal therapy [COG, (MCP842)] have shown equivalent results with less than 1% incidence of CNS relapses. RT is not recommended.[74-78]

Recently conducted international ALCL99 study has shown that high-dose methotrexate (HD-MTX) (3 g/m^2 intravenously over 3 hours) is sufficient to protect the CNS in CNS-negative patients in the absence of additional intrathecal chemotherapy and addition of vinblastine during induction and as maintenance for a total treatment duration of 1 year did not reduce the risk of failure.[77-78] Thus, disseminated ALCL may be managed with six cycles (6 months) of B-cell type regimen using short infusion HD-MTX.

B-Cell Lymphoma (Table 12)

Treatment of Limited Stage B-Non-Hodgkin Lymphoma

Children with limited stage B-cell NHL (stage I or stage II, BFM R1/R2 or FAB-A group) have a good prognosis with an estimated 5-year EFS of 90–95% with minimal chemotherapy (range 6 weeks to 4 months). There are several multiagent chemotherapy regimens that have resulted in this excellent outcome as shown in Table 12. In the most recent BFM study (BFM-95), it was shown that reducing the dose or duration of methotrexate infusion did not affect the results for localized disease.[55-60,68]

Treatment of Advanced B-Non-Hodgkin Lymphoma

The prognosis of advanced B-NHL has improved significantly over the past decade with the use of use of short intensive chemotherapy regimens such as FAB/LMB96 (FAB), Orange (CCG) or BFM NHL90-95 with more than 90% 5-year DFS except in patients with CNS disease. Recent studies have demonstrated that cranial irradiation can be eliminated in patients with CNS-positive disease with the

TABLE 12: Treatment and outcome of B-cell non-Hodgkin lymphoma (B-NHL)

Protocol	Number	Stage	EFS (%)	Duration/number of cycles
COMP	57 135	I/II III/IV	84 53	6 months
LMB89	52 386 123	Group A Group B Group C	98 92 84	Group A: Two cycles, No IT Group B: Five cycles Group C: Eight cycles
FAB-LMB96	136 760 238	Group A Group B Group C	98 90 79	Group A and C: As LMB89 Group B: Four cycles with reduced dose cyclophosphamide
BFM-95	98 233 82 142	R1 R2 R3 R4	94 94 85 81	R1: Two cycles R2: Four cycles R3: Five intensified cycles R4: Six intensified cycles
CHOP	266	I/II	90	Six cycles
Orange (CCG)	34	III/IV	77	5–7 months

Abbreviations: COMP, cyclophosphamide oncovin methotrexate prednisone; LMB89, mature B-cell lymphoma 89; FAB-LMB96, French-American-British 96; BFM95, Berlin-Frankfurt-Munster-95; CHOP, cyclophosphamide, hydroxydaunorubicin, oncovin, prednisone; CCG, children's cancer group.

substitution of more aggressive high-dose methotrexate and additional intrathecal chemotherapy.[55-60,68] Recently conducted FAB/LMB96 study showed that intermediate-risk patients (group B) with good response to prophase COP can be treated with reduced intensity therapy with four courses but high-risk patients should receive standard FAB/LMB therapy (eight courses).[59-60] Rituximab, a mouse/human chimeric monoclonal antibody targeting the CD20 antigen, has shown good responses in relapsed B-NHL and a promising response rate of 41.4% in a phase II window study in newly diagnosed B-Cell NHL. Based on results of a recent COG pilot study (ANHL01P1), which showed it is feasible and safe to include rituximab in the current chemotherapy backbone, current studies are evaluating rituximab in high-risk B-NHL patients.[79]

Primary mediastinal DLBCL: The response to chemotherapy is slow and outcome is poor in PMBL. In the BFM study of 30 children, the 5-year EFS was 70% using chemotherapy alone. In FAB-LMB96 study of stage III PMBCL, the 5-year EFS was 66% versus 85% for adolescents with nonmediastinal DLBCL. Recently, a single-arm study in adults showed excellent EFS of 93% utilizing the DA-EPOCH-R regimen (dose-adjusted etoposide, doxorubicin, cyclophosphamide, vincristine, prednisone, and rituximab; usually six cycles) with filgrastim and no RT. This is currently being tested in pediatric clinical trials. Early mediastinal irradiation in incomplete initial responders may be considered.[80]

Management of Relapse

Relapse is a significant obstacle to long-term survival for children with advanced-stage NHL. In LL, most relapses occur within 2 years of diagnosis and the outcome after salvage chemotherapy is poor for children with advanced-stage disease at initial presentation. However, survival rates of 30–50% have been reported after allogeneic stem cell transplantation (SCT).[81-82]

The outcome of relapsed patients with BL is dismal because most relapses tend to occur early during active chemotherapy, and drug resistance is a major obstacle to successful salvage. Current protocols combine chemotherapy with rituximab followed by allogeneic or autologous SCT. The outcome is more favorable for patients who achieve a second remission before proceeding to SCT.[81] Children with relapsed DLBCL are often treated with salvage chemotherapy regimens such as ICE, GDP (gemcitabine, dexamethasone and cisplatinum) and DECAL (dexamethasone, etoposide, cisplatin, HD cytarabine, and L-Asp) with rituximab followed by autologous SCT. The outcome is quite favorable for those children who have chemosensitive disease at the time of relapse.[81]

The survival after relapse of ALCL is relatively favorable in contrast relapsed LL and BL. A French study demonstrated excellent responses to single-agent vinblastine followed by some very durable second remissions. A survival rate of 69% at 3 years with courses of CCNU, vinblastine, bleomycin or cytarabine followed by autologous HSCT in some of the patients has been reported.[83] Even in high-risk patients with on-therapy relapse or relapse after autologous SCT, long-term remissions have been observed after allogeneic SCT.[84] The potential benefit of vinblastine and anti-CD30 antibody combined with either an APO or BFM-like regimen is currently under investigation. Phase 1 study of ALK oncogenic tyrosine kinase inhibitor (crizotinib) in pediatric patients with ALCL has shown response rate of 88% in ALCL (ALK+) patients.[85] Brentuximab vedotin is a novel antibody-drug conjugate that targets CD30, a cell surface antigen expressed by HL and ALCL. A phase II trial in adults with relapsed ALCL has shown CR rates of approximately 55–60% and PR rates of 29%.[86]

Conclusion

Refinements in systemic chemotherapy fuelled by better understanding of NHL biology in children have led to cure in approximately 80–85% of all patients. This improved outlook for childhood NHL, however, has come with a certain price. The use of intense chemotherapy has resulted in late effects, such as sterility, cardiomyopathy, and secondary malignancies. Consequently, the emphasis for the near future is to decrease the therapy in good risk patients as well as better identification and development of new therapeutic approaches for high-risk cases. In future, as the molecular pathogenesis of the malignant lymphomas is better elucidated, it is likely that targeted therapy will substitute for some of the toxic chemotherapy and thereby maximize the chance for cure while avoiding both acute and chronic toxicities of chemotherapy. This novel molecular biologic information will also be valuable for developing more sensitive diagnostic tools, measurement of early response to therapy as well as submicroscopic disease and for identifying new prognostic subgroups.

REFERENCES

1. Glaser SL, Hsu JL. Hodgkin's disease in Asians: incidence patterns and risk factors in population based data. Leuk Res. 2002; 26(3):261-9.
2. Grufferman SL, Delzell E. Epidemiology of Hodgkin's disease. Epidem Rev. 1984;6:76-106.
3. Correa P, O'Conor GT. Epidemiologic patterns of Hodgkin's disease. Int J Cancer. 1971;8:192-201.
4. Çavdar AO, Pamir A, Gözdasoglu S, et al. Hodgkin's disease in children: clinicoepidemiologic and viral (Epstein-Barr virus) analyses. Med Pediatr Oncol. 1999;32:18-24.
5. Sackmann-Muriel F, Zubizarreta P, Gallo G, et al. Hodgkin's disease in children: results of a prospective randomized trial in a single institution in Argentina. Med Pediatr Oncol. 1997;29:544-52.
6. Westergaard T, Melbye M, Pedersen JB, et al. Birth order, sibship size and risk of Hodgkin's disease in children and young adults: a population-based study of 31 million person-years. Int J Cancer. 1997;72 (6):977-81.
7. Arora RS, Eden OB, Kapoor G. Epidemiology of childhood cancer in India. Ind J Cancer. 2009;46:264-73.
8. Dinand V, Arya LS. Epidemiology of childhood Hodgkin's disease: is it different in developing countries? Indian Pediatr. 2006;43(2):141-7.
9. Yeole BB, Advani SH, Sunny L. Epidemiological features of childhood cancers in greater Mumbai. Indian Pediatr. 2001;38(11):1270-7.
10. Naresh KN, Johnson J, Srinivas V, et al. Epstein-Barr virus association in classical Hodgkin's disease provides survival advantage to patients and correlates with higher expression of proliferation markers in Reed-Sternberg cells. Ann Oncol. 2000;11:91-6.
11. Hjalgrim H, Askling J, Rostgaard K, et al. Characteristics of Hodgkin's lymphoma after infectious mononucleosis. N Engl J Med. 2003;349 (14):1324-32.
12. Dinand V, Arya LS, Dawar R. Hodgkin's disease in North Indian children: prevalence and significance of Epstein-Barr virus Latent Membrane Protein-1 detection in Hodgkin's and Reed Sternberg cells. Indian J Medical Res. 2005;121:157.
13. Swerdlow SH, Campo E, Harris NL, et al (Eds). World Health Organization Classification of Tumors of Hematopoietic and Lymphoid Tissues. Lyon: IARC Press; 2008.
14. Krikorian JG, Portlock CS, Mauch PM. Hodgkin's disease presenting below the diaphragm: a review. J Clin Oncol. 1986;4:1551-6.
15. Olsson H, Brandt L. Relief of pruritus as an early sign of spinal cord compression in Hodgkin's disease. Acta Med Scand. 1979;206:319-25.
16. Stefanato CM, Reyes-Mugica M. Masked Hodgkin's disease: the pruriginous disguise. Pediatr Hematol Oncol. 1996;13:293-6.
17. Cavalli F. Rare syndromes in Hodgkin's disease. Ann Oncol. 1998;9(Suppl 5):S109.
18. Callahan BC, Coe R, Place HM. Hodgkin disease of the spine presenting as alcohol-related pain: a case report and review of the literature. J Bone Joint Surg Am. 1994;76:119-23.
19. Sills RH. The spleen and lympvh nodes. In: McMillan JA, Feigin RD, DeAngelis C, Jones MD (Eds), Oski's Pediatrics. Principles and Practice, 4th edition, Philadelphia: Lippincott, Williams & Wilkins; 2006. p. 1717.
20. Heiberg E, Wolverson MK, Sundaram M, et al. Normal thymus: CT characteristics in subjects under age 20. AJR Am J Roentgenol. 1982;138:491-5.
21. Murphy SB. The national impact of clinical cooperative group trials for pediatric cancer. Med Pediatr Oncol. 1995;24:279-85.
22. Mahoney DH, Schreuders LC, Gresik MV, et al. Role of staging bone marrow examination in children with Hodgkin disease. Med Pediatr Oncol. 1998;30:175-9.
23. Schellong G, Potter R, Bramswig J, et al. High cure rates and reduced long-term toxicity in pediatric Hodgkin's disease: the German-Austrian multicenter trial DAL-HD-90. J Clin Oncol. 1999;17;3736-44.

24. Rühl U, Albrecht M, Dieckmann K, et al. Response-adapted radiotherapy in the treatment of pediatric Hodgkin's disease: An interim report at 5 years of the German GPOH-HD95 trial. Int J Radiat Oncol Biol Phys. 2001;51:1209-18.
25. Donaldson SS, Hudson MM, Lamborn KR, et al. VAMP and low-dose, involved-field radiation for children and adolescents with favorable, early-stage Hodgkin's disease: Results of a prospective clinical trial. J Clin Oncol. 2002;20:3081-7.
26. Nachman JB, Sposto R, Herzog P, et al. Randomized comparison of low-dose involved-field radiotherapy and no radiotherapy for children with Hodgkin's disease who achieve a complete response to chemotherapy. J Clin Oncol. 2002;20:3765-71.
27. Kung FH, Schwartz CL, Ferree CR, et al. POG8625: a randomized trial comparing chemotherapy with chemoradiotherapy for children and adolescents with Stages I, IIA, IIIA1 Hodgkin Disease: a report from the Children's Oncology Group. J Pediatr Hematol Oncol. 2006;28(6):362-8.
28. Hudson MM, Donaldson SS. Hodgkin's disease. In: Pizzo PA, Poplack DG (Eds). Principles and Practice of Pediatric Oncology, 5th edition. Philadelphia: Lippincott Williams & Wilkins; 2006. pp. 695.
29. Donaldson SS, Link MP, Weinstein HJ, et al. Final results of a prospective clinical trial with VAMP and low-dose involved-field radiation for children with low-risk Hodgkin's disease. J Clin Oncol. 2007;25:332-9.
30. Tebbi CK, Mendenhall N, London WB, et al. Treatment of stage I, IIA, IIIA1 pediatric Hodgkin disease with doxorubicin, bleomycin, vincristine and etoposide (DBVE) and radiation: a Pediatric Oncology Group (POG) study. Pediatr Blood Cancer. 2006;46:198-206.
31. Mauz-Körholz C, Hasenclever D, Dörffel W, et al. Procarbazine-free OEPA-COPDAC chemotherapy in boys and standard OPPA-COPP in girls have comparable effectiveness in pediatric Hodgkin's lymphoma: the GPOH-HD-2002 study. J Clin Oncol. 2010;28:3680-9.
32. Dörffel W, Rühl U, Lüders H, et al. Treatment of children and adolescents with Hodgkin lymphoma without radiotherapy for patients in complete remission after chemotherapy: final results of the multinational trial GPOH-HD95. J Clin Oncol. 2013;31:1562-9.
33. Shankar A, Visaduraki M, Hayward J, et al. Clinical outcome in children and adolescents with Hodgkin lymphoma after treatment with chemotherapy alone: the results of the United Kingdom HD3 national cohort trial. Eur J Cancer. 2012;48: 108-16.
34. Friedman DI, Wolden S, Constine L, et al. AHOD0031: a Phase III Study of Dose-Intensive Therapy for Intermediate Risk Hodgkin Lymphoma: a Report from the Children's Oncology Group. Blood. 2010;116:766.
35. Schwartz CL, Constine LS, Villaluna D, et al. A risk-adapted, response-based approach using ABVE-PC for children and adolescents with intermediate- and high-risk Hodgkin lymphoma: the results of P9425. Blood. 2009;114:2051-8.
36. Kelly KM, Sposto R, Hutchinson R, et al. BEACOPP chemotherapy is a highly effective regimen in children and adolescents with high-risk Hodgkin lymphoma: a report from the Children's Oncology Group. Blood. 2011;117:2596-608.
37. Mauz-Körholz C, Gorde-Grosjean S, Hasenclever D, et al. Resection alone in 58 children with limited stage, lymphocyte-predominant Hodgkin lymphoma-experience from the European network group on pediatric Hodgkin lymphoma. Cancer. 2007;110:179-87.
38. Appel B, Chen L, Hutchison RE, et al. Treatment of pediatric lymphocyte predominant Hodgkin lymphoma (LPHL): a report from the Children's Oncology Group. J Clin Oncol. 2013;31:613s.
39. Shankar A, Hall GW, Gorde-Grosjean S, et al. Treatment outcome after low intensity chemotherapy (CVP) in children and adolescents with early stage nodular lymphocyte predominant Hodgkin's lymphoma: an Anglo-French collaborative report. Eur J Cancer. 2012;48:1700-8.
40. Pellegrino B, Terrier-Lacombe MJ, Oberlin O, et al. Lymphocyte-predominant Hodgkin's lymphoma in children: therapeutic abstention after initial lymph node resection: a Study of the French Society of Pediatric Oncology. J Clin Oncol. 2003;21: 2948-56.
41. Murphy SB, Morgan ER, Katzenstein HM, et al. Results of little or no treatment for lymphocyte-predominant Hodgkin disease in children and adolescents. J Pediatr Hematol Oncol. 2003;25: 684-92.
42. Lieskovsky YE, Donaldson SS, Torres MA, et al. High-dose therapy and autologous hematopoietic stem-cell transplantation for recurrent or refractory pediatric Hodgkin's disease: results and prognostic indices. J Clin Oncol. 2004;22:4532-9.
43. Harris RE, Termuhlen AM, Smith LM, et al. Autologous peripheral blood stem cell transplantation in children with refractory or relapsed lymphoma: results of Children's Oncology Group study A5962. Biol Blood Marrow Transplant. 2011;17:249-56.
44. Johnston WT, Lightfoot TJ, Simpson J, et al. Childhood cancer survival: a report from the United Kingdom Childhood Cancer Study. Cancer Epidemiol. 2010;34:659-68.
45. Ng AK, Bernardo MP, Weller E, et al. Long-term survival and competing causes of death in patients with early-stage Hodgkin's disease treated at age 50 or younger. J Clin Oncol. 2002;20:2101-12.
46. Voss SD, Constine LS, Chauvenet A, et al. Surveillance computed tomography imaging and detection of relapse in intermediate- and advanced-stage pediatric Hodgkin's lymphoma: a report from the Children's Oncology Group. J Clin Oncol. 2012;30(21):2635-40.
47. Castellino SM, Geiger AM, Mertens AC, et al. Morbidity and mortality in long-term survivors of Hodgkin lymphoma: a report from the Childhood Cancer Survivor Study. Blood. 2011;117:1806-16.
48. Reiter A. Diagnosis and treatment of childhood non-Hodgkin lymphoma. Hematology Am Soc Hematol Educ Program. 2007:285-96.
49. Percy CL, Smith MA, Linet M, et al. Lymphomas and reticuloendothelial neoplasms. In: Ries LA, Smith MA, Gurney JG, et al (Eds). Cancer incidence and survival among children and adolescents: United States SEER Program 1975-1995. Bethesda, Md: National Cancer Institute, SEER Program, 1999. pp. 35-50.
50. Naresh KN, Srinivas V, Soman CS. Distribution of various subtypes of non-Hodgkin's lymphoma in India: a study of 2773

lymphomas using REAL and WHO Classifications. Annals of Oncology. 2000;11(Suppl 1):S63-S7.

51. Sandlund JT, Downing JR, Crist WM. Non-Hodgkin's lymphoma in childhood. N Engl J Med. 1996;334(19):1238-48.
52. Oschlies I, Salaverria I, Mahn F, et al. Pediatric follicular lymphoma: a clinicopathological study of a population-based series of patients treated within the non-Hodgkin's Lymphoma--Berlin-Frankfurt-Munster (NHL-BFM) multicenter trials. Hematologica. 2010;95:253-9.
53. Claviez A, Meyer U, Dominick C, et al. MALT lymphoma in children: a report from the NHL-BFM Study Group. Pediatr Blood Cancer. 2006;47:210-4.
54. Nakatani K, Nakamoto Y, Watanabe K, et al. Roles and limitations of FDG PET in pediatric non-Hodgkin lymphoma. Clin Nucl Med. 2012;37:656-62.
55. Patte C, Auperin A, Michon J, et al. The Societe Francaised Oncologie Pediatrique LMB89 protocol: highly effective multiagent chemotherapy tailored to the tumor burden and initial response in 561 unselected children with B-cell lymphomas and L3 leukemia. Blood. 2001;97:3370-9.
56. Reiter A, Schrappe M, Tiemann M, et al. Improved treatment results in childhood B-cell neoplasms with tailored intensification of therapy: a report of the Berlin-Frankfurt-Munster Group Trial NHL-BFM 90. Blood. 1999;94:3294-306.
57. Woessmann W, Seidemann K, Mann G, et al. The impact of the methotrexate administration schedule and dose in the treatment of children and adolescents with B-cell neoplasms: a report of the BFM Group Study NHL-BFM95. Blood. 2005;105: 948-58.
58. Gerrard M, Cairo MS, Weston C, et al. Results of the FAB LMB 96 international study in children and adolescents (C+A) with localized, resected B cell lymphoma [large cell lymphoma (LCL), Burkitt's lymphoma (BL) and Burkitt-like lymphoma (BLL)]. J Clin Oncol. 2003;22:795-801.
59. Patte C, Auperin A, Gerrard M, et al. Results of the randomized international FAB/LMB96 trial for intermediate risk B-cell non-Hodgkin lymphoma in children and adolescents: It is possible to reduce treatment for the early responding patients. Blood. 2007;109:2773-80.
60. Cairo MS, Gerrard M, Sposto R, et al. Results of a randomized international study of high-risk central nervous system B non-Hodgkin lymphoma and B acute lymphoblastic leukemia in children and adolescents. Blood. 2007;109:2736-43.
61. Le Deley MC, Reiter A, Williams D, et al. Prognostic factors in childhood anaplastic large cell lymphoma: results of a large European intergroup study. Blood. 2008;111:1560-6.
62. Cairo MS, Sposto R, Gerrard M, et al. Advanced stage, increased lactate dehydrogenase, and primary site, but not adolescent age (≥ 15 years), are associated with an increased risk of treatment failure in children and adolescents with mature B-cell non-Hodgkin's lymphoma: results of the FAB LMB 96 study. J Clin Oncol. 2012;30: 387-93.
63. Poirel HA, Heerema NA, Swansbury J, et al. Cytogenetic analysis of 238 pediatric mature B-cell non-Hodgkin lymphoma (NHL) cases from the randomized international FAB LMB96 trial identities several patterns of chromosomal abnormality and new prognostic factors. Pediatr Blood Cancer. 2006;46:835-42.
64. Mussolin L, Pillon M, d'Amore ES, et al. Minimal disseminated disease in high-risk Burkitt's lymphoma identifies patients with different prognosis. J Clin Oncol. 2011;29:1779-84.
65. Damm-Welk C, Busch K, Burkhardt B, et al. Prognostic significance of circulating tumor cells in bone marrow or peripheral blood as detected by qualitative and quantitative PCR in pediatric NPM-ALK-positive anaplastic large-cell lymphoma. Blood. 2007;110:670-7.
66. Cairo MS, Coiffier B, Reiter A, et al. Recommendations for the evaluation of risk and prophylaxis of tumor lysis syndrome (TLS) in adults and children with malignant diseases: an expert TLS panel consensus. Br J Hematol. 2010;149:578-86.
67. Anderson JR, Jenkin RD, Wilson JF, et al. Long-term follow-up of patients treated with COMP or LSA2L2 therapy for childhood non-Hodgkin's lymphoma: a report of CCG-551 from the Childrens Cancer Group. J Clin Oncol. 1993;11:1024-32.
68. Link MP, Shuster JJ, Donaldson SS, et al. Treatment of children and young adults with early-stage non-Hodgkin's lymphoma. N Engl J Med. 1997;337:1259-66.
69. Reiter A, Schrappe M, Ludwig WD, et al. Intensive ALL-type therapy without local radiotherapy provides a 90% event-free survival for children with T-cell lymphoblastic lymphoma: a BFM group report. Blood. 2000;95:416-21.
70. Amylon MD, Shuster J, Pullen J, at al. Intensive high-dose asparaginase consolidation improves survival for pediatric patients with T cell acute lymphoblastic leukemia and advanced stage lymphoblastic lymphoma: a Pediatric Oncology Group study. Leukemia.1999;13:335-42.
71. Eden OB, Hann I, Imeson J et al. Treatment of advanced stage T-cell lymphoblastic lymphoma: results of the United Kingdom Children's Cancer Study Group (UKCCSG) protocol 8503. Br J Hematol. 1992;82:310-6.
72. Patte C, Kalifa C, Flamant F, et al. Results of the LMT81 protocol, a modified LSA2L2 protocol with high dose methotrexate, on 84 children with non-B-cell (lymphoblastic) lymphoma. Med Pediatr Oncol. 1992;20:105-13.
73. Burkhardt B, Woessmann W, Zimmermann M, et al. Impact of cranial radiotherapy on central nervous system prophylaxis in children and adolescents with central nervous system-negative stage III or IV lymphoblastic lymphoma. J Clin Oncol. 2006;24:491-9.
74. Seidemann K, Tiemann M, Schrappe M, et al. Short-pulse B-non-Hodgkin lymphoma-type chemotherapy is efficacious treatment for pediatric anaplastic large cell lymphoma: a report of the Berlin-Frankfurt-Munster Group Trial NHL-BFM 90. Blood. 2001;97:3699-706.
75. Brugières L, Le Deley MC, Pacquement H, et al. CD30 (+) anaplastic large-cell lymphoma in children: analysis of T- and NK-cell lymphomas in children and adolescents of 82 patients enrolled in two consecutive studies of the French Society of Pediatric Oncology. Blood. 1998;92:3591-8.
76. Williams DM, Hobson R, Imeson J, et al. Anaplastic large cell lymphoma in childhood: analysis of 72 patients treated on The

United Kingdom Children's Cancer Study Group chemotherapy regimens. Br J Hematol. 2002;117:812-20.

77. Brugières L, Le Deley MC, Rosolen A, et al. Anaplastic large cell lympoma (ALCL) in children: equal efficacy but greater toxicity of chemotherapy including methotrexate (MTX) 1g/m^2 in 24-hour infusion with intrathecal injection (IT) than chemotherapy with MTX 3g/m^2 in 3-hour infusion without IT: results of the ALCL99–R1 randomized trial [abstract]. Blood. 2006;108:122a.

78. Le Deley MC, Rosolen A, Williams DM, et al. Vinblastine in children and adolescents with high-risk anaplastic large-cell lymphoma: results of the randomized alcl99-vinblastine trial. J Clin Oncol. 2010;28:3987-93.

79. Meinhardt A, Burkhardt B, Zimmermann M, et al. Phase II Window Study on Rituximab in Newly Diagnosed Pediatric Mature B-Cell Non-Hodgkin's Lymphoma and Burkitt Leukemia. J Clin Oncol. 2010;28:3115-21.

80. Seidemann K, Tiemann M, Lauterbach I, et al. Primary mediastinal large B-cell lymphoma with sclerosis in pediatric and adolescent patients: treatment and results from three therapeutic studies of the Berlin-Frankfurt-Munster Group. J Clin Oncol. 2003;21:1782-9.

81. Attarbaschi A, Dworzak M, Steiner M, et al. Outcome of children with primary resistant or relapsed non-Hodgkin lymphoma and mature B-cell leukemia after intensive first-line treatment: a population-based analysis of the Austrian Cooperative Study Group. Pediatr Blood Cancer. 2005;44:70-6.

82. Burkhardt B, Reiter A, Landmann E, et al. Poor outcome for children and adolescents with progressive disease or relapse of lymphoblastic lymphoma: a report from the berlin-frankfurt-muenster group. J Clin Oncol. 2009;27:3363-9.

83. Brugières L, Pacquement H, Le Deley MC, et al. Single-drug vinblastine as salvage treatment for refractory or relapsed anaplastic large-cell lymphoma: a report from the French Society of Pediatric Oncology. J Clin Oncol. 2009;27:5056-61.

84. Woessmann W, Zimmermann M, Lenhard M, et al. Relapsed or refractory anaplastic large-cell lymphoma in children and adolescents after Berlin-Frankfurt-Muenster (BFM)-type first-line therapy: a BFM-group study. J Clin Oncol. 2011;29:3065-71.

85. Mossé YP, Lim MS, Voss SD, et al. Safety and activity of crizotinib for pediatric patients with refractory solid tumors or anaplastic large-cell lymphoma: a Children's Oncology Group phase 1 consortium study. Lancet Oncol. 2013;14(6):472-80.

86. Pro B, Advani R, Brice P, et al. Brentuximab vedotin (SGN-35) in patients with relapsed or refractory systemic anaplastic large-cell lymphoma: results of a phase II study. J Clin Oncol. 2012;30:2190-6.

60 Adult Lymphomas

Manju Sengar

INTRODUCTION

Lymphomas are malignancies of immune system and are derived from lymphocytes at various stages of their development. They are a heterogeneous group of malignancies in terms of histology, clinical presentation and outcomes. The two broad subtypes are—Hodgkin and non-Hodgkin lymphomas (NHL). Hodgkin lymphomas constitute approximately 10% of all lymphomas whereas remaining 90% are NHL. Lymphomas can have a wide variety of clinical presentation and can present to any specialist based on the site of involvement. It often shares clinical features of infectious disorders like tuberculosis thus resulting in delays in diagnosis and appropriate management.

NON-HODGKIN LYMPHOMA

Approximately 65,540 new cases were diagnosed in USA in year 2007 and 20,210 patients died due to NHL in 2008. Incidence of NHL is gradually increasing all over the world including India. Due to improvements in treatment and supportive care the survival rates have also improved over the years. Since immunosuppression is one of the risk factors, increasing incidence of acquired immunodeficiency syndrome is considered as one of the reason for the rising incidence. Increased use of pesticides has also been linked to the increased incidence. Other causative factors, which have been linked to the development of NHL, include—infectious agents like Epstein-Barr virus, hepatitis C virus, *Helicobacter pylori* and autoimmune disorders.

Non-Hodgkin lymphomas include a wide spectrum of cancers some being indolent and compatible with survival for years without therapy whereas others being highly aggressive need urgent treatment. Based on morphology, immunophenotype, genetic abnormalities and cell of origin WHO 2008 classification for hematolymphoid neoplasms (Table 1) classifies NHL into various subtypes, Approximately 85–90% are B-cell NHL whereas remaining are T-cell NHL.[1] Distribution of various subtypes of NHL varies across different geographic regions. In India, diffuse large B-cell NHL is the most common subtype followed by follicular NHL.[2] T-cell NHL are common in Asia and in India, approximately 16% of NHL are of T-cell type.

Clinical Features

Clinical features are variable and are based on site of disease and lymphoma subtype. The most common presentation is peripheral lymphadenopathy—single site or multiple sites. In most cases it is painless and gradually progressive. It may result in compressive symptoms based on its size or location – limb edema, pain, superior vena cava obstruction, jaundice, etc. Generalized lymphadenopathy is more common amongst low grade NHL. Extranodal disease can involve gastrointestinal (GI) tract, testis, breast, orbit or bone. Extranodal involvement is common in diffuse large B-cell NHL, (DLBL) and T-cell NHL. Involvement of central nervous system at diagnosis is less than 5% and mostly seen in patients with BL, involving testis, breast, paraspinal region, paranasal sinuses or multiple extranodal sites. Weakness, fatigue or bleeding manifestations can occur due to anemia

TABLE 1: WHO 2008 classification of lymphomas

Chronic lymphocytic leukemia/small lymphocytic lymphoma
B-Cell prolymphocytic leukemia
Splenic marginal zone lymphoma
Hairy cell leukemia
Lymphoplasmacytic lymphoma • Waldenstrom macroglobulinemia
Heavy chain disease • Alpha heavy chain disease • Gamma heavy chain disease • Mu heavy chain disease
Plasma cell myeloma
Solitary plasmacytoma of bone
Extraosseous plasmacytoma
Extranodal marginal zone B-cell lymphoma of mucosa—associated
Lymphoid tissue (MALT lymphoma)
Nodal marginal zone B-cell lymphoma (MZL)
Follicular lymphoma
Primary cutaneous follicle center lymphoma
Mantle cell lymphoma
Diffuse B-cell lymphoma (DLBCL), not otherwise specified
Lymphomatoid granulomatosis
Primary mediastinal (Thymic) large B-cell lymphoma
Intravascular large B-cell lymphoma
Primary cutaneous DLBCL, leg type
ALK+ large B-cell lymphoma
Plasmablastic lymphoma
Primary effusion lymphoma
Large B-cell lymphoma arising In HHV8 –associated multicentric Castle man's disease
Burkitt lymphoma
B-cell lymphoma, unclassifiable, with features intermediate between diffuse large B-cell lymphoma and burkitt lymphoma
B-cell lymphoma, unclassifiable, with features intermediate between diffuse large B-cell lymphoma and hodgkin lymphoma
Hodgkin lymphoma
Nodular lymphocyte—predominant Hodgkin lymphoma
Classical Hodgkin lymphoma
Nodular sclerosis classical Hodgkin lymphoma
Lymphocyte—rich classical Hodgkin lymphoma
Mixed cellularity classical Hodgkin lymphoma
Lymphocyte—depleted classical Hodgkin lymphoma

and thrombocytopenia, secondary to bone marrow involvement. The propensity to involve bone marrow varies based on the subtype of NHL—higher in patients with low grade NHL like small lymphocytic lymphoma, follicular NHL and marginal zone NHL. In addition constitutional symptoms like fever, weight loss (B symptoms—fever > 38°C, weight loss > 10% in last 6 months and drenching night sweats) are seen in varying proportion of patients and may indicate the need for therapy in low grade NHL or may upstage the lymphomas.

Diagnostic Work Up

Biopsy

The most important investigation is biopsy of the node or the clinically involved extranodal site in absence of clinically significant lymphadenopathy. The biopsy should preferably be excisional and from the most representative site. Making a diagnosis on fine-needle aspiration should be strongly discouraged. In case of bulky nodes where excision would lead to significant morbidity or major surgery an incisional biopsy is recommended. If there are no peripheral lymph nodes, core needle biopsy of abdominal or mediastinal node can be considered. The biopsied tissue should be bisected and stored in 10% formalin immediately to avoid fixation artefacts or autolysis. In case, if any molecular studies are needed on fresh tissue appropriate instructions should be obtained from the pathologist before doing the biopsy. The biopsy is subjected to morphological examination and immunohistochemistry to diagnose and subtype lymphomas.

Imaging

Either a contrast enhanced CT (CECT) chest, abdomen (Figs 1 and 2) and pelvis or a Positron emission tomography (PET)-CT (Fig. 3) can be done to assess various disease sites, involvement of spleen, liver and other extranodal sites. In most high-grade lymphomas (diffuse large B-cell, mantle cell, Burkitt, lymphoblastic), which are known to be FDG-avid both are acceptable options. In lymphomas with variable FDG avidity (marginal zone, follicular,

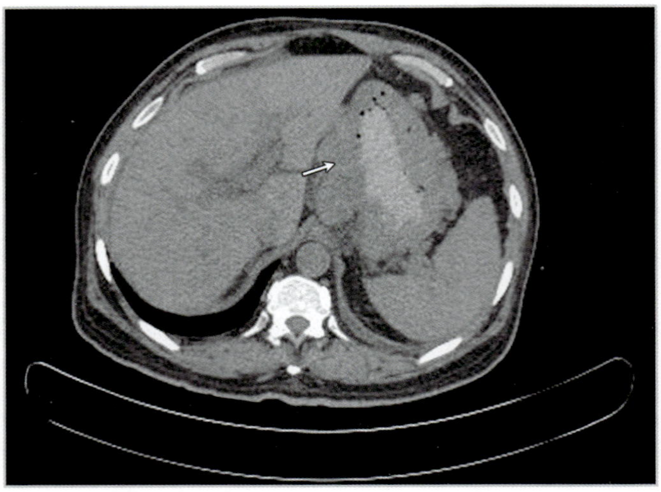

Fig. 1: CT abdomen shows diffuse gastric wall thickening in a known case of diffuse large B cell NHL (arrow)

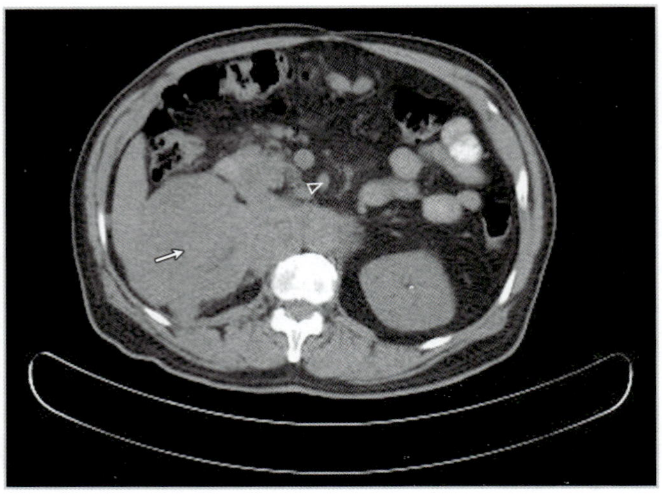

Fig. 2: CT abdomen shows right kidney deposit (arrow) and retroperitoneal lymphadenopathy (arrowhead) in a patient with NHL

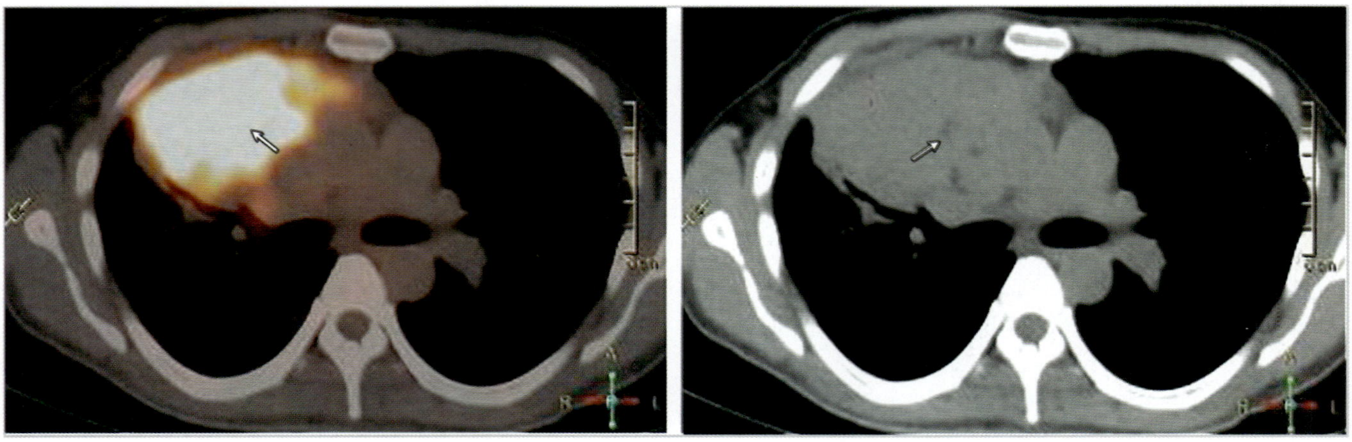

Fig. 3: PET-CT shows FDG avid anterior mediastinal mass with infiltration of right lung upper lobe (arrow) in a case of Hodgkin's lymphoma

small lymphocytic) PET-CT should be done at baseline only if the response evaluation is to be done with PET-CT otherwise CECT alone is sufficient. PET-CT helps in upstaging in approximately 15% of cases whereas it can downstage the disease in 8% of cases; however, its impact on change in treatment plan and overall outcome is not clear.[3,4] Other imaging modalities like MRI or bone scan are considered only in cases with central nervous system involvement, cord or root compression or bone lymphomas.

Bone Marrow Biopsy

In all cases of NHL bone marrow biopsy and aspiration is necessary to rule out the involvement of the marrow except in cases where there is involvement of peripheral blood (peripheral blood spill).

Body Fluid Examination

In patients with pleural effusion, ascites or pericardial effusion cytological examination of fluid is important to rule out involvement as it upstages the lymphoma to stage IV. Examination of cerebrospinal fluid is done in patients with clinical/radiological features of central nervous system (CNS) involvement or in cases which have high risk of CNS involvement as discussed earlier.

Peripheral Smear Examination

Baseline complete blood counts and peripheral smear is mandatory in all patients with suspected lymphomas. In cases with peripheral blood lymphocytosis—morphological features and flow cytometry can help making the diagnosis of lymphomas for example chronic lymphocytic leukemia, follicular lymphoma (FL), hairy cell leukemia, splenic marginal zone lymphomas.

Endoscopic Evaluation

Lymphomas involving GI tract - marginal zone lymphoma, mantle cell lymphoma (MCL) or primary DLBL or BL of GI tract will need upper GI endoscopy or colonoscopy for biopsy and evaluation of extent of disease.

Molecular Studies

Certain lymphomas have pathognomonic genetic abnormalities which help in establishing the diagnosis (c-myc translocation in BL, t(11;14) in mantle cell). Fluorescent in situ hybridization (FISH) studies on paraffin block of tissue or bone marrow can help in making the diagnosis.

Blood Biochemistry

Evaluation of organ functions to assess the suitability for therapy—liver function, renal function and cardiac evaluation are required before beginning the therapy.

Staging

In adults, non-Hodgkin and Hodgkin lymphomas are staged as per Cotswold modification of Ann-Arbor stage (Table 2).

Prognostication

For diffuse large B-cell NHL, international prognostic index (age > 60 years, > 1 extranodal sites, raised lactate dehydrogenase (LDH), performance status > 1, stage III/IV disease) has been used to prognosticate patients (Table 3). This index was derived in a retrospective analysis of aggressive NHL who was treated with chemotherapy only; however, it still holds value even in rituximab-chemotherapy era. The prognostic index used for FL lymphoma is mentioned in Table 4.[5]

Histopathology and Treatment of Various Subtypes of NHL

Lymphoblastic lymphoma (LBL): This is a highly aggressive subtype of NHL and if left untreated patients can succumb

TABLE 2: Ann Arbor staging classification for Hodgkin and non-Hodgkin lymphomas

Stage I	Involvement of a single lymph node region (I) or of a single extralymphatic organ or site (IE)
Stage II	Involvement of two or more lymph node regions or lymphatic structures on the same side of the diaphragm alone (II) or with involvement of limited, contiguous extralymphatic organ or tissue (IIE)
Stage III	Involvement of lymph node regions on both sides of the diaphragm (III) which may include the spleen (IIIS) or limited, contiguous extralymphatic organ or site (IIIE) or both (IIIES)
Stage IV	Diffuse or disseminated foci of involvement of one or more extralymphatic organs or tissues, with or without associated lymphatic involvement

All cases are subclassified to indicate the absence (A) or presence (B) of the **systemic "B"** ***symptoms*** of significant unexplained fever, night sweats, or unexplained weight loss exceeding 10% of body weight in last 6 months

TABLE 3: International prognostic index

Age over 60 years	
Serum lactate dehydrogenase concentration above normal	
Eastern cooperative oncology group (ECOG) performance status ≥ 2	
Ann Arbor stage III or IV	
Number of extranodal disease sites >1	
Score	*Risk group*
0-1	Low risk
2	Low-intermediate risk
3	High-intermediate risk
4 to 5	High risk

TABLE 4: Follicular lymphoma international prognostic index (FLIPI) score

Age over 60 year	
Ann Arbor stage III-IV	
Hemoglobin level < 12 g/dL	
Raised lactate dehydrogenase level (more than upper limit of normal) ≥4 nodal sites	
Score	*Risk group*
0-1	Low risk
2	Intermediate risk
≥3	High

within few weeks. It constitutes 2% of all NHL. Most often it affects younger adults and males. Most of these patients present with advanced stage of disease, B-symptoms and raised LDH levels. T-LBL commonly presents with mediastinal masses whereas B-LBL commonly involves extranodal sites and skin. Morphologically both T and B-LBL appear similar with medium-sized neoplastic cells with high nuclear-cytoplasmic ratio and fine chromatin (blastic). The T-subtype shows positivity for CD3, and other Pan T-cell antigens (CD2, CD5 and CD7). B-subtype shows cytoplasmic CD10, CD79a, CD19 and variable CD20 expression. The hallmark of LBL is nuclear Tdt positivity. Treatment of LBL is same as acute lymphoblastic leukemia with multiagent chemotherapy used during induction, consolidation, early and late re-intensification, CNS prophylaxis and maintenance. Use of consolidative mediastinal radiotherapy remains controversial. The cure rates are variable (45–72%) among different reported series.[6]

Diffuse Large B-Cell Lymphoma

It constitutes approximately 30–40% of NHL. It can affect any age group. DLBL can be de-novo or develop as transformation of low-grade NHL. Most commonly DLBL presents as localized nodal mass or can present at extranodal site like stomach, bone, testis or CNS. Morphologically, it is characterized by diffuse growth pattern with complete effacement of nodal architecture. Neoplastic cells are large with prominent nucleoli and scanty cytoplasm. These cells express CD19, CD79a, CD20 along with CD10, CD30 and CD5 in small proportion of cases. DLBL are a heterogeneous group of lymphomas and have been divided into three categories based on their gene expression profile—germinal center, activated B-cell and primary mediastinal subtype. Separation of these three entities has prognostic relevance; however, immunohistochemistry with CD10, Mum-1 and Bcl-6 have had variable success in identifying these subtypes. Treatment of DLBL has seen major advances since the introduction of rituximab-anti-CD20 monoclonal antibody. Combination of rituximab with CHOP chemotherapy has benefited both young and elderly patients with localized and disseminated disease.[7] Radiotherapy is used after completion of chemotherapy in patients with bulky disease and extranodal site at presentation. High dose chemotherapy and autologous stem cell transplant is reserved for patients with chemosensitive relapse.

Burkitt Lymphoma

Burkitt lymphoma consists of three subtypes—endemic, sporadic and immunosuppression related. Endemic subtype is seen in pediatric population in Africa and mostly involves facial bones. Sporadic cases are seen in adults and mostly have extranodal presentations—GI tract, breast, kidneys and gonads. Immunosuppression-related BL is seen in patients with HIV/AIDS and can have disseminated presentation. It consists of uniform, monotonous population of medium-sized neoplastic cells with basophilic cytoplasm and nucleus with fine chromatin. The tumor may show starry-sky pattern due to macrophages which have phagocytized the cell debris. It has very high number of mitoses and apoptotic cells due high proliferation rates. BL is characterized by c-myc rearrangement secondary to translocation involving c-myc and heavy or light chain gene [t(8;14),(8;22), (2;8)]. Treatment of BL is based on multi-agent short course, non-cross resistant intensive chemotherapy. In addition, all patients need CNS prophylaxis with intensive intrathecal chemotherapy. The cure rates vary between 30% and 70% based on stage.[8]

Follicular Lymphoma

It accounts for approximately 20% of all NHL. The median age at presentation is 60 years in western countries. It commonly presents with generalized lymphadenopathy. Most of the patients are asymptomatic at presentation. Involvement of liver and bone marrow is seen in 50–70% of patients. FL is characterized by effacement of architecture of lymph node with closely stacked expanded follicles. The neoplastic cells resemble the germinal center cells—centrocytes and centroblasts. Based on the number of centroblasts per high power field, FL is graded in three types—Grade 1 to 3 (Fig. 4). These cells express CD10, Bcl-2, CD20 and CD79a. The majority of the cases have t(14;18) with Bcl-2 gene rearrangement. Significant proportions of these patients are asymptomatic and can be kept under observation or watchful waiting.[9] Presence of constitutional symptoms, cytopenias, bulky nodes, symptomatic organomegaly, organ dysfunction and compressive symptom warrants therapy in FL. At present chemoimmunotherapy with bendamustine and rituximab is considered as standard of care.[10] Patients can be given maintenance rituximab if they achieve complete or partial response after initial chemotherapy to prolong the progression free survival. In case of FL grade 3b or transformation to high-grade lymphomas R-CHOP becomes the treatment of choice. Newer therapies like radioimmunotherapy have been tested as consolidation therapy or for treating relapsed disease. Use of autologous stem cell transplant is limited to relapsed setting with high relapse rates.[11]

Small Lymphocytic Lymphoma

Small lymphocytic lymphoma (SLL) and chronic lymphocytic leukemia are same disease with different clinical manifestations. Most of these patients are elderly and have lymphocytosis or asymptomatic nodal enlargement is detected coincidentally while undergoing investigations for some unrelated disorder. Lymph node architecture is replaced by sheets of small lymphocytes. Peripheral smear shows mature lymphocytes along with smudge cells. Neoplastic cells show positivity for B-cell markers along with CD5, CD23 with weak CD20 and surface immunoglobulin expression. As in FL, these patients can be kept under watchful waiting in absence of symptoms. If therapy is indicated then chemoimmunotherapy is used. Chemotherapy varies from fludarabine and cyclophosphamide or chlorambucil based on comorbidities and age.[12]

Mantle Cell Lymphoma

It constitutes less than 2% of all NHL. Median age at presentation is 58 years. It can have clinical features like chronic lymphocytic leukemia with predominant bone marrow and blood involvement with indolent course. However, in most of the patients, it presents with generalized lymphadenopathy and GI involvement and have aggressive natural history. The histology can show nodular pattern to diffuse areas (Fig. 5). Neoplastic cells are larger than mature lymphocytes, monomorphic, with irregular nuclei and scant cytoplasm. They express B-cell markers—CD20, CD79 along with CD5 and cyclin D1. The characteristic

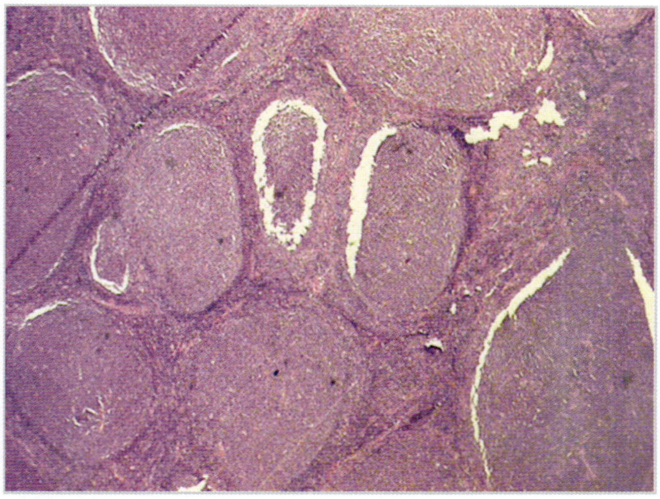

Fig. 4: Low grade follicular lymphoma with nodules or neoplastic follicles scattered uniformly throughout the node. H and E: 4x

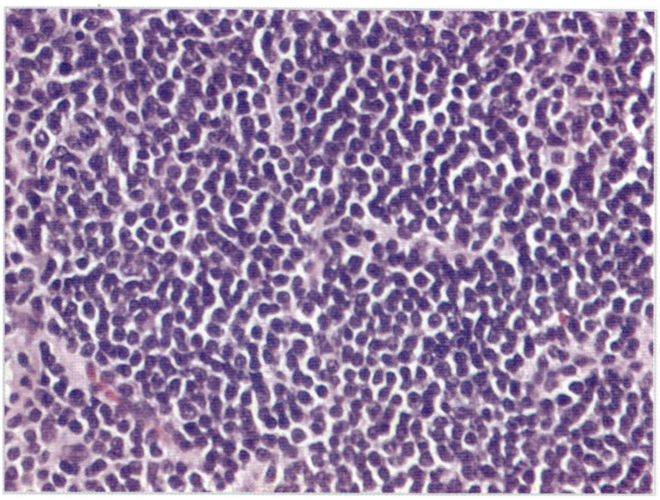

Fig. 5: Diffuse effacement of a node by monotonous small cells in a mantle cell lymphoma. H and E 20x

chromosomal translocation is t(11;14) resulting in overexpression of cyclin D1. These patients if young should be treated with intensive chemoimmunotherapy (preferably cytarabine based) followed by autologous stem cell transplant.[13] Patients who are not candidate for transplant can be given R-CHOP or bendamustine-R followed by rituximab maintenance.[14] Relapses are inevitable. Current therapies have improved the median survival to 5–7 years.

Splenic Marginal Zone NHL (SMZL)

These patients have predominant splenomegaly and lymphocytosis. Involvement of lymph nodes is uncommon. *Splenic marginal zone NHL* (SMZL) usually have indolent course and incurable with available therapies. Histology shows expansion of marginal zone of white pulp resulting in nodular growth pattern. The circulating lymphocytes show villous cytoplasmic projections giving rise to the nomenclature—splenic lymphoma with villous lymphocytosis. The tumor cells are positive for B-cell markers and surface immunoglobulin (Ig). Treatment options include observation in asymptomatic patients to splenectomy or rituximab monotherapy or rituximab and chemotherapy.[15]

Extranodal Marginal Zone NHL

It can involve any epithelial organ but the most common site includes stomach followed by salivary glands, lacrimal gland, thyroid and lung. Most of these cases occur secondary to chronic antigen stimulation caused by either infectious agents like *H. pylori, Chlamydia psittaci, Borrelia burgdorferi* or autoimmune diseases like Hashimoto's thyroiditis and Sjogren's syndrome. The histology shows perifollicular and interfollicular growth with marked expansion of marginal zone and involvement of adjacent mucosa. The characteristic feature is presence of lymphoepithelial lesions. The neoplastic cells are small, monocytoid B-cells. The neoplastic cells show positivity for CD19, CD20 and CD22. The most common cytogenetic abnormality is t(11;18) followed by t(1;14). In cases with disease localized to gastric mucosa anti-*H. pylori* therapy is potentially curable.[16] Other patients can be treated with radiotherapy with prolonged disease free period. In cases with symptomatic and disseminated disease, chemoimmunotherapy is treatment of choice.

T-cell NHL

T-cell NHL includes peripheral T-cell lymphoma – NOS, NK-T cell lymphoma, hepatosplenic lymphoma, subcutaneous panniculitis like T-cell lymphoma, enteropathy-associated T-cell lymphoma. These patients present with advanced stage, B symptoms, and extranodal site of involvement. Chemotherapy results in poor responses with high frequency of relapses in all subsets.[17]

Hodgkin Lymphoma (HL)

It was first described in 1832 by Dr Thomas Hodgkin. As opposed to NHL incidence of Hodgkin lymphoma (HL) has remain unchanged over the years. Incidence of HL is approximately 2.7 per 100,000 per year. It is more common in men as compared to women. HL comprises of classical HL and nodular lymphocyte predominant HL. Classical HL has four subtypes—lymphocyte predominant, nodular sclerosis, mixed cellularity and lymphocyte-depleted (Fig. 6).

Clinical features

Clinical presentation varies among different subtypes of HL. It commonly presents as lymphadenopathy- the most common site being cervical. B symptoms are seen in 25% of patients. Patients with nodular sclerosis are usually young females and have mediastinal mass. Patients with lymphocyte-depleted histology have predominantly infradiaphragmatic disease. Involvement of bone marrow is seen in 5–8% patients.

Diagnostic work up

The diagnosis and staging of HL is similar to NHL. PET-CT has been evaluated in HL more extensively and considering the emerging data on role of interim PET-CT in management of HL it becomes imperative to

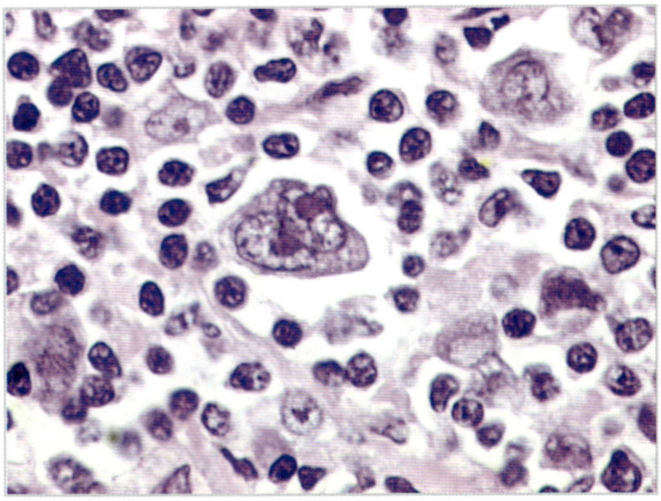

Fig. 6: The typical Reed-Sternberg cell in a Hodgkin lymphoma. H and E: 100x

TABLE 5: International prognostic score (IPS) for HL

Age over 45 years
Male gender
Stage IV disease
WBC > 15,000/mm^3
Absolute lymphocyte count < 600/mm^3 or < 8% of WBC
Albumin > 4 g/dL

have baseline PET-CT to interpret the interim PET-CT results. In patients with early stage HL with normal blood counts and no other risk factors bone marrow biopsy is not needed.

Prognostication

Several cooperative groups have divided patients with HL as early favorable, early stage unfavorable and advanced stage disease based upon several factors; bulk, mediastinal mass, number of nodal areas, B symptoms, erythrocyte sedimentation rate (ESR), age and gender. This stratification helps in individualizing therapy to improve the cure rates and minimization of long-term toxicity. In advanced stage disease international prognostic score (IPS) has been used to predict the prognosis.[18] It is based on seven laboratory and clinical parameters (Table 5). Addition of each factor results in 8% decline in 5-year freedom from treatment failure. In several retrospective analysis, interim PET-CT emerges as one of the most important prognostic tool irrespective of IPS.

Treatment

Combined modality therapy with ABVD (doxorubicin, bleomycin, vinblastine and dacarbazine) and radiotherapy has become the standard of care for early stage HL. For early favorable group, 2–4 cycles of ABVD followed by 20 Gy involved field radiotherapy is the recommended therapy.[19] For early unfavorable disease, 4 cycles ABVD followed by 30 Gy involved field radiation is the standard of care in most centers. Six cycles of ABVD are used for treatment of advanced stage disease. Some of the centers recommend escalated BEACOPP as the chemotherapy regimen for patients with unfavorable and advanced stage disease.[20] However, both short-term and long-term toxicities remain a concern. Role of radiotherapy in advanced stage disease remain unclear.

Nodular Lymphocyte-Predominant Hodgkin Lymphoma (NLPHL)[21]

It is a rare subtype of HL and accounts for approximately 5% of all HL cases. NLPHL forms a distinct entity in terms of its histology, clinical presentation and natural history. It has a more indolent course as opposed to classical HL. Treatment for classical HL has evolved over the years with the help of several large randomized controlled trials. On the contrary, management of NLPHL has been based on small case series or retrospective data due to rarity of disease. A large majority of times NLPHL is treated on the lines of classical HL as seen in German Hodgkin study group recommendations. However, it is relevant to understand the differences between these two entities as NLPHL is characterized by early stage at presentation and late relapses and most of these relapses can be treated successfully resulting in excellent long-term survival. Given the longevity of these patients (young age at diagnosis and excellent overall survival) one should consider therapies which should not have excessive toxicities resulting in treatment related deaths. The treatment options of early stage NLPHL include radiation, combine modality therapy and surgery (rarely). Advanced stage disease is treated on similar lines of classical HL.

REFERENCES

1. Swerdlow SH, Campo E, Harris NL, et al. WHO classification of tumors of haematopoietic and lymphoid tissues, 4th edition. Lyon, France: IARC Press; 2008.
2. Naresh KN, Srinivas V, Soman CS. Distribution of various subtypes of non-Hodgkin's lymphoma in India: a study of 2773 Lymphomas using REAL, and WHO Classification. Ann Oncl. 2000;11(suppl 1):63-7.
3. Newman JS, Francis IR, Kaminski MS, Wahl RL. Imaging of lymphoma with PET with 2-[F-18]-fl uoro-2-deoxy-D-glucose:correlation with CT. Radiology. 1994;190:111-6.
4. Zinzani PL, Magagnoli M, Chierichetti F, et al. The role of positron emission tomography (PET) in the management of lymphoma patients. Ann Oncol. 1999;10:1181-4.
5. Solal-Céligny P, Roy P, Colombat P, et al. Follicular lymphoma international prognostic index. Blood. 2004;104:1258-65.
6. Sehn LH, Donaldson J, Chhanabhai M, et al. Introduction of combined CHOP plus Rituximab therapy dramatically improved outcome of diffuse large B-cell lymphoma in British Columbia. J Clin Oncol. 2005;23:5027-33.
7. Sweetenham JW, Borowitz MJ. Lymphoblastic lymphoma: precursor cell lymphomas in B and T cells. In: Armitage JO, Mauch PM, Harris NL, Coiffi er B, Dalla-Favera R, (Eds). Non-Hodgkin lymphomas, 2nd edition. Philadelphia, PA: Wolters Kluwer and Lippincott Williams and Wilkins. 2010;185-95.
8. Gascoyne RD, Magrath IT, Sehn L. Burkitt lymphoma. In: Armitage JO, Mauch PM, Harris NL, Coiffi er B, Dalla-Favera R, (Eds). Non-Hodgkin lymphomas, 2nd edition. Philadelphia, PA: Wolters Kluwer and Lippincott Williams and Wilkins. 2010; 334-57.
9. Ardeshna KM, Smith P, Norton A, et al. Long-term effect of a watch and wait policy versus immediate systemic treatment for asymptomatic advanced-stage non-Hodgkin lymphoma: a randomised controlled trial. Lancet. 2003;362:516-22.
10. Morschhauser F, Radford J, Van Hoof A, et al. Phase III trial of consolidation therapy with yttrium-90-ibritumomab tiuxetan compared with no additional therapy after first remission in advanced follicular lymphoma. J Clin Oncol. 2008;26:5156-64.
11. Deconinck E, Foussard C, Milpied N, et al. High-dose therapy followed by autologous purged stem-cell transplantation and doxorubicin-based chemotherapy in patients with advanced follicular lymphoma: a randomized multicenter study by GOELAMS. Blood. 2005;105:3817-23.
12. Hallek M, Fischer K, Fingerle-Rowson G, et al. Addition of rituximab to fludarabine and cyclophosphamide in patients with chronic lymphocytic leukemia: a randomized, open- label, phase 3 trial. Lancet. 2010;376:1164-7.
13. Geisler CH, Kolstad A, Laurell A, et al. Long-term progression-free survival of mantle cell lymphoma after intensive front-line immunochemotherapy with in vivo-purged stem cell rescue: a nonrandomized phase 2 multicenter study by the Nordic Lymphoma Group. Blood. 2008;112:2687-93.
14. Howard OM, Gribben JG, Neuberg DS, et al. Rituximab and CHOP induction therapy for newly diagnosed mantle-cell lymphoma: molecular complete responses are not predictive of progression-free survival. J Clin Oncol. 2002;20:1288-94.
15. Oscier D, Owen R, Johnson S. Splenic marginal zone lymphoma. Blood Rev. 2005;19:39-51.
16. Bayerdorffer E, Neubauer A, Rudolph B, et al. for the MALT lymphoma study group. Regression of primary gastric lymphoma of mucosa-associated lymphoid tissue type after cure of *Helicobacter pylori* infection. Lancet. 1995;345:1591-4.
17. Vose J, Armitage J, Weisenburger D, et al. International peripheral T-Cell and natural killer/T-Cell Lymphoma study: pathology findings and clinical outcomes. J Clin Oncol. 2008;26:4124-30.
18. Hasenclever D, Diehl V. A prognostic score for advance Hodgkin's disease. International Prognostic Factors Project on Advance Hodgkin's Disease. N Engl J Med. 1998;339:1506-14.
19. Noordijk EM, Carde P, Dupouy N, et al. Combined-modality therapy for clinical stage I or II Hodgkin's Lymphoma: long term results of the European Organization for Research and Treatment of Cancer H7 randomized controlled trials. J Clin Oncol. 2006;24:3128-35.
20. Engert A, Diehl V, Franklin J, et al. Escalated-Dose BEACOPP in the treatment of patients with advance-stage Hodgkin's Lymphoma: 10 years of follow-up of the GHSG HD9 study. J Clin Oncol. 2009;27:4548-54.
21. Xing KH, Savage KJ. Modern management of Lymphocyte predominant Hodgkin lymphoma. Br J Hematol. 2013;161: 316-29.

61 Evidence-based Medicine in Oncology: Problems, Challenges and Opportunities

Praful Desai

INTRODUCTION

Evidence-based medicine (EBM) and "standard of care" are the current buzzwords in medicine. Almost up to the end of the last century, by far and large, medicine was globally practiced, based on one's experience, expertise, belief and studies based on literature. It depended also on lessons learnt at academic medical meetings. This learning process by the medical fraternity and its clinical application, in general, served the society well.

The advent of the internet era, communication boom and the enthusiasm of academically inclined individuals (medical) ushered in a practice changing era. Many randomized clinical trials, well conducted on a voluminous number of patients, continued to be published. This was the era of mid 1980s, soon after the publication of classic trials of Bonadonna and Veronesi in Italy (1970) and Fisher in the United States (US), National Surgical Adjuvant Breast and Bowel Project (NSABP). Slowly and steadily, the era of "evidence-based clinical medicine" emerged particularly in the US and Europe. The gradual spread of EBM as a norm for therapy and its concept is a welcome addition to medicine as a whole.

There is always a historical background to all major breakthroughs in science and medicine. The genesis of this thought process of EBM is attributed to Dr Gordon Guyatt from Ontario, Canada who coined the term "scientific medicine" around 1992–1994.[1] An academic senior as he was, and concerned with treatment lapses around him, he tried to tread an untrodden path. Uproar and outrage from colleagues was the consequence of this thought process and the word "EBM" was accepted as a kind of consensus which must have satisfied the "naysayers". Any new idea always meets with opposition, protest and discontent as changing conventional ways and habits is often difficult; nevertheless, over a period of time at least in the larger academic institutions and medical centers in India, EBM was slowly being considered as a necessary step towards the practice of scientific medicine.

The objective and purpose of EBM is to exhibit and offer a standard of medical (or other) care which is based on a scientific analysis of collated therapeutic experiences, appropriately and statistically evaluated. This is a major coalition of science and medicine. No greater medical benefit could be bestowed on a patient than to exhibit EBM therapies, in a given clinical setting. It is indeed, a combination of clinical professional expertise with best external evidence supported by clinical research (patient centered) which will include diagnostic tests and therapeutic efficacy leading to an end result over a period of months to years. It is not a "cook book" of medicine, as often labelled by the sceptics. Severe criticism of EBM referred to it as an "old hat, dangerous innovation", perpetrated by the arrogant to serve cost cutters and suppress clinical freedom.[1]

PROBLEMS AND CHALLENGES

The main components and ingredients required to practice EBM are trained and enthusiastic professionals (doctors, nurses, academic scientists and statisticians) and a technical infrastructure with a conducive environment, which will be able to change our established procedures. Contrariwise, the main components of problems and impediments to introduce EBM are socioeconomic issues related to the patient population and the institution. Non-updated professionals, uninformed patients and smaller institutions are major reasons why EBM will be difficult to implement. In a large country like India, with a rural and semiurban population component of 65–70%, even well informed and enthusiastic professionals will find it difficult to implement EBM. Guidelines for its implementation are not always easy or practical. The danger of EBM becoming a legal document can be a major source of concern and anxiety to the medical fraternity, as medicine still remains a science of opinions, and experience and to practice EBM beyond major institutions and private medicine is going to be an uphill task.

The importance of EBM and its benefits, however, cannot be overemphasized by the example that we now have in the treatment of cancers of breast, cervix, colon, prostate and even lung.[2] These are all based on EBM developed after decades of study. No major studies on routine screening for lung cancer are available until now; a study of early lung cancer action project (ELCAP) of 5,000+ US based Japanese population, found 23% of solitary lung (noncalcific nodule), of which 12% were found to be malignant.[2] Though a significant finding, its implementation is difficult for a population based screening program for lung cancer.

The contribution of neo-adjuvant chemotherapy, cyclophosphamide, etoposide and platinum (CEP) and surgery versus surgery alone for lung cancer shows a 5 year survival rate of 0% with surgery alone and 17% with surgery and neo-adjuvant chemotherapy.[2] Similarly, lobectomy versus segmental resection of a localized cancer in the lung in the aged (more than 75 years) population has been shown by EBM that the former has a higher chance of cure than the latter because of increased local recurrences.[3]

Evidence-based medicine can often be equated with "academic excesses" which are difficult to implement even at secondary or tertiary centers. For example, according to EBM, a stage IIIA lung cancer will have to undergo (Box 1) six to seven steps of investigations before finally deciding on either to offer exploratory surgery or radiotherapy.

Box 1: The CONUNDRUM–EBM protocol Academic Excesses? Lung cancer stage IIIA (T1-3N2) mediastinal nodes

- Prove histology – mediastinoscopy
- Neoadjuvant chemotherapy
- Prove down-staging (imaging)
- Repeat mediastinoscopy (if negative)
- Restaging thoracotomy
- Repeat PET/CT
  - Exploratory thoracotomy (Resection), or
  - Radiotherapy

After multidisciplinary consult

Abbreviations: PET, positron emission tomography; CT, computed tomography

It would be logical and wise, therefore, that until many of these steps above and techniques are validated prospectively, they should not replace the judgment, the art and the skill of the treating pulmonologist and the surgeon to decide which patients should proceed with surgery or otherwise, following induction chemotherapy.

Patient and tumor heterogeneity, surgical expertise and individual preferences of a reluctant, balanced or a diehard surgeon; variable tumor responses (complete response, partial response or no response) to chemotherapy and subsequent decisions often have to be individualized where EBM implementation is not always feasible or practical. EBM, therefore, like the laboratory, is an excellent guide for the experienced clinician, but a poor master. *I would certainly like to be guided by EBM but not be governed by the EBM.*

The advent of EBM in India was the initiation of Indian Cancer Cooperative Network (ICCN) in 2005 by a group of countrywide oncologists at a major conference in Jaipur. It did not reach its logical endpoint due to vastness

TABLE 1: Alternatives to evidence-based medicine obstacles to overcome

Basis for discussions	*Marker*	*Measuring device*	*Units of measurement*
Evidence	Randomized clinical trials	Meta-analysis	Odds ratio
Eminence	Radiance of gray hair	Luminometer	Optical density
Vehemence	Levels of stridency	Audiometer	Decibels
Eloquence/Elegance	Smoothness of eloquence or nap of suit	Teflometer	Adhesion score
Diffidence	Level of gloom	Nihilometer	Sighs
Nervousness	Litigation phobia	Every conceivable test Defensive medicine	Bank balance
Confidence (over)	Bravado	Sweat test	No sweat

Source: Isaacs D, Fitzgerald D. Seven alternatives to evidence-based medicine. BMJ. 1999;319(7225):1618.

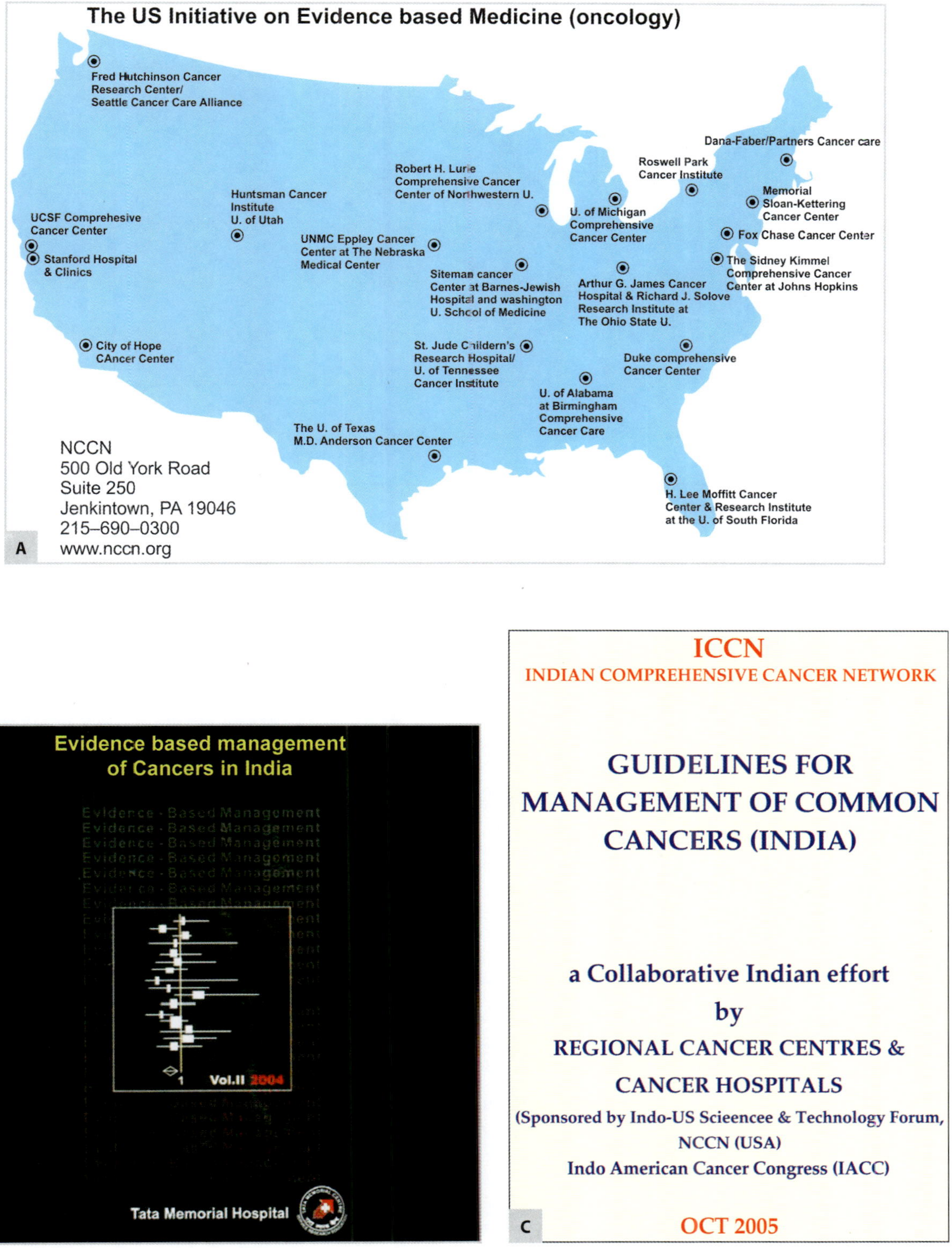

Figs 1A to C: Initiatives for EBM in the US and India

of the country to be able to create a national document. EBM conferences convened once in 2 years by the Tata Memorial Center, provide useful roadmaps for appropriate guidelines in diagnosis and management of cancers in India. The National Cancer Cooperative Network (NCCN) from the US is currently the international document of general guidelines for EBM in oncology. Figures 1A to C show initiatives for EBM in the US and India.

The concluding Table 1 offers an interesting and a humorous side to our current approach to EBM.

REFERENCES

1. Sackett DL, Rosenberg WM, Gray JA, et al. Evidence-based medicine: What it is and what it isn't. BMJ. 1996:312(7023):71-2.
2. Rolh JA, Fossella F, Komaki R, et al. A randomized trial comparing perioperative chemotherapy and surgery with surgery alone in resectable stage IIIA non-small-cell lung cancer. J Natl Cancer Inst. 1994;86(9):673-80.
3. Rosell R, Gómez-Codina J, Camps C, et al. A randomized trial comparing preoperative chemotherapy plus surgery with surgery alone in patients with non-small-cell lung cancer. N Engl J Med. 1994:330(3):153-8.

62 General Principles in Oncologic Anesthesia

Sateesh Gupte

INTRODUCTION

Cancer affects almost all organs in the body. Depending on the site and organ affected, it can compromise the function of vital organs. This is usually by either pathophysiological changes in the organ or mechanical pressures on vital structures. Distant metastases caused by cancer can also affect other organs as primary cancer. Though rare, many general paraneoplastic disturbances occur along with cancer. They include endocrinologic, neurologic, renal, hematologic, gastrointestinal and miscellaneous syndromes. All these can cause interference in the management of the patient during anesthesia. Main treatment modalities of cancer consist of surgery, chemotherapy and radiotherapy and the latter two can pose problems in the conduction of anesthesia due to their metabolic effects on the patient. Management of anesthesia for cancer patients requires knowledge of the above mentioned effect of cancer on the human system. This would enable the anesthesiologist to take proper precautions during anesthetic management. These factors which affect management of anesthesia will be discussed.

Age

Cancer is not restricted to any particular age group and this is borne out by the incidence of cancer in children and young adults. However, majority of patients are in the older age group. Age is a more specific risk factor for anesthesia and surgery.[1] The elderly have higher morbidity rates because of declining physiologic functions[2] and increased presence of cardiovascular, pulmonary and renal symptoms that affect the perioperative and postoperative risks in the patient. Tiret et al.[3] have shown in a prospective study the increase in the anesthetic complications attributed to advancing age. Consequently, when dealing with elderly cancer patients, the anesthesiologist must take into consideration the higher risks these patients are prone to. He must take adequate precautions to anticipate, and prevent potential cardiovascular and pulmonary complications and use drugs with care and caution.

GASTROINTESTINAL

Problems with anorexia, weight loss and cachexia are common in cancer patients.[4,5] Anorexia, cachexia, loss of body tissue, and inability to conserve normal regulatory function of metabolism, has no relation to size, site or type of neoplastic tissue.[6] Often anorexia and cachexia appear before malignancy is detected and disappear when malignancy is resected or controlled. It could be owing to the molecules produced by the tumor causing a metabolic chaotic state.[7] In addition to anorexia and cachexia, protein losing enteropathies are very common with malignancies. More than 90% of cancer patients have low serum protein and albumin levels.[8] Metabolic studies show that it could be due to decreased albumin synthesis or abnormal distribution of albumin in effusion fluids, or increased loss in gastrointestinal tract (protein losing enteropathy).[9] This hypoproteinemia will cause edema. In some cases, these are the early signs of the presence of malignancy. In many cases diarrhea is an early sign of malignancy. When patients with these effects of malignancy come up for surgery, the anesthesiologist must evaluate the total effect of this on the body physiology by estimating the serum proteins, electrolytes, hemoglobin, liver and kidney function. He must also undertake adequate corrective action by crystalloids, protein infusion or hyperalimentation before surgery. Dosage of anesthetic drugs should be reduced proportionally.

FEVER

Fever may frequently accompany cancer. Certain tumors are associated with fever. Major associations are with Hodgkin's disease, myxomas, lung cancers, hypernephromas, osteogenic sarcomas and variety of other tumors. This fever may sometimes be due to infection in the tumor or breakdown of toxic products from the tumors, which are pyrogenic. The fever usually goes away when the offending malignancy is treated.[8] The anesthesiologist should bring the temperature down before taking up the patient for surgery.[10]

HEMATOLOGICAL ABNORMALITIES

Anemia is a frequent accompaniment of cancer. There are many causes of anemia, like anemia of chronic disease, blood loss, bone marrow invasion, suppression of bone marrow by chemotherapy and radiotherapy, vitamin and iron deficiency.[11] Sometimes erythrocytosis is observed in some cancers like renal and hepatic malignancies. Granulocytosis is often observed in leukemia, gastric, pancreatic and lung malignancies as well as melanomas and other cancers. Granulocytopenia is usually due to chemotherapy and radiotherapy and other toxic drugs. Neutropenia alone may develop with marrow involvement by carcinoma, lymphoma, myeloma, or leukemia. However, pancytopenia is more common. These conditions should be treated by steroids and appropriate blood fractions when available. In these circumstances, patients are in an immunocompromised state, and care should be taken regarding asepsis in the theater. Thrombocytosis may occur in some cases, no specific treatment is generally needed. Thrombocytopenia in cancer patients is usually found in cases with leukemia and disseminated intravascular congestion (DIC), as well as in cases where patients have received chemotherapy and radiation. This condition responds to steroids and splenectomy.[8] Thrombophlebitis, migratory thrombophlebitis and DIC respond to the removal of cancer. DIC should be treated with fresh frozen plasma and platelet transfusions. Hematologic complications should be treated with steroids and appropriated blood fractions but real relief comes to the patient after removal or treatment of the offending cancers.[8] The anesthesiologist has to try to get the patient in the best possible condition to stand the surgical procedure.

HYPOGLYCEMIA

This is usually due to insulinomas, yet more than 250 cases of hypoglycemia associated with non islet cell tumors have also been reported.[12] Fibrosarcoma, leiomyomas, rhabdomyosarcomas, liposarcomas and hepatomas contribute to more than 75% of the tumors causing hypoglycemia. These tumors might be secreting substances with insulin-like activities, thereby accelerating glucose catabolism and causing hypoglycemia.[8] The symptoms are dizziness, weakness, nausea, seizures and coma. This is an emergency situation and intravascular (IV) glucose and glucagons should be used to keep the blood sugar at optimum level. During surgery for these tumors, the possibility of hypoglycemia should be kept in mind and wide swings in the blood sugar levels avoided by frequent blood glucose estimations together with adequate and fast glucose infusions when necessary.

HYPERCALCEMIA

This condition is common in cancer patients. Primary hyperparathyroidism and metastatic cancer are the most common causes of hypercalcemia and both diseases are prevalent. This could be due to local osteolytic activity in the secondaries in the bones or ectopic hormone activity in cancers of the lung, kidney, ovary and multiple myeloma. In patients with severe hyperparathyroidism, markedly elevated calcium levels are seen.[13] Hypercalcemia commonly presents with fatigue, constipation, nausea, polyuria and lethargy which can lead to coma. There is severe dehydration due to obligatory water loss on account of excessive excretion of calcium and vomiting. Intravenous hydration is the sheet anchor of therapy. Isotonic saline should be used to avoid dilutional hyponatremia. Volume expansion increases renal blood flow and therefore helps in excretion of calcium. Rate of fluid is to be adjusted according to the initial degree of dehydration, cardiac function and renal excretory capacity.[8] Serum electrolytes, calcium and creatinine should be checked regularly along with urine, and a watch should be kept for congestive failure and potassium and magnesium losses. Along with this, diuretics, oral and IV phosphorus, corticosteroids and calcitonin can be used.[8] After correcting the serum calcium levels, patient can be taken up for surgery.

RENAL DYSFUNCTION

The paraneoplastic abnormality of the renal system is deposition of tumor antibody-antigen complexes on the glomerular membrane which cause nephrotic syndrome-like condition.[8] The kidney can also be affected in malignancy by amyloid infiltration, renal vein thrombosis and neoplastic infiltration of the kidneys, and also by primary malignant tumors of the kidney. Other renal abnormalities in cancer could be due to obstruction of the ureters by pelvic tumors, electrolyte and fluid imbalances induced by the tumor or its therapy, hypercalcemia, uric acidosis, consumptive coagulopathy all of which can lead to glomerular abnormalities. Many of these abnormalities are potentially reversible. Thorough investigation of electrolytes, serum creatinine and urea is necessary and corrective action should be taken with drugs, restriction or infusion of fluids and crystalloids. In case of obstruction to ureters, where possible insertion of double J catheters in the ureters is the first line of action, if this fails nephrostomy is indicated till the obstruction is removed. In case of renal malignancy in one kidney, if the renal function is normal on the other side, the patients do not pose any special problems during anesthesia when they undergo radical surgery for nephrectomy on the affected side. Careful use of drugs, especially relaxants and nephrotoxic drugs and restricted use of fluids, crystalloids is important. In advanced cases, repeated creatinine estimation is essential. When kidney function is affected considerably, dialysis should be at hand.

ENDOCRINOLOGIC

Paraneoplastic syndrome is comparatively common and has to be differentiated from malignancy of an endocrine organ, secondary involvement of the endocrine gland by malignancy, alteration of the hormone production by medicines, and benign pathology of endocrine glands.[8] Hormone production in paraneoplastic syndrome will be independent of normal regulatory mechanisms as the hormone produced in these cases will be from the tumor. The effects of this syndrome will disappear when the offending tumor is removed. Thus, lung cancer of all types can present as Cushing's syndrome due to abnormal production of adrenocorticotropic hormone (ACTH). Also in lung cancer due to abnormal production of parathyroid hormone, hypercalcemia can be encountered. Association of hyponatremia in lung cancer lead Schwartz and associates to postulate in 1957 that there was a "syndrome of inappropriate secretion of antidiuretic hormone" (SIADH), antidiuretic hormone (ADH), arginine, vasopressin (AVP), caused by stimulation of posterior pituitary, to secrete AVP in the presence of lung tumor.[14,15] It was later demonstrated by Amatruda and associates in 1963, to be related to tumor production of AVP.[16] In lung, ovary and adrenal malignancies, secretion of gonadotropins can give rise to precocious puberty, gynecomastia and virilization. In medullary thyroid carcinoma, secretion of thyrocalcitonin can cause hypocalcemia, and hypoglycemia can be caused by retroperitoneal tumors secreting insulin. If the anesthesiologist is aware of these metabolic dysfunctions, he can look for the presence of these abnormal functions and investigate the patient and then he is able to take appropriate action in conduction of anesthesia in patients who exhibit these abnormalities.

NEUROLOGIC

Specific neurological syndromes develop commonly in cancer patients. In patients, where no known cancer is present, presence of these syndromes can indicate a possibility of malignancy and should be investigated for the same. These syndromes are subacute cerebellar degeneration, dermatomyositis in elderly, subacute motor neuropathy, dorsal root ganglionitis, and Eaton-Lambert syndrome. Subacute cerebellar degeneration usually occurs with lung cancer and sometimes with other malignancies. It presents with ataxia, hypotonia, dysarthria and pendular reflexes,[17,18] and dementia may occur. Other syndromes include limbic encephalitis and optic neuritis. In optic neuritis there is decreased vision and papilledema. In dermatomyositis and polymyositis patients, a high percentage of these end up developing cancer. These conditions affect proximal muscles, the progressive muscle weakness stabilizes after certain period.[8] Muscle biopsy shows necrosis. Eaton-Lambert syndrome also known as myasthenic syndrome, is associated with small cell carcinoma of the lung, and causes prolonged response to non-depolarizing muscle relaxants. This possibility should be kept in mind when anesthetizing cases for lung cancer and these drugs used carefully.

LACTIC ACIDOSIS

This is usually associated with acute myelogenous or lymphatic leukemia, Hodgkin lymphoma and other lymphomas. This condition responds to bicarbonate therapy, and responds in parallel with tumor regression to therapy.[19]

ANESTHETIC PROBLEMS IN SPECIFIC OPERATIONS

A general idea will be given in the following paragraphs. Generally, when any patient comes up for surgery, certain baseline investigations should be done preoperatively. They include routine urine examination, complete blood count, chest X-ray, electrocardiogram, liver and kidney function tests, 2D ECHO for cardiac function and also serum electrolytes and proteins should be estimated, and other relevant investigations, done depending upon the site of cancer.

Anesthesia for Head and Neck Surgery

In these cases, there might be trismus and tumors blocking the nasopharynx, pharynx and larynx and cause difficulty in intubation. When the approach to the larynx or the larynx itself is partially blocked, it is better to assess the difficulty preoperatively and do a tracheostomy first and then induce anesthesia. If the difficulty in intubation is obvious, and not due to tumor obstructing the airway, an attempt should be made to intubate the patient awake by use of local anesthesia and sedation, and then induce anesthesia. If this fails, fiberoptic flexible laryngoscope will help in intubating most cases. Preoperative tracheostomy should be used for cases where all the above procedures will not succeed; where fragile bulky tumor is obstructing the airway, and where there is obvious respiratory distress. In an emergency, where general anesthesia is induced, and attempts at intubation fail, and the patient shows sign of hypoxia, a thick needle should be inserted through cricothyroid membrane and oxygen given through it and then proceed with tracheostomy. Bleeding in the mouth and aspiration are real dangers at the end of the operation. Patients should be well awake at the end of the operation with all reflexes active or the tube should be kept in position till the patient wakes up. Nodes in the neck can press on the carotid bifurcation. A watch should be kept on the carotid sinus reflex and slowing of the heart. Intravenous atropine, local application of xylocaine will correct the slowing. Blood loss should be measured accurately and replaced. Care of eyes is important when the patient is covered with towels during surgery.

Lung Surgery

Many paraneoplastic syndromes accompany lung malignancy. Fever and anorexia are common. Hypercalcemia, hyponatremia, Cushing's syndrome, myasthenic syndrome, subacute cerebellar degeneration, non-bacterial thrombotic endocarditis, DIC, and nephrotic syndrome should be looked for and the possibility of one or more of these being present should be kept in mind. If suspicion exists, appropriate tests should be carried out. When the growth in the lung is pressing or infiltrating major vessels or the trachea, sudden bleeding is possible and adequate blood and fluids should be kept at hand, including a big size vein canulated for transfusion and also central-line. When there is involvement of the trachea or carina, it will be known preoperatively from the MRI and CT scan, and in some rare cases, cardiopulmonary bypass may be required. Patients should be checked for all other medical problems and treated adequately before taking up for surgery. The four risk factors that influence the outcome of thoracic surgery are the: (1) patient's age; (2) preoperative status of the respiratory system; (3) accompanying cardiovascular disease; and (4) extent of pulmonary resection.[20] Pulmonary function tests should be performed in all cases. This gives an idea of the postoperative adequacy of pulmonary function. If FEV1 is 2.5 liters or more, these patients usually tolerate pneumonectomy well, but when FEV1 is less than one, there is contraindication for pneumonectomy. In many centers a double lumen endobronchial tube is used to facilitate surgical exposure, to allow selective collapse of the operative non-dependent lung, and allow suctioning of both the lungs.[21] This collapse of the nondependent lung reduces the lung manipulation, retraction and trauma, all of which can impair postoperative gas exchange. Absolute indication for separating the lung include massive hemorrhage, lung abscess, bronchopleural fistula, giant lung cysts or bulla and unilateral bronchopleural lavage;[20] all other indications are relative. Both right and left sided endobronchial tubes are available; left sided tube is preferred to avoid inadvertent occlusion of the right upper lobe bronchus, which is common with a right sided tube.[22] After confirming the position of the double lumen tube, the patient is turned in lateral position; this itself can alter the patient's ventilation perfusion ratio (V/G ratio). The nondependent upper lung is well ventilated while the dependent lower lung is well perfused. Ventilation of the dependent lung is further reduced by weight of the mediastinum and abdominal contents pressing on the diaphragm. In spite of the theoretical possibility of absorption atelectasis and oxygen toxicity, the benefits of oxygenating the dependent lung with 100% oxygen far exceed the risks.[21] The high $FI0_2$ should be avoided in patients treated with bleomycin to avoid lung toxicity. It is safer to give high inspiratory oxygen than to risk effects of hypoxia. In spite of this, if there is hypoxia, it is better to revert back to two lung anesthesia. Blood gas analysis should be done preoperatively and usual monitoring of Sa2, capnography, ECG, central venous pressure (CVP) and blood pressure should be carried out. Generally, postoperatively intermittent positive pressure respiration (IPPR) of the lungs is avoided, lest it should force open the bronchial sutures. Care is taken when using anesthetic drugs, especially relaxants, so that reversal of the patient is complete. In rare cases, when reversal is not satisfactory, there should be no hesitation in instituting IPPR, for the required period.

TUMORS OF ENDOCRINE GLAND

Preoperative evaluation and anesthetic management of endocrine tumors require knowledge of the physiology of the glands and the effects of dysfunction caused by their tumors. Surgery may be needed in these cases for the tumor or some other condition where such tumors co-exist.

In pituitary adenomas, there is excess secretion of growth hormone which produces acromegaly. This causes distorted facial features and prognathism, which may cause difficult mask fit, enlarged tongue, epiglottis and cords, and may cause difficulty in visualizing the larynx for intubation. Adequate assessment is required before starting anesthesia and fiber optic laryngoscope should be used to secure adequate airway, and then induce anesthesia.[23] Hypertension, hepatomegaly and cardiac enlargement may also be present. They should be treated before taking up the patient for surgery.

ADRENAL

Adrenal cortical adenomas, when small are usually benign. Larger tumors are malignant. They produce hypercortisolism. Large tumors can produce adrenogenital syndromes.[24] Adenomas producing Cushing's syndrome respond well to surgery. Excessive ACTH production by pituitary causes hyperplasia of both the adrenal cortices and cause Cushing's syndrome like symptoms. These adrenal tumors present with diabetes, hypokalemia, hypertension, sodium retention, obesity and mental disturbances. After resection, it is good practice to continue with corticosteroid supplement and replacement therapy. In Conn's disease, primary aldosteronism is due to solitary adenomas. After resection, mineralocorticoid replacement is not required. In Cushing's syndrome, the diabetes, hypertension and hypokalemia is corrected preoperatively. Ectopic ACTH producing tumors-like small cell carcinoma of the lungs, carcinoid tumors of the bronchus, carcinoma of the thymus and medullary carcinoma of thyroid can also present as Cushing's syndrome. Adrenal insufficiency is due to relative deficiency caused by involvement of adrenal gland by metastases and can also be caused by excess use of steroids. Steroids cover during surgery is essential. Signs of insufficiency are weakness, anorexia, hyperpigmentation and postural hypotension. Hydrocortisone sodium succinate, 100 mg eight-hourly should be given.

Pheochromocytoma

Pheochromocytoma arises from the chromaffin cells in the adrenal medulla and sometimes their ectopic sites in the abdomen. It secretes catecholamines. It causes hypertension, which is episodic or sustained, along with tachycardia, arrhythmias and cardiomyopathy. There is vascular bed constriction with decreased plasma volume. The hypertension can cause sudden death due to an acute hypertensive crisis. Diagnosis is clinched by estimation of catecholamines in the urine and blood. Symptoms can be controlled by the use of alpha blockade and later on by beta blockade. Phenoxybenzamine is very effective alpha blocker. Blockade with this drug for 10–15 days prior to surgery brings back the intravascular volume to normal levels. Beta blockers are added to this therapy after 10 days. Beta blockers should never be given before alpha blocker treatment, lest it causes cardiac failure. This therapy reduces the occurrence of unmanageable swings in the blood pressure and avoids cardiac or cerebral complications and also the syndrome of vascular collapse after the removal of the tumor. For surgery, premedication should be with tranquilizers, avoiding atropine and opioids. Arterial line, CVP, capnography, oxygen saturation must be monitored. One infusion with sodium nitroprusside and another with noradrenaline should be ready and used depending on the blood pressure. Intravenous beta blockers, alpha blockers, cortisone and xylocaine should be ready in the syringes. Hypotensive response, postoperatively, should be managed with volume infusions and if necessary, dopamine. Transfusions during surgery should be aggressive. Intraoperative hypertension, arrhythmias are common during induction and manipulation of the tumor and are managed with sodium nitroprusside and xylocaine 50–100 mg. Central venous pressure and urine output are the best guides to postoperative vascular status. The patient should be monitored in the intensive care unit for the first twenty-four hours.

Carcinoid Tumors

Carcinoid tumors arise from enterochromaffin cells mainly in the small bowel and appendix but are also found in the bronchi, thymus, head and neck, urinary tract and other tissues. These tumors secrete serotonin, histamine and prostaglandins. In about 5% of the cases, the released vasoactive substances cause symptoms which require treatment (carcinoid syndrome).[25,26] The main clinical effects are cutaneous flushing, diarrhea, asthma, facial telangiectasis and valvular heart disease. The hypovolemia and electrolyte imbalances should be corrected preoperatively. Manipulation of the tumor and other stimuli can precipitate severe hypotension, hypertension, bronchospasm and tachycardia.[23] Stomatostatin or octreotide are the most useful drugs which block the effects of released vasoactive substances. Somatostatin is administered intravenously prior to surgical manipulation of the tumor. Central venous pressure, arterial line for blood pressure reading and other monitoring is essential. Smooth induction and avoidance of drugs that release histamines or activate sympathetic nervous symptoms, are ways to avoid intraoperative carcinoid crisis.[26] It is the best to avoid hypotensive anesthesia like spinal, epidural and halothane. Opioids should be avoided as they release serotonin.

Parathyroid

Excessive secretion of parathyroid hormone due to parathyroid hyperplasia, benign adenoma of parathyroid or parathyroid carcinoma results in primary hyperparathyroidism.[27] The main risk in these cases during anesthesia is arrhythmias due to hypercalcemia. Hypercalcemia should be corrected as best as possible before surgery. Adequate hydration and urine output during surgery is important.[23] Postoperative hypocalcemia is treated with intravenous calcium.

Thyroid

Following thyroidectomy for medullary carcinoma, injury to the recurrent laryngeal nerve can cause upper respiratory obstruction, and aspiration due to injury to the superior laryngeal nerve. Sometimes this lesion is accompanied by pheochromocytoma. During surgery, care should be taken to avoid carotid sinus reflex, air embolism and pneumothorax.

Insulinomas

Pancreatic beta cell insulinomas produce large quantities of insulin. The important thing during anesthesia is to avoid wide swings in the blood sugar levels. A glucose infusion and meter to estimate blood sugar should be handy. Manipulation can cause profound fall in blood sugar levels during surgery and hyperglycemia after removal of the tumor.

CANCER CHEMOTHERAPY

Anesthetic management of a cancer patient who comes for surgery after chemotherapy, needs a clear knowledge of the side effects of the drugs used in this therapy. Most chemotherapeutic agents act by interfering with the enzymes, which relate most often to DNA synthesis or function.[28] Along with the effect on cancer cells these drugs affect the functioning of the normal cells, and cause the toxic effects. A detailed preoperative assessment of such patient is necessary before surgery. This should include a thorough chemical examination. All routine tests like complete blood count, urine analysis, blood sugar, electrolytes, coagulation profile, serum creatinine and urea, serum bilirubin and liver function tests, chest X-ray, ECG and 2D echocardiography should be carried out. Preoperative blood gas analysis should also be done. Any abnormality in the investigations should be submitted to suitable corrective treatment and brought to normal as far as possible. The toxic effects of cancer chemotherapy, which concerns the anesthesiologist are nausea, vomiting, diarrhea, bone marrow depression causing leukopenia, thrombocytopenia, anemia, thrombosis, renal and cardiac, pulmonary, hepatic and neurologic toxicities. Most of these drugs cause immunosuppression and demand strict aseptic techniques during anesthesia.

These anticancer drugs may be classified as alkylating agents, antimetabolites, plant alkaloids, antibiotics, nitrosoureas, enzymes and random synthetics. The commonly used alkylating agents are busulfan, chlorambucil, cyclophosphamide, melphalan, thiotepa and ifosfamide. Bone marrow suppression is the dose limiting factor and also hemolytic anemia. Inhibition of plasma cholinesterase by this drug may result in prolonged response to succinylcholine, but succinylcholine has been given to these patients usually without prolonged effects.[29] Bulky tumors sensitive to these drugs can cause purine and pyramidine breakdown leading to uric acid nephropathy.[30] To avoid this, adequate fluid intake and alkalization of urine are helpful. These drugs also carry the potential for pneumonitis and pulmonary fibrosis; vomiting is common.

Commonly used antimetabolites are methotrexate, mercaptopurine, thioguanine, flurouracil and 5-azacytidine; they affect bone marrow and gastrointestinal epithelial cells. Majority of these drugs are immunosuppressants and can occasionally cause renal tubular necrosis and rarely hepatotoxicity.

Plant alkaloids include vincristine and vinblastine. Bone marrow depression causing leukopenia is major toxic effect. Neurologic toxicity causes encephalopathy and peripheral neuritis.

The antibiotic group includes adriamycin, daunorubicin, bleuomycin, dactinomycin, mithramycin and mitomycin-C. About 49% of the drug is metabolized in the liver, therefore any compromise of hepatic function will increase toxicity of the drug.[31] Bone marrow depression and cardiac toxicity are the dose limiting factors. The cardiac toxicity is in the form of cardiomyopathy causing congestive heart failure. The first sign of this is dry cough, which progresses to congestive failure. Patients who have received high doses of radiation to the chest area, and those who along with these drugs are given cyclophosphamide therapy, are susceptible to cardiac failure. Failure is also more likely to happen with pre-existing heart disease. The profound cardiac and ventricular failure is resistant to cardiotropic drugs and mechanical ventricular assistance.[32] Diagnostic merit of the conspicuous diminution in QRS complex voltage, suggesting the diffuse character of the myocardial damage, is limited because of the lack of its specificity,[33] as this occurs in many other conditions. Echocardiography has been used to diagnose cardiotoxicity before the clinical damage takes place.[34] Nonspecific ECG changes occur during chemotherapy and disappear in a month or two. They include supraventricular tachyarrhythmias, premature ventricular contractions, abnormalities of conduction, left axis deviation, decreased QRS voltage and variety of non-specific ST-T segment abnormalities.[32] These abnormalities occur during therapy irrespective of the schedule, and except for the decreased QRS voltage, resolve in one or two months after the therapy is over.[32] Cytotoxic action of bleomycin and radiation may act synergistically during simultaneous therapy. Pulmonary toxicity is the most serious drug limiting effect reported in 10–25% of the patients. Elderly patients on higher dose of this drug, those who have taken radiotherapy to lungs and those who have existing lung pathology, are more likely to get this toxicity. It has been postulated that previous bleomycin therapy sensitizes the lung to higher oxygen concentrations, which in normal circumstances is harmless. These patients are more at risk after anesthesia and surgery, for adult respiratory distress syndrome.[35-39] Fluid replacement during surgery with colloids rather than crystalloids will reduce the incidence of pulmonary edema.[39] Mithramycin can cause hepatorenal dysfunction and also hemorrhagic diathesis, which is fatal and can occur in 1–5% of the patients.[40] Mitomycin is highly toxic and can cause pulmonary fibrosis and nephrotoxicity. Nitrosoureas cause pulmonary toxicity leading to fibrosis; hepatotoxicity is mild and transient.

In the enzyme group, L-Asparaginase causes coagulopathy and hepatotoxicity and also hemorrhagic pancreatitis. In the random synthetics group, cisplatinum is a highly toxic drug; myelosuppression and renal toxicity are the dose limiting factors. Peripheral neuropathies, seizures and hypercalcemia can occur.

From the above description of toxicity of chemotherapeutic drugs, the anesthesiologist will be able to choose the drugs to be used in anesthesia and those to be avoided and precautions to be taken for minimizing the toxic effects of the chemotherapeutic drugs. In case where the drug causes hepatotoxicity, certain inhalational agents like halothane and relaxants, which are metabolized by the liver, should be avoided. In cases where renal toxicity is expected, the patients should have balanced salt solutions with mannitol to increase the perfusion of the kidneys. Watch should be kept on the urine output during and after the surgery and nephrotoxic drugs avoided. CVP monitoring and watch on the electrolyte replacement is necessary. Myelosuppression is totally reversible and the counts come back in 3–6 weeks after stoppage of chemotherapy. If anemia is present, whole blood replacement or blood components should be transfused as necessary before surgery. Pulmonary fibrosis and pneumonitis caused by bleomycin, methotraxate, mitomycin-C and other drugs should be properly investigated with chest X-ray and pulmonary function tests, when a patient comes with dyspnea. Blood gas analysis should be done preoperatively. Where possible, the operation should be delayed and supportive treatment with steroids, breathing exercises and antibiotics should be given to improve the patient's condition. Excessive high oxygen concentrations should be avoided as they may cause toxicity. Postoperative ventilator support should be kept ready and acute respiratory distress syndrome (ARDS) should be watched for and treated. Cardiotoxicity may occur in patients treated with adriamycin, cisplastin, doxorubicin and some other agents in this group. ECG and ejection fraction will help in the diagnosis and extent of cardiomyopathy. Congestive failure caused by these drugs should be treated with digitalis, diuretics and oxygen. Cardiac depressant anesthetics should be avoided.

These patients pose quite a problem to anesthesiologist and should be treated with utmost care and caution with exact fluid and blood replacement, and drugs like beta-blockers and xylocaine to treat arrhythmias. Usual operation theater monitoring is mandatory with central venous pressure and, where possible, pulmonary arterial and wedge pressure recording in bad risk cases. Diarrhea and vomiting should be treated with fluids and supportive therapy and electrolyte levels brought to normal before surgery.

Radiation of the vital organs of the body can cause side effect, which can be serious and troublesome. Mediastinal radiation for Hodgkin's disease has caused pericarditis. This is dose dependent. Newer shielding methods reduce the incidence and severity of this complication. The most common form of radiation induced complication of heart are chronic and acute pericarditis and myocardial fibrosis. The acute pericarditis comes within one year of radiation. It can cause mild to severe degree of tamponade requiring pericardiocentesis or a pericardial window.[41] The incidence of coronary artery disease due to radiation is dependent on internal thickening and atheromatous deposits in the coronary artery.[42] These effects of radiation take some months to years to affect the organ and so do not pose a problem when surgery is performed immediately after radiation. However, when a patient gives history of having radiation to the chest, the anesthesiologist should investigate the cardiac status by ECG, 2D ECHO, stress test and institute treatment where possible. The incidence and severity of radiation damage to lungs are related principally to the volume of lung tissue irradiated, the total dose, the rate of its delivery and the quality of radiation.[43] Acute radiation pneumonitis becomes evident usually 2–3 months after radiation is over; this slowly leads to fibrosis of the lung in some cases. Progressive dyspnea is the only clinical finding. Knowledge of this fact will help the anesthesiologist to investigate, treat and take precautions during anesthesia. Pulmonary function tests will show restrictive disease; X-ray will show the radiated area differently and in some cases, the blood gas analysis will show less concentrations. Radiation in the region of the neck can cause edema of the glottis and cause difficulty in intubation; a smaller size tube carefully passed will avoid damage to the larynx. In the case of toxicity of chemotherapeutic drugs and radiation, discontinuation of the treatment by these modalities is not always desirable or possible, but knowledge of the effects of these treatments forewarns the anesthesiologist what to expect during the conduction of anesthesia. He can then take appropriate action to reduce the effects of these complications.

REFERENCES

1. Thomas FR, Jones RL. Risks and outcome in oncology patients undergoing anaesthesia and surgery. Int Anaesthesiol Clin. 1998;36(3):141-9.
2. Miller RD. Anaesthesia for the elderly. In: Miller RD (ed). Anaesthesia. 5th ed. Chiedeniff-Livingstone.
3. Trite L, Desmonts JM, Hatton F, et al. Complications associated with anaesthesia, prospective survey in France. Can Anaesth Soc J. 1986;33:336-44.
4. De Wys WD. Working conference on anorexia and cachexia of neoplastic disease. Cancer Res. 1970;30:2816-8.
5. Gold J. Cancer cachexia and gluconeogensis. Ann NY Acad Sci. 1974;230:6-13.
6. Waterhouse C. How tumors affect host metabolism. Ann NY Acad Sci. 1974;230:86-93.
7. Theologides A. The anorexia, cachexia syndrome, A new hypothesis. Ann NY Acad Sci. 1974;230:14-22.
8. De Vita V Jr, Hellemam S, Rosenberg SA. Cancer, principles and practice of oncology, 3rd Edition. JB Lippincot Co; Philadelphia: 1989. pp. 1896-933.
9. Walldman TA, Broder S, Strober W. Protein losing enteropathies in malignancies. Ann NY Acad Sci. 1974;230:306-17.
10. Bodel P. Tumours and fever Ann NY Acad Sci. 1974;230:6-13.
11. Berlin NI. Anaemia of cancer. Ann NY Acad Sci. 1974;230:209-11.
12. Papaioanwou AN. Tumours other than insulinoma associated with hypoglycaemia. Surg Gynecol Obst. 1966;123:1093-109.
13. Heath HH III, Hidgson SF, Kennedy MA. Primary hyperparathyroidism, incidence, morbidity and potential economic impact on the community. N Eng J Med. 1980;302:189-93.
14. Winklev WA, Cranshaw OF. Chloride depletion in conditions other than Addison's disease. J Clin Invest. 1938;17:1-6.
15. Swartz WDF, Bennet W, Curelop S, et al. A syndrome of renal sodium loss and hyponatraemia, probably resulting from inappropriate secretion of Anti Diuretic Hormone. Am J Med. 1957;23:529-42.
16. Amatruda TT, Murlow PJ, Gallaghar JC. Carcinoma of the lung with inappropriate dieresis. N Engl J Med. 1963;269:544-49.
17. Brain WR, Wilkinson M. Subacute cerebellar degeneration associate with neoplasms. Brain. 1965;88:465.
18. Paone JF, Jayasingam K. Remission of cerebellar dysfunction after pneumonectomy for bronchogenic carcinoma. N Engl J Med. 1980;302:156-7.

19. Nadiminti Y, Wang JC, Chou, et al. Lactic acidosis associated with Hodgkin's disease, response of therapy. N Engl J Med. 1980;303:15-7.
20. Benumof J. Anaesthesia for thoracic surgery. Philadelphia. Pa: WB Saunders; 1987. pp. 126-53.
21. Mohindra P, JM Yacob. Anaesthetic management of the cancer patient undergoing noncardiac thoracic surgery. Int Anaesthsiol Clin. 1998;36(3):45-9.
22. Smith A, Hirch N, Ehrenwerth J. Placement of double lumen endobronchial tubes. Br J Anaesth. 1986;58:1317-20.
23. Dougherty TB, Cronan LH Jr. Anaesthetic implications for surgical patients with endocrine tumours. Int Anaesthesiol Clin. 1998;36(3):31-44.
24. Hough AJ, Hollified JW, Page DL, et al. Diagnostic factors in adrenal cortical tumours. Am J Clin Pathol. 1979;72:390.
25. Weidner FA, Ziter FMH. Carcinoid tumours of the gastrointestinal tract. JAMA. 1981;245:1153-5.
26. Oates JA. The carcinoid syndrome. N Eng J Med. 1966;315:702-4.
27. Stoelting RK, Dierdorf SF. Endocrine disease in anaesthesia and coexisting disease, 3rd Edition. New York NY: Churchil Livingstone; 1993. pp. 339-73.
28. Selvin BL. Cancer chemotherapy: Implications for the anaesthesiologist. Anaes Analg. 1981;60:425-34.
29. Dillman JB. Safe use of succinylcholine during repeated anaesthesia in a patient treated cyclophosphamide. Anaes Analg. 1987;66:351-3.
30. Rundles RW, Wyngaarden JB, Hitchings GH, et al. Drugs and uric acid. Annu Rev Pharmacol Toxicol. 1969;9:345-62.
31. Benjamin RS, Clinical pharmacology of Adriamycin (NSC123127). Cancer Chemotherapy Rep. 1975;6:183-5.
32. Lefrak EA, Pitha J, Roseinham S, et al. Adriamycin cardiomyopathy. Cancer Chemother Rep. 1975;6:203-8.
33. Minow RA, Gottlieb JA, Freireich RJ. Electrocardiogram QRS voltage changes in adriamycin cardiopathy. Proc Am Assoc Ancer Res. 1975;16:87.
34. Jouse SE, Ewy GA, Groves BM. Echocardiographic detection of adriamycin heart disease. Proc Am Assoc Ancer Res. 1975;16:228.
35. Young DM. Pathologic effects of adriamycin in experimental systems. Cancer Chemother Rep. 1975;6:159-75.
36. Jorgensen SJ. Time dose relationships in combined bleomycin treatment and radiotherapy. Eur J Cancer. 1972;8:531-4.
37. Blum RH, Carter SK, Agre KA. A chemical review of bleomycin–a new antineoplastic agent. Cancer. 1973;31:903-14.
38. Rudders RA, Mensley GT. Bleomycin pulmonary toxicity. Chest. 1973;63:626-8.
39. Goldiner PR, Carlon G, Cvitkovic E, et al. Factors influencing post-operative morbidity and mortality in patients treated with bleomycin. Br Med J. 1978;1:1644-7.
40. Montow RW, Talley RW, Caldwell MJ, et al. Observations on the mechanism of haemorrhagic toxicity in Mithramycin therapy. Cancer Res. 1969;29:697-703.
41. Stewart JR, Fazardo LF. Radiation induced heart disease, clinical and experimental aspects. Radiol Clin North Am. 1971;9:511-31.
42. Kohn KE, Stewart JR, Fazardo LF, et al. Heart disease following radiation. Medicine. 1967;46:281-98.
43. Devita V Jr, Hellman S, Rosenberg SA. Cancer, Principles and Practice of Oncology, 3rd Edition. Lippincot and Co; Philadelphia: 1989; pp. 2162-3.

63 Cancer Pain Management

Kailash Sharma, Parmanand Jain

INTRODUCTION

Cancer and its related pain is a universal phenomenon affecting patients around the globe. Many international bodies have stated that 80% of patients with cancer pain can be successfully treated, despite the fact cancer pain often is inadequately controlled world over. Extraordinary breakthroughs in our understanding of cancer pain have recently ushered into opening newer treatment options. The neurobiology of bone pain has changed the way we treated primary or metastatic bone lesions. The neuronal changes underlying chemotherapy-induced painful peripheral neuropathy is better understood. As the underlying mechanisms of cancer pain unraveled, newer treatments shall be targeted, e.g. anti-nerve growth factor monoclonal antibodies like tanezumab reducing activation of sensory nociceptors or reducing bone pain by reducing osteoclastic activity by osteoprotegerin. Assessment of pain is the key to successful pain management. Patients with cancer pain can be best managed with a multidisciplinary approach. The goal of cancer pain therapy in patients undergoing active therapy is to provide them with sufficient relief to tolerate the diagnostic and therapeutic procedures required for treatment. Opioids remain crucial to the management of cancer pain. However, obstacles to global pain relief remain primarily issues of access to clinicians and medications which are scarce in developing countries. Many physicians are still fearful of using opioids due to side effects, mainly addiction, respiratory depression or tolerance which are not clinically relevant. In patients with advanced cancer, control of pain with easy access to opioids should allow them to function at a level they choose and to die relatively free of pain. Control of other symptoms and treatment of psychological distress are equally important as it greatly affects the entire pain experience and may lead to severe suffering and existential distress.

EPIDEMIOLOGY

Pain is experienced by one third of all cancer patients despite the availability of efficacious analgesics. Pain is the first symptom in 20–50% of all cancer patients. Approximately 30–50% patients suffer pain during active cancer treatment and 75–95% suffer pain during advanced disease due to failed treatment, chemotherapy, tumor progression or associated pathology in tumor tissue. Pain in advanced cancer is described as moderate to severe in approximately 40–50% and excruciating in 25–30% patients. Pain limits daily activity in 41% patients who have mild-moderate pain and in 94% patients with severe pain. About 33% cancer survivors also suffer pain, e.g. post-mastectomy or post-thoracotomy pain. Pain can be due to tumor or cancer treatment or may be unrelated to cancer. Direct involvement by tumor is the most common cause of pain. Patients with cancer often have multiple causes of pain and multiple sites of pain (Table 1).

In a 10-year prospective study, Zech et al.[1] reported on localization, etiology and type of pain syndromes. Pain was most often localized to lower back, lumbar spine, sacrum and coccyx (36%) followed by abdominal region (27%), thoracic region (24%), lower limbs (22%). In 85% of patients, cancer was the most common cause of pain. Somatic (35%) and somatic-neuropathic (21%) were not common pathophysiologic types of pain.

TABLE 1: Cancer pain syndromes

Pain syndromes associated with tumor infiltration
• Cranial neuralgia
• Glossopharyngeal, trigeminal neuralgia
• Base of skull metastasis
• Orbital, parasagittal, middle fossa and sphenoid sinus metastasis
Tumor infiltration of plexus
• Intercostal neuropathy, peripheral neuropathy
• Cervical, brachial, lumbosacral plexopathy
• Leptomeningeal metastases
Tumor infiltration of epidural space
• Epiduro-spinal cord compression
• Pain syndromes associated with cancer therapy
• Post-chemotherapy pain syndromes
Pain syndromes associated with cancer therapy
Post-chemotherapy pain syndromes
• Peripheral neuropathy, steroid pseudorheumatism and acute herpetic neuralgia
Postsurgical pain syndromes
• Post-mastectomy, post-radical neck dissection, post-thoracotomy and phantom limb pain
Postradiation pain syndromes
• Radiation fibrosis of brachial, lumbosacral plexus, radiation myelopathy

Caraceni et al.[2] published a study involving prospective, cross-sectional, international survey of pain specialists, and their patients. This study also incorporated data from Tata Memorial Center, Mumbai, India. They reported that somatic pain occurred in 39.7% of patients with major pain syndromes comprised of skeletal lesions (41.7%), other types of visceral lesions (28.1%) and soft tissue infiltration (27.8%). More than 76% had Karnofsky performance score of less than 70%. Almost 25% of patients experienced two or more types of pain. A large majority of patients (92.5%) had one or more types of pain and 20.8% of patients suffered pain due to cancer therapies.

DEFINITION AND TYPES OF PAIN

International Association for the Study of Pain has defined pain (1986)[3] as "pain is an unpleasant sensory and emotional experience associated with actual or potential tissue damage or described in terms of such damage". In cancer patients, presence of pain usually implies presence of pathology rather than a delusion or masked depression.

Depending on the "pathophysiology", three types of pain have been described.

1. *Somatic pain*: Well-localized pain due to activation of nociceptors in cutaneous or deep tissue. Metastatic bone pain, musculoskeletal pain and postsurgical incision pain are common examples of somatic pain.
2. *Visceral pain*: Deep, squeezing and pressure like; it is poorly localized or dull aching. Visceral pain is often referred to cutaneous sites remote for the site of lesion. It results from the activation of nociceptors arising from infiltration, compression, extension or stretching of the thoracic, abdominal or pelvic viscera. It is often accompanied by signs of activation of autonomic nervous system such as nausea, vomiting and diaphoresis.
3. *Neuropathic pain*: Burning, shock or current-like pain or dysesthesia. It is most common in areas of sensory loss and may be associated with hypersensitivity to noxious and non-noxious stimuli. It results from the injury to the peripheral or central nervous system (CNS) as a result of tumor compression or infiltration of peripheral nerves or spinal cord. Surgery, radiation therapy or chemotherapy may also cause injury to nerves. Paclitaxel, vincristine or oxaliplatin are commonly used chemotherapeutic agents which may cause painful peripheral neuropathies. Brachial or lumbosacral plexopathies and lesion in spinal cord and CNS may also cause severe neuropathic pain.

Temporal characteristics: Pain may also be classified according to its temporal distribution. Acute pain is characterized by a well-defined temporal pattern of pain onset, generally associated with subjective and objective physical signs and with hyperactivity of autonomic nervous system like hypertension and tachycardia. Acute pain is usually self-limited and responds to treatment with analgesics and to treatment of precipitating cause. It can be further subdivided into subacute or episodic. Chronic pain is persistence of pain for more than 3 months with a less well-defined temporal onset. As the autonomic nervous system adapts, these patients will lack the objective signs commonly seen with acute pain. Chronic pain is associated with significant changes in personality, lifestyle and functional ability.

"Breakthrough pain" is often referred to as incident pain. It is defined as the sudden flare of pain in a setting of a controlled background pain.[4] Breakthrough pain has got multiple characteristics. In some patients, it characterizes pain onset or marked worsening of pain at the end of dosing interval of the regularly scheduled analgesic.

Cancer pain can also be classified as pain due to tumor, cancer treatment or unrelated to it.[5]

- *Tumor-related pain:* Pain may be the major symptom, prompting medical consultation and the diagnosis of cancer. Recurrent pain during the course of illness or after successful therapy has the immediate implication of a recurrent disease
- *Pain due to cancer therapy:* Post-surgery pain like phantom limb pain, post-thoracotomy or post-mastectomy pain, post-chemotherapy pain or pain due to radiation neuropathy are few examples
- *Pain unrelated to cancer:* Patients may have pain due to diabetic neuropathy, post-herpetic neuralgia, cardiac pain or joint pain due to osteoarthritis.

PRACTICAL APPROACH TO A PATIENT WITH CANCER PAIN

Clinical Assessment of Pain

Adequate clinical assessment of pain is a critical component for defining the appropriate therapeutic strategy for each individual patient.

- Believe the patient's complaint of pain
- Take careful clinical history. Nature and quality of pain with exacerbating and relieving factors, response to previous and current analgesic therapy including the details of cancer therapy
- Perform a careful medica and neurologic examination
- *Review the appropriate diagnostic studies*: Computed tomography (CT) scan, magnetic resonance imaging (MRI), bone scan and tumor markers often help to differentiate the primary site of the tumor and the metastatic involvement
- *Evaluate the patient's psychological state*: Depression may occur in as many as 25% patients.[5]
- Individualize the therapeutic approaches and discuss advance directives with patient and family.

Measurement of Pain

It is difficult to measure the exact quantum of pain because of its subjective nature. What patient says "hurts" is pain. There are several scales available. Visual Analogue Scale (VAS) has been used where there is a 10 cm line anchored on either end by two points: "no pain" and "worst possible pain" experienced by a patient. The patient is asked to mark the intensity of pain on the line. Numeric rating scales is a commonly used scale, asking patients to rate their pain experience on a 0–10 number scale where 0 is no pain and 10 is worst possible pain. Verbal (categorical): None, mild, moderate, severe, excruciating. However, pain rating scales are unimodal assessment. Quality of life assessment in a multimodal way includes pain questionnaire charts described in the literature are as follows:

- *Brief Pain Inventory*: The Wisconsin Brief Pain Questionnaire (BPQ) is a self-administered, easily understood method to assess pain.[6]
- *McGill Pain Questionnaire*: The McGill Pain Questionnaire (MPQ) is extensively used pain assessment instrument that produces scores on four empirically derived dimensions, as well as several summary scores.[7] The MPQ offers a methodological approach to assess the sensory, affective and evaluative component of pain.
- *Memorial Pain Assessment Card*: This scale[8] was devised by Analgesic Study section of Memorial Sloan-Kettering Cancer Center to assess the relative potency of analgesic drugs. This scale consists of three visual analog scales that measures pain intensity, pain relief and mood.

PHARMACOLOGICAL MANAGEMENT OF CANCER PAIN

The management of cancer pain involves analgesic therapy along with anesthetic, neurosurgical, rehabilitative, psychologic and psychiatric methods. The treatment must be tailored to suit the individual needs and should be titrated to effective pain relief. All oncologists should have a working knowledge of pain management and the use of drug therapy should be within the armamentarium of any physician or nurse who cares for the patient with cancer pain. The use of specific anesthetic and neurosurgical technique often require trained medical personnel who have clinical experience in managing cancer pain. Such approaches may require referral to specialty center.

Analgesic Drug Therapy

Principles

Most cancer pain can be controlled, in most patients at most of the times. The priorities of the patient care are as follows: (1) to render a pain-free night which is nearly always possible, (2) to ensure pain-free at rest, which is usually possible and (3) to control incident pain (related to physical activity or movement) which is much more difficult to achieve. Various guidelines in the management of cancer pain have been issued by various organizations and researchers. All of them have emphasized that oral analgesic drug therapy is the mainstay of treatment and all have focused on the aims of drug therapy to achieve adequate pain relief safely within an acceptable time frame, to minimize the side effects and to provide ongoing analgesic therapy by the most convenient and least noxious route available.

WHO Three-Step Analgesic Ladder

The World Health Organization (WHO) analgesic ladder was recommended in 1986[9] which is a conceptual approach widely used as a clinical and educational tool. This simple guideline recommends oral analgesics which can be prescribed as per the severity of pain (mild, moderate and severe) from step one to three (Table 2). Analgesic potency gets escalated from non-opioid to weak-to-strong opioid-like oral morphine. Opioid is combined with adjuvant analgesics which are used to enhance pain relief and reduce the side effects. Adjuvant drugs can be prescribed at any stage of the treatment.

There are several important aspects missing from the above WHO three-step ladder model, such as newer analgesic approaches [e.g. N-methyl-D-aspartate (NMDA) antagonists], oncological methods, bisphosphonates, surgical interventions, nerve blocks, etc. Therefore, European Organization for Research and Treatment of Cancer (EORTC) has suggested a three-dimensional pyramid approach which involves four basic approaches to cancer pain control: (1) surgery and physical methods, (2) psychological and behavioral methods, (3) analgesics, and (4) anti-cancer therapies.

TABLE 2: Guidelines for use of analgesics in the management of cancer pain[5]

• Start with a specific drug for a specific type of pain
• Know the relative potency, duration, and side effects of the drug
• Administer analgesic on regular basis
• Choose the route of administration as per the patients needs—oral, rectal, subcutaneous, intravenous, sublingual, transdermal, intraventricular
• Use a judicious combination of drugs to provide analgesia
• Anticipate and treat the side effects like sedation, nausea, vomiting and constipation
• Provide management of the tolerant patient
• Prevent and treat acute withdrawal
• Anticipate complications like overdose, psychologic dependence.

Non-opioid Analgesics

The non-opioid analgesics include acetaminophen and the nonsteroidal anti-inflammatory drugs (NSAIDs). The NSAIDs are believed to provide analgesia through a peripheral mechanism related to inhibition of the enzyme cyclo-oxygenase (COX), thereby reducing the inflammatory mediators. These drugs are most commonly used orally and their analgesia is limited by a ceiling effect, so that increasing the dose beyond a certain level does not increase the analgesic effect. Most common toxicity associated with the use of NSAIDs is gastrointestinal toxicity. Factors which contribute to high risk of gastrointestinal complications are advanced age, use of high doses, concomitant administration with corticosteroids and history of acid peptic disorder. A recent critical review reported that the role of paracetamol and NSAIDs still remain controversial and there is no evidence to show that they should be used to start pain treatment as step one drugs and after how long an opioid should be added on top. Paracetamol is devoid of any benefit if given in less than 4 g per day dose. NSAIDs could be given with opioids after evaluating their response to justify the prolonged use.[10] NSAIDs are especially beneficial to provide effective pain relief in bone metastasis pain which occurs most commonly in cancer breast, prostate or lung. The gold standard for bone pain is palliative radiotherapy but NSAIDs are adjuvants to further enhance the pain relief due to their anti-inflammatory activity (Table 3).

Opioid Analgesics (Tables 4 and 5)

Opioid analgesics are mainstay in the management of cancer pain. During last 2 decades, there has been a dramatic increase in our knowledge of the sites and mechanism of action of opioids. These drugs produce their analgesic effects by binding to discrete opiate receptors in the peripheral and central nervous system. In contrast to non-opioids, opioid analgesics (pure agonists) do not appear to have ceiling effect, i.e. as the dose is escalated, analgesia also increases and the increment in analgesic is linear to the point of loss of consciousness.

Effective use of opioids requires the balancing of the most desirable effects of pain relief to the undesirable effects of nausea, vomiting, mental clouding, constipation, tolerance and physical dependence. These undesirable effects impose a practical limit on the dose useful for a particular patient. The selection of an opioid analgesic is based on the need to treat the severity of pain from moderate to severe pain. The morphine-like opioid drugs represent one end of the spectrum, which includes all other opioids.

TABLE 3: Commonly available nonsteroidal anti-inflammatory drugs (NSAIDs)

Name	Half-life (hours)	Dosing interval	Starting dose (mg/day)	Maximum dose (mg/day)
Acetaminophen	2–4	4–6	1,000	4,000
Aspirin	3–12	4–6	1,000	6,000
Ibuprofen	3–4	4–8	1,200	4,200
Naproxen sodium	12	12	500	1,000
Ketoprofen	2–3	6–8	150	300
Indomethacin	4–5	8–12	75	150
Diclofenac	2–4	6	75	200
Ketorolac	4–6	4–6	150	300
Piroxicam	24	24	20	40
Cyclo-oxygenase (COX)-2 inhibitor	6–8	12–24	20	60

TABLE 4: Opioid analgesics commonly used in India for cancer pain management

Drug	Equianalgesic	Starting oral dose (mg)	Duration of action (hours)
Morphine	10	30–60	4
Codeine	130	200	2–4
Buprenorphine	0.3	0.3	6–8
Fentanyl	0.1	--	1–3
Fentanyl-transdermal	--	--	72

TABLE 5: Principles of opioid use

- Choose a well-tolerated opioid
- Use morphine as drug of choice for moderate to severe pain
- Avoid opioid which are difficult to use (methadone), produce excess side effects (codeine)
- Use round-the-clock dosing
- Identify indications for alternative or novel routes of administration
- Quantity analgesic response and duration
- Review opioid doses regularly until pain is controlled
- Identify dose limiting side effects
- Anticipate constipation and psychological side effects
- Diagnose opioid resistant pain syndromes
- Be aware of the equianalgesic dose of opioids

Pure Agonists

- Morphine: Although, the oral bioavailability varies from 35% to 75%, its plasma half-life is somewhat shorter than its duration of analgesia, which limits its accumulation. The pharmacokinetic properties contribute to safe use of morphine. Morphine-6 glucuronide (M6G) is an active metabolite of morphine that is eliminated by kidney. Recent studies have demonstrated that M6G will accumulate in patients with renal insufficiency. Based on single dose studies in patients with acute or chronic pain, the relative potency of intramuscular to oral morphine is 1:6. However, with repeated administration when patients are dosed on a regular schedule, the intramuscular to oral ratio is reduced to 1:2 or 1:3. The controlled-release morphine preparations (Morcontin) provide analgesia with a duration of 8–12 hours and allow the cancer patients a freedom from repetitive dosing especially during night. The patient should be initially titrated on immediate-release morphine and once stabilized, converted to controlled-release morphine preparations. The management of "breakthrough pain" by rescue medication is done traditionally by immediate release morphine (10% daily dose); however, fentanyl may be considered which is used through novel routes of administration (transmucosal, transbuccal, sublingual in cream, spray, or tablet form), allowing faster action and of short duration that is just ideally cover breakthrough pain episodes. Patients who have sustained moderate-severe pain can be better controlled on fentanyl transdermal patches (25, 50, 100 g) which is especially useful in patients who have oral tumors, trismus, vomiting, intestinal obstruction where oral morphine is an impractical choice. There are several factors which lead to clinical opioid dose escalation: disease progression, psychological reasons (anxiety, depression), pharmacokinetic reasons (poor absorption, drug interaction), opioid refractory pain, e.g. neuropathic pain or tolerance due to several reasons: (1) pharmacodynamic tolerance: (a) cellular tolerance, (b) tolerance at systems level: (i) adaptive processes: upregulation of pro-nociceptive systems, non-opioid receptors like NMDA, antiopioid peptides, (ii) activation of immune system; (2) pharmacokinetic tolerance (liver metabolism, poor absorption).

Anticipation and Treatment of Side Effects

The side effects of the opioid analgesics often limit their effective use. The most common side effects are sedation, respiratory depression, nausea, vomiting, constipation, multifocal myoclonus and seizures. Sedation and drowsiness vary with the drug, dose and may occur after both single and repeated administration. Respiratory depression is the most serious adverse effect of the opioids, however, rare in opioid-dependent patients. It occurs most commonly after short-term administration of an opioid and is usually associated with other signs of CNS depression including sedation and drowsiness. This can be reversed by giving the short-acting opioid antagonist naloxone. It should be titrated carefully to prevent the precipitation of withdrawal symptoms. The incidence of nausea and vomiting is high in ambulatory patients. Nausea with one drug does not mean that other opioids will also have the same effect. Switching to alternative opioid analgesic or using an antiemetic together with the opioid are the best ways to obviate these effects. Constipation results from the actions of these drugs at multiple sites in the bowel motility, which is far more difficult to manage. When opioid analgesics are prescribed, a regular bowel regimen including cathartics and stool softeners should be started.

Adjuvant Drugs

These are commonly used to (1) provide analgesia for certain types of pain viz. neuropathic pain or somatic bone pain, (2) treat opioid side effects and (3) treat other symptoms associated with pain or to potentiate the analgesia of the drugs in a synergistic manner. These adjuvants are the integral part of WHO three-step ladder guidelines.

The adjuvant analgesics can be divided into (1) antidepressants, (2) anticonvulsants, (3) neuroleptics, (4) corticosteroids and (5) oral muscle relaxants, antihistaminic and sympatholytic drugs.

- *Antidepressants*: The tricyclic antidepressants (TCAs) may be the most useful group of psychotropic drugs used in the management of cancer pain. Their analgesic effects are mediated by enhancement of serotonin activity. The starting dose of tablet amitriptyline should be 10–25 mg at night and to be increased gradually in 2–4 weeks periods. TCAs are the firstline therapeutic approach for neuropathic pain and it should be tried for several weeks before discontinuing it. They may require almost a week for a proper clinical effect.
- *Anticonvulsants*: Anticonvulsants medication has become widely accepted in the treatment of chronic cancer pain. The role of these drugs in management of neuropathic pain is based on the fact that they stabilize the membrane and suppress the paroxysmal discharge and reduce the neuronal hyperexcitability. The most commonly used drugs are phenytoin, carbamazepine, sodium valproate, clonazepam, gabapentin and pregabalin.
- *Corticosteroids*: It is used as a multipurpose drug.[11] It is used in patients with advanced disease leading to transient improvement in appetite, analgesia and mood. The major indications for corticosteroids are refractory neuropathic pain, bone pain and headache due to raised intracranial tension. In cancer pain syndromes such as epidural spinal cord compression (ESCC),[12] 85% of the patients receiving 100 mg of dexamethasone reported significant pain relief associated with marked reduction in analgesic requirement. Corticosteroid is effective in brachial and lumbosacral plexopathy. A loading dose of 16 mg and maintenance with 4 mg/day of dexamethasone is often effective in advanced cancer patients with pain.
- *Other adjuvant drugs*: There are wide varieties of adjuvant drugs such as clonidine, benzodiazepine, neuroleptics and NMDA antagonists used in the management of neuropathic pain. Use of ketamine infusion has been found to be effective in certain cases of refractory neuropathic pain. Metastatic disease to bone is the most common cause of pain in patients with advanced cancers of breast, lung and prostate. The drugs viz. bisphosphonates compounds, radionucleotides, e.g. strontium 89, samarium 153 have been found to be effective in the treatment of pain with multifocal metastatic bone disease. The current bisphosphonates used for the treatment of bone pain include pamidronate and clonidronate. Strontium 89 is indicated in patients with refractory multifocal pain due to osteoblastic lesion, who have a life expectancy greater than 3 months and have sufficient bone marrow reserves.

INTERVENTIONS IN PAIN MANAGEMENT

When symptoms are not controlled adequately with medications and other conservative therapy and when life expectancy is limited, neurolytic blocks can be employed. Anesthetic and neurosurgical approaches are most effective in treating patients with well-defined, localized pain. These procedures are often not very effective in managing neuropathic pain except for the use of local anesthetics and most useful in managing the somatic and visceral pain. However, cancer patients often have a mixed somatic, visceral and neuropathic pain syndrome, the selection for these procedures become difficult at later stage of the disease.[13] These procedures should be tried at an earlier stage to have maximal advantage and better quality of life. Intrathecal therapy by pump implant, neurolytic celiac plexus or superior hypogastric or ganglion impar block, spinal neurolysis, vertebroplasty and image-guided tumor ablation are some of the interventional procedures. About 8–11% patients can benefit substantially from these procedures to reduce the side effects of analgesics. A temporary diagnostic block using a local anesthetic should always precede a neurolytic block. Some cancer pain syndromes are more amenable to neurolytic block, e.g. celiac plexus block for cancer pancreas and paravertebral somatic block for post-thoracotomy pain syndrome. Often the best results are obtained in patients who are blocked at an early stage of their illness.

Peripheral Nerve Block

Peripheral neurolysis has a definite role, although limited, in the management of pain of malignant origin. To ensure effective analgesia, neural blockade is planned proximal to the source of nociception. In case of anterior chest wall pain, a more proximal intercostals or paravertebral may be useful or rarely subarachnoid block can be used if skill and expertise is available. Many peripheral nerves are of mixed function. Local anesthetic is essential to evaluate the impact of concomitant motor deficit. This technique is also limited by the fact that each peripheral nerves subserves sensory function over many levels, and usually several nerves must be blocked to provide analgesia.

- *Cranial nerve blocks*: Pain caused by head and neck malignancies often poses the most challenging management problem to the pain specialist. Conventional analgesic therapy may prove inadequate in part because of failure of physiologic splinting, a normal coping strategy, unavailable when pain is aggravated by the act of swallowing, eating, talking and movement of head. Cephalic pain is rarely limited to the distribution of a single nerve because of overlapping sensory innervations (cranial nerves VII, IX and X). In selected patients, the blockade of the involved cranial or upper cervical nerves is of great value. Lasting pain relief is difficult to achieve with discrete nerve block because of sensory overlap. Technical difficulties may also be encountered because of the tendency for tumors in these regions to erode and destroy surrounding tissues. Malignant cancer pain limited to the distribution of the trigeminal nerve or one of its branches may be amenable to thermal or chemical interruption of the involved nerve. If extension of analgesia is necessary, consideration may be given to blocking the 2 and 3 cervical roots and/or the IX and X cranial should not be attempted as it causes paralysis of pharyngeal and laryngeal muscles.
- *Sacral nerve block*: Pain due to pelvic or rectal malignancies in whom bladder and bowel functions are still intact, selective sacral nerve root blocks through sacral foramina, is useful to determine the pathways involved in transmission of pain. The 2 and 3 sacral roots are most commonly implicated in maintenance of bladder function and unilateral predominance of innervation of detrusor reflex activity have been observed.
- *Subarachnoid and epidural neurolysis*: Most of these procedures have gone into archives of pain treatment and are no longer used. However, authors feel that in developing and low resource countries these techniques can be very useful to provide long-term pain relief without incurring much cost. Epidural and intrathecal neurolytic blocks using absolute alcohol or phenol 6% (aqueous or heavy), have been used primarily to manage patients with far advanced disease whose pain is either unilateral in the chest or abdomen or midline in the perineum. These approaches are less useful in managing upper and lower limb pain associated with brachial and lumbosacral plexopathy because of the high risk of motor weakness. The advantages of neurolysis can be realized by a proper case selection with ease of performance, sufficient duration of pain relief, and repetition when necessary. Neurolytic neuraxial block produces pain relief by chemical rhizotomy. Alcohol and phenol both cause an indiscriminate neurolysis regardless of size of the nerve fibers. Epidural phenol neurolysis offers pain relief over wide distribution. Despite the considerations noted above the main disadvantages with epidural neurolysis are short duration and less intensity of analgesia.

Sympathetic Nerve Block

Sympathetic block is effective in conditions with vaso-motor or viscera-motor hyperactivity. This hyperactivity accompanies many of the cancer-related pain syndromes such as visceral pain of plexopathies.

- *Cervicothoracic ganglion block (stellate ganglion block)*: It is useful for pain in the face, upper neck and hemicranium. Usually local anesthetics are used in serial order to have good results. Corticosteroids can be used. Neurolytics are fraught with danger of complications as recurrent laryngeal and vagus nerves are in close vicinity and also vertebral artery.
- *Lumbar sympathetic block*: It may provide significant relief from intractable pain of urogenital origin and pain due to carcinomatous invasion of local nerves and plexus in the perineum and lower extremity.
- *Neurolytic celiac plexus block (NCPB)* has received widespread recognition as it has excellent potential to relieve upper abdominal and referred back pain caused by malignancy involving the upper abdominal structure (pancreas, stomach, duodenum, liver and gallbladder). Currently, endoscopic ultrasound (EUS) has been used to perform celiac plexus block (CPB). C-arm guided NCPB can be performed with 50% alcohol. Side effects may include hypotension, diarrhea, and uncommonly pneumothorax and rarely paraplegia. Good to excellent relief was reported in 89% patients during first 2 weeks after CPB and partial-complete relief in 90% patients at 3 months. Reported side effects were local pain (96%), diarrhea (44%), and hypotension (38%). No influence of type of imaging on pain relief was found.[14-16]
- *Superior hypogastric plexus block*: Pelvic pain can be due to malignancy of rectum, vagina, cervix and other pelvic organs. The pain is often somatic, visceral or a combination of both as the pelvic organs is innervated by somatic and sympathetic fibers.[17] A select group of patients can be benefited when other modalities fail to relieve intractable pain. The technique requires the support of biplanar radiological facilities. Ganglion impar block can be given through the sacrococcygeal joint in perineal pain of cancer cervix, rectum and prostate.

Currently various invasive continuous infusion techniques using programmable pumps and epidural ports have been used to provide long-term pain relief. Radiofrequency denervation and dorsal column stimulation (DCS) have also been successfully used in selected cases. Physiatric and psychologic methods are used as good complimentary tools in relieving pain. The situation may also be improved by suggesting modifications to the patient's way of life by using various rehabilitative methods.

REFERENCES

1. Zech DL, Grond S, Lynch J, et al. Validation of World Health Organization Guidelines for cancer pain relief: a 10-year prospective study. Pain. 1995;63(1):65-76.
2. Caraceni A, Portenoy RK. An international survey of cancer pain characteristics and syndromes. IASP Task Force on Cancer Pain. International Association for the Study of Pain. Pain. 1999;82(3):263-74.
3. Pain terms: a list with definitions and notes on usage. Recommended by the IASP Subcommittee on Taxonomy. Pain. 1979;6(3):249.
4. Portenoy RK, Hagen NA. Breakthrough pain: definition, prevalence and characteristics. Pain. 1990;41(3):273-82.
5. Foley KM. Supportive care and quality of life. In: Devita VT, Hellman S, Rosenberg SA (Eds). Cancer: Principles and Practice of Oncology, 5th edition. Philadelphia: Lippincott-Raven Publishers; 1997. pp. 2807-41.
6. Daut RL, Cleeland CS, Flanery RC. Development of the Wisconsin Brief Pain Questionnaire to assess pain in cancer and other diseases. Pain. 1983;17(2):197-210.
7. Graham C, Bond SS, Gerkovitch MM, et al. Use of the McGill Pain Questionnaire in the management of cancer pain: replicability and consistency. Pain. 1980;8(3):377-87.
8. Fishman B, Pasternak S, Wallerstein SL, et al. The Memorial Pain Assessment Card. A valid instrument for the evaluation of cancer pain. Cancer. 1987;60(5):1151-8.
9. Cancer pain relief and palliative care. Report of WHO Expert Committee. World Health Organ Tech Rep Ser. 1990;804:1-75.
10. Mercadante S, Giarratano A. The long and winding road of non steroidal anti-inflammatory drugs and paracetamol in cancer pain treatment: a critical review. Crit Rev Oncol Hematol. 2013;87(2):140-5.
11. Bruera E, Roca E, Cedaro L, et al. Action of oral methylprednisolone in terminal cancer patients: a prospective randomized double blind study. Cancer Treat Rep. 1985;69(7-8):751-4.
12. Greenberg HS, Kim JH, Posner JB. Epidural spinal cord compression from metastatic lesions: results with new treatment protocol. Ann Neurol. 1980;8(4):361-6.
13. de'Courcy JG. Interventional techniques for cancer pain management. Clin Oncol (R Coll Radiol). 2011;23(6):407-17.
14. Jain PN, Shrikhande SV, Myatra SN, et al. Neurolytic celiac plexus block: a better alternative to opioid treatment in upper abdominal malignancies: an Indian experience. J Pain Palliat Care Pharmacother. 2005;19(3):15-20.
15. Eisenberg E, Carr DB, Chalmers TC. Neurolytic celiac plexus block for treatment of cancer pain: a meta-analysis. Anesth Analg. 1995;80(2):290-5.
16. Negels W, Pease N, Bekkering G, et al. Celiac plexus neurolysis for abdominal cancer pain: a systematic review. Pain Med. 2013;14(8):1140-63.
17. Plancarte R, Amescua C, Patt RB, et al. Superior hypogastric plexus block for pelvic cancer pain. Anesthesiology. 1990;73(2):236-9.

64 Palliative Care and Quality of Life in Advanced Cancer

Mary Ann Muckaden, Jayita Deodhar, Shrikant Atreya

INTRODUCTION

All over the world, management strategies for cancer include maximum efforts towards prevention, early detection and scientific treatment. Yet, data from WHO[1] shows "Cancer is a leading cause of death worldwide and accounted for 7.6 million deaths (around 13% of all deaths) in 2008. About 70% of all cancer deaths occurred in low- and middle-income countries. Deaths from cancer worldwide are projected to continue to rise to over 13.1 million in 2030. Palliative care is treatment to relieve, rather than cure, the symptoms caused by cancer. Palliative care can help people live more comfortably; it is an urgent humanitarian need for people worldwide with cancer and other chronic fatal diseases. It is particularly needed in places with a high proportion of patients in advanced stages where there is little chance of cure."

Palliative care provided at the appropriate time, i.e. early within this disease trajectory; is evidenced based;[2,3] in fact, WHO recognizes it as an exercise in prevention of untold suffering; while relief of suffering is the 4th phase of cancer prevention,[4] WHO recommends that Palliative care should be initiated as soon as possible; as do National Comprehensive Cancer Network (NCCN) guidelines.[5] When active treatment should cease, and palliative care measures continued, should be a joint decision between oncologists, palliative care physicians, patient and family.

Being faced with a life-threatening or advanced disease is a crisis that affects patient and family alike. Though some people may grow from the experience; it remains distressing for all.[6]

INCIDENCE OF ADVANCED CANCERS

Cancer is a leading cause of death worldwide, with 7.6 million deaths (around 13% of all deaths) in 2008. Half of all cancer deaths each year are due to lung, stomach, liver, colorectal and female breast cancers.[1]

Rationale of Treatment when Disease is Advancing

With the advent of newer modalities of anti-cancer therapy; palliative chemotherapy, radiation and surgery form an integral component of treatment for advanced cancers and are covered elsewhere.

- Radiation-tumor-static, short-term, high daily dose fractionation schedules
- Chemotherapy-sensitive tumors, simple schedules, commonly oral "metronomic", easy to administer at home.
- Surgery-amputations (toilet mastectomy, extremities), diversions, stents.

The National Comprehensive Cancer Network guidelines[5] are specific for shared care between oncologist, palliative care teams and other professionals like mental health specialists, social services and others, including community services whatever available. They elaborate that this would ensure better "Quality of life" by reducing symptoms and psychological distress. Ongoing communication between all professionals involved in care pathway, patient and family can lead to ongoing review of care at every step. It is important to have some discussions on "advanced care planning" as soon as feasible.

DEFINITION OF PALLIATIVE CARE

Palliative Care is defined by WHO as an approach that improves the quality of life of patients and their families facing the problem associated with life-threatening illness, through the prevention and relief of suffering by means of early identification and impeccable assessment and treatment of pain and other problems, physical, psychosocial and spiritual. NCCN guidelines include the role of family needs, values, beliefs and cultures in the provision of the same.

GOALS OF CARE

Palliative Care

- Provides relief from pain and other distressing symptoms
- Affirms life and regards dying as a normal process
- Intends neither to hasten or postpone death
- Integrates the psychological and spiritual aspects of patient care
- Offers a support system to help patients live as actively as possible until death
- Offers a support system to help the family cope during the patients illness and in their own bereavement
- Uses a team approach to address the needs of patients and their families, including bereavement counseling, if indicated
- Will enhance quality of life, and may also positively influence the course of illness
- Is applicable early in the course of illness, in conjunction with other therapies that are intended to prolong life, such as chemotherapy or radiation therapy, and includes those investigations needed to better understand and manage distressing clinical complications.

PHYSICAL SYMPTOMS AND THEIR CONTROL

Robert Twycross[6] states that 'Care of the Dying goes far beyond pain and symptom management'. Support is not only for patient but also for families. He goes on to call this "one of the most rewarding of their responsibilities".

Holistic care of patients should be individually planned. This is dependent on the suffering and governed by prevalence of symptoms. In a systematic review of 44 studies looking at symptom prevalence, the authors[7] identified five most common symptoms at presentation. These symptoms (fatigue, pain, lack of energy, weakness, and appetite loss) occurred in more than 50% of the patients weight loss occurred significantly more often closer to the end of life.

Good symptom control is an essential component of effective palliative care and is based on the 5 principles of EEMAA:[6]

- **E**valuation—Diagnosis of each symptom before treatment
- **E**xplanation—To the patient before treatment
- **M**anagement—Individualized treatment
- **M**onitoring—Continuing review of the impact of treatment
- **A**ttention to detail—No unwarranted assumptions

Adhering to such a systematic approach helps not only in better symptom control but increases compliance and Holistic care.

GASTROINTESTINAL SYMPTOMS

Nausea and Vomiting

One of the common symptoms experienced by patients with advancing cancer. Caused by anti-cancer therapy, drugs or obstruction; either within or outside lumen of gut.

It is important to identify the receptor, which is being stimulated, so as to treat appropriately.

Some generic guidelines:

- Reverse the causes where feasible
- Check plasma levels of creatinine, digoxin, calcium
- Drug by receptor stimulated by causative factor.

Management

General

- Check plasma levels of creatinine, digoxin, calcium.
- Consider stopping gastric irritant drugs, e.g. antibiotics, corticosteroids, NSAIDs
- Reverse cause where feasible, e.g. bisphosphonates for hypercalcemia
- Drugs depending on receptor stimulation
- May need to start with subcutaneous route and switch to oral as soon as possible
- Where IV route is available; IV followed by oral
- Rectal route efficacious, should be used where indicated
- Maintain hydration.

Specific

- Haloperidol: 1–3 mg × q24 hour at night, metoclopramide, domperidone: 10–20 mg × 8 hourly

		Area	*Receptor*	*Trigger*
A	Chemoreceptor trigger zone (CTZ)	Area postrema (Base of 4th ventricle)	D2, 5-HT_3, Substance P	Drugs (Morphine, digoxin), hypercalcemia, uremia
B	Cerebral cortex	Higher center	GABA, 5HT	Anxiety
C	Vestibular system	Inner ear	ACh or H_1 receptors	Movement, vertigo
D	Gut and serosal surfaces in the viscera	GI tract	$5HT_3$ receptors	Radiotherapy, chemotherapy, intestinal distention

Stimulation of any of the receptors sends message to vomiting center (located in brainstem but within blood-brain barrier)

↓

Gastric atony, retroperistalsis, thoracic and abdominal muscle contractions

↓

Vomiting

Fig. 1: Receptors and triggers involved in the mechanism of nausia and vomiting induced by anti-cancer therapy

- Anti-anxiety drugs, e.g. lorazepam, alprazolam
- Drugs for vertigo, e.g. dimenhydrinate, meclizine
- Ondansetron: 4–8 mg q8 × h, granisetron: 1–2 mg × 12 hourly (Fig. 1).

Other Broad Spectrum Drugs Include

- Cyclizine and levomepromazine are drugs of choice (not available in India)
- Olanzapine is another broad spectrum drug which in low doses helps in intractable vomiting[8]
- Prokinetic drugs like metoclopramide or mosapride induce peristalsis; propel food distally, relieving sensation of nausea and vomiting
- Copious secretions should be reduced. Drugs of choice are octreotide or somatostatin. Some studies have shown effectiveness of glycopyrrolates.
- Subcutaneous route is ideal. This can be done using a syringe driver or 'Butterfly' fixed subcutaneously and bolus medication injected every 4 hours, and can be managed at home by trained relatives
- Rarely IV is used initially; for both; oral should be started as early as possible.

Constipation

Very common in patients with advanced cancer due to:

- Patients with advancing disease are often immobile
- Loss of appetite with dehydration
- Lack of privacy to use toilet
- Iatrogenic (morphine, NSAIDs, Anti-5HT3 drugs, e.g. ondansetron, vincristine).

Management

Non-drug measures

- Increase oral intake
- Encourage fluids
- Mobilize patient where feasible
- Provide privacy and access to toilet.

Drugs

Different class of drugs is usually combined for optimum effect. Commonly used preparations are:

- Bulk forming: Mineral oils: Liquid paraffin—30 mL × HS, isabgol powder: 5 grams × HS
- Surfactants like lactulose syrup—30 mL × HS and milk of magnesia—30 mL × HS
- Intestinal motility agents: Senna—10 mg × HS, Sodium picosulfate—10 mg × HS

With severe constipation of 5–7 days; manual evaluation is necessary. Softening of stool with arachis oil or glycerine overnight, is followed by a gentle manual evacuation to loosen the impacted fecal lump. This is followed by a high phosphate enema (pain S/W enema will have no yield due to impaction and hurt the mucosa).

Diarrhea

It is uncommon. Subacute intestinal obstruction, leading to spurious diarrhea, needs to be ruled out. Anti-motility drugs like loperamide for symptomatic relief are helpful. Where clinically suspicious of infection; appropriate anti-boitic should be started. Hydration is essential but should be given orally or S/C (1 liter can be given a day by hypodermoclysis); there is usually no need for IV, as patient is being cared for at home.

Anorexia and Cachexia Syndrome

Definition: Anorexia is the loss of appetite or desire to eat. Cachexia is considered as an involuntary, ongoing loss of bodyweight (>5%), accompanied by other factors which most often but not always occur such as anorexia, muscle strength decline or inflammation.[9]

Diagnosis of cachexia: Weight loss of greater than 5% over the last 6 months. Weight loss should be ongoing in the last 1–2 months. In patients with significant fluid retention, large tumor mass or obesity significant muscle wasting may occur in the absence of weight loss.[9]

Pathophysiology (Fig. 2)

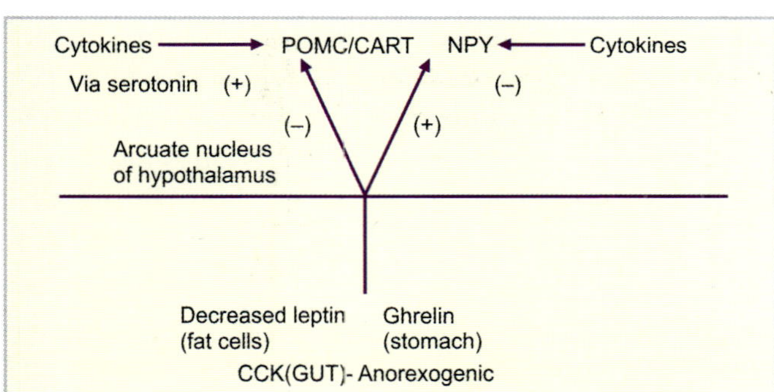

Fig. 2: Pathophysiology of anorexia-cachexia syndrome

Management

- Correct the correctable cause where appropriate:
  - Malabsorption, depression, and anxiety, nausea or vomiting, mucositis, xerostomia, dysphagia
  - Protein loss: Paracentesis, nephritic syndrome, prolonged inactivity and hypogonadism.

Nonpharmacological management

I. *Nutritional Advice:* Improves calorie and protein intake and in one study reported to have halted the progressive weight loss following nutritional advice and liquid oral supplementation like branched chain amino acids, vitamin D and zinc.

II. *Enteral or Parenteral Feeding:* Benefits only small subset of population like those undergoing chemotherapy, mechanical obstruction of the GI tract, dysphagia due to non-malignant conditions like motor neurone disease (MND). However, the place of aggressive nutrition management on malignant disease remains ill defined.

III. Physical activities.

Pharmacological management

I. *Corticosteroids:* These are known to improve appetite, sensation of well-being, performance status. However, the effect is limited to 4 weeks. There is no evidence that on glucocorticoid is superior to the other.[10]
   - Starting Dose: Oral dexamethasone 4mg or prednisolone 30 mg in the morning. Consider need for a proton pump inhibitor.
   - Side-effects: Fluid retention, candidiasis, myopathy, insomnia, gastritis.
   - Prescribe for 1 week, if no benefit, stop. If helpful, reduce to lowest effective dose; review regularly and withdraw if no longer improving symptoms.

II. *Progestational drugs:* These are known to:
   - Improve appetite and increase weight in patients with cancer.
   - Take up to 2 weeks to take effect but benefit more prolonged than steroids.
   - More appropriate for patients with a longer prognosis.
   - **Megestrol acetate:** Starting dose 160 mg orally daily for one month, then review. Dose range (160–800 mg). No evidence for optimal dose.[11]
   - Side-effects: Nausea, fluid retention, increased risk of thromboembolism.

   Reduce dose gradually if used for more than 3 weeks (adrenal suppression).

III. *Prokinetic agent:*
   - Used for early satiety, delayed gastric emptying, gastroparesis or nausea.
   - Metoclopramide 10 mg or domperidone 10–20 mg (less long-term side-effects) given three times a day, half an hour before meals.

IV. *Other medications:*
   - **Non-steroidal anti-inflammatory agents:** Non-steroidal anti-inflammatory drugs alone seem to offer little benefit. NSAIDs may be more effective as part of a multi-modal intervention.[10]
   - **Thalidomide:** This is an anti-inflammatory, antiangiogenic and anticytokin agent. This is known to increase fat-free mass as well as appetite.[12]

- **Selective androgen receptor modulator (Ostarine):** This drug has demonstrated promising results in phase I and II clinical trials, increasing total lean body mass, enhancing functional performance and decreasing total tissue percent fat.[13]
- Olanzapine/Clozapine: The drugs are known to increase the IL6 levels in the body. There is increase in the BMI. This is also reflected by the reflux increase in the leptin levels.[14]
- **Drugs under clinical trial:** Ghrelin, gluconeogensis inhibitor (metformin), creatine, myostatin antagonists.

Fatigue and Asthenia

Definition

- Easy tiring and reduced capacity to maintain performance
- Generalized weakness, defined as the anticipatory sensation of difficulty in initiating a certain activity
- Mental fatigue, defined as the presence of impaired mental concentration, loss of memory and emotional liability
- Multiple factors interact with each other and contribute to fatigue:[15]
  - Direct effects: Lipolytic factors, tumor degradation factors, proteolytic factors, invasion of brain or pituitary gland by tumor
  - Induce host factors: IL1, IL6, TNF
  - Accompanying factors: Psychological issues, anemia, cachexia, infection, metabolic disorders, endocrine disorders, paraneoplastic syndrome.

Management

- Non-pharmacological management: Counseling, physiotherapy, occupational therapy.
- Pharmacological management:
  - Corticosteroids (as above)
  - Megestrol acetate.

  Other management as described in cachexia:
  - Psychostimulants: Methylphenidate and modafanil are known to promote a sense of well being, reduce fatigue and alleviate depression. Methylphenidate is also known to reverse opioid induced fatigue and sedation.
- Specific measures:
  - Correction of anemia: Blood transfusion as and when needed[16]
  - Midodrine, specific alpha 1 sympathomimetic agent can be used autonomic failure in diabetic and neurological disorder
  - Counseling and antidepressants for treating major depression
  - Correction of metabolic disorders like hyponatremia, hypercalcemia, hypokalemia, hypoxia, dehydration
  - Treatment of endocrine abnormality like Addison's disease, hypothyroidism, hypogonadism.

Bowel Obstruction

Pathophysiology should be well understood before management options are decided.[17] Common feature but very distressing feature of advanced abdomino-pelvic cancer especially if there has already been previous surgery and/or radiation. Traditionally, management has tended towards insertion of a Ryle's tube, and nil orally with IV fluids to keep the gut quiescent. However, an alternate philosophy has been considered more humane and effective. Baines et al.[18]in 1985, first described a study on 38 patients managed at St Christopher's hospice with symptomatic management by the subcutaneous route. This has been replicated in a number of studies done all over the world. The management depends on the stage of the obstruction. In subacute obstruction, there is still a small passage allowing liquid bowel contents to pass; which is recognized by the presence of increased bowel sounds. Treatment includes short-term steroids and prokinetic drugs. Buscopan 10 mg for colicky pain is used, if indicated. The patient can still have small feeds. When obstruction is complete, bowel sounds are absent. The patient would have symptoms of colicky pain, regular pain due to stretching of the capsule of distended organs and fecal vomiting due to stasis. Pain is managed as per the WHO ladder. Invariably the patient is already on step 3 drugs like morphine, which cause gastric and intestinal stasis. This fact is exploited here to further cause relaxation. This will relieve the non-colicky pain and lead to less vomiting. The subcutaneous route is best, using a syringe driver or the Edmonton injector.[19] Gastric and intestinal secretions are reduced with glycopyrrolates and octreotide or somatostatin. The patient can, therefore, be cared for at home and allowed small sips of water or any other fluid if desired. Ice cubes if sucked, keep thirst away. Small quantities of fluids up to 1 liter can be transfused (thermolysis) through the subcutaneous route.

Parenteral Nutrition

Its role in patients with limited lifespan is controversial as quality of life has to be balanced against hypoproteinemia. There is adequate evidence against its routine use for patients with less than 3 months estimated survival and side effects are well known. Options should be discussed with patient and family by professionals before instituting such treatment.[20-22]

Dyspnea

There are many causes of dyspnea in patients with advanced malignancy.

- Primary causes include:
  - Central—Carcinoma lung and mediastinal tumors causing airway obstruction
  - Peripheral—Lymphangitis carcinomatosis
- Secondary causes include:
  - Local—Pleural or peritoneal effusions
  - Infections
  - Systemic causes include anemia, hypoproteinemia, etc.

Management

Non-drug

- Oxygen therapy is useful only where PO_2 levels are very low.
- Position, relaxation therapy, breathing techniques, psychological support aid in management.

Drug

- Any anti-cancer intervention is appropriate when the life- expectancy is in weeks or months and symptom benefit outweighs burden
- Same is true for any intervention to lessen symptom, e.g. tapping of pleural effusion, pericardial pig tail or window
- Bronchodilators and steroids where appropriate: Nebulized or oral
- Low-dose morphine (2.5–5 mg q4h for opioid naïve or 50% escalation for those already for pain) reduces awareness of dyspnea in terminal phase
- Benzodiazepines reduce anxiety. Lorazepam 0.5–1 mg × 4 hourly orally and PRN.

Delirium

It is common when entering terminal phase and can be very distressing.

Management

- Reverse cause: Dehydration, hypercalcemia, bladder or bowel distension
- Maximize non-pharmacological interventions: Safe environment, quiet room, familiar and professional staff.
- Haloperidol 0.5–5 mg oral × 4–24 hourly (IV if agitated till controlled)
- Olanzapine oral 2.5-7.5 mg × 4–8 hourly (max 30 mg/d)
- When severe, add lorazepam 0.5-2 mg × hourly SQ/IV
- Support relatives.

Bleeding

May be from surface wound or body cavity. It is usually caused by erosion of capillary; rarely erosion can affect veins or even arteries. In stool, the color can guide origin. Black stools indicate gastric bleed.

Management

- External bleed:
  - Local sustained pressure, local application of ethamsylate or tranexamic acid tabs 500 mg crushed and mixed in xylocaine jelly; change every 24 hour

    or
  - Gauze soaked in nor-adrenaline (1:1000)
  - When severe, consider oral ethamsylate or tranexamic acid tabs 500 mg q × 8 h for 3–5 days, till bleeding stops
  - Vaginal bleeding vaginal pack using diluted nor-adrenaline (1:1000) changed every 24 hour. Systemic therapy where appropriate.
- Laser, cryo, brachytherapy where appropriate
- Gastroscopy or colonoscopy with laser may be helpful
- Artery ligation, amputation, if justified, where benefit outweighs medical futility
- Massive bleeds from major vessels are life threatening.

Moving patient is futile as collapse is imminent. Preparation with presence of dark towels, sedation for patient and preparation of family are essential.

PSYCHOLOGICAL CARE

Personalized medical care has been consistently proven in literature as contributing to the maintenance of psychological balance and quality of life in patients suffering from chronic conditions.[23] The most common psychological distress includes depression and anxiety; severe distress is manifested by feelings of helplessness, worthlessness, lack of role in family and society. In severe cases, this may lead to suicidal ideas/attempts; a clinical feature oncologists need to recognize when dealing with patients whose cancer is incurable.

Loss/grief is part of living with advanced cancer. The "stages of grief" have been immortalized by Kubler-Ross.[24]

However, newer models suggest living with the grief and moving forward; ever gazing backward.[25] The concept of anticipatory loss/grief is also well recognized.

Psychological support is provided for every patient and their family by the palliative care team at first referral. Empathy and active listening are essential ingredients in provision of such support, which can be part of general counseling to discussions regarding prognosis with trained personnel. These routine services range from active listening and general counseling to prognosis explanations by trained personnel. The relevance of good communication skills cannot be over-emphasized here. Patients and families are encouraged to talk to each other and jointly address problems with the help of the multiprofessional palliative care team in an environment of confidentiality, trust, privacy and adequacy of time.

The aim is self-help, with active support provided at the right times; through the entire disease trajectory and into the bereavement process. The role of support groups is proven. Family collusion, where present, has to be handled with culture specific skills, especially when there are obvious indications that the patient is interested in knowing his or her own prognosis. It is important to illicit their help, rather than antagonize their feelings, as these mostly emerge from a feeling of over-protectiveness. Where the team is unable to take care of the psychological distress, the patient may be referred to a clinical psychologist or psychiatrist, where psychological therapies including behavior modifying therapies[19,20] may be used. To be able to provide this continuity of care, training of palliative care workers has proved to be effective[26] and needs to be ongoing.

Social Issues and their Relevance to Care

Care of social issues is very cultural specific. Some important issues covered are rehabilitation of the patient to live as normal a life as possible; financial help for devices, financial aid for medications, etc. Families too, need to be given the aid required to achieve normalcy, either when the patient is unable to provide for their family or after the bereavement. The aim is to create a network of care as close to the patients home as feasible. This involves using existing resources and adding to them where necessary. A very important aspect of continuity of care is Government and NGO cooperation.

PLACE OF CARE

Hospital versus Home care versus Hospice care should be the choice of patient and family. Though patient choice is always respected, and often it is the home, the care provided should be adequate. Family members often feel inadequate and are one of the main reasons they prefer hospital care. Arrangement with local family physicians is the alternative to community nurses of the developed countries. Home care for patients with advanced cancer has been shown to be cost effective; yet can only be effective if home care teams can provide effective holistic care.[27] Studies have shown the importance of family physicians or hospice rapid response teams[28] for provision of "out of hours care". Place of care may change many times during the disease trajectory.

Hospice care takes care of patients where symptom control is difficult at home or adequate family support is not available. Hospice care in a country like India is an option, not often exercised, as family units are strong and provide sufficient care with the help of the professionals. Patients like to be surrounded by their family and care-givers need to be at home to care for the rest of the family.

SPIRITUAL CARE

Care for patients and families suffering from spiritual distress is one of the difficult, yet imperative areas of care. It is important to distinguish between religion and spirituality. Care for spiritual distress in Western countries is taken care of by chaplains. In countries where religion is a way of life, the two may be more intertwined and interdependent. Care for spiritual distress falls upon palliative care teams. Wright[29] expands on the role of spirituality and palliative care as "spirituality has come to be regarded as an essential feature of hospice and palliative care. While only 20% in Western Europe and 14% in Eastern Europe claimed to attend a religious service on a weekly basis, beliefs had not been discarded: seven out of ten adults still claimed to believe in God. Paradoxically, the journey into death is sometimes considered to be the ultimate vehicle for spiritual discovery".

Narayanasamy[30] states "Empirical evidence suggests that spiritual support may act as an adjunct to the palliative care of those facing advanced diseases and end of life".

A Consensus Conference in 2009, led by Puchalski C,[31] was based on the belief that spiritual care was a fundamental component of quality palliative care. One prominent finding was "spiritual care models offer a framework for healthcare professionals to connect with their patients; listen to their fears, dreams, and pain; collaborate with their patients as partners in their care; and provide, through the therapeutic relationship, an opportunity for healing." Details are present in the report.

ETHICS AND PALLIATIVE CARE

A compilation of views from all over the world has brought out the following issues as relevant to ethics in palliative care:[32,33]

- A duty to alleviate suffering
- Respect for persons
- Autonomy
- Non-maleficience
- Beneficence
- Utility
- Justice
- Human rights.

These concepts are crucial to decision making; requiring trust between doctor and patient. This can only develop over time, using adequate communication skills. Thus, the view that Palliative Care should be introduced as early in the trajectory of illness as necessary gets strengthened. The evidenced based treatment results should always be foremost in helping patients with decision making.

END-OF-LIFE CARE

World Health Organization (1998) defines end-of-life care as *"the active, total care of patients whose disease is not responsive to curative treatment"*. National Institute of Health (2004) states that 'the underlying disease process should be irreversible, and that the symptoms or impairments resulting from it, require either professional, or informal family/volunteer care in the time leading up to death.

Some features for recognition are:

- Becomes increasingly weary, weak, and sleepy;
- Becomes less interested in getting out of bed or receiving visitors;
- Becomes less interested in things happening around him/her;
- Often becomes confused, occasionally with features of agitated anguish.

Care at this time is as challenging, as it is rewarding, especially if patient preference is respected and advanced care planning is practiced.[34,35] Medical futility needs to be considered for every medical decision.[36] Any form of intervention, e.g. stents for symptom control, nasogastric feeding and medication versus parenteral nutrition should be decisions taken by patient and family; supported by professionals. NCCN guidelines show lack of benefit of such interventions when death is estimated in weeks.

The route of medication is important; as absorption from the stomach or small intestine is slowing down. An alternate route has to be considered. Some drugs are well absorbed sublingually, e.g. morphine, buprenorphine, hyoscine, and lorazepam. The subcutaneous route allows ease of administration at home (cocktail can be prepared for 24 hour and administered by self or relatives). The rectal and transdermal route are also preferred at this stage. Only essential medications are used at this time; all unnecessary medications, e.g. antihypertensives and corticosteroids should be stopped. Only essential medications should be continued and reviewed regularly.

All treatment decisions should be shared decision making between patient, family and professionals. This also includes decisions like place of death; this should be where patient and family are best supported.

ETHICS IN END-OF-LIFE CARE

Decisions for interventions are based on the "total clinical goal" for every patient and not just on the immediate consequence. Quality of life is paramount; yet varies with each individual and thus should be based on joint decisions between physician and family. This forms the basis of "medical futility"[37] and is extended to decision-making regarding "withholding and withdrawing" unnecessary interventions, e.g. vasopressors, dialysis, ventilator support and assisted nutrition and hydration.[38] Though medically sound, such decisions are difficult. Physicians should seek guidance and collaboration from colleagues, higher authorities and even the court, where decision making is in conflict.

Advance directives or living will is a written decision made by a patient what is her/his wish for terminal care. This helps in decision making and aids in a "do not resuscitate" order (withhold CPR).

Euthanasia is defined as "the deliberate and painless termination of life of a person afflicted with an incurable and progressive disease leading inexorably to death. Euthanasia in this chapter means the administration of death to the dying" and should not be confused with cessation of treatment. For a palliative care physician many of these decisions would depend on the ability to communicate with dying patients.

BEREAVEMENT SUPPORT

An integral component of palliative care and is offered by all palliative care teams till such time, the next of kin is able to move on in life. Normal grief is experienced in 90% of families. Prolonged, delayed or excessive depression can be life-threatening and prolonged intervention may be necessary to prevent the same. Studies have shown that intervention too soon by palliative care teams can even be detrimental and should be preserved only for those families showing abnormal grief.[39] Optimum timing of a bereavement visit is also a topic of research and there are conflicting reports in literature.

RESEARCH AND PALLIATIVE CARE

As in any other branch of clinical medicine, there is a need for evidence based research.[40,41] Traditionally, sick patients being managed at home or hospice precluded efforts. However, the last 10 years has seen an outpouring of research, though not many are level 1 or 2. It is interesting to note that there is as much effort in this from nurses as from doctors.

PEDIATRIC PALLIATIVE CARE

In Western literature, the incidence of children needing Palliative care in Canada was 14.7/10,000 children between 1984 and 1994. Similarly, in Australia, the crude average incidence was found to be 13.8/10,000 under the age of 15.[42] Unfortunately, there are no accurate estimates for developing countries which include India—children die more from acute conditions and malnutrition.

Hynson[43] speculates that the spectre of death is ever present in the cancer disease trajectory, as a consequence of infection or any other complication. The presence of the palliative care physician from the inception of therapy has been referred to as "upstream palliative care" where the seriousness of the situation is revisited at regular intervals.

In many of the conditions requiring palliative care in children, transition to Palliation may come after years of treatment, e.g. acute lymphatic leukemia. The spectre of sudden death is a reality. For this scenario, the presence of the Palliative care team provides supportive care or holistic care taking care of physical symptoms while providing psychological and social support to the family. The child and family become familiar with the palliative care team who assist in taking care of every need. As the disease progresses, the involvement of the palliative care team in the care increases and the transition is smooth.

At the Tata Memorial Center, presence of a palliative care clinician in every joint clinic ensures discussion regarding every treatment option. Children enter the palliative care pathway while continuing with some form of palliative chemotherapy. This helps the family come to terms with the situation; the palliative care team supporting through whole process. When chemotherapy is no longer beneficial, family support continues, enabling a smooth transition into palliative care only.

COMMUNITY-BASED PALLIATIVE CARE

The rising trend in chronic degenerative diseases, increasing disability, rapidly increasing medical cost, commercialization, poor accessibility to primary healthcare and poverty preclude utilization of majority of the medical services by the population.[44,45]

In the country, Palliative care caters only to a small minority of the population. The major challenges for the palliative care practitioners in developing countries is to develop a culturally and socioeconomically appropriate and acceptable system that is accessible to every needy in the community.[46]

This could be achieved in following manner:

1. **Education of the medical and paramedical staff in palliative care:** Rural palliative care providers are usually generalists who may be lacking the knowledge and skills needed to competently care for palliative care patients and families. These patients often comprise a small, infrequent portion of their workload, making it challenging to maintain competency in this specialized area of practice. Providing continuing education opportunities to rural palliative care providers is thus considered essential in increasing a rural community's capacity to deliver palliative care, by keeping providers abreast of changes in best practice and helping them to translate current research findings into practices.[47]
2. **Patient care and empowerment of patient and family:** This includes provision of palliative care through a multiprofessional approach. This should also include empowerment of patients and relatives towards treatment and support.
3. **Continuity of care:** Home based care that is inclusive of doctor, nurses and social workers work in the context of poverty by attempting to retain a holistic approach, acknowledging patients' physical and social needs, and providing psychological and spiritual support.[48]

4. **Community empowerment:** This ensures that emotional and social support, which is as important as physical continues to be provided. This could be achieved by empowering the local organizations and voluntary groups. The stakeholders in the community that include community based organizations, faith healers, gram panchayat, village leaders, self-help groups could be an important resource for social and psychological support for patients and caregivers.[49]

CONCLUSION

Thus community-based palliative care that envisages providing a holistic care could only be achieved through a multi-thronged approach and must be configured to the local needs and customs. It should be community based and integrated with local health and social care, with accessible referral pathways. They also must be responsive to changing individual and population needs and to shifts in local and national health structures between and across services. A public health approach with integration into government policy and core health service provision is necessary to significantly impact the national burden of palliative care needs.

EPILOGUE

Praful Desai

"Palliative care at the end of life" in cancer patients is a major issue that is often neglected and relegated to the family with minimal scientific inputs from a family doctor. Abandonment by actively practicing oncologists in terminal phase is a major setback for patient's physical and mental equilibrium. This reflects poor medicine and poor human values. The time to hand-over the patient to a palliative medicine specialist should be the function of the treating oncologist in consultation with the family and even the patient some of whom even expect the scenario and even wish to cease active therapy onslaughts by the oncologist.

This is science itself with highest human values and only the best human doctors are capable of handling palliative care assisted by the paramedical team. Just as the beginning of a life is probably the most beautiful and sublime event in human existence, passing into the unknown, and an eternal event for all of us, should be transformed into a dignified, peaceful and painless event, however difficult to accept. We need to learn and accept that death is an eventual passage after life.

In an era of overwhelming science, medicine and technology, prolongation of lives can become the ultimate motto of all of us involved in this business. Unregulated, science, medicine and technology's final destination could be "**The Conquest of Mortality**".

Should we proceed towards this ultimate goal?

These are too important issues to be tackled without the involvement of the society and the powers that are and that be. In its ultimate analysis, the true value of a humane medicine is to weigh our success against our failures, the benefits versus risks and the value of old treatment against new practices. Only our conscience can ultimately decide the right course of action in a given clinical scenario.

REFERENCES

1. Global factsheet International Agency for Research on Cancer. World Health Organisation, World Cancer factsheet. Copyright August; 2012. Cancer Research UK.
2. Dennis K, Librach SL, Chow E. Palliative care and oncology: integration leads to better care. Oncology. 2011; 25(13):1271-5.
3. Kamal AH, Swetz KM, Carey EC, et al. Palliative care consultations in patients with cancer: a mayo clinic 5 year review. J Oncol Pract. 2011;7(1):48-53.
4. MacDonald N. Palliative Care-the fourth phase of cancer prevention. 1991;15:253-5.
5. NCCN Clinical Practical Guidelines in Oncology (NCCN Guidelines) Version 2. 2013 nccn.org.
6. Symptom Management in Advanced Cancer, 4th edn. Robert G. Twycross , Wilcock A, Claire (Eds). Palliative drugs.com, Limited 2009.
7. Saskia CCM. Symptom Prevalence in Patients with advanced Cancer—A systematic review. J Pain and Symptom Management. 2007;34(1):94-104.
8. Gupta M, Davis M, Legrand S, et al. Nausea and vomiting in advanced cancer—"The Cleveland Clinic Protocol" J Support Oncol. 2012. pii: S1544-6794(12)00173-5.
9. Florian S. Classification and Pathophysiology of Anorexia-Cachexia Syndrome. In: Geoffery H, Nathan C, Nicholas A C, et al (eds). Oxford Textbook of Palliative Medicine, 4th edn. London: Oxford University Press; 2010. pp 888-907.
10. Brown JK. A systematic review of the evidence on symptom management of cancer related anorexia and cachexia. ONF. 2002; 29(3):517-30.
11. Berenstein EG, Ortiz Z: Megestrol acetate for the treatment of anorexia-cachexia syndrome. Cochrane Database Syst Rev. (2005) CD004310.

12. Gordon JN, Trebble TM, Ellis RD, et al. Thalidomide in the treatment of cancer cachexia: a randomised placebo controlled trial. Gut. 2005;54(4):540-5.
13. Zilbermint MF, Dobs AS. Nonsteroidal selective and rogen receptor modulator ostarine in cancer cachexia. Future Oncol. 2009;5(8):1211-20.
14. M Schuld A, Schacht A, Himmerich H, et al. Effects of clozapine and olanzapine on cytokine systems are closely linked to weight gain and drug-induced fever. Psychoneuroendocrinology. 2009;34(1):118-128.
15. Yennurajalingam S, Bruera E. Fatigue and Asthenia. In: Geoffery H, Nathan C, Nicholas A C, et al (Eds). Oxford Textbook of Palliative Medicine, 4th edition. Londom: Oxford University Press; 2010. pp 916-27.
16. Munch TN, Zhang T, Willey J, et al. The association between anemia and fatigue in patients with advanced cancer receiving palliative care. Journal of Palliative Medicine. 2005;8:1144-49.
17. Jatoi A, Podratz KC, Gill P, et al. Pathophysiology and palliation of inoperable bowel obstruction in patients with ovarian cancer. J Support Oncol. 2004.,2(4):323-34.
18. Baines M, Oliver DJ, Carter RL. Medical management of intestinal obstruction in patients with advanced malignant disease. Lancet. 1985;2:990-3.
19. Fainsinger R , Spachynski K, Hanson J, et al. Symptom control in terminally ill patients with malignant bowel obstruction (MBO). J Pain Symptom Manage. 1994;9(1): 12-8.
20. Acreman S. Nutrition in palliative care.Br J Community Nurs. 2009;14(10):427-8.
21. Bachmann P, Marti-Massoud C, Blanc-Vincent MP, et al. Standards, options and recommendations: nutritional support in palliative or terminal care of adult patients with progressive cancer. Bull Cancer. 2001;88(10):985-1006.
22. Geppert CM, Andrews MR, Druyan ME. Ethical issues in artificial nutrition and hydration: a review. J Parenter Enteral Nutr. 2010;34(1):79-88.
23. Reeve J, Lloyd-Williams M, Dowrick C. The psychologic distress in patients with cancer. Nurs Clin North Am. 2001;36(4):809-25.
24. Kübler-Ross, E. On Death and Dying, Routledge, 1969. ISBN 0-415-04015-9
25. Moules NJ, Simonson K, Prins M, et al. Making room for grief: walking backwards and living forward. Nursing Inquiry. 2004;11(2):99-107.
26. Lloyd-Williams M, Reeve J, Kissane D. Distress in palliative care patients: developing patient-centred approaches to clinical management. Eur J Cancer. 2008;44(8):1133-8.
27. Artherholt SB, Fann JR. Psychosocial care in cancer. Curr Psychiatry Rep. 2012;4(1):3-9.
28. Communication skills training for health care professionals working with cancer patients, their families and/or carers. Cochrane Database Syst Rev. 2004;(2): CD003751.
29. Wright M. Hospice care and models of spirituality. Eur J Palliative Care. 2004;11(2) 75-8.
30. Narayanasamy A. Palliative care and spirituality. Indian J Palliat Care. 2007;13:32-41.
31. Puchalski C. Improving the quality of spiritual care as a dimension of palliative care: the report of the consensus conference Journal of palliative medicine 2009; 12:885-904. DOI: 10.1089/jpm.2009.0142
32. Hudson P. Home-based support for palliative care families: challenges and recommendations. Med J Aust. 2003.15;179(6 Suppl): S35-7.
33. Butler C, Holdsworth LM, Coulton S, et al. Evaluation of a hospice rapid response community service: a controlled evaluation. BMC Palliative Care. 2012;11:11.
34. Fins JJ, Nilson EG. Withholding and withdrawing life-sustaining care. In: Hanks G, Cherny NI, Christakis NA, Fallon M, Kaasa S, Portenoy RK (Eds.) Oxford Textbook of Palliative Medicine, 4th edn. Oxford University Press, UK, 2009:320-32.
35. Boyle DK, Miller PA, Forbes-Thompson SA. Communication and end-of-life care in the intensive care unit: patient, family, and clinician outcomes. Crit Care Nurs. Q2005;28(4):302-16.
36. Cairns R. Advance care planning: thinking ahead to achieve our patients' goals. Br J Community Nurs. 2011;427:16.
37. Jox RJ, Schaider A, Marckmann G, et al. Medical futility at the end of life: the perspectives of intensive care and palliative care clinicians. J Med Ethics. 2012;38(9):540-5.
38. Lorenz KA, Lynn J, Dy SM, et al. Evidence for improving palliative care at the end of life: a systematic review. Ann Intern Med. 2008;148(2):147-59.
39. Schut H, Stroebe MS. Interventions to enhance adaptation to bereavement. Journal of Palliative Medicine. 2005; 8(1), S140-8.
40. Aziz NM, Miller JL and Curtis JR. Palliative and end-of-life care research: Embracing new opportunities. Nurs Outlook. 2012;60(6):384-90.
41. Connor SR. Hospice and palliative care: The essential guide, second edition. Journal of Social Work in End-Of-Life and Palliative Care. 2012;8(2):199-201.
42. Lenton S, Goldman A, Eaton N, Southall D.' Development and Epidemiology'. In:Goldman A, Hain R, Liben S. Oxford Textbook of Paediatric Palliative care for Children ed 1. London Oxford University. 2006;3-13.
43. Hynson LJ. The child's journey:Transition from health to ill-health'. In: Goldman A, Hain R, Liben S. Oxford Textbook of Paediatric Palliative care for Children 1st edn. London Oxford University Press. 2006;14-27.
44. World Health Organization—NCD Country Profiles. 2011.
45. Hung PM, Dzung TV, Dahlgren G, et al. In: Evans T, Whitehead M, Diderichsen F, Bhuiya A, Wirth M (Eds). Challenging inequalities in health. From ethics to action, Vietnam: efficient, equity oriented financial strategies for health, 2001. New York: Oxford University Press. 2001;296-306.
46. Ajithakumari K, Kumar S , Rajagopal MR. Palliative home cared the Calicut experience. Palliat Med. 1997;11:451-4.
47. Kelley ML, Habjan S, Aegard J. Building capacity to provide palliative care in rural and remote communities: does education make a difference? J Palliat Care. 2004;20:308-15.
48. Grant L, Brown J, Leng M, et al. Palliative care making a difference in rural Uganda, Kenya and Malawi: three rapid evaluation field studies. BMC Palliative Care. 2011;10:8.
49. Suresh KK. A Regional Community-Based Palliative Care Model. J Pain and Sympt Managem. 2007;33(5):623-27.

65 Microbial Pathogens and Infection Control in Immunocompromised Cancer Patients

Rohini Kelkar

INTRODUCTION

Microbial pathogens continue to be a serious cause of morbidity and mortality in patients with neoplastic diseases.

The compromised host defenses play a major role as determinants of infection. The introduction of more and more aggressive chemotherapeutic regimens with the resultant prolonged and profound neutropenia is one of the most significant factors in promoting invasion by microbes. Other factors include widespread use of long-term venous access devices and the use of antimicrobial agents for prophylaxis.[1] The cancer patient is thus drowned in a sea of microbes. Most often, these infections are of bacterial etiology. Gram-positive bacteria are a common cause of sepsis in patients with intravascular devices. In India, Gram-negative organisms remain a common cause of infections.

The availability of broad spectrum Gram-negative cover has resulted in the emergence of infections by multidrug resistant microorganisms as well as several unusual infections by new emerging pathogens. The progress made in the treatment of established infection has not paralleled the strategies for prevention. This highlights need to strengthen the preventive strategies, which in turn necessitates continuous monitoring of infection trends. These trends differ at different points in time, from institute to institute, and are dependent on the type of malignancy and the treatment modality. Thus, keeping track of microbiologically documented infections is an important component. The emergence of antimicrobial resistance, globally, over the past few decades has become a matter of increasing concern.

ETIOLOGY

Establishing the etiology of an infectious episode is a difficult exercise in the immunocompromised cancer patient. Since most infections are due to commensal or opportunistic microorganisms, the isolation of a microorganism on culture may not necessarily prove it to be the cause of illness. For example, the isolation of a coagulase negative *Staphylococcus* species from a blood culture may indicate that it is the causative agent of sepsis, or it may be a culture contaminant from the skin. It is also often difficult to recognize the site or origin of an infection. This is particularly so in two settings:

1. The critically ill patient
2. The neutropenic patient.

These patients lack the key signs of inflammation. For example, in spite of extensive infection in the lung parenchyma, the neutropenic patient fails to mount an inflammatory response so as to create a density recognizable on a chest radiograph.

The origin of an infectious episode may be:

- *Endogenous:* Majority of infections are endogenous in origin from the gastrointestinal tract. These can be attributed to breaches in the mucosal barrier. Other endogenous sites include pulmonary lesions caused by Candida or Aspergillus, particularly during neutropenic episodes in leukemia and other solid tumors.
  The urinary tract is a common site in critically ill patients as a source of sepsis. Yeast infections can disseminate and lead to fatal sepsis in such patients.
- *Exogenous infections:* Colonization of vascular access devices by commensal flora from the skin is a common

occurrence. The coagulase negative Staphylococci and other slime producing microorganisms are involved. Surgical site infections (SSI) may be due to the use of inadequately sterilized instruments, inadequate skin preparation or due to lapses in aseptic precautions by the operating surgeon. Rarely, this may be due to the use of contaminated irrigation fluids or intravenous fluids. The environment, as a source of exogenous infection, has a very small role to play.

Causative Agents

A variety of microorganisms can cause infections in cancer patients, but the most common pathogens are bacteria. It is worthwhile noting that the incidence of fungal infections in this population is on the rise in the developed world and in the developing countries as well (Box 1).[2-12]

Polymicrobic infections, i.e. multiple bacterial as well as mixed infections can also occur.

Pathogenesis of Infections in Patients with Neoplastic Disease

The factors involved in the pathogenesis of infections may be due to the disease itself or iatrogenic. In both instances the prime factor is a defect in the host defenses. The extent and duration of neutropenia is the most frequent predisposing factor. Neutropenia significantly increases the risk of bacterial, fungal and viral infections. Candidemia is important in patients with prolonged neutropenia and mucosal damage. Infections with filamentous fungi like *Aspergillus*, *Scedosporium* species, *Fusarium* species, *zygomycetes* and the dematiaceous fungi develop in patients with prolonged and profound neutropenia. Herpes simplex infection may be reactivated in neutropenic patients with leukemia.

Specific immune defects in certain malignancies predispose to certain infections. Patients with chronic lymphocytic leukemia and multiple myeloma have hypogammaglobulinemia, leading to increased susceptibility to infections with encapsulated bacteria like *Streptococcus pneumoniae*. Patients with hairy cell leukemia have T-cell abnormalities, which predispose them to opportunistic nontuberculous mycobacterial (NTM) infections. High dose corticosteroids affect the functions of the immune system, blunt local signs of infections and such patients are at increased risk of common bacterial infections as well as infection with *Pneumocystis carinii, Nocardia* species, mycobacteria and opportunistic fungi and viruses.

Box 1: Comprehensive list of the documented infections

Bacteria
- Gram Positive
  - *Staphylococcus aureus* (including MRSA)
  - Coagulase-negative staphylococci
  - *Streptococcus pneumonia*
  - Group A beta hemolytic streptococci
  - *Corynebacteria*
  - Enterococci
  - *Listeria*
  - *Bacillus* species
- Gram negative:
  - *Enterobacteriaceae: (E. coli, Klebsiella, Enterobacter)*
  - Pseudomonas aeruginosa
  - *Non-aeruginosa Pseudomonas* species, *Stenotrophomonas maltophilia and Burkholderia* species
  - *Acinetobacter baumannii*
  - *Proteus* species
  - *Serratia marcescens*
  - *Flavobacterium* species

Anaerobic bacteria:
- Bacteroides
- Fusobacteria
- *Peptococcus*
- *Peptostreptococcus*
- *Clostridia*

Mycobacteria:
- *Mycobacterium tuberculosis*
- Nontuberculous Mycobacteria

Viruses:
- Cytomegalovirus
- Herpes viruses [Herpes simplex virus (HSV), varicella zoster Virus (VZV)]
- Enteroviruses
- Influenza viruses
- Respiratory syncytial virus, H1N1

Fungi:
- *Candida* and other yeasts
- *Aspergillus*
- Zygomycetes like *Rhizopus*
- *Fusarium*
- *Geotrichum*
- *Histoplasma capsulatum*
- *Penicillium*
- *Pneumocystis carinii*

Protozoa:
- *Toxoplasma gondii*
- *Cryptosporidia*
- *Plasmodium*
- *Giardia lamblia*
- *Ascaris lumbricoides* and other intestinal helminths

Abbreviation: MRSA, methicillin-resistant *Staphylococcus aureus*

Patients with febrile neutropenia are initially predisposed to bacterial infections. With prolonged and profound neutropenia they are at risk of developing fungal and viral infections.[16,17]

In most patients, immune defects are iatrogenic, in the form of impairment of humoral (B cell) and or cell mediated (T cell) functions or neutropenia induced by chemotherapy or radiation therapy.

Breaches in the continuity of the skin or mucus membranes are often a portal of entry for microorganisms. The extensive use of antibiotics suppresses the normal flora and results in the overgrowth of resistant microorganisms. Sometimes a tumor mass may obstruct a vital organ, impair circulation and provide a nidus for infection. Thorough knowledge of the effects of chemotherapy also helps to identify high-risk group of patients. Not all cytotoxic drugs are immunosuppressive. Steroids do not cause neutropenia but inhibit T lymphocyte activity. Surgical patients with large tumors and extensive resections are also a high risk group.

The use of indwelling catheters as vascular access devices for treatment and in critical care units are important factors in many infectious in cancer.[13,21,22]

EPIDEMIOLOGY

The epidemiology of infections differs depending on the type of treatment. Many of these infections in the severely immunocompromised patient are caused by the normal flora of the skin and mucous membranes. Hospitalization, antimicrobial prophylaxis (AMP) and use of empiric antibiotics results in colonization with "hospital flora".

These patients may remain colonized with this acquired flora for prolonged periods of time. The immune-suppressed state results in infections due to some unique/rare opportunistic microorganisms and healthcare associated or nosocomial infections. These patients are also prone to community-acquired infections seen in immune competent hosts.[13-15, 18-20]

LABORATORY DIAGNOSIS

With several advances made in diagnostics, the microbiology laboratory plays an important role. Meaningful contribution by a clinical microbiology laboratory is possible only if an appropriate specimen is sent for processing. When a specimen is sent for culture, it is essential to exclude the normal contaminating flora.[23]

Blood Culture

This is the most useful investigation, particularly in the febrile neutropenic patient. The recovery of microorganisms from blood in a bacteremic patient depends on the timing of the culture, ongoing antibiotics, method of collection and method of processing. Aseptic precautions during collection are essential to prevent the isolation of contaminating skin flora. Automated blood culture systems have virtually replaced earlier manual systems. Automated systems that are available emit signals indicating growth. Thus, the detection is rapid and the time required for identification and susceptibility testing is reduced. These systems are capable of detecting the minimum inhibitory concentrations (MICs), of antimicrobials which are important for the management of patients. There are several commercial sources. Many laboratories in India continue to use manual systems for blood cultures. In patients with indwelling catheters quantitative cultures from peripheral and catheter are helpful in evaluating whether the catheter is a source of bacteremia. This can be proven if the same microorganism is isolated from the peripheral vein and the catheter.

Cultures from Sterile Body Sites and Fluids

The isolation of pathogenic microorganisms or repeated isolation of an opportunistic pathogen is of significance. These fluids may also be incubated in the automated blood culture systems for a rapid diagnosis and early recovery of microorganisms.

Surveillance Cultures

This practice consists of screening the patients' oropharynx, stool and skin. This provides information on microbial colonization rather than disease and is sometimes an indicator of a future episode of infection, although it is rare to find the same flora as the etiologic agent in an episode of infection. Surveillance cultures including nasal swabs, axillary swabs and perianal swabs are recommended for screening of patients known to be colonized or suspected to be colonized, with methicillin-resistant *Staphylococcus aureus.* Stool surveillance cultures are an indicator of colonization with multidrug resistant organisms like extended spectrum beta lactamase (ESBL) producers or vancomycin-resistant enterococci (VRE). The isolation of *Aspergillus* from the nasal swab of a patient undergoing treatment for leukemia may serve as a useful predictive indicator of a future episode of aspergillosis. Some protocols for work up of patients undergoing hematopoietic stem cell transplant (HSCT) include surveillance cultures from various sites.

Sputum/Respiratory Tract Cultures

Respiratory tract cultures should be interpreted along with the clinical and radiological findings. In non-neutropenic patients, the presence of significant numbers of pus cells (> 25/lpf) in a gram stain of the specimen is a useful indicator of infection. If the results of culture are considered in isolation, the end result may be treating "bacteria" rather than an infection. Further, hospitalized, or critically ill patients get colonized with hospital flora within 24 hours of hospitalization.

Antimicrobial Susceptibility Testing

The isolation of a pathogenic microorganism on culture is followed by testing for antimicrobial susceptibility. The results are reported as Susceptible (S), Resistant (R) or Intermediate (I). The interpretation of a resistant result is absolute. A susceptible result is a guideline for choosing an antimicrobial. The MIC is a more accurate result for the institution of therapy.

Direct Examination

This is the first step in processing all clinical material. It is particularly useful in certain situations like: skin vesicles of unknown etiology can be processed as follows:

- Gram stain for bacteria
- Potassium hydroxide mount/calcofluor white fluorescent stain for fungus
- Tzanck smear for herpes type giant cells.

The absence of any of these may indicate that the vesicle is a drug eruption. Direct examination of sterile body fluids like cerebrospinal fluid serves as a useful tool for the detection of Cryptococci with an India ink preparation. Stool examination is useful for the detection of parasites and a hanging drop preparation for motility can help in the diagnosis of suspected cases of cholera.

Differential Stains

Acid-fast stain is used for the direct visualization of mycobacteria and nocardia in respiratory tract and pus samples. Toluidine blue "O" and Giemsa is used for the rapid examination of respiratory specimens for *Pneumocystis carinii*. Giemsa stain is a useful stain to identify the multinucleated "herpes" type giant cells from Tzanck smears which are scrapings from the base of a skin vesicle. Kinyoun's cold acid fast stain is performed on stool specimens for the detection of cryptosporidia or isospora.[23]

Tissue Diagnosis

The oncology patient poses a diagnostic dilemma in several situations. Lung infections are a typical example of such a situation. Differentiation between malignancy alone, malignancy with an infection or an infection alone is often a difficult decision. Invasive procedures may not be possible in patients with immunosuppression and specimens like nondirect bronchoalveolar lavage or bronchoalveolar lavages (BAL) may be collected. Open lung biopsies are rarely possible but offer the most accurate tissue diagnosis. Many times, material from suspicious lesions is collected only for histopathology. The microbiologist may have to depend on special stains and his/her own skills to diagnose an infection. It is possible to identify the nature of the agent on histology; however, speciation of a fungus is not possible on the basis of morphology of the fungal mycelia that are visualized, except in sections showing yeasts with the morphological features of *cryptococci* which can be reliably identified. Isolation on culture, therefore, remains the gold standard with all agents of infectious diseases. Lymph node lesions are another difficult situation where establishing the etiology of an infectious agent in the absence of malignancy/metastasis is elusive. In cases with mycobacterial lymphadenopathy, the direct visualization of acid fast organisms is often negative. Majority of these aspirates/tissue on culture, are known to yield positive results.

VIRAL INFECTIONS

The commonly encountered viral infections consist of herpes viruses, cytomegalovirus (CMV), hepatitis B and hepatitis C viruses and HIV. In the recent years cases with H1N1 and severe acute respiratory syndrome (SARS) have been documented during the respective outbreaks. Due attention needs to be paid to the other endemic and epidemic viruses like hepatitis E and A. Serological tests to detect antibodies of the IgG and IgM class were the mainstay for the diagnosis of these infections. There are several limitations of these assays, because immunocompromised patients do not mount sufficient response to antigenic stimulation and clinical infections may not be detectable by such assays alone. Molecular techniques are available for the diagnosis of CMV, hepatitis B virus (HBV), HCV and HIV, HEV, HAV, H1N1 and SARS. These have replaced the older methods. The real time quantitative polymerase chain reaction (RT-PCR), is now routinely available for the diagnosis and monitoring the treatment of infections with CMV and hepatitis B virus and HIV infections.

Similar assays are available for the diagnosis of other viral infections. These tests may, however, be beyond the reach of many healthcare facilities in the developing countries.

FUNGAL INFECTIONS[32,33,36-44]

These pose a major threat to cancer patients and remain a diagnostic dilemma for laboratories. In most situations, the diagnosis is clinical, supplemented with radiological signs and the treatment is empirical. The probability of isolation of a fungus from blood cultures is less than 1%. Morphologic diagnosis of a fungal infection should be supplemented with cultures. Not all fungi are responsive to antifungals and drug resistance is on the rise. The diagnosis of a fungal infection in the cancer patient consists of:

A high index of clinical suspicion in patients with prolonged and profound neutropenia not responding to antibacterial agents

- Collection of appropriate material with a request for rapid methods like direct examination in case of pus/BAL, etc. using the calcofluor fluorescent stain
- Culture
- Identification of the fungus
- Susceptibility testing to antifungal agents, now included in most laboratories as a routine practice due to availability of standardized methodology and increasing reports of antifungal drug resistance.

Rapid assays for the detection of fungal antigens and nucleic acids by the PCR are available for some common agents like *Candida* and *Aspergillus*.

Blood culture for fungus: A blood culture yielding fungal growth is a certain test of systemic fungal infection in a patient. The main disadvantage is that it is relatively slow (the process takes days), is insensitive and requires specialized expertise for species determination. About 50% of patients with autopsy-proven disease have negative blood cultures antemortem. For detection of *Aspergillus* in blood, at least two (each 10 mL) aerobic blood cultures should be collected. If patients have a central venous access device, then cultures should be obtained through the catheter as well. The currently used methods (Bactec Mycosis-IC/F Medium, Bast-T-Alert, etc.), detect *Candida* species. in up to 60% of all fungemia within 2–5 days. Blood cultures have a very poor yield in patients with invasive aspergillosis and the results are often negative even in patients with disseminated disease. Thus, a lack of positive culture does not rule out the diagnosis of invasive aspergillosis.

Fungal Serology

Patients with fungal sepsis show few distinctive clinical signs, and microbiological techniques frequently fail to isolate the causative organism. Diagnosis by serological testing has received considerable attention. Recent efforts have been directed toward the rapid diagnosis of the mycoses by the detection of circulating fungal antigens and metabolites. Among these markers are mannan, galactomannans and beta D glucan which have been shown to be useful in the diagnosis of invasive candidiasis and aspergillosis respectively.

Invasive Aspergillosis

Galactomannan, a polysaccharide component of the *aspergillus* cell wall, is one of the first antigens detected in body fluids of experimental animals and patients with invasive aspergillosis. It has been studied extensively and has been shown to correlate with clinical diagnosis and response to antifungal therapy. Three different techniques have been evaluated to detect galactomannan in body fluids of patients namely, latex agglutination (with a detection limit of 15 ng/mL), radioimmunoassay (with a detection limit of 10 ng/mL) and enzyme-linked immunosorbent assays (with a detection limit of 4–5 ng/mL), marketed as Platelia *Aspergillus* (Bio-Rad, Marnes-la-Coquette, France). This test is one of the most sensitive methods currently available to detect galactomannan with the lower limit of detection being 0.5–1.0 ng per mL of serum. The Platelia *Aspergillus* test is now included in the consensus definitions for the diagnosis of systemic fungal infections (SFI) issued jointly by the European Organization for Research and Treatment of Cancer and the National Institute of Allergy and Infectious Diseases Mycoses Study Group and have been accepted as part of the standard of care for patients with hematolymphoid malignancies at high risk of fungal infections.

The Platelia *Aspergillus* assay has a false-positive rate ranging from 1% to 18% with serum samples. Despite the drawbacks, the Platelia *Aspergillus* assay represents a marked improvement in the serological diagnosis of patients at risk for aspergillosis. Galactomannanemia is transient and therefore it is recommended that weekly testing be performed in high risk patients. Confirmation of suspected invasive aspergillosis should be obtained by additional radiological and/or microbiological examinations.[45-52]

Approach to Laboratory Diagnosis of an Infective Episode

- High index of suspicion
- Collection of appropriate material
- Preliminary reporting on direct examination with special stains/procedures
- Isolation of the etiology agent on culture
- Identification and antimicrobial susceptibility testing
- Interpretation of results in the clinical context
- Serologic diagnosis
- Rapid detection of the antigens/metabolites
- Management issues.

Monitoring of Infections

One of the most important strategies for control of infections is keeping track of the pattern of infections. Infections can be classified by site. It is also possible to calculate infection rates. Active surveillance permits recognition of trends in infection rates, antimicrobial resistance among pathogens and identification of out breaks. Surveillance data serves as a quality indicator of patient safety and care. Site specific infections/rates are useful parameters for monitoring. The Center for Disease Control, Atlanta, Georgia has a surveillance system for monitoring nosocomial infection (NNIS, i.e. National Nosocomial Infections Surveillance). A similar scheme can be followed for monitoring infections in oncology. The following sites can be monitored:

- Bloodstream infections (BSI)
- Surgical site infections
- Lower respiratory tract infections
- Urinary tract infections
- Line-associated infections or catheter-related BSI.

Bloodstream Infections

The detection of living microorganisms in blood cultures is the most important indication of a serious infection.

In oncology practice differences in causative agents are often seen between different patient groups. Moreover, global differences are also evident.

Thus, varying patterns are seen in leukemia and solid tumors and surgical patients. Critically ill patients also show a different pattern. This highlights the need for continuous monitoring of trends in infections.[29-31]

Bloodstream infection trends at Tata Memorial Hospital over 3 decades.

Studies of septicemias in the 80's[24] revealed that *Pseudomonas aeruginosa* and *Klebsiella* were the commonest etiologic agents. A similar study in 1990 showed that *Pseudomonas* was the commonest isolate followed by *Staphylococcus aureus* and *Acinetobacter* species. In 1994, the pattern of BSI showed a predominance of *Staphylococcus aureus*.

Figure 1 shows that there are differences in the pattern of Gram-negative infections between 2000 and 2012.

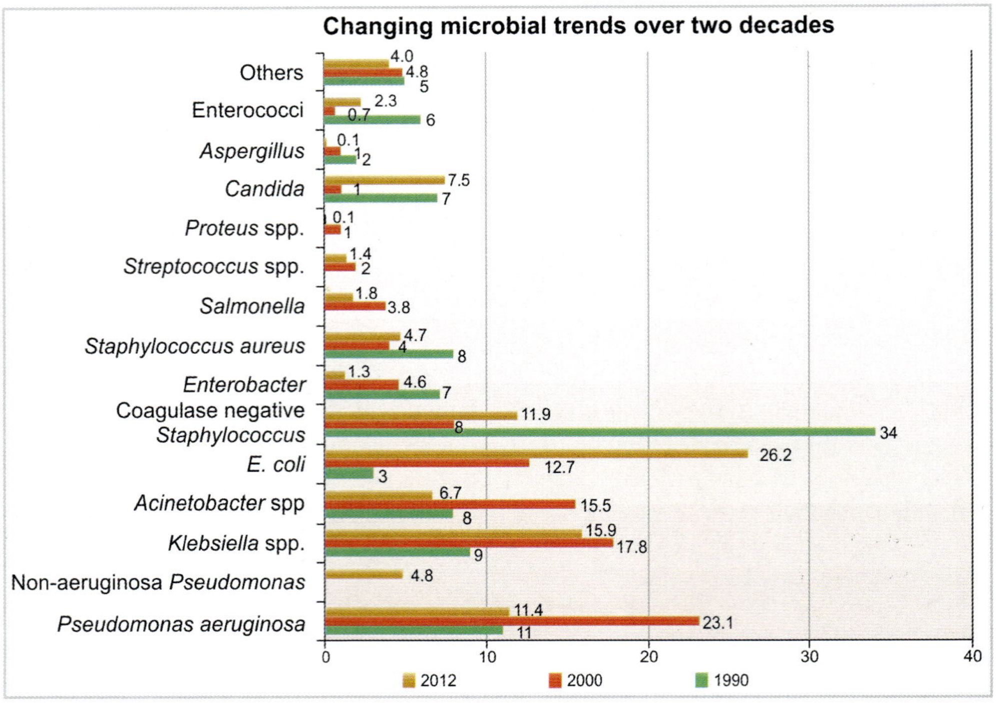

Fig. 1: The pattern of bloodstream infection over 2 decades

There is a rise in the percentage isolation of *Pseudomonas aeruginosa* and non-*aeruginosa Pseudomonas* species and *Escherichia coli*.

Further, there is a sharp rise in the number of the Gram-negative multidrug resistant *Enterobacteriaceae* isolates. This includes 13% of the Enterobacteriaceae being positive for ESBL production, 23% being Carbapenem-resistant Enterobacteriaceae, 50% of the *Acinetobacter baumannii* isolates being Carbapenem-resistant Acinetobacter baumannii, 2% MRSA, 1% VRE and 5% of the isolates were *Candida* species. Global trends have shown a changing pattern, revealing an increase in the incidence of Gram-positive infections and fungal infections. The NNIS data has shown a high rate of fungal infections in medical oncology 8.9–10.6 infections per 1,000 discharges. *Candida albicans* was the most frequently isolated fungal pathogen. A later study of 249 episodes Candidemia in cancer patients[49] showed a predominance of non *albicans Candida spp.* Aspergillosis outbreaks have been classically associated with construction activities. The source of infection is airborne spores and the proximity of these to the patients' airway is an important factor in infection.[50-53]

Fungal Infections in Indian Scenario

In the last 50 years, the incidence of fungal infections in cancer has increased more than tenfold. Majority of these isolates are from patients with leukemia. Not only has the frequency of isolation increased but also they tend to occur earlier during the course of the underlying malignancy. The use of fungemia (i.e. positive blood cultures) as an indicator of incidence leads to an underestimation of the frequency (Fig. 2).

The data reveals that *Candida* and *Aspergillus* are the most important etiological agents, with a predominance of non-albicans *Candida* species. However, several emerging opportunistic fungi are now being documented. Identification of all mycelia fungi is difficult for a routine diagnostic laboratory (Figs 3 and 4).

The numbers indicated in the bars are absolute numbers.

In 1993, yeast isolates were predominant, thereafter, a tendency toward mycelial fungal predominance is observed with time. Majority (76%), of these fungi isolated are from medical oncology. Another interesting finding is

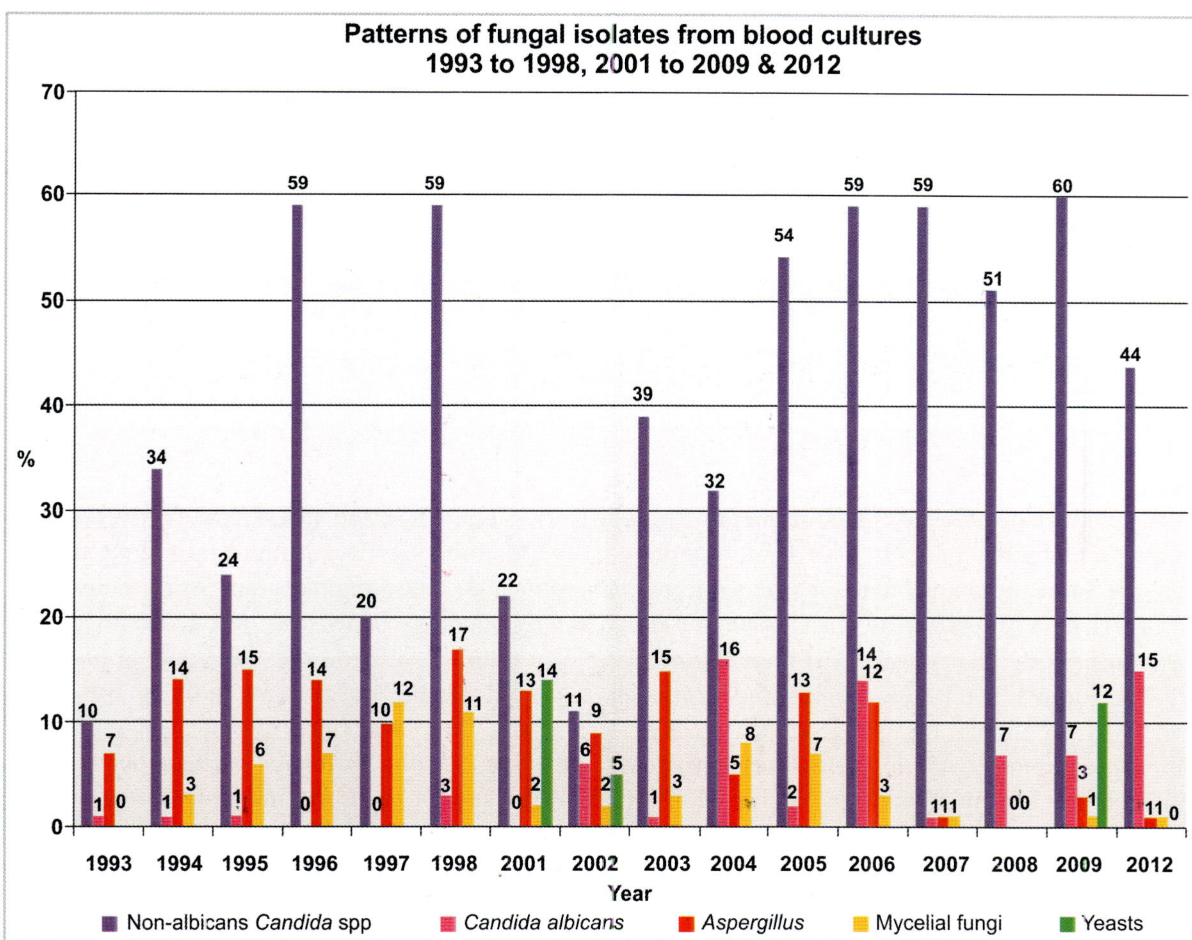

Fig. 2: The pattern of fungal isolates from blood cultures at the Tata Memorial Hospital

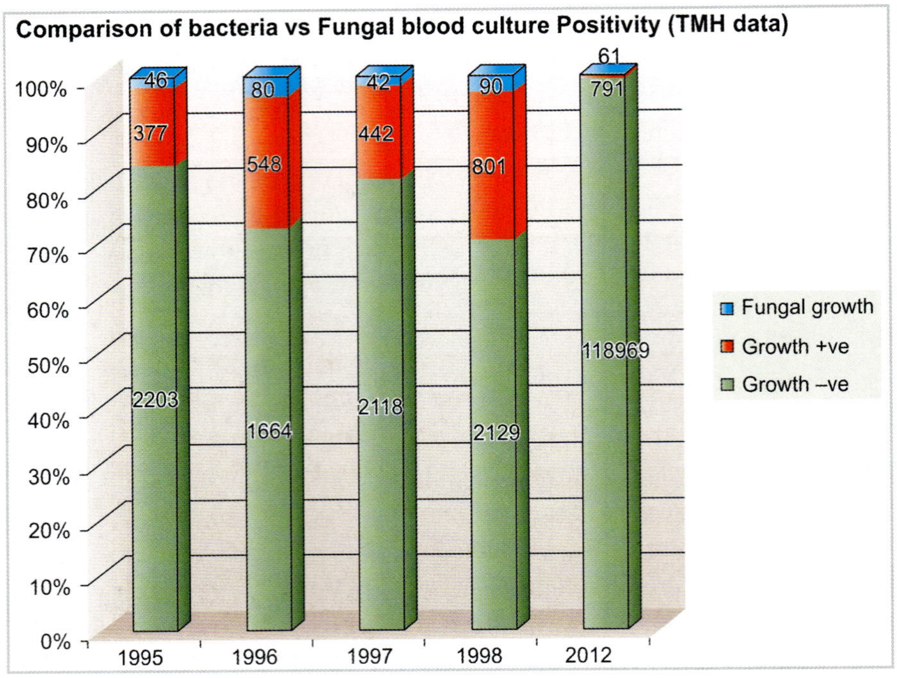

Fig. 3: The bacterial versus fungal blood culture positivity over three decades

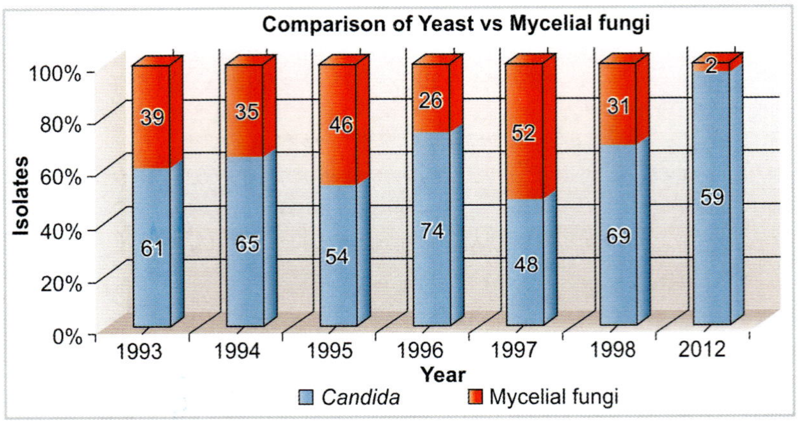

Fig. 4: The comparison of yeast versus mycelial fungal isolates at Tata Memorial Hospital

that patients with acute myeloid leukemia are more prone to Aspergillosis whereas patients with acute lymphatic leukemia are more prone to infections Tata Memorial Hospital (TMH) data. The pattern of yeast isolates observed at Tata Memorial Hospital has also been different from that reported.[43-44] Worldwide, *Candida albicans* predominates. However, TMH experience reveals *Candida tropicalis* to be the most predominant isolate. There is a clear increase in the incidence of fungal infections in cancer. Moreover, there is a change in the trend from yeast predominance to mycelial fungal predominance. This changing trend can be attributed to the improved antimicrobial cover resulting in a selection of other opportunistic pathogens.

A total of 58,136 blood cultures were processed in the Microbiology Department from 2001 to 2009. There were 9,027 blood samples from which pathogenic isolates were obtained. Thus, the overall positivity was 15.5%. The number of blood cultures yielding fungi as isolates was 551, i.e. 6.1% of positive cultures. The overall fungal positivity is 1% with majority of the isolates being *Candida* species. The non-albicans *Candida* species predominate with *Candida tropicalis* and *Candida parapsilosis* being the common species. *Aspergillus* species is the most common mycelial isolate.

There is a difference in the pattern of SFI in patients with leukemia where yeast infections predominate (83%)

and the solid tumors where 30% of SFI are due to mycelial fungi. Fungal infections in the surgical services are on the rise. Candidemia is an important cause of mortality and morbidity. We have documented some rare entities like *Fusarium, Rhizopus, Cladosporium, Saccharomyces cerevisiae, Geotrichum* and *Trichosporon* species from blood cultures and cases of cutaneous aspergillosis.

MYCOBACTERIAL INFECTIONS

These cannot only mimic cancer but can coexist with a malignancy. The use of more aggressive treatment protocols is bringing to light new infectious complications. The incidence of documented (culture positive) mycobacterial infections at TMH has been increasing since 1990. It was 0.56% of the total registered patients whereas in 1998 it was 1.12%.[43,44] The highest incidence being among patients with head and neck malignancy. Of 50 mycobacteria isolated from cancer patients 30% were found to be nontuberculous mycobacteria, *Mycobacterium fortuitum* chelonei complex being the most frequent.

Majority of the NTM, isolates are from BAL and lymph node aspirates. Data analyzed in the next decade from 371 culture positive cases, shows that a third of the culture positive cases were pulmonary samples from lung cancers, 17% from cases with lymphadenopathy, 8% from leukemias, 6% had a malignancy with pyrexia of unknown origin. Two-thirds of the isolates were from pulmonary sites. The incidence of multiply drug resistant (MDR) tuberculosis is found to be 6% over the last 2 decades. Molecular epidemiology of mycobacterial infections is currently under investigation and will be a useful tool for tracking transmission of infections in healthcare settings.[54-63]

Hepatitis and Cancer

Hepatitis B

Hepatitis B virus infections pose a serious threat to the oncology patient. Since the 1980s, we have observed a high incidence of hepatitis B surface antigen positivity in patients with acute lymphoblastic leukemia. Several avenues to control this infection have failed. With the availability of the recombinant DNA vaccine double dose immunization was attempted in this patient population. However, seroconversion to antibody positive status was very poor and only 10% of immunized children showed protective antibody titers. Measures taken to prevent transmission of HBV include screening of donor blood, single dose injectables and the reinforcement of sterilization practices. The HBV is a highly transmissible virus and a very small microscopic quantity (0.4 μL) of infected blood can transmit infection. Thus, horizontal transmission from infected household contacts is possibly through exposure to infected blood/body fluid via scratches, bites on skin lesions plays a significant role in perpetuating this infection.[106-109]

The overall prevalence of Hepatitis B surface antigen positivity in the screened cancer population during the last 5 years is 5.9%.

Hepatitis C

Hepatitis C infections are now beginning to pose problems in cancer patients. The real impact of this virus in cancer population in India is just beginning to be experienced. Since long-term follow-up of patients is not available and it may take up to 2 decades for the disease itself to manifest in the form of chronic hepatitis. Data on the incidence of HCV infections in the general population in India and the developing world is now available. The prevalence in the Asian countries is 1.5–6% in comparison with the United States which has a low prevalence (< 2%).[108-109] Transmission of HCV is most often percutaneously through blood or blood products. It has therefore become an important etiologic agent as a cause of hepatitis in cancer patients. Screening of blood and blood products for antibodies is now mandatory. This will greatly lower the risk of transmission via contaminated blood in the future (the risk in the developed world being < 0.1%).[109]

The overall prevalence of hepatitis C antibody positivity in the screened cancer population at TMH during the last 5 years is 1.9%.

HIV and Cancer

HIV infection predisposes to certain malignancies namely, Kaposi's sarcoma, Non-Hodgkin's lymphoma and cervical cancer. Screening of high risk patients for HIV infections is being practiced at many centers where the prevalence of HIV seropositivity is above 1%. The HIV positive status of patients with malignancies often alters the course of management of cancers. Further, they are predisposed to infections that are common in AIDS like cryptococcal meningitis and cryptosporidiosis.

CYTOMEGALOVIRUS INFECTIONS

These are common infections affecting most of the population and viral acquisition occurs early in life. This is an important complication following hematopoietic stem cell transplantation (HSCT). This virus is known to remain in the latent state at multiple sites in the body. Three types of infection are known: primary infection in seronegative individuals, secondary infection due to reactivation of a latent infection, post-transplantation and superinfection or reinfection. CMV infection causes a wide range of clinical manifestations. Mild infections manifest as prolonged fever with myalgias and arthritis. CMV-induced pneumonia; gastrointestinal disease and colitis are common manifestations. An important effect of CMV infection is increased susceptibility to opportunistic superinfection with *Pneumocystis carinii*, *Aspergillus* and bacteria.

Diagnosis of cytomegalovirus infection: Serology is useful for determining past history of CMV infection before the transplant, since infected patients rarely mount sufficient antibody titers for a diagnosis.

Currently used tests include:

- pp65 antigenemia assay
- In-situ hybridization assays
- Real time PCR-based quantitative assays are the most useful for prognosis and the detection of drug resistance
- Shell vial and other viral cultures are cumbersome.

At TMH, we started the in situ hybridization and pp65 antigenemia assay in 2004 and found that the hybridization assay was superior. From 2008 onward we have shifted to the quantitative real time PCR-based assay which is highly sensitive and useful to gauge the response to treatment. The assays are performed twice a week on all the post-transplant cases.[105] The two commonly used antiviral agents for treatment are ganciclovir and valganciclovir. New antiviral drugs are under investigation.

INFECTIONS IN SURGICAL ONCOLOGY: SURGICAL SITE INFECTIONS[64-102]

The principles of antisepsis were introduced in the late 1860s by Joseph Lister. This transformed surgery, a discipline associated with infection and death to one that could eliminate suffering and prolong life SSI's are the third most commonly reported nosocomial infection in the US.[110] They account for 14–16% of all nosocomial infections among hospitalized patients. They also result in increased hospital stay by approximately 10 days and an additional cost of $ 2,000.[27, 28]

Surgical site infections can be classified into:

- Superficial incisional
- Deep incisional
- Origin/space.

Despite several advances in infection control practices SSI's remain a substantial cause of morbidity in hospitalized patients. The surgical oncology patient poses as an ideal candidate for SSI and many of these are preventable. The important variables include the patient, the surgical team and the environment.

Microbiology of Surgical Site Infections

Although the trend has not changed drastically there has been a distinct rise in the number of infections caused by MRSA. There is also a noticeable increase in the non-aeruginosa, *Pseudomonas* species which includes *Stenotrophomonas maltophilia* and *Burkholderia* species. *Acinetobacter baumannii* has established itself as a nosocomial pathogen. These are all emerging bacterial pathogens. There is also a dramatic rise in the number of resistant microorganisms (Fig. 5).

MULTIDRUG-RESISTANT ORGANISMS: CURRENT SCENARIO[34]

The problem of drug resistance and "multiply drug resistant organisms" (MDRO) is a growing concern worldwide. In India, the threat is more serious because antibiotics are available "across the counter" sometimes without prescription and resultant misuse. Indiscriminate use of antimicrobials is common and antibiotics prescriptions are often based on information provided by medical representatives, rather than on the clinical condition of the patient and knowledge of pharmacology. Medical practitioners feel safe under the "antibiotic umbrella" has proven to be a myth. In many instances viral infections are treated with antimicrobials and to save costs in inappropriate doses, promote development of resistance.

The development of antibiotic resistance is related to their use. The mechanisms of drug resistance and the transfer of these resistance factors in bacteria are complex. In some instances resistance has been shown as soon as an antibiotic is introduced for use. Some of the genes responsible for drug resistance are called "jumping genes" because they are transferred from one bacterium to another even of two different genera.

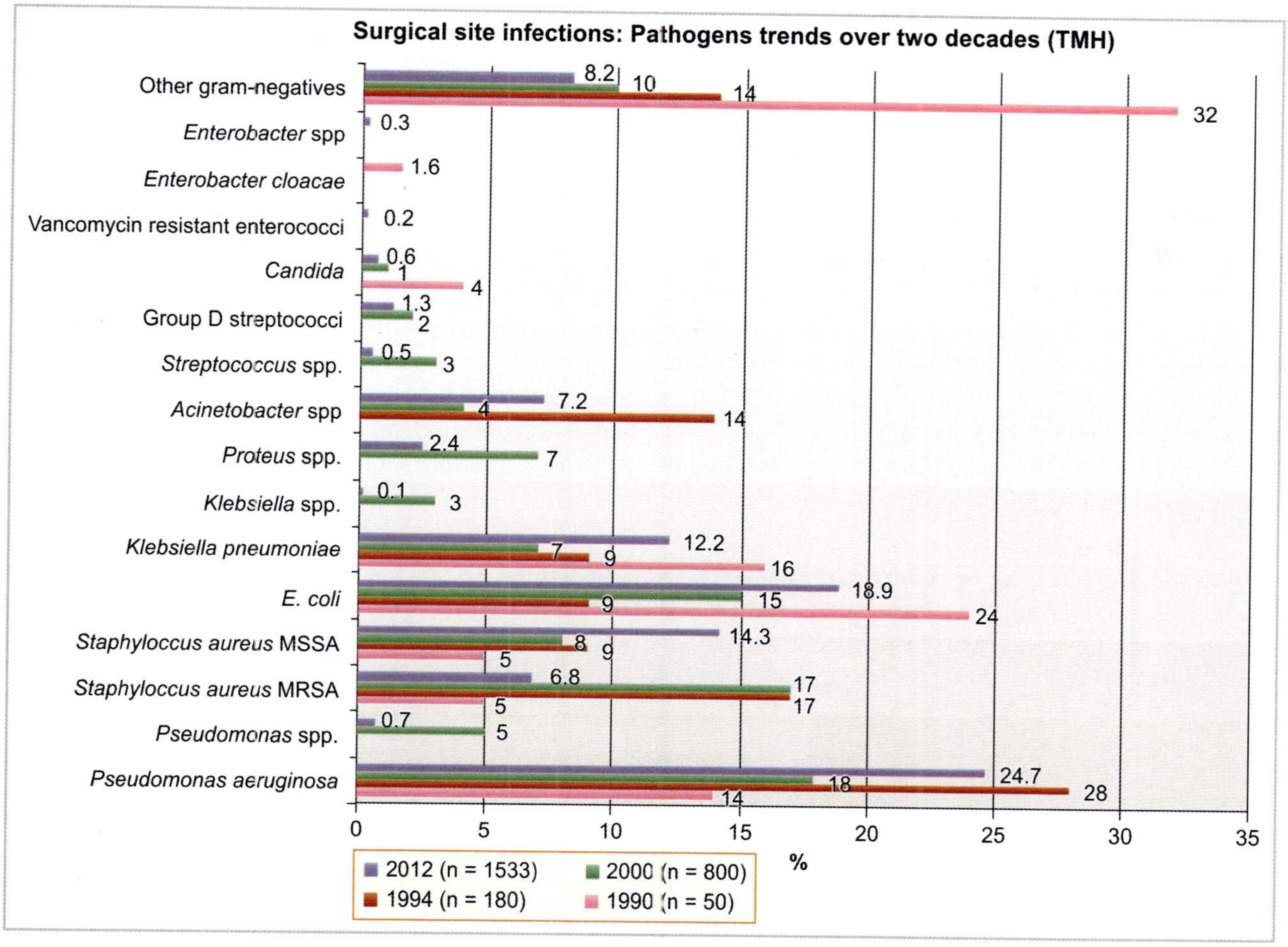

Fig. 5: The pattern of isolates from surgical site infection over 2 decades

By virtue of the extensive use of antimicrobials in hospitals, they are considered the "epicenters" of drug-resistant microorganisms. The patients who harbor these organisms carry them to the "community". In both hospitals and in the community, these organisms once introduced, can spread like fire. The single most effective means of controlling this spread from person to person is by augmenting simple infection control measures like "hand hygiene".

The current rate of increase in resistance to antimicrobials is alarming. The pace of antimicrobial drug development has markedly slowed in the last 20 years (US FDA approval of new antibacterial agents decreased 56% from 1983 to 2002). The time ripes for a new awakening and it is imperative to make the best use of the currently available antimicrobials. A rational approach to this huge problem is through an effective *"antibiotic policy"* or better described today by the medical community as *"antimicrobial stewardship program".*

These policies and programs focus on the judicious use of antimicrobials to provide better patient outcomes (results), better patient safety through reduced risk of side effects (adverse effects), cost effective treatment and reduction or stabilization in the levels of drug-resistant microorganisms. Antimicrobial stewardship programs include interventions that promote the rational use of antimicrobials through education of healthcare providers and patients, clinical guidelines defining the appropriate use of specific antimicrobials for specific conditions and organisms. They also involve processes to review antibiotic prescriptions by doctors, restrictive use of certain antimicrobial agents in hospitals only on approval, computer-based support and the cycling of antibiotics. The clinical microbiologist plays a pivotal role and is responsible for the timely delivery of reports on the cause of an infection and the choice of the antimicrobial agent. Local data on the prevalence of multidrug-resistant organisms forms the backbone of the policy.

Infection control is important to prevent the spread of these MDRO from one case to another and from the healthcare provider to the patients. Any antimicrobial stewardship program should be integrated with the infection control program which helps reduce antimicrobial resistance, evaluate the efficacy of the program and improve patient outcomes. The following Figure 6 shows the isolation rates of multidrug-resistant organisms from SSI.

The numbers in the bars are absolute numbers.

The following two Figures 7 and 8 show the sample wise isolation rates of methicillin-resistant and sensitive *Staphylococcus aureus*, i.e. MRSA and MSSA.

It is clear that the threat of antimicrobial-resistant bacteria is now a reality. These infections are more often fatal, result in prolonged illness and a greater chance for resistant organisms to spread to other people and finally increased costs of care, due to newer and more expensive drugs.

In order to contain drug resistance and contain it to hospitals, it is essential to use the correct antimicrobial administered by the best route, in the right dosage, at optimum intervals for the appropriate period. These are essentially the guidelines for surgical AMP.

PRINCIPLES OF ANTIMICROBIAL PROPHYLAXIS IN SURGICAL ONCOLOGY

Surgical AMP, refers to a brief course of an antimicrobial agent initiated just before an operation begins.[110-112] It is used to reduce the microbial burden of intraoperative contamination to a level that can be contained by host defenses. The mode of delivery should be by intravenous infusion and the agent should be bactericidal and cover the most probable intraoperative contaminants. Therapeutic levels of the antimicrobial agent should be maintained in both the serum and tissues throughout the operation. Thus, AMP has to be tailor made to suit the surgical procedure. AMP is not indicated for contaminated

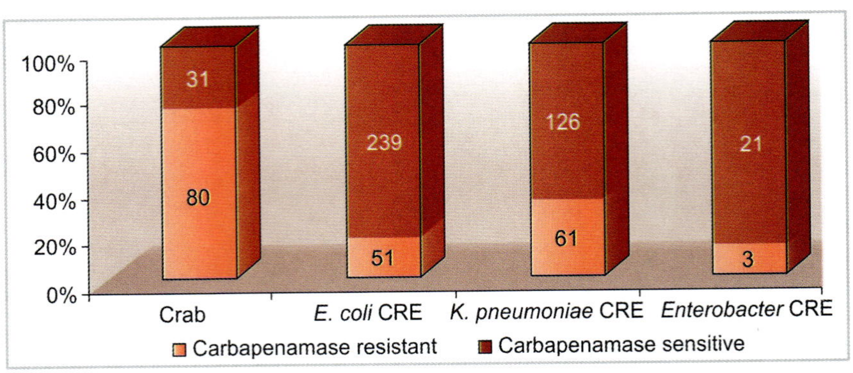

Fig. 6: The prevalence of carbapenem-resistant isolates from surgical site infection at Tata Memorial Hospital (The numbers in the bars are absolute numbers)

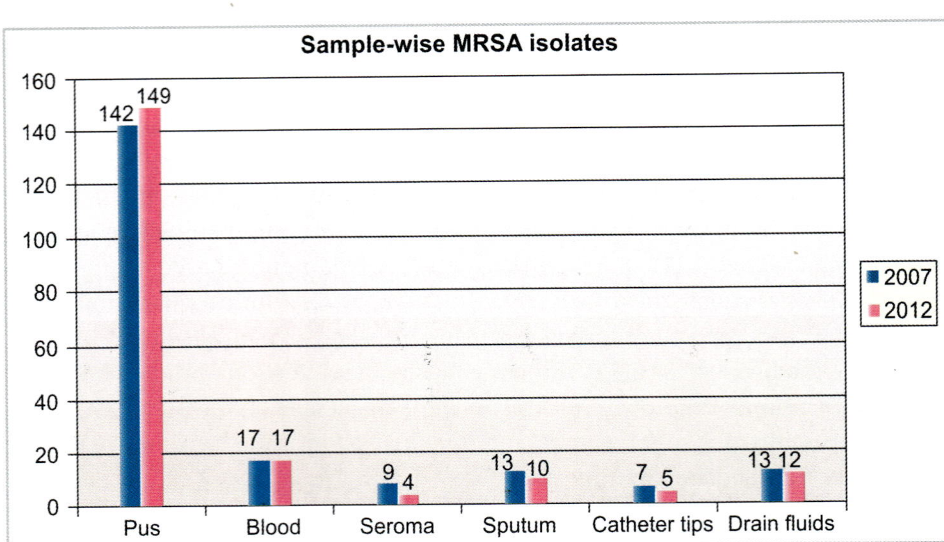

Fig. 7: The isolation of methicillin-resistant *Staphylococcus aureus* from different samples

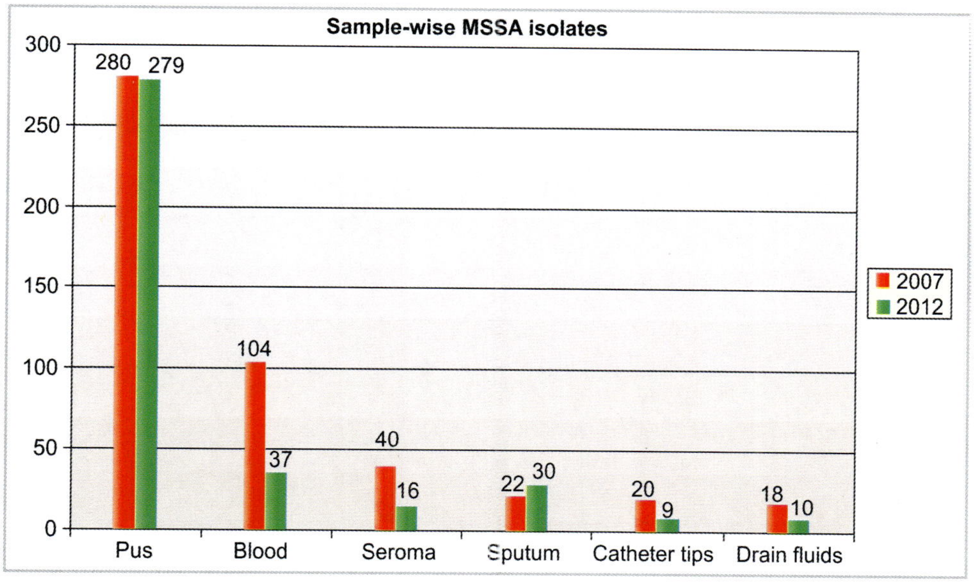

Fig. 8: The isolation of methicillin-sensitive *Staphylococcus aureus* from different samples (Majority of the isolates of *Staphylococcus aureus* are from pus cultures followed by blood cultures)

or dirty wounds since these patients are recipients of therapeutic antimicrobials. Cephalosporins are the most frequently used agents for AMP.[112] Intestinal surgeries require an agent with anaerobic coverage. The routine use of vancomycin for prophylaxis is not recommended. The time of administration is critical and should be with induction of anesthesia.

INFECTIONS IN HEMATOPOIETIC CELL TRANSPLANT RECIPIENTS

The program for bone marrow transplantation has been an education on the multitude of infections that may be encountered. During the first year following transplant recipients typically follow a predictable pattern of immune system deficiency and recovery, unfortunately the range of microbes is not as predictable. During the first month the deficits include impaired phagocytosis and damaged mucocutaneous barriers with the additional burden of indwelling intravenous catheter. These serve as a portal of entry for opportunistic pathogens. Besides coagulase negative Staphylococci we have encountered *Candida* Species and methicillin-resistant *Staphylococcus aureus*. Providing quality care of vascular catheters is of primary importance (Fig. 9).

Opportunistic Pathogens

Three phases are described:

Phase I

Pre-engraftment: During the first month, there are two critical risk factors prolonged neutropenia and breaks in the mucocutaneous barrier. Hence, the oral, gastrointestinal and skin flora are sources of infection *Candida* species and later *Aspergillus* infections are known to occur. Herpes simplex virus reactivation can also occur.

Phase II

Post-engraftment: This phase is dominated by impaired cell-mediated immunity. CMV is a critical pathogen and at 30–100 days after transplant can cause pneumonia, hepatitis and colitis. This also potentiates super infection with opportunistic pathogens, *Toxoplasma gondii, Pneumocystis carinii* and *Aspergillus* infections are also common. We have documented a fatal lung infection with a *Microsporidium* species. along with *Candida* in a female patient who underwent bone marrow transplant for chronic myeloid leukemia. She died on day 22 post-transplant and the diagnosis of this rare infection was only made at autopsy.[113]

Phase III

Late phase: Cell-mediated and humoral immune defects make patients at risk for certain infections including CMV varicella zoster and encapsulated bacteria like *Streptococcus pneumoniae*. The infections encountered in our setting include *Aspergillus, Candida*, CMV, Herpes

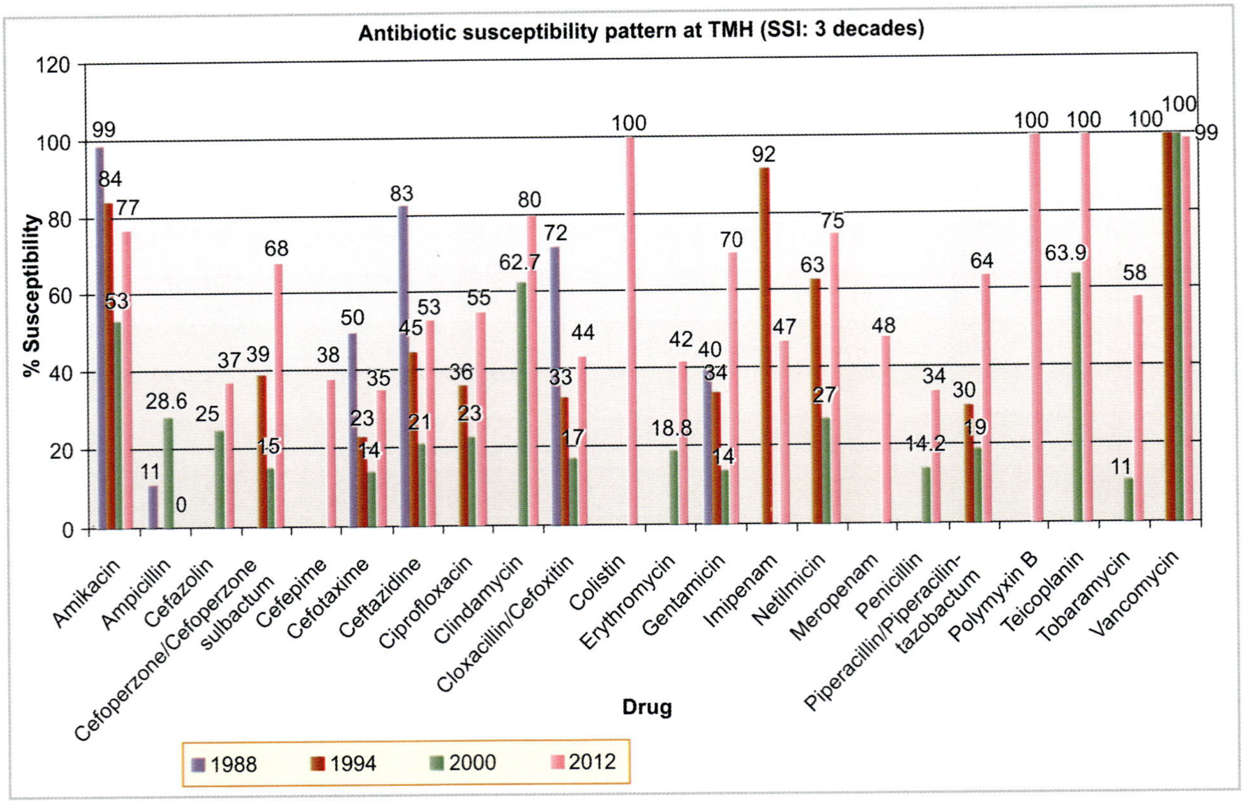

Fig. 9: The antimicrobial susceptibility pattern of pathogens isolated from "surgical site infection" from 1988 to 2012

zoster and mycobacteria. In a developing country, it is necessary to prevent these infections by reinforcing hygienic standards.

MANAGEMENT PRINCIPLES

In oncology practice, there are three issues in the management of infections:

1. Empirical treatment of an infection in febrile neutropenia
2. Management of a documented infection
3. Surgical antimicrobial prophylaxis.

The occurrence of fever in a neutropenic patient is a common event and it is essential to commence antimicrobials without delay. However, the use of antimicrobials should be guided by scientific evidence. Bacteremia in these patients is most frequently due to aerobic Gram-positive cocci, (*Staphylococcus*/CNS) or aerobic Gram-negative bacilli (*Pseudomonas aeruginosa*, *E. coli* and *Klebsiella pneumoniae*)

In patients already on broad spectrum antibiotics fungal infections are common although fungi may also be a cause of primary infection. The signs of inflammation in many of these patients are muted making these patients difficult to evaluate. A single oral temperature greater than or equal to 38.3°C is considered as fever. Neutrophil counts less than 1,000 cells/mm result in increased susceptibility to infections and the risk of infections increases substantially with counts falling below 500 with the highest risk less than or equal to 100/mm. A neutrophil count less than 500 cells/mm for 10 days is a major risk factor for impending infection. Empirical administration of broad spectrum antibiotics is necessary. However, a thorough patient evaluation for a possible site of infection as well as collection of appropriate specimens for culture is essential.

GUIDELINES FOR ANTIMICROBIAL THERAPY[104]

Initial Therapy

All febrile neutropenic patients with counts less than 500 should promptly be started on broad spectrum antibiotics. The choice of antibiotic regimen should be guided by local data on lines, frequency and susceptibilities of bacterial isolates in the facility. In patients with vascular access devices, catheter-related sepsis should be considered, catheter removal is advisable in certain unusual/

nonresponsive infections.[35] The initial regimen needs to be continued for at least 3 days to determine the efficacy. If the patient becomes afebrile, the further course depends on whether the etiology is identified or not If the etiology is identified, shift to appropriate treatment. If not, depending on the patient risk factor, a change to oral antibiotics (low risk) or continuation of the same regimen (high risk) is recommended.

Antibiotic treatment should be continued for a minimum of 7 days, or until culture results become negative for causative organisms and all sites of infection have resolved. The neutrophil count should be more than 500/mm before antibiotics are stopped. In the absence of documentation of the infective episode antibiotics should be continued for 7 days and the duration of therapy extended if neutropenia persists. It must be borne in mind that variations are often required in the clinical situation. If fever persists after 3 days treatment the patient needs to be reassessed for the following:

- Resistant bacterial infection
- Assessment of serum antibiotic levels
- Investigation for rare infections like *Toxoplasma gondii*, herpes simplex, CMV, mycobacteria, etc.

If reassessment still does not indicate a cause one of three choices are suggested:

1. Continue initial antibiotics
2. Change or add antibiotics
3. Add an antifungal to the regimen with or without change of antibiotics.

Vancomycin should be added whenever there is a suspicion of or documentation of site-specific isolates of coagulase negative Staphylococci. Vancomycin resistance is now increasing and VRE need to be considered when treatment with linezolid is indicated. The empiric addition of antifungal therapy is indicated in patients who remain febrile and have profound neutropenia for 1 week despite the administration of broad spectrum antibiotics in adequate doses. Several new antifungals have been added namely, caspofungin, posaconazole, anidulafungin and the new echinocandins. Liposomal amphotericin has replaced amphotericin.

Duration of Antimicrobial Therapy

The patients' neutrophil count is the single most important factor. Once the count is more than 500 and the patient is afebrile antibiotic therapy may be stopped. However, the picture is unclear once amphoterin B is started empirically. It has been suggested that 2 weeks is appropriate and ampho B can be stopped if no discernible clinical lesions are detected by clinical evaluation, chest X-rays and CT of abdominal organs. In patients with fungal systemic infections the splenic, hepatic or renal lesions sometimes become apparent as the neutrophil count increases. Antiviral agents are not justified for empiric use in the treatment of febrile neutropenia unless there is evidence of a viral infection. Acyclovir is indicated for herpes simplex or varicella zoster infections. CMV infections are treated with ganciclovir.

Antibiotic Prophylaxis for Afebrile Neutropenic Patient

Patients with neutrophil counts less than 100 cells/mm are a high risk of developing infections. They also have additional risk factors like mucosal breaks/breaches and indwelling catheters as well as the disease status itself. Each case must be received on an individual basis. Chemo prophylaxis has included oral absorbable antibiotics like trimethoprim, sulfamethoxazole (TMP-SMZ) and the quinolones. Opinions differ on the routine use of TMP SMZ during neutropenia. In situations with a high risk of *Pneumocystis carinii* infections it may be indicated.

Antifungals

Fluconazole prophylaxis is recommended in bone marrow transplant patients. However, this too can result in an increase in the fluconazole-resistant *Candida* like *Candida krusei*. Itraconazole prophylaxis has not resulted in a reduction in the incidence of aspergillosis.

PREVENTION AND CONTROL OF INFECTIOUS COMPLICATIONS[115-117]

The need for infection control:

In an era where long-term survival following treatment for malignancies has become a reality, life-threatening infectious complications is an ever present danger. Healthcare-associated infections are rapidly increasing and so also the threat of drug-resistant microorganisms. This is reflected in the form of prolonged hospitalization, increased length of stay and the costs that go with it. Thus, there is an acute need to have a functional infection control program in all healthcare institutions and even more so in cancer centers. Infection control programs not only reduce morbidity but are also helpful for preventing outbreaks caused by multidrug resistant organisms such as MRSA, ESBL producers or Carbapenem-resistant Gram-negative bacilli. There is a definite need for establishing good infection control practices and integrate them with cancer care.

There are three basic principles for the prevention and control of healthcare-associated infections, namely, hygiene, cleanliness and sterility. The common goal of all practices is to minimize the risk of infectious complications to both patients and healthcare workers.

A successful strategy is based on the following principles:

- Understanding the modes of transmission of infectious diseases
- Implementation of universal precautions and barrier protection to break the chain of disease transmission
- Establishing standards of hygiene
- Use of standard procedures for sterilization, disinfection and antisepsis
- Surveillance of healthcare-associated infections
- Appropriate use of antibiotics.

Such a program needs to be structured. In clinical oncology, there are some critical areas that call for attention:

- Prevention of SSI
- Prevention of infections in critical care
- Prevention of infections in HSCT and during febrile neutropenia
- Prevention of device-related infections.

Handwashing is the single most important measure for preventing the spread of infection. Hands must be washed before significant contact with any patient and after activities likely to cause contamination. Social handwash utilizes a neutral Ph soap whereas hygienic and surgical handwash utilize antiseptics.

Universal precautions are meant to protect hospital personnel from transmissible blood borne pathogens. They consist of the use of handwashing and protective barriers like gloves, masks, appropriate handling and disposal of sharps and other infectious wastes and the use of aseptic techniques. Additional precautions include respiratory precautions to prevent transmission of respiratory pathogens like respiratory syncytial virus, sputum positive pulmonary tuberculosis. Isolation precautions are required to contain epidemiologically significant infections like methicillin-resistant *Staphylococcus aureus*.

Immunocompromised host precautions are essential for the protection of bone marrow transplant patients and neutropenic patients with high risk of infections. The specifications here include:

- Isolation in single rooms
- Use of masks for all persons entering the room
- Plants and flowers should not be allowed into the room
- Good handwashing before each patient contact
- All equipment brought to the room must be cleaned prior to use
- Patients should wear a mask when traveling to other areas of the hospital.
- Universal precautions to be enforced.

PREVENTION OF SURGICAL SITE INFECTIONS[118-121]

There are certain risk factors that have been identified by multivariate analysis in epidemiological studies. These are known to have a significant independent association with the development of SSIs after a specific operation. Knowledge of these factors allows targeted prevention before certain operations for example, if a patient has known skin colonization with *Staphylococcus aureus* (MRSA), he should be treated prior to the surgical procedure. Preventive measures in contrast are actions intentionally taken to reduce the risk of a SSI. Many of these actions are directed toward reducing microbial contamination of the tissues or sterile surgical instruments. The factors that may influence the risk of SSI development include patient characteristics like age, nutritional status, diabetes and smoking, colonization with microorganisms, immune-compromised status and length of preoperative stay.

The operative factors include:

- Duration of surgical scrub
- Skin antisepsis and preoperative skin preparation
- Preoperative shaving
- Duration of surgery
- Antimicrobial prophylaxis
- Operating room characteristics like ventilation
- Introduction of foreign material in the surgical site
- Sterility of instruments
- Factors related to surgical techniques.

Some of the salient factors are considered here:

Operative Characteristics

Preoperative Issues

- *Preoperative antiseptic showering*: has been shown to reduce microbial counts. In a developing country where overall hygienic standards are poor, this practice should be advocated.
- *Preoperative hair removal*: Preoperative shaving of the surgical site the night before the operation is known to be associated with a higher risk of SSI than either

the use of depilatory agents or no-hair removal. This is attributed to the microscopic cuts resulting from shaving, which serve as foci for bacterial multiplication. Clipping hair immediately before an operation has been associated with a lower risk of SSI than shaving or clipping the night before the operation.

- *Patient skin preparation in the operating room*: Chlorhexidine gluconate and Iodophors have a broad spectrum of antimicrobial activity and are recommended. Chlorhexidine gluconate (4%) achieves a greater reduction in skin microflora than did povidone-iodine (10%). Current recommendations show that alcoholic chlorhexidine is approved for skin antisepsis.
- *Preoperative hand antisepsis*: The antiseptics used for the surgical scrub, the method and duration of scrub as well as the drying of hands are important in reducing the transient microflora of the operating team. The choice of agents lies between chlorhexidine gluconate (4%) and povidone-iodine (7.5%). No clinical trials have evaluated the impact of a choice of scrub agents on SSI risk.
- Antimicrobial prophylaxis has already been dealt with.

Intraoperative Issues

Operating rooms should be maintained at positive pressure with respect to adjacent areas. Ventilation systems should have two filter beds with the efficiency of the first filter being greater than or equal to 30% and that of the second filter bed being greater than or equal to 90%.[114] The essential parameters for operating rooms include a temperature of 20–23°C, relative humidity 30–60%, with air changes of a minimum of 15 total air changes per hour with three air changes of fresh air. The above conditions are necessary to inhibit bacterial multiplication. Ultraclean air is recommended for high risk surgeries like orthopedic procedures with implantable devices. Several guidelines discuss the details of planning of operating rooms with reference to the ventilation systems. Environmental monitoring sampling is recommended only during the investigation of outbreaks. In a developing country like India, microbiological sampling serves as a monitor of the cleaning practices. With the current status of operating facilities in developing countries it is of utmost importance that each facility should have rigid norms for maintenance of hygiene and discipline in the operating room.

Environmental surfaces should be cleaned according to the following schedule:

- Prior to the first surgery
- After each case and particularly in case of blood/body fluid spills
- At the end of the day
- Thorough cleaning on weekends including maintenance of the air handling units.

Sterilization of Surgical Instruments

Inadequate sterilization of surgical instruments has resulted in outbreaks of SSI. Surgical instruments may be sterilized by steam, ethylene oxide or plasma or other approved methods. The most important aspect is monitoring the quality of the sterilization procedure. Thus, it is mandatory to use biological indicators to monitor the performance of a steam sterilizer.

Surgical Attire and Drapes

It is known that microorganisms are shed from hair, exposed skin and mucous membranes of operating room personnel. Although very few clinical trials have evaluated the role of surgical attire and SSI, it seems prudent to use these barriers to minimize patient exposure from microorganisms. Moreover, surgical attire also protects the surgical team members from exposure to blood borne pathogens.

Asepsis and Surgical Technique

All scrubbed personnel must adhere to the principles of asepsis. Good surgical technique also reduces the risk of SSI. Hypothermia, foreign body and drains can all contribute to SSI. Postoperative incision care and surveillance for SSI are the last two factors that require monitoring. Every oncology center should have a surveillance system for monitoring SSI.

Prevention of Intravascular Device-related Infections

Intravascular devices are being increasingly used in clinical oncology practice. They may be long-term or short-term devices and have varied purposes from administration of intravenous fluids to monitoring the hemodynamic status of critically ill patients. Device-related infections have become a major cause of concern. Catheter-related BSI are particularly important being associated with increased morbidity and mortality. It is also observed that BSI rates are higher among individuals with intravascular devices than among those without. The potential sources of contamination of intravascular devices consist of colonization of the hub, hands of medical personnel, skin flora of the patient, contaminated fluids/medications and contamination during insertion of the device. All these can lead to hematogenous spread of the infection.

Coagulase negative Staphylococci and other Gram-positive skin colonizers are frequent. Other emerging pathogens like enterococci, *candida* species and other fungi also should be considered. Colonization of healthcare workers with pathogens is important. Contaminated fluids may result in infections with Gram-negative organisms like *pseudomonas, acinetobacter* or *Serratia marcescens*. Establishing the clinical diagnosis of a catheter-related infection is often difficult. Both clinical and laboratory criteria for diagnosis have significant limitations. The introduction of semiquantitative methods for obtaining cultures of catheters has greatly enhanced the ability to diagnose catheter-related infections.[103,122] A variety of local infection complications are also known. In long-term catheters, exit site, tunnel or pocket infections can occur.

Strategies for Prevention

- Healthcare workers should be trained for the insertion, use and maintenance of intravascular devices
- Surveillance for catheter-related infections should include palpation of the insertion site, visual inspection of the site and monitoring catheter-related BSI
- Hand washing while handling catheter and barrier precautions during insertion and care
- Proper aseptic precautions and regimentation of catheter site dressings
- Appropriate replacement of intravascular devices. Removal of the device when its use is no longer clinically indicated.

Proper care of intravascular devices by trained personnel and strict asepsis is the key to success in controlling device-related infectious complications.

REFERENCES

1. Schimpff SC, Young VM, Greene WH, et al. Origin of infection in acute nonlymphocytic leukemia. Significance of hospital acquisition of potential pathogens. Ann Intern Med. 1972;77(5):707-14.
2. Singer C, Kaplan MH, Armstrong D. Bacteremia and fungemia complicating neoplastic disease: a study of 364 cases. Am J Med. 1977;62(5):731-42.
3. Wade JC, Schimpff SC, Newman KA, et al. *Staphylococcus* epidermidis: an increasing cause of infection in patients with granulocytopenia. Ann Intern Med. 1982;97(4):503-8.
4. Mayo JW, Wenzel RP. Rates of hospital-acquired bloodstream infections in patients with specific malignancy. Cancer. 1982;50(1):187-90.
5. Robinson GV, Tegtmeier BR, Zaia JA. Brief Report: nosocomial infection rates in a cancer treatment center. Infect Control. 1984;5(6):289-94.
6. Neu HC. Infections due to gram-negative bacteria: an overview. Rev Infect Dis. 1985;7 Suppl 4:S778-82.
7. Anaissie E, Kantarjian H, Jones P, et al. Fusarium. A newly recognized fungal pathogen in immunosuppressed patients. Cancer. 1986;57(11):2141-5.
8. Rotstein C, Cummings KM, Nicolaou AL, et al. Nosocomial infection rates at an oncology center. Infect Control Hosp Epidemiol. 1988;9(1):13-9.
9. Walsh TJ, Pizzo PA. Nosocomial fungal infections: a classification for hospital-acquired fungal infections and mycoses arising from endogenous flora or reactivation. Annu Rev Microbiol. 1988;42:517-54.
10. Bodey GP, Elting LS, Rodriguez S, et al. *Klebsiella* bacteremia: A 10-year review in a cancer institution. Cancer. 1989;64(11):2368-76.
11. Pfaller MA. Nosocomial candida infections. In: Doebbeling BN, Herwaldt LA, Nettleman MD, et al (Eds). Hospital-acquired infections: new challenges. Kalamazoo: UpJohn; 1991.
12. Schwarz RE, Groeger JS, Coit DG. Subcutaneously implanted central venous access devices in cancer patients: a prospective analysis. Cancer. 1997;79(8):1635-40.
13. Wright WL, Wenzel RP. Nosocomial *Candida*. Epidemiology, transmissions, and prevention. Infect Dis Clin North Am 1997; 11:411-425.
14. Kenneth V I Rolston et al. Infections in patients with cancer Holland-Frei Cancer Medicine. 5th edition. Hamilton (ON): BC Decker; 2000.
15. Bodey GP, Rodriguez V. Infections in cancer patients on a protected environment-prophylactic antibiotic program. Am J Med. 1975;59(4):497-504.
16. Bodey GP, Vartivarian S. Aspergillosis. Eur J Clin Microbiol Infect Dis. 1989;8(5):413-37.
17. Beck-Sague C, Jarvis WR. Secular trends in the epidemiology of nosocomial fungal infections in the United States, 1980-1990. J Infect Dis. 1993;167(5):1247-51.
18. Viscoli C, Girmeniz C, Marinus A, et al. Candidemia in cancer patients: factors associated with etiology (albicans vs. non-albicans) and survival (abstract 31). Infectious Diseases Society of America, 34th Annual meeting: New Orleans; 1996.
19. Arnow PM, Anderssen RL, Mainous PD, et al. Pulmonary aspergillosis during hospital renovation. Am Rev Respir Dis. 1978;118(1):49-53.
20. Lentino JR, Rosenkranz MA, Michaels JA, et al. Nosocomial aspergillosis: a retrospective review of airborne disease secondary to road construction and contaminated air conditioners. Am J Epidemiol. 1982;116(3):430-7.
21. Pizzo PA. Considerations for the prevention of infectious complications in patients with cancer. Rev Infect Dis. 1989;11 Suppl 7:S1551-63.
22. Rhame FS. Lessons from Roswell Park bone marrow transplant aspergillosis outbreak. Infect Control. 1985;6(9):345-6.

23. Opal SM, Asp AA, Cannady PB, et al. Efficacy of infection control measures during a nosocomial outbreak of disseminated aspergillosis associated with hospital construction. J Infect Dis. 1986;153(3):634-7.
24. Manual of Clinical Microbiology, 6th Edition: American Society for Microbiology; 1995. pp. 3-50.
25. Athanikar N, Advani SH, Ahuja HG, et al. Septicemia in hematological malignancies (analysis of 50 patients). Ind J Hematol. 1986;4:24-9.
26. Shannon Smiley et al. Epidemiology and management of opportunistic infections in immunocompromised patients with cancer. Abstr Hematol Oncol. 2005;8(3):20-30.
27. Cruse P. Wound infection surveillance. Rev Infect Dis. 1981;3(4):734-7.
28. Cruse PJ, Foora R. The epidemiology of wound infection: a 10 year prosmecture study of 62, 939 wounds. Surg Chin North Am. 1980;60(1):27-40.
29. Management issues in seriously ill patients with nosocomial infections. Excerpta Medica. Asia Pacific Congress Series No. 81. Proceedings of a round table.
30. Pizzo PA. Practical considerations for the management of fever and infections in neutropenic patients. Clin Oncol. 1985;4:405-33.
31. Bodey GP. Infection in cancer patients. A continuing association. Amer J Med. 1986;81(1A):11-25.
32. Hawkins C, Armstrong D. Fungal infections in the immunocompromised host. Clinics in Haemat. 1984;13(3):597-630.
33. Gold JW. Opportunistic fungal infections in patients with neoplastic disease. Am J Med. 1984;76(3):459-63.
34. Prabhash K, Medhekar A, Biswas S, et al. Comparison of in vitro activities of ceftazidime, piperacillin-tazobactam and cefoperazone-sulbactam and the implication on empirical therapy in patients with cancer. Ind J Cancer. 2009;46(4):318-22.
35. Advani SH. Indian Guidelines in Febrile Neutropenia. The Indian Society of Medical and Pediatric Oncology. ISMPO. 2004 p.25.
36. Reinhart K, Bauer M, Riedemann NC, et al. New approaches to sepsis: molecular diagnostics and biomarkers. Clin Microbiol Rev. 2012;25(4):609-34.
37. Brown AE. Overview of fungal infections in cancer patients. 1990;17(3 Suppl 6):2-5.
38. Bodey G, Bueltmann B, Duguid W, et al. Fungal infections in cancer patients: an international autopsy survey. Eur J Clin Microbiol Infect Dis. 1992;11(2):99-109.
39. Hawkins C, Armstrong D. Fungal infections in the immunocompromised host. Clin Haematol. 1984;13(3):599-630.
40. Wenzel RP, Pfaller MA. Candida species: emerging hospital bloodstream pathogens. Infect Control Hosp Epidemiol. 1991;12(9):523-4.
41. Brown AE. Overview of fungal infections in cancer patients. Semin Oncol. 1990;3(Suppl 6):2-5.
42. Walsh TJ, Pizzo PA. Nosocomial fungal infections. Ann Rev Microbiol. 1988;42:517-45.
43. Thakkar N, Kelkar RS. Study of pathogenic fungi isolated from cancer patients. MSc Thesis; 1999.
44. TMH data. Polymerase chain reaction assay for the early and rapid diagnosis of fungal infections in high risk cancer patients on aggressive chemotherapeutic protocols (PhD thesis); 2011.
45. Hopwood V, Johnson EM, Cornish JM, et al. Use of the Pastorex aspergillus antigen latex agglutination test for the diagnosis of invasive aspergillosis. J Clin Pathol. 1995;48(3):210-3.
46. Stynen D, Goris A, Sarfati J, et al. A new sensitive sandwich enzyme-linked immunosorbent assay to detect galactofuran in patients with invasive aspergillosis. J Clin Microbiol. 1995;33(2):497-500
47. De Paul B, Walsh TJ, Donnelly JP, et al. European Organization for Research and Treatment of Cancer/Invasive Fungal Infections Cooperative Group; National Institute of Allergy and Infectious Diseases Mycoses Study Group (EORTC/MSG) Consensus Group (2008)—Revised definitions of invasive fungal disease from the EORTC/MSG Consensus Group. Clin Infect Dis. 2008;46(12)1813-21.
48. Bretagne S, Costa JM, Bart-Delabesse E, et al. Comparison of serum galactomannan antigen detection and competitive polymerase chain reaction for diagnosing invasive aspergillosis. Clin Infect Dis. 1998;26(6):1407-12.
49. Sulahian A, Tabouret M, Ribaud P, et al. Comparison of an enzyme immunoassay and latex agglutination test for detection of galactomannan in the diagnosis of invasive aspergillosis. Eur J Clin Microbiol Infect Dis. 1996;15(2):139-45.
50. Verweij PE, Stynen D, Rijs AJ, et al. Sandwich enzyme-linked immunosorbent assay compared with Pastorex latex agglutination test for diagnosing invasive aspergillosis in immunocompromised patients. J Clin Microbiol. 1995;33(7):1912-4.
51. Maertens J, Verhaegen J, Lagrou K, et al. Screenig for circulating galactomannan as a noninvasive diagnostic tool for invasive aspergillosis in prolonged neutropenic patients: a prospective validation. Blood. 2001;97(6):1604-10.
52. Maertens J, Van Eldere J, Verhaegen J, et al. Use of circulating galactomannan screening for early diagnosis of invasive aspergillosis in allogeneic stem cell transplant recipients. J Infect Dis. 2002;186(9):1297-306.
53. Rohini K. Opportunistic fungal and mycobacterial infections in cancer. In: Mahajan RC, Therwath A (Eds). Multidrug Resistance in Emerging and Re-emerging Disease. Narosa Publishing House. 2000 p.235-42.
54. Canetti G, Fox W, Khomenko A, et al. Advances in techniques of testing mycobacterial drug sensitivity tests in tuberculosis control programmes. Bull World Health Org. 1969;41(1):21-43.
55. Frieden TR, Sterling T, Pablos-Mendez A, et al. Drug resistant tuberculosis in New York city. N Eng J Med. 1993;328(8):521-6.
56. Hardas UD, Jayaraman VS. Pattern of drug resistance in tuberculosis. Ind J Tuber. 1984;31:168-70.
57. Mukherji AK. Tuberculosis control program in India: Progress and prospects. Ind J Tub. 1995;42:72-85.
58. Murillo J, Wells GM, Barry DW, et al. Gastrointestinal tuberculosis mimicking cancer-a reminder. Am J Gastroenterology. 1978;70 (1):53-7.
59. Ramakrishnan CV. The problem of drug resistance in tuberculosis. Lung India. 1990;8:44-52
60. Sepkowitz KA, Raffalli J, Riley L, et al. Tuberculosis in the AIDS era. Clin Micro Rev. 1995;8:180-94.
61. Snider DE, La Montagne JR. The neglected global tuberculosis problem: a report of the 1992 World Congress on Tuberculosis. J Inf Dis. 1994;169(6):1189-96.

62. The global challenge of tuberculosis Editorial. Lancer. 1994;344(8918):277-9.
63. Cohen T, van Helden PD, Wilson D, et al. Mixed-strain *Mycobacterium tuberculosis* Infections and the Implications for Tuberculosis Treatment and Control. Clin Microbiol Rev. 2012;25(4):708-19.
64. Garner JS, Favero MS. CDC Guidelines for Handwashing and Hospital Environmental Control, 1985. In Infection Control. 1986;7(4):231-43.
65. Garner JS. CDC guideline for prevention of surgical wound infections 1985. Supercedes guideline for prevention of surgical wound infections published in1982. (Originally published in 1995). Revised. Infect Control. 1986;7(3):193-200.
66. Simmons BP. Guideline for prevention of surgical wound infections. Infect Control. 1982;3:185-96.
67. National Nosocomial Infections Surveillance (NNIS) report, data summary from October 1986-April 1997, issued May 1997. A report from the NNIS System. Am J infect Control. 1997;25(6):477-87.
68. Emori TG, Gaynes RP. An overview of nosocomial infections, including the role of the microbiology laboratory. Clin Microbiol Rev. 1993;6(4):428-42.
69. Cruse P. Wound infection surveillance. Rev Infect Dis. 1981;4(3):734-7.
70. Cruse PJ, Foord R. The epidemiology of wound infection: a 10-year prospective study of 62,939 wounds. Surg Clin North Am. 1980;60(1):27-40.
71. Martone WJ, Jarvis WR, Culver DH, Haley RW. Incidence and nature of endemic and epidemic nosocomial infections. In: Bennett JV, Brachman PS (Eds). Hospital Infections, 3rd edition. Boston: Little, Brown and Co; 1992. pp. 577-96.
72. Vegas AA, Jodra VM, Garcia ML. Nosocomial infection in surgery wards: a controlled study of increased duration of hospital stays and direct cost of hospitalization. Eur J Epidemiol. 1993;9(5): 505-10.
73. Consensus paper on the surveillance of surgical wound infections. The Society for Hospital Epidemiology of America; The Association for Practitioners in Infection Control; The Centers for Disease Control; The Surgical Infection Society.. Infect Control Hosp Epidemiol. 1992;13(10):599-605.
74. National Nosocomial Infections Surveillance (NNIS) report, data summary from, October 1986-April 1996, issued May 1996. A report from the National Nosocomial Infections Surveillance (NNIS) System. Am J Infect Control. 1996;24(5):380-8.
75. Jarvis WR. Epidemiology of nosocomial fungal infections, with emphasis on Candida species. Clin Infect Dis. 1995;20(6):152-30.
76. Cruse PJ. Surgical wound infection. In: Wonsiewicz MJ (Ed). Infectious Diseases. Philadelphia: WB Saunders Co; 1992. pp. 758-64.
77. Altemeier WA, Culbertson WR, Hummel RP. Surgical considerations of endogenous infections-sources, types, and methods of control. Surg Clin North Am. 1968;48(1):227-40.
78. Velasco E, Thuler LC, Martins CA, et al. Risk factors for infectious complications after abdominal surgery for malignant disease. Am J Infect Control. 1996;24(1):1-6.
79. Edwards LD. The epidemiology of 2056 remote site infections and 1966 surgical wound infections occurring in 1865 patients: a four year study of 40,923 operations at Rush-Presbyterian-St. Luke's Hospital, Chicago. Ann Surg. 1976;184(6):758-66.
80. Dineen P, Drusin L. Epidemics of postoperative wound infections associated with hair carriers. Lancet. 1973;2(7839):1157-9.
81. Ford CR, Peterson DE, Mitchell CR. An appraisal of the role of surgical face masks. Am J Surg. 1967;113(6):787-90.
82. Barber GR, Miransky J, Brown AE, et al. Direct observations of surgical wound infections at a comprehensive cancer center. Arch Surg. 1995;130(10):1042-7.
83. Cruse PJ, Foord R. A five year prospective study of 23,649 surgical wounds. Arch Surg. 1973:107(2):206-10.
84. Haley RW, Culver DH, Morgan WM, et al. Identifying patients at high risk of surgical wound infection. A simple multivariate index of patient susceptibility and wound contamination. Am J Epidemiol. 1985;121(2):206-15
85. Culver DH, Horan TC, Gaynes RP, et al. Surgical wound infection rates by wound class, operative procedure, and patient risk index. National Nosocomial Infections Surveillance System. Am J Med. 1991;91(Suppl 3B):152S-7S.
86. Garibaldi RA. Prevention of intraoperative wound contamination with chlorhexidine shower and scrub. J Hosp Infect. 1988;11(Suppl B):5-9.
87. Paulson DS. Efficacy evaluation of a 4% chlorhexidine gluconate as a full-body shower wash. Am J Infect Control. 1993;21(4):205-9.
88. Hayek LJ, Emerson JM, Gardner AM. A placebo-controlled trial of the effect of two preoperative baths or showers with chlorhexidine detergent on postoperative wound infection rates. J Hosp Infect. 1987;10(2):165-72.
89. Hamilton HW, Hamilton KR, Lone FJ. Preoperative hair removal. Can J Surg. 1977;20(3):269-71, 274-5.
90. Hardin WD, Nichols RL. Handwashing and patient skin preparation. In: Malangoni MA (Ed). Critical Issues in Operating Room Management. Philadelphia: Lippincott-Raven; 1997. pp. 133-49.
91. Association of Operating Room Nurses. Recommended practices for skin preparation of patients. AORN J. 1996;64(5):813-6.
92. Shirahatti RG. Joshi RM, Vishwanath YK, et al. Effect of preoperative skin preparation on post-operative wound infection. J Postgrad Med. 1993;39(3):134-6.
93. Larson EL. APIC guideline for handwashing and hand antisepsis in health care settings. Am J Infect Control. 1995;23(4):251-69.
94. Ayliffe GA. Surgical scrub and skin disinfection. Infect Control. 1984;5(1):23-7.
95. DiPiro JT, Cheung RP, Bowden TA, et al. Single dose systemic antibiotic prophylaxis of surgical wound infections. Am J Surg. 1986;152(5):552-9.
96. Trilla A, Mensa J. Perioperative antibiotic prophylaxis In: Wenzel RP (Ed). Prevention and Control of Nosocomial Infections, 2nd edition. Baltimore: Williams and Wilkins; 1993. pp. 665-82.
97. Nichols RL. Surgical antibiotic prophylaxis. Med Clin North Am. 1995;79(3):509-22.
98. Polk HC, Wilson MA. Systemic antibiotic prophylaxis in surgery. In: Fry DE (Ed). Surgical Infections, Boston: Little, Brown and Co; 1995. pp. 127-33.
99. Ayliffe GA. Role of the environment of the operating suite in surgical wound infection. Rev Infect Dis. 1991;13(Suppl 10):S800-4.

100. Hambraeus A. Aerobiology in the operating room-a review. J Hosp Infect. 1988;11(Suppl A):68-76.
101. Mitchell NJ, Hunt S. Surgical face masks in modern operating rooms-a costly and unnecessary ritual? J Hosp Infect. 1991;18(3):239-42.
102. Olson MM, Lee JT. Continuous 10-year wound infection surveillance. Results, advantages, and unanswered questions. Arch Surg. 1990;125(6):794-803.
103. Maki DG, Weise CE, Sarafin HW. A semiquantitative culture method for identifying intravenous catheter-related infection. N Engl J Med. 1977;296(23):1305-9.
104. Hughes WT, Armstrong D, Bodey GP, et al. 1997 Guidelines for the use of antimicrobial agents in neutropenic patients with unexplained fever. J Infect Dis. 1997;25(3):551-73.
105. Meijer E, Boland GJ, Verdonck LF, et al. Prevention of cytomegalovirus disease in recipients of allogeneic stem cell transplants. Clinic Microbiol Review. 2003;16(4):647-57.
106. .Goyal S, Pai SK, Kelkar R, et al. Hepatitis B vaccination in acute lymphoblastic leukemia. 1998;22(2):193-5.
107. Nag S, Vaidya S, Pai S, et al. Hepatitis B viral infection in acute lymphoblastic leukemia. Ind J Hematol. 1995;13-150.
108. WHO Hep C: global prevalence. Weekly Epidemiological Record. 1997;46:341-3.
109. Conry-Cantilena C, VanRaden M, Gibble J, et al. Routes of infection, viremia and liver disease in blood donors found to have hepatitis C virus infection. 1996. M Eng J of Med. 1996;334(26):1691-6.
110. Schulz TF. Cancer and viral infections in immunocompromised individuals. Int J Cancer. 2009; 125(8):1755-63.
111. Emori TG, Goupies RP. An overview of nosocomical infections including the role of the Microbiology laboratory. Clin Microbial Rev. 1993;6(4):428-42.
112. Nichols RC. Surgical antibiotic prophylaxis. Med Clin Morth AM. 1995;79(3):509-22.
113. Kelkar R, Sastry PS, Kulkarni SS, et al. Pulmonary microsporial infection in a patient with CML undergoing allogeneic marrow transplant BMT. 1997;19(2):179-82.
114. American Institute of Architects guidelines for design and construction of hospital and health care faculties Washington (DC); American Institute of Architect Press; 1996.
115. Kelkar RS. Infection Control in paediatric oncology practice. Practical Paediatric Oncology (Reference Manual), 1st edition; 1998. pp. 102-6.
116. Shaw K, Sungkhobol D, Kelkar R, Munshi N, Vasta M, kumari S, Senaratana W, Bhatia R, Velmonte M. Practical guidelines for Infection Control in Health Care facilities; WHO SEARO Regional Publications No 41, WHO, 2004.
117. Kelkar R. Guidelines on Prevention and Control of Hospital Associated Infections. WHO, Regional Office for South-East Asia, SEA-HLM-343; 2002.
118. Kelkar R. Consensus guidelines for the prevention of infections in the operating room: Hospital Infection Society-Mumbai Forum; 2005.
119. Kelkar R, Nataraj G (Eds). Best Practice Guidelines for the reuse of single use devices: Hospital Infection Society, Mumbai Forum; 2007.
120. Who Guidelines on Hand Hygiene in Healthcare. CDC Hand Hygiene in Healthcare Settings; 2009.
121. O'Grady NP, Alexander M, Dellinger EP, et al. Guidelines for the prevention of intravascular catheter-related infections. Centers for Disease Control and Prevention. MMWR Recomm Rep. 2002;51(RR-10):1-29.

SELECTED READINGS

1. Centers for Disease Control and Prevention; Infectious Disease Society of America; American Society of Blood and Marrow Transplantation. Guidelines for preventing opportunistic infections among hematopoietic stem cell transplant recipients. MMWR Recomm Rep. 2000;49(RR-10):1-125, CE1-7.
2. Association of Operating Room Nurses. Standards, Recommended Practices, Guidelines. Denver: Association of Operating Room Nurses; 1999.
3. Larson EL. APIC guideline for handwashing and hand antisepsis in health care settings. Am J Infect Control. 1995;23(4):251-69.
4. Recommended practices for skin preparation of Patients. Association of Operating Room Nurses. AORN J. 1996;64(5): 813-6.
5. Rutala WA. APIC guideline for selection and use of disinfectants. Am J Infect Control. 1990;18(2):99-117.
6. Favero Medical Superintendent, Bond W. Sterilization, disinfection and antisepsis in the hospital. In: Balows A, Hausler WJ, Herrmann KL, Isenberg HD, Shadomy HJ (Eds). Manual of Clinical Microbiology, 5th edition. Washington (DC): American Society for Microbiology; 1991. pp. 183-200.
7. American Institute of Architects Committee. Guidelines for design and construction of Hospital and health care facilities. Washington (DC): American institute of Architects Press; 1996.
8. Platt R. Guidelines for perioperative antibiotic prophylaxis. In: Abrutyn E, Goldmann DA Scheckler WE (Eds). Saunders Infection Control Reference Service. Philadelphia: W3 Saunders Co; 1997. pp. 229-34.
9. Wong ES. Surgical site infections. In: Mayhall CG (Ed). Hospital Epidemiology and Infection Control. Baltimore: Williams and Wilkins; 1996. pp. 154-74.

66 Cancer Control in Developing Countries

Praful Desai, Bhagwan Nene, Madan Chauhan

INTRODUCTION

Cancer continues to challenge the skill, ingenuity and resources of the human mind, science and technology even in the 21st century. Rising rapidly toward the number one killer in many Western countries, it is preceded only by stroke and cardiovascular diseases. Owing to its large population, the developing countries share a major burden of new and prevalent burden of cancer. Projected World Health Organization (WHO) figures for 2020 estimate a global burden of new cases as 20 million, of which 14 million will be in the developing countries, forming 70% of the total cancer load. It is significant to compare 1985 figures which showed an incidence of 7.6 million new cases, of which 52% were in the developing world. As the global population grows (6 billion) and ages more, cancer will reign supreme and continue to claim a very major component of our resources, energy, research, technology and tragedies in the years to come. The simplest and the most effective way to counteract this oncoming deluge is PREVENTION and EARLY DIAGNOSIS, which is possible only through education at appropriate levels.

Seventy percent of the Indian population lives in rural and semiurban areas. Admittedly, the scenario in these regions is steadily progressing, albeit at a very slow pace. In most developing countries, health and disease are major socioeconomic problems. Rural population based on personal experience, have a tremendous native intelligence; however, socioeconomic problem prevents or limits their access to appropriate health care. Priorities in health care vary widely in developed and developing countries and the powers in control of health in developing regions often have to prioritize their resources according to the needs. Infectious diseases, tuberculosis, malaria, infant mortality and malnutrition will naturally claim for greater attention of the state and the Central Ministries of Health in a country like India. Globally, there is a strong inversely proportion relationship between socioeconomic status and cancer incidence.

A sample study of 200 consecutive patients (from rural and semiurban areas) attending the outpatients at Tata Memorial Hospital (1988) showed socioeconomic problems in 75% (finances, distances to travel, family issues, staying in a metropolitan area, etc). There were disease-related physiologic disabilities in 20%; 43% could not complete treatment, though 57% went through the therapy. Long-term follow-up was feasible in only one-third of the patients. The scenario after a quarter of a century has indeed improved; more facilities, improving economic status and the health-related infrastructure and education has helped; yet a countrywide concerted effort by a strong partnership between Government and Private enterprises, and Cancer Societies is needed. Nongovernmental Organizations (NGOs) and Medical Colleges need to address to training and education of professionals and paramedical staff. The importance of prevention and early diagnosis and access to proper therapy cannot be overemphasized. Public education by media and other sources is imperative.

METHODOLOGY—LOW COST/LOW TECHNOLOGY EFFORT—A REPLICABLE MODULE

A simple practical approach envisages—most importantly:

- Education about prevention; based on lifestyle and habits

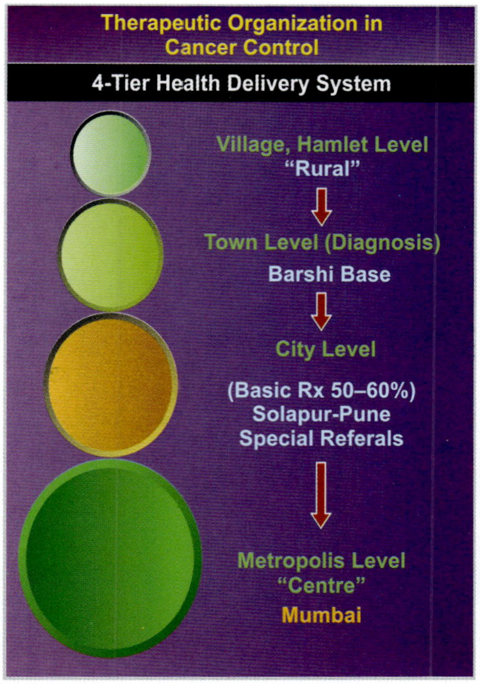

Fig. 1: Mutually supportive and interactive system for cancer care

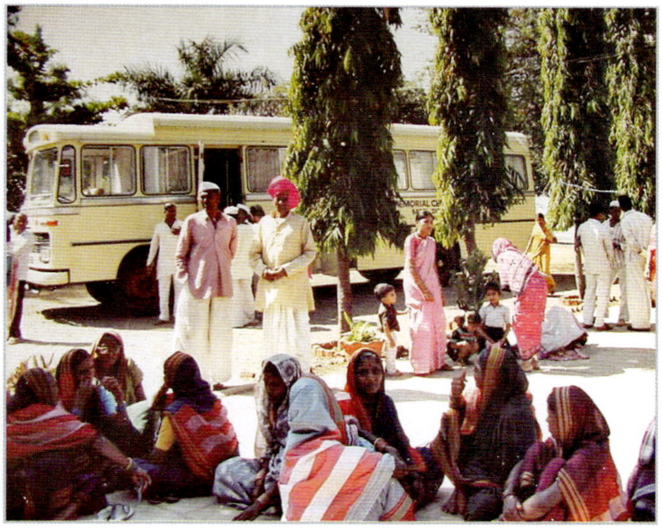

Fig. 2: Self-contained diagnostic van with villagers waiting for their turn for examination

- Facilities for simple clinical examinations
- Minimal diagnostic facilities for imaging and laboratory studies
- Ability to offer therapy to at least 75% of patients who require average therapeutic support of surgery, radiotherapy, chemotherapy and rehabilitation support system.

The need for support from NGOs, Cancer Societies and voluntary organizations is important in such an effort (Fig. 1).

COMPREHENSIVE CANCER CENTERS

The need for Comprehensive Cancer Centers (CCC) is vital; it has to be the citadel of cancer effort in the country. Clinical and basic cancer research, professional education of the highest standard and the ability to effectively offer the state-of-the-art therapy at a tertiary level are major components. Effective support to secondary centers for technology transfer in diagnosis, therapy and training professionals are important functions of a CCC. Depending on the size of the country, e.g. India, 8–10 CCCs may adequately satisfy the need of a population of 1.2 billion. The primary effort has to be service, education and research (basic and clinical), the CCC spearheads the technology transfer efforts across the country.

COMMUNITY CANCER CENTERS

The major vehicle to effectively drive the cancer effort is the Community Cancer Center. It should have the resources to treat even the more complicated and technology-oriented therapy. Professional training of a high caliber is necessary requisite. Interactive and mutually supportive strategies with two higher and lower level institutes are the necessary ingredients. Community cancer center plays a very major role in an effort of a large country like India. Each of the larger states in India should have a Community Cancer Center. The town level and the village level (Fig. 2) support system form the basic needs for a very large majority of population, providing the most basic forms of treatment support in their own environment. Important facilities for routine screening programs [Pap smears, chest X-rays, sonography, mammograms—when indicated (Figs 3 and 4)] need to be organized at these levels. Basic laboratory facilities are mandatory. Education at all levels should become a priority (Figs 5A and B).

The Barshi model (town level) (Figs 6A to E) offers a practical approach toward cancer control in India which seems to have had a significant impact on the population. From a humble effort of a simple outpatient *primary care it grew into a sprawling Community Cancer Center over almost three decades.* Training and education at all levels

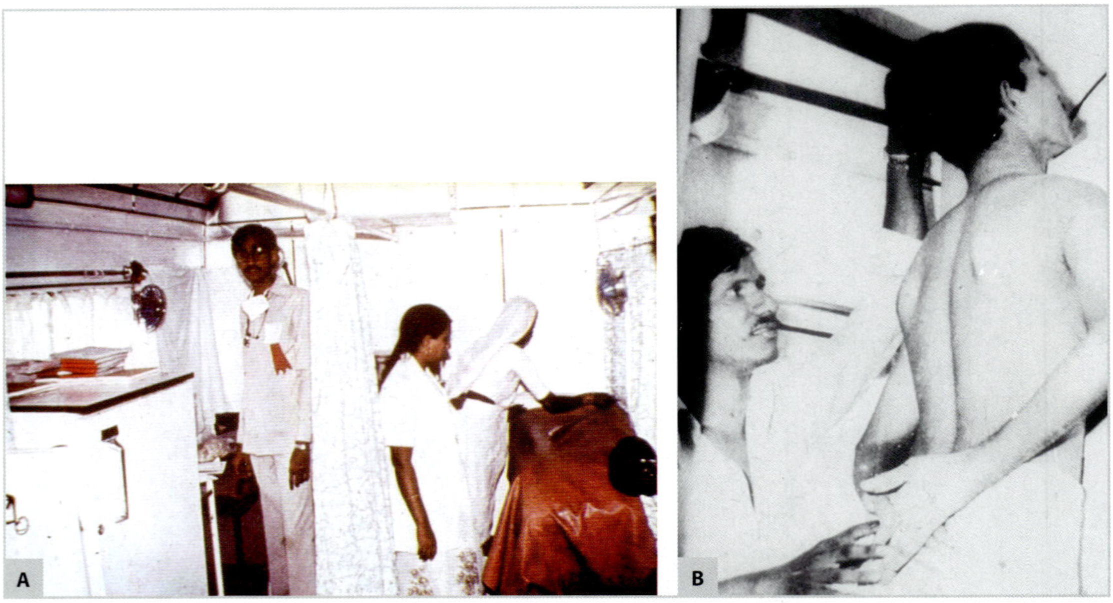

Figs 3A and B: Inside of the van (A) Facilities for clinical examination, (B) For diagnostic X-rays and Pap smears

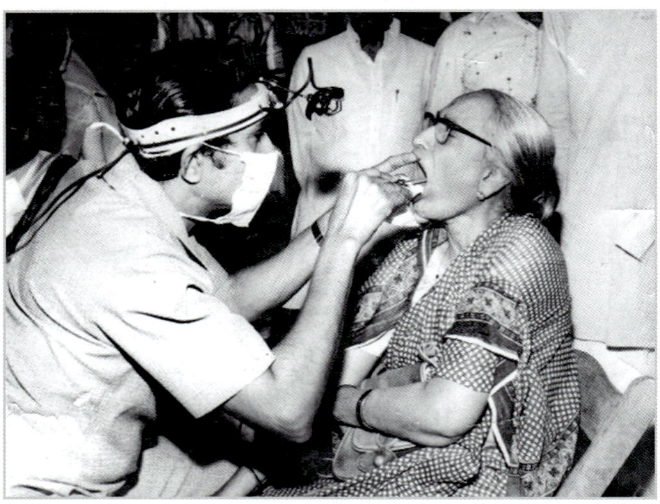

Fig. 4: Clinical examination in the outpatient department (OPD) during a rural camp at Barshi

has been at the core by manual and technical transfer of technology through the CCC (Tata Memorial Hospital, Mumbai, India) to the town level. The effort began as a small outpatient set up is now a major Community Cancer Center (Figs 6A to E). Apart from being recognized as a model by the WHO as a low-cost technology effort for developing countries, it has since then been the recipient of large government and philanthropic grants including a $ 5 million (Bill and Melinda Gates Foundation, United States of America) project for early diagnosis and prevention of

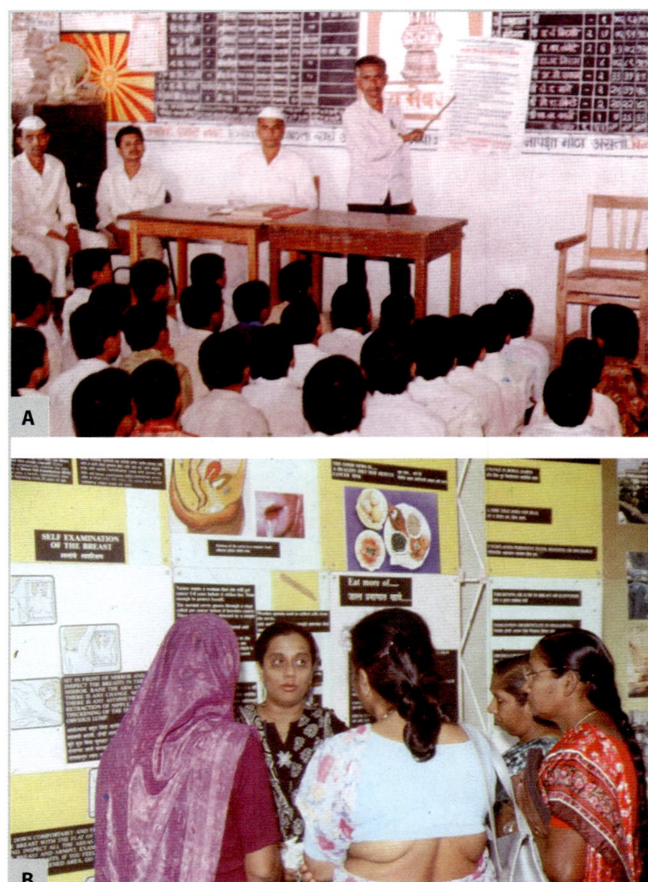

Figs 5A and B: Education for (A) children and (B) women on cancer prevention and early diagnosis

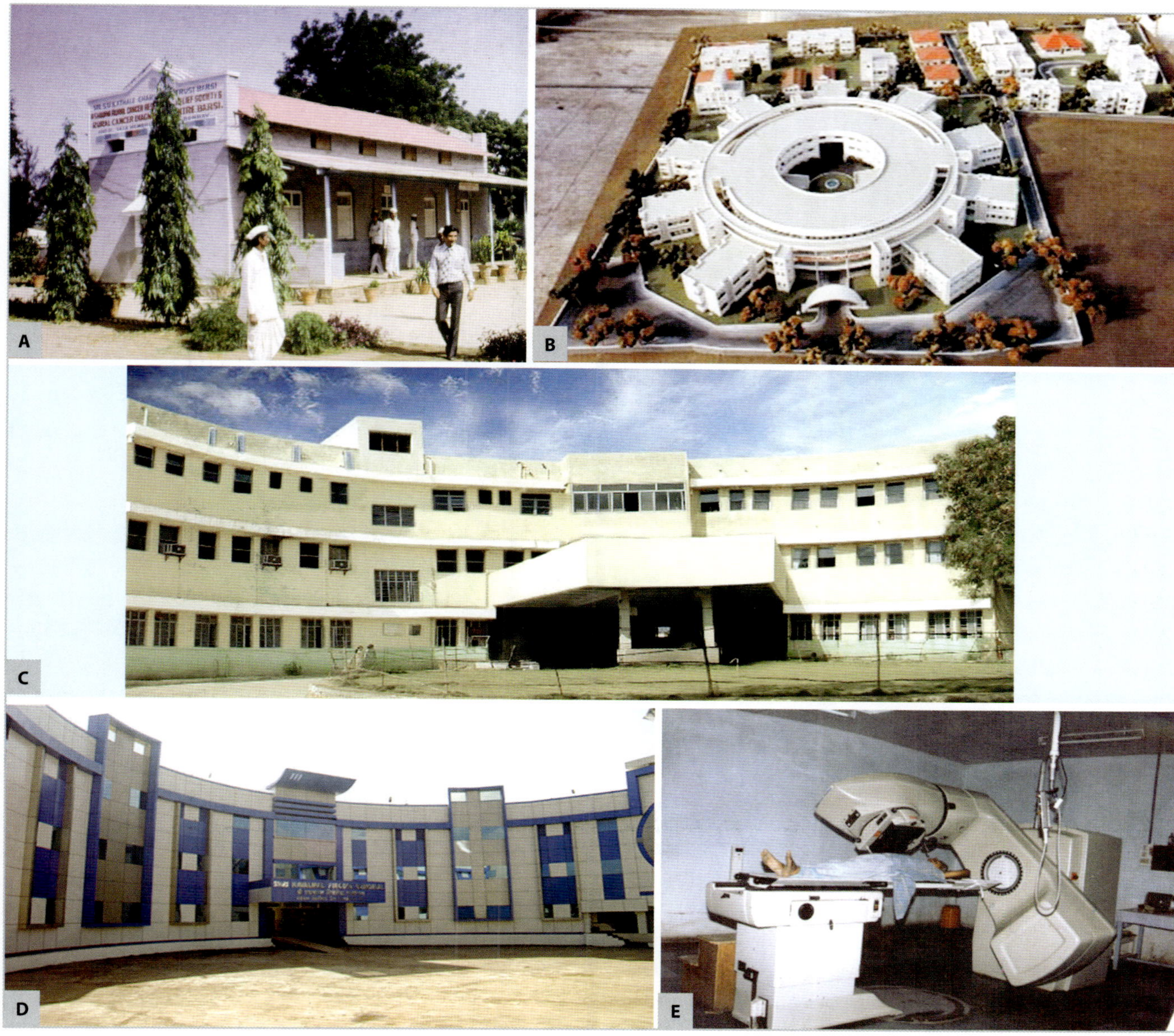

Figs 6A to E: (A) A gentle start (1982) with only an outpatient department (OPD); (B) The vision—the proposed model; (C to E) A robust end with all modern facilities for diagnosis and treatment (a well-organized community cancer center)

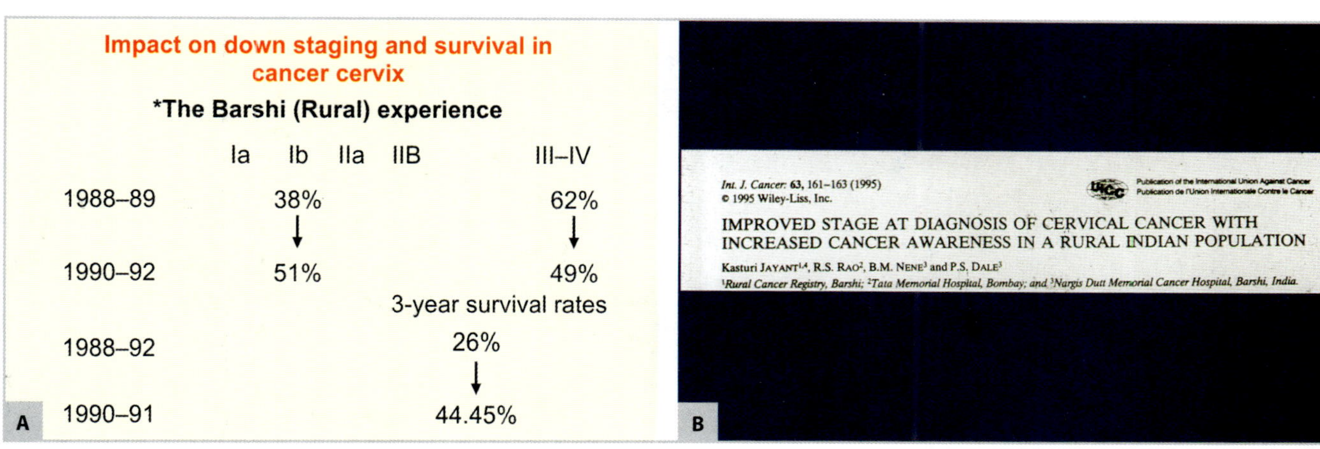

Int. J. Cancer: **63**, 161–163 (1995)
© 1995 Wiley-Liss, Inc.
Publication of the International Union Against Cancer
Publication de l'Union Internationale Contre le Cancer

IMPROVED STAGE AT DIAGNOSIS OF CERVICAL CANCER WITH INCREASED CANCER AWARENESS IN A RURAL INDIAN POPULATION

Kasturi JAYANT[1,4], R.S. RAO[2], B.M. NENE[3] and P.S. DALE[3]
[1]*Rural Cancer Registry, Barshi;* [2]*Tata Memorial Hospital, Bombay; and* [3]*Nargis Dutt Memorial Cancer Hospital, Barshi, India.*

Figs 7A and B: Scientific data on (A) Downstaging of cervical cancer with (B) a scientific publication in International Journal of Cancer

TABLE 1: Genesis of a rural cancer facility to a major Community Cancer Center

Year	*Events*
1980-81	Registration of Trust and Society
1982	Mobile van-commissioned: Tata Memorial Hospital/BARSHI Cancer Center started
1983	Outpatient department (OPD)
1984	Indoor patient department
1986-87	X-ray and ultrasonography unit and cancer registry
1992	Radiotherapy unit
1995	Medical oncology plus fiber optic scopes
1999	CT Scan/IARC: Cervical Cancer Prevention Project
2000	Colposcopy, HPV and cytology laboratories
2001	Training Program for Government Medical Officers
2002	Telepathology
2005-06	Mammography and nuclear medical imaging (gamma camera)
2009	Cervical Cancer Vaccination Project
2011	Major project on cervical cancer
2011	MRI: Sponsored by Indo-US Health Care, Hyderabad, India
2011	Linear Accelerator: Donation from Firodiya Trust, Pune, India
2012	Ayurveda department
2012	"Rajiv Gandhi Arogya Yojana" by Government of Maharashtra

Abbreviations: CT, computed tomography; IARC, International Agency of Research in Cancer; HPV, human papillomavirus; MRI, magnetic resonance imaging

cervical cancer. The illustrations provide a tiny glimpse of a catalytic effort through a Comprehensive Cancer Center (Tata Memorial Hospital Cancer Center) to this village and town area. It is a classic example of the combined efforts, through the support of Government of India (the Atomic Energy Commission) and the philanthropy of the house of TATAs and most importantly the outstanding local effort of highly dedicated local professionals from BARSHI.

Comprehensive Cancer Centers across the country need to act as catalytic forces to disseminate knowledge, experience and expertise, clinical and basic research ethos, to the lower tires of the cancer control pyramid for developing countries. These are low-cost technology models which can slowly and steadily develop into major and effective cancer control institutes across the country (Table 1).

A GENTLE START TO A ROBUST END

67

The Future: Cure, Control or Peaceful Coexistence?

Praful Desai

The global society at large is concerned as much, if not more, than the oncologic community (scientists, researchers and clinicians) as to the time frame when cancer will be completely decoded and a "cure" will emerge. The most feared and probably the most serious disease to afflict our civilization continues to exercise the skill and ingenuity of the human mind for more than a century and beyond. Even the most intensive, vigorous and combined efforts of science, medicine, research, politics and social activists have not been able to completely comprehend the finer nuances of the cancer cell. It would be naïve, however, to say that no progress has been made. Probably, the present and the upcoming decades are likely to be the most exciting periods toward the rapid progress in understanding and decoding the mystery of the cancer cells. The trenches of medicine and science are never faultless; the progress of science, irrespective, is painfully slow. To use a Churchillian phrase cancer is indeed a riddle, wrapped in a mystery inside an enigma; a phrase used at the time of the discovery of the DNA by Watson and Crick in 1953.

The progress made toward the cure and control of cancer in the last four decades is shown in Table 1. This is the result of complementary efforts of all oncology disciplines. The ability to code genomic sequences, education regarding prevention and early diagnosis, imaging techniques, science and technology, appropriate combination therapies, after care and rehabilitation, all have had a share in whatever progress has resulted in the last quarter of a century. It would be just to say that more progress has resulted in the last 30 years than the previous 70 years of the last century; however, it is only from the past that we weave the fabric of our present and the future.

Let us look and review the present and its likely impact on the coming decades in our onward journey to contain, control and cure cancer by understanding cancer. We know that the way we practice medicine today is way different than it was just 10 or 20 years ago. Today's medicine, of necessity, has to be preventive (only way we can "cure" cancer today),[6] personalized (targeted, individualized), proactive and patient participative. Add "evidence based" to this list and we have the current scenario of how medicine should be practiced in our secondary and tertiary therapeutic institutions.

We now know that genetic changes are the fundamentals at the core of carcinogenesis in most, if not all cases. The sequencing and decoding of the human genome in the last 10 years, it is envisaged, will change the entire landscape of medicine but none more than in oncology. The present is enshrined in the luster of the past and it was Theodor Boveri[7] who first proposed that chromosomal alterations lead to cancer in 1914. Bishop and Varmus[8] identified human proto-oncogenes (1976) and oncogenes in 1985. The launch of **Human Genome Project (1990)**[7]

TABLE 1: Five-year relative survival rates

Site of cancer	*1970s*	*1980s*	*1990s*	*2000s*
Breast	75%[5]	79%[1]	51.4%[5]	77%[4]
Cervix	70%[5]	68%[1]	46.1%[5]	71%[1]
Lung	13%[5]	7.2%[3]	13.5%[5]	16%[1]
Colon	52%[5]	36.6%[2]	32.3%[5]	56%[1]
Rectum	49%[5]	42.2%[2]	33.6%[5]	69%[1]
Kidney	51%[5]	56%[1]	36.0%[5]	70%[1]

and its completion in 2003[8]—by two parallel groups (Craig Venter and Francis Collins) herald a new era in medicine recalling the past history of DNA discovery (1953). The discoveries were not without the ugly face of competitive science. By 2011, 142586[7] mutations were known in cancer gene census.

Today's science is the medicine of tomorrow; the captured knowledge of today will very likely and hopefully impact on the cancer scenario of the future: Prevention, prediction, targeted personalized therapies; currently, the scenario in biomedical research and its possible impact, particularly in cancer, is too exciting to envisage.

The heterogeneity of every tumor can now be studied in most tumors; breast cancer may be, say 10–15 different types of lesions based on its morphology and biologic studies; the same is true of many other cancers. We now know that before this knowledge, breast cancer with negative hormone receptors and strong HER2 positivity was a lethal cancer; however, today early stage HER2 with node positivity and negative receptors can be cured up to 90% by targeted (Herceptin®) therapy. Even with metastatic, Her2-positive lesions, the chances of recurrences are minimal. Targeting the epidermal growth factor receptor (EGFR) and KRAS mutations in colon, stomach and lung cancers by appropriate tyrosine kinase inhibitors [cetuximab (Erbitux®)] and use of bevacizumab (Avastin®) to prevent angiogenesis are classic examples of translational research leading to longer remissions and toward disease-free survivals, though, in an incremental fashion. Understanding mutational chromosomal landscapes in difficult tumors will allow us to predict clinical behavior and allow precise targeted therapies in each tumor.

As and when available, plasma-based DNA analysis[9] may even allow us to study the determinants of cancer and how to prevent them. This may be routinely employed in the future. Genetically engineered T-cells may become a major revisitation to stimulate immunogenic processes in the system and open up new vistas in immunology. All these are scientific outflows of collective and individual brilliance of our scientific, technologic and clinical researchers.

Despite this exciting scenario for the future, we have to dwell into the present. Too many cancers are diagnosed late, particularly in developing countries and death rates are not rapidly declining. Metastases, despite adequate therapy, are frequent; based on the biologic behavior, even an early cancer may metastasize rapidly and locally advanced cancer may happily surprise us by a prolonged survival. Tumor biology is the king, selection of therapy is the queen and technique of therapy is the prince in oncology.[10] The mirage of cancer cure is visible, but its pursuit and conquest will require our continued efforts, perseverance, persistence and patience in the coming decades.

The increasing remissions and disease-free survivals that we now witness in many cancers with an improved quality of life are directly dependent on our present markedly improved diagnostic and therapeutic process. This in itself is a major achievement and breakthrough in the present cancer scenario.

We now know, based on solid fundamental science, that cancer is deeply entwined within ourselves and our genetic framework. External and internal stimuli, genetic interactions with the environment and within the cells, chromosomal mutations and alterations are ultimately at the base of carcinogenesis, steadily unraveling under the unremitting efforts of scientists and researchers; however, to unravel it completely is to understand life and nature in all its nuances, to understand the complexity of birth, growth, disease and death is not going to be easy as the entire landscape of natural phenomenon including life itself is and may remain unconquerable. "Cure" for cancer continues to remain a mirage in the far away horizon, though visible it surely is.

The sequence of cancer—control—remission—recurrence—further treatment and longer remissions—recurrences, metastasis—and still further therapy with another remission with a better quality of life and significant life prolongation is a significant milestone and victory of sorts against cancer.[11] These efforts toward prolonged cancer control are rapidly pushing cancer into a chronic medical condition like diabetes, hypertension, asthma, arthritis, etc, which are compatible with a reasonably comfortable and coexistence with our system.

In the words of an outstanding recent cancer biographer, Siddhartha Mukharjee[11] "given what we know about cancer, even this would represent a technological victory unlike any other in our history. "It would be a victory over our own inevitability—a victory over our genomes".[11]

REFERENCES

1. Altekruse SF, Kosary CL, Krapcho M, et al. (Eds). SEER Cancer Statistics Review, 1975–2007. Bethesda, MD: National Cancer Institute. [online] SEER website. Available from: http://seer.cancer.gov/csr/1975_2007 [Accessed January, 2014].
2. Yeole BB, Sunny L, Swaminathan R, et al. Population-based survival from colorectal cancer in Mumbai, (Bombay) India. Eur J Cancer. 2001;37(11):1402-8.
3. Mathers CD, Boschi-Pinto C, Lopez AD, et al. Cancer incidence, mortality and survival by site for 14 regions of the world. Global Programme on Evidence for Health Policy Discussion Paper No. 13; World Health Organization, 2001.
4. Ganesh B, Talole SD, Dikshit R, et al. Estimation of survival rates of breast cancer patients—a hospital-based study from Mumbai. Asian Pac J Cancer Prev. 2008;9(1):53-7.
5. Yeole BB, Kurkure AP, Sunny L. Cancer survival in Mumbai (Bombay), India, 1992–1999. Cancer Survival in Africa, Asia, the Caribbean and Central America IARC Scientific Publications No. 162. International Agency for Research on Cancer, Lyon, 2011.
6. Mukharjee S. Prevention is the cure. The Emperor of All Maladies. London: Fourth Estate, 2011.
7. Samuels Y, Bardelli A, Lopez-Otin C, et al. The cancer genome. In: DeVita VT, Lawrence TS, Rosenberg SA, DePinho RA, Weinberg RA (Eds). DeVita, Hellman, and Rosenberg's Cancer: Principles and Practice of Oncology, 9th edition. Philadelphia: Lippincott Williams & Wilkins; 2011. p. 2-22.
8. Bishop JM, Varmus HE. The fruits of our long-term endeavor. In: Siddhartha Mukharjee (Ed). The Emperor of All Maladies.
9. Baselga J. Personal comment—advances in medical oncology—Memorial Sloan-Kettering Cancer Center (MSKCC).
10. Blake C. Aphorisms for Surgeons.
11. Mukharjee S. The Emperor of All Maladies. New York: Scribner (Simon and Schuster Inc.); 2010.

68 The Conquest of Mortality: Science, Medicine and Technology's Final Destination?

Praful Desai

We are living in exciting times. The progress of the human race in the last 30 years has far exceeded that of the previous 300 years. Every sphere of human endeavor is witnessing gargantuan changes far beyond our expectations of even 20 years ago. Be it science, communications, technology, business, industry—you name it and the scenario is changing by the year. The science fiction of Robotic and Bionic (electronically engineered) man as we see in the movies is closer to truth than mere fiction. Medicine is no exception as "robotic surgery" and "telemedicine" are now established procedures. The sea-change in the way we now practice medicine today is technology dependent and vastly different than it was, say, just about 10 to 15 years ago. Whether we accept it or otherwise, the Art of Medicine is almost—totally being replaced by a technical craft due to the tremendous progress of technology. The incredible advantages of technology in medicine have reaped tremendous benefits for the society when appropriately used. Many people live today because of this progress but it would be simplistic and naïve to assume that there is no negative spin off as a consequence of this technologic impact in medicine. Quite a few have succumbed due to inappropriate use, abuse, or overuse of technology. Man has conquered the stars and the seas, mastered the skies, has split the atom, understood the biologic nuances of the human system in health and disease; however, one thing man has NOT been able to achieve is the "conquest of death and mortality" due to disease and natural processes of aging.

Our present and future is steeped very much in the past. Four hundred years ago Rene Descrates and Francis Bacon, leading philosophers of that age gave a calling to eradicate disease, and eliminate death from human civilization—a call referred to as the "Baconian" theory. This has, forever remained the calling of the medical profession ever since. Aldous Huxley in 1934 wrote a futuristic novel "A Brave New World", in which he envisaged and predicted a genetically engineered society, laid the visions of in vitro fertilization (IVF) by laboratory techniques—an idea which was severely criticized by the "Puritans" of the time and yet what has happened in the succeeding decades is now history. James Watson and Francis Crick in 1953 broke the genetic code of the DNA, which makes every individual a distinctive entity quite apart from the other and held out a promise that knowledge in Genetics could be a panacea for the human race. These ideas and discoveries have laid the foundation for the current thrust on "biologic" understanding of the human system. If the last century was appropriately known as the Century of Physics (Einstein's theory; splitting of the atom, fusion technology for unlimited energy—which is yet a dream, optical physics, etc.) the present millennium is well on its way to be recognized as a century of Biology or Biogenetic Technology; if the present state of biogenetic technology is any indication, this thinking indeed has a sound basis.

Today's science is tomorrow's medicine. Just as technology in different fields (including medicine) is unstoppable the progress in the "conquest over disease and death" is and will be unstoppable. While we are excited at the possibility of genetic engineering, robotic surgery and telemedicine (which will do away with the need of doctors and paramedics), which have almost come to stay, the science laboratories around the world (mainly in advanced countries) are grappling with gene manipulations to increase lifespan, prevent or defy senescence and create a genetically-engineered world in which there is eternal life sans disease, sans sadness or happiness, sans emotions and sentiments, no love or hate where everyone lives a mechanical life, a kind of situation controlled by the state.

What we are able to do and achieve in the practice of medicine today is nothing compared to what is happening and will happen in the future in the laboratories. Just as technology is not going to stop in its onward march, the scientists in the laboratory are not going to restrain themselves from their dreams of progress in science. Cloning of animals in the laboratory is now history since "Dolly" the sheep was cloned in 1997. Sheep, rabbits, mice have been cloned already; men are not far away. Scientists in Harvard are waging a war with the powers that are to win approval to clone humans from embryonic stem cells and sooner or later they will win. The tremendous debates about the pros and cons of "stem cell research" (already on in many countries including India)—will become a thing of the past and when in full swing, readymade body parts be it liver, lungs, heart, kidney, brain, etc.—will be available off the shelf for the asking. The mad rush for procuring "organs" for transplant by fair means or foul will become a thing of the past; however; wait a minute; human and scientific ingenuity will procure organs from headless mice in the laboratories.

Does All This Sound Utopian? Not Quite.

The genetic basis of human life has been well established and the genes and the chromosomes, which from the basis of DNA are now well defined by mapping of the "genome" by the scientists (private and government) in the US. Craig Venter and Francis Collins working in a private and government set-up respectively were in an unholy war to outdo the other in trying to complete the human "genome". Presidential restraint had to be used to cool the war between the two scientific groups. The reasons are not far to seek why this is not an uncommon scenario in science or medicine. Both move by market forces due to the environment in which we live and so did the race of mapping the human genome.

We now know—based on scientific facts, that the genes control everything—our personality, structure, behavior, lifespan and intelligence, though our environment does have a significant impact. Human beings are the product of the genes they inherit from their parents but are often the result of the environment in which they live.

Two groups of scientists almost simultaneously from the University of Texas (USA) and University of Bath (UK)—over a period of 4 years (1994–1998), created in the laboratories, headless mice and the other group created headless tadpoles. Researchers found the gene that tells the embryo to produce the head and they deleted it. They did this in a thousand of mice embryos, four of which were born. Having no way to breathe the mice died instantly. Why create them in the first place? The Texas researchers want to learn how the genes determine embryo development; but you do not have to be a genius to see the true utility of manufacturing headless creatures; indeed, for their organs, fully formed, perfectly useful, and ripe for plundering to market forces. Why should we panic? Simply because headless humans are next.

Princeton biologist Lee M Silver says (London Times): "It would almost certainly be possible to produce human bodies without a forebrain." Thus, by deleting genes (responsible for developing the forebrain which is responsible for personality, emotions, memory, consciousness, etc.) in a legal sense, therefore, these creatures will not be "persons" and therefore it is perfectly permissible legally to keep them "alive" as a "future source of organs". "Alive"—never have a pair of quotation marks loomed so ominously. Take the "mouse frog technology", apply it to humans, combine it with cloning, and you become a "GOD"; delete the "forebrain" gene from the human embryonic stem cells, let the hindbrain gene remain (responsible for respiratory and cardiovascular system) and implant the cells in a female womb (much like in vitro fertilization) and allow it to grow to full term and you will have created a headless human (with intact respiratory and cardiovascular system) yet with no consciousness, no personality, no emotions. There are of course, technical hurdles along the way; suppressing the equivalent head gene in man and incubating tiny infant organs to grow into larger ones that adults could use. And creating artificial wombs (as per Aldous Huxley), given that it might be difficult to recruit sane women to carry headless fetuses to their birth/death.

It will not long, however, before these technical barriers are breached. In fact, as early as 1998 a Chicago physicist assembled a team to produce the first human clone, which had at that time occasioned yet another wave of "Brave New World" anxiety. The ethical barriers are already cracking. Lewis Wolpert, Professor of Biology at the University College, London, finds producing headless humans "perfectly distasteful" but given the shortage of organs, does not think distaste is a sufficient reason NOT to go ahead with something that would save lives, and Professor Silver not only sees "nothing wrong, philosophically or rationally" about producing headless humans for organ harvesting; and he wants to convince a skeptical public that it is perfectly OKAY.

When prominent scientists are prepared to acquiesce in—or indeed encourage—the deliberate creation of deformed and dying quasi-human life you know we are facing a bioethical abyss. There is no grosser corruption of biotechnology than creating a human mutant and disemboweling it at our pleasure for spare parts. The headless clone solves the facsimile problem. It is the gateway to the ultimate vanity: IMMORTALITY.

This kind of progress in scientific laboratories leaves you breathless and gasping. And the basis of our current scientific abilities will create waves of progress (?) in clinical medicine, which we are very likely to witness with the advancing human genomic discoveries.

Nicholas Wade, a highly reliable science writer in 'Nature' and 'Science', in his recent book on "Transformation of Medicine based on Human Genomic Discoveries" writes about the three waves of medicine, which he refers to as "conventional", "germ line" and "life extending".

In "conventional" wave of medicine, "gene chips" will be able to scan your genome and detect your vulnerability to various diseases over a lifespan giving you the opportunity to prevent it by "genetic engineering" by deleting the abnormal gene (a distinct possibility in the next two or three decades). Instead of helping people to live longer with disease (as it is today) medical science will harness the process of stem cells (research currently on) to grow into any number of replacement parts and organs. Livers, brains, kidneys, hearts—indeed any other organ, in fact, can be replaced with easily available organs developed from embryonic stem cells. This will, as Wade concludes "lead to the fulfillment of conventional medicine's ultimate goal—good health to the end of one's days, which will add up to, on an average, around 120 years".

The second wave of "progress" will be "germ line (genetic) manipulation of the human genome" or "germ line therapy", which will help to repair clear cut genetic defects (understandable and acceptable) but will also have the ability to "enhance" you—by gene manipulation/mutation techniques by which you can increase your height, your IQ, or intelligence (achieved in the laboratory in experimental animals)—any takers?

The "life-extending" wave of medicine will allow the scientists to achieve the utopian dream—the ultimate—of radically increasing the "natural" lifespan of the human species. Scientists have extended the lifespan of round worms, mice, fruit-flies already manifold. Wade points out that if the same is accomplished in humans the extension in human lifespan could be from 80 years to 320 years.

Indeed, Aldous Huxley in 1932 envisaged the possibilities of such a "Brave New World"—never mind the tremendous and insoluble socioeconomic complexities of such a new world order, this will be the crowning achievement of scientists in the laboratories and the medical professionals in the clinics. The consequences of such an upcoming scenario is difficult to comprehend and too devastatingly complex to imagine. Scientists, technologists, medical professionals will press ahead in their quest for progress to satisfy their egos to convince themselves and others about their limitless capabilities.

It is for these reasons that science is probably too important a subject to be left to the scientists alone, just as war is too important a matter to be left to the Generals.

Apart from the horrendous social consequences of limitless life and genetically altered body structure, artificially enhanced intelligence (which has been achieved in the laboratory) the eternal beauty of normal life will vanish; the beauty of a rose is because it is going to whither and human mortality does matter; indeed it is sacrosanct—we have deadlines to meet, milestones to achieve, seeing grandchildren graduating, love, joy, sadness, emotions, sentiments and excitements to be experienced. All this will vanish in the "Brave New World" where scientific monstrosity will devour normal human strength and fragility brought forth by normal evolutionary biological forces after a trial and error of millions of years of human existence. Do we have a right to disrupt such natural events just to satisfy our scientific ego? The time therefore appears rife to debate fiercely what is right and what is wrong in our scientific research. No easy answers to that. Can we also, on the other hand, prevent research in embryonic stem cells, which, as is claimed, may help in Alzheimer's or other neurological disorders, cardiac dysfunction, cancer and other chronic diseases? *The supreme objective of science (biology) is to defeat disease and conquest of mortality.*

There is however, a flip side to this frighteningly positive scenario. Writing in a highly controversial book "The End of Science", John Horgan states that based on the current scientific prowess in the laboratory (stem cells, genomic discoveries, cloning, etc.) the end point in applied biology is therefore, nothing less than human immortality. The strong possibility that scientists can identify and then arrest the mechanism underlying senescence is a perennial favorite of science writers; one might have more confidence in scientists' ability to crack the riddle of senescence if they had more success with a presumably simpler problem, CANCER. We still cut cancer with surgery, burn it with radiation and poison it with chemotherapy. May be cancer—and by extension "mortality" is simply too complex a problem to solve.

Horgan further states that, "Ironically, biology's inability (as of now) to defeat death and conquest of mortality may be its brightest hope. Harvey Sapolsky, a professor of Social Policy at the MIT noted that the major justification of funding science was (in USA) National Security or more specifically, the cold war. Now that scientists have no longer to worry about the "evil empire" (cold war) to justify their huge budgets, Sapolsky asked, what other opponent can serve as a substitute? The answer he came up with was "mortality". Most people think that living longer and possibly forever, is desirable (?) he pointed out. And the best thing about making IMMORTALITY the primary goal of science, Sapolsky added, is that it is almost certainly unattainable, so scientists can keep getting funds for more research forever.

As the genius of science and medicine extends the horizon of what we can do, we are increasingly confronted complex questions about what we should do.

Despite the awesome strength and possibilities of our current scientific and medical prowess, do we have the moral, ethical, legal and social right to disrupt the natural evolutionary biological forces of millions of years to alter "life" as we live today: simply and beautifully with all its joys and sadness, triumphs and tragedies, winning and losing and trying to achieve our small deadlines that make our lives so meaningful and eternally livable.

GUIDE TO FURTHER READING

I acknowledge the help from the following publications and are grateful to their respective authors and publishers:

1. John Horgan. The End of Science. New York: Broadway Books; 1996.
2. William Kristol, Eric Cotien. The Future is Now. Rowman & Littlfield Publishers; 2002.
3. Aldous Huxley. A Brave New World. HarperCollins Publishers Inc; 1932.
4. Charles Krauthammer. Of Headless Mice…And Men. "Time"; Jan 1998.
5. Adam Wolfson. Biodemocracy in America. The Public Interest; Winter 2002.
6. Nicholas Wade. Life Script: How the Human Genome Discoveries Will Transform Medicine and Enhance Your Health. Genomic Discoveries & Medicine; 1998.

Index

Page numbers followed by *f* refer to figure and *t* refer to table.

A

Abbe-Estlander flap 153
Abdominal wall reconstruction 601
Abdominoperineal resection 125, 130
Abiraterone 484
Abnormal mitoses 145
Accelerated fractionation 68
Acetaminophen 670
Acinetobacter baumannii 691
Acoustic neuroma 91
Acetate dehydrogenase 635
Acute
  lymphoblastic leukemia 62
  respiratory distress syndrome 663
Adenocarcinoma 183, 252, 265, 383, 405, 489
  of stomach 203
Adenoid
  basal carcinoma 383
  cystic carcinoma 183, 383
Adenoma 250, 446, 450
  of parathyroid 662
  tubular adenomas 250
  villous adenomas 250
Adenomatous
  polyp with high-grade dysplasia 252*f*
  polyposis coli 439
Adenosquamous carcinoma 383, 405
Adequate regional dissection 226
Adjuvant
  chemoradiation 173*f*
  chemotherapy 240, 353, 372, 390, 413, 497
  concurrent chemoradiotherapy 413
  drugs 671
  external beam radiotherapy 400
  postoperative radiation therapy 391
  radiation therapy 412
  radiotherapy after subtotal excision 571
  therapy 262, 412, 465
    in pancreatic cancer 319
  treatment for GBC 299
Adrenal 661
  androgen production 484
  carcinoma 445
  cortical carcinoma 448
  cysts 446
  glands 444*f*
  mass 445
  tumors 445
Adrenocortical carcinoma 91
Adrenocorticotropic hormone 79, 407, 444, 446, 588
Adriamycin 340, 628, 629, 630, 631
Adult lymphomas 644
Advanced
  cancers, incidence of 674
  germ cell tumors 506
  nonseminoma 508
  ovarian cancer 372
  seminoma 508
  stage
    disease 390
    lymphoblastic lymphoma 638
Airway obstruction 611
  symptoms 612
  treatment 612
Albicans Candida spp 691
Alcohol 234
Alendronate 556
Alpha fetoprotein 59, 507
American
  Cancer Society 113, 331*t*
  College of Radiology Imaging Network 332
  Joint Committee on Cancer 406, 461*t*
  Society
    for Radiation Oncology 556
    of Clinical Oncology 357
  Urological Association 121
Aminoglutethimide 484
Amphipathic polyethylene glycol 104
Ampulla 205
  of vater 209
Ampullary adenoma 213
Anal
  canal tumor 130
  carcinoma 62
  intraepithelial neoplasia 265
Analgesic drug therapy 668
  principles 668
Anaphylactic reactions to chemotherapeutic agents 610
Anaplastic
  astrocytoma 563, 567
  carcinoma 187
  large cell lymphoma 634, 634*f*, 637, 638
  lymphoma kinase 64, 403, 456, 634
  oligoastrocytoma 561, 567
Anastomotic stricture at esophagogastric junction 217*f*
Anatomic areas within oropharynx 171*f*
Anatomical regions in hypopharynx 174*f*
Anatomy of pharynx 169*f*
Ancillary techniques 28
Andreas Vesalius 2*f*
Androgen
  deprivation therapy 483
  receptor 484
    modulator 678
Anesthesia for head and neck surgery 660
Anesthetic problems in specific operations 660
Aneurysmal bone cyst 537
Angiosarcomas of chest wall 438
Ann Arbor
  classification of Hodgkin lymphoma, modified 627*t*
  staging classification for Hodgkin and non-Hodgkin lymphomas 647*t*
Anorexia 657
  cachexia syndrome, pathophysiology 677*f*
  of syndrome 677
Anterior
  exenteration in females 494*f*
  U cut 131
Antiandrogen withdrawal syndrome 80
Anti-angiogenesis therapy to control hematogenous metastasis 240*f*
Antibiotic prophylaxis for afebrile neutropenic patient 699

Antibody scan 44
Anticipation and treatment of side effects 671
Antidiuretic hormone 659
Anti-estrogen therapy 354
Antimicrobial
prophylaxis in surgical oncology 696
susceptibility testing 688
therapy, duration of 699
Antral adenocarcinoma 206*f*
Arcelona-clinic liver cancer staging 281*t*
Aromatase inhibitors 339, 346
Arterial blood gas analysis 441
Asbestos 404
Ascites 126
Asepsis and surgical technique 701
Asia-Pacific Association for liver treatment hepatocellular carcinoma 282
Aspergillus 689, 694
Scedosporium species 686
species 692
Aspirin 670
Asthenia 678
Asthma 662
Atypical
alveolar hyperplasia 405
lobular hyperplasia 338
small acinar proliferation 476
teratoid rhabdoid tumor 570
Autogenous reconstructions 605
Autoimmune diseases 650
Autologous bone marrow transplant 5
Automated DNA sequencing 95
Axillary lymph node 340, 342*t*
dissection 339, 342, 344, 352*f*
Axillary staging 340

B

Bacillus Calmette-Guérin therapy 492
Bacterial versus fungal blood culture positivity over three decades 692*f*
Balloon
dilation ablation 215*f*
dilation done 217*f*
Barium study of patient with lesion in ascending colon 253*f*
Barrett's
esophagus 202, 203*f*, 210
mucosa with polypoidal ulcerated adenocarcinoma 203*f*
Barriers to optimal
outcome in childhood cancers 621*f*
treatment of childhood cancers in India 621
Basaloid squamous carcinoma 382
Base tongue 171*f*
B-cell
lymphoma 57, 638
non-Hodgkin lymphoma, treatment and outcome of 637, 639*t*
BCG failure 493
Beatson-hormonal manipulation 339
Benign
and intracranial extra-axial tumors, management of 570
fibrous histiocytoma 537
lesions 436, 446
tumor 429
of follicular 186
Bereavement support 682
Beta-human chorionic gonadotropin 60, 503
Bevacizumab 63, 242, 415
Bilateral
breast cancer 346
gillies fan-flaps 593
nasolabial flap for submucous fibrosis 594*f*
ovarian tumors 369*f*, 375*f*
Bile duct 205
resection 299
Biliary
malignancies 291
stenting on of pancreaticoduodenectomy, effect of 312
Biological therapy 240
Biopsy 440, 646
interpretation 145
of bone tumors 538
or not to biopsy 280
Bipolar energy 127, 128
Birt-Hogg-Dube syndrome 454
Bismuth-corlette classification for hilar cholangiocarcinoma 302
Bisphosphonates 558
Bladder
cancer 488
carcinoma 62
Bleeding 679
management 679
Bleomycin 507, 509, 628, 629
Blood
biochemistry 647
culture 687
for fungus 689
loss 497
Bloodstream infection 690
trends 690
Bloom syndrome 90, 539
Blue dye 342
B-non-Hodgkin lymphoma, treatment of
advanced 638
limited stage 638
Body
fluid examination 647
mass index 363
Bone
and soft tissue 536
tumors 53
cuts for segmental 151*f*
forming neoplasm 35*f*
infarcts 537
marrow
aspiration and biopsy 627
biopsy 647
metastases 55, 59
sarcoma 91
scans 46, 47
tumors and soft tissue sarcomas 536
Borderline
ovarian tumors 375
resectable pancreatic cancer 318
Borrelia burgdorferi 650
Bortezumib 64
Bowel
leak and fistulae 497
obstruction 678
Brachytherapy 70, 71, 355, 357*f*, 483
in nutshell 71*t*
Brain
metastasis 581
management of 577
radiotherapy for multiple metastases, whole 580
tumor introduction 560
Brainstem gliomas 570
Branch vein umbilical fissure 297*f*
Breast 59, 711
cancer 44, 46, 62-64, 76, 77, 91, 325, 326, 358*t*, 364, 438
and pregnancy 349
screening 18, 88, 93
conservation
surgery 338-340, 341*f*, 345, 350, 357
therapy 603
conservative surgery, reconstructive surgery 603
conserving therapy 343, 352
imaging reporting and data system 334
implants 605

MRI 333
reconstruction 603
mastectomy 603
self-examination 19, 331
ultrasound 331
Bricker's
ileal conduit 495
technique 519
Brief pain inventory 668
Broad
spectrum drugs include 676
tongues of cohesive malignant hepatocytes wrapped by peripheral endothelium 280*f*
Bronchoalveolar carcinoma 405
Bruton's tyrosine kinase 64
Buprenorphine 670
Burden of hereditary cancers 84
Burkholderia species 694
Burkitt lymphoma 62, 633, 633*f*, 648

C

Cachexia syndrome 677
Cancer
anal canal 265*f*
antigen 59*f*, 349
cervix 380
chemotherapy 61, 662
control in developing countries 706
curable with combination chemotherapy 62
esophagus, radiotherapy response in 230*t*
for adult cancers 615*t*
for childhood cancers 615*t*
from an unknown primary site 585
of anal canal 250, 264
introduction 264
etiology 264
pathology 265
treatment 265
of colon 250
of esophagus 222
of head and neck region 62
of hypopharynx, staging of 176
of larynx 160
diagnosis 161
introduction 160
of pharynx 168
general features 168
goals of treatment 170
nasopharynx 169
results of treatment 171
surgical anatomy 168
of rectum 250
of thyroid
adjuvant radioactive iodine 191
etiology 186
introduction 186
investigations 188
management of neck nodes 190
pathology 186
staging 188
treatment 188
pain
analgesics in management of 669*t*
management 666
practical approach to a patient with 668
syndromes 667*t*
rectum variations in metropolitan cities 251
registry hub 15
research 112
type of 615
Candida 689
albicans 691
predominates 692
parapsilosis 692
species 689, 702
tropicalis 692
Carcinoembryonic antigen 349, 350, 365, 586
Carcinogenic embryonic antigen 59, 60
Carcinoid
crisis 534
tumors 662
Carcinoma 192
antigen 125 369
cervix 52
in situ 382, 384, 406, 488, 489, 490, 493, 504
of buccal mucosa 592*f*
of cervix 379
of colon 250
of rectum 255
etiology 255
introduction 255
surgery 257
concept of total mesorectal excision in rectal surgery 257
hand-sewn 257
of thyroid 186
stomach 233
epidemiology 233
introduction 233
Carcinosarcoma anterior lower gum with minimal cortical erosion 149*f*
Cardiac
dysfunction 390
failure 612
symptoms 612
treatment 612
multigated acquisition 44
problem 598
tamponade 612
symptoms 612
treatment 612
Cardioesophageal junction 236*f*
Cases of submucous fibrosis 593
Castration resistant prostate cancer 79, 484
Cat's eye reflex 621
Catecholamine receptor scanning 46
Causative agents 686
Cecostomy 518
Celiac
axis nodal clearance 225*f*
plexus
block 673
neurolysis 202, 215
Cell
carcinoma of esophagus 203
cycle
nonspecific agents 61*f*
progression 76
regulatory molecules 75
in mantle cell lymphoma 649*f*
in sarcomatoid pattern 187
lack nuclear features of papillary carcinoma 187
Cellular and nuclear pleomorphism 145
Celomic epithelium 365
Central
brain tumor registry of united states 560
nervous system 467, 624, 636, 637
tumors 560
venous pressure 661
Centralization of pancreatic resections 318
Cervical
axillary lymphadenopathy 407
cancer 62, 381
screening and prevention 15
esophagus 176
intraepithelial neoplasia 16, 380, 384
nodes 226
Cervicothoracic ganglion block 673
Cervix 711
Cetuximab 63, 416
Chemoradiotherapy 240, 387
definitive treatment 229

Chemosensitive tumors 441
Chemotherapy 60, 68, 229, 240, 353, 389, 428, 552
and hormonal therapy 558
and targeted therapy 565
cancer esophagus 230*t*
for locally advanced breast cancer 353
for metastatic breast cancer 353
induced nausea and vomiting 62
regimens in children with Hodgkin lymphoma 628
surgery-chemotherapy 238
Chernobyl disasters 186
Chest
radiography 440
wall postexcision reconstruction with goretex mesh repair 601*f*
wall reconstruction 598
wall resections and reconstructions 440
X-ray 425
Chevassu's maneuver 503*f*
Child with non-Hodgkin lymphoma 635*t*
Childhood
cancers, burden of 614
non-Hodgkin lymphomas 632*t*
Child-Pugh classification 278*t*
Children with non-Hodgkin lymphoma 635
Children's cancer group 629, 637, 639
Chlamydia psittaci 650
infections 635
Cholangiocarcinoma 299
introduction 299
Chondroblastoma 537
Chondroma 436, 537
Chondromyxoid fibroma 537
Chondrosarcoma 437, 441, 537, 542, 543*f*
Chordoma 537
Choriocarcinoma 59, 62367, 502
Choroid plexus tumor 91
Chromophobe 455
Chronic
hypercalcemia 194
lymphoblastic leukemia 64
lymphocytic leukemia 64, 647
myelogenous leukemia 63
myeloid leukemia 64, 86, 95
Circumferential margins 257
in surgery for rectal cancer 259*f*
Cisplatin 507, 509
Cladosporium 693
Classical
Hodgkin lymphoma 626, 645
seminoma 501
Classification of
carcinoma of breast 326
diffuse large B-cell lymphoma 32*f*
germ cell tumors of testis 501
lymphedema 352*t*
pap smear 384*t*
surface epithelial tumors 365*t*
Clear cell 367
adenocarcinoma 396
carcinoma 383
Clinical breast examination 19, 331
CNS tumors
complications of 564
histology of 561
Codeine 556, 670
Codman's triangle 35*f*, 539, 539*f*
Collecting duct tumors 455
Collimator shaped beam 66*f*
Colon
and rectal cancer 125
and rectum 50
cancer 63
Colonic and rectal nets 532
Colorectal cancer 27*f*, 126, 207, 364
surveillance 207
Colostomy 526
in infant or child 526
Colposcopy 384
Combination
chemotherapy 415
therapy for carcinoma stomach 240
Combined oral contraceptives 394
Common
malignant tumors 59*t*
symptoms, management of 564
Commonly occurring tumors of small bowel 245*t*
Community
based palliative care 682
cancer centers 707
empowerment 683
Complete response 563
Completion of
extensine D_3 dissection 237*f*
total thyroidectomy 44
Complex heterogeneous mass in left kidney 457*f*
Complications of
BCG 493
colonic surgery 255
pancreaticoduodenectomy 314
Composite left cheek-mandible defect 154*f*
Comprehensive
cancer centers 707
list of documented infections 686*f*
Computed tomography 37, 39*f*, 42, 50*f*, 53, 71, 341, 345, 368, 440, 445, 502, 507, 509
scan 36, 36*f*, 368*f*, 369*f*, 408*f*, 447, 452*f*, 453*f*, 458*f*, 466*f*
of paraganglioma 452*f*
Concurrent chemotherapy 390
Condyloma 265
Condylomatous carcinoma 382
Confocal laser endomicroscopy, techniques of 203
Conformal radiotherapy 72
Conservation breast surgery 339
Constipation 676
management 676
non-drug measures 676
Contemporary
chemotherapy regimens for children with hodgkin lymphoma 629*t*
imaging modalities 561
management of bladder cancer 492
Continent urinary diversion 495
Continuity of care 683
Contralateral breast 604
Contrast
enhanced CT scan of chest 425
MRI of thorax 425
Controlled radial expansion 216
Conventional
clear cell 455
carcinoma 455
radical cystectomy 494
Core needle biopsy 335
over fine needle aspiration cytology 25
Corticosteroids 671
Cowden syndrome 88
Cranial nerve blocks 672
Craniopharyngiomas 571, 572
Creation of loop ileostomy 519*f*
Cribriform pattern with high-grade cytologic atypia 252*f*
Criteria of unresectability of HCC 284
Crizotinib 64, 640
Crohn's disease 127
Cumulative survival in locally advanced gastric cancer 239*f*
Cuncurrent chemoradiotherapy 69
Cushing's syndrome 405, 407, 432, 446, 533, 661
Cutaneous manifestations 589
Cyclin dependent kinases 75
Cyclo-oxygenase inhibitor 670
Cyclophosphamide 4, 339, 340, 628, 629, 630, 631, 639
oncovin methotrexate prednisone 639

Cylindroma 183
Cystectomy in males 494*f*
Cystitis cystica and glandularis 489
Cystocopy 385
Cystosarcoma phyllodes 347
Cystourethroscopy and transurethral resection 491
Cytogenetic analysis 586
Cytomegalovirus infections 693, 694
Cytoreductive surgery 371
Cytotoxic T-lymphocyte antigen 63

D

D'Amico risk stratification of carcinoma prostate 482*t*
Dacarbazine 448, 628
Deep
  lobe 182*f*
  vein thrombosis 407, 589
De-epithelized skin flaps 602
Dehydroepiandrosterone 77, 444
  sulfate 445
Delayed gastric emptying 316
Delirium 679
  management 679
Delivery of
  hydrophobic drugs 104
  nucleic acids 105
Deltopectoral flap 591*f*
Denonvilliers' fascia 130
Denosumab 556, 558
Dental rehabilitation 150*f*
Deoxyribonucleic acid 43, 60, 67, 85, 112, 358, 404, 625
Depiction of morphology of three classes of cholangiocarcinoma 301*f*
Dermoid cyst 367
Desmoids tumors 437
Desmoplastic fibroma 537
Determinants of nodal metastasis 199
Development of video capsule endoscopy 202
Diabetes and hypertension 395
Diagnosis and pretherapy workup 264
Diagnosis of digestive cancers 206
Diagnostic staging laparoscopy 210
Diarrhea 662, 677
Diclofenac 556, 670
Diet 234
  and lung cancer 405
  and obesity 476
Diethylstilbesterol 379, 381
Different neck compartments 191*f*
Diffuse
  gastric body 206*f*
  large B-cell
    lymphoma 633, 648
    NHL 644
  large cell lymphoma 634*f*
Digestive
  anastomosis 314
  tract cancers 202
Digital
  per-rectal examination 256
  rectal examination 478, 478*f*
Dihydrotestosterone 79
Dilation done with controlled radial expansion balloon 217*f*
Disease
  burden 15, 18, 20
  free survival 121, 341, 552
  free survival 226
  of remaining colon 526
Dissection of
  pararectal space 131
  rectovaginal space 131
  ureteric tunnel 132
Distant metastasis 126, 163
Division of
  mediastinum 424*f*
  rectum distal to tumor 130*f*
Donor sites 600
Dose of cetuximab 263
Double
  balloon 207
  strand break 67, 68
Doxorubicin 340, 629
Drop shaped rete ridges 145
Duct carcinoma in situ 327, 336
Ductal carcinoma in situ 19, 328*f*
Dysgerminoma 367
  of left ovary 60*f*
Dysplastic lesions of digestive tract 203
Dyspnea 679
  management 679
    non-drug 679

E

Early
  cardioesophageal lesion 224*f*
  colon cancer 212
  gastric cancer 212
  menarche and late menopause 395
Elastofibroma dorsi 439
Electron microscopy 586
Eligibility criteria for using anti-EGFR drugs 263
Embryonal
  carcinoma 60*f*, 367, 501, 502
  rhabdomyosarcoma 62
Emergencies in oncology 609
Encapsulated tumor with cells in follicular pattern 187
Encasement of mesenteric vessels 248*f*
End colostomy 517
End ileostomy 518, 527
End of life care 572
Endocrine
  and neuroendocrine tumors 44
  combination therapy 81
Endocrinologic 659
End-of-life care 681
Endometrial
  cancer 91, 394, 396
  hyperplasia 396
Endometrioid
  adenocarcinoma 383, 383*f*, 396*f*
  carcinoma 366*f*
Endoscopic
  evaluation 647
  mucosal resection 202
    technique
      injection + band application 211*f*
      injection + hood application 211*f*
      injection + snaring 211*f*
  palliative treatment 214
  resection 211
  submucosal dissection 202
    steps of 212*f*
  treatment 210
    of postoperative 216
  ultrasonography 202
  ultrasound 408
Endothelial growth factor receptor 102
Endothelial-cell killing 566
Enneking system for malignant tumors 538*t*
Enteral feeding 677
Enterobacteriaceae 691
Enzyme cyclo-oxygenase 669
Eosinophilic granuloma 437
Ependymomas 570
Epidemiology for
  cholangiocarcioma 300
  gallbladder carcinoma 291
Epidermal
  cells 183
  growth factor receptor 5, 31, 33, 44, 60, 63, 64, 115, 580
Epidural
  neurolysis 672
  spinal cord compression 671
Epithelial dysplasia 142
Epithelioid type 274*f*
Erlotinib 416

Erythroplakia 142, 143
Esophageal
  cancer 62, 214, 222
  nets 532
Esophagus 122, 205, 206
Estrogen
  and breast tumor 76
  receptor 75, 76, 345, 351
Ethics
  and palliative care 681
  in end-of-life care 681
Ethnicity 235
  diagnosis 235
  genetics 235
  investigations 235
  pathology 235
  symptomatology 235
  treatment 236
    lymph node dissection 237
    surgery 236
Etoposide 507, 509, 629
  plus cisplatin 507
Euronet pediatric Hodgkin's lymphoma 630
European
  Organization for Research and Treatment of Cancer 563
  Society for Medical Oncology 468
Evaluation of hereditary cancers 87
Event-free survival 637
Evidence-based medicine in oncology 653
Ewing's sarcoma 25, 438, 441, 536, 537, 541, 615
  of femur 541*f*
Exogenous infections 685
Extended spectrum beta lactamase 687
Extension into parapharyngeal space 182*f*
Extent of lymph node dissection 388
External beam
  radiation therapy 65, 356, 391
  radiotherapy 400, 483
Extra-abdominal muscles 603
Extracranial course of facial nerve 181*f*
Extrahepatic 260
Extranodal marginal zone NHL 650
Extraperitoneal
  radical cystectomy 495*f*
  retrograde cystectomy 494
Extra-platysmal flaps 184
Extrathoracic metastases on positron emission tomography 51*f*

F

Facial telangiectasis 662
Familial
  adenomatous polyposis 87, 89, 207
  forms of large bowel cancer 252
    familial adenomatous polyposis 252
    hereditary nonpolyposis colorectal cancer 252
  papillary RCC 454
  retinoblastoma 537
Fanconi anemia 90
Fentanyl 670
  transdermal 670
Fertility drugs 364
Fever 658
Fiberoptic bronchoscopy 409
Fibroma 367, 501, 537
Fibromatosis 439
Fibrosarcoma 537
Fibrous dysphasia 436, 537
Fibula 597
  graft
    front face 156*f*
    open mouth 156*f*
    profile 156*f*
Final transection area 297*f*
Fine needle aspiration 425
  biopsy 202
  cytology 25, 188, 192, 335, 369
    gastrointestinal stromal tumor 275*f*
  of moderately differentiated hepatocellular carcinoma 280
Fisher hypothesis 339
Five-year relative survival rates 711*t*
Flaps 602
  donor site selection 596
  elevation 599
  requirements 599
Fluid-attenuated inversion recovery 565
Fluorescent in situ hybridization 25, 94
Fluorine-18 estradiol receptor scan 48
Fluorodeoxyglucose 37, 46
Follicle stimulating hormone 77
Follicular
  adenoma 187
    and carcinoma 186
  lymphoma 57, 647, 649
    international prognostic index score 648*t*
  type 186
Front face 155*f*
Functional
  adrenal mass 446
  magnetic resonance imaging 38*f*
  role of larynx 160*f*
Fungal
  infections 689
    in Indian scenario 691
  serology 689
Fusarium 693

G

Galen's theory 1
Gallbladder 205
  cancer before operation 295
  carcinoma 291
    introduction 291
    with duodenal infiltration 294*t*
Gamma camera 43
Ganglioneuromas 446
Gardner syndrome 89
Gastric
  cancer 50, 62, 214
  carcinoids 62, 534
  fundus with central ulcer and bleed 209*f*
  pull-up 179*f*
  tube conduit prepared for anastomosis 225*f*
  ulcer 206
Gastrinoma 45
Gastroendocrine pancreatic neuroendocrine tumors 56
Gastroesophageal
  junction 125*f*
  reflux disease 223
Gastrointestinal 657
  cancers 12, 50
  carcinoids 533
  lymphoma 209
  stromal 252
    tumors 25, 53, 64, 95, 209, 273, 589
      introduction 273
      management 275
      pathology 273
      pathology gross 273
      pathology investigations 275
  symptoms 675
  tract 532
Geftinib 64
Gender adaptation 629
Gene expression profiling 28, 95
General principles in oncologic anesthesia 657
Genesis of rural cancer facility to major community cancer center 710*t*

Genetic
and cancer 84
disease 84
of sporadic and hereditary cancers 84
predisposition 625
syndrome 88, 89
testing 91
Genitourinary cancers 52
Geotrichum species 693
Germ cell 365
tumors 62, 367, 428, 500, 501, 537
Gerota's fascia 127
Gleason scoring 476
of prostate cancer 476
Glioblastoma 561, 565
in elderly patients 568
multiforme 563
Gliomatosis cerebri 567
Global burden of cancer 363
Glucagonoma 45
Glucose uptake ratio 53
Goals of care 675
Gonadal
stromal tumors 501
tumors 615
Gonadoblastoma 501
Gonadotropin releasing hormone therapy 484
Gorlin's syndrome 91
Grading of
breast carcinoma 328
human epidermal growth factor receptor 2 329*t*
Grafts material for structural support 600
Granulomatous carcinoma 346
Granulosa cell tumor 367, 501
Gross appearance of familial adenomatous polyposis 252*f*
Growing teratoma syndrome 508
Growth signal inhibitors 63
Guidelines for relative risk of malignant behavior 274*t*
Gynecologic surgery 364
Gynecological tract cystectomy with neobladder in females 495*f*
Gynecology oncology group 391

H

Hairy cell leukemia 647
Hand-assisted laparoscopic surgery 125
Hand-Schuller-Christian disease 437
Harmonic scalpel 127, 128
Harrington's classification for spinal metastases 557*t*
Hashimoto's thyroiditis 650
Head
and neck
cancer 53, 63
reconstruction techniques in 591
region, reconstructive options for 593
squamous cell carcinoma 67
Helicobacter pylori 203, 644, 650
infection 635
Hemangiomas 437
Hematological abnormalities 658
Hematopoietic stem cell transplant 687, 694
Hemi-body irradiation 556
Hemoclips applied 153*f*
Hemostasis achieved 207*f*
Hepatic malignancies 277
introduction 277
investigation 278
natural history of hepatocellular carcinoma 278
pretherapy work-up 278
biochemistry 278
radiological imaging 279
tumor markers 279
staging 281
Hepatitis
and cancer 693
B 693
virus 688
C 693
Hepatocellular carcinoma 51, 277
introduction 277
with arterial enhancement and washout 279*f*
Herceptin 242
Hereditary
breast
cancer syndromes 326
ovarian cancer 91
syndrome 85, 88
cancer 84
syndrome 91*f*
leiomyoma RCC 454
nonpolyposis colon cancer 85, 91
syndrome 88, 89
retinoblastoma 90, 91, 539
High chance of high-grade dysplasia 203
High dose rate 71
High grade
prostatic intraepithelial neoplasia 476
squamous epithelial lesion 384, 385
High intensity focused ultrasound and cryotherapy 483
High nuclear grade 328
High prostate-specific antigen 37
High-dose methotrexate 638
Hilar 299
Hiroshima disasters 186
HIV and cancer 693
Hodgkin's
and non-hodgkin lymphoma 624*t*
disease 39*f*, 62, 63, 186
lymphoma 25, 62, 624, 628, 644, 646*f*, 650
classification of classical 626*t*
in children 631*t*
treatment of
high-risk classical 630
intermediate-risk classical 630
low-risk classical 630
reed-sternberg 625
Homogenous leukoplakia 142
Hopkins verbal learning test-revised 581
Hormonal
dependence of malignant cells 74
therapy 353, 354, 399, 484
Hormone
and contraceptives 394
and ovarian cancer prediction study 364
deprivation 75
in prostate cancer 79
induced cancers 80*f*
interference 75
receptor 329
replacement therapy 19
therapy 364
Hospice life care 572
Hounsfield units 445
HPV vaccination 17
Human
chorionic gonadotropin 507
epidermal growth factor receptor 345
immunodeficiency virus 380
papillomavirus 17, 142
infection 379
related lesions 265
testing 17
Huntington's disease 626
Hürthle cell 187
Hydroxydaunorubicin 639
Hypercalcemia 610, 658
pathophysiology 610
symptoms 610
treatment 610
Hypercalcemic crisis 195
Hyperthermic intraperitoneal chemotherapy 261, 374, 374*f*

Hyperviscosity syndrome 612
symptoms 613
treatment 613
Hypofractionation 68
Hypogammaglobulinemia 427
Hypoglycemia 589, 658
Hyponatremia 613
symptoms 613
treatment 613
Hypopharyngeal cancers
classification of 175
clinical features 175
epidemiology 175
incidence 175
physical findings 175
Hypopharynx
advanced disease 176
and cervical esophagus 174
introduction 174
early cancer 176
reconstruction 177
results of treatment 179
Hypothalamo-pituitary-gonadal axis 484
Hypoxia imaging 55

I

Ibrutinib 64
Ibuprofen 556, 670
Ifosfamide 507, 509
Ilium 596
donor site 598
Image-guided radiation therapy 37
Imatinib 64
Immature teratoma 367
Immune dysregulation 625
Immunocompromised cancer 685
Immunohistochemistry 24, 28, 274, 586
Important nodal groups 198*f*
In situ hybridization 28, 29, 531
In vitro fertilization, visions of 714
Incidence of stomas 512
Incidental carcinoma of gallbladder 295
Incision plan 177*f*
Increased nuclear-cytoplasmic ratio 145
Indian Cancer Cooperative Network 654
Individual tumors, management of 565
Indomethacin 670
Infections in
hematopoietic cell transplant recipients 697
patients with neoplastic disease 686
surgical oncology 694
Infective episode, diagnosis of 690
Inferior vena cava 444, 452*f*, 551
Infiltrating duct carcinoma 346
Inflammatory breast cancer 345, 346*t*
Infradeodenal common bile duct stricture 208*f*
Inhomogeneous leukoplakia 142
Inoperable
hilar cholangiocarcinoma 216*f*
midesophageal malignant stricture 214*f*
Insulinomas 45, 662
Intensity modulated
arc therapy 72
radiation therapy 4, 37, 71, 355, 356*f*, 391
techniques 401
radiotherapy 71
Intermediate cells 183
Internal mammary nodes 342, 355
International
Adjuvant Lung Cancer Trial 413
atomic energy agency 57
cancer genome consortium 95
collaborative ovarian neoplasm 373
Germ Cell Cancer Collaborative Group 507, 509
prognostic
index 648*t*
score for HL 651*t*
study group on pancreatic fistula definition of postoperative pancreatic fistula 315*t*
Interventions in pain management 672
Intestinal stoma surgery 515
Intracellular accumulation of nanoparticles 106*f*
Intractable pain 215
Intraductal
carcinoma 328
ultrasonography 208
Intraepithelial stage 382*f*
Intrahepatic cholangiocarcinoma 287
Intraoperative frozen section 304
Intraoral view 156*f*
Intraperitoneal chemotherapy 373
Intratubular germ cell neoplasia 500, 501
Intravascular
congestion, disseminated 658
device-related infections, prevention of 701
Intravenous pyelogram 496*f*
Intravesical therapy 492
Introduction of hormone therapy 63
Invasive
aspergillosis 689
breast cancer 326, 339, 352, 352*t*
carcinoma of cervix 385
ductal carcinoma 327*f*, 328*f*
lobular carcinoma 327
Iodine-131 metaiodobenzylguanidine therapy 56
Ionizing radiation 404
Ipilimumab 63
Irradiated chest wall 601
Irregular epithelial stratification 145
Irrigation 526, 527*f*
Irritable bowel syndrome 526
Ischemia of stoma 520
Isotope therapy of neuroendocrine tumors 56
Issues in salivary gland surgery nonsurgical treatment 185
Italian Association for Pediatric Hematology and Oncology 637
Ivor-Lewis technique 123

J

Janus kinase inhibitor 64
Jejunal ulcerated leiomyoma with bleed 153*f*
Jejunum in place 178*f*

K

Karapandzic technique 153, 153*f*
Karnofsky performance score 563
Ketoconazole 484
Ketoprofen 670
Ketorolac 670
Kidney 711
disorders 524
Killian's dehiscence 174
Kinesin spindle protein 106
Koch's lesion 49*f*
Kocher maneuver 125
Krukenberg's tumor 351, 375
Kudo's pit pattern 204*f*

L

Lactate dehydrogenase 368, 502, 503, 636, 637
Lactic acidosis 659
Lamina propria 490
Laparoscopic
assisted surgery 126
low anterior resection 127, 128
pancreatic resections 318
radical
hysterectomy 131
nephrectomy 462
right hemicolectomy 126

surgery 213
trans-hiatal esophagectomy 123, 123*t*
Large
cell carcinoma 405
gastrointestinal stromal tumor 209*f*
rectal villous adenoma 208*f*
ulcerated ampullary adenocarcinoma with intraductal extension 209*f*
Laryngeal
cancer 62
general principles 162
management of relapse and treatment failure 164
cavity, middle part of 161
Laryngopharyngectomy specimen 177*f*
Laryngopharynx 174, 593
Late toxicity, avoidance of 629
Latent membrane protein-1 626
Lateral mobilization of rectum 129*f*
Latissimus dorsi
muscle 599
myocutaneous flap 605
Layer of buccopharyngeal fascia 174
Left
gastric artery 225*f*
ilio-obturator lymph node dissection 132*f*
pararectal space 132
thoracoabdominal approach 224*f*
ureteric tunnel dissection 132*f*
Lesion in
buccal mucosa seen during surgery 592*f*
lower rectum postchemoradiotherapy 257*f*
Letterer-Siwe disease 437
Leukemia 501, 615
Leukokoria 621
Leukoplakia 142, 143
Leydig cell tumor 367, 501
Li-Fraumeni syndrome 86, 88, 91, 537, 539, 545
Ligation of
ileocolic vessels 128*f*
inferior mesenteric pedicles 129*f*
Lip split with cheek flap 150*f*
Lipoma 437
Liposarcoma 438
Lips 593
Liver 59
and pancreas 51
function tests 56
metastasis in colorectal cancers 260
resection 282
closure 284
drainage 284
postoperative care in cirrhotic patients 284
exposure and mobilization 283
for gallbladder cancers 296
inflow control 283
operative technique modifications for hepatic resection in cirrhotic patients 283
parenchymal transection 283
surgical principles for hepatic resection 282
transplantation 285, 306
LN dissection 132
Lobectomy versus total thyroidectomy in thyroid cancers 191
Lobular
carcinoma in situ 328, 338
neoplasia 328
Local
recurrence of rectal cancers 260*t*
tumor invasion 303
Localized esophageal cancer 224
Locally advanced breast cancer 48, 337, 339, 340, 344, 345, 345*f*
Locoregional therapy 285
Loop
colostomy 517
ileostomy 519, 527
Loss of
heterozygosity 85, 455
intercellular adherence 145
polarity of basal cells 145
Low
cervical 225
dose-involved-field radiation therapy 631
glomerular filtration rate 464
grade
dysplasia 208*f*
follicular lymphoma with nodules 649*f*
gliomas 567
intramedullary osteosarcoma 540
squamous epithelial lesion 384
molecular-weight heparin 564
nuclear grade 328
tumors of rectum 130
Lumbar sympathetic block 673
Lung 585, 711
cancer 48, 91, 407, 439
surgery 660
Luteinizing hormone releasing hormone 75, 102
Lutetium-177 dotatate therapy 56
Lymph node 121
biopsy 627
Lymphadenectomy 398
extent of 299
Lymphatic
dissemination 405
drainage
in ovarian cancer 370*f*
of stomach 237*f*
spread of laryngeal cancer 162*f*
Lymphedema 344, 351
Lymphoblastic lymphoma 634, 634*f*
Lymphocyte-predominant Hodgkin lymphoma, treatment of nodular 630
Lymphoma 59, 439, 501, 537, 615
in children 624
Lymphorrhea 497
Lynch syndrome 89, 394

M

Magnetic resonance imaging 37, 39, 42, 330, 341, 368, 375*f*, 385, 408, 437, 440, 459*f*, 479, 479*f*, 502, 533*f*, 537
of breast 335*f*
Malabsorption of vitamin B_{12} 524
Male breast cancer 91, 347
Malignant
colorectal obstruction 215
fibrous histiocytoma 537, 546
germ cell tumors 429
lesions 437, 438, 445
liver tumors, classification of 277*t*
melanoma 63, 265
mixed Müllerian tumor 367, 397
mixed tumor 183
peripheral nerve sheath tumor 91
salivary gland tumors 183*f*
schwannoma 431
Mammalian target of rapamycin 468
Mammogram 352
Mammography 18, 35, 331
Management of
breast cancer 339
early stage I and II cancer of larynx 165
germ cell tumors of testis 504
laryngeal cancer 162
locally advanced breast cancer 345
lung cancer 403

metastatic
disease 547
neck 200
muscle invasive carcinoma bladder 494
pancreaticoduodenectomy 314
prostate cancer 486
recurrent disease 372
skeletal metastases 553
stage III and stage IV cancer of larynx 166
tumors of hypopharynx 176
Mandibular reconstructions 595
Mantle cell lymphoma 649
Marginal mandibulectomy 151*f*, 152*f*
Margins of resection 28
Maryland's forceps 132
Mastectomy 339*f*
site 604
Mature b-cell lymphoma 89 639
Mature cystic teratoma 367
McGill pain questionnaire 668
Mechlorethamine 628
Mediastinal
ganglioneuromas 431
tumors 424
Medical management of brain metastasis 579
Medicine obstacles to overcome 654*t*
Medullary
carcinoma 346, 455
thyroid cancer 45, 59, 64, 91
Medulloblastoma 568
Melanoma 64
Memorial
pain assessment card 668
sloan-kettering cancer center classification for hilar cholangiocarcinoma 302*t*
Mendelian
autosomal dominance 189
disorder 84
Meningiomas 570
Mesenchymal tumors 430
Mesna 507
Mesothelioma 439, 585
Metabolic
acidosis 524
scan 43
Metachronous bilateral breast cancer 346
Metaiodobenzylguanidine 532
scan 46*f*
Metastatic
and recurrent tumors 498
axillary nodes 336*f*
bone disease 57
brain tumors 577
breast cancer 350
disease 304, 484
neck 197
anatomy of fascia 197
anatomy spaces of neck 197
clinical features 199
introduction 197
N0 neck 200
N1 neck 200
N2 neck 200
N3 neck 200
neck levels 198
staging 199
triangles of neck 197
renal cell carcinoma 466
setting 262
Methicillin-resistant *Staphylococcus aureus* 686, 700
from different samples 696*f*
Methods of
reconstruction 595
skeletal stabilization 601
Methotrexate 339, 631
Methylguanine-methyl-transferase 562
Microbial pathogens and infection control in immunocompromised cancer patients 685
Microbiology of surgical site infections 694
Microinvasive squamous carcinoma 382
Microsatellite instability 94
Microsporidium species 697
Microsurgical breast reconstruction 606
Microvascular free
flaps 600
tissue transfer 594
Middle hepatic vein apex of transection 298*f*
Minimal
access surgery 135, 136*f*
in surgical oncology 138
deviation adenocarcinoma 383
invasive surgery 120, 259*f*, 482
for bladder cancer 498
Mini-mental state examination 564
Mirel's scoring system 557*t*
Mixed
adenocarcinoma 396
cellularity classical hodgkin lymphoma 645
tumors 501
Mode of
dissemination 405
spread 369
Modified
FIGO grading system 396
median lip split with Z's 151*f*
radical
mastectomy 339, 358
neck dissection 201
Scarff-Bloom-Richardson grading system 329
Molecular
biologic techniques 531
biology 310
of medulloblastoma 563
revolution 339
profiling 586
scan 44
targeted therapy 428
taxonomy of cancers 93
Monodermal teratoma 367
Mononuclear phagocyte system 104
Morphine 556, 670
Mouth opening 155*f*
Mucinous breast cancer 346
Mucoepidermoid carcinoma 183
Mucosa-associated lymphoid tissue 635
type lymphoma 186
Mucosal hyperplasia lower end of self-expandable metal stent in esophagus 215*f*
Mucous secreting cells 183
Multicentric disease 340
Multileaf collimators 72
Multinodular goiter 192
Multiple
basal cell carcinoma 91
daily fractions 68
endocrine neoplasia 90, 91, 186, 194
full-term pregnancies 381
myeloma 64
pulmonary metastases 460*f*
ligation-dependent probe amplification 91
Muscle flap 599
Musculocutaneous flaps 599, 603
Musculofascial flaps 602
Musculoskeletal tumor society 538
Mutually supportive and interactive system for cancer care 707*f*
Myasthenia gravis 426
Mycobacteria 686
Mycobacterial infections 693
Mycobacterium
fortuitum chelonei 693
tuberculi 4

Mycosis fungoides 589
Myelofibrosis 64
Myelolipoma 446, 450
Myeloma 537
Myocutaneous flap 602
Myoma screw 131

N

N0 neck 200
Nanotechnology application in cancer therapy 102
Naproxen sodium 670
Narrow band imaging
  Kudo's IIIL pattern, malignant adenomatous polyp 204*f*
  ulcerated dysplastic barrett's mucosa with stricture 203*f*
Nasogastric tube 125
Nasopharyngeal cancer 62
Nasopharynx 169*f*, 170
National
  cancer
    data base, evaluation of 191
    Registry Programme 12
  Institute of Health 114
  nosocomial infections surveillance 690
  Surgical Adjuvant Breast and Bowel Project 339, 340, 653
Natural orifice transluminal endoscopic surgery 137, 139, 202, 213
Nausea 675
  management 675
Neck
  levels 198*f*
  residue and lymph node metastasis 55
Need for neoadjuvant chemoradiotherapy 256
Neoadjuvant
  approaches in pancreatic cancer 319
  chemotherapy 240, 263, 339, 369, 371, 389, 414, 497
    contribution of 654
    in colonic cancers 255
  therapy 413
  three-drug chemotherapy 176
  treatment for GBC 299
Nephrogenic adenoma 489
Nephron sparing surgery 463
Neurilemoma 431
Neuroblastoma 45, 59, 431, 446, 615, 617
  management algorithm in 618*f*
  risk stratification in 618*f*
Neuroendocrine
  carcinoma 383, 529
  tumors 44, 59, 252, 529
    of gastrointestinal tract 531
    of jejunum 246*f*, 534*f*
    of lung 532
Neurofibroma 431, 437
Neurofibrosarcomas 439
Neurogenic tumor 431, 437
Neurologic 659
Neurolytic celiac plexus block 673
Neuromuscular disorders 589
Neuropathic pain 667
Neurosurgery, principles of 564
Neutropenic sepsis 609
  pathophysiology 609
  symptoms 609, 610
  treatment 609, 610
Newer concepts in pancreatic cancer 318
Nicotine derived nitrosamine ketone 404
Nipple
  areola reconstruction 607
  creation 607
  discharge 349
N-methyl-D-aspartate 669
Nocardia species 686
Nodal
  dissection 226
  staging and fluorodeoxyglucose-positron emission tomography 49
Nodular
  hyperplasia 446
  lymphocyte-predominant Hodgkin lymphoma 626, 651
  pattern of hepatocellular carcinoma on gross examination 283*f*
Nomenclature of neck dissections 200
Non-aeruginosa pseudomonas species 691
Non-albicans *Candida* 692
  species 691
Non-germ cell tumors 501
Non-Hodgkin's lymphoma 62, 63, 624, 644
Nonhomologous end joining 67
Non-HPV cancers 171
Noninvasive
  breast cancer 336
  papillary carcinoma 490
Non-muscle invasive bladder cancer 492
Non-opioid analgesics 669
Nonseminoma 501*f*
Non-seminomatous germ cell tumor 430, 500, 501, 505, 505*t*, 507
Non-small cell
  carcinoma 64
  lung carcinoma 32, 48, 62, 101, 404, 580
Non-steroidal
  anti-inflammatory
    agents 677
    drugs 555, 669, 670*t*
  estrogen diethylstilbestrol 78
Nontuberculous mycobacterial 686
Normal cellular function 86
N-staging for all head and neck sites except thyroid 148*t*
Nuclear factor-kappa-B pathway 626
Nulliparity and infertility 395
NWTSG approach 619

O

Obesity 234, 363, 395
Obstructive
  jaundice in resectable pancreatic head 312
  rectal cancers 260
Odor 522
Oligo brain metastasis, management of 580
Oligodendroglioma 567
Oncocytoma 446, 450
Oncologic surgery, major 590
Oncology and hematology-Hodgkin lymphoma 630
Oncoplastic surgery 603
Oncovin 628, 630, 631
  prednisone 639
Opening of peritoneum 127*f*
Opioid
  analgesics 669
  use, principles of 670*t*
Optic pathway glioma 91
Oral cancers 147
  anatomical boundaries and subsites 147
  approach to treatment 149
    cheek flap 149
    peroral 149
    visor flap 150
  cheek and gum 153
  chemotherapy 159
  floor of
    mouth 157
    tongue 157
  general features 147
  introduction 147
  lips 153
  managing mandible 150
  mandible 154
  radiotherapy 159

retromolar trigone 157
surgical approaches 149
Oral
cavity, subsites 147*f*
chemotherapy 262
contraceptives 381
lesions 145
lichen planus 142, 144
premalignant lesions 142
Oropharyngeal walls 171*f*
Oropharynx 171
clinical features 172
introduction 171
management 172
representative case 172
staging 172
Orthopantomogram of fibular reconstruction for mandibular defect 597*f*
Orthopantomograph weeks 157*f*
OSLO tomosynthesis screening trial 331
Osteoblastoma 537
Osteochondroma 436, 537
Osteogenic sarcoma 59, 62, 496*f*
Osteoid osteoma 537
Osteosarcoma 35*f*, 437, 441, 537, 538, 539*f*
Ovarian
cancer 52, 62, 91, 363, 364
screening 88, 93
tumors 351
Ovary 585

P

Paget's disease 347, 537, 539
Pain
measurement of 668
syndromes with
cancer therapy 667
tumor infiltration 667
to cancer therapy 668
types of 667
Palliation 229, 306
in pancreatic cancer 319
of intrathoracic disease 416
Palliative care 299, 572, 674, 675
definition of 675
Palliative chemotherapy 415
Pancreas 59, 205
cancer 62
Pancreatic
anastomosis 313
body and tail cancer 316
cancer, staging of 311
head 312
malignancies 310
Pancreaticobiliary 207
cancer 215
Papanicolaou smears 383
Papillae with characteristic nuclear features 187
Papillary
carcinoma 187, 346, 455
urothelial neoplasia 489
Papilloma 489
Paracetamol 556
Parafollicular cells 187
Paraganglioma 45
Paramedian mandibulotomy 152*f*
approach for lateral base tongue tumors 173*f*
Paranasal sinuses
orbit base 593
skull base 593
Paraneoplastic syndromes 425, 588
in cancer 588
Parastomal hernia 521, 526
and mesh repair 522
Parathyroid 662
adenoma of left inferior gland 196*f*
carcinoma 662
tumors 194
clinical features 194
introduction 194
investigations 194
management 194
Parenteral
feeding 677
nutrition 678
Paris classification 211*f*
Parosteal osteogenic sarcoma 540, 540*f*
Parotid gland 181*f*
Pars membranacea 125
Partial
breast
irradiation 339
radiation 355
response 563
Patch pharyngoplasty with adequate luminal diameter 177*f*
Pathology and patterns of spread 300
Pectoralis
major
muscle 600
myocutaneous flap 591
Pediatric
B-cell non-Hodgkin lymphoma 636*t*
cancer
unit model of care for childhood cancers in India 622*f*
units, creation of 621
CNS tumors, management of 568
Hodgkin lymphoma 624
risk stratification in 628*t*
treatment of 630
non-Hodgkin lymphoma 632
definitive therapy of 636
oncology 614
group 629, 637
palliative care 682
Pedicle latissimus dorsi flap 442*f*
Pelvic
and abdominal gist in male 276
lymph node dissection 480
lymphadenectomy 482
wall 259*f*
Peptide receptor radionuclide therapy 56
Percutaneous
ethanol injection 285
fine-needle aspiration 409
Periampullary cancer 312
Perineal radical prostatectomy 483
Perioperative chemotherapy 240
Periosteal osteogenic sarcoma 540
Peripheral
inserted central catheters 62
nerve
block 672
tumors 436
smear examination 647
vascular complication 497
Peristomal skin
lesions 522
protection 523*f*
Peritoneal
carcinomatosis 261
in stomach cancer 238
Peroral resectiion 149*f*
Peutz-Jeghers syndrome 87-89, 207
Pharmacological management of cancer pain 668
Pharyngeal walls 174*f*
Pheochromocytoma 45, 59, 91, 445, 446, 451*f*, 611, 661
pathophysiology 611
symptoms 611
treatment 611
Phyllodes tumor 347, 347*t*
Piece meal polypectomy done 208*f*
Pilocytic astrocytoma 561
Piroxicam 670
Pituitary
adenomas 571
tumors 45

Platelet-derived growth factor receptor 562
Pleomorphic xanthoastrocytoma 561
Pneumatic compression stocking 497
Pneumocystis carinii 686, 688, 694
Poly methyl methacrylate 441*f*
Polyaromatic hydrocarbons 404
Polycythemia 589
Polyembryoma 501
Polymerase chain reaction 28, 30, 95
Polymeric nanoparticles 105
Polymethyl methacrylate 441
Polypoidal lesion in transverse colon 254*f*
Polyps adenomas 260
Port positions 122*f*
Portal vein
embolization 304
resections 305
touch technique 305
Positron emission
mammography 46, 48
tomography 39, 39*f*, 42, 43, 46*f*, 53, 341, 345, 425, 440, 448, 480
scan 46, 47*f*, 368, 440, 458, 502
Post nasolabial flap 594*f*
Postchemotherapy
management 508
pain syndromes 667
Postcolonic endoscopic submucosal dissection for intramucosal cancer 213*f*
Postcricoid pharynx 174*f*
Post-cystectomy urinary diversion 495
Posterior
lesion of tongue and oropharynx 152*f*
mediastinal tumors 432
U cut 131*f*
Postmastectomy radiation therapy 357*t*
Postoperative
dental rehabilitation 598
ileus 497
neck residual tissue 55
pancreatic fistula 315
radiation 400
radiotherapy 400, 412
Post-pancreatectomy hemorrhage 314
Post-radiotherapy
complex rectosigmoid resistant stricture 217*f*
complications 216
Postsurgical pain syndromes 667
Pouch of Douglas 129
Pramidronate 556
Preauricular skin crease 184
Precancerous squamous lesions 382
Precursor
B-lymphoblastic 632
t-lymphoblastic 632
lymphoma 637
Prednisone 628, 629, 630, 631
Premalignant
conditions 205
of digestive tract 203
Preoperative
biliary drainage 304
downstaging of rectal cancer 256
hand antisepsis 701
radiation therapy 413
Pretherapy work-up and investigation 223
Prevention
and management of anastomotic leaks 228
and surveillance 287
of colorectal cancer 202
Primary
abdominal tumor and nodal metastases 46*f*
bone tumors 536
brain tumors
imaging of 561
management of 560
breast reconstruction using latissimus dorsi flap and implant 606*f*
chemotherapy 62, 506
chondrosarcoma 542
hyperparathyroidism 194
inflammatory breast cancer 346
lymphoma with nodal mass in ileum 248*f*
malignant liver tumors 287
mucosal reapproximation 150*f*
neuroendocrine tumor 533*f*
Primitive neuroectodermal tumor 536
Principles of
hormone treatment in
breast cancer 78
prostate cancer 81
nuclear imaging 43
Procarbazine 628, 631
lomustine 567
Procedure loop electro excision 385
Progesterone receptor 345, 351
Prognostic
factors for survival in high-grade gliomas 563
indices for brain metastasis 579*t*
Prokinetic agent 677
Proliferative
inflammatory atrophy 476
verrucous leukoplakia 142, 143*f*
Prophylactic surgery 365
Prostate 59
cancer 29*f*, 52, 62, 474, 476*f*, 477
inflammatory atrophy 476
specific antigen 59, 478, 482, 486, 586
density 478
velocity 478
Protocols of chemotherapy 263*t*
Pseudomonas 702
aeruginosa 690, 691, 698
Pseudomyxoma peritonei
chemotherapy 271
introduction 269
pathology 269
treatment 269
conservative approach 271
cytoreductive surgery 269
hyperthermic intraperitoneal pseudomyxoma peritonei chemotherapy 269
tumor
around transverse colon 271*f*
infiltration in transverse mesocolon 271*f*
P-staging 26
Psychological care 679
Pulmonary
artery 411, 440*f*
function test 441
metastases 55
osteoarthopathy 407
problem 598
Pylorus preserving pancreaticoduodenectomy versus classic whipple 313
Pyriform sinus 174*f*

Q

Quality of life in advanced cancer 674
Quantum
dots 100, 101
of node retrieval 226

R

Radiation therapy 340, 355, 387
oncology group 164, 563
Radiation-tumor-static 674
Radical
mastectomy 7, 339
neck dissection 200
nephrectomy 466*f*
prostatectomy 482, 482*f*
Radio sensitizer 68
Radioactive colloid 342
Radioembolization 57
Radio-frequency ablation 51, 202, 285, 415, 464

Radioiodine
scan of thyroid 45*f*
therapy for thyroid cancer 55
Radiology oncology system 33
Radiosurgery alone versus SRS with WBRT for oligo metastases 581
Radiotherapy 374, 391, 399, 427, 497, 556
Radius 596
Rare lymphomas in children 635
Rare primary liver tumors 288
Rationale for combination chemoradiotherapy 68
Rationale of treatment disease advancing 674
Recent advances in delivery of WBRT 581
Recessive hereditary colon cancer 89
Reconstruction
by bipaddled pectoralis major flap 154*f*
of chest wall 441
Reconstructive surgery in oncology 590
Rectum 711
Rectus abdominis muscle 602
Recurrent
carcinoma of
cervix 388
ovary 372*f*
disease 350, 485
glioblastoma, treatment of 568
laryngeal nerve 188
metastatic disease 240
Recursive partitioning analysis 563, 563*t*
Red cell aplasia 427
Reed-sternberg cells 625
Re-exploration complications of pancreaticoduodenectomy 316
Refractory disease 630
Regional lymph nodes 163, 504
Relapsed disease 630
Renal
and bladder cancer 52
cell carcinoma 454, 458*f*
dysfunction 659
failure 194
glomerular filtration rate 44
nephropathies 589
Results with surgery 238*f*
Retinoblastoma 91, 562, 615, 620
protein phosphorylation 75
Retroperitoneal
lymph node dissection 60, 371*f*, 506*f*
node dissection 506
sarcomas 550
Retropubic radical prostatectomy 480
Reverse transcription polymerase chain reaction 28
Rhabdomyosarcoma 438, 441
Rhizopus 693
Ribonucleic acid 105, 112
Right
and left hemicolectomy 125
cardinal ligaments 132*f*
hepatectomy specimen of large metastatic lesion 261
hepatic resection for hepatocellular carcinoma 283
lateral approach of superior mesenteric artery first technique 318*f*
posterior portal vein clamp 297*f*
Wilm's tumor, typical scan 619*f*
Rituximab 63
Road map after completion of dissection 133*f*
Robotic
open surgery for cancer rectum 259
pancreatic resections 318
surgery 125, 714
Role of
adjuvant chemoradiation 241
chemotherapy 399, 579
fulvestrant 354
oophorectomy 354
oral chemotherapy in adjuvant setting 262
prophylactic anticonvulsants 579
steroids 579
targeted therapy in
brain metastasis 580
management of colorectal cancer 263
metastatic cancer of stomach 242
Rothmund-Thomson syndrome 539
Rudolph Virchow 2*f*

S

Saccharomyces cerevisiae 693
Sacral nerve block 672
Sagittal anatomy of larynx 161*f*
Saline implants 605
Salivary gland surgery 185
facial nerve 185
Salivary glands tumors 180
diagnosis 181
introduction 180
management of neck 184
surgical anatomy 180
Salivary tumors
distribution 180
classification of 183
Salvage therapy 509
Sandwich technique 441*f*
Sarcomatoid carcinoma 382
Scapula 597, 598
Scintimammography 46
Sclerosing stromal tumor 367
Secondary
chondrosarcoma 543
to inoperable carcinoma head pancreas 208
Secretion of antidiuretic hormone 588
Segment of jejunum 178*f*
Segmental resection with clear margins 156*f*
Selection of surgical approach for mid-lower rectal cancers 260
Selective neck dissections 201
Self-expandable metal stent placed 216*f*
to alleviate jaundice 208*f*
to relieve dysphagia 214*f*
Seminoma 429, 501, 501*f*, 504
Sentinel lymph node 340, 343*f*, 344*f*
biopsy 338, 338*f*, 344
retrieval in breast cancer 343
Sentinel node mapping 46
Sequential chemoradiation 69
Seroma 344, 598
Serous
carcinoma 366*f*
papillary
adenocarcinoma 383
carcinoma 396, 397*f*
Sertoli
cell tumor 367, 501
Leydig cell tumor 367
Serum creatinine 56
Several hereditary cancer syndromes 91
Severe
acute respiratory syndrome 688
malena 126
Sex cord 365, 367, 501
Sexually transmitted diseases 476
Sigmoid loop colostomy 527
Silicone implant 605
reconstruction 601
Simplified classification system for common bone tumors 537*t*
Simulator training 136
Single
balloon 207
fan shaped structure 132*f*
hemoclip applied, hemostasis achieved 209*f*
incision laparoscopic surgery 137
nucleotide polymorphisms 92
photon emission computer tomography 42
port surgery 125

strand break 68
walled carbon nanotubes 102
Sjogren's syndrome 650
Skeletal
reconstruction 599
support, indications for 600
Skin
flaps 602
grafts 602
Sleeve lobectomy 409, 410
Small
bowel 206
carcinoids 534
enema of 246*f*
nets 532
cell
carcinoma 405
lung cancer 45, 405
lymphocytic lymphoma 649
malignant lesions 593
round cell tumors of childhood 616*t*
tissue 28
Smooth muscle tumors 252
Soft
palate 171*f*
tissue 91
sarcomas 25, 62, 545
tumors 615
Solitary
adrenal metastases 412
nucleotide polymorphisms 112
plasmacytoma 438
pulmonary nodule 48
thyroid nodule management algorithm 191
Somatic pain 667
Specimen of
esophagectomy with two-field dissection 227*f*
opened to mucosal extent of lesion 275*f*
total laryngopharyngectomy 179*f*
total thyroidectomy 189
Speckled leukoplakia 143*f*
Spermatocytic seminoma 561
Spinal
accessory nerve 197
cord compression 612
symptoms 612
treatment 612
hemangioblastoma 91
Spindle cell
carcinoma 382
type 274*f*
Spiritual care 680
Splenic marginal zone 650
lymphomas 647
NHL 650
Sporadic cancer 84
Spread of
metastases to brain 578
ovarian cancer 369*f*
Squamous
carcinoma 382
invading molar area of mandible 156*f*
lower lip 153*f*
cell carcinoma 206, 222, 265, 396, 405, 489
intraepithelial lesion 382
Stages of ovarian carcinoma 370*t*
Stagewise management of prostate cancer 486*t*
Staging
laparoscopy 304
of cancer of larynx 162
of digestive cancers 206
of lung cancer 406*t*
of neck based upon size, laterality and multiplicity 199*t*
of tumor, nodes and metastases 449*t*
Standard
median lip split incision 151*f*
resection versus adequate regional 227*f*
lymphadenectomy 227*f*
uptake value 47
versus extended lymphadenectomy 313
Staphylococcus
aureus 687, 700
species 685
Stapler anastomosis 257
Stellate ganglion block 673
Stenotrophomonas maltophilia 694
Stereotactic
ablative radiotherapy 412, 415
conformal radiotherapy 571
radiation 68
Sterile body sites and fluids, cultures from 687
Stoma retraction 521
Stomach 205, 206
cancer 63
Stomal
prolapse 521, 526
stenosis 521
Streptococcus pneumoniae 686
Stromal tumors 365, 367
Subarachnoid neurolysis 672
Subclassification of depth of superficial esophageal cancer 210*f*
Subependymal giant cell astrocytoma 91
Submandibular
and sublingual glands 182*f*
incision with access to anterior mandible 151*f*
salivary gland 180
Submucous fibrosis 142, 143, 593
resolution of 594*f*
Superficial esophageal cancer 211
Superior
hypogastric plexus block 673
sulcus tumors 411
vena cava 411
syndrome 611, 634
symptoms 611
treatment 611
Superparamagnetic iron oxide nanoparticle 101, 102
Supervoltage therapy 339
Supportive care 572
Supra-azygous mobilization of esophagus 125*f*
Supraglottic larynx 160
Supravital staining 143*f*
Surface
epithelial tumors 365
with electrocautery 297*f*
Surgery
for pancreatic cancer 312
for rectal cancer 259*f*
types of 603
Surgical
anatomy of
hypopharynx 174
larynx 160
nasopharynx 169
oropharynx 172
attire and drapes 701
coronal anatomy of larynx 161*f*
resection in hilar cholangiocarcinoma, principles of 304
treatment of hepatocellular carcinoma 281
Surveillance cultures 687
Survival rates 357, 395
Sympathetic nerve block 673
Synchronous bilateral breast cancer 346
Syndrome of inappropriate
antidiuretic hormone 405
secretion of antidiuretic hormone 659
Synthetic material for structural support 600

System for childhood non-Hodgkin lymphoma 635*t*
Systemic therapy
- for colorectal cancer 261
- of breast cancer 352
- of epithelial ovarian cancer 371
- of recurrent or metastatic disease 399
- of uterine carcinoma 399

T

T2-weighted heterogeneously hyperintense lesion in left temporal region 578
Talcum powder 364
Tamoxifen 63
Targeted biological therapy 240
Targeted therapy 28, 63*t*, 64*t*, 287, 263, 263*f*, 353, 354, 415, 468
Taxanes 68
T-cell
- lymphomas, management of 637
- NHL 650

Technical modifications of
- distal pancreaticosplenectomy 317
- pancreaticoduodenectomy 313

Technique of
- creation of stoma 516
- identification of sentinel lymph nodes 342*f*

Telemedicine 714
Temporary colostomy 526
Tensin homolog 562
Teratomas 429, 501, 502
Testes 484
- sparing surgery 504

Testicular
- cancer 52
- intraepithelial neoplasia 500, 504
- tumors 500, 501*t*

Thalidomide 677
Thecoma 367, 501
Therapeutic
- endoscopy in digestive tract malignancies 202
- exploitation of mutations 86
- impact of tumor markers in cancer 59
- nuclear oncology 55

Therapy algorithm of colorectal cancer 264
Thermal ablation treatment of cancer 106
Thoracoscopic transthoracic esophagectomy 123
Thoracoscopy 122, 409
Thoracotomy 409
Thrombocytosis 589
Thrombophlebitis 589
Thrombotic manifestations 589
Thymic carcinoma 428
Thymoma 426
Thymus 426
Thyroglobulin 188
Thyroid 662
- cancer 44
- gland 186
- stimulating hormone 44, 192
- tumor composed of C-cells 187

Tissue diagnosis 688
TNM
- classification of
  - CRCs 253*t*
  - extrahepatic bile duct tumors 302*t*
  - prostate cancer 481*t*
- staging
  - of testicular tumors 504*t*
  - of thymic tumors 427*t*
  - system 538

Tobacco 234
Toluidine blue staining 21
Tomosynthesis 339
Tomotherapy 72
- devices 72

Tonsillar pillars 171*f*
Tonsils 171*f*
Total
- laryngectomy specimen 165
- mesorectal excision 259*f*
- pelvic exenteration 388
- proctocolectomy 125

Toxicities of aromatase inhibitors 354
Toxoplasma gondii 697, 699
Tracheoesophageal fistula 231
Tramadol 556
Trans-activating transcriptional activator 106
Transanal
- endoscopic microsurgery 260
  - adjuvant radiotherapy 260

Transarterial
- chemoembolization 40, 40*f*, 286
- radioembolization 286

Transbronchoscopic needle aspiration 409
Transesophageal ultrasonography 426
Transitional
- carcinoma 489
- cell 367
  - carcinoma 382, 488

Trans-oral robotic surgery 121
Transrectal ultrasound 486
- guided biopsy of prostate 479*f*
- guided needle biopsy 478

Transthoracic esophagectomy 123*t*
Transurethral resection 337, 489, 492
Transverse rectus abdominis myocutaneous flap 606
Trastuzumab 63, 242
- emtansine 63

Treatment
- goals and alternatives 184
- of advanced disease 241
- of localized renal cell carcinoma 462
- of lung cancer 409
- of primary tumor 503
- of renal cell carcinoma 64
- schedule 281*t*

Treponema pallidum 4
Trichosporon species 693
Tricyclic antidepressants 671
Trophoblastic tumor 501
T-staging for tumors of lip and oral cavity 148*t*
Tuberculosis of ascending colon 127
Tuberous sclerosis 87, 90, 91, 454
Tubular
- adenoma composed of tubular glands 251*f*
- carcinoma 346

Tumor
- angiogenesis imaging 55
- drug resistance imaging 55
- exhibiting
  - c-cell differentiation 187
  - follicular differentiation: specific types 186
- imaging in vivo 102
- induced hypoglycemia 611
  - symptoms 611
  - treatment 611
- induced osteomalacia 589
- infiltration of plexus 667
- invades
  - deep muscle 490
  - muscle 490
    - layer 259*f*
  - perivesical tissue 490
  - subepithelial connective tissue 490
  - superficial muscle 490
- lysis syndrome 609
- markers 349, 502, 586
- necrosis factor 105, 626
- node metastasis 461, 480, 481, 486

Node Metastasis
classification 163t, 172t
of cancers of hypopharynx 176t
of cancers of nasopharynx 170t
Staging 461t
system 162
of adrenal gland 444
of central nervous system 560
of chest wall 436
of endocrine gland 661
of small bowel 245
carcinoid tumors 245
clinical presentation 245
diagnostic work-up 245
etiology 245
introduction 245
treatment 246
adenocarcinoma 247
lymphoma 247
metastatic 248
sarcoma 247
related pain 668
spread in gallbladder cancer 293
suppressor genes 86
and oncogenes 86t
Type of
anastomotic disruptions 228
brachytherapy 71
endometrial carcinoma 397t
nuclear scans in oncology 43
Typical hypervascular hepatoma 40f
Tyrosine kinase inhibitor 32, 468, 579, 640

U

Ultrasonography 36, 333
guided celiac plexus block 215
of breast 334f
Uncommon pancreatic tumors 319
Undifferentiated carcinoma 187
Ureteral stenosis 524
Urinary tract infection 478, 523
Urostomy 519, 527
Urothelial cancers 488
Use of methylene blue stain 204
Usual sequence of events for development of mucosal cancers 205
Uterine artery and vein 132f

V

Vaccination 18
Vancomycin-resistant enterococci 687
Various premalignant conditions of digestive tract 205t
Vascular
anastomosis complete 178f
endothelial growth factor 5, 63, 106, 468, 562
resections 314
stroma and amyloid 188
Vemurafenib 64
Verrucous carcinoma 143f, 382
Vestibular schwannoma 571
Video-assisted thoracoscopy 409
Villoglandular papillary adenocarcinoma 383
Villous adenoma composed of villiform structures 251f
Vinblastine 628, 629, 631
Vincristine 567, 628, 629, 630, 631
Viral infections 688
Virtual reality simulators 136
Visceral pain 667
Vision 122, 514
Visor flap 151f
Volumes radiation therapy 401
Vomiting 675
management 675
Von Hippel-Lindau
disease 87, 90, 91, 454
factor 64

W

Warty carcinoma 382
Werner syndrome 539
Wertheim-Meigs radical hysterectomy 386f
Whipple's procedure 532
White light endoscopy 203
pink mucosa above Z-line 203f
WHO
2008 classification of lymphomas 645t
three-step analgesic ladder 669
Whole brain radiotherapy 565, 579
Wilms' tumor 62, 615, 619
management algorithm in 620f
Wound dehiscence 497

X

Xeroderma pigmentosum 87, 90
X-ray chest 408

Y

Yolk sac tumor 367, 501, 502

Z

Zoledronic acid 556, 558
Zonal anatomy of prostate 475f
Zones of adrenal cortex, adrenal medulla and adrenal hormones 444f